D1608553

Clinical Monitoring

Clinical Monitoring

Practical Applications for Anesthesia and Critical Care

Carol L. Lake, M.D., M.B.A.
Professor and Chair
Associate Dean for Continuing Medical Education
Department of Anesthesiology
University of Louisville School of Medicine
Louisville, Kentucky

Roberta L. Hines, M.D.
Professor and Chair
Department of Anesthesiology
Yale University School of Medicine
New Haven, Connecticut

Casey D. Blitt, M.D., D.A.B.A., F.A.C.A.
Clinical Professor of Anesthesiology
University of Arizona Health Sciences Center
Risk Manager and Medical Director
Perioperative Services
Old Pueblo Anesthesia
Tucson Medical Center
Tucson, Arizona

W.B. SAUNDERS COMPANY
A Harcourt Health Sciences Company
Philadelphia London New York St. Louis Sydney Toronto

W.B. SAUNDERS COMPANY
A Harcourt Health Sciences Company

The Curtis Center
Independence Square West
Philadelphia, Pennsylvania 19106

Library of Congress Cataloging-in-Publication Data

Lake, Carol L.
    Clinical monitoring: practical applications for anesthesia and critical care / Carol L.
Lake, Roberta L. Hines, Casey D. Blitt.—1st ed.

        p.   ;   cm.

    Includes bibliographical references and index.

    ISBN 0–7216–8698–2

    1. Anesthesia.   2. Critical care medicine.   3. Patient monitoring.   I. Hines, Roberta L.
II. Blitt, Casey D.,   III. Title.
    [DNLM: 1. Monitoring, Physiologic—methods. 2. Anesthesia. 3. Critical Care.
    WB 142 L192c 2001]

RD82.L345   2001   617.9′6—dc21   00-023912

Acquisitions Editor: Allan Ross
Project Manager: Edna Dick
Production Manager: Frank Polizzano
Illustration Specialist: Lisa Lambert

CLINICAL MONITORING: Practical Applications for Anesthesia
and Critical Care   ISBN 0–7216–8698–2

Printed in the United States of America.

Last digit is the print number: 9   8   7   6   5   4   3   2   1

Contributors

Carlos U. Arancibia, M.D.
Professor and Interim Chair
Department of Anesthesiology
Virginia Commonwealth University
Medical College of Virginia
Director of Surgical Services
Medical College of Virginia Hospitals
Richmond, Virginia
Monitoring Intracranial Pressure

Solomon Aronson, M.D., F.A.C.C., F.C.C.P.
Professor and Director
Division of Cardiovascular Anesthesia
The University of Chicago Department of Anesthesia and
  Critical Care
Chicago, Illinois
Perioperative Echocardiography

Kornel D. Balon, Jr., M.D.
Director of Cardiovascular Anesthesia
Central DuPage Hospital
Staff Anesthesiologist
West Central Anesthesiology Group
Winfield, Illinois
Perioperative Echocardiography

Steven J. Barker, M.D., Ph.D.
Department of Anesthesiology
University of Arizona
Health Sciences Center
Tucson, Arizona
Monitoring of Oxygen

Robert F. Bedford, M.D.
Anesthesia Service
James A. Haley Veterans Affairs Medical Center
Tampa, Florida
Invasive and Noninvasive Blood Pressure Monitoring

Charlotte Bell, M.D.
Yale University Medical Center
New Haven, Connecticut
Monitoring in Unusual Environments

Casey D. Blitt, M.D., D.A.B.A, F.A.C.A
Clinical Professor of Anesthesiology
University of Arizona Health Sciences Center
Risk Manager and Medical Director
Perioperative Services
Old Pueblo Anesthesia
Tucson Medical Center
Tucson, Arizona
History and Philosophy of Monitoring

Marc J. Bloom, M.D., Ph.D.
Clinical Associate Professor of Anesthesiology
New York University School of Medicine
Director
Neuroanesthesia and Neurophysiology Programs
New York University Hospital Center
New York, New York
*Electroencephalography and Monitoring of Anesthetic
  Depth*

Peter C. Brath, M.D.
Assistant Professor
Cardiothoracic Anesthesiology and Critical Care Medicine
Department of Anesthesiology
Wake Forest University School of Medicine
Winston-Salem, North Carolina
*Electrocardiographic Monitoring for Ischemia and
  Arrhythmias*

Douglas B. Coursin, M.D.
Professor of Anesthesiology and Internal Medicine
University of Wisconsin-Madison
Associate Director
Trauma and Life Support Center
University of Wisconsin Hospital and Clinics
Madison, Wisconsin
Biochemical and Metabolic Indicators

Charles G. Durbin, Jr., M.D., F.C.C.M.
Professor of Anesthesiology
University of Virginia School of Medicine
Medical Director
Respiratory Care
University of Virginia Health System
Charlottesville, Virginia
Arterial Blood Gas Analysis and Monitoring

Jan Ehrenwerth, M.D.
Professor of Anesthesiology
Yale University School of Medicine
Attending Physician
Yale–New Haven Hospital
New Haven, Connecticut
Electrical Safety

John H. Eichhorn, M.D.
Professor and Chairman
Department of Anesthesiology
University of Mississippi School of Medicine
Chairman
Department of Anesthesiology
University of Mississippi Medical Center
Jackson, Mississippi
Monitoring and Patient Safety

Mark H. Ereth, M.D.
Assistant Professor of Anesthesiology
Mayo Medical School
Consultant in the Department of Anesthesiology
Mayo Clinic/Mayo Foundation
Rochester, Minnesota
*Monitoring Coagulation and Hemostasis: Perioperative
  Assessment of Coagulation and Platelet Function*

David M. Gaba, M.D.
Director
Patient Safety Center of Inquiry
Anesthesia Service
VA Palo Alto Healthcare Systems
Palo Alto
Professor of Anesthesia
Department of Anesthesia
Stanford University School of Medicine
Stanford, California
Simulators

Thomas J. Gal, M.D.
Professor of Anesthesiology
University of Virginia School of Medicine
Attending Anesthesiologist
University of Virginia Health System
Charlottesville, Virginia
Monitoring the Function of the Respiratory System

Hugh C. Gilbert, M.D.
Assistant Professor
Northwestern University Medical School
Chicago
Senior Attending
Evanston Northwestern Healthcare
Evanston, Illinois
Point-of-Care Monitoring and Analysis

Michael Griffin, M.B., M.R.C.P.I., F.F.A.R.C.S.I.
Assistant Professor
Department of Anesthesiology
Yale University School of Medicine
New Haven, Connecticut
Pulmonary Artery Catheterization

H. Russell Harvey, M.D.
Fellow in Critical Care
University of Wisconsin-Madison
Attending Physician
University of Wisconsin
Hospital and Clinics
Madison, Wisconsin
Biochemical and Metabolic Indicators

James D. Helman, M.D.
Staff Anesthesiologist
Cardiac Anesthesiology and Pain Management
Virginia Mason Clinic
Seattle, Washington
Monitoring Pain Management Procedures

Roberta L. Hines, M.D.
Professor and Chair
Department of Anesthesiology
Yale University School of Medicine
New Haven, Connecticut
Pulmonary Artery Catheterization

Daniel J. Kennedy, M.D.
Assistant Professor
Cardiothoracic Anesthesiology and Critical Care Medicine
Department of Anesthesiology
Wake Forest University School of Medicine
Winston-Salem, North Carolina
*Electrocardiographic Monitoring for Ischemia and
  Arrhythmias*

Jonathan T. Ketzler, M.D.
Assistant Professor of Anesthesiology and Internal Medicine
University of Wisconsin-Madison
Attending Physician
University of Wisconsin Hospital and Clinics
Madison, Wisconsin
Biochemical and Metabolic Indicators

Carol L. Lake, M.D., M.B.A.
Professor and Chair
Associate Dean for Continuing Medical Education
Department of Anesthesiology
University of Louisville School of Medicine
Louisville, Kentucky
Monitoring of Temperature and Heart and Lung Sounds

Arthur M. Lam, M.D., F.R.C.P.C.
Professor of Anesthesiology and Neurological Surgery
  (Adjunct)
University of Washington School of Medicine
Attending Anesthesiologist and Head
  Division of Neuroanesthesia
Harborview Medical Center
Seattle, Washington
Specialized Neurophysiologic Monitoring

Robert G. Loeb, M.D.
Associate Professor of Anesthesiology
University of Arizona Health Sciences Center
Tucson, Arizona
Principles of Pressure Monitoring

Wayne K. Marshall, M.D.
Professor
Department of Anesthesiology
The Pennsylvania State University College of Medicine
Hershey, Pennsylvania
Monitoring Intracranial Pressure

Jerry McCoy, Ph.D., M.D.
Assistant Professor of Clinical Anesthesiology and Critical Care
University of Arizona Health Sciences Center
Tucson, Arizona
Principles of Pressure Monitoring

Timothy McCulloch, M.B.B.S., F.A.N.Z.C.A.
Acting Assistant Professor of Anesthesiology
University of Washington School of Medicine
Attending Anesthesiologist
Harborview Medical Center
Seattle, Washington
Specialized Neurophysiologic Monitoring

Melinda Mingus, M.D.
Medical Director
Ambulatory Surgery Unit
Mount Sinai–New York University Medical Center Health
  Systems
New York, New York
Monitoring in Office-Based Anesthesia

S. S. Moorthy, M.D.
Professor of Anesthesia
Department of Anesthesia
Indiana University School of Medicine
Chief of Anesthesia
Richard L. Roudebush Veterans Affairs Medical Center
Indianapolis, Indiana
Evoked Potentials

George Mychaskiw II, D.O.
Assistant Professor and Director
Cardiac Anesthesiology
University of Mississippi School of Medicine
Jackson, Mississippi
Monitoring and Patient Safety

Gregory A. Nuttall, M.D.
Assistant Professor of Anesthesiology
Mayo Medical School
Consultant in the Department of Anesthesiology
Mayo Clinic/Mayo Foundation
Rochester, Minnesota
Monitoring Coagulation and Hemostasis: Perioperative Assessment of Coagulation and Platelet Function

William C. Oliver, Jr., M.D.
Assistant Professor of Anesthesiology
Mayo Medical School
Consultant in the Department of Anesthesiology
Mayo Clinic/Mayo Foundation
Rochester, Minnesota
Monitoring Coagulation and Hemostasis: Perioperative Assessment of Coagulation and Platelet Function

Richard C. Prielipp, M.D.
Professor
Department of Anesthesiology and Critical Care Medicine
Wake Forest University School of Medicine
Winston-Salem, North Carolina
Monitoring of the Neuromuscular Junction

R. V. Reddy, M.D.
Associate Professor of Neurology
Department of Neurology
Indiana University School of Medicine
Attending Physician
Richard L. Roudebush Veterans Affairs Medical Center
Indianapolis, Indiana
Evoked Potentials

J. Richard Roskam, M.D., M.B.A.
Assistant Clinical Professor
Indiana University School of Medicine
Informatics Fellowship Director
Richard L. Roudebush Veterans Affairs Medical Center
Indianapolis, Indiana
Information Systems

William T. Ross, Jr., M.D., M.B.A.
Professor of Anesthesiology
University of Virginia School of Medicine
University of Virginia Health System
Medical Director
Virginia Ambulatory Surgery, Inc.
Charlottesville, Virginia
Monitoring the Anesthesia Machine and Respiratory Gases

Roger L. Royster, M.D.
Professor and Vice-Chairman
Cardiothoracic Anesthesiology and Critical Care Medicine
Department of Anesthesiology
Wake Forest University School of Medicine
Winston-Salem, North Carolina
Electrocardiographic Monitoring for Ischemia and Arrhythmias

Paula J. Santrach, M.D.
Assistant Professor of Laboratory Medicine and Pathology
Mayo Medical School
Co-Director of Hospital Clinical Laboratories and Consultant in the Division of Transfusion Medicine
Mayo Clinic/Mayo Foundation
Rochester, Minnesota
Monitoring Coagulation and Hemostasis: Perioperative Assessment of Coagulation and Platelet Function

Jeffrey J. Schwartz, M.D.
Associate Professor
Department of Anesthesiology
Yale University School of Medicine
Attending Physician
Yale–New Haven Hospital
New Haven, Connecticut
Electrical Safety

Nitin Shah, M.D.
Associate Clinical Professor and Director, Ambulatory Anesthesia
University of California at Irvine
Irvine Medical Center
Orange
Staff Anesthesiologist and Chief
Surgical ICU
Long Beach Veterans Affairs Healthcare Systems
Long Beach, California
Invasive and Noninvasive Blood Pressure Monitoring

Kirk Shelley, Ph.D., M.D.
Associate Professor of Anesthesia
Yale University School of Medicine
New Haven, Connecticut
Pulse Oximeter Waveform: Photoelectric Plethysmography; Monitoring in Unusual Environments

Stacey Shelley, B.S.N.
New Haven, Connecticut
Pulse Oximeter Waveform: Photoelectric Plethysmography; Monitoring in Unusual Environments

Brian E. Smith, M.D.
Clinical Assistant Professor
Department of Anesthesia
Stanford University School of Medicine
Staff Anesthesiologist
El Camino Hospital
Mountain View, California
Simulators

Kevin K. Tremper, M.D., Ph.D.
Professor and Chair
Department of Anesthesiology
University of Michigan Medical School
Chairman
Department of Anesthesiology
The University of Michigan Hospitals

Ann Arbor, Michigan
Monitoring of Oxygen

Rebecca S. Twersky, M.D.
Associate Professor of Anesthesiology and Vice-Chair for
    Research
SUNY Health Science Center at Brooklyn
Medical Director
Ambulatory Surgery Unit
The Long Island College Hospital
Brooklyn, New York
Monitoring in Office-Based Anesthesia

Jeffery S. Vender, M.D., F.C.C.M.
Professor of Anesthesiology
Northwestern University Medical School
Chicago
Chairman
Department of Anesthesiology and
    Director
Medical-Surgical Intensive Care
Evanston Northwestern Healthcare
Evanston, Illinois
Point-of-Care Monitoring and Analysis

Michael H. Wall, M.D.
Assistant Professor
Department of Anesthesiology and Critical Care Medicine

Wake Forest University School of Medicine
Winston-Salem, North Carolina
Monitoring the Neuromuscular Junction

Charles L. Williams, M.D.
Assistant Professor
Division Head of Neuroanesthesia
Virginia Commonwealth University
Medical College of Virginia
Richmond, Virginia
Monitoring Intracranial Pressure

Andrew M. Woods, M.D.
Associate Professor of Anesthesiology
University of Virginia
Medical Director
Postanesthesia Care Unit and Surgical Admissions
University of Virginia Health System
Charlottesville, Virginia
Maternal and Fetal Monitoring in Obstetrics

Christopher J. Young, M.D.
Clinical Instructor
Southwestern Missouri State University School of Anesthesia
Director of Cardiovascular Anesthesia
St. John's Regional Health Center
Springfield, Missouri
Perioperative Echocardiography

Preface

As the title states, this new monitoring book has been designed to be both clinical and practical. In addition, we have attempted to ensure that the information is current, and more importantly, useful to the reader. All of these editors have years of experience in monitoring patients during anesthesia and critical care. This new edition combines and updates the clinical knowledge presented in Hines and Blitt, *Monitoring in Anesthesia and Critical Care Medicine*, 3rd edition, and Lake, *Clinical Monitoring in Anesthesia and Critical Care*, 2nd edition. We hope we have avoided duplication and overlap of information, but apologize in advance if there is some. We hope that the book is readable and user friendly, and contains information that is worthwhile to the reader's practice. We sincerely thank all of the contributors for sharing their outstanding expertise and knowledge. We also thank the staff and management at W.B. Saunders and Harcourt Health Sciences for their efforts in creating this text. Thanks to families, colleagues, and others for their support and encouragement. We hope that this book will help improve the quality of patient care and patient safety.

CAROL L. LAKE, ROBERTA L. HINES, AND CASEY D. BLITT

Contents

PART ONE

General Principles

1 History and Philosophy of Monitoring

Casey D. Blitt, M.D.

Monitoring is crucial to the practice of the medical specialty of anesthesiology: it provides us with information to facilitate timely therapeutic intervention. Monitoring should reduce the frequency of undesirable outcomes and thereby improve patient safety. Where monitoring started is unclear. All practitioners, however, from Crawford Long to William T. G. Morton, have needed some yardstick to gauge "how the patient is doing." Fundamentally, monitoring is data collection.

Data may be collected by utilizing the senses or by utilizing instrumentation. Utilizing the senses includes "finger on the pulse" and visual observations such as the color of the blood and movement of the chest or a reservoir bag to assess respiration and ventilation. Movement of the patient is also used to assess depth of anesthesia. Early devices (instrumentation) included the stethoscope and the manual blood pressure cuff. The stethoscope was modified to provide auditory information concerning the movement of gas in the airway, and it was taught that cardiac function could be assessed with stethoscopy by listening to the "quality" of the heart tones. While the heart rate clearly could be determined via a modified stethoscope, myocardial contractility probably could not be adequately assessed using such a stethoscope.

Since monitoring is data collection, the data may be collected manually by the aforementioned senses or automatically. In order to be of value, the data must be processed, usually in the brain of the anesthesia practitioner. Automatic data collection methods are most desirable because they usually provide continual information and allow the practitioner more time for cognitive decision making. While automatic data collection involves the potential of annoyance because of false alarms, errant data display, and even occasional malfunction in the electrically hostile operating room environment, it is my opinion that the safe, clinical practice of the medical specialty of anesthesiology requires the availability of certain basic automatic data collection devices.

Monitoring instrumentation encompasses a variety of modalities, from the basics to the more sophisticated devices. The basic automatic data collection devices are (1) the pulse oximeter, (2) the oscilloscopic electrocardiograph, (3) the automatic noninvasive blood pressure instrument, and (4) infrared (or other mechanism) measurement of exhaled carbon dioxide.

More sophisticated and specialized instrumentation includes devices for measuring somatosensory evoked potentials, transesophageal echocardiography, near-infrared spectroscopy, bispectral index (BIS), and invasive pressure monitoring.

Vigilance is the motto of the American Society of Anesthesiologists (ASA), and no other single word best describes the task of the anesthesiologist. Monitoring enhances vigilance and allows the anesthesiologist to be the guardian angel of the patient. The dictionary provides multiple definitions of a monitor or monitoring. The word originally comes from the Latin *monere,* to warn. Monitor may be used as both a noun and a verb. As a noun, a monitor is (1) one who admonishes, cautions, reminds, or advises; (2) a pupil who assists a teacher in routine duties; (3) any device used to record or control a process; (4) an articulated device holding a rotating nozzle used in firefighting and mining; (5) a heavily ironclad warship of the 19th century with a low flat deck and one or more gun turrets, specifically the first such ship, the Union vessel *Monitor,* which fought the Confederate ironclad *Merrimac* on March 9, 1862; and (6) any tropical carnivorous lizard ranging in length from several inches to 10 ft.

As a transitive verb, including the forms *monitored, monitoring,* and *monitors,* to monitor means (1) to check (the transmission quality of the signal) by means of a receiver; (2) to test (a surface) for radiation intensity; (3) to keep track of by means of an electronic device; (4) to check by means of a receiver for significant content (sending messages during war); (5) to scrutinize or check systematically with a view to collecting certain specified categories of data; and (6) to keep watch over, supervise (monitoring an examination). As an intransitive verb, to monitor means "to act as a monitor."

In my opinion, monitoring and vigilance are interrelated. Monitoring provides us information to enhance our vigilance and facilitate therapeutic intervention. Monitoring modalities fall into three categories, which may be formulated as: (1) You absolutely have to have it. (2) I'd like it but can live without it. (3) It's extra and not needed.

Special situations require specialized monitors and specialized applications. Can monitoring eliminate critical incidents or sentinel events in anesthetic and critical care areas? Can monitoring eliminate hypoxic accidents, drug overdoses, and equipment failures? I believe that monitoring per se cannot eliminate these events, but it can substantially improve early recognition of situations of esophageal intubation, anesthetic circuit disconnections, errors in gas supplies or flow, loss of airway, and drug excess so as to permit early intervention. Multiple backup and redundant modalities may be desirable because the more systems you have to tell you that your patient is hypoxemic, the greater chance you have to receive input if one system fails and to take appropriate therapeutic action.

Many parallels, comparisons, and similarities have been made between the administration of anesthesia and piloting an airplane. Repetitive tasks, boredom, fatigue, and the sudden need to act quickly to avoid disaster are common grounds for the anesthesiologist and the airline pilot. Pilots have a very standardized workplace, and they are extremely familiar with this workplace. Anesthesiologists also should have a standardized workplace with which they are very familiar. Pilots are allowed to fly only a certain number of hours without time off. Anesthesiologists, in my opinion, should not be allowed to administer anesthesia around the clock without rest. Patient safety is a primary concern, and accidents may occur.

All monitoring modalities fit into a continuum of invasive versus noninvasive. "Invasive" is a relative term and is somewhat dependent on the eye of the beholder. It is not my intent to promote or denigrate any monitoring modality on the basis of invasiveness or lack thereof. The cost of monitoring is important simply because economic considerations are important to the practice of medicine. Unfortunately, the cost-benefit ratios for most monitoring devices are not known. Special situations require specialized applications of monitors. The reader will encounter many of these in this book. There is clearly a difference between qualitative and quantitative information that is obtained from monitoring devices. When possible, quantitative information is preferable. In addition to providing information, documentation of information in the medical record is an important consideration in anesthesia. Automated record-keeping systems are currently available that *approach* a degree of sophistication and user-friendliness to be applicable for widespread utilization in anesthesia. Clearly, automatic data collection is more easily stored, retrieved, and displayed in automated record-keeping systems. Communication between practitioners via monitored data also is facilitated by automatic data collection methods.

What are the reasons for monitoring? That is, why monitor our patients? In my opinion, it provides better patient care, early diagnosis and treatment of untoward conditions, and protects the practitioner. Whether monitoring can truly decrease the frequency of adverse outcomes will never be known. Can appropriate monitoring modalities reduce the cost and frequency of adverse outcomes in other areas such as the postanesthesia care unit (PACU)? Can monitoring improve operating room utilization or lower pharmacy costs? The answer to these questions is not yet known, but we may find information regarding these issues in the future. The question is frequently asked, Can the expenditure for purchase of equipment be justified by decreasing adverse outcomes? Again, I believe that this question is frequently unanswerable.

A distinct value of automated record-keeping systems and data collection is the ability to re-create and revisit a catastrophe or sentinel event. That is, a "black box" exists to help us analyze the event and see what happened. The fear of such a black box is that the information may not be able to be protected from discovery in a legal action. Automated systems that can collect data, store, and retrieve it so as to reconstruct the "event" are extremely valuable and in my opinion a necessary ingredient of any automated record-keeping system. A frequent question that is asked is, Who is responsible for the data collection system—the practitioner, the healthcare facility, or even the insurance carrier? Probably, all three entities are responsible. Who is responsible for monitoring and for implementing the correct responses to the data collected? Clearly, the responsibility for responding correctly rests with the practitioner. Monitoring and data collection are useless if the practitioner is not able to react to and treat the condition that is diagnosed or facilitated by the monitors.

What monitors should be selected and used by the practitioner? Medical judgment, good medical practice, and personal preference all become factors. Even if we cannot prove conclusively that certain monitors are beneficial, it is clear that certain minimal monitoring guidelines must be met, especially with regard to preplanned anesthetics given in designated anesthetizing locations. Everywhere that the medical specialty of anesthesia is practiced, monitoring should be the same. The only exception is if there are physical conditions, for example, the magnetic resonance imaging suite, that would preclude or render useless certain monitoring modalities. Institutional guidelines should delineate the monitors to be used. If minimum guidelines cannot be met, appropriate written documentation must explain *why* they cannot be met. The ASA has established minimum monitoring standards that are continually being revised.[1]

All published standards address the issue of "presence" of qualified personnel in a location where the anesthetic care is being given.[1, 2] Thus, we have a standard in place that the anesthesiologist or a healthcare provider under the medical direction of an anesthesiologist must be physically present in the anesthetizing area from the start of the anesthetic to the safe transfer of the patient to a recovery area. This "presence of personnel" statement implies that monitors probably are not of great value if there is no one to observe the information obtained. Regardless of the minimum monitoring standards that have been established, no guarantee exists that practicing according to these published standards will result in a favorable outcome.

Documentation of monitoring is extremely important. Good documentation is of value in three primary areas: (1) educational, (2) historical, and (3) medicolegal. The historical and educational aspects of the anesthesia record should be clear to any practitioner. Good documentation facilitates the learning process and enables us to learn the effects of medications, physiologic interventions, and so forth, on the course of the anesthetic. The historical aspect allows subsequent practitioners to learn "what went on before," and hopefully facilitate continual improvement in patient care. The medicolegal aspect is extremely important. It often has been said that "the only time someone looks at the anesthesia record is when something has gone awry." In a legal action, the anesthesia record will be scrutinized and dissected. Since memories fade rapidly, it is frequently the only method whereby anyone can tell what sort of anesthetic care was rendered to the patient. Your anesthesia record can be your greatest ally or your greatest enemy in a legal action. The better your record is, the greater ally it becomes. The admonition, "If it wasn't written down, it wasn't done" turns out to be true more often than not.

The following represents my opinion of what constitutes minimum monitoring guidelines. These guidelines may be exceeded at any time based on the judgment of the involved anesthesia personnel. Monitoring should be tailored to the specific operative procedure, the patient's risk factors, and coexisting medical conditions.

The preoperative check of anesthesia apparatus and equipment is important to the safe conduct of the anesthetic. I recommend the anesthesia apparatus checkout procedure endorsed by the ASA or a reasonable equivalent that is approved by the department of anesthesia at any specific institution.[3] The checkout procedure is a guideline that users should be encouraged to modify to accommodate differences in equipment design and variations in local clinical practice. This anesthesia apparatus checkout is periodically updated in conjunction with the Food and Drug Administration (FDA), and can be obtained either from the FDA or the ASA. Once the preoperative check and the presence of personnel criteria have been satisfied, I recommend the following monitors for patients undergoing general anesthesia:

A. Cardiovascular system
1. Pulse oximeter
2. Automatic blood pressure measurement
3. Oscilloscopic electrocardiogram
B. Respiratory system
1. Pulse oximeter
2. Exhaled gas flow measurement (ventimeter or other respirometer equivalent), when a circle system is used
3. Infrared or comparable gas analysis to measure exhaled carbon dioxide, inhaled and exhaled oxygen, and other gaseous or volatile anesthetics in the circuit
4. Circuit low pressure alarm if mechanical ventilation is used
C. Ability to monitor temperature

If the patient is undergoing regional anesthesia, I recommend the following monitoring modalities or equivalents:

A. A readily available oxygen source with an artificial ventilation support system
B. Cardiovascular system
1. Pulse oximeter
2. Automatic blood pressure measurement
3. Oscilloscopic electrocardiogram
C. Respiratory system
1. Pulse oximeter
D. Ability to monitor temperature

For limited procedures (the practitioner must define "limited") that include but are not restricted to conscious sedation, deep sedation, monitored anesthesia care, and so forth, I recommend the following modalities:

1. Pulse oximeter

2. Automatic blood pressure measurement

3. Oscilloscopic electrocardiogram

One may ask, Why does the precordial stethoscope not appear in any of the aforementioned recommendations? In my opinion, the precordial stethoscope, while a valuable monitoring modality for many years, has been essentially replaced by more sophisticated devices such as the oscilloscopic electrocardiogram, pulse oximeter, and exhaled gas monitors. This does not mean that the precordial stethoscope may not be of value, but I think that it has been replaced by better technology. The reader also will note that I am recommending monitoring of anesthetic gases and vapors. In my opinion, this is essential to our practice in the new millennium.

Which monitors are "standard of care" and which are not is a matter of intuition. Since standard of care is an opinion expressed by either experts or practitioners, certain arguments obviously can be made as to whether certain monitors are or are not standard of care. Minimum monitoring guidelines would clearly be thought by most practitioners to constitute standard of care.

Monitoring outside the operating room is becoming increasingly important. Patients are being cared for by personnel other than anesthesiologists, and patients are being cared for in office practices as well. All patients who are sedated or otherwise have an altered state of consciousness should be appropriately monitored regardless of the location. Healthcare facilities, offices, and so on should develop protocols for monitoring patients, and anesthesiologists should be willing to provide input into these monitoring protocols. Pulse oximetry, oscilloscopic electrocardiography (when indicated), and intermittent noninvasive blood pressure determination would seem to be of unquestionable value in these circumstances. Pulse oximetry would seem to be particularly valuable. In circumstances such as these, costs should not be an issue; patient safety should be paramount. The issue frequently arises as to what should be done if a piece of monitoring equipment is either nonfunctional or unavailable. It is easy to create rationalizations, but in my opinion the prudent healthcare professional should simply decline to provide care, except in truly emergent conditions, when appropriate monitoring equipment is nonfunctional or unavailable. To proceed without appropriate monitoring equipment compromises patient safety and should be avoided despite pressures to push ahead.

Failure to monitor is occasionally cited as a reason why a desired outcome was not achieved (i.e., an undesirable outcome has resulted), and failure to monitor thus becomes an issue in a legal action. It is important to remember that monitoring in and of itself cannot guarantee any given outcome and the failure-to-monitor allegation may or may not be appropriate. Situations in which failure to monitor has been alleged to be causative include injuries related to the positioning of the patient and the development of peripheral nerve injuries perioperatively. Once the patient has been properly positioned for an operation, it may be difficult or impossible to continually monitor the patient to ensure that a "position-related injury" does not occur. The allegation of "failure to monitor" after a patient has been properly positioned and all the usually acceptable clinical precautions have been taken to ensure that position-related injuries do not occur is unreasonable. While peripheral nerve injuries may sometimes be related to positioning, failure to monitor as a causative factor in the development of peripheral nerve injuries is in most circumstances inappropriate. Many perioperative peripheral nerve injuries occur as a result of patient predisposition in combination with other factors that are frequently beyond the control or domain of the anesthesiologist. This does not mean that proper care should not be taken in positioning patients during surgery; it is merely meant to reinforce the concept that all peripheral nerve injuries do not occur in the operating room or PACU.

As a certified healthcare risk manager, I feel obligated to share with you some thoughts that integrate monitoring, risk management, and patient safety. It is my opinion that a right atrial catheter tip location for a central venous pressure (CVP) line is perfectly acceptable, and leaving a catheter in such a position is in accordance with "standard of care." Standardization of the anesthesia workplace or workstation is necessary. Nothing is more disconcerting than to go from anesthetizing location to anesthetizing location and find that nothing is in the same place. Standardization of the anesthetic workplace has great potential for minimizing human error. Interfacing of monitoring equipment and ancillary devices is improving, but there is still room for improvement.

It would appear that most practitioners are currently using standardized color-coded labels for medicines. The multiplicity of vendors and continual packaging changes make labeling of medicine very important. In nonanesthesia situations, medication errors have been frequently reported.[4] The relationship of these medication errors to labeling is unclear. We must not succumb to production pressure. "The need to get the case done" should not supersede the issue of *patient safety.* We must continue to be vigilant and watch over activities in the PACU. While there are no standards or guidelines for appropriate monitoring in the PACU, it is clear that under most circumstances pulse oximetry, oscilloscopic electrocardiography, and automated blood pressure measurement are the cornerstones of PACU monitoring.

Where do we go from here? Properly trained, concerned, educated practitioners with the medical knowledge necessary to make diagnoses and therapeutic decisions are the key to the future of safety in monitoring while the patient sleeps. I believe that aggressive risk management and peer review have the ability to reduce the incidence of anesthesia-related sentinel events.[4] Monitoring and risk management go hand in hand because risk management involves monitoring of the practice of anesthesiology. "We watch over you while you sleep" is a slogan. Monitoring and risk management are means to achieve an end—that is, to make anesthesia as safe as possible for every patient.

REFERENCES

1. American Society of Anesthesiologists Standards for Basic Intraoperative Monitoring. December 1986, revised 1988, 1992, 1998, 1999.
2. Eichhorn JH, Cooper JB, Cullen DJ, et al: Standards for patient monitoring during anesthesia at Harvard Medical School. JAMA 1986; 256:1017.
3. American Society of Anesthesiologists Anesthesia Apparatus Checkout Recommendations. October 1986, revised 1993.
4. Gawande A: When doctors make mistakes. New Yorker: Feb 1, 1999, pp 40–55.

2 Information Systems

J. Richard Roskam, M.D., M.B.A.

The anesthesiologist's work environment has become increasingly computerized. Computerization began with the integration of patient monitoring equipment and computers in the operating theatre and postsurgical care units in the 1970s. It has continued with the development and use of electronic medical record systems, advanced computer-based monitoring and data input devices, digital imaging systems, anesthesia information management systems (AIMSs), and clinical decision support tools.

The first efforts to automatically record and print the course of anesthesia as part of the paper medical record date to the 1970s. Since then the AIMS has evolved into desktop computer–based systems that can assist with the preoperative evaluation, anesthesia course, and postoperative outcome and quality analysis.[1] This chapter includes a discussion of computerized patient records (CPRs), computerized AIMSs, information systems for the operating room (OR), and computer-assisted preoperative testing.

One of the major challenges facing the anesthesiologist today is acquiring the skills to master the increasing number of computerized medical devices and electronic medical record systems in use. The major challenges for designers of computerized medical equipment and electronic medical record systems are to develop products that are intuitive and easy to operate, that improve (or at least do not interfere with) the anesthesia process of care, and that can be easily integrated with existing and future clinical and administrative information systems.

The Computerized Medical Record

Overview

Patient records are a primary source of information for clinical activities. In the broadest sense, the computerized patient record is a system for computer-based data collection, storage, and retrieval in any clinical setting. The computerized patient record may consist of records stored in an information database as unstructured text, but generally it implies that data are stored in a database structure allowing easy retrieval when needed.

The Paper Medical Record

Accurate and detailed records form an integral part of the practice of anesthesia. The ever-increasing complexity of modern anesthetic techniques and equipment may leave little time to record observations and chart physiologic variables as frequently and accurately as one would like.[2, 3] Few would argue the point that adequate anesthesia care requires ready access to pertinent medical information, such as allergy history, medical history, or current medications, in addition to the physiologic and observational data evaluated during the anesthetic procedure. This information has traditionally been contained in the paper medical record kept with the patient in the OR and on the paper anesthesia record.

What Is Wrong With the Paper Record?

There are many shortcomings in the paper medical record. It is often physically cumbersome to use, incomplete due to filing errors or lost pages, or illegible. More important, searching through a paper medical record for specific information can be time-consuming. Paper medical records are accessible to only one provider and in one location at a time. The time lag to file information into the paper record can result in crucial information being unavailable to clinicians at the time and point of care. Misplaced records require that care be provided without any information other than what can be obtained from the patient or family. This level of information can frequently be inadequate for optimal medical decision making.

The Computerized Patient Record

Increasingly, medical care providers are turning to electronic medical record systems to overcome the drawbacks of the paper-based medical record and to provide real-time access to patient information. In addition, electronic medical records provide the anesthesiologist with new views of information, such as the ability to review longitudinal data in summarized form, as well as access to computerized clinical data sets for quality improvement and provider profiling.

Electronic medical record systems vary tremendously in scope and capability. They may consist of electronic repositories of text entries or progress notes contained in a portable computing device such as a personal digital assistant (PDA) carried by the anesthesiologist. Or they may be highly integrated and scalable network systems that make a wide variety of medical, financial, and demographic information available at the point of care and to many different providers simultaneously in geographically dispersed locations.

Definition

Hospitals have traditionally used departmental computerized systems for patient registration and billing, laboratory values, material management, and financial management. These systems generally function as separate "islands of automation," often created by different vendors or running on different computer platforms. Until recently, these separate information database and management systems could not exchange data or be easily integrated with each other. From the clinician's viewpoint, the electronic medical record results when the desired clinical data, such as text reports and progress notes, laboratory studies, images, and patient demographics, converge into a single interface available at the point of care.

History

The earliest attempts at the electronic medical record were limited by the available computer and display technology, which consisted of a mainframe or minicomputer system and character-based display terminals (so-called dumb terminals) directly connected to the main computer (Fig. 2–1). Clerical staff or data entry technicians entered the data. Clinicians were able to retrieve and view only a limited amount and types of data. Most data were quickly moved to magnetic tapes to be archived. Archiving on magnetic tape effectively made data unavailable at the point of care owing to the amount of time and effort required to locate and retrieve the archived information.

With the introduction during the 1980s of the personal computer by IBM and the development of local area networks (LANs) and affordable high-capacity optical storage devices, many paper documents could be scanned and

stored as images. This system of information storage, however, was primarily used to archive paper-based records and never achieved significant use as a point-of-care, real-time clinical electronic medical record.[4] The reasons for this include the high personnel cost of scanning documents, the slow response time to retrieve images from optical archives to the clinician's desktop computer, and the inconvenience of paging through and reviewing optically stored documents.

Today, the electronic medical record interface is limited primarily by the imagination of designers and by the needs of users. New database tools, faster computers, graphical interfaces, and automated instruments have significantly advanced the state of the art in patient care information systems. Typically, the clinician views and enters data from a desktop workstation connected through a computer LAN to server computers holding one or more databases. These databases represent the core data of the clinical patient information system. The actual electronic medical record software (called the interface) controls the look and feel of the user interface. The complexity and capability of the electronic medical record system is determined not only by the user interface but also by the ability of the interface to connect the user to other clinical information databases, legacy systems, and applications.

Hardware

Most new-generation electronic medical records systems are designed to run on desktop computer workstations using

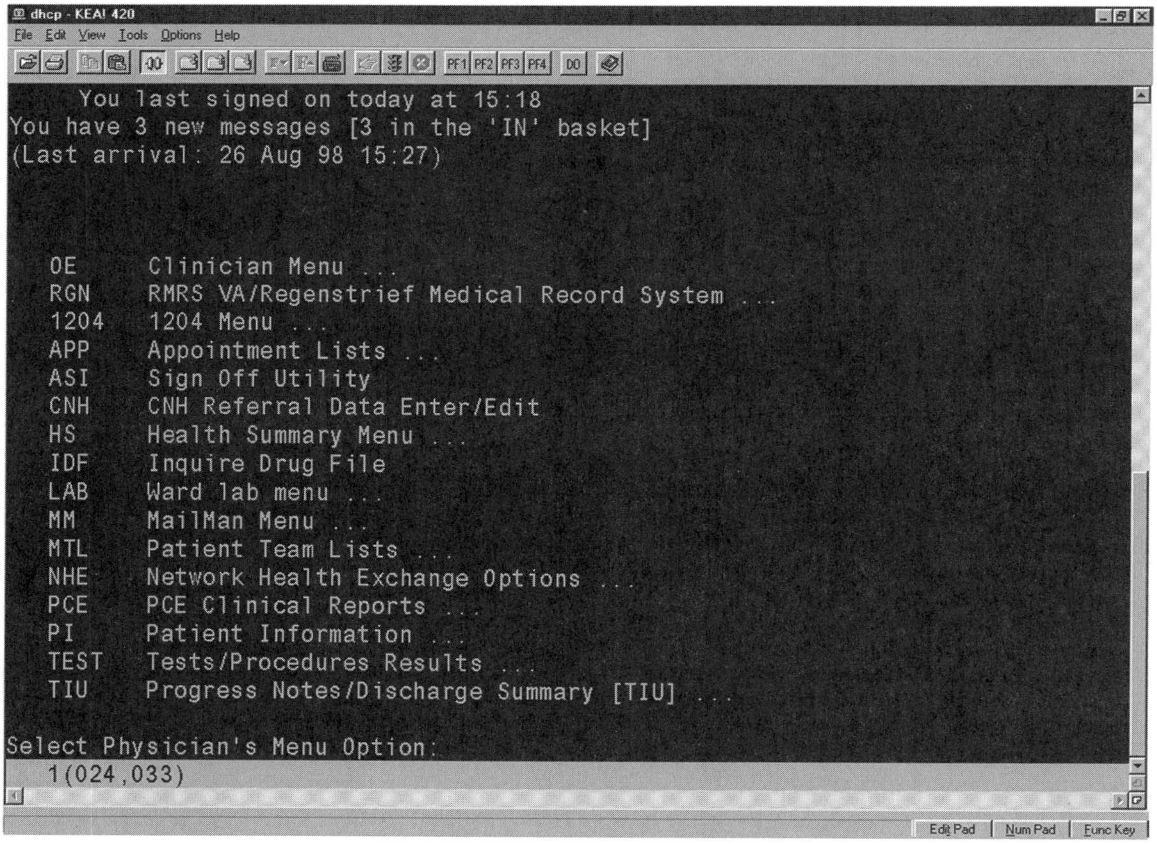

Figure 2–1. Dumb terminal screen output of a VAX/VMS minicomputer patient information system. Note the character-based user interface, with menu-driven navigation through the components of the patient information system. (Courtesy of Roudebush VA Medical Center, Indianapolis.)

client-server architecture. The client computer (also called a workstation) is accessed at the point of care (Fig. 2–2). It consists of a video display unit, microprocessor unit, keyboard, and pointing device. Other data input devices may be connected to the workstation, including a light pen, digitizing board, touchscreen, or monitoring equipment (Fig. 2–3).

Client workstations communicate through a central administrative server (computer) whose network operating system routes the communication of data between the client workstation and other database servers or legacy information system. In the client-server architecture, applications are divided between the client workstation and the server. Both the client and server operate together to execute the application. Examples of database servers include SYBASE, Oracle, and Microsoft SQL (structured query language).

The server operating system controls how quickly the server can complete client requests. The leading server operating systems are (1) UNIX, developed in the late 1960s, a multiuser, fully preemptive multitasking operating system; (2) Windows/NT, an operating system for Intel and RISC processors; and (3) Novell Netware, a server operating system with features like those of UNIX and Windows/NT.

Middleware

Client/server interactions should be transparent to users and applications. The clinician wants to view and record information without having to manage the data exchange transactions or networking system. To manage client-server interactions, a common set of interfaces has been developed. Together, these are known as *middleware*. Information from one device or system is shared with another device or system through an agreed-on method of representing the data. There are three communication standards that govern all but a few health information exchange situations: HL7, IEEE P1073 MIB, and DICOM (Fig. 2–4). Each standard was originally intended for a specific purpose, and therefore has both strengths and limitations.

HL7

HL7 (Health Industry Level 7 interface standard) was developed in the United States to promote communication between information systems (applications) within the hospital environment.[5] HL7 enables electronic data exchange between healthcare applications provided by different vendors, using different computer processors, programming languages, and operating systems. Since HL7 can, in principle,

enable communication between any system regardless of its computer architecture, HL7 supports communication between new and existing systems.[6]

HL7 defines transactions for transmitting data about patient registration, admission, discharge and transfers, insurance, charges and payers, orders and laboratory results, tests, image studies, nursing and physician observations, pharmacy orders, and master files. An example of the use of the HL7 interface standard would be the connection of a cardiac catheterization computer system to a narrative storage archive in the computerized patient record. Using the HL7 standard, the catheterization report can be transmitted to the narrative archive, even if the two computers are of different design and use different operating systems and programs.

Medical Information Bus

The IEEE P1073 Medical Information Bus (MIB) standard was created to provide communication among bedside devices in a medical environment. MIB was designed for the automation of the recording and the entry of information from medical instruments, primarily in ORs and critical care units, where instruments are typically mixed and matched. These standards are ongoing, having first been developed by the Institute of Electrical and Electronic Engineers (IEEE) in 1984.

MIB is an object-oriented design model. The medical device data language (MDDL) defines virtual medical objects, such as patient, host, and clinician, as well as common system actions, such as set, query, and report. MIB objects define the data, what to do with the data, and how other computer programs can access it.

The important feature of the MIB interface is that it is designed for the movement of bedside devices common in medical settings. Devices are "plug and play," and the MIB interface associates the device with the patient, allows real-time and remote access to data, and enables any manufacturer's device to be used without a custom interface.[7]

DICOM

The Digital Imaging and Communications in Medicine (DICOM) standard was developed to allow manufacturers and users of medical imaging equipment to connect all the various devices needed, such as storage archives, review and display workstations, and printers. DICOM is covered in more detail in the discussion of imaging information systems later in this chapter.

Other middleware interfaces have been developed. The

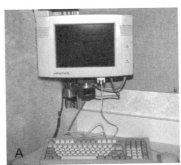
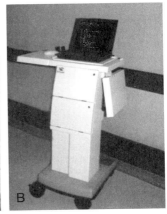

Figure 2–2. Point-of-care clinical workstations: *A,* Unit with integrated color liquid-crystal display screen and central processing unit in one case designed to save space in a typical examination room. *B,* For mobile applications on an inpatient ward, the clinical workstation is a laptop computer mounted on a battery stand and connected to the local area network via a radiofrequency wireless PCMCIA network card and wall-mounted wireless transceiver. (Courtesy of Diana Baxter, Roudebush VA Medical Center, Indianapolis.)

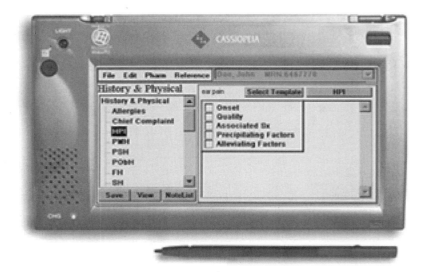

Figure 2-3. Example of an electronic medical record system designed for hand-held computing devices. This system runs on the Windows CE operating system. A wireless transponder option provides real-time connectivity with the host system. The unit measures 0.8 × 7.0 × 4.5 in., weighs less than 1 lb, and uses a pen input device on a "virtual" keyboard or handwriting recognition. (Courtesy of Physix, Inc., Houston.)

Common Object Request Broker Architecture standard (CORBA) was developed in 1989 by the Object Management Group (OMG), a nonprofit consortium of over 700 software vendors, developers, and users. The Distributed Healthcare Environment (DHE) is a middleware architecture permitting data sharing between end-user applications, including legacy systems.

Networking Infrastructure

The client workstations and server operate on a LAN. A LAN is an interconnected group of computers that can communicate with each other in a limited geographic area and share

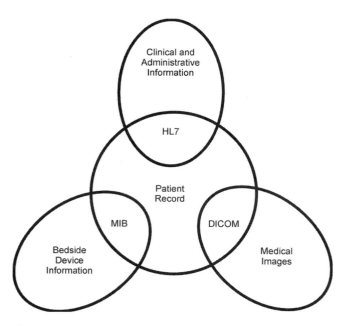

Figure 2-4. Communication standards allow for the exchange of information between different devices and information systems. These three standards provide for almost any data communication. HL7, Health Industry Level 7; MIB, Medical Information Bus; DICOM, Digital Imaging and Communications in Medicine. (Courtesy of Diana Baxter, Roudebush VA Medical Center, Indianapolis.)

information and resources (such as files and printers). A wide area network (WAN) allows users to communicate with each other over a geographically diverse area, such as within a multifacility system spread out over several cities or states. A high bandwidth telecommunications channel, such as T1, T2, telephone-switched packet service, or ISDN (integrated services digital network) line, links the individual facilities.

Between the client workstation and the central administrative server and other database servers is a system of cabling, hubs, routers, and switches that control data transmission across the network. While there are many highly technical issues involved in the design of efficient and reliable networks, the most important issue for users is the speed at which data can be transmitted, as this affects data retrieval and storage response time. Speed increases as the capacity and throughput of the cables, hubs, routers, and switches is increased.

Although wired networks have lower investment costs, wireless networks are approaching the same data transmission rates (Fig. 2-5). The primary difference between a wired and wireless network is the method of transmitting signals between the client workstation or input device and the network routers or server. This requires the placement of a wireless network adapter card in the client workstation and transceivers located throughout the hospital or clinic. Client workstations can be used up to several hundred feet from the transceiver stations.

Mobile and remote computing is of interest to the busy clinician, allowing access to patient information from any location, using wired or cellular phones. Wireless, mobile networks require telephone carriers to transmit and receive the data-carrying signals. This can be done using cellular networks, satellite networks, or packet-radio communication. While this form of connectivity offers convenience, it is slow. Transmission rates are typically 8000 to 19,000 bytes per second, compared to rates of 10 to 100 million bytes per second (MBps) in wired networks. The cost of mobile telephone service can be high, and so mobile data communication is best suited for medical applications where it is crucial or highly necessary to communicate simple patient information in real time when the clinician is not physically located in the hospital or clinic.

An interesting capability of some computerized patient record systems is the ability to transmit messages to alphanumeric pagers, using existing radio paging service (Fig. 2-6).

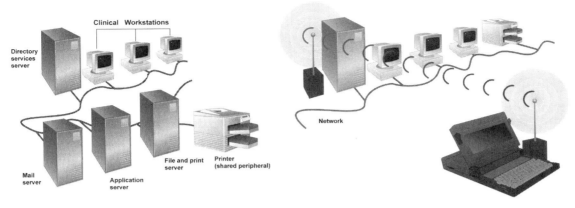

Figure 2-5. A graphic view of a combined wired and wireless local area network. (Courtesy of Diana Baxter, Roudebush VA Medical Center, Indianapolis.)

For example, the clinician can receive information, such as critical laboratory results, directly on the pager. One such system, Pageman, developed at the Roudebush VA Medical Center, Indianapolis, provides compatibility with standard numeric and alphanumeric paging protocols. A decision support system built into the hospital's clinical information system generates automated clinical alerts when trigger events occur (these are easily programmed in the decision support query language). The alerts can be set to be transmitted as alphanumeric pager messages, e-mail, or computer login messages.

Requirements

One essential requirement of any electronic medical record system, however advanced, is that it represent a change in the way work is done in clinical practice (Fig. 2-7). Given the disruptive nature of change, the basic requirement for any electronic medical record system can be answered by the simple question, Can I do my work more easily and better than I could before?

An acceptable electronic medical record system should have six design prerequisites according to Metzger and Teich[8]:

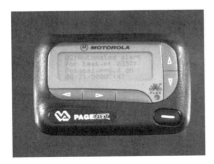

Figure 2-6. Alphanumeric radiofrequency pager linked to the computerized patient record. Note the message display showing a clinical notification created by the decision support protocol for hyperkalemia critical values. Message text reads: "Automated alert for test,pt 0357: Potassium = 6.4 on 08/21/98 @ 07:41." (Courtesy of Diane Baxter, Roudebush VA Medical Center, Indianapolis.)

1. Patient care information systems must be available whenever users need them to manage patient care.

2. Patient care information systems must be available wherever decisions about care are made.

3. Patient care information systems must provide quick and value-added access to information.

4. Patient care information systems must be designed to fit actual patient care processes and work situations.

5. Patient care information systems must be so easy to use that they require little or no training.

6. Involving physicians with direct data entry requires minimizing time and maximizing incentives.

When electronic medical record systems do not meet all or some of these requirements, physician resistance is likely. Users will feel overburdened by the additional workload imposed by a poorly designed system.

Advantages

For many care settings, the electronic medical record offers the clinician advantages over the traditional paper-based record. Most significantly, information can be accessed or inputted at the point of care, an important logistical consideration in some care settings, such as the intensive care unit (ICU) or OR, where the clinician may need to remain at the patient's bedside for extended periods. Data retrieval and display speeds have continued to improve, with many systems designed to display large volumes of data within 500 ms of request, on average. In addition, the graphical user interface (GUI) of the modern desktop computer has dramatically increased ease of use and lowered training requirements (Fig. 2-7).

New views of data are available with electronic medical record systems. Data that would be spread among many pages or reports in a paper record can be easily formatted to a single page or monitor screen, allowing the clinician to review longitudinal information, such as changes in laboratory values, at a glance. Graphing of numerical data points, such as blood pressure or heart rate over time, can also be displayed easily.

Integration of disparate data elements is possible in the electronic medical record through database queries and data

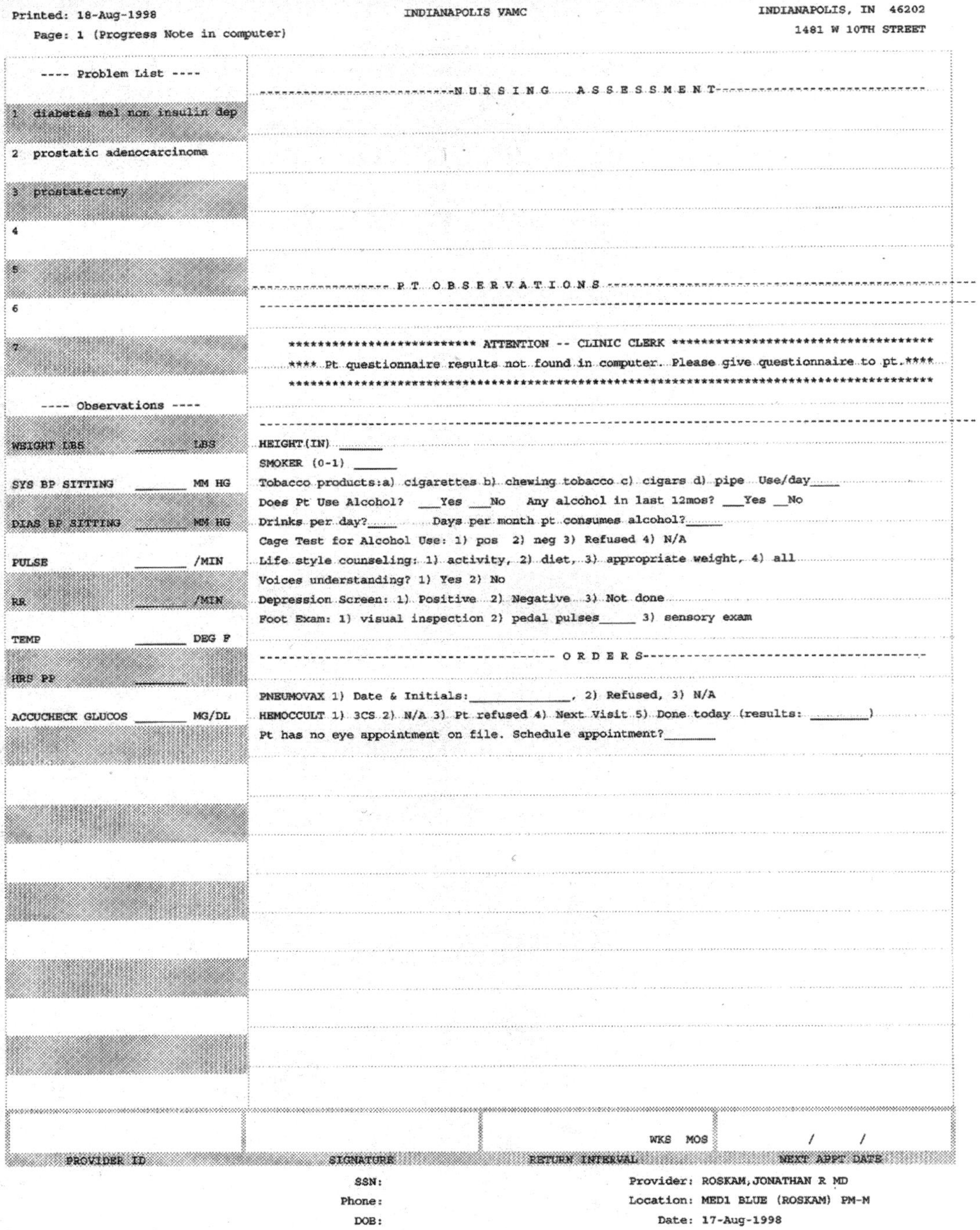

```
Printed: 18-Aug-1998                    INDIANAPOLIS VAMC              INDIANAPOLIS, IN  46202
    Page: 1 (Progress Note in computer)                                    1481 W 10TH STREET

 ---- Problem List ----      ----------------------N U R S I N G   A S S E S S M E N T----------------------

 1 diabetes mel non insulin dep

 2 prostatic adenocarcinoma

 3 prostatectomy

 4

 5                           ------------------- P T  O B S E R V A T I O N S -----------------------------
                            -------------------------------------------------------------------------
 6

 7                           *************************** ATTENTION -- CLINIC CLERK *************************
                            **** Pt questionnaire results not found in computer. Please give questionnaire to pt.****
                            ****************************************************************************

 ---- Observations ----     -------------------------------------------------------------------------

 WEIGHT LBS        LBS      HEIGHT (IN)
                            SMOKER (0-1)
 SYS BP SITTING    MM HG    Tobacco products:a) cigarettes b) chewing tobacco c) cigars d) pipe  Use/day
                            Does Pt Use Alcohol?  ___Yes ___No   Any alcohol in last 12mos? ___Yes ___No
 DIAS BP SITTING   MM HG    Drinks per day?_____  Days per month pt consumes alcohol?_____
                            Cage Test for Alcohol Use: 1) pos  2) neg 3) Refused 4) N/A
 PULSE             /MIN     Life style counseling: 1) activity, 2) diet, 3) appropriate weight, 4) all
                            Voices understanding? 1) Yes 2) No
 RR                /MIN     Depression Screen: 1) Positive  2) Negative  3) Not done
                            Foot Exam: 1) visual inspection 2) pedal pulses_____ 3) sensory exam
 TEMP              DEG F
                            --------------------------------- O R D E R S----------------------------
 HRS PP
                            PNEUMOVAX 1) Date & Initials:_____, 2) Refused, 3) N/A
 ACCUCHECK GLUCOS  MG/DL    HEMOCCULT 1) 3CS 2) N/A 3) Pt refused 4) Next Visit 5) Done today (results: _____)
                            Pt has no eye appointment on file. Schedule appointment?_____

 PROVIDER ID          SIGNATURE           RETURN INTERVAL    WKS  MOS     /    /
                                                                        NEXT APPT DATE
              SSN:                              Provider: ROSKAM,JONATHAN R MD
              Phone:                            Location: MED1 BLUE (ROSKAM) PM-M
              DOB:                              Date: 17-Aug-1998
```

Figure 2-7. Sample clinic encounter form generated by an electronic medical record system. This "hybrid" system uses paper encounter forms and structured data input. Data are entered from the problem list, vital signs, and patient observation sections. Note the patient-specific clinical reminders which are the output of the encounter-based decision support system. (Courtesy of Roudebush VA Medical Center, Indianapolis.)

summary reports. This makes evaluating and understanding interrelated but separately collected data relatively easy. Further, database analysis across patient populations or over time is possible with the electronic medical record. The importance of this capability in the managed care environment, to assist in the evaluation of quality, cost, and outcomes, is an important factor driving the widespread adaptation of the electronic medical record.

Decision Support Capabilities

Most currently available or developed electronic medical record systems are limited to the storage and retrieval of information. However, the most advanced systems include decision support capabilities (Fig. 2-8). This is one of the most significant potential benefits to clinicians using computerized records. Decision support tools amplify the experience and judgment of clinicians. Using rules-based expert engines, it is possible to provide to the clinician real-time, point-of-care, and patient-specific information such as drug-drug interactions, allergy warnings, critical laboratory values, drug monitoring requirements, and needed interventions. While all of this knowledge may be practiced by the expert clinician, the speed, breadth, and consistency of a computer decision support system far exceed those of the most dedicated and expert clinician.

In computerized patient record systems that include on-line clinician order entry, a decision support system can allow the real-time display of messages at the point of care and prior to ordering. This has been shown to improve both the quality and cost-effectiveness of the clinician's care, as well as increase the satisfaction of clinical users with the computerized patient record system.

Imaging Information Systems

Picture archiving and communication systems (PACSs) provide for the acquisition, storage, and retrieval of digital images. PACS technology has been under development since the early 1980s.[9] Digital images are generated by imaging modalities such as computed tomography (CT) scanners, magnetic resonance imaging (MRI) equipment, ultrasound machines, or endoscopes, as examples. PACS are highly scalable, meaning that many imaging modalities may be added to the system (Fig. 2-9).

In the computerized patient record, PACS images can become integrated with other patient information to create a multimedia patient record. However, even though the technology to implement PACS continues to decrease in cost and increase in capability, PACS images typically are initially used to replace the radiology information system (RIS) and are limited to filmless radiology imaging. One reason for this is that PACS technology is complex and difficult to achieve.[10] Functional integration of a PACS into an existing computerized patient record system has been done successfully only rarely.

To overcome the problem of interfacing different imaging modalities, the American College of Radiology and the Na-

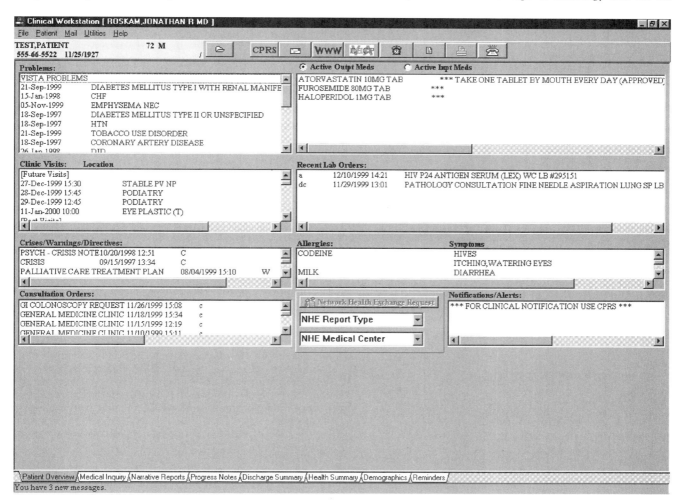

Figure 2-8. Graphical user interface for a comprehensive computerized patient record system. The user interface is written in Delphi 3.0 for Windows and communicates with a host database system written in MUMPS. The interface uses a "tabbed" chart format, with tabs displayed at the bottom of the chart. (Courtesy of Roudebush VA Medical Center, Indianapolis.)

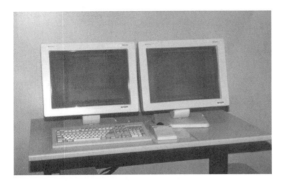

Figure 2–9. PACS (picture archiving and communication system) viewing workstation installed in an intensive care unit charting room. For comparison of prior films, two displays are used side by side. (Courtesy of Diana Baxter, Roudebush VA Medical Center, Indianapolis.)

tional Equipment Manufacturers Association (NEMA) jointly developed the DICOM 3.0 standard. The DICOM 3.0 standard interface governs the way the imaging modalities send and receive data over the LAN to the PACS server.

The goal of a PACS is to manage digital images for radiologists and other clinicians and make them available on display workstations at the point of care, such as in the ICU or OR. Acquisition of patient images is accomplished by transmitting the digital image(s) from the imaging modality using the DICOM 3.0 interface standard onto the LAN and then to one or more interpretation quality gray-scale workstations. The images are archived on an optical jukebox, and the archive workstation registers the DICOM data on its relational database. The archive workstation maintains a relational database management system for locating and archiving image files and associated patient data.

The radiologist or other clinician uses a viewing workstation to retrieve and display images. Prior examinations archived on the optical jukebox can be requested and downloaded onto the user's workstation. A properly functioning PACS can improve availability of old images, minimize lost films, and maintain high output.[11]

PACS technology requires high-capacity file servers for the large number of patient images to be stored. For example, MRI examinations may produce over 400 images in a single study. A radiology department performing 120,000 examinations per year would generate about 3.25 terabytes (1 terabyte is 1×10^{12} bytes) per year of data to be archived. Current digital image archiving systems have a capacity of from 10 to 100 terabytes.

In the future, continued emphasis on total integration of all components of the patient care information system means the merger of the RIS, PACS, CPR, and financial information systems into one integrated whole.

The Internet as a Clinical Information System

The Internet is predicted to become the most important communication medium in the future information society. In healthcare, the Internet provides potential access to information within a hospital, within a network of medical centers, physicians' offices and homes, and throughout the world. The important property of the World Wide Web (WWW) is that it provides a uniform operating environment that allows computer platforms of any configuration to communicate with each other. Any user with any computer and modem can access the Internet and communicate with any other user. The Internet permits assembling a virtual patient record without actually moving the underlying data until they are needed. Applications can now reach across networks and into legacy systems to gather patient information just in time, obviating the current practice of consolidating everything in one repository (in practice, this is challenging to accomplish outside of a single site).

The Internet is a communications system initially created by the U.S. Department of Defense Advanced Research Projects Agency as a medium for secure and uninterrupted global data transmission. It is now used worldwide by the private sector for commerce, education, research, and entertainment.

There are many medical uses of the Internet. For example, a recent report was published detailing the use of the Internet as a teleconferencing medium for anesthesiologists who conduct "virtual grand rounds."[12] An Internet-based decision support system for evaluating chest pain is in use at a California medical center.[13]

In what is among the most ambitious efforts to communicate medical information, the Euromed Project seeks to create a global telemedical society based on the WWW.[14] Euromed has introduced a new global standard called Virtual Medical Worlds (VMW) to reduce the complexity of searching the Web for related patient information. Hyperlinks are used to create the patient's medical record (a hyperlink jumps the user from one Web page location to another). Although information that comprises the patient's medical record may be dispersed in many different computers all over the Web, all the data are potentially accessible from a single HTML (hypertext markup language) Web page which forms the electronic health card of the patient.

The VMW standard consists of several components: medical images in DICOM 3.0 format stored on a PACS, reconstructed medical pictures in VRML 2.0 format stored on WWW servers and medical applications (that use the X Windows protocol). Medical providers linking to the patient's dispersed records will have a computer on the Internet configured as a WWW server.

Personal Computerized Patient Record

In the VMW scheme, every patient will be able to have a personal home page (PHP) as the "repository" of his or her patient record. The PHP will be located on a unique WWW VMW server. The clinician will be able to trace all of the medical history related to the patient from hyperlinks on the PHP. Clinicians anywhere will be able to access this patient information as they provide care. Before this system of interconnectivity and global access to a patient's personal medical history can become widespread, issues of data security and user access, uniform data representation models, and patient self-reporting of medical information will need to be addressed.

Challenges

Healthcare providers all want electronic medical record systems. However, electronic medical record systems are difficult to develop because existing data sources, such as laboratory systems, pharmacy systems, and registration and billing systems, are separated by different database and coding sys-

Table 2–1. Message Standards for Different Data Types

Data Type and Source	Message Standards
Laboratory tests	Health Industry Level 7 (HL7) ORU, American Society for Testing and Materials (ASTM) 1238, Comité Européean de Normalisation (CEN) ENV 1613
Images	Digital Imaging and Communications in Medicine (DICOM)
Electrocardiograms	CEN
Gastrointestinal endoscopy, etc.	HL7
Obstetrics ultrasound, etc.	HL7
Admission, discharge, transfer registration information	HL7, CEN ENV 12538
Pharmacy	HL7 and National Council for Prescription Drug Programs (NCPDP)

tems. Thus the electronic medical record continues to lack complete integration with all of the hospital information systems that contain clinically useful information. The development of message standards has essentially solved the challenge of transmitting patient clinical information from one system to another.[15] Table 2–1 shows what standards are available for common medical information.

The development of standard codes and vocabularies for basic clinical concepts continues to be a challenge. A familiar example of codes is the International Classification of Diseases (ICD-9) system. Other codes and vocabularies include the National Drug Code (NDC) in the United States, Logical Observations Identifiers Names and Codes (LOINC) for laboratory tests and clinical measurements, Standardized Nomenclature of Medicine (SNOMED), Read codes, and the MED (medicine), all broad code systems in use.

One last problem to overcome is the efficient capture of clinician information in coded form understandable by a computer. Physicians tend to record their observations as free text. Translating free text into computer-interpretable codes and structure is very challenging. Entering structured data instead of free text places significant time and training demands on clinicians, and is generally not acceptable. Thus, complete coding of data into the entire medical record will not happen in the near future.

Government Computerized Patient Record

A major new initiative is under way in the United States to develop a government computerized patient record (GCPR). Cooperation between the Department of Veterans Affairs, Department of Defense, and Indian Health Service began formally in January 1998. The aim of this project is to develop the infrastructure to allow organizations with different computerized patient record systems to share patient data without having to move to a common user interface or underlying health information system. A large-scale data representation model, data translation service, and data exchange infrastructure are planned to create a fully integrated computerized patient record system that can effortlessly access and provide clinical data from any patient information system.

Security

There are significant security issues related to the computerized patient record. Security issues fall into three main categories: (1) intrahospital use, (2) interinstitutional use, and (3) storage.[16] These issues are summarized in Table 2–2.

There are several common security issues. Authentication is the step whereby computer users "prove" who they are to gain access. Logins that require only an access code and password offer less efficient security than systems requiring both a password and token (such as an employee ID card with magnetic stripe or bar code). Users may distribute their password to others, reducing the security of the system.

Access control means the institution decides which data an individual or user class may access. This can be accomplished by assignment of "keys" for each category of data that needs to be controlled. Access logs that require the user to provide justification for requesting information before the data are transmitted are helpful. Many institutions have strict limited-access policies for sensitive patient information, such as human immunodeficiency virus (HIV) testing and psychiatric records.

Table 2–2. Security Issues in Various Uses of the Computerized Patient Record

	Security-Related Issues	Examples	Available Technology
Intrahospital use	Access control	How to prevent file access by unauthorized persons	Password or token
	Outside intrusion	How to prevent access by outside intruders	Firewall
Interhospital use	Integrity	How to prove the integrity of data sent via the network	Message digest
	Leakage	How to prevent leakage of data during transmission	Encryption
	Authentication	How to prevent reception of transmitted data by unauthorized persons	Public and private keys
Storage	Identity	How to guarantee the stored data are the same as the original	Digital signature
	Modification	How to prevent or detect modification of data after storage	Digital signature
	Long-term storage	How to guarantee safe storage in the long term	Frequent reading of the archive
	Destruction, loss, theft, etc.	How to prevent loss, destruction, or theft of data stored	Physical security
	Readability	How to guarantee the long-term readability of stored data with changing technology	

Data from Kaihara S: Realisation of the computerised patient record: Relevance and unsolved problems. Int J Med Inform 1998; 49:1–8.

Computer security education programs and random audits of user access logs also increase the security of the information management system. Inappropriate browsing of patient records can be discouraged with such methods.

Data Integrity

Although a paper-based manual medical record may be criticized for data omissions and inaccuracies, the same can be said of electronic medical record systems. Without a paper trail, it is vital that those entering data electronically are adequately trained and that data validation procedures are in place. When direct input of data by physicians is required, the time needed for such work should be as minimal as possible. Otherwise, the system is unlikely to be accepted by physicians. Software interfaces should be designed in such a way as to minimize errors in data entry. Human coding (converting written observations into computer-understandable codes for computer data entry) is error-prone and expensive, potentially reducing data integrity.

Data Evaluation Features

One of the emerging capabilities of the electronic medical record is the creation of large patient databases for healthcare outcome and economic research. After only several years of use, many electronic patient databases can contain extensive records on tens of thousands of patients.[17] By 1996, one of the oldest electronic medical record systems in continuous use had extensive data on 1.4 million patients, including more than 6 million prescription records, millions of orders, nearly 200,000 electrocardiogram tracings, and 100 million coded patient observations and test results.[18]

Data Warehousing

With the accumulation of large amounts of structured patient medical information into data warehouses, it becomes possible to provide the information resource for data mining and knowledge discovery. Patient outcomes, disease factors, and economic or treatment variables can be studied reliably within the large set of patient records provided by the data warehouse. This kind of resource promises to improve health policy, research, and the evaluation of medical treatments.

Profiling Information Systems

Measuring the performance of individual clinicians, health plans, and hospitals is becoming increasingly popular in the healthcare system in the United States. With managed care, great emphasis has been placed on developing healthcare "report cards" and other means to compare the quality or cost of care provided by health plans or practitioners. A healthcare profiling information system provides the data sets and analytic methods that allow for comparisons based on quantitative or qualitative measures. Such measures may include the cost of service, patient satisfaction ratings, mortality rates, preventive health intervention rates, or appointment availability. Generally, such profiling is performed within the context of comparison to other service providers, peers, or competitors.

The Joint Commission for the Accreditation of Healthcare

Organizations (JCAHO) has developed many performance standards for hospital organizations. The Indicator Measurement System (IMSystem) was developed beginning in 1987.[19] It is a comparative performance measurement system that is intended to measure meaningful patient outcomes. The JCAHO anesthesiology (perioperative) indicator-based performance standards are outlined as follows[20]:

1. *Numerator:* Patients developing a central nervous system (CNS) complication within 2 postprocedure days of procedures involving anesthesia administration

2. *Numerator:* Patients developing a peripheral neurologic deficit within 2 postprocedure days of procedures involving anesthesia administration

3. *Numerator:* Patients developing an acute myocardial infarction within 2 postprocedure days of procedures involving anesthesia administration

4. *Numerator:* Patients with a cardiac arrest within 2 postprocedure days of procedures involving anesthesia administration

5. *Numerator:* Intrahospital mortality of patients within 2 postprocedure days of procedures involving anesthesia administration

Profiling must be performed using the best statistical methods. However, commonly used profiling information systems have several deficiencies, including ignoring important relevant information, such as case mix, using statistical standards when medical standards would be more appropriate, and ignoring differences in workload.[21] Additionally, debate over the usefulness of profiling systems includes concerns over (1) the quality of the data, (2) patient risk stratification (3) outcome industry standards, and (4) data and report standardization.[22]

The scope and accuracy of profiling systems vary. The first national "quality" assessment was released by the Healthcare Financing Administration in 1987. It reported on the observed and expected mortality rates of each hospital in which Medicare patients underwent coronary bypass surgery. Publication of this data was later suspended because of concerns that the data analysis was misleading and inadequate.

Other governmental agencies have released health report cards in the public interest with varying success. The 1993 New York State Department of Health report on coronary artery bypass graft surgery listed mortality data and profile statistics for 31 hospitals.[23] Christiansen and Morris[21] evaluated the effect of risk adjustment on reducing unfair profile evaluations. Using case mix adjustment of the New York data, they showed that for two hospitals with "comparable" mortality rates of 4.48% and 4.55%, the risk-adjusted mortality rates were 8.77% and 5.77%, respectively.

A number of public interest and private organizations are producing health report cards or profiling information systems for managed care. The most prominent is the National Committee for Quality Assurance (NCQA), established in 1979 by the Group Health Association of America and the American Managed Care and Review Association. The NCQA accredits over 600 health maintenance organizations. In 1991 the NCQA released the first Health Plan Employer Data and Information Set (HEDIS), a tool to allow purchasers of healthcare to compare the performance of provider organizations. The latest version of HEDIS (3.0) reports on over 60 standardized indicators of cost, access, financial stability, membership, and patient satisfaction. HEDIS 3.0 focuses on outcomes as well as process to measure quality. It includes measures for Medicare and Medicaid populations, increases the scope of healthcare reported on, and standardizes the patient satisfaction survey process.[24] Importantly, however, HEDIS 3.0 does not adjust for differences in population health risk. The value of a health report card system such as HEDIS is that it specifies how a provider organization should calculate performance measures, allowing meaningful comparisons.

Anesthesia Information Management Systems

The anesthesia record is intended to provide information in three broad categories: clinical care, historical data, and retrospective data for quality improvement and physician profiling. As the practice of anesthesia has changed in response to advances in the technology of physiologic monitoring, pharmacology, biomedical engineering, and surgical technique, a significant increase in the quantity and type of data to be recorded in the anesthesia record has resulted. This increase in the amount of data to be responded to and documented has, in turn, increased the complexity of transcribing a completely accurate picture of the patient's perioperative course.

Computerized AIMSs are being used increasingly to facilitate the efficient management of anesthesia departments as well as to improve the process of documenting and facilitating the patient's entire anesthetic course, including preoperative, intraoperative, and postoperative care. AIMSs can also provide significant management and clinical data for economic, quality, and academic analysis.[25] Efforts at developing computerized AIMSs began in the 1970s, primarily at academic medical centers with informatics development capabilities.[26] Today both hospital-developed and commercial AIMS products are in use. Many of these computerized systems represent the second and third generation of development.

Even when data in the anesthesia record are captured at only 5-minute intervals, the anesthesiologist faces considerable difficulty in keeping up with all of the physiologic data typically transcribed unless an assistant is available solely for manual record-keeping purposes.[27, 28] In all but the simplest cases, the plethora of data has exceeded the ability to manually record it. During anesthesia, the anesthesiologist can watch over 30 interrelated metrics to determine the physiologic condition of the patient.[29] Given the challenges of using the traditional manually recorded anesthesia record, significant interest and effort have been expended to automate the collection and recording of data.

History of the Anesthetic Record

Early anesthetic records date back to 1894 when Ernest Codman and Harvey Cushing, while medical students at the Massachusetts General Hospital, developed "ether charts" to learn more about the delivery of ether and improve patient outcomes. These charts were simple compared to modern anesthesia records, and included only the pulse, respiration, and temperature, as well as brief comments about the patient, procedure, and ether dose administered. It was not until 1902 that Cushing recommended the inclusion of routine blood pressure monitoring as part of the anesthesia record.[30]

Since then the anesthetic record has become significantly more complex, although the basic principles have remained

similar to those described by Cushing. Some of the historical efforts to improve the anesthetic record and allow for the analysis of the data in it are noteworthy.

The development of mechanized methods of data collection and data compilation were the first efforts at improving the written anesthesia record. The Hollerith punch card method was advocated by the American Society of Anesthesiologists (ASA) in the 1940s.[31]

This system required the use of cards with holes punched in columns of numbers. Each column represented some anesthesia data element, such as operation type, diagnosis, patient demographics, time unconscious, complications, and so on.[32] A specially fabricated mechanical tabulator read the punch cards.

To allow for the retrospective analysis of simple manually collected anesthesia record data, a modification of the Hollerith card was developed in England. The Nosworthy card was an 8- by 5-in. punch card that contained a brief preoperative history on the front and a small graphic representation of the anesthesia procedure on the back[33, 34] (Fig. 2–10). All around the edge of the card's front were a series of printed circles, each one representing a category of information, such as anesthetic agent or site of operation. The anesthesiologist would write a comment next to the applicable circle, which would later be punched out past the card's edge, leaving a U-shaped defect. To sort through a stack of Nosworthy cards by a single parameter (punched-out area), a thin metal wire was pushed through the desired position allowing all the nonpunched cards to be removed. The remaining cards all contained the same punched-out data element.

Full-page anesthesia record formats were also developed and used frequently, including the Chicago Keysort anesthesia record.[35] Much later, the Committee of Clinical Anesthesia Study of the ASA developed a new punch card type of anesthesia record.[36] This record, used from the 1960s, contained not only documentation of the anesthetic course but also preoperative and postoperative information. Although

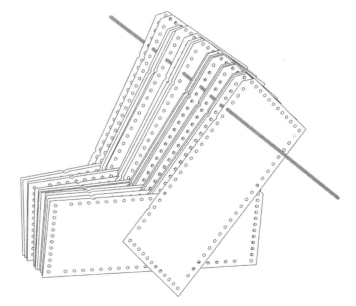

Figure 2–10. Card sorting method with Nosworthy punch cards. The punched-out cards remain behind when the needle is lifted. (Courtesy of David E. Gregory, Roudebush VA Medical Center, Indianapolis.)

the system was easy to use and allowed for the later collation and analysis of anesthesia data, it required the use of trained coders to enter the data in the punch card format.

Limitations of the Manual Anesthetic Record

Many authors have argued that the typical written anesthesia record is less than optimal for understanding the events leading up to anesthesia- or surgery-related intraoperative catastrophe.[37] This contention may be due to a combination of factors. Manual anesthetic records are more likely to contain errors in data entry, data omissions, and legibility problems compared with computer-assisted records. During anesthetic administration, the anesthesiologist spends a significant amount of time viewing the monitors that display patient information, evaluating the displayed data to determine whether they are normal, deciding whether the data (if abnormal) are accurate, and responding to abnormal data. The observed data are entered manually into the anesthesia record. Much of this activity is repetitive and routine and may predispose to data transcription errors or omissions.

At other times the anesthesiologist may be fully occupied with other aspects of patient care, finding it difficult to precisely record anesthetic data every 5 minutes as recommended by the ASA. In such situations, when the anesthesiologist's attention is diverted from more important tasks by the need to record data in the anesthesia record, the use of memory recall and time pressures can cause transcription errors and omissions that would otherwise not occur.

Handwritten anesthesia records can contain inaccuracies related to observer bias, falsification, or recall errors.[38, 39] In one confidential study of the accuracy of manual anesthesia records, the rate of occasional data omission or falsification was 55%.[40] Observer bias can result in the "smoothing" of recorded data and has been reported in multiple studies comparing handwritten with automated anesthesia records. The computer-assisted recording of data is completely objective and reflects the expected transient fluctuations in physiologic indicators precisely. Perhaps because the anesthesiologist may fear that such recorded fluctuations would require more explanation, manually entered data, such as a low systolic blood pressure, may be inflated to produce a more "acceptable" record.

In comparing hand-entered and computer-entered physiologic data, investigators found that low values for blood pressure and heart rate and high values for end-tidal CO_2 were recorded significantly more often using a computerized record system than with manual data recording.[37] This smoothing bias has been found in other studies.[41] Characteristically, there is little discrepancy between automated and manually entered readings when the values of systolic and diastolic blood pressure and heart rate are in the normal range. However, as these values exceed either the upper or lower limit of normal, the discrepancy between automated readings and manually recorded readings increases.[42] High readings are lowered, and low readings are elevated in the manual record.

In today's managed care environment, there are significant additional problems with the handwritten anesthesia record. Even small-scale retrospective assessments of anesthesia care must be based on time-consuming and resource-intensive chart reviews, rather than relying on more efficient and less costly computerized reporting. With paper-based anesthesia records, the lack of detailed documentation of resource use, including personnel time, medications, equipment, and supplies, makes cost assessments and provider profiling more problematic.

An important additional consideration is the use of anesthetic records for medicolegal purposes. In this setting, accuracy, legibility, completeness in recording details, and the quality of comments become surrogates for the quality of the anesthetic care. Missing data or poorly kept data open the door to conjecture and interpretation, increasing potential liability for the anesthesiologist.

This is not to say that handwritten anesthetic records have no advantages. Indeed, the written record is easy to learn, simple to use, permits considerable individual variation in style of completion, takes up very little OR space, is highly portable, is inexpensive, and requires little maintenance. The challenge in moving to a computer-assisted anesthesia record or computerized anesthesia information management system is to preserve these positive attributes without unduly burdening the anesthesiologist with the inputting of data.

Anesthesia Workflow

The workflow processes of anesthesia care are an important determinate of whether a computerized system will be acceptable and efficient to use. As with other computerized information management systems, the clinician must be able to perform work better and more easily than before.

What goes on during the intraoperative period? The anesthesiologist performs any number of tasks, including properly positioning the patient, placing noninvasive and invasive monitors, and inducing and maintaining anesthesia. Besides these procedural tasks, the anesthesiologist watches the monitors and other patient status indicators, constantly observing, evaluating, and reacting to that information. Drugs, fluids, and possibly blood products are administered. Verbal communication with the surgeon and other OR staff occurs. Only some of this information is recorded on the anesthesia record and only as time permits.

Studies using videotape recordings have shown that the anesthesiologist spends between 6% and 15% of the available time in record-keeping.[43] About 25% of the anesthesiologist's time may be spent in monitoring.[44] Several factors contribute to the effect of automated anesthesia record-keeping on the amount of time available to directly observe the patient, instead of manually entering data. These include the overall ease of use of the automated system, the familiarity of the anesthesiologist with the system, and the ergonomics of the AIMS intraoperative components. The failure of one commercial AIMS in a major academic center was partially due to crowding of the OR, requiring placement of the AIMS unit on the right side of the anesthesia machine.[45] This nonergonomic equipment layout resulted in the patient being out of the anesthesiologist's field of view when the AIMS was used.

Approaches to Computerized Anesthesia Information Management Systems

Historically, the computerized AIMS was developed within a single institution and as an "island of automation" to meet the immediate information needs of the anesthesiologist. Integration with other hospital and clinical information systems was accomplished infrequently. There continues to be significant transition among commercial vendors of computerized AIMSs, with companies entering and exiting the market.

However, the latest commercial products have greatly benefited from the tremendous recent advances in computerized medical records (data communication standards, data standardization, integration tools for legacy systems, and hardware advances). This should add some stability to the commercial market, giving the products longer useful lives and making them more attractive to acquire.

What would the ideal computerized AIMS look like? It would be only one component of a fully functioned computerized patient record system. The ideal AIMS would be integrated with every other hospital and clinical information system. It would bring into one user interface all of the information necessary for preoperative assessment, instant recall of past anesthesia records, intraoperative record-keeping, integrated monitor displays with artifact filtering, postoperative care, clinical decision support, and structured data for outcomes research. All the data would be available in real time and at the point of care. In addition, the system would be integrated with the OR information system used for case scheduling and inventory control. There would be seamless information exchange with all the other hospital information systems, including pharmacy, radiology, charge capture and billing, registration, and outpatient systems. It would provide a paperless system that allows the anesthesiologist to perform better and more efficiently than in a manual system. Powerful database analytic tools and reporting would be easily available to every user. Such a system does not exist today.

Current computerized AIMSs have two basic components. The intraoperative record-keeper uses interfaces with monitoring equipment to provide automated data acquisition and produces a computer-assisted paper or electronic anesthesia record. The database component integrates the record-keeping function with information stored during preoperative assessments and intraoperative and postoperative care. The database allows retrieval of past anesthesia records and the creation of various management workload and quality reports. Off-line data acquisition, including data entry, data display, data storage and retrieval, and anesthesia record production, varies depending on the manufacturer or developer. Due to the past limitations of commercial AIMSs, systems have been developed by anesthesiologists and informatics departments in hospitals to better meet their needs.

History of Computerized Anesthesia Information Management Systems

One of the first efforts at the development of a noncommercial computerized AIMS was the Duke Anesthesia Monitoring Equipment (DAME) system. Development of DAME by the department of anesthesiology at Duke University began in 1972, with installation of the system in 10 ORs, in 1980.[46] Users never fully accepted the system, and it was discontinued in 1983. Many of the reasons for discontinuation provide insight into evaluating a computerized AIMS for purchase or development.

Conceived as an automated record-keeping and database system, DAME introduced many innovative concepts later adopted by commercial systems. It both displayed and automatically recorded monitored vital signs. Other data, including drug and surgical events, could be inputted for the anesthesia record printout and for storage into the archive database. Drug and event entries were made using light pen and bar code input devices. A computer video monitor and keyboard were also provided, in addition to the primary monitoring screen.

Very few features, such as the automated blood pressure component of the monitor, were liked by the users. There were many serious shortcomings. Frequent network problems, software bugs, and monitor system crashes made DAME unreliable. The use of bar codes for the entry of drugs and events proved to be unworkable. Some codes were too long and were frequently read incorrectly. If the bar code source pages disappeared or became soiled, data entry was not possible. Ergonomic issues resulted because the equipment was heavy and cumbersome, and could not always be positioned optimally for the anesthesiologist. Some features, such as the electrocardiographic wiring and temperature channel, were either disliked or not used.

Computer-Assisted Anesthesia Record-Keeping

Other early attempts at computerized anesthesia information systems were less ambitious than DAME and focused on computer-assisted record-keeping. Some information was entered automatically (vital signs) and some manually (such as drugs and anesthesia events). The computer-assisted anesthetic record (CARR) developed at Emory University in the 1970s used plotter-entered data over a preprinted anesthesia record to produce clean "handwritten" records.[47] The semiautomated anesthesia record keeper (SARC) was developed by the University of Florida and the Datascope Corporation (Paramus, NJ).[48] It combined a clipboard-based plotter printing on only part of the form from behind the preprinted anesthesia record, allowing the anesthesiologist to enter handwritten comments and data on the other portion of the form. In addition, SARC plotted the automated vital signs vertically from top to bottom of the left half of the form. This allowed the user to write comments, drugs, and events on horizontal lines on the unused right half of the page so that they were time-aligned with the plotted vital sign trend data.

One major problem with automated monitor data sampling is artifact. The curves of heart rate and arterial blood pressure are prone to show outliers caused by surgical cauterization or arterial line flushing. Computerized AIMSs may include an "artifact" filter using algorithms to suppress the recording of outlier data.[49]

Diatek Arkive System

A commercial computerized AIMS, the Diatek Arkive "Organizer" System, illustrates both the benefits and problems associated with converting from a manual to automated anesthesia information system. Development of the Arkive system began in 1982 by Diatek Corporation of San Diego. Five successive versions of the AIMS were produced before the product was discontinued in 1995.

The later designs used a high-resolution flat-panel gas plasma display screen with pressure-sensitive touchscreen. The screen display mimicked the anesthesia record and was attached to the "organizer" cart positioned to the anesthesiologist's right, between the anesthesia machine and the patient. A removable boom over the breathing circuit hoses allowed the screen to be repositioned according to the anesthesiologist's preference. The cart had adjustable shelving for patient monitors, and modules allowed for the interfacing of monitor equipment through their analog or digital outputs. Case data were stored on a data diskette. The anesthesia record was printed using a dot matrix printer mounted on the back of the cart. Entry of data required the anesthesiologist to use the display panel touchscreen or a limited number of keys. For text entry, a keyboard was displayed on the touch panel. For numeric entry, a keypad was displayed. As an alternative to "typing" on the touch panel, voice entry of drugs and comments was possible. Boilerplate notes could be used for preconfigured cases. Preconfigured cases allowed the anesthesiologist to customize the monitor display, drugs, and notes for each type of case. Finally, a module was available to handle intravenous infusions. Improvements continued to be made by the manufacturer, including software revisions, support for network laser printing of anesthesia records, and redesign of the screen display to allow the boom to be mounted on the anesthesia machine.

The Arkive system required substantial user training.[45] Other problems included loss of power when the battery system discharged, difficulty positioning the organizer cart in some ORs, printer paper jams, and the requirement to be able to touch-type to be efficient (this was particularly noted for operations lasting less than about 45 minutes). The Arkive system did have many advantages over a manual anesthesia information system. Benefits included legible anesthesia records, automatic data acquisition, electronic access to previous cases, and complete data recording during critical episodes (Table 2–3).[50]

Hospital-Developed Computerized Anesthesia Information Management Systems

A recent hospital-developed computerized AIMS is in use at the Buccheri La Ferla hospital in Palermo, Italy.[17] Development there began in 1986 on a system that includes preoperative visit information as well as an intraoperative automated record-keeper. Preoperative data are collected at the patient's bedside or outpatient visit and entered into a portable computer in real time. Case information is entered by the

anesthesiologist into a personal computer (PC) workstation during anesthesia. Automated data monitoring is performed, with a trend output at 1-minute intervals. Patient data are stored in coded format and codes can be customized (heart is stored as "76"). This allows the resulting patient record to be independent of language. Postoperative orders can be entered into and printed from the system.

Additional features added to this system include an online help function to assist in pharmacologic calculations and drug administration, a centralized user interface-display, and a mail-messaging feature to send data and messages between anesthesia workstations. Finally, the designers included the ability to display any patient's trend data from a remote location via modem connection to the networked system.

Commercial Anesthesia Information Management Systems

In addition to hospital-developed AIMSs, an increasing number of commercial AIMSs are being marketed. Several such systems will be described to illustrate the approach commercial vendors have taken (no endorsement of these systems is intended). Many of the commercial systems available have been developed by manufacturers of anesthesia workstations, OR monitoring equipment, or anesthesia machines, and have varying degrees of integration with the company's medical equipment product line. In addition, the degree of integration with other clinical and hospital information systems varies. In many cases, integration with existing information systems represents the greatest implementation requirement, long-term cost, and barrier to effectiveness of such systems.

Recall Anesthesia Information Management System

Currently available in Europe, the Recall Anesthesia Information Management System marketed by Drägerwerk AG provides for preoperative records, intraoperative automated record-keeping, quality assurance and cost reporting, and an integration pathway for other hospital information systems. The Recall "chart" module is used to create a complete electronic anesthetic record. All relevant perioperative information is available to the anesthesiologist in a single display.

The automated record-keeping function provides preconfiguration setups of drug, dose, route, materials, and methods. Automatic recording of monitored vital signs, recording of all times, events, routes, and material usage, and encoding of diagnoses, procedures, events, and complications complete the record-keeping.

The database system allows for later analysis of records, including routine reports on OR usage, length of anesthesia, drug usage, and reasons for cancellations. User-specific queries allow customized reports.

Saturn Information System

The Saturn Information System (North American Dräger, Telford, PA) represents a newer generation of commercial AIMSs. Designed to provide an integrated perioperative system and OR information system, the Saturn user interface is integrated with OR SUITE (IntegraSys, San Diego) which provides OR case scheduling, inventory control, perioperative charting, clinical pathways, and OR management reporting functions.

The Saturn Information System is a 32-bit application for the Windows NT client-server environment. The Sybase SQL

Table 2–3. Data Acquired by the Arkive System

Type of Data	Automatic Insertion	Manual Insertion
Physiologic data	yes	yes
Heart rate	yes	
Invasive arterial blood pressure	yes	
Noninvasive arterial blood pressure	yes	
Pulmonary arterial blood pressure	yes	
Central venous pressure	yes	
Cardiac output (intermittent)	yes	
Mixed venous oxygen saturation	yes	
Arterial oxygen saturation	yes	
Respiration	yes	
End-tidal carbon dioxide	yes	
Temperature	yes	
Electroencephalography	yes	
Blood loss	no	yes
Urine output	no	yes
Equipment used	no	Text entry
Notes	no	Text entry
Events (preconfigured)	Via touch screen	
Drug and fluid (preconfigured)	Via touch screen	

Data from Coleman RL, Stanley T III, Gilbert WC, et al: The implementation and acceptance of an intraoperative anesthesia information management system. J Clin Monit Comput 1997; 13:121–128.

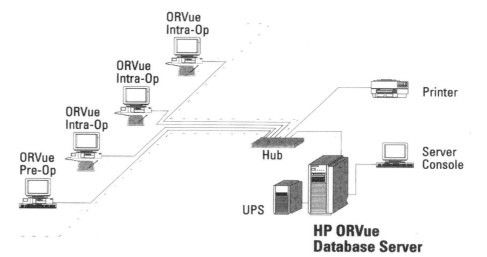

Figure 2–11. Schematic diagram of the ORVue client-server system, showing the point-of-care peripherals and central server. (Courtesy of Hewlett-Packard, Palo Alto, CA.)

database is ODBC*-compliant, which supports SQL queries and allows it to be integrated with other hospital information management systems. The graphical interface features "flat" navigation, allowing data input or retrieval with no more than two user steps (the anesthesiologist uses a touch-sensitive flat-panel color display or mouse). Case preconfiguration is accomplished by extensive lists and templates to customize the software at a department or individual clinician level. The initial version released in September 1998 includes a preoperative component, intraoperative anesthesia record-keeper with the ability to include postoperative care notes, and a limited database management reporting system of predefined reports.

To meet the needs of the OR environment, the hardware components are splashproof. The hardware system is designed to be nonproprietary, so that any anesthesia monitor can be used (plug and play) after initial setup.

ORVue Anesthesia Information Management System

The ORVue Anesthesia Information Management System (Hewlett-Packard, Palo Alto, CA) was designed to address many of the information needs of the anesthesiologist (Fig. 2–11). It includes a preoperative module, intraoperative automatic record-keeper, SQL database system for quality and cost analysis, and interfaces for monitoring equipment outputs and importing of laboratory information. It is a client-server application running on HP UNIX. A newer version, designed for the Windows NT client/server environment and featuring additional functionality, including better integration with the company's CareVue clinical information system, was released in October 1998 (produced by another vendor but marketed by Hewlett-Packard). Many of the features of the current product were carried over in concept and are

instructional as examples of a commercial approach to the AIMS (Table 2–4).

The preoperative assessment system provides on-line and printed records. It differs from other systems in its graphical interface patient questionnaire, designed to be used in real time by the anesthesiologist while interviewing the patient. Clerical staff, nurses, or anesthesiologists can perform data entry. Previous case records can be reviewed on-line, and all information is available for intraoperative review. Structured data input increases completeness and consistency of documentation. The preanesthesia evaluation progress note is accessible to multiple users, including clerks, nurses, and the anesthesiologist, to enter information.

The intraoperative record-keeper module automates the acquisition of patient monitoring data and allows for easy entry of anesthesia data (drugs, infusions, events, comments). The anesthesiologist enters data with an input tablet and pen device, usually with one or two pen clicks. Events are entered by clicking the event key to display a customizable list (such as intubation, operation start/end, or aspiration). The software is configurable for both the department and individual anesthesiologist. It can function as a stand-alone product or as one component of the complete AIMS. A filtering process reduces artifact.

To accommodate those situations when the anesthesiologist has insufficient time to record all the details about the course of anesthesia, a MARK EVENT key is used. Clicking this key places a marker to which the anesthesiologist may return later to add details.

The central server and database system is SQL-based, allowing open exchange of information with other hospital information systems, such as billing, registration, scheduling,

---

*OBDC or open database connectivity standard provides a high-level interface that applications can use to communicate with other databases. In this case the Sybase SQL database can use ODBC to communicate with foreign databases, such as Microsoft SQL running on Windows NT, DB/400 on an AS/400, or Oracle on a UNIX system.

Table 2–4. Functional Components of the HP ORVue AIMS

ORVue PreOp	Preoperative documentation and record generation
ORVue Intra-Op	Computer-assisted record keeping with automated monitoring data input
ORVue Database	SQL server and database system
ORVue Statistics	Database analysis tool for quality, cost, and utilization

and laboratory. Up to 4000 patient records can be stored before archiving.

The database analytic tool comes with a comprehensive set of predefined queries and reports, displayed as charts or tables. The MS Query user interface allows creation of custom queries and reports.

Required Features of Anesthesia Information Management Systems

There are several characteristics of computerized AIMSs that are important to users. These include easy manual data entry, real-time data retrieval, accurate automated data entry from monitors, and easy interfacing with existing equipment and hospital information systems.

Manual data entry into the computer interface must be easy to be acceptable to the clinician. Ideally, entry of data into the computer system should approximate the time required to record the same information on paper. Keyboard entry can be problematic for long text inputs, and other means of data input, such as quick menus, pick lists, and predefined datasets, are desirable.

Physiologic data must be readily available in a format that is easy to read and interpret. Graphically represented trend plots are the easiest to understand and the most acceptable to users.[51]

Information automatically entered from monitoring equipment must be accurate, free of artifact, and provided at appropriate intervals for the anesthesia record. Acquiring data at less than 5-minute intervals is often unnecessary, and rapid sampling can produce a large data file during long cases. Data compression techniques may then be necessary. Sampling rates should be easily adjustable (more frequent) when critical events occur.

The end-user interface should be customizable for each anesthesiologist and for routine cases. Greater integration of the information system display with other monitoring equipment and medical devices can save space, an important consideration in most ORs.

Integration

Major limitations occur when the computerized AIMS is not adequately integrated with existing clinical and hospital information systems. An example of the need for integration is the patient identifier. A master patient index should be used to accurately identify the patient in all care settings and across different information systems. Unless the computerized AIMS is integrated with the hospital's registration system (master patient index), the patient identifier must be hand-entered into the AIMS or fed by another system. This requires duplicate effort, can lead to errors in the entry of the patient identifier (with potentially devastating results), and makes it impossible to reliably import clinical data from other hospital information systems. Without access to the master patient index, each system must be manually updated whenever patient identifier information is changed (such as a name change or correction). The logistics of accomplishing this completely are demanding.

Integration is also important to allow for communication of information from different systems and to reduce duplicate data entry, which is unacceptable to clinicians. Despite a manufacturer's claims of integration, the typical hospital will likely spend more time and expense in integrating a new computerized AIMS with existing information systems than in purchasing the new system and training users.

Planning for a Computerized Anesthesia Information Management System

Prior to the purchase or design of a computerized AIMS, all potential users should be consulted, including clinicians, OR staff, and the hospital departments that are expected to feed information to the AIMS. Design requirements must include the infrastructure needed to operate a computer client-server network, such as the number of computer workstations; the location of network ports, printers, and the network wiring capacity; integration with other information systems; and standardization of data terms. Commercial off-the-shelf products are unlikely to be able to provide a turnkey-integrated solution without significant on-site customization.

Sanderson and Reves[52] have identified eight steps for system integration of computerized AIMS once the basic functional requirements have been agreed upon:

1. Analysis of workflow diagrams and the existing trail of paper forms
2. Mapping the data models of each of the interacting systems
3. Identifying common data elements in the data models, enforcing the principle of never entering the same data twice
4. Redesigning the application forms to match new workflows, staff expectations, and ergonomics
5. Redesigning the workflow diagrams according to the new plans
6. Verifying that changes to forms and staff practices meet professional, legal, and administrative regulatory needs
7. Communicating the desired forms to the vendors involved
8. Retraining the appropriate staff in expectation of new work practices

The authors recommend that at least the first three steps be performed before the purchase decision.

Information Systems for Preoperative Evaluation

The preanesthetic patient evaluation provides important information. It influences the selection of anesthetic agents and techniques and identifies patients who may require special precautions during the anesthesia course or perioperatively. Obtaining a thorough evaluation is often difficult, as when the patient presents emergently. With the shift to ambulatory surgery, the lead-time to perform the preanesthetic evaluation can be limited. The handwritten preanesthesia evaluation may be illegible or incomplete. Even when an evaluation has been performed and neatly documented, it may not always be available at the time of anesthesia if the patient's medical record cannot be obtained. In such a case the clinician is forced to rely on memory.

Computerized AIMSs that include the record of preanesthesia evaluation have several advantages. Information from previous procedures can be available in real time. Anesthetic risks documented in prior records but buried in old volumes of the medical record are accessible, avoiding critical incidents when the anesthesiologist does not have ready access to this information.[53] A computer-assisted preanesthetic record can be more detailed and clinically useful than the handwritten record.[54]

Further, computerization of the preanesthesia evaluation allows the use of structured data input by the clinician. Structured data input guides the data collection process, reducing the clinician's potential omission of information. It allows standardization of the data collected and adherence to content guidelines through computer-generated reminders or templates. Electronic data storage permits later research and quality analysis on the preanesthesia information database. Finally, the additional diagnosis information obtained from computerized preanesthetic records increases billing efficiency.[56]

Operating Room Information Systems

The traditional focus of OR computerized information management systems has been on computerized scheduling and materials management.[55] However, the use of information systems for the OR is changing to encompass all the processes of care provided in the OR, as well as to improve communication between surgeons, OR nurses, and anesthesiologists. Further, OR information systems are intended to ensure clinical quality and financial efficiency through management report and query capability. OR information systems are of interest to the anesthesiologist, particularly as they relate to improvement in the efficiency of case scheduling, patient movement tracking, and production of meaningful cost and quality data.

Design Issues

The design of any computerized OR information system must address the complexity of the workflow and processes of care in the OR. It should meet both the clinical and administrative data needs of users. An optimal system would fully integrate patient scheduling, materials management, clinical notes, flow sheets and record-keeping (nurses, anesthesiologists, surgeons), patient movement tracking, billing, and analysis of quality, cost, and efficiency.

Operation of the OR is both complex and expensive, accounting for as much as 9% of a hospital's budget.[56] In 1996, the cost of OR time at the Stanford University Medical Center was reported as $8.13 per minute (Table 2-5).[57]

Approaches to Operating Room Information Systems

Manual information systems for the OR continue to be used today but are unacceptable for many reasons. Hand entry of data is time-consuming and tends to be complete only if OR staff have sufficient time. Manual reporting of case times is generally based on estimates. Scheduling can be inefficient based on subjective or inaccurate estimates by surgeons or staff of the amount of time required. The costs incurred in the OR area cannot be easily assessed systematically and continuously with manual data collection and storage methods. The efficient management of supplies and ordering is difficult using manual inventory control methods.

Commercial off-the-shelf (COTS) scheduling and material management systems are available. The make or buy decision

Table 2–5. Operating Room Costs per Minute for a University OR

Source of Operating Room Costs	Costs ($/min)	%
Nurses and technicians in each room	$2.42	28
Basic supplies (linens, etc.)	$1.69	21
Control desk clerks, housekeeping, etc.	$1.27	16
Hospital administration, medical records, etc.	$2.93	36
TOTAL	$8.13	

Data from Dexter F, Macario A: Applications of information systems to operating room scheduling (editorial). Anesthesiology 1996; 85:1232–1234.

depends on several factors including (1) the ability to integrate the system with other information systems in the hospital, (2) multidisciplinary assessment of the specific needs of the OR environment, (3) the software development capability of the institution, (4) the time frame in which the system is desired, and (5) the relative costs of design and implementation compared to buying and implementation. Commercial materials management systems alone can easily exceed $300,000 in initial capital expense for the average hospital.[58, 59] These systems can, however, easily pay for themselves through greater efficiency within 1 to 2 years. Finally, commercial systems may not address the needs of academic and training programs, in which data collection must include information for residency requirements, board certification, and graduate medical education.

Scheduling and Efficiency

Scheduling surgical procedures is a major and complex process. It requires use of scheduling guidelines, credentials, accurate estimates of case length, anesthesia provider availability lists, and support personnel work schedules, as well as the availability of the correct surgical equipment and supplies. Inaccurate scheduling can result in underutilization of the OR suite. When case lengths are underestimated, unplanned overtime or cancellations occur. OR utilization rates tend to be low overall, ranging from 40% to 60%.[60]

Computerized OR scheduling systems enable users to "block-schedule" using historical case length data by surgeon and procedure. They provide for the capture of time stamps for events (e.g., when the patient arrives, when induction occurs, beginning and ending of surgery). They should accommodate the various ways that surgeons schedule patients. The schedule database allows reports to be generated on surgical suite utilization, cancellation rates, reasons for delays, and procedures. The scheduling system may provide decision support, such as estimating case duration for a given surgeon and procedure. The predictive scheduling ability of one commercial software system was found to be less accurate than estimates given by the surgeons.[60] Thus, more work needs to be done in the area of predictive modeling to determine the optimal elective surgery time.

Material Management

Maintaining the correct inventory of supplies and equipment is important. Excess inventory costs are considerable, as is the cost of canceling cases when needed supplies and equipment are not on hand. Supply costs can be as much as 50% of OR variable expenses. Inefficient inventory systems may result in hundreds of thousands of dollars worth of supplies in reserve.[61]

The computerized approach to inventory control involves providing inventory tracking (usually using bar coding equipment), just-in-time or predictive ordering, and analytic tools to reduce overall materials acquisition, storage, and usage costs. Analytic tools report on inventory turnover rates, par levels (the desired minimum inventory level of each item needed for efficient operation), and comparative costs. In integrated solutions, the computerized material management system provides billing information or communicates electronically with the hospital's patient billing system.

Electronic data interchange (EDI) allows for varying levels of integration of the materials management information system with suppliers and the hospital's accounting department. With EDI, requests for quotations, purchase orders, shipping notices, invoicing, and order status updates can be communicated electronically between the hospital's purchasing or supply department and vendors. The hospital's accounting department can also be integrated into the system to provide electronic fund transfers. EDI helps reduce inventory, or move to just-in-time inventory or stockless inventory systems, and reduces the need for warehouse space. Alternatively, some hospitals have "outsourced" their entire central supply departments to prime contractors using EDI. Vanderbilt University Hospital reported saving $1.5 million over 2 years by outsourcing.[56]

Quality Improvement

Analysis of information contained in an OR information system database can improve quality, lead to workflow process improvements, and reduce costs. Development of OR clinical pathways that both lower costs and improve care depends on studying historical data. Documentation for outside review organizations, such as JCAHO or NCQA, can be included in the OR data collection system and made available as reports. Improvements in scheduling efficiency, use of supplies and personnel, and time performance are maximized when accurate time and event data are entered and readily accessible. Precise costing of procedures and processes is possible only when data are collected and stored in a standardized format. This generally can be accomplished only with computerized inventory and cost accounting systems.

Anesthesia Simulators

A relatively recent information technology development is the use of anesthesia patient simulators for training and certification. Anesthesia simulators are of two types: (1) full-scale computer-based manikin systems and (2) graphic, screen-based systems. The full-scale manikin systems are designed for a simulator facility, where the training room resembles a fully equipped modern operating theatre, complete with anesthesia machine, monitoring equipment, and OR personnel to maximize the realism of the training experience (see Chapter 3). Events are controlled from an operator's console. The manikin allows for intubation, ventilation via the anesthesia machine or mask (with physiologic gas exchange readings based on actual airflow), and administration of drugs with computer-simulated response. Two manikin simulators are commercially available, the Eagle Patient Simulator (Eagle Simulation, Inc., Binghamton, NY) and METI Human Patient Simulator (HPS) (Medical Education Technologies, Inc., Sarasota, FL).

Graphic, screen-based simulators run on desktop PCs, requiring the user to interact with the multimedia software program only, and are significantly less expensive. PC-based simulators are available from Anesoft Corporation (Issaquah, WA) and Advanced Simulation Corporation (Point Roberts, WA).

Uses of simulators include basic procedures training, dealing with specific crises or events, practicing skills, and crisis management. Mathematical models of cardiovascular physiology, respiratory physiology, and pharmacology determine the "patient" response. Anesthesia simulators can simulate many anesthesia critical events, including myocardial infarction, arrhythmia, anaphylaxis, and malignant hyperthermia.

REFERENCES

1. Merritt WT: Automation and anesthesia information management. *In* Blitt CD, Hines RL (eds): Monitoring in Anesthesia and Critical Care Medicine, ed 3. New York, Churchill Livingstone, 1995, p 639.
2. Prentice JW, Kenny GNC: Microprocessor-based anaesthetic record system. Br J Anaesth 1984; 56:1433–1437.
3. Yagiela JA, Graef TR, Hooley JR: Computer-assisted validation of observer-recorded data in patients receiving intravenous sedation. Anesth Analg 1992; 74:S359.
4. Sidelli RV, Johnson SB, Clayton PD: Full-text document storage and retrieval in a clinical information system. Top Health Inform Manage 1993; 3:36–50.
5. Blobel B, Holen M: Comparing middleware concepts for advanced healthcare system architecture. Int J Med Inform 1997; 46:69–85.
6. Beeler GW: HL7 Version 3—An object-oriented methodology for collaborative standards development. Int J Med Inform 1998; 48: 151–161.
7. Dain SL: Medical device to computer networking: Past, present, and future. Int J Intensive Care 1998; vol. 5(suppl):S41–S44.
8. Metzger JR, Teich JM: Designing acceptable patient care information systems. *In* Drazen E (ed): Patient Care Information Systems: Successful Design and Implementation. New York, Springer-Verlag, 1995, p 84.
9. Templeton AW, Dwyer SJ III, Johnson, JA, et al: An on-line digital image management system. Radiology 1984; 152:321–325.
10. Dwyer SJ III: Imaging system architecture for picture archiving and communication systems. Radiol Clin North Am 1966; 34: 445–450.
11. Bryan S, Weatherburn G, Watkins J, et al: Radiology report times: Impact of picture archiving and communication systems. AJR 1998; 170:1153–1159.
12. Ruskin KJ, Allan Palmer TE, Hagenouw RR, et al: Internet teleconferencing as a clinical tool for anesthesiologists. J Clin Monit Comput 1998; 14:183–189.
13. Anderson MF, Moazamipoir H, Hudson DL, et al: The role of the Internet in medical decision making. Int J Med Inform 1997; 47: 43–49.
14. Marsh A: The creation of a global telemedical information society. Int J Med Inform 1998; 49:173–193.
15. McDonald CJ, Overhage JM, Dexter P, et al: What is done, what is needed and what is realistic to expect from medical informatics standards. Int J Med Inform 1998; 48:5–12.
16. Kaihara S: Realisation of the computerised patient record: Relevance and unsolved problems. Int J Med Inform 1998; 49:1–8.
17. Lanza V: Automatic record keeping in anaesthesia—a nine-year Italian experience. Int J Clin Monit Comput 1996; 13:35–43.
18. McDonald CJ: The barriers to electronic medical record systems and how to overcome them. J Am Med Inform Assoc 1997; 4: 213–221.

19. 1987 Joint Commission Standards for Healthcare Organizations. Oakbrook Terrace, IL.
20. www.JCAHO.org
21. Christiansen CL, Morris CN: Improving the statistical approach to health care provider profiling. Ann Intern Med 1997; 127: 764–768.
22. Swamidoss CP, Sorin JB, Watrous G, et al: Health-care report cards and implications for anesthesia. Anesthesiology 1998; 88: 809–819.
23. Coronary Artery Bypass Surgery in New York State. Albany, New York State Department of Health, 1993.
24. Spoeri RK, Ullman R: Measuring and reporting managed care performance: Lessons learned and new initiatives. Ann Intern Med 1997; 127:726–732.
25. Reich DL: Computerized recordkeeping and information management in cardiothoracic and vascular anesthesia. J Cardiothorac Vasc Anesth 1997; 11:543–544.
26. Coleman RL, Stanley T III, Gilbert WC, et al: The implementation and acceptance of an intra-operative anesthesia information management system. J Clin Monit Comput 1997; 13:121–128.
27. Thrush DN: Automated anesthesia records: Are they better? Anesth Analg 1991; 72:S296.
28. Logas, WG, McCarthy RJ, Narbone RF, et al: Analysis of the accuracy of the anesthetic record. Anesth Analg 1987; 66:S107.
29. Michel P, Gravenstein D, Westenkow DR: An integrated graphic data display improves detection and identification of critical events during anesthesia. J Clin Monit Comput 1997; 13:249–259.
30. Cushing H: On the avoidance of shock in major amputations by cocainization of large nerve-trunks preliminary to their division: With observations on the blood-pressure changes in surgical cases. Ann Surg 1902; 36:312.
31. Saklad M: A method for the collection and tabulation of anesthesia data. Anesth Analg 1940; 19:184.
32. Tovell RM, Dunn HL: Anesthesia study records. Anesth Analg 1932; 11:37.
33. Nosworthy M: A method of keeping anesthetic records and assessing results. Br J Anesth 1943; 18:160.
34. Pender JW: A combined anesthesia record and statistical card. Anesthesiology 1946; 7:606–610.
35. Conroy WA, Cassels WH, Stodsky B: The Chicago keysort anesthesia record. Anesthesiology 1948; 9:121–133.
36. Crawford OB, Stephen CR, Pender JW: A comprehensive simple anesthesia record. Anesthesiology 1960; 21:557–563.
37. Thrush DN: Automated anesthesia records and anesthetic incidences. J Clin Monit Comput 1992; 8:59.
38. Cook RI, McDonald JS, Nunziata E: Differences between handwritten and automatic blood pressure records. Anesthesiology 1989; 71:385–390.
39. Galletly DC, Rowe WL, Henderson RS: Accuracy of text entries within a manually compiled anaesthetic record. Br J Anaesth 1992; 68:381–387.
40. Galletly DC, Rowe WL, Henderson RS: The anaesthetic record: A confidential survey on data omission modification. Anaesth Intensive Care 1991; 19:74–78.
41. Block FE: Normal fluctuation of physiologic cardiovascular variables during anesthesia and the phenomenon of "smoothing." J Clin Monit Comput 1991; 7:141.
42. Hollenberg JP, Pirraglia PA, Williams-Russo P, et al: Computerized data collection in the operating room during coronary artery bypass surgery: A comparison to the hand-written anesthesia record. J Cardiothorac Vasc Anesth 1997; 11:545–551.
43. Drui AB, Behm RJ, Martin WE: Predesign investigation of the anesthesia operational environment. Anesth Analg 1973; 52:584.
44. McDonald JS, Dzwonczyk RR: A time and motion study of the anaesthetist's intraoperative period. Br J Anaesth 1990; 64:582.
45. Block FE, Reynolds BA, McDonald JS: The Diatek Arkive "Organizer" patient information management system: Experience at a university hospital. J Clin Monit Comput 1998; 14:89–94.
46. Block FE, Burton LW, Rafal MD, et al: Two computer-based anesthetic monitors; the Duke Automatic Monitoring Equipment (DAME) system and the MicroDAME. J Clin Monit Comput 1985; 1:30–51.
47. Frazier WT, Odom SH: Spatial orientation of a computer-assisted anesthetic record. In Gravenstein JS, Newbower RS, Ream AK, et al (eds): The Automated Anesthesia Record and Alarm Systems. Boston, Butterworth, 1987, p 67.
48. Paulus DA, ver der Aa JJ, Mclaughlin G, et al: Semi-automated anesthesia record keeping. In Gravenstein JS, Newbower RS, Ream AK, et al (eds): The Automated Anesthesia Record and Alarm Systems. Boston, Butterworth, 1987, p 153.
49. Petry A: Computer aided monitor-data processing (CAMP). J Clin Monit Comput 1998; 14:101–112.
50. Coleman RL, Stanley T III, Gilbert WC, et al: The implementation and acceptance of an intra-operative anesthesia information management system. J Clin Monit Comput 1997;13:121–128.
51. Chase CR, Ashikaga T, Mazuzan JE: Measurement of user performance and attitudes assists the initial design of a computer user display and orientation method. J Clin Monit Comput 1994; 10:251–263.
52. Sanderson IC, Reves J: Implementing an anaesthesia information management system in a complex hospital network. Int J Intensive Care 1998; 5(suppl):S45–S49.
53. Gibby GL, Paulus DA, Sirota DJ, et al: Computerized pre-anesthetic evaluation results in additional abstracted comorbidity diagnosis. J Clin Monit Comput 1997; 13:35–40.
54. Essin DJ, Dishakjiian R, deCiutiis VL, et al: Development and assessment of a computer-based preanesthetic evaluation system for obstetrical anesthesia. J Clin Monit Comput 1998; 14:95–100.
55. Bird LJ: Computerization in the OR. AORN J 1997; 66:312–317.
56. Gordon T, Paul S, Lyles A, et al: Surgical unit time utilization review: Resource utilization and management implications. J Med Syst 1988; 12:169–179.
57. Dexter F, Macario A: Applications of information systems to operating room scheduling (editorial). Anesthesiology 1996; 85:1232–1234.
58. Sandrick K: Information management systems in the OR: Making a commitment. Bull Am Coll Surg 1997; 82:15–18.
59. Westbrook ML, Dunn SE, Wilcox-Riggs SW: Development of a comprehensive surgical information system at Madigan Army Medical Center. Mil Med 1996; 161:154–158.
60. Wright IH, Kooperberg C, Bonar BA, et al: Statistical modeling to predict elective surgery time. Anesthesiology 1996; 85:1235–1245.
61. Regnier SJ: Symposium explores information management in the OR. Bull Am Coll Surg 1997; 82:53–57.

3 Simulators

Brian E. Smith, M.D.
David M. Gaba, M.D.

Simulation

Simulation is a powerful technique for the refinement of human performance. A medical resident rehearsing his discussion of bad news with a patient, or a surgical intern tying sutures on her scrubs while on call is using simulation to improve his or her subsequent real-world performance. While these simple techniques of simulation have been in use for some time, recent technological improvements have allowed for the adaptation of more advanced simulation techniques from other industries. This development has opened a rapidly expanding field of highly realistic simulations of patients and entire medical environments, providing much greater fidelity and broader use than previously possible.

Simulation can be defined as the artificial replication of sufficient elements of a real-world domain to achieve a specified goal. Simulation typically refers to the replication of a broad range of an environment; replication of only a very narrowly defined subdomain is usually referred to as a "part-task trainer." *Fidelity* refers to the accuracy with which the simulation reproduces the domain, both in the number of elements that the simulator presents and in the faithfulness of those datastreams to their real-world behavior. The fidelity required for a particular application depends on the specific goal: tying sutures on one's scrub pants may provide a realistic enough simulation of suturing a superficial laceration but would be inadequate practice for performing a coronary artery graft anastomosis. The highest possible fidelity would be a simulation so accurate that the person in the simulator could not distinguish it from the real thing. Such a simulation could be said to pass the famous Turing* test posed for artificial intelligence.

Interest in medical simulation has increased dramatically as emphasis on patient safety and its relation to human performance, the work environment, and human error has become more prominent. Simulation provides critical advantages in the area of training and evaluation of personnel and for the investigation of human performance-shaping factors in the medical workplace.

Simulation is most valuable when the actual behaviors to be practiced are risky, expensive, rare, and highly dynamic. Combat has been the driving force for many simulators. Good and Gravenstein[1] pointed to the use of the quintain in the Roman Empire as an early example of simulation-based training. This device delivered a blow to the practicing lancer who failed to hit the target correctly during tilting exercises. All aspects of modern warfare are widely practiced on advanced simulators by the best-equipped militaries of the world today. Although the nuclear power, shipping, and chemical manufacturing industries have recognized the value of simulation-based training and research, no industry has embraced it as pervasively as commercial aviation.

Aerospace Simulation

Although a number of aircraft simulators were built between 1910 and 1927, none of them could provide the proper feel of the aircraft because they could not dynamically reproduce its behavior.[2] Modern aviation simulators can trace their origin to the Link Trainer, patented by Edward Link in 1930. This small "blue box" used pneumatics to simulate the sensation of flying an aircraft in response to the operator's controls. It was widely used to train new pilots during World War II. Early aircraft simulators were used exclusively to teach novice pilots the basics of aircraft control. Aviation simulation has steadily improved over the last 70 years with the addition of electronic controls, computer model–driven responses, and realistic graphic displays. The simulation fidelity is now high enough that commercial pilots may be certified to fly a new type of aircraft with simulator experience only. Aircraft on trans-Pacific commercial flights often carry four pilots; given work-hour restrictions, the long flights, and the redundancy of four pilots on the flight deck, it is not uncommon for a copilot to have logged more takeoffs and landings in the simulator than in the actual aircraft.[3]

Types of Medical Simulators

Medical simulators now in use are quite varied in their characteristics and fidelity. At the lowest fidelity (and correspondingly lowest cost) are computer-assisted instruction programs that represent certain portions of the anesthesiologist's work environment on-screen. Higher fidelity can be

---

Substantial portions of the text are adapted, sometimes with minimal revision, from Gaba DM. The human work environment and anesthesia simulators. In Miller RD (ed): Anesthesia, 5th Edition, New York, Churchill Livingstone, 1999. In the electronic format, those sections are designated by blue type.

*Turing was a famous computer scientist who proposed a test to tell if computers were "thinking" or "intelligent." If you converse with a person and with a computer via a keyboard and a screen, if you can tell which is which, the computer is "intelligent."

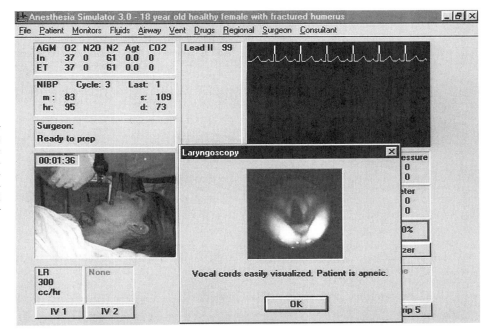

Figure 3–1. The Anesthesia Simulator 3.0 is a menu-driven program that uses additional pop-up windows to illustrate physical findings. Vital signs are updated continuously in the main window, and some monitor sounds are audible. The program display is in full color. (Courtesy of Anesoft Corporation, Bellevue, WA.)

achieved by actual physical devices or space designed to replicate portions of the domain. Physical simulations can range from narrowly limited part-task trainers to full-scale operating suites or intensive care units (ICUs). Virtual reality (VR)–based simulation is still in its infancy. This exciting approach uses a virtual, computer-generated space with multiple sensory feedback mechanisms to simulate the work environment of the anesthesiologist with the potential for very high fidelity, low operating costs, and a broader range of datastreams than is possible with physical simulators.

Screen-Based Simulations

Screen-based simulators typically use a standard personal computer (PC) to represent selected visual and auditory components of the environment, usually providing dynamic clinical data in real time from physiologic and pharmacologic models. The predominant advantages of such a system are the widespread availability of the platform and the low cost associated with distributing software once developed.

Sleeper and Body Simulation

Smith and associates in San Diego have modeled the cardiopulmonary system and drug distribution.[4-6] They developed a set of linked physiologic and pharmacologic models that accurately reproduced major elements of a patient's clinical course. The early work had used analog and hybrid computers; more recently the systems have used standard PCs. When the models were combined with an appropriate graphic representation of the patient and clinical data on the computer screen, and a graphical user interface for the input of clinically relevant actions, the system became a complete screen-only simulator, known originally as SLEEPER.[7] SLEEPER used a complex transport model to deal with gas exchange and drug distribution. This model provided the opportunity to demonstrate the behavior of "drugs" with characteristics unlike those of any existing drug, as well as

the ability to predict the concentration of drugs in specific anatomic regions (e.g., myocardium or gray matter).

In collaboration with GE Marquette Electronics, Inc. (Milwaukee, WI), the SLEEPER software evolved into a new program called BODY Simulation. In addition to extensions to the original transport and physiologic models, a unique feature of BODY is that the monitoring equipment and anesthesia delivery equipment can be high-resolution computer screen replicas of actual GE Marquette monitors. This feature lends additional realism to the system and allows it to test the user interface of the clinical equipment. BODY is now available in a Windows NT 32-bit compatible version for about $1000 (Advanced Simulation Corporation, Point Roberts, WA). The physiologic and pharmacologic models used in BODY are available as a Windows Dynamic Link Library (DLL), allowing custom interfaces to be built in a variety of programming environments to develop new simulation programs. An example is the Research Triangle Institute's Virtual Medical Trainer/Trauma Patient Simulator.

Anesthesia Simulator

At the University of Washington, Seattle, Howard Schwid, M.D. (formerly a research fellow with N. Ty Smith, M.D., University of California, San Diego) and programmer Daniel O'Donnell developed a screen-based simulator originally called the Anesthesia Simulator Recorder (ASR, trademark Anesoft Corporation, Bellevue, WA).[8-10] This simulator evolved ultimately into Anesthesia Simulator (AS), which is now in version 3.0. It was specifically geared to *training* anesthetists to manage patients, with more emphasis on critical incidents and less on pharmacologic and physiologic plotting (although this is possible with AS 3.0). This system provides graphic representations of mock monitoring displays and clinical equipment, and photographs to display the patient and actions taken on the patient (Fig. 3–1). Interaction with this system also uses a desktop pointing device. The AS uses traditional pharmacokinetic and pharmacodynamic models drawn from the pharmacology literature to track drug levels and effects of more than 80 drugs as opposed to the physical transport models used in SLEEPER and BODY Simulation. A unique feature of AS is that 80 cases have been contributed by nationally recognized experts. Critical events can be preselected by the user or selected at random by the system, and on-line expert advice is available during the case. Continuing medical (CME) and nursing education (CNE) credits can be arranged through the University of Washington for use of the simulator. A critical care simulator has been derived from the project as well, featuring 20 ICU- and emergency room (ER)-based scenarios.[11] The original anesthesia-based program has been extended to an advanced cardiac life support (ACLS) simulator, a critical care version, a hemodynamic simulator, and a sedation simulator, with a total of over 28,000 copies distributed.

Schwid and his collaborators[9] conducted evaluations of the original ASR with 44 anesthesia residents and faculty at several teaching institutions in the United States. The results showed that the ASR was easy to learn to use, was reasonably realistic, and was rated as an outstanding teaching device. The group more recently published a study suggesting that clinicians retain ACLS guidelines better after training on the ACLS simulator than after studying the ACLS textbook for a similar period of time.[12]

Virtual Reality Simulations

VR describes a technique whereby a computer-generated space and objects within it are presented to the user in a three-dimensional representation with multiple sensory feedback cues. Visual data can be presented via goggles or a computer screen, and auditory information is presented via earphones. Often, tactile (haptic) feedback is delivered to allow the realistic manipulation of objects and devices within the virtual environment. The computing power necessary is at the leading edge of available graphic workstations. VR could theoretically be used in a hybrid simulator, with a VR patient "laid over" a real clinical environment.

A complete VR patient simulator would be very complicated to produce because it requires

- A complete computer model of the patient, the environment, and the *function* of every object in the environment that might be utilized (such as monitoring devices, carts, and the like)

- A means of tracking visual, audio, and touch fields of the user to determine what is to be displayed and to identify the physical actions that are being performed

- Appropriate display hardware for every sensory modality and appropriate input hardware for each action pathway (e.g., touch, speech, and so on)

- Hardware to compute all the models, conduct the tracking, and produce all the outputs to the display hardware *in real time*

VR is still a developing field. There is intense interest in VR in a number of domains, particularly the military and entertainment. Although the potential of this approach is very exciting, practical VR simulators are currently quite limited in capability, are extremely expensive to produce, or in many cases, both limited and expensive. As of this writing there has been no publicly demonstrated VR system providing complete auditory, visual, and sensory feedback with a dynamic, realistic representation of a patient and OR environment.

Components of Comprehensive High-Fidelity Simulators

The high-fidelity patient simulators now in use have many common characteristics. Foremost is a physical representation of the patient, which has multiple output modalities generated from real-time physiologic and pharmacologic models. The available simulators are distinguished primarily by their control logic, the subset of datastreams selected for simulation, and the operator interface.

Control Logic

Early simulators required input from an operator to change states or variables represented. In essence, the physical simulator allowed the operator to manifest an internal, mental simulation. Since many physiologic states can be modeled using simple algebraic formulas or differential equations that can be solved easily in real time, more recent simulators have sought to run continuous internal models of organ systems, normal as well as pathologic, that respond automatically to inputs from the operator, the physical environment, or variables from other organ system models running in parallel.

However, not all states or changes in a patient can be modeled using differential equations. For example, ventricular fibrillation is a totally different state of heart rhythm that does not evolve continuously from normal rhythms. No model can predict *exactly* when a patient will suffer a myocardial infarction or when an ischemic heart will begin to fibrillate. A model can predict only those factors that increase the likelihood of such events. Thus, most simulators incorporate other modeling techniques in addition to the basic physiologic and pharmacologic mathematical equations, including finite-state models, instructor initiation of abnormal events, and even manual modulation of modeled parameters. In finite-state models, different underlying clinical states are defined, each of which has appropriate entry conditions as well as transition conditions to other states. When an entry or transition condition is met, a new state becomes active that may directly trigger new observable phenomena (e.g., ventricular fibrillation) or may alter constants in the mathematical models, which then evolve in time.[8-10]

Datastreams

To be successful, a simulator must provide a realistic enough representation of the clinician's experience with a real patient that the subject identifies and accepts the data being presented. Once past the acceptance threshold, the subject tends to associate that clinical cue with prior experiences with the same datastreams obtained in the real world and tends to ignore infidelities that are otherwise readily apparent. For example, a blood pressure cuff may be placed on the arm of the simulator manikin above an arterial line site, yet few clinicians have seemed to recall that the arterial tracing is dampened by the inflation of the cuff. If used as a part-task trainer on pulses and blood pressure determination, this would be a readily identified artifact, but when embedded in a broader simulation of the patient during surgery, the variety of datastreams presented simultaneously makes such artifacts immaterial. Some datastreams are nearly obligatory, including electrocardiography (ECG), pulse oximetry and plethysmography, noninvasive and invasive vascular pressures, spontaneous respiration, heart and lung sounds, palpable pulses, speech, response to neuromuscular blockade monitoring, and expiration of CO_2. A wide variety of additional clinical cues is supported by the various simulators, and new features are developed regularly, but nowhere in simulation is the cost-realism tradeoff so evident as in the selection and implementation of clinical datastreams.

Interface

The control logic of realistic simulators is manipulated via the instructor/operator's station(s) (IOS), which allows the instructor to create or select specific patients, to select and implement abnormal events and faults, and to monitor the progress of the simulation session. There may also be a remote-control hand-held IOS in addition to the main IOS. The IOS typically provides logs of physiologic changes and the subject's responses and may provide graphics to support the analysis of a simulation run. Displays of data from the underlying state variables generated by the mathematical models can be used for instruction in the simulator even when these data could never be acquired in a real patient. Some screen-based simulators provide advice and tutorials linked to the management of simulated events. With realistic simulators, detailed records of the simulation and the actions taken may also be made using video and audio recording of the subjects working in the simulator.

Realistic Simulators

Sim One

Sim One, the first realistic simulator for the training of anesthesiologists, was created in the late 1960s by the Sierra Engineering Company based on specifications from Abrahamson and Denson at the University of Southern California.[13-15] The goal was to construct a simulated patient for learning the induction of anesthesia along with the skill of tracheal intubation. The system consisted of a patient manikin including head, neck, thorax, upper abdomen, and arms. The manikin and the table upon which it was permanently mounted contained electromechanical and pneumatic actuators for a variety of clinical features. Appropriate to the era, Sim One did not stimulate any electronic monitors; its datastreams were palpable pulses, heart sounds, and movement. Sim One had a variety of electronic sensors to detect the clinicians' actions. Placement of the mask on the manikin's face was sensed by tiny reed relays embedded in the plastic flesh of the face. A special magnetic endotracheal tube was constructed with iron molded into the plastic. Its position could be determined by magnetic sensors. Sim One could automatically recognize the identity and amount injected of four drugs: thiopental, succinylcholine, methoxamine, and ephedrine. This system depended on each drug being administered using a specific size of needle, and thus it could not be expanded to identify a larger number of drugs. A standard anesthesia machine was specially instrumented to report gas flow rates (but not the concentration) of volatile anesthetic.

A mainframe computer program provided the control logic. The program would respond to drugs based on dose-time-effect curves, but there was no true modeling of pharmacokinetics or pharmacodynamics. The Sim One IOS provided readouts of the system's internal status and external outputs. Chart recordings of multiple variables could be produced. The IOS provided toggle switches or buttons to actuate a variety of preprogrammed events, including cardiac arrest, bucking, increased and decreased blood pressure or heart rate, changes in respiratory rate, and occlusion of a mainstem bronchus.

Produced in 1968 as a single handcrafted unit, Sim One was a technological marvel, costing approximately $100,000 (on the order of $500,000 today). It incorporated many features of today's patient simulators, and even included a number of desirable features that are not currently implemented. Sim One was used for several training purposes of which only a few involved anesthesiologists. The investigators used the simulator to speed the training of anesthesia residents in tracheal intubation.[16] Ten novice residents were randomly allocated to receive either no additional training or special training in intubation using Sim One (between 5.5 and 9.5 hours of training over a 2-week period). The investigators attempted to measure the proficiency at intubation of the 10 residents by scoring blinded copies of the residents' anesthetic records. The scoring for each record was a binary decision ("plus" or "minus") as to whether "On the basis of what you see on this chart, would you be willing to trust the anesthesiology resident in an operating room without supervision?" Performance criteria were set as (1) 4 consecutive plus ratings, (2) 7 of 8 consecutive cases with a plus rating, and (3) 9 of 10 consecutive cases with a plus rating. There was a statistically significant difference between the groups in the number of cases (and the number of days, 45.6 vs. 77 days), to achieve the 9-out-of-10 criterion. There was no difference in the time to achieve the other criteria.

Although the investigators' intent was admirable, this study was seriously flawed. The simulator group received special one-on-one attention, which the control group did not receive. The scoring system for the anesthetic records was poorly defined and ambiguous. The performance criteria they established were completely arbitrary. Appropriate statistical techniques were not utilized to evaluate the results. In another publication,[17] the investigators stated that residents cut their number of errors in anesthesia induction by half and reduced the average time to perform an induction by one third after training with Sim One; however, no details of these experiments were provided. They also listed other training uses, including teaching nurses to perform "ventilator application" (perhaps this referred to intermittent positive pressure breathing [IPPB] treatments), intramuscular injection, recovery room care, and pulse and respiration measurement. They discussed the cost-effectiveness of Sim One in terms of decreased faculty time to impart specific skills, improvements in student performance, and potential reduction in patient discomfort and risk. In many ways long before their time they stated that

> the effectiveness of simulation depends on the instructional method with which simulation is being compared. For example, if there is no alternative training method available . . . the effectiveness of a simulation device probably depends on the simple fact that the device provides some kind of learning experience as opposed to none. When a simulation device is compared with conventional on-the-ward training, however, the device's effectiveness seems related to the degree to which learning a given task is facilitated by systematic presentation of that task. Systematic presentation is not easily achieved on the wards, whereas simulation devices can provide a number of systematic patterns, such as graduation of difficulty level or complexity.[17]

The Sim One project drifted into oblivion (a planned Sim Two was never built) for a number of reasons.[18] It was clearly ahead of its time technologically, although changes in anesthesia and monitoring techniques have outstripped Sim One's ability to replicate important aspects of the anesthesia work environment. Sim One was costly, and many anesthetists of the time viewed computers and technology with suspicion. Finally, both the investigators and the profession as a whole did not have sufficient understanding of the relevant issues of human performance for which simulator training, testing, and research would be an ideal tool. Thus, although we can now see that Sim One had great potential for teaching personnel about the management of a variety of challenging perioperative situations, its use in anesthesia then was focused primarily on standard inductions and tracheal intubation. We now know that although simulator training in intubation can be helpful (and simulator training in complex airway management may be even more useful), most residents rapidly acquire reasonable skill at intubation through clinical experience. To be truly useful the simulator must be targeted at a different set of skills. Thus, for these and for many other reasons lost in time, the legacy of Sim One essentially disappeared.

The Reinvention of Patient Simulators for Anesthesiology

Several of the modern realistic patient simulators trace their roots back to the mid-1980s, when for the first time technological advances in the computer industry provided considerable computational power at reasonable cost. These simulators were developed independently of each other, and, in fact, most teams had no direct knowledge of Sim One. The potential for screen-based simulators in anesthesia probably followed the development of popular screen-based flight and driving simulators. Off-the-shelf waveform generators became available that gave realistic simulators the ability to stimulate electronic clinical monitors under computer control. Most important perhaps, improvements in pharmaceuticals, equipment, and monitoring decreased anesthetic morbidity and mortality considerably, unmasking the issues of human factors and ergonomics in the evolution of medical mishaps.[19-23] It was these *human factors* that made the use of simulation technology so prevalent and visible in civil aviation, the space program, military applications, and the nuclear power industry, making its adaptation to medical use a logical progression.

The feature set of each of the available simulators changes rapidly. Because of the delay inherent in publishing, the features noted here for each model are likely to be incomplete. For a current description of the simulator feature sets, the reader is advised strongly to contact the manufacturers of the simulators described.

Comprehensive Anesthesia Simulation Environment

Development. In 1986 Gaba and DeAnda[24] at VA Palo Alto and Stanford University began developing the Comprehensive Anesthesia Simulation Environment (CASE) series of anesthesia simulators with a primary goal of conducting research into decision making by anesthetists. (The first transcript of an anesthetist responding to a simulated intraoperative crisis was obtained in spring 1986.) The architecture of the first generation CASE 1.2-1.3 simulator used commercially available clinical waveform generators to provide signals to actual clinical instruments. Other devices, such as the automated noninvasive blood pressure cuff, were "simulated" using a computer program on a Macintosh Plus computer acting as a virtual instrument.[24]

The CASE 1.2-1.3 manikin was modified to enable occlusion of the left mainstem bronchus, infusion of CO_2, and the insertion of intravenous (IV) lines. This manikin allowed mask ventilation, incubation, and auscultation of breath sounds but did not have palpable pulses or spontaneous ventilation. The behavior of all of the waveform generators

and actuators was coordinated using a central control computer. The control logic of CASE 1.2 was provided by an operator typing commands at the IOS based on a written script describing the appropriate changes for a variety of anticipated actions on the part of the subject in the simulation. An experienced anesthesiologist typically observed the activities of the subject and directed the simulator operator using a private headset intercom. This control logic and IOS enabled the simulator to respond to any actions on the part of the subject, not just those that were previously anticipated.

The CASE 1.2 system was evaluated by residents[24] (and later faculty and private practitioners) and was rated as very realistic, except for the plastic manikin. The success of such a crude system, which lacked physiologic models, lies in the exceptional variability of actual patients and in the ability of anesthetists to "suspend disbelief" if placed in a plausible clinical scenario. No anesthetist can predict the exact behavior of a *specific patient* in response to drugs and actions. The responses of the simulator only have to be plausible for the situation to appear very realistic. This is especially true for critical-event training situations, in which plausible but unusual events are presented. On the other hand, physiologic and pharmacologic models do offer substantial advantages, including greater consistency and reproducibility of scenarios, the ability to handle multiple physiologic changes simultaneously, and greater automation of the simulation process.

In 1989 CASE 2.0 featured a major redesign that incorporated a physiologic model of the cardiovascular system.[25] Waveforms and electronic datastreams, including heart sounds, were generated directly from the cardiovascular model. CASE 2.0 was used extensively in the conduct of the Anesthesia Crisis Resource Management training program described later in this chapter.

Commercialization of CASE. In 1992-1993 the CAE-Link Corporation, a manufacturer of military aviation and spaceflight simulators, licensed technology from David Gaba and Howard Schwid's groups as part of its development of a commercial anesthesia simulator system. The medical simulation division of CAE-Link has subsequently evolved into MedSim Advanced Medical Simulation.*

This simulator was originally called the Virtual Anesthesiology Training Simulator System, but the name was later changed to the PatientSim (Fig. 3-2). It is completely operated by physiologic, pharmacologic, and finite-state models. The PatientSim contains complete models of cardiovascular, pulmonary, fluid, acid-base-electrolyte, neuromuscular, and thermal physiology. It includes computer-controlled electromechanical lungs with dynamically changeable compliance that are embedded totally within the manikin's thorax so that the patient manikin can be moved onto an operating room (OR) table, ICU bed, or ER gurney. The thorax can withstand full-force cardiopulmonary resuscitation (CPR), which is automatically detected. The airway allows a variety of management techniques, including mask ventilation, use of a laryngeal mask airway (LMA), oral or nasal insertion of

---

*One of us (D.M.G.) and his partner received a payment from CAE-Link to license our simulator technology, and we receive a royalty on the sale of each anesthesia simulator by MedSim-Eagle. Both authors of this chapter are periodically paid consultants to MedSim-Eagle Simulation, Inc. on patient simulator development.

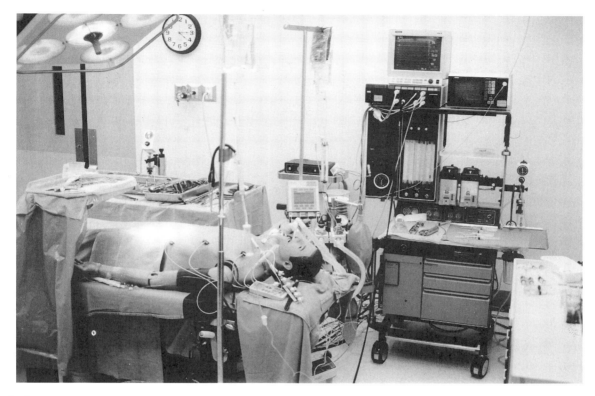

Figure 3–2. The MedSim Patient Simulator, configured in an operating room environment at the Simulation Center for Crisis Management Training, VA Palo Alto Health Care System. The operating room environment is duplicated in nearly every detail.

an endotracheal tube, transtracheal jet ventilation (TTJV), and use of a Combitube, cricothyrotomy, and fiberoptic or retrograde wire intubation. The airway can be dynamically modified by pneumatic bladders to simulate a difficult airway or laryngeal spasm. Quantitative physical elimination of CO_2 through the lungs is provided so that a clinical gas analyzer can be used in its usual manner. Other gases wash in and wash out appropriately, but there is no uptake and distribution of O_2, N_2O, or volatile agents in the standard unit. The interface components are housed in a rolling cart that can be placed underneath or beside the patient's bed.

The manikin provides electronically generated heart sounds and breath sounds, dynamically changeable airway anatomy, palpable carotid and radial pulses, and a thumb twitch responding to stimulation by actual nerve stimulators. Full hemodynamic monitoring is supported, including ECG, plethysmography, noninvasive blood pressure determinations, arterial and pulmonary artery pressures, pulmonary capillary wedge pressure, and thermodilution cardiac outputs. The cardiovascular model can generate and model the hemodynamic consequences of a variety of dysrhythmias, CPR, or defibrillation. The simulator includes a cardiopulmonary bypass (CPB) model so that cardiac surgery scenarios can be presented, including initiation and weaning from bypass.

Additional datastreams include eyelids that open and close, and pupils that constrict or dilate in response to light, drugs, or neurologic injuries. Arm movements support response to painful stimuli or spontaneous movement in the awake patient. Traumatic injuries can be simulated and procedures common in trauma settings (such as placement of a chest tube) are possible, with automatic detection of thoracostomy and relief of tension pneumothorax, if present. An

optional trauma module allows simulation of compartment syndrome resulting from a midshaft femur fracture, with displacement of the distal femur, dynamic swelling of the thigh and calf, and occlusion of pedal pulses.

The IOS in the PatientSim uses a graphical user interface (GUI) (Fig. 3–3) to provide a rich set of tools for the instructor to choose from and implement different events (up to five events can run *simultaneously*), different simulated patients, and complete scenarios. The instructor can tailor each event in advance, altering features such as the onset time, severity, and manifestations of the event. Tailored events can be saved under different names, allowing the creation of an unlimited library of events or scenarios. The IOS can be controlled remotely by a simple hand-held liquid-crystal display (LCD) device, or via a battery-powered tablet computer with a touchscreen interface and a cordless ethernet connection to the main IOS.

Many inputs to the device are automatic. A gas analyzer recognizes all inspired gases and passes their values to the pharmacologic models. An automated drug recognition system detects the drug and dosage administered through an electronically coded ring affixed to each syringe in conjunction with an instrumented stopcock manifold. The system can track the kinetics and dynamics of more than 90 different drugs. Using a drug editor, new drugs can be added to the library, or if desired, the kinetics or dynamics of existing drugs can be altered. The PatientSim also logs simulator outputs, state changes, and actions by the subject, which are input to the simulator.

MedSim has demonstrated a SmartStethoscope system that utilizes an instrumented stethoscope to receive auditory cues transmitted from the manikin based on automatic detection of stethoscope location. This system allows generation of a

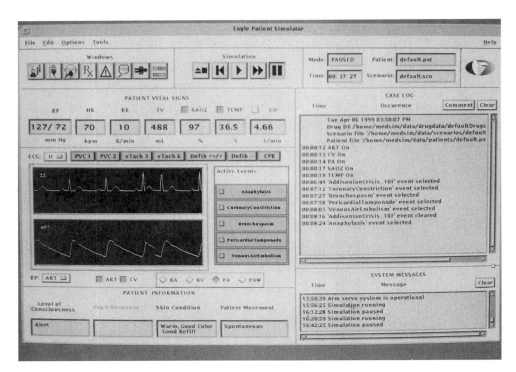

Figure 3–3. The graphically oriented interface of the MedSim Patient Simulator Instructor/Operator Station (IOS).

wider variety of different sound characteristics based on location, as well as higher-fidelity, artifact-free sound reproduction in the stethoscope.

An exciting new technology demonstrated publicly in 1999 incorporates transesophageal echocardiographic data via an esophageal echo probe that can be placed in the manikin. The echo image is generated on the basis of the settings on the probe and the location and orientation of the probe tip, as determined by sensors adjacent to the esophagus. Full integration of the images to reflect the dynamic physiologic models has not yet been implemented.

Gainesville Anesthesia Simulator

Shortly after the CASE simulator was developed, a similar simulator was produced at the University of Florida, Gainesville, by a team headed by Gravenstein and Good.[1] This system, called the Gainesville Anesthesia Simulator (GAS), also used commercially available waveform generators under the control of a central computer, along with a manikin and real OR equipment. GAS could stimulate noninvasive blood pressure measurement devices and provide palpable pulses. Unlike CASE, it was capable of spontaneous ventilation using a mechanical lung placed inside the operating table on which the manikin was mounted. An interesting component of GAS was an anesthesia machine modified to incorporate a variety of mechanical faults that could be triggered electronically.

Over time other important features have been added to GAS, including a complex quantitatively accurate physical simulation of multiple gas exchange. The lung concentrations of O_2, N_2O, N_2, and one volatile anesthetic could be physically made to match the alveolar gas content predicted by a mathematical model of gas exchange and anesthetic uptake and distribution. Another first for GAS was a moving thumb that responds appropriately to stimulation from a nerve stimulator, based on the level of neuromuscular blockade. The Gainesville group then developed a simulator control system using physiologic and pharmacologic models.

Commercialization of GAS. GAS was also commercialized, initially with Loral Data Systems and later via an independent spinoff company, with Loral Data Systems as a minority shareholder, Medical Education Technologies, Inc. (METI, Sarasota, FL). The METI Human Patient Simulator (HPS) (Fig. 3–4) also uses full physiologic and pharmacologic mathematical models. Its manikin supports numerous clinical cues and interventions such as pulses, breath sounds, heart sounds, invasive airway management, and so on. It provides outputs for nearly all modalities of invasive and noninvasive monitoring. Like its predecessor GAS, it continues to provide quantitative physical modeling of uptake and distribution of several gases. The newest version of the HPS has moved the lung system to a remote interface cart, thus freeing the manikin from its table, and allowing for full-force CPR chest compressions. The HPS includes a genitourinary system that allows user-selectable urine output, Foley catheterization (the manikin contains interchangeable genitals to provide for either sex) and an automatic drug recognition system that uses a bar-code scanner embedded in the stopcock manifold assembly (a design sketched but not implemented for CASE 3.0).

The IOS of the HPS runs on a PC and allows real-time control of parameters and scenarios. A pen-based remote PC can be used as the IOS. The user interface primarily involves selection of files from menus and is somewhat less graphically oriented than the user interface on the PatientSim. The HPS allows for graphic display of pharmacokinetic data in real time for educational uses.

Leiden Anesthesia Simulator

At the 1992 World Congress of Anesthesiologists, a group from Leiden, the Netherlands, led by Chopra and Bovill, unveiled the Leiden Anesthesia Simulator.[26, 27] This simulator used the same architecture as CASE 1.2 and replicated many of its features as well as some of GAS. (In fact, the Leiden simulator was derived in part from technical information provided to the Leiden group by the Stanford investigators

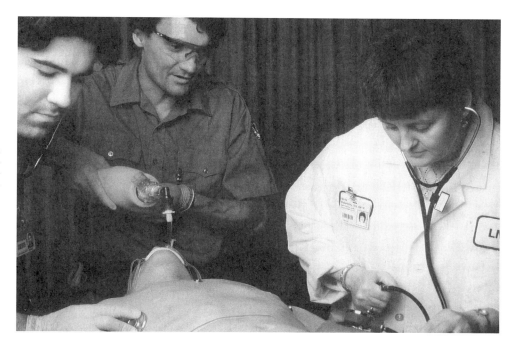

Figure 3-4. The METI Human Patient Simulator, in use as a training device for a team of healthcare personnel. (Courtesy of Medical Education Technologies, Inc., Sarasota, FL.)

led by Gaba and Schwid.) Like GAS, the Leiden simulator incorporated a mechanical lung capable of spontaneous ventilation. The Leiden simulator is now driven by physiologic and pharmacologic models, has a new user interface, and features state-of-the-art digital lung sounds. The Leiden simulator is now operated as the Skills Lab Anesthesiology, which will soon be charged with training every anesthesia resident in the Netherlands. There is a proposal currently under review to use the center for performance evaluation of all residents.

The SIMA Project

The Anaesthesia Simulator Sophus was developed by a group of anesthesiologists and scientists in Denmark (Herlev Hospital, Roskilde University, and Risø National Laboratory). All necessary physiologic parameters are animated and controlled by signals from the computer. Simulation of human response to anesthesia is based on detailed mathematical models of pharmacokinetic and dynamic processes and the cardiovascular system. Now in version 3, Anaesthesia Simulator Sophus does not yet appear to be quite as comprehensive as the MedSim PatientSim or the METI HPS. The SIMA project builds on the Sophus simulator; a collaborative group from academia and industry plans to enhance the software and hardware of Sophus and release it commercially. The Sophus simulator is also in use at the University of Basel, Switzerland, where it has been adapted to form the Wilhelm Tell simulator. A unique feature of Wilhelm Tell is the addition of perfused bovine or porcine organs from a slaughterhouse, upon which surgeons can perform laparoscopic procedures while anesthesiologists manage the patient.

PATSIM-1, ACCESS

A realistic simulator dubbed PATSIM-1 was developed at Stavanger College, Stavanger, Norway. While not supporting the breadth of datastreams that the commercial simulators do, it has an impressive list of features for a noncommercial simulator. It stimulates real OR or ICU monitors, has a variety of

controls over ventilation parameters, and has some unique features, for example, patient movement under light anesthesia. The PATSIM team aspires to simulate all datastreams to interface directly with actual clinical equipment in the usual way, for example, arterial waveforms come from hydraulic pressure waves in a simulated artery on the manikin, not an electronic waveform generator in the simulator computer. The simulator includes the unique features of regurgitation, aspiration, and perioral cyanosis. It is not yet model-driven, and relies on operator inputs for simulated patient variables. ACCESS (Anesthesia Computer Controlled Emergency Situation Simulator), a less realistic system developed at the University of Wales, is essentially a computer screen–based simulator with the addition of a manikin. The manikin is a standard resuscitation dummy and supports a very limited feature set. ACCESS is now in use at 10 separate hospitals in the United Kingdom.

Aftermarket Augmentation

Many simulator laboratories have creatively augmented the function of the commercially available patient simulators to add features of particular interest. A few examples follow.

The METI simulator has been adapted to respond physiologically to complex ventilatory parameters, including the addition of positive end-expiratory pressure (PEEP), pressure support, and inverse ratio ventilation, using sensors and an external computer interfaced with the simulator via the Human Patient Simulator Internal Data Exchange Protocol (HIDEP).[28] Also taking advantage of the METI simulator's use of the HIDEP protocol, a novel graphic display of simulator physiology has been developed that collects and organizes model-driven, operator-selected, and measured variables.[29] An intracranial pressure (ICP) model was developed using the temperature, $PaCO_2$, PaO_2, systolic (SBP) and diastolic blood pressures (DBP), and central venous pressure (CVP) variables outputted from the HPS, displaying cerebral blood flow, volume, cerebral metabolic rate of oxygen ($CMRO_2$), and ICP in real time.[30]

A MedSim PatientSim in use at the University of Pittsburgh has been modified to more realistically accept an LMA, has been fitted with dentures that simulate dental damage during laryngoscopy, and can become diaphoretic (J. Schaefer, M.D., personal communication, 1996).

At the VA Palo Alto Health Care System, a reservoir of fake blood is placed in the OR table, accessible to the surgeon-actor for simulated hemorrhage; additional blood can be pumped from the control room to the reservoir to produce a virtually limitless volume of shed blood. Urine is pumped in a similar manner to the manikin's Foley catheter via a calibrated IV infusion pump; the color of the urine can be altered by addition of dye. The patient's arm is instrumented with a system of tubes, one-way valves, and a source of fake arterial blood to allow arterial blood sampling and flushing of the arterial line. The Center for Medical Simulation in Boston has successfully simulated a seizure using a system of piano wires attached to the manikin's limbs (Dan Raemer, personal communication, 1999).

Uses of Realistic Simulators

Simulators can provide more than an introduction to anesthetic techniques. As in aviation, simulation is increasingly being used for education, training of personnel for catastrophic system failures, research, risk management, public relations evaluation and improvement of the human-machine interface, assessment of operator performance, and investigation of accidents. There is an enormous breadth of simulation activities worldwide, and new and more imaginative uses are continually being developed. The simulator is an excellent tool for a diverse set of applications and is adapted to fit the needs of the local environment and users.

Education and Training

For our purposes, we draw a distinction between *education,* which involves teaching conceptual knowledge, and *training,* which involves teaching specific skills. Using the simulator as a tool to assist in imparting principles of physiology and pharmacology is *education;* using the simulator in its highest-fidelity mode in concert with a realistic clinical environment to learn or practice clinical skills and behaviors is *training.*

Simulators have been used for community outreach programs to expose high-school students to medicine as a potential career.[31] A common educational use of simulators is for introduction to anesthesia principles for medical students and starting anesthesia residents. Courses can be adapted to any level; most simulators can be configured with as little or as much complexity as desired. Undergraduate and preclinical medical students can learn experientially about pharmacology, physiology, physical examination skills, and monitoring in the simulator. During their anesthesia or ICU rotations they can discuss cardiovascular physiology and experiment on the simulator at the same time.[32, 33] Lee[33] succinctly stated the benefits of simulator-based medical student teaching programs:

- The ability to bring clinical applicability to medical students early in their training
- The ability to teach topics that are difficult to teach in a purely didactic form
- The provision of a safe and natural bridge between didactic and clinical work

- An introduction to anesthesiology early in a student's career
- An ability to provide a service that increases the standing of anesthesiologists in the local and national medical community

Training

Clinical medical or nursing students can learn procedural skills, get a chance to manage an unstable patient on their own, and learn to handle dynamic situations using a simulator. However, most training applications are targeted at the graduate and postgraduate clinician for whom more intensive and more advanced training is appropriate.

Anesthesia Crisis Resource Management

While analogies between aviation and anesthesia have been widely used, it has been only a decade since the medical community began to take serious notice of the striking similarities between the work environment in dynamic medical domains and in industries such as aviation. These domains are similar because they share the cognitive profile of intense time pressure, high risk, continually shifting and competing goals, and complex human-machine interactions.

An analysis of the evolution of critical events in the early simulator prototype suggested gaps in the training of anesthesiologists concerning several aspects of decision making and crisis management that were not systematically taught during standard residency.[21, 22, 24, 34-37] Crew (originally Cockpit) Resource Management (CRM), a system of training aircrews to perform effectively during crises, was first adapted to medicine between 1988 and 1990, when, armed with their new realistic simulator, Gaba, Howard, and Fish began teaching these concepts at VA Palo Alto and Stanford University.[38] The course, termed Anesthesia Crisis Resource Management (ACRM), deals with technical aspects of managing critical events, but more important, addresses the behavioral skills that correlate with effective performance. These skills cannot otherwise be practiced and cannot be learned by osmosis; they often are contrary to the individualistic "unassuming" work style of many anesthesiologists. Anesthesiologists, often used to working alone, must learn to work effectively as a crew with other anesthesia providers and as a team working with other crews such as nurses and surgeons.

The ACRM course, as taught at VA Palo Alto/Stanford, begins with an introduction to CRM principles, team-building exercises, and practice at accident analysis of trigger videos using the principles of CRM. Most of the 1-day course is then spent alternating highly realistic simulations of critical incidents with detailed videotape debriefings. The realistic simulations make use of trained actors who play the roles of surgeons, nurses, and other personnel. Participants get the opportunity to be in the "hot seat," as well as be a "first responder," who remains blinded to the scenario but may be allowed to be summoned as help by the hot seat trainee. The course syllabus eventually evolved into a textbook,[39] which has been translated into German and Japanese. Key points applied throughout the course include the following:

- *Allocate attention wisely:* manage distractions and competing tasks
- *Use all available information:* check additional datastreams to filter out artifact
- *Avoid fixation errors:* reevaluate often

- *Distribute the workload:* work as a manager as much as possible
- *Utilize all available resources:* be creative
- *Communicate effectively:* state orders or queries clearly to specific individuals
- *Resolve conflicts quickly:* concentrate on *what* is right rather than *who* is right

Since the inception of this course in 1990, the response has been quite positive. The ACRM curriculum has been formally adopted as a major focus of training at several major teaching institutions—the Boston Center for Medical Simulation; the Canadian Simulation Centre (Toronto); University of Pittsburgh; University of Alberta (Edmonton); Washington University (St. Louis); Southern Health Care Network (Melbourne, Australia); Royal Perth Hospital (Perth, Australia; Chelsea and Westminster Hospital, and St. Bartholomew's and the Royal London School of Medicine and Dentistry (London, UK). Several variant curricula similar to ACRM were developed based on the textbook and on firsthand observation of early ACRM training courses at the VA Palo Alto/Stanford center. These variants include the Rational Anesthesia curriculum in Denmark (which has been given to the majority of Danish anesthesiologists and anesthetic nurses), and simulation training courses in Brussels, Belgium.

ACRM training is mandatory for anesthesia trainees at our institution. The curriculum is fully staged through the residency; completely different ACRM II and ACRM III courses are given to second- and third-year anesthesia residents, respectively. The advanced courses emphasize increasing safety culture in the OR for residents soon to graduate to the practice of anesthesia. The residents use ACRM concepts as they debrief their peers and themselves after real-life critical incidents.

The ACRM III course features a unique scenario in which the patient is allowed to die. This complication is absolutely avoided in the basic courses because it carries with it a profound emotional effect on the participant that interferes with effective debriefing. In ACRM III, it is exactly those issues with which we deal: how to recover from a disastrous outcome, how to notify and recruit help from the correct hospital personnel, and how to impound the OR if an equipment-related problem is suspected. After the anesthesiologist, in conjunction with the surgeon, decides to suspend resuscitation efforts, the trainee is led by the surgeon to a waiting area where an actor plays the role of a family member, and the trainee gets the opportunity to practice delivering bad news. The OR scenario and subsequent family conference are videotaped for detailed debriefing. Residents' comments on this activity have been very positive, remarking on the fact that training in this difficult aspect of practice has rarely been offered. An analysis is currently under way on the trainee's performance during the family conference.

ACRM training is very complex and requires skills and considerations that are unique. For that reason, special training for ACRM instructors has been developed by the Working Group on Crisis Management Training in Health Care, comprising the three pioneering centers in the development of ACRM (the VA Palo Alto/Stanford Simulation Center, the Boston Center for Medical Simulation, and the Canadian Simulation Centre). The Working Group has developed and tested a 3-day ACRM instructor training course and has produced a 150-page training manual for ACRM instructor candidates. Experience with the instructor training course suggests that the most difficult aspect of ACRM instructing is debriefing, and that new instructors require a significant period of experience, preferably under supervision by more senior instructors, before they are ready to be fully independent ACRM instructors. ACRM instructor training continues at these three centers under the auspices of the Working Group.

The concepts of ACRM apply to many healthcare environments outside the OR, and many investigators have been actively working to extend it to radiology,[40, 41] and to in-hospital resuscitation "code" teams[42] and OR teams, including surgeons and nurses.[43] Lou Halamek, a neonatologist at Stanford, has developed a CRM course to train pediatricians and neonatal ICU (NICU) nurses for delivery room and NICU crises. The course can be adapted to provide a measure of combined team training, incorporating obstetricians and anesthesiologists.[44, 45]

Team Oriented Medical Simulation

Team Oriented Medical Simulation (TOMS) is another curriculum whose roots are in aviation and CRM. It was developed independently of ACRM, by Hans Gerhard Schaefer and Robert Helmreich.[46] It has many characteristics in common with ACRM but includes more emphasis on the social psychology of team interactions in the OR and is always conducted with combined teams of anesthetists, surgeons, nurses, and ancillary personnel. Communication skills between crews are heavily emphasized.

What are the advantages and disadvantages of, and obstacles to, attempting combined team training? The advantages clearly include

- The ability to foster team interaction
- Cross-training (or at least cross-discipline understanding) of personnel
- Exploration of actual team interactions rather than scripted interactions
- Training the teams as teams rather than training the individuals to work in teams

On the other hand, disadvantages and obstacles include

- The political difficulties of bringing all crews on board simultaneously for combined training
- The expense and political difficulties of withdrawing an entire team from actual patient care for training
- Current lack of highly realistic work for surgeons to perform. The Wilhelm Tell simulations can encompass only a few surgical procedures, and thereby exclude many surgical specialties
- Inability to cover technical and cognitive issues fully for each crew
- Inability to present a full spectrum of teamwork challenges

We foresee that eventually both approaches will be utilized. ACRM-like approaches allow focused training for specific disciplines about cognitive issues of resource management and specific teamwork issues pertaining to that discipline while allowing for discussion of relevant technical matters. Combined team training, like TOMS, would then provide a supplementary training experience specifically focused on interdisciplinary teamwork issues.

Other Examples of Simulation-Based Training

The American Society of Anesthesiologists (ASA) Difficult Airway Algorithm provides a cognitive framework for managing one of the most challenging clinical scenarios. However, performing procedures from memory for the first time under intense time pressure on a desaturating patient is not optimal. Skills that are used rarely, but expected to be performed rapidly and flawlessly, must be practiced. The simulator provides a perfect setting: a realistic airway, the necessary equipment, and a fully realistic environment in which to practice those skills. A study of 18 anesthesiology residents before and after a simulation-based difficult airway course showed a significant improvement in performance, based on the clinical outcome predicted by the simulator models (i.e., whether or not the simulated patient died of hypoxia).[47] There was a high degree of acceptance of the course, and 93% of residents thought the training would improve subsequent performance. There was, however, no control group given a lecture, book, or traditional manikin-based course for comparison.

In concert with the Food and Drug Administration (FDA), Glaxo Wellcome Pharmaceuticals decided to provide extensive training to clinicians on the new opiate remifentanil as a part of its introduction to clinical use. Real-time clinical simulation was an ideal training forum for that training because

- Remifentanil has unusual kinetics, which many simulators can illustrate effectively using model-driven real-time plots simultaneously with clinical cues.
- Total intravenous anesthesia (TIVA) is a technique requiring skills and considerations different from those of inhalation anesthesia and involves new and potentially unfamiliar equipment and principles that can be practiced in the simulator before use.
- Safety measures geared toward ensuring ventilation of the patient also help ensure anesthetic delivery; TIVA removes some or all of that tight linkage and thus has a different set of safety elements that necessitate careful consideration and training.

Several curricula were developed using simulators to train clinicians to use remifentanil safely. Murray et al.[48] reported on perhaps the largest of these programs and found a very high degree of simulator acceptance among the participants, who were mostly (79.9%) new to patient simulation. There was a significant increase in the comfort level of participants using the drug, and all of the participants rated the simulator as an "excellent" or "good" means to learn about new agents such as remifentanil.

Several simulation centers conduct training for personnel from companies that produce and sell pharmaceuticals and medical devices. The University of Florida, Gainesville has run such courses for many years, and the course at the Boston Center for Medical Simulation has the engaging title of Anesthesia for Amateurs. These curricula allow sales representatives and executives to achieve a better firsthand understanding of the challenges of the clinical environments in which their products are used.

Research

The realistic simulator is an excellent laboratory for the study of human performance and performance-shaping factors, for investigations into the cognition of clinical decision making, and for evaluation of equipment and the human-machine interface (Table 3-1).

The Study of Critical Incidents in Anesthesia

In 1989 Gaba and DeAnda[34] published the first of a series of papers on the response of anesthesiology trainees, faculty,

Table 3-1. The Pros and Cons of Simulation

Features Making Simulation an Excellent Investigative Tool
There is never risk to a real patient
Rare critical events can be simulated at will
Error evolution can be allowed without intervention
Cases can be repeated in an identical manner to multiple subjects
The causes of faults or pathologic processes can be definitively known
The environment and subjects can be highly instrumented
Invasive probes may be inserted into the scenario
Archival records allow reanalysis of events

Features Limiting the Usefulness of Simulation
Subjects know they are being evaluated; they may exhibit artifactual behaviors such as hypervigilance or a cavalier attitude
Simulator fidelity may be inadequate to probe specific errors
The simulations may not include the underlying organizational systems and constraints of real clinical environments that might affect performance
Time in simulation laboratories is expensive

and private practitioners to critical incidents using a realistic simulator. Using incidents that varied in type and severity, they measured the latency to detection and correction of the event. The subjects were asked to "think aloud" to gather information about their detection and management strategies.

For each incident there was considerable interindividual variability in detection and correction times, in the information sources used, and in the actions taken. In each experience group there were "outliers" who required excessive time to solve the problem or who never solved it. In each experience group at least one individual made major errors that could have had a substantial negative impact on a patient's clinical outcome. For example, one faculty never used electric countershock to treat ventricular fibrillation. One private practitioner treated an endobronchial intubation as if it were "bronchospasm" and never assessed the symmetry of ventilation. One resident never found an airway disconnection.

The average performance of the anesthetists tended to improve with experience, although this varied by incident. The performance of the experienced groups was not definitively better than that of the second-year residents (who were in their final year of training at that time). Many (but not all) novice residents performed indistinguishably from more experienced subjects. The elements of suboptimal performance were both technical (choosing defibrillation energies appropriate for internal paddles when using external paddles; ampule swap; failure to inflate the endotracheal tube cuff resulting in a leak) and cognitive (failure to allocate attention to the most critical problems, fixation errors).

Schwid and O'Donnell[49] from the University of Washington used the screen-based Anesthesia Simulator Consultant to perform a similar experiment. This technique in some ways allowed a more detailed analysis of the subject's actions but suffered from using the screen-based OR environment. Like Gaba and DeAnda, they found major errors and omissions at all experience levels in both event detection and treatment. Fixation errors were noted, and subjects failed to use operational knowledge they had about diagnosis and treatment of specific problems. For example, 60% of subjects did not make the diagnosis of anaphylaxis when confronted with heart rate, blood pressure, peak inspiratory pressure, and skin rash data.

Botney et al.[50, 51] analyzed videotapes from 18 different simulator training sessions on crisis management. In one event a volatile anesthetic vaporizer had been left on at 4%

and was hidden beneath a printout from the noninvasive blood pressure (NIBP) device. Simultaneously, there was a mechanical failure of the capnograph, making it impossible to confirm endotracheal intubation using CO_2 measurements. This event purposely presented an opportunity for the subject to become fixated on the endotracheal tube while ignoring other relevant information. Five of 18 subjects never discovered the volatile anesthetic overdose despite catastrophic effects on blood pressure and heart rate and clear evidence that the endotracheal tube was correctly placed. Of those who did detect the vaporizer setting the average time to detection was nearly 4 minutes, with some subjects taking more than 12 minutes.

In the second event studied there was a loss of pipeline O_2 supply while an anesthetist was assuming the care of a critically ill patient who required an FIO_2 of 100% to achieve satisfactory blood oxygenation. The oxygen cylinder on the machine was empty (i.e., it had not been checked by the initial anesthetist who left the case after becoming ill). Although the pipeline failure was quickly detected (19 seconds), the responses to it were extremely variable and showed several problems. Five of 18 subjects closed the anesthesia circuit (which preserves the existing O_2 in the circuit), but all 5 subsequently switched to ventilation with a self-inflating bag using room air, or to mouth-to-tube ventilation. Five of 18 subjects could not open the reserve O_2 cylinder because they could not locate the tank wrench attached to the machine (it tended to rest between two gas cylinders). Several teams had trouble in mounting a new tank on the anesthesia machine; problems with the gasket disk were frequent. The anesthesiologists did not appear to have a well-formulated plan for managing this event, and they did not optimally coordinate their actions with their assistants or with the other OR personnel.

Devitt et al.[52] studied the response of anesthesia residents and faculty to five matched pairs of simulated intraoperative events embedded in two scenarios. They evaluated response on a 3-point scale (described in more detail later under Performance Assessment). Although faculty scored higher than residents overall, they scored lower on two events: "sinus bradycardia during peritoneal traction," and "coronary ischemia." In both cases residents executed a "corrective treatment" more frequently than did faculty. These two and several other events showed low "internal consistency" in this study (the rank-order pattern of response across subjects for these events did not match that of the other events). However, the lower performance of faculty on two events of apparent clinical importance was unexplained. Were faculty less likely to execute a corrective action in these events because they were more willing to assess the situation over time or because they were less vigilant or less decisive? This study did not answer these troubling questions.

Performance- and Ventilation-Related Events

The performance of clinicians using standard monitors and displays during simulated critical ventilation-related events was investigated using a realistic simulator. Latency to diagnosis, means of diagnosis, and latency to treatment were recorded. Following the simulations, subjects were interviewed for metacognitive information. In general, subjects made incomplete use of crucial datastreams in monitoring and diagnosing ventilation-related problems. Poor instrument design was implicated as a contributing cause.[53–55]

Simulation technology can be used to investigate the utility of monitors or techniques that would be impossible to validate in the real world owing to the infrequent and unpredictable nature of certain types of incidents, and the ethical issue of withholding techniques from the control group that are thought to increase patient safety. For example, Lampotang et al.[56] were able to demonstrate a reduction in the time to diagnosis of a ventilation-related critical incident in a group randomized to utilize oximetry and capnography in the simulator, as compared with a control group going through otherwise identical simulations without those monitoring modalities.

Workload and Performance

Byrne et al.[57] reported on the use of charting accuracy during critical incidents in a moderate-fidelity simulator as a fully embedded secondary probe, using this measure of spare capacity as a proxy for performance. The study has been criticized[58] because of the authors' assumptions about the relationship between the primary task (taking care of the patient), the secondary task (charting fidelity), and "performance." A good performance on the secondary task does not necessarily ensure a good performance with respect to the patient—in fact, one might argue that an effective strategy for good "performance" would be to sacrifice charting accuracy temporarily to concentrate on managing a critical incident! Further, the relatively low fidelity of the simulations (no surgeons or nurses, the presence of a friendly "tutor" who was an investigator), the unusual chart presented to the subjects (2.5-minute time intervals), and the short duration of the simulations (three critical incidents in 25 minutes) make these findings questionable.

Performance-Shaping Factors

In the most comprehensive simulation-based experiment performed to date by the VA Palo Alto/Stanford group, the performance of anesthesia residents was measured under two carefully controlled and highly disparate conditions: acutely fatigued and sleep-extended. In the fatigued condition, subjects were kept awake and busy with anesthesia-related tasks for 24 hours prior to the simulated case; in the sleep-extended condition, subjects were required to extend their sleep each morning by at least 2 hours for 4 days prior to the case. Subjects kept a sleep log, wore a wrist activity monitor, and wore ambulatory electroencephalographic (EEG) devices during the sleep deprivation phase and the simulated cases.

Performance measures were in three categories: pure laboratory tests of vigilance (the psychomotor vigilance task [PVT]); fully embedded and partially embedded secondary probes; and full clinical patient care (of a simulated patient). Subjects had to conduct a complete anesthetic (duration, approximately 4 hours), including preoperative assessment, pre-use checkout of key equipment, and induction and maintenance of anesthesia. During the assessment and machine checkout, as well as the case, the investigators embedded a variety of technical and clinical faults that had to be recognized and handled appropriately.

The key findings of these studies can be summarized as follows:

- Sensitive laboratory tests of psychomotor vigilance detected large decrements in reaction time in the fatigued state versus the sleep-extended state. The decrement was greatest early in the morning following sleep deprivation.[59]
- Performance of the preanesthetic equipment checkout was very poor in both groups of residents; no difference between groups was detected.[60]
- Most subjects preserved performance[61] and vigilance while acutely sleep-deprived during care of the simu-

lated patient, but there were subtle indicators of impairment during the fatigued state. When fatigued, subjects seem to focus their attention on patient monitoring and reduce their other activities.

- Some subjects had a high incidence of microsleeps in the sleep-deprived state.[62] A few subjects (approximately 16%) had significant periods (minutes) of profound complete sleep during the care of the simulated patient. During these periods vigilance and performance can be assumed to be zero. In the few instances when a clinical probe or vigilance probe coincided with such a sleep period, the measured performance was in fact zero. Interestingly, this did not result in catastrophe to the simulated patient, for several reasons:
  1. During the maintenance phase of anesthesia during straightforward surgery in healthy patients, acute changes are possible but uncommon. Thus, it is possible for an anesthetist to fall asleep for several minutes or longer and have nothing untoward occur in the interim.
  2. Our clinical vigilance probes "timed out" after 3 minutes if not detected. Furthermore, the vital signs "ramp" probes leveled out at abnormal but noncatastrophic values. Had the vital signs continued to change without detection, a clinical catastrophe would have eventually occurred.
  3. We had few clinical events. By chance, only one occurred while a subject slept, and several events were missed by nonsleeping subjects and by sleep-extended subjects.
- Clinical performace varied strongly between and within individuals over time. The subjects in the sleep-extended state made a surprising number of errors in detecting or acting upon abnormalities and in responding to vigilance probes. Clearly, sleep deprivation and fatigue are not the only factors responsible for suboptimal performance.

Other Research Uses

The realistic simulator has been used to evaluate a new equipment checkout regimen[63] and to compare the performance of clinicians with an artificial intelligence system for postoperative cardiac surgery.[64] Other ongoing investigations the authors are aware of include

- Holter monitoring of clinicians during simulated critical events[65, 66]
- Analysis of teamwork and the effects of demeanor on communication and team performance
- Use of a head-mounted camera to study dynamic decision making in OR personnel during realistic simulations of critical incidents

Ancillary Uses of Simulation?

Clearly, education, training, and research constitute the major applications of patient simulation, but there have been a number of other interesting uses. The simulation center has been used as a "film studio" to create realistic clinical vignettes for films (e.g., three in the ASA patient safety videotape series) and for medicolegal defense. The simulator has been used for preprocurement testing of clinical equipment (including new devices that could not be evaluated in clinical use because they did not yet have FDA approval), and as part of the training of clinicians to use new equipment. Similarly, simulators have been used by manufacturers to test the usability of prototype devices.

Effectiveness

The most important question concerning simulator-based training in anesthesiology is its cost-effectiveness. This is a complicated question that has two relatively independent components. The first component is, What is the impact and benefit of the training on the performance abilities of participants? The second is, What does it cost to achieve that impact? In principle, simulation has many advantages as a training tool[24]:

- There is no risk to a patient.
- Exercises in routine procedures can be repeated intensively, while scenarios and events involving uncommon but serious problems can be presented at will.
- Participants can learn to use actual complex devices (with a hands-on simulator).
- The same scenario can be presented independently to multiple subjects for evaluating individual or group performance.
- Errors can be allowed to occur that in a clinical setting would require immediate intervention by a supervisor.
- The simulation can be frozen to allow discussion of the situation and its management, and it can be restarted to demonstrate alternative techniques.
- Recording, replay, and critique of performance are facilitated, since there are no issues of patient safety or confidentiality.

The fidelity required of the simulator and thus the choice between screen-only and realistic simulators depends on the intended goals of the training and the relevant target population. A broad spectrum of computer-based training programs is available and is in use at many institutions. Computer-assisted instruction programs and part-task trainers are used to teach basic concepts and technical material, such as the uptake and distribution of inhaled anesthetics or pharmacokinetics of IV drugs. These will be appropriate for students, novices, and advanced residents and experienced practitioners. Screen-only simulators are inexpensive and easy to use. They allow the presentation of, and practice with, the concepts and procedures involved in managing normal and abnormal case situations. They too will be valuable for a large number of user populations. Realistic simulators can be used to capture the full complexity of the real-task domain, including the human-machine interactions and the complications of working with multiple personnel. Although they can do double duty in roles where less sophisticated simulators might suffice, their strength will be in the training of residents and experienced practitioners in a variety of domains. Regardless of the device used, the simulator is only a teaching tool that must be coupled with an effective curriculum for its use.

The evaluations conducted so far suggest that a variety of simulator-based training curricula are powerful techniques that students as well as novice residents and experienced anesthetists believe to be highly beneficial to their education and training. Questionnaires[67-69] and structured interviews[70] have documented that participants and instructors alike believe that simulation training has improved the participants' clinical skills. One clinician[71] ascribed her success in managing a cardiac arrest on an airline flight to skills learned during ACRM.

Good et al.[72] reported on a randomized study of the effect of simulator-based training on novice resident performance. Twenty-six beginning residents, matched for previous training and gender, were randomized to receive either daily simulator training sessions or daily lectures on 10 predefined learning objectives during weeks 2 and 3 of the residency. Resident performance was assessed both by a written test and by evaluations of clinical ability by supervisors at weeks 1, 3, 8, and 13 of training. There was no difference in performance on the written test. While there was a trend of improvement in the overall raw clinical ability scores for the simulator group at weeks 3 and 8, this was not statistically significant. However, the change in clinical score was significantly greater for the simulator group than for the lecture group at weeks 3 and 8, but not at week 13, by which time the change in clinical score was identical for the two groups. This study suggests that there may have been somewhat faster improvement in clinical ability when simulator-based training was used, but that by 3 months of anesthesia experience all residents had improved their ability by the same amount. It was noted that additional work is needed to refine and coordinate the clinical and simulator curricula and also that continuing simulator exercises may have benefits over the single "bolus" of training over 2 weeks.

As the developers of Sim One pointed out, when simulation provides an opportunity to teach material that cannot be taught in another way, as for the systematic instruction of anesthesiologists in handling critical events such as cardiac arrest, anaphylaxis, or malignant hyperthermia (MH), there is *nothing* with which to compare the simulator.

Assessing whether the actual outcome of patients can be affected by this or any other training modality will be extremely difficult and expensive. Those investigating simulator-based training do not believe that such an outcome study is logistically feasible.[36] Determining the impact of a given type of simulator training on the intermediate variables of "performance" and "ability" is feasible but will not be easy. The Leiden group has provided data supporting the contention that simulation training improves performance on handling an MH situation. However, there is a potential for substantial bias when an attempt is made to measure the impact of the simulator training by using performance in the simulator as a criterion. The control procedures as used by the Leiden group alleviate this bias but cannot eliminate it.[73]

Perhaps of even greater importance, there is currently no gold standard methodology for measuring the clinical performance of anesthetists in actual practice. Ironically, the simulator itself provides a tool for presenting the same calibrated scenario to multiple anesthetists and may thus be crucial to developing such performance measures. The work to date on performance assessment using simulation is encouraging in that the measures already tried appear to be as good as or better than those now used by the profession for credentialing and peer review. However, it may be necessary to further validate the performance assessment tools. Definitive studies of these tools and of the impact of various training curricula can be designed, but they will be very costly owing to the high interindividual variability (requiring a large number of subjects) and the complexity of both conducting realistic simulation scenarios and conducting fair and thorough objective and subjective performance assessments. There is now in place a large enough network of simulation centers to support such a definitive multicenter study, but it is uncertain whether any funding agency will be willing to support the costs of this complex study.

Other factors complicate the assessment of the effectiveness of simulator-based training. Studying the impact of a single session of a course that uses a new technology and a new approach to training may underestimate the course's impact were it to be used on a regular and repetitive basis. For example, it is widely believed in commercial aviation that CRM training must begin with the initial training of pilots and be continued throughout their career. Social psychologists Robert Helmreich and H. Clayton Foushee, two of the main architects of CRM training, have written: "Data indicate that even intensive initial CRM training constitutes only an awareness phase and introduction to the concepts, and that continuing reinforcement is essential to produce long-term changes in human factors practice."[74] Similarly, United Airlines states in its CRM manual: "Command/Leadership/Resource management (United's terminology for CRM) cannot be a one-shot approach. It has to be a coordinated long range program. It must therefore be an integral part of the entire training effort: new hire training, transition and upgrade programs, and recurrent training"[75]

If these data are valid, it makes no sense to delay a decision to implement a long-term program of this type of training while awaiting definitive proof of its effectiveness, because that proof can come only from very long-term evaluations after the training is fully deployed. The decision to implement such long-term programs, whether in aviation or in healthcare, must be made largely on the basis of face validity and imperfect empirical data.

Finally, simulation training must be viewed within the context of an integration of educational and training experiences. Although the simulator offers important opportunities to target training situations that cannot be safely presented any other way, real-world experience has a much larger cumulative impact. The same principles and procedures taught in training must be reinforced within the real-world operational environment. Simulator-based safety training can be totally negated if production pressures or latent failures in the workplace create disincentives to implement its teachings effectively. In such settings it could appear that simulation training is failing to yield higher patient safety when in reality it is other factors that are eroding safety. Any long-term studies of the impact of simulation training will need to control for potent confounding variables.

Costs of Patient Simulation

A key question concerning the use of simulators is the cost of simulator-based training. The costs depend on many of the same factors that determine the curriculum to be used:

- Types of training involved, ranging from technology in-service to training in basic anesthesia skills, critical incidents management, or crisis resource management
- Target populations for the training, whether equipment technicians, medical students, novice residents, experienced residents, nurse anesthetists, teaching faculty, or private practitioners
- Organizational and financial characteristics of the institution

The hardware and software cost of the screen-only simulator is quite low (as low as $1500), while the equivalent cost of a complete hands-on simulator is relatively high. The prices of commercial simulators can be over $200,000 depending on features (contact the manufacturer for detailed information), and this does not include the necessary clinical and ancillary equipment and space. However, even these large expenditures do not dominate in the cost equation because the capital equipment and space renovation can be amortized over a relatively long useful life, with appropriate provisions for service and upgrades.[76] The dominant cost to any department using the simulator is likely to be that of providing expert instructors and of contributing to the professional direction of the simulation center. While a credible expert must oversee the curriculum and the operation of the center, the type of training and the target population will determine the actual amount of expert instruction that is required per participant. For example, a single faculty member can review the summaries of exercises performed by residents on a screen-only simulator in a few hours per resident per year. A single instructor can use the simulator to demonstrate pulmonary or cardiovascular physiology to a whole class of medical students. When training novice residents in basic anesthesia skills it might be possible to have senior residents or fellows conduct the sessions at a low marginal cost or to use faculty in 1- to 2-hour blocks without requiring extensive additional expenditures. However, when training experienced residents and practitioners in complex material, such as the handling of critical events, there is likely to be no substitute for expert instructors. The cost of expert instruction will depend on the organizational arrangements of the institution, which vary widely.

Another organizational factor that affects the cost has to do with making trainees available for what can be complex, exhausting, and lengthy training sessions. Removing residents from revenue-producing work for training purposes is expensive. On the other hand, if simulator training could allow residents or other anesthetists to work more safely and more efficiently, the benefit could outweigh the cost. Furthermore, many programs have used simulation training as a recruiting tool, both to attract students to anesthesiology and to attract the best candidates to a specific residency. In the long run, if simulator-based training is found to be desirable, innovative changes in organization will evolve to allow it to occur.

Simulation Centers

Although one can install a simulator in a laboratory or conference room, many institutions have equipped complete simulation centers. Typically these centers provide a separate control room to allow complex simulations to be presented without an instructor intruding on the simulated case. The center also provides a debriefing room where videotapes of the simulation session can be reviewed. Some centers have elaborate computer-controlled audiovideo systems allowing the recording of multiple views with real-time annotation of the tapes and rapid search to marked portions of the tape. Dedicated centers facilitate all types of research and training applications of simulators but are especially important for intensive activities such as ACRM. Typically, a technician, anesthesia fellow, or administrator manages the center, coordinating scheduling and logistics as well as assisting the experienced clinicians in conducting training and research.

The costs of a simulator training program can be shared between the anesthesia departments of multiple institutions. Even more frequently today, the cost is shared between departments within a single institution because the simulator is a resource tool for training in other areas besides anesthesia. The patient simulator has proved to be a suitable platform for the training of physicians, nurses, technicians, and other medical and technical personnel, both in intradisciplinary groups and in combined teams.

At this time, despite the lack of definitive cost-effectiveness data, training with realistic simulators is under way at well over one hundred sites around the world, with many of them choosing to conduct fairly high-end crisis management and critical incident training sessions. These programs have already "voted with their feet" on the issue of cost versus benefit, judging that the many varied opportunities afforded by patient simulation outweigh the initial and recurring costs. With so many centers exploring the realities of simulation training, we can expect to see additional data on efficacy and cost within the next few years, although definitive studies may never be available.

Performance Assessment

Several research groups have been investigating performance assessment tools for use during simulation sessions. The most common assessment is to evaluate the quality of the technical management of the situation presented, that is, which clinical actions were taken in response to an abnormality. Simulation offers some benefits in assessing technical performance. Because the nature and cause of the critical incident is known, one can, in advance, construct a list of essential or appropriate technical activities with relative weights of importance. For example, in assessing technical performance in managing MH, terminating the trigger agent and administering IV dantrolene would be crucial, even essential, items, whereas cooling measures, hyperventilation, and bicarbonate therapy would be among many appropriate (but less vital) technical responses. One can also specify in advance the technical pitfalls to look for. For MH these might include diluting dantrolene with the wrong diluent (not sterile water) or an insufficient quantity of diluent. These are pitfalls known to plague those unfamiliar with MH therapy.

Technical Assessment

Chopra et al.[73] assessed technical performance in simulations of MH and anaphylaxis for anesthesiologists using a checklist of appropriate actions. However, the authors used only a single rater and could not measure the variability between raters.

The University of Toronto (Canadian Simulation Centre) has demonstrated good interrater reliability (kappa = 0.96) between two raters of a very basic performance assessment rating system using a simple 3-point scale of the response of an anesthesiologist working alone to a simulated clinical anomaly: 0 = no response; 1 = compensating intervention; 2 = definitive management.[77] The raters produced scripted test tapes in which an anesthesiologist-actor responded at each of the three predetermined levels of performance to 10 different clinical problems ranging in difficulty from very simple (bradycardia during peritoneal traction) to very difficult (anaphylaxis). This strong interrater reliability must be interpreted with caution. The scenarios were acted out to demonstrate clearly different levels of performance, consistently over the duration of each clinical problem. Further, raters might have discerned that each problem was portrayed exactly once at each performance level.

A subsequent analysis of the rating system showed that there was poor internal consistency between the diffferent anesthetic problems presented in the scenarios.[52] This suggests that the items acted "independently, reflecting different aspects of anesthesia care." When aggregated across the five problems, the results were affected by the "level of importance placed on each problem by individual subjects."[52]

However, the same group has shown that a slightly modified simulator test can discriminate between several broad practice categories,[78] both in terms of the score on the 3-point scale and in rapidity of response.[79] This group also showed that a six-event simulator test yielded good interrater reliability and good correlation between clinical evaluations, written tests of knowledge, and simulation performance for fourth-year medical students.[80] Kurrek's group[81] subsequently compared scores from raters viewing live performances in the simulator with performances viewed on videotape and found good interrater reliability, with the weighted kappa statistic not significantly different at $P < .05$. This study again used a relatively simple 3-point scale.[81]

The VA Palo Alto/Stanford group assessed the technical performance of 14 anesthesia teams, each managing two different complex critical events (MH and cardiac arrest).[82] Scoring was based on a predefined checklist of appropriate medical and technical actions for recognition, diagnosis, and therapy. Point values for successful implementation of each action were assigned subjectively by the investigators in advance. Some items were rated as "essential items" whose absence resulted in a net score of zero points. Raters recorded the presence or absence of each action during a scenario and then summed the point values for all actions recorded as present. Each technical score was expressed as the fraction of the maximum possible score (100 for cardiac arrest, 95 for MH).

In this study, three raters agreed frequently concerning the presence or absence of checklist items, and the interrater variability was good (approximately 0.6).[82] The teams scored well technically, usually accruing over 80% of the available points, and never missing an essential item. This performance should not be surprising because of three factors: (1) participants had at least 2 years of postgraduate medical training and all had previously received ACLS certification; (2) the scenarios portrayed in this study have well-known treatment protocols and the most crucial items could be accomplished by only one or two individuals who knew exactly what to do; and (3) the ACRM training paradigm in which the simulations were conducted encourages distribution of workload and mobilization of help, tending to level out the technical performance.

Behavioral Processes in the Management of Abnormalities

A complementary evaluation used by some groups is to assess the quality of the cognitive and behavioral processes used by individuals and teams to recognize the abnormality and to direct the implementation of the technical management. The behavioral component of crisis management must, however, be assessed subjectively. Two research groups (VA Palo Alto/Stanford and University of Basel) are studying adaptations of the anchored subjective rating scales developed by the NASA (National Aeronautics and Space Administration)/University of Texas Aerospace Crew Performance Project.

The VA Palo Alto/Stanford group also studied the interrater variability of subjective ratings of behaviors on 5-point anchored scales.[82] Again, several tests of interrater reliability were used. With the most stringent test (S_{av}—equivalent to the kappa statistic), "fair" (0.2 to 0.4) to "moderate" (0.4 to 0.6) agreement was found for the behaviors considered most crucial in crisis management (e.g., leadership, workload distribution, primary anesthesiologist overall, team overall). Other interrater reliability statistics showed even greater agreement. Although there was some difficulty in agreement on the operational definitions of each type of behavior, the

investigators stated that the largest problem in achieving agreement was the high variability of each behavior over the course of a simulation scenario. For example, an anesthesiologist might show evidence of good communication at one instant, only to be shouting ambiguous orders into thin air at the next. Aggregating these behaviors into a single rating was extremely difficult, even for bounded time segments of the scenario. The investigators also showed that combining scores from any two raters had a very low probability of differing from the mean of five raters by more than 1 rating point, whereas any single rating could differ by that amount 14% of the time.

Using the mean of all five raters' scores, there was much higher variability between teams in their crisis management behaviors.[82] Several teams (14% for cardiac arrest, 28% for MH) had mean overall team ratings at the level of "minimally acceptable" or below—1 or 2 on the 5-point rating scale—and the performance of the primary anesthesiologist was rated at or below this level even more frequently (21% for cardiac arrest, 35% for MH). The ratings for specific crisis management behaviors showed similar patterns.

The Danish group has also given a preliminary report on their attempts to validate subjective and objective evaluation parameters, a technique they call PEANUTS (*p*erformance *e*nhancement in *an*esthesia *u*sing the *t*raining *s*imulator).[83]

The interrater reliability of ratings of crisis management behaviors was not as strong as was hoped. However, these are assessments of very complex behaviors and actions, and it should not be surprising that ratings are difficult. In fact, the VA Palo Alto/Stanford results given above are considerably better than those found in recent assessments of the interrater reliability of mock oral examinations[84] (data from the actual American Board of Anesthesiology examinations are not available), and the VA Palo Alto/Stanford interrater reliability results are approximately the same as those found among peer reviewers (before any discussion) of actual clinical care in cases "previously judged to involve a perioperative indicator (an event or action that leads to an adverse outcome)."[85] Thus the reliability of simulator-based ratings of crisis management behaviors appears to be on a par with those measures currently representing the standard of performance assessment in the anesthesiology profession.

Simulator Patient Outcome as a Measure of Performance

Can the "clinical" outcome of the simulator's mathematical physiology predict how a real patient would have fared under that individual's care? In extreme cases this is likely to be true. A subject who demonstrates totally erroneous decision making (e.g., failure to defibrillate a simulated patient with ventricular fibrillation) will quickly allow the patient's state to deteriorate. However, the mathematical models are not sufficient to predict what would happen to any actual patient after complex sequences of therapy and more subtle patient care judgments. Thus, the clinical outcome of the simulated patient is one datum that can be used to assess the performance of the anesthetist on a simulation scenario, but for the foreseeable future any credible performance measurement technique must involve subjective and semiobjective judgments by clinical experts.

The results from the various simulation groups suggest that it should be possible to develop a reasonable set of performance measures of anesthetist skill using the simulator as a tool to present standardized patient scenarios. This set of tools would not be perfect but would be likely to be as good as the tools currently used to make decisions regarding board certification and peer review of adverse events. A definitive study of these tools can be done in principle but would require a large number of subjects rated by multiple raters and would thus be complex and costly. No funding agency has yet come forward to support such a definitive study. Incidentally, no existing performance measurement in healthcare has been subjected to such a costly, complete, and public validation.

Can Simulators Be Used for the Evaluation and Testing of Residents or Practitioners?

Anesthetists have discussed the possibility of using the simulator as a tool for examinations, either for graduation from a residency or for board certification. This use would require further evaluation of the simulation scenarios and of the predictive power of the performance assessment tools used. A difficulty with using simulation for board certification testing is that the OR equipment would rarely be the same as that used by the candidate, and the OR staff's operational protocols might differ from those familiar to the candidate. In the training situation these difficulties can be overlooked as part of the global "suspension of disbelief" needed to maximize the benefits of simulator training. In the test situation these differences can be a disadvantage for some candidates. Perhaps this could be overcome by providing practice time to candidates in a standardized simulation setup identical to that of the testing center.

Despite these difficulties, it is likely that as the use of patient simulators becomes more widespread, anesthesiologists and other clinicians will become more interested in using them to assist in evaluating performance. The existing system of performance evaluation, which uses a relatively haphazard combination of subjective judgments of clinical competency in residency along with written or oral examinations, has itself never been validated. Many believe that the written examination does not correlate well with clinical ability, and the degree to which the oral examination process tests actual clinical skill is unknown. Simulation could offer candidates the ability to demonstrate their clinical abilities in a controlled clinical domain while still demonstrating their consulting and language skills through oral examination.

The first trials of evaluation using simulators may occur in situations for which the evaluation is a nonthreatening critique or is graded pass-fail. Another situation would be the evaluation of residents who have been placed on probation or for whom dismissal from the residency is already a distinct possibility. For these residents the burden of proof is on them to demonstrate their skills. The simulator might offer a more controlled environment for them to do so. The same could be true for practitioners who wish to return to clinical work after a hiatus.

The Future of Patient Simulation in Anesthesia

The use of patient simulators has now grown beyond its initial phase as a purely experimental technology and modality to enter a new period of growth and consolidation. Although many questions remain unanswered about the impact of the technology, there now seems little question that simulation will be a significant technique for education, training, and research within anesthesiology and in many other domains in healthcare. At the level of basic healthcare education, simulators have already begun to make their mark in applications aimed at professional students (e.g., medicine and nursing). The expansion of clinical training beyond anesthesiology, for resident physicians and for experienced clinicians (physicians, nurses, and combined teams), has been an important development. Not only has this brought the benefits of simulation-based training to these other healthcare settings, it has also brought anesthesiologists to the forefront of issues related to education, training, and performance assessment. As the specialty of anesthesiology seeks to redefine its role within healthcare, the emergence of anesthesiologists both as experts in the use of simulation and as experts in the cognitive skills of complex dynamic decision making adds another important role for the profession.

Over the last few years directors of many anesthesia training programs have asked whether they need a simulator and can afford it. Probably half the training programs in the United States have simulators or have negotiated access for at least some of their trainees to other programs' simulators. With so many programs having simulators, officials of other institutions who have been reluctant in the past are beginning to see the value in acquiring them. The question now asked is whether the institution as a whole can benefit from the applications of simulation. In general, both new and existing simulation centers are based on multidisciplinary applications and cost sharing, although often anesthesiologists play the dominant role in running the center. It is likely that simulation-based training, led largely by anesthesiologists, will become a routine part of the initial and recurrent training of *all* clinicians who work in settings involving high complexity and dynamism.

The simulators themselves are undergoing a steady stream of enhancements and improvements. Although cost is a major impediment to achieving all the enhancements that are technically feasible, the feature list will probably expand without enormous changes in cost. There is a vigorous competition between multiple manufacturers of simulators at varying levels of fidelity and complexity. However, there are some fundamental limits to how exact the simulators can become. Unlike aeronautical engineers, physicians do not design and build the system they wish to model. The fundamental differential equations of fluid mechanics and aerodynamics are firmly established, allowing supercomputers to provide technically meaningful simulations as replacements for many wind tunnel tests. Furthermore, there still are wind tunnel tests as well as test flights of actual prototype aircraft. Sophisticated instrumentation can be built into test structures to define their behaviors accurately. Physicians and simulator engineers will never have this kind of knowledge about the human body.

The early 21st century will probably see VR simulations take over from computer screen and realistic simulations. However, the pace of VR development continues to be relatively slow. There is not yet a robust inexpensive platform for developing complex virtual worlds. Until such platforms are developed, perhaps for entertainment applications, VR systems will probably remain too complex and expensive to take over from current simulation modalities. In order to fully take over for the kinds of applications currently being performed with hands-on simulators, VR systems will have to allow nearly complete immersion into a multiperson artificial world, with replication of tactile, visual, and auditory stimuli. Nonetheless, within one or two decades reasonably priced VR systems *will* allow full immersion, at which time VR may become the norm for training in many complex work fields. VR technology could also change the nature of work itself.

REFERENCES

1. Good ML, Gravenstein JS: Anesthesia simulators and training devices. Int Anesthesiol Clin 1989; 27:161–168.
2. Rolfe J, Staple K: Flight Simulation. Cambridge, UK, Cambridge University Press, 1986, p 4.
3. Carley WM: Pull Up! United 747's Near Miss Initiates A Widespread Review of Pilot Skills. New York, The Wall Street Journal, Eastern Ed, Mar 19, p A1, 1999.
4. Smith N, Zwart A, Beneken J: Interaction between the circulatory effects and the uptake and distribution of halothane: Use of a multiple model. Anesthesiology 1972; 37:47–58.
5. Zwart A, Smith NT, Beneken J: Multiple model approach to uptake and distribution of halothane: The use of an analog computer. Comput Biomed Res 1972; 5:228–238.
6. Fukui Y, Smith N: Interactions among ventilation, the circulation, and the uptake and distribution of halothane—use of a hybrid computer multiple model: II. Spontanous vs. controlled ventilation and the effects of CO_2. Anesthesiology 1981; 54:119–124.
7. Smith N, Sebald A, Wakeland C, et al: Cockpit simulation—will it be used for training in anesthesia? Presented at Anesthesia Simulator Curriculum Conference, Rockville, MD, 1989.
8. Schwid HA: A flight simulator for general anesthesia training. Comput Biomed Res 1987; 20:64–75.
9. Schwid HA, O'Donnell D: The Anesthesia Simulator-Recorder: A device to train and evaluate anesthesiologists' responses to critical incidents. Anesthesiology 1990; 72:191–197.
10. Schwid H, O'Donnell D: Educational computer simulation of malignant hyperthermia. J Clin Monit Comput 1992; 8:201–208.
11. Schwid H: Critical Care Simulator, Anesthesia Simulator. Vol. 1999. Anesoft, Inc., 1999.
12. Schwid H, Rooke GA, Ross BK, et al: Use of a computerized and advanced cardiac life support simulator improves retention of advanced cardiac life support guidelines better than a textbook review. Crit Care Med 1999; 27:821–824.
13. Denson J, Abrahamson S: A computer-controlled patient simulator. JAMA 1969; 208:504–508.
14. Carter D: Man-made man: Anesthesiological medical human simulator. J Assoc Adv Med Instrum 1969; 3:80–86.
15. Abrahamson S: Sim One—a patient simulator ahead of its time. Caduceus 1997; 13:29–41.
16. Abrahamson S, Denson J, Wolf R: Effectiveness of a simulator in training anesthesiology residents. J Med Educ 1969; 44:515–519.
17. Hoffman K, Abrahamson S: The "cost-effectiveness" of Sim One. J Med Educ 1975; 50:1127–1128.
18. Good M, Gravenstein J: Training for safety in an anesthesia simulator. Semin Anesth 1993; 12:235–250.
19. Cooper J, Newbower R, Long C, et al: Preventable anesthesia mishaps: A study of human factors. Anesthesiology 1978; 49:399–406.
20. Cooper JB, Newbower R, Kitz R: An analysis of major errors and equipment failures in anesthesia management: Considerations for prevention and detection. Anesthesiology 1984; 60:34–42.
21. Gaba D, Maxwell M, DeAnda A: Anesthetic mishaps: Breaking the chain of accident evolution. Anesthesiology 1987; 66:670–676.
22. Gaba D: Human error in anesthetic mishaps. Int Anesthesiol Clin 1989; 27:137–147.
23. Weinger M, Englund C: Ergonomic and human factors affecting anesthetic vigilance and monitoring performance in the operating room environment. Anesthesiology 1990; 73:995–1021.
24. Gaba DM, DeAnda A: A comprehensive anesthesia simulation environment: Re-creating the operating room for research and training. Anesthesiology 1988; 69:387–394.
25. Gaba D, Williams J: CASE simulation system status report 9/89. Presented at Anesthesia Simulator Curriculum Conference, Rockville, MD, 1989.
26. Chopra V, Engbers F, Geerts M, et al: The Leiden anesthesia simulator: A high fidelity system for anesthesia training (abstract). Presented at 10th World Congress of Anesthesiologists, The Hague, Netherlands, 1992.
27. Chopra V, Engbers F, Geerts M, et al: The Leiden anaesthesia simulator. Br J Anaesth 1994; 73:287–292.
28. Shekter I, Ward D, Stern D, et al: Enhancing a patient simulator to respond to PEEP, PIP and other ventilation parameters. Presented at Meeting of the Society for Technology in Anesthesia, San Diego, 1999.
29. Westenskow D, Bonk R, Sedlmayr M: Enhancing a human simulator with a graphic display of physiology. Presented at Meeting of the Society for Technology in Anesthesia, San Diego, 1999.
30. Thoman W, Lampotang S, Gravenstein D, et al: An ICP model for the human patient simulator. Presented at Meeting of the Society for Technology in Anesthesia, Tucson, 1998.
31. Murray W, Schneider A: Teaching high school students. In Henson LC, Lee AC, Basford A (eds): Simulators in Anesthesiology Education. New York, Plenum Press, 1998.
32. Fried E: Integration of the human patient simulator into the medical student curriculum: Life support skills. In Henson LC, Lee AC, Basford A (eds): Simulators in Anesthesiology Education. New York, Plenum Press, 1998.
33. Lee A: Simulators for medical students and anesthesia resident education. In Henson LC, Lee AC, Basford A (eds): Simulators in Anesthesiology Education. New York, Plenum Press, 1998.
34. Gaba DM, DeAnda A: The response of anesthesia trainees to simulated critical incidents. Anesth Analg 1989; 68:444–451.
35. Gaba D: Human performance issues in anesthesia patient safety. Probl Anesth 1991; 5:329–350.
36. Gaba D: Improving anesthesiologists' performance by simulating reality (editorial). Anesthesiology 1992; 76:491–494.
37. Gaba D: Dynamic decision-making in anesthesiology: Cognitive models and training approach. In Evans D, Patel V (eds): Advanced Models of Cognition for Medical Training and Practice. Berlin, Springer-Verlag, 1992, pp 122–147.
38. Gaba D, Howard S, Fish K, et al: Anesthesia crisis resource management training (abstract). Anesthesiology 1991; 75:A1062.
39. Gaba D, Fish K, Howard S: Crisis Management in Anesthesiology. New York, Churchill Livingstone, 1994.
40. Raemer D, Barron D, Blum R, et al: Teaching crisis management in radiology using realistic simulation. Presented at Meeting of the Society for Technology in Anesthesia, Tucson, Jan. 14–17, 1998.
41. Sica GT, Barron DM, Blum R, et al: Computerized realistic simulation: A teaching module for crisis management in radiology. AJR 1999; 172:301–304.
42. Raemer D, Maviglia S, Van Horne C, et al: Mock codes: Using realistic simulation to teach team resuscitation management. Presented at Meeting of the Society for Technology in Anesthesia, Tucson, Jan. 14–17, 1998.
43. Kurrek M, Devitt J, Ichinose F, et al: Simulator team training: A concept beyond anesthesia. Presented at Meeting of the Society for Technology in Anesthesia, Tucson, Jan. 14–17, 1998.
44. Halamek L, Howard S, Kaegi D, et al: The simulated delivery room as a laboratory for the study of human performance (abstract). J Invest Med 1998; 46:167A.
45. Halamek L, Howard S, Smith B, et al: Development of a simulated delivery room for the study of human performance during neonatal resuscitation. Pediatrics 1997; 100 (suppl): 513–524.
46. Helmreich R, Schaefer H: Team performance in the operating room. In Bogner M (ed): Human Error in Medicine. Hillsdale, NJ, Erlbaum, 1994, pp 225–253.
47. Schaefer J, Dongilli T, Gonzalea R: Results of systematic psychomotor difficult airway training of residents using the ASA Difficult Airway Algorithm & Dynamic Simulation (abstract). Anesthesiology 1998; 89:A60.
48. Murray W, Good M, Gravenstein J, et al: Novel application of a full human simulator: Training with remifentanil prior to human use (abstract). Anesthesiology 1998; 89:A56.
49. Schwid H, O'Donnell D: Anesthesiologists' management of simulated critical incidents. Anesthesiology 1992; 76:495–501.
50. Botney R, Gaba D, Howard S, et al: The role of fixation error in preventing the detection and correction of a simulated volatile anesthetic overdose (abstract). Anesthesiology 1993; 79:A1115.
51. Botney R, Gaba D, Howard S: Anesthesiologist performance during a simulated loss of pipeline oxygen (abstract). Anesthesiology 1993; 79:A1118.
52. Devitt JH, Kurrek MM, Cohen MM, et al: Testing internal consistency and construct validity during evaluation of performance in a patient simulator [see comments]. Anesth Analg 1998; 86:1160–1164.

53. Sowb Y, Loeb R, Smith B: Cognitive performance during simulated ventilation-related events. J Clin Monit Comput 1998; 14: 535.

54. Sowb Y, Loeb R, Moore P: Competence analysis of intraoperative critical events. J Clin Monit Comput 1998; 14:535–536.

55. Sowb Y, Loeb R, Smith B: Clinicians' response to management of the gas delivery system. Presented at Meeting of the Society for Technology in Anesthesia, San Diego, Jan. 20–23, 1999.

56. Lampotang S, Gravenstein JS, Euliano TY, et al: Influence of pulse oximetry and capnography on time to diagnosis of critical incidents in anesthesia: A pilot study using a full-scale patient simulator. J Clin Monit Comput 1998; 14:313–321.

57. Byrne AJ, Sellen AJ, Jones JG: Errors on anaesthetic record charts as a measure of anaesthetic performance during simulated critical incidents [see comments]. Br J Anaesth 1998; 80:58–62.

58. Howard S, Gaba D: Factors influencing vigilance and performance of anesthetists. Curr Opin Anesthesiol 1998; 11:651–657.

59. Howard S, Smith B, Gaba D, et al: Performance of well-rested vs. highly-fatigued residents: A simulator study (abstract). Anesthesiology 1997; 87:A981.

60. Smith B, Howard S, Weinger M, et al: Performance of the preanesthesia equipment checkout: A simulator study. Presented at Meeting of the Society for Technology in Anesthesia, San Diego, Jan. 20–23, 1999.

61. Smith B, Howard S, Weinger M, et al: Fatigue effects on clinical performance during simulated intraoperative events. Presented at Meeting of the Society for Technology in Anesthesia, San Diego, Jan. 20–23, 1999.

62. Howard S, Keshavacharya S, Smith B, et al: Behavioral evidence of fatigue during a simulator experiment (abstract). Anesthesiology 1998; 89:A1236.

63. Berge JA, Gramstad L, Grimnes S: An evaluation of a time-saving anaesthetic machine checkout procedure. Eur J Anaesthesiol 1994; 11:493–498.

64. Larsson J, Hayes-Roth B, Gaba D, et al: Evaluation of a medical diagnosis system using simulator test scenarios. Artif Intell Med 1997; 11:119–140.

65. Kaegi D, Halamek L, Van Hare G, et al: Effect of mental stress on heart rate variability: Validation of virtual operating and delivery room training modules. Presented at Society for Pediatric Research, San Francisco, 1999.

66. Kaegi D, Halamek L, Dubin A, et al: Heart rate variability as a marker for workload during neonatal resuscitation (abstract). Pediatrics 1998; 102:766–777.

67. Howard SK, Gaba DM, Fish KJ, et al: Anesthesia crisis resource management training: Teaching anesthesiologists to handle critical incidents. Aviat Space Environ Med 1992; 63:763–770.

68. Holzman RS, Cooper JB, Gaba DM, et al: Anesthesia crisis resource management: Real-life simulation training in operating room crises. J Clin Anesth 1995; 7:675–687.

69. Kurrek MM, Fish KJ: Anaesthesia crisis resource management training: An intimidating concept, a rewarding experience [see comments]. Can J Anaesth 1996; 43:430–434.

70. Small S: What participants learn from anesthesia crisis resource management training (abstract). Anesthesiology 1998; 89:A71.

71. Leith P: Crisis management training helps young anesthesiologist successfully manage mid-air passenger cardiac arrest. J Clin Monit Comput 1997; 13:69.

72. Good M, Gravenstein J, Mahla M, et al: Can simulation accelerate the learning of basic anesthesia skills by beginning anesthesia residents (abstract)? Anesthesiology 1992; 77:A1133.

73. Chopra V, Gesink B, De Jong J, et al: Does training on an anaesthesia simulator lead to improvement in performance? Br J Anaesth 1994; 73:293–297.

74. Helmreich R, Foushee H: Why crew resource management? In Wiener E, Kanki B, Helmreich R (eds): Cockpit Resource Management. San Diego, Academic Press, 1993, pp 3–46.

75. Orlady H: Airline pilot training today and tomorrow. In Wiener E, Kanki B, Helmreich R (eds): Cockpit Resource Management. San Diego, Academic Press, 1993, pp 447–478.

76. Kurrek M, Devitt J: The cost for construction and maintenance of a simulation centre. Can J Anaesth 1997; 44:1191–1195.

77. Devitt JH, Kurrek MM, Cohen MM, et al: Testing the raters: Inter-rater reliability of standardized anaesthesia simulator performance [see comments]. Can J Anaesth 1997; 44:924–928.

78. Devitt J, Kurrek M, Cohen M: Can a simulator based evaluation be used to assess anesthesiologists (abstract)? Anesthesiology 1998; 89:A1172.

79. Kurrek M, Devitt J, Cohen M: Relationship between response time and performance score during clinical competence evaluation in the simulator (abstract). Anesthesiology 1998; 89:A1179.

80. Morgan PJ, Cleave-Hogg D: Evaluation of medical students' performances using the anesthesia simulator. Acad Med 1999; 74: 202.

81. Kurrek M, Devitt J, Cohen M, et al: Inter-rater reliability between live scenarios and video recordings in a realistic scenario. Presented at Meeting of the Society for Technology in Anesthesia, San Diego, Jan. 20–23, 1999.

82. Gaba D, Howard S, Flanagan B, et al: Assessment of clinical performance during simulated crises using both technical and behavioral ratings. Anesthesiology 1998; 89:8–18.

83. Jacobsen J, Jensen PF, Osterfaard D, et al: Performance enhancement in anesthesia using the training simulator Sophus (PEANUTS). In Henson L, Lee A (eds): Simulators in Anesthesiology Education. New York, Plenum Press, 1998, pp 103–106.

84. Klock P, Jacobsohn E, Group OBE: Inter-rater reliability of oral board examinations with American and Canadian examiners (abstract). Anesthesiology 1998; 89:A66.

85. Levine R, Sugarman M, Schiller W, et al: The effect of group discussion on interrater reliability of structured peer review. Anesthesiology 1998; 89:507–515.

4 Monitoring and Patient Safety

George Mychaskiw II, D.O.
John H. Eichhorn, M.D.

Improved monitoring of both the patient and the anesthesia delivery system over the last 15 years has significantly helped make anesthesia for surgery much safer. The occurrence of intraoperative catastrophes solely attributable to problems with anesthesia care causing death, cardiac arrest, and permanent brain damage has been greatly reduced.

The strategies and behaviors associated with attempting to make operative anesthesia safer are referred to as "safety monitoring,"[1] a term coined to distinguish this specific program for prevention of major anesthesia accidents from the other types of monitoring best characterized as "physiologic monitoring." This distinction is important. "Monitoring" is often correctly associated with the use of an intra-arterial cannula for direct continuous systemic blood pressure measurement, a pulmonary artery catheter for pressure measurements, and, now, transesophageal echocardiography for evaluation of left ventricular wall motion (all of which are thoroughly discussed in this book). These types of monitors allow continuous fine-tuning of anesthetic management and physiologic parameters under evolving conditions during surgery. As important as this is, it is secondary in a circumstance of, for example, an unrecognized disconnection of the breathing circuit from the endotracheal tube connector in a patient under full muscle relaxation being mechanically ventilated who, as a result, is *not* ventilated, becomes hypoxemic, and has a cardiac arrest. Such occurrences were alarmingly common relatively recently. Safety monitoring evolved in response to such events.

Purpose of Safety Monitoring

"Better monitoring would have prevented this accident!" is a well-meaning but poorly stated conclusion of many investigators and speakers analyzing major anesthesia-related adverse incidents.

This type of pronouncement dramatically illustrates one of the most difficult aspects of the recent revolution in anesthesia practice in general and the safety of intraoperative anesthesia care in particular: the relationship between human behavior and technology. Put as simply as possible, technology (in this case, monitoring) *never* "prevents" anything. Behaviors (specifically, the correct response to a much earlier warning of an adverse development during the course of an anesthetic) can and do prevent severe intraoperative anesthesia accidents.

It is well recognized that there is a finite amount of time in the evolution of an anesthesia "critical incident" (a set of circumstances that, if left unchecked, produces patient injury[2]) for the anesthesia provider to recognize that there is a problem, diagnose it correctly, and act definitively to prevent an adverse event. It had been almost a time-honored tradition in anesthesia that the recognition of a severe, even life-threatening, problem came quite late in the development of a clinical scenario with the surgeon calling up over the draped ether screen, "Hey! The blood looks a little dark down here!" Of course, at this point, the patient had become significantly hypoxemic, as evidenced by the hemoglobin desaturation. There was precious little time to intervene before brain and heart ischemia led to injury or even death. The strategic underpinning of safety monitoring acknowledges that critical incidents will *always* occur. Given the nature of the complex technical environment in which anesthesia is administered today and the fallibility of humans functioning in that environment, it is impossible even to suggest that critical incidents will be eliminated, or even dramatically reduced. These critical incidents occur at a rate of about 1 in 15 anesthetic procedures performed.[3] This rate of over 6% is significant and underscores the necessity for sensitive monitoring capability, vigilance of the anesthesia provider to interpret these monitors, and training of that provider in the management of critical incidents. It has been shown that there is only a 0.53% morbidity rate associated with these incidents, further emphasizing the importance of rapid detection and early management.[3] In fact, the presence of an anesthesia provider throughout the procedure is the most important component of the existing widely accepted standards for monitoring.

In spite of the many advances, breathing system connectors will still become accidentally disconnected from endotracheal tubes, esophageal intubations will occur, breathing system tubing and endotracheal tubes will become kinked or internally obstructed, and oxygen supplies will occasionally fail. There will be threats to patient safety during anesthesia.

The central concept of safety monitoring is to provide the earliest possible warning of an untoward development (such as the breathing circuit becoming disconnected from the endotracheal tube), thus maximizing the time available to diagnose and treat the event and thus prevent patient injury. Given the fascination with, and investment in, high-level technology of modern medicine, it is not surprising that the emphasis is on the technology—the electronic machines. However, safety monitoring is one of the best examples that illustrate the circumstances in which the machines, the monitors, themselves do nothing but extend the human senses. They facilitate the behaviors—make the human behaviors easier for the humans. Those monitoring behaviors that lead to the earliest possible warning and the maximum time for intervention can be accomplished without electronic machinery. This was clear in the original Harvard monitoring standards[4] and must be understood to separate human behavior from technology and to expose the essence of safety monitoring. It is certainly true that performing the behaviors of safety monitoring is easier when correctly applied and functioning electronic monitors such as capnography, pulse oximetry, noninvasive blood pressure (NIBP) measurement, and electrocardiography (ECG) are used. It is even legitimate to say that effective use of these instruments is the *best* way to implement the behaviors of safety monitoring, particularly the continuous (as opposed to intermittent) nature of the monitoring tasks. This does not diminish the need to emphasize behaviors first and technology second. In the last 15 years, monitoring has progressed to a level that leaves no significant physiologic system unattended. This is especially true in safety monitoring and engineering. Although most modern anesthesia systems have evolved to a state of near perfection of engineering and performance, critical incidents continue to occur at rates in excess of what can be attributed to mechanical failure. As in aviation, human error is responsible for most anesthetic misadventures. The trend of the future is more emphasis on the human factors of anesthesia safety—that is, the engineering of monitoring systems to facilitate proper use and interpretation data to permit early detection of critical incidents and training in management of critical incidents. Anesthesia simulators, again taking the lead from aviation, have shown promise in improving the human element in anesthesia safety.[5]

Thus there are two separate but related points regarding the role of safety monitoring. First, monitoring does not prevent injury-causing anesthesia accidents. These accidents are prevented by the information generated by the monitoring behaviors leading to earlier identification of untoward developments and consequent correct intervention. Second, while sophisticated electronic monitors may be the best way to implement safety monitoring behaviors, precisely how this earliest possible information is obtained is irrelevant as long as there is effective intervention in time to prevent patient injury.

Epidemiology of Catastrophic Anesthesia Accidents

It would seem relatively simple to be able to collect statistics about adverse outcomes caused by anesthesia care. If a patient has an intraoperative event that involves the anesthetic rather than the surgery and there is a catastrophic outcome such as cardiac arrest, permanent central nervous system (CNS) damage, or death, this would be registered in a database as an anesthesia accident. Reputable academic investigators could then examine the data collected, assemble information about risk factors and complication rates, and try to offer suggestions for improvements in practice. However logical this may sound, it has not happened and likely never will. For many years, until quite recently, information has been lacking about even the most basic safety statistics in anesthesia care. Many authors published series of patients experiencing anesthesia complications and these have been reviewed from a historical perspective.[6-8] Prior to the 1980s, virtually all of these reports were anecdotal and retrospective. There was and is extremely little information about rates of major anesthesia complications among large populations undergoing surgery.

The paucity of information about severe anesthesia accidents exists for several reasons. One central factor is the sheer physical difficulty of organizing the collection of such data. Serious adverse anesthesia outcomes were and (even more so now) are very rare. Therefore, meaningful incidence figures require the collection of information about massive numbers of anesthesia care, far more than any one institution or local system of institutions can assemble in a reasonable period of time. In the United States, no national repository of statistical data exists about adverse patient outcomes caused by medical care. Even if such a database existed and reporting were mandatory under federal law, ensuring full compliance by practitioners and hospitals would be extraordinarily difficulty at best. In fact, it is virtually impossible to imagine there could ever be such a system in the United States. However, an international convention dedicated to the investigation and prevention of anesthetic mortality has been proposed.[9] Such organizations exist in aviation, as exemplified by the International Civil Aviation Organization (ICAO), the Federal Aviation Administration (FAA), and the National Transportation Safety Board (NTSB). Although the development of a "Federal Anesthesia Administration" seems unlikely to most U.S. anesthesia providers, tort reform coupled with globalization of the healthcare industry and multinational trade agreements places the creation of such a body within the realm of possibility. At this time, however, the field still suffers for lack of genuine information.

Further, definitions of what exactly constitutes an anesthesia accident have varied from study to study, often making the aggregation of statistics from multiple studies impossible. As noted, several papers reporting series of anesthetic mishaps have been published, but each without a valid denominator. Even if the authors believe that all the adverse events during a delineated interval have been captured by them and could constitute a valid numerator for an incidence calculation, it is not possible to calculate a rate without the total number of anesthesia procedures in that time period as a denominator. For a rate to have any meaning, the denominator would need to be many millions, and no system or person has the resources to assemble such a massive database accurately.

Finally, the characteristics of the medicolegal system in the United States virtually guarantee that there will never be widespread reporting of detailed accurate information about adverse medical outcomes—particularly anesthesia catastrophes—because these are almost always associated with the potential for lawsuits and the possibility of large monetary settlements or awards. Because the financial stakes are extremely high, malpractice insurance carriers fiercely guard all clinical information in any way associated with a case that has not been "closed" (come to financial conclusion one way or another). Very often, when a malpractice lawsuit is settled by the insurance company without a trial, one of the stipulations is that the record is sealed, and no one will ever know what the testimony would have been. This prevents academic anesthesiologists from studying the case and gathering information that could help prevent similar accidents in the future. Fortunately, in the mid- to late 1980s, there was some modification of the strict denial of access to insurance company files in that the American Society of Anesthesiologists (ASA) Committee on Professional Liability organized the ASA Closed Claims Study and secured information from several malpractice insurers about claims associated with anesthesia after the subject files were permanently closed. Although this was a valuable step, it constituted only a very limited look at a subset of anesthesia-related accident cases. No incidence data could be generated because no denominators existed. Several very interesting conclusions of this study are discussed below.

From the mid-1950s through the early 1980s, there was a widely accepted axiom in the anesthesiology profession that the death rate associated with anesthesia care was 1 to 2 per 10,000 patients.[10] Immediately upon mention of such a statistic, problems arise. Does this include all patients, regardless of preoperative physical status and type of surgery? Is this consideration the same from study to study? (The widely differing definitions of anesthesia mortality that were used have been noted.[6]) Should patients with high risks from their surgical conditions be excluded? Should only "healthy" patients (such as ASA physical status I and II)[1] be included in such calculations to focus attention exclusively on the role of anesthesia care? What would this do to the resultant calculated incident rates? However valid these questions are, they cannot be answered; not enough information exists. Therefore, the "baseline" mortality figures so widely quoted must be interpreted with caution; however, the idea of approximately a 1/10,000 anesthesia mortality rate was so widely accepted for so long that it is as reasonable a starting point as any. Then, two questions eventually to be addressed here are: What has happened to the anesthesia accident rate? and, How is monitoring and, specifically, safety monitoring involved in this—past, present, and future?

Refreshingly, certain themes were consistent and meaningful in the earlier reports of anesthesia accidents. Multiple reviews exist,[11] but in searching for a common focus in many reports, it is clear that unrecognized hypoventilation due to a long list of potential causes is, *by far,* the most common cause of intraoperative anesthesia catastrophes. This reflects and correlates with the original critical incident study,[2] in which the most common cause of anesthesia critical incidents (events that did cause or would have caused patient injury if left to evolve without intervention) was breathing system disconnection. As noted, the classic list of causes of unrecognized hypoventilation goes on to include esophageal intubation, kinking or obstruction of tubes or tubing, incorrect ventilator settings, and simple inadequate spontaneous or assisted ventilation during anesthesia. A 1985 classic study of cardiac arrests due to anesthesia[12] cited "failure to ventilate" as both the most common cause of arrest and one that is completely preventable. In 1990, the ASA Closed Claims Study consistently cited "respiratory" causes as the most common of major adverse events, and among respiratory causes, "inadequate ventilation" leads the list.[13] A major, although less frequent (yet never to be forgotten), cause of intraoperative anesthesia catastrophe is inadequate delivery of oxygen in the fresh gas flow. (It is relevant to note that one of us [J.H.E.] was introduced to and became involved in the field of anesthesia patient safety by being involved in the investigation of a set of catastrophic anesthesia accidents due to the delivery of an anoxic fresh gas, argon, to the central oxygen supply at a small rural hospital in which the anesthesia machine oxygen monitors were not functioning on the day of the event.) Keeping in mind the role and purpose of safety monitoring outlined above, it is not surprising that the monitoring of patient ventilation and oxygenation forms the cornerstone of the principles of safety monitoring.

Monitoring Standards and Their Impact on Safety Monitoring

The adoption of anesthesia safety monitoring behaviors in the mid- and late 1980s was profoundly accelerated by formal published standards of practice for anesthesia that prescribed safety monitoring principles. Prior to this time, many anesthesia practitioners had already incorporated some or most of the basic ideas and used precordial or esophageal stethoscopes to auscultate breath sounds and heart tones,

sometimes even continuously, and applied an ECG monitor to most patients. Formal published standards codified these behaviors, most importantly, promoted the idea of genuinely continuous monitoring (as opposed to the usual intermittent, checks), and coincided in time with new technology—the widespread availability of capnography and pulse oximetry as well as new awareness of oxygen monitors with lower-limit alarms and also ventilator disconnection monitors. These standards promoted development of new monitoring strategies in a manner unparalleled in the history of anesthesia practice.

It is worth noting that the original impetus for formal standards of practice grew out of a risk management committee at Harvard Medical School formed in response to a significant concern from Harvard's malpractice insurance company about the great expense of anesthesia-caused patient injury and death claims. Anesthesia patient safety was not good, according to insurance claims statistics. In 1984, the committee reviewed all the claims and incidents on file since the company was founded in 1976. Among healthy patients (ASA status I and II patients who should reasonably expect no adverse outcome related to anesthesia), the rate of severe intraoperative accidents was already comparatively low (1/75,700), but the patterns seen in the analysis of the accidents that did occur was clear.[1] Unrecognized hypoventilation was again, by far, the cause most frequently associated with intraoperative catastrophes (cardiac arrest, permanent CNS damage, or death). There was also a death involving failure of oxygen delivery from an anesthesia machine that did not have an oxygen analyzer. These patterns correlated with those previously identified in the literature.

Because of the findings and the consequent desire to counteract the problems, the Harvard Anesthesia Risk Management Committee devised the set of simple strategies that later helped define safety monitoring.[4] Believing that mere suggestions, guidelines, or even recommendations did not convey the necessary sense of urgency, the group sought a mechanism to make the behaviors mandatory and the concept enforceable. As a risk-management initiative, use of the medicolegal implications of publishing formal standards of practice was chosen. This created an environment in which there was a powerful incentive to adopt the behaviors prescribed by the standards. In early 1985, all nine Harvard teaching hospitals adopted the original standards. There was relatively little opposition, due in large measure to the desirable goal of fewer and less severe patient injuries, the lack of major disruption in that many practitioners were already meeting the standards, and the potential for lowered malpractice premiums if the initiative was successful in saving the insurance company money.

In October 1985, the ASA established a Committee on Standards of Care. This was significant because in 1976 a proposal from a few individuals to consider formulating standards for obstetric anesthesia was received negatively. The new ASA standards committee evaluated all relevant material, including the Harvard monitoring standards, and sought broad-based input from the ASA membership. The original ASA Standards for Basic Intraoperative Monitoring were adopted unanimously by the ASA in 1986. Whether times had simply changed since 1976 or there was no opposition because of the inherent reasonableness of the standards cannot be known. The ASA monitoring standards paralleled in part the prior effort at Harvard. There have been several key amendments and modifications since then, and the 1998 version is reprinted in Figure 17-4.

The original 1986 ASA monitoring standards capture the essence of the concept of safety monitoring. They depend on behaviors to generate information. The standard mandating the presence of qualified anesthesia personnel throughout the conduct of an anesthetic was questioned by some as being so obvious as to be unnecessary. Its inclusion reflected the still-extant and sad but true circumstances in which patients were left unattended after the institution of regional anesthesia or left fully anesthetized and on a mechanical ventilator during intervals in which the anesthesia provider would take a break. It was believed that clearly stipulating the unacceptability of these behaviors might not influence the offenders directly but would help create an atmosphere in which all members of the team would exert pressure on negligent anesthesia providers to cease intraoperative absences. Further, the strong emphasis on the provider rather than electronic machines as the central element of safety monitoring set the intended priorities.

Timing figured so prominently in the ASA standards that it was necessary to define the words *continually* and *continuous* in the context of monitoring behaviors. This was deemed necessary because of the inevitable medicolegal implications of the interpretation of the document by plaintiffs' attorneys. A crucial element in these standards was the shift from the often-observed habit of the intermittent check of vital signs and delivery system function with potential lapses of attention in between to a continuous process of monitoring that is maintained at a consistently high level of attention. This is the basis for believing that earlier warnings of untoward developments will result from these practices. Specific applications of "continuous" use of ECG, an oxygen analyzer with a lower-limit alarm, and, during mechanical ventilation, a disconnection monitor with an alarm are illustrations of this thinking.

The modifications since 1986 center on behavior versus technology. The original ASA standards referred to the observation of *qualitative* clinical signs to verify adequate blood oxygenation. Importantly, there is reference to the desirability of the addition of *quantitative* assessment, and pulse oximetry is "encouraged." As the technology of pulse oximetry evolved and became ubiquitous, it became clear to the ASA standards committee, and ultimately to the ASA membership, that this quantitative assessment, applied continuously, was effective and superior. Accordingly, the behavior of ensuring adequate blood oxygenation was married to the applicable emerging technology, and quantitative assessment (effectively, pulse oximetry) was made mandatory during all anesthesia procedures starting at the beginning of 1990.

Similarly, the original ASA standards "encourage" the use of capnography to verify the correct placement of an endotracheal tube and then to monitor ventilation throughout the procedure. After 1986, it was thought by those administering the ASA Closed Claims Study that unrecognized esophageal intubations were the source of catastrophic anesthesia accidents least favorably influenced by the adoption of the standards. Accordingly, the objective identification of exhaled carbon dioxide as verification of correct placement of an endotracheal tube was changed from "encouraged" to mandatory, effective in 1991. Because only the filter paper color-change indicator is a means to do this, the change effectively required the use of a capnograph. Continuous capnography during general anesthesia with an endotracheal tube was upgraded and emphasized as "strongly encouraged" in 1992, but it was not instituted as an official standard. This was modified slightly but importantly in the standards effective July 1999, in which the statement has been considerably strengthened, and quantitative monitoring methods such as capnography, capnometry, and mass spectroscopy are mandated.

It is interesting to note a reciprocal of this issue in the case of temperature monitoring. In the original standards, availability of a means to continuously measure temperature is mandated and the actual monitoring of temperature is required when "changes in body temperature are intended, anticipated or suspected. . . ." This facilitates the desired behavior in the maintenance of appropriate body temperature. At least three organized attempts have been made to amend the standards to make temperature measurement mandatory during the conduct of all anesthetics, the principal arguments being that this will help identify patients who develop malignant hyperthermia and also patients who accidently become hypothermic. These proposals for another shift toward requiring technology for the implementation of a mandated behavior have been rejected by the ASA, the reasoning being that it does not involve the same degree of safety. The initial diagnosis of malignant hyperthermia rarely depends on temperature measurement, especially today with the extensive use of capnography. Support for the diagnosis by applying the technology required when temperature change is suspected is appropriate, but depending on mandatory measurements in intraoperative diagnostic screening has not been thought to be indicated by the ASA, which places reliance on the behavior of the practitioner rather than on reflex adoption of technology simply because it exists. The implication is less clear regarding prevention of the potential ill effects of hypothermia, and efforts to require temperature monitoring persist.

The role of formal published standards of care in influencing anesthesia outcome has been examined[14, 15] with the monitoring standards studied as the prototypic example. It is very important not to overemphasize the standards themselves. The standards can only initiate behaviors that then must be translated by practitioners into beneficial actions. Further, standards of care represent only one component of the so-called safety movement in anesthesia that began in the mid-1980s.[16] While published safety standards may be the most visible component, there are many others: expanded research into patient safety (including newly developed quality assurance and quality improvement mechanisms); improving the "quality" of trainees entering the field of anesthesiology; improvements in education (longer residency, more and better textbooks and journals); better equipment (reliability, design, ergonomics); improved medications; and increased awareness of anesthesia safety issues by patients and practitioners alike (promoted by the profession itself through its organizations and foundations as well as by the medicolegal and insurance establishments). The monitoring standards have evolved as the most discussed and the best-recognized element of the safety movement. This must not obscure the fact that there have been several other components evolving simultaneously, each with its own contribution to improved anesthesia patient safety. Dissecting out the exact role of each part is likely to be difficult.

The published standards both symbolize and prescribe safety monitoring principles and promote their application through specific mandated behaviors, best implemented today with the technology of modern electronic monitoring devices. It is important to understand that monitors cannot "prevent" adverse anesthesia events, as claimed by many. There are unstated but crucial critical assumptions in such statements. Monitors themselves do not prevent anything. Monitors can only provide information that allows the actuation of the behaviors of safety monitoring. It is reasonable to hypothesize that the earliest possible warning of an untoward development (such as a disconnection of the breathing system from the endotracheal tube being revealed instantly by the capnogram waveform and signaled in seconds by the associated alarm as well as by the ventilator disconnection alarm, be it pressure- or volume-activated) alerts the practitioner to the incident and provides the maximum amount of time possible to make the correct diagnosis and intervene appropriately (reconnect the breathing system to the endotracheal tube) and prevent patient injury. The actions, prompted by safety monitoring and initiated and supported by electronic monitor–generated information, prevent major anesthesia accidents.

Potential Emerging Standards: Simulators, Certification, Bispectral Index

Recently, use of anesthesia simulators for training in the management of critical incidents has been emphasized. As technology continues to develop, it is likely that a significant portion of future anesthesiology training will be conducted on patient simulators, providing the advantage of exposure to rare events such as disconnections or malignant hyperthermia. This will undoubtedly improve the human component in anesthesia safety. Additionally, there is increased awareness that certification to an objective standard of competence is an element of anesthesia safety. Both the ASA and the American Association of Nurse Anesthetists recognize the need for certification and continuing education and recertification in anesthesia practice and, by extension, in anesthesia safety. Board certification is analogous to periodic maintenance of an anesthesia machine to ensure safe operation. Board certification, and especially periodic recertification, will improve anesthesia patient safety.

In the last 5 years there has been an increasing emphasis on intraoperative patient awareness during general anesthesia as an anesthetic complication. The rate of awareness is estimated to be 0.1% to 2.0%.[17] Patient advocacy groups have been formed to promote recognition of awareness as a significant problem that can have devastating psychological consequences. Although the true incidence and consequence of this phenomenon are still debated, it is universally acknowledged that it should be avoided. Previously, measurement of the intraoperative level of unconsciousness or hypnosis had been cumbersome, relying on complicated equipment and data which are difficult to interpret, such as multichannel processed EEG and midlatency auditory evoked potentials. A monitor has been developed which, through a proprietary algorithm, measures a single-channel EEG and produces an indexed value, known as the bispectral index (BIS) (Fig. 4–1) (Aspect Medical Systems, Natick, MA). A processed EEG that produces a BIS of less than 60 correlates with unconsiousness and a significantly decreased probability of intraoperative recall. A value greater then 70 correlates with a significant probability of recall. Further investigation into the usefulness of the BIS monitor is ongoing, but it is currently the best and most user-friendly method of monitoring the level of unconsciousness (hypnosis) under anesthesia. The BIS monitor straddles the line between being a physiologic monitor and a safety monitor. From the physiologic standpoint it is used to titrate dosages of anesthetics to optimize operating room and postanesthesia care unit efficiency, while as a safety monitor it helps to ensure adequate hypnosis to prevent awareness and recall. Again, the significance of the magnitude of awareness as a problem is debatable, but it is likely that patient demand will make BIS monitoring a de facto standard of care.

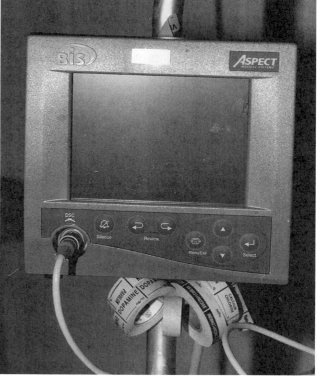

Figure 4–1. The bispectral index (BIS) monitor (Aspect Medical Systems, Natick, MA), now in use at every anesthetizing location at the University of Mississippi Medical Center, Jackson.

Has Safety Improved? Does Safety Monitoring Make a Difference? Is It Cost-Effective?

Because safety monitoring is closely associated with publishing standards of anesthesia care, extensive evaluations of the possible impact of the monitoring standards have been carried out.[18, 19] The simple answers to the questions posed above are (1) yes, anesthesia safety has improved; (2) yes, it appears that safety monitoring does make a difference; and (3) yes, it is cost-effective, although the relevant factors are somewhat difficult to sort out.

For those who demand a clear statistical answer of "$P < .05$" to define truth in all cases, there will be some difficulty in addressing these questions. The epidemiology of rare events is not easy to deal with, both conceptually and statistically. Further, the lack of consistent definitions and experimental designs among investigations from different times and institutions makes comparisons problematic. Finally, it seems impossible that there will ever be a prospective study to settle the question once and for all of whether safety monitoring makes a difference. In countries and institutions with institutional review boards or "human experimentation subjects" committees, there is no ethical way to justify a "no monitoring" control group. Because of the evolution of anesthesia practice standards prescribing the principles of safety monitoring as a minimum level of care in most industrialized countries, proposals to omit this care in the interest of scientific investigation would meet extraordinary opposition and it is unlikely that any reputable investigator would propose such a study. Similarly, because of the impossibility of being certain that a particular problem is being prevented, it is difficult to estimate the cost benefit of safety monitoring. Reduction in insurance premiums and lower awards to injured plaintiffs are difficult to quantitate, as opposed to the actual cost (capital and operating) of a pulse oximeter, for example.

Therefore, two additional thinking patterns emerge. The first is that, in regard to this particular type of question, alternative definitions of "truth" must be considered. In spite of the hard-core traditionalists, it is possible that a conclusion may be valid even when there is no means to obtain the $P < .05$ proof that physicians have been conditioned to respect since the first day of medical school. Such alternative thinking takes place frequently in academic anesthesiology departments during case conference presentations. From evaluation of all the available information from all possible sources, the group hearing the case presented discusses what has been heard and eventually comes to a conclusion as to what caused the event being presented, even if there are conflicting accounts from different people involved and gaps in the story. The group comes to a collective definition of the truth with which it is satisfied and upon which it bases recommendations for future action. This is the type of thinking that can be applied when traditional studies and statistics simply do not work for one reason or another.

The second point is even more relevant. Even if there were a possible study or other mechanism of determination, it is not necessary to "prove" that safety monitoring in and of itself caused a measurable incremental improvement in the outcome and cost of anesthesia care. In fact, to attempt to make such a claim is unrealistic, given all the other factors evolving simultaneously. These other factors have had an impact on anesthesia care. It is not necessary to attempt to isolate improved monitoring as the only cause of improved outcome because it would be difficult or impossible to dissect out contributions from the various components of anesthesia care. Even acknowledging the traditionalists' strong desire for single variable analysis and statistical proof, it may be necessary to recognize a multivariate situation with a consensus accepted as the conclusion. It is reasonable to acknowledge safety monitoring as the most dramatic and most visible component of the safety movement and the one that best symbolizes what has changed in intraoperative anesthesia care in the last decade or so. The extremely strong association in time of the development of the ideas for behaviors to make anesthesia safer, the implementation of those behaviors (especially with new and greatly facilitative technology), and the coincident decrease in the number and severity of intraoperative anesthesia catastrophes together stands as the source of a consensus-derived conclusion that safety monitoring has improved anesthesia care. It follows then that improved care leads to better outcome and lower costs. However, it is impossible to compare rigorously the cost of monitoring with the cost of not monitoring because the economic consequences of poor outcomes are highly variable.

It is appropriate to explore this suggestion from several different perspectives. These include retrospective case analyses, retrospective epidemiologic studies, one prospective epidemiologic study, and insurance industry information.

Among retrospective case analyses, the ongoing ASA Closed Claims Study is the most comprehensive. Each case analyzed in this large study was reviewed by independent reviewers who rendered several opinions about the case material, one of which concerned whether "better monitoring would have prevented the adverse outcome." One pass through the databank yielded a report that focused specifically on respiratory events.[13] Among the adverse outcomes associated with respiratory events, 72% were judged by the reviewers as being preventable with better monitoring, and nearly all of the "inadequate ventilation" and "esophageal intubation" cases would have been prevented. This is not the best language to express this judgment. It would be better to state that the information generated from better monitoring would give significantly earlier warning of the untoward development and, assuming a reasonable response from the responsible practitioner, the adverse outcome would have been prevented. In any case, the point is clear that a battery of independent reviewers believed after a retrospective case review that the principles of safety monitoring would have improved anesthesia outcome.

Another consideration of the ASA Closed Claims Study database, of which the respiratory events were a subset, considered the role of monitoring in mishap prevention.[20] The characteristics of cases classified as "preventable with better monitoring" by the reviewers were delineated. The "severity of injury score" averaged at the top of the scale for preventable injuries and near the middle for those judged not preventable. Similarly, the cost of the insurance settlement or judgment for the preventable injuries was over 10 times that of the nonpreventable ones. Table 4–1 shows the breakdown of this database by type of negative outcome experienced and shows that over half of all (not just respiratory) cases of death and brain damage were considered preventable with better monitoring. Predictably, the "proper use" of pulse oximetry and capnography was "deemed useful" in preventing the adverse outcome in over half the total cases (Table 4–2).

Analysis of the Harvard data[1] had two purposes, the first of which was a retrospective case analysis. In a manner similar to that later adopted by the ASA Closed Claims Study, a retrospective analysis was carried out of available data relative to all major intraoperative anesthesia accidents (death, permanent CNS damage, cardiac arrest with eventual

Table 4–1. ASA Closed Claims Study: Preventability of Complications

Complication	Negative Outcome Considered Preventable by Additional Monitors (no. of cases)	Negative Outcome Considered Not Preventable by Additional Monitors (no. of cases)
Death	241 (57.1%)	158 (37.4%)
Nerve damage	1 (0.6%)	164 (92.1%)
Brain damage	83 (58.4%)	51 (35.9%)

Percentages do not necessarily add to 100 because of cases in which there was insufficient information to judge preventability.
From Tinker JH, Dull DL, Caplan RA, et al: Role of monitoring devices in prevention of anesthetic mishaps: A closed claim analysis. Anesthesiology 71: 541, 1989.

recovery) among "healthy" (ASA physical status I and II, specifically limited to this population because of the reasonable expectation of no adverse outcome) patients over a 12-year period through mid-1988. Taking all possible evidence (including confidential insurance files) into account, decisions were made by the author as to whether the events would have been preventable by the application of safety monitoring principles. Of the 11 cases, 7 involved unrecognized hypoventilation. These 7 and the additional case of the incorrect fresh gas flow setting leading to anoxia were judged preventable via the safety monitoring process (earlier warnings eliciting correct responses in time to prevent injury). Again, by implication, this suggests a positive impact on anesthesia outcome from the attitudes and behaviors (including the use of technology) mandated by the monitoring standards. This analysis has been criticized by authors[21] who take a narrow view of the purpose of these case studies. It is acknowledged that there were "associated issues" such as the degree of supervision of residents or nurse anesthetists, but it must be emphasized that this in no way diminishes the concept that earlier warning of an untoward development—to any provider with any level of training—should maximize the chance of correct diagnosis and intervention early enough to prevent injury.

Retrospective epidemiologic studies address the question of the value of safety monitoring from a slightly different aspect. As noted, it must be accepted that there are associated variables. Several investigators have found associations in time of the advent of safety monitoring with an improve-

ment in anesthesia outcome for various populations. Although there is no specific reference to safety monitoring in the discussion, one of the most impressive studies by far is the mammoth British Confidential Enquiry Into Perioperative Deaths.[22] This was the first indication that a change was evolving from the long-accepted idea that the anesthesia mortality rate was 1/10,000 to 1/20,000. In this 1987 publication, Lunn and Devlin found that the death rate solely attributable to anesthesia was 1/185,000, fully an order of magnitude lower than that previously believed.[22] A different and less rigorous large-scale study of anesthesia death rates in Massachusetts[23] depended on retrospective data gathering from different sources, thus potentially suffering from the potential pitfalls of nonparallel definitions mentioned earlier. Nonetheless, Zeitlin suggested that the anesthesia death rate in that population was 1/4630 in 1965 and an extrapolated 1/62,500 in 1989. He noted several possible causative factors, the principles of safety monitoring being the most prominent.

Another type of retrospective analysis came when Keenan and Boyan[24] (possibly inspired by some earlier groundbreaking work[25]) considered intraoperative anesthesia-related cardiac arrest. They compared 107,257 anesthesia procedures in the period 1969 to 1978 with 134,677 procedures during the period 1979 to 1988. In the first period, the risk of preventable cardiac arrest was 1/6711; the rate of arrest caused by respiratory events was 1/11,905. In the second period there were statistically significant decreases in both rates, to 1/14,925 for preventable arrests and to 1/66,666 for arrests with respiratory causes. Pulse oximetry was introduced at their institution (Beth Israel) in 1984 and, following that, there had been no arrests from respiratory events.[24]

The other component of the analysis of the Harvard data[1, 26] is a retrospective epidemiologic evaluation. This constituted a functionally prospective examination of the incidence rate of major intraoperative accidents discovered among healthy patients. The Harvard monitoring standards were implemented in July 1985. As shown in Table 4–3, the rate of major intraoperative anesthesia accidents decreased more than fivefold thereafter through mid-1990. Statistical comparison of extremely rare events (very low rates) is difficult. However, the appropriate 2 × 2 Fisher's Exact Test reveals that the post-standards rate of 1/392,000 patients with major intraoperative accidents attributable solely to anesthesia care approaches statistical significance with $P = .08$. Importantly, it is fully acknowledged that many positive developments in anesthesiology were occurring simultaneously with the concept of safety monitoring and published stan-

Table 4–2. ASA Closed Claims Study: Monitors Deemed Useful in Cases of Preventable Injuries or Deaths

Monitors	Overall (n = 346)[a]	Regional (n = 51)	General (n = 290)
Pulse oximetry	138 (40%)	41 (80%)	93 (32%)
Capnometry	8 (2%)	1 (1%)	7 (2%)
Pulse oximetry plus capnometry	176 (51%)	8 (16%)	168 (58%)
Other	18 (5%)	0 (0%)	17 (6%)
Not specified	6 (2%)	1 (1%)	5 (2%)

[a]In five cases the type of anesthesia employed was not specified.
From Tinker JH, Dull DL, Caplan RA, et al: Role of monitoring devices in prevention of anesthetic mishaps: A closed claim analysis. Anesthesiology 71: 541, 1989.

Table 4–3. Harvard Medical School Rates for Major Anesthesia Accidents and Deaths Among Healthy Patients Before and After Adoption of Monitoring Standards

Dates	ASA P.S. I and II Patients	Intraoperative Accidents	Associated Deaths
Jan. 1976–June 1985	757,000	10 (1/75,700)	5 (1/151,400)
(Note: Original monitoring standards adopted July 1985.)			
July 1985–June 1990	392,000	1 (1/392,000) $P = .08$*	0 0 $P = .12$*

*By Fisher's Exact Test.

dards of care. It is simplistic to say that safety monitoring alone reduced anesthesia accidents. Rather, these principles and the published standards codifying them reflect widespread changes in attitudes and practices. This conclusion is emphasized in an epidemiologic review of the potential impact of pulse oximetry and capnography on anesthesia risk.[27] This evaluation includes the French anesthesia risk data,[28] which were generated just before safety monitoring was publicized and used for comparison purposes. The prospect for risk reduction is shown in Table 4–4. The review suggested that anesthesia appears to be safer, but this cannot be attributed to improved monitoring alone because other, simultaneous events occurred. The usual plea for more and better epidemiologic studies of anesthesia care and outcome is included.

The only truly prospective trial of any part of the principles of safety monitoring is the Danish study of pulse oximetry in 20,802 patients.[29] This effort focused specifically on pulse oximetry and whether there would be any difference in outcome in approximately 10,000 patients who had pulse oximetry used during and following their anesthetics versus 10,000 who did not. The rate of diagnosis of hypoxemia, of course, was much higher in the monitored group but, fundamentally, there was no major statistically significant improvement in outcome in the monitored group. Does this mean that pulse oximetry is worthless and should be abandoned, or at least removed from the formal, published standards of care? No. While the work involved in collecting data on over 20,000 patients is massive and admirable, the fundamental difficulty is immediately apparent. An accompanying editorial[30] notes that the authors never expected results oriented toward the question of the of rate of catastrophic anesthesia outcome because the power analysis done before the study was undertaken showed that demonstrating a difference in the rate of already extremely rare events such as intraoperative anesthesia catastrophes would require a patient population vastly larger than that used in this study. There were some suggestive points, such as rate of intraoperative cardiac arrest: 12 in the unmonitored group versus 8 in the monitored group. However, the incidence of postoperative coma was higher in the monitored group, and this was ascribed to random variations, as could also be the case with the cardiac arrest data. Critics of technology, safety monitoring, standards, and modern developments in general may seize upon this study, but incorrectly so. While certainly provocative, the Danish study clearly reinforces the previously stated notion that it is physically impossible at this time to carry out a definitive prospective study to evaluate safety monitoring in traditional terms. Alternative definitions of "truth," beyond $P < .05$, must be sought.

Some of the initial impetus in the United States for the investigations and efforts that led to the concepts of anesthesia safety monitoring came from the insurance industry and its concern about costs. It is appropriate to consider the subsequent events regarding anesthesiologists' malpractice insurance losses and premiums. There have been multiple articles in the U.S. lay press concerning the fact that in the last few years, there has been a general reduction across the board for all specialties in the number and amounts of medical malpractice insurance claims. Anesthesiology in almost all cases has had the most dramatic of these reductions among medical specialties. Further, in a great many locations, insurance premiums have been significantly reduced for anesthesiologists, much more so than for other specialists. Dramatic examples come from the Harvard experience. In the period 1976 to 1985, the insurer's dollar loss per anesthetic was $5.24. In 1986, it fell to $2.00; in 1987, to $1.84; and, in 1988, the insurance loss per anesthetic was $0.78.[31] This represents a fall of more than sevenfold in a very short period.

Another common measure in the insurance industry is the so-called relativity rating, or the degree of insurance risk for a given group of practitioners compared to the lowest-risk medical specialty, usually primary care internal medicine. In 1985 at Harvard, anesthesia's relativity rating was 5.2. By 1989 it had fallen to 2.5, while that for general surgery decreased slightly from 5.2 to 4.8, and that for obstetrics and gynecology had increased from 7.2 to 7.5. It is extremely unlikely that plaintiffs' attorneys are ignoring cases of major damage allegedly due to anesthesia. Further, malpractice insurance company actuaries and officials are not charitable people; they are not going to reduce their companies' income from premiums unless there are good reasons to do so.

All these data suggest strongly that anesthesia-caused injuries are now fewer and less severe. Similarly and importantly, in the period 1986 to 1991, combining the avoidance of increases and actual reductions (including a 32% reduction in 1989), malpractice insurance premiums paid by anesthesiologists at Harvard decreased more than 60%. Premium reductions for anesthesiologists have also taken place in many other locations across the country. Premiums can be reduced only when there is a surplus of reserves over the need to pay claims. Does this indicate that the principles of safety monitoring have improved anesthesia outcome? Not exactly. However, it must be accepted that anesthesia care is safer than it was only a few years ago. It is only logical to suggest again that safety monitoring constitutes one important component (if not the most important, but here, again, is the difficulty of dissecting one out) of the milieu that has

Table 4–4. Estimate of Potential Risk Reduction by Monitoring

| | Risk (per 10,000) | | Risk Reduction | | Number Needed |
Origin	CONTROL	TREATED[a]	RELATIVE[b]	ABSOLUTE[c]	to be Treated[d]
Keenan[19]	0.67	0.00	100%	0.67	14,925
Eichhorn[12]	0.16	0.031	80.6%	0.129	77,519
Tiret[18]	1.25	0.00	100%	1.25	8,000

[a]Assumes that all cardiac arrests are preventable by universal application of monitoring.
[b]Relative risk reduction: the reduction of adverse events achieved by a treatment, expressed as a proportion of the control rate.
[c]Absolute risk reduction: difference in event rates between control and treatment groups.
[d]Number to be treated: the number of patients who must be treated to prevent one adverse event (mathematically equal to the reciprocal of the absolute risk reduction).
From Duncan PG and Cohen MM: Pulse oximetry and capnography in anaesthetic practice: An epidemiological appraisal. Can J Anaesth 38:619, 1991.

led to improved anesthesia care and lower cost of management of complications.

There are, of course, those who are skeptical about some of the points made here about safety monitoring. Orkin[32] believes that certain of the analyzed accident cases that would have been prevented by correct functioning of the principles of safety monitoring reveal generally poor quality of care and "very poor judgment" on the part of the anesthesia providers. He wonders whether adherence to minimal monitoring standards can compensate for this and implies that it is simplistic to expect correct responses (even to very early warnings of threatening developments) by the small but definite number of inadequate practitioners who are inherently dangerous to patients. Also noted by Orkin is the multifactorial general trend to better care. He suggests that there has been a tendency toward better anesthesia outcome for some time, antedating the development and adoption of the principles of safety monitoring and reflecting the generalized improvements in the many factors related to overall anesthesia care. Because of the general improvements in care and his belief in the importance of nonanesthesia factors to anesthesia outcome, Orkin expects monitoring alone to have a minimal effect. Further, he stresses the already very low rate of events that the monitoring is intended to detect. Because of the unlikely occurrence of preventable events, Orkin suggests that "before and after" statistics supporting a change are more the result of very rare and thus essentially random events rather than an impact on anesthesia outcome by monitoring. Additionally, he notes that the standards codify what in most cases was already routine practice. While this is used as an argument to minimize the potential impact of the standards, he does not address the stated intention of the standards to encourage good practice by those already so engaged and to target for improvement the small minority of questionable practitioners by providing guidelines for action and the requisite peer pressure to force a change in behavior. Orkin incorrectly extracts monitoring out of the larger context outlined previously and functionally sets it up as a strawman. This is done effectively but requires attributing claims for the efficacy of safety monitoring and the associated standards that were never intended in any way by their creators. In conclusion, Orkin makes the universally applicable and appropriate plea for more definitive outcome studies to better evaluate the impact of practice standards and, by implication, safety monitoring.

Keats[33] on the other hand, gives a sweeping critique of the reasoning (or lack of it) behind many practices in anesthesiology, not just limited to monitoring or the associated standards. Generally, he challenges many modern habits, from ECG monitoring through scavenging systems and up to pulse oximetry with the fundamental thesis that there is no valid evidence for the efficacy of any of these measures. He hypothesizes that there are many fully accepted standards of care, including for monitoring, that have no demonstrated benefit at all for the patient and that may, in fact, create new risks. Further, Keats believes there is no statistically valid evidence that anesthesia mortality has improved at all in the last several decades. He cites the "error-blame bias" and the common discomfort with ignorance as the reasons behind what he sees as essentially an irrational drive toward conclusions and actions. His plea for valid data is more specific in that he carefully outlines the desired studies both of the hazards of current "improvements" and of graded outcomes among stratified patient populations. Absent this, he concludes, "we will never know, for all our technical sophistication, if we are improving the outcomes of anesthesia care."[33]

Discussion

Critics aside, it is reasonable to attempt to correlate safety monitoring with anesthesia patient safety. In keeping with the analogy to an anesthesia case conference presentation and the resultant consensus definition of truth that shapes future action, the weight of the evidence can be examined.

Until the last few years, major intraoperative anesthesia "critical incidents" (such as an esophageal intubation or the disconnection of the breathing system from the endotracheal tube connector underneath the drapes) often went unrecognized until there was marked cyanosis followed quickly by arrhythmias and preterminal bradycardia. Because the "event" had developed so far by then, this left very little time to diagnose and treat the problem before patient injury occurred. The intention and value of the behaviors of safety monitoring are to create a "system" that dependably alerts the anesthesiologist much earlier to the development of an adverse event and thus to allow much more time for problem analysis and effective intervention before the patient is damaged. Review of the information presented above reveals that there can be no doubt that this purpose is facilitated by safety monitoring.

Critical incidents such as esophageal intubations and tubing disconnections will always occur because of both human error and the complexity of mechanical equipment, particularly in the environment of anesthesia delivery and the monitoring workstation. The purpose of safety monitoring is to prevent as many as possible (it is hoped virtually all) of these critical incidents from evolving into anesthesia catastrophes.

The principles of safety monitoring stress behavior over technology and this is articulated in the monitoring standards. The behaviors of genuinely continuous monitoring of oxygenation, ventilation, and circulation are the heart of the standards. The utilization of pulse oximetry and capnography may, in fact, be the most effective and efficient way to execute the behaviors of truly continuous monitoring. However, again, it cannot be emphasized strongly enough that these technologies are not a substitute for human behavior. There is a misperception that both monitoring standards and safety monitoring focus and depend on technology. That simply is not true. The first monitoring standard included in all the sets published (including in the "Recommended Minimal Standards for Anesthesia Care" developed by the International Task Force of Anaesthesia Safety and adopted as world standards by the World Federation of Societies of Anesthesiologists at the 10th world congress in June 1992[34]) mandates the continuous presence of a qualified anesthesia provider, emphasizing that the continuous vigilance of the person administering the anesthetic is the absolute cornerstone of intraoperative safety.

Consistently, throughout the modern study of intraoperative anesthesia accidents, unrecognized hypoventilation has been identified as by far the most common cause. "Hypoxemia" as the cause of cardiac arrest, CNS damage, or death is often listed in reports or reviews, but the actual number of cases of inadequate fresh O_2 are small in number compared to the great many in which failure of ventilation eventually causes hypoxemia. The single most important component of safety monitoring is genuine continuous monitoring of ventilation, including (and perhaps even especially) during regional anesthesia and monitored anesthesia care. Although there have been some persistent warnings that capnography can occasionally give misleading information or can be misinterpreted in various situations (and, until 1999, this had prevented it from becoming mandated as an official ASA monitoring standard of care), it is the best way during general anesthesia to verify adequate ventilation. A pretracheal or precordial stethoscope affording attention to breath sounds is valuable, but it is qualitative as opposed to the more definite quantitative nature of capnography. Pulse oximetry is, of course, helpful in a wide variety of situations and it is a very useful safety monitor, but not as much so as many practitioners think. Desaturation is detected before the profound cyanosis and bradycardia are obvious. However, the patient exhibiting definite desaturation (such as to 85% when the default alarm sounds) may be well along on the downward spiral when attention is called to the situation by this particular monitor. Reiterating that the goal of safety monitoring is the earliest possible warning of danger and that most serious incidents involve ventilation, a capnograph or other method of continuous ventilation monitoring is the most effective safety monitor.

Reviews suggest a decreasing incidence of intraoperative anesthetic mishaps. One particularly comprehensive and thoughtful review by Keenan[10] concludes:

> To summarize the evidence since 1985, major changes in safety awareness and the widespread adoption of improved monitoring methods (especially of oxygenation and ventilation) during anesthesia, in all likelihood, have led to a substantial reduction in anesthetic mortality and major morbidity. While epidemiologic studies documenting these changes are yet to be published, case collection and critical incident studies have been reported that suggest anesthesia outcome is improving. . . .

The majority of anesthesia practitioners with at least a decade's experience apparently believe that intraoperative anesthesia is safer today. Although no one can or should claim that this is solely the result of advances in monitoring, it is reasonable to suggest that the principles of safety monitoring (both in general and as implemented through the standards) have contributed significantly to this, along with improvements in the education and skill of anesthesia practitioners, the tools and medications available to them, and the ongoing research on how to best use these.

An important testimony to the decrement in adverse anesthesia-related occurrences (which has been "caused," as noted, by a great many concurrent factors that are perhaps best symbolized by the concepts of safety monitoring) is the specific selective reduction of malpractice insurance premiums for anesthesiologists. Because neither insurance companies nor plaintiffs' attorneys are charitable, this must reflect the fact that there is less patient damage caused by anesthesia today—precisely the goal of safety monitoring. Because the insurance industry is cyclic and because attorneys are creative and innovative in pursuing medical liability claims, we should not be surprised at future increases in malpractice insurance premiums.

It is, of course, understandable that there are some (many?) who believe that almost everything in life is random and there have been no real changes in anything. A thorough examination of all the material presented here (particularly the often-repeated qualification that while monitoring may be the most visible and dramatic component, it is not just new and better monitoring that is responsible for the relatively recent improvement in anesthesia outcome) leads to the belief that anesthesia is safer today than it was even relatively recently and that improved monitoring—structured through the principles of safety monitoring—has had a significant role in this improvement.

In the future, more emphasis should be placed on improving the human aspect of anesthesia safety. A timely and appropriate response to the warnings of monitors is as important, if not more so, than the monitors themselves. It is a tired old analogy that administering anesthesia is similar to piloting a commercial jetliner, and it certainly does not apply in many situations, but the comparison is applicable to safety monitoring. The lessons learned from commercial aviation, in cockpit resource management and human interaction with complex mechanical, electronic, and personnel systems, apply to the administration of anesthesia.

Finally, it is not incomprehensible that a governmental or quasi-governmental agency will eventually come into being for the purpose of investigation and study of anesthesia accidents. A "National Anesthesia Safety Board" would greatly facilitate a true accounting of the rate and nature of anesthesia critical incidents and would promote improved safety related to the human element of anesthesia systems.

REFERENCES

1. Eichhorn JH: Prevention of intraoperative anesthesia accidents and related severe injury through safety monitoring. Anesthesiology 1989; 70:572.
2. Cooper JB, Newbower RS, Long CD, et al: Preventable anesthesia mishaps: A study of human factors. Anesthesiology 1978; 49:399.
3. Spittal MJ, Findlay GP, Spencer I: A prospective analysis of critical incidents attibutable to anaesthesia. Int J Qual Health Care 1995; 7:363–371.
4. Eichhorn JH, Cooper JB, Cullen DJ, et al: Standards for patient monitoring during anesthesia at Harvard Medical School. JAMA 1986; 256:1017.
5. Sigurdsson GH, McAteer E: Morbidity and mortality associated with anesthesia. Acta Anaesthesiol Scand 1996; 40:1057–1063.
6. Duberman SM, Bendixen HH: Mortality, morbidity and risk studies in anaesthesia, In Lunn JN (ed): Epidemiology in Anaesthesia. London, Edward Arnold, 1986, p 37.
7. Desmonts JM: Outcome after anaesthesia and surgery: Epidemiological aspects. Baillieres Clin Anaesthesiol 1992; 6:463.
8. Keenan RL: Anaesthetic mishaps: Outcome and prevention. Baillieres Clin Anaesthesiol 1992; 6:477.
9. Faunce TA, Rudge B: Deaths on the table: Proposal for an international convention on the investigation and prevention of anaesthetic mortality. Med Law 1998; 17:31–54.
10. Keenan RL: What is known about anesthesia outcome. Probl Anesth 1991; 5:179.
11. Pierce EC, Cooper JB: Analysis of anesthetic mishaps. Int Anesthesiol Clin 1984; 22:190.
12. Keenan RL, Boyan CP: Cardiac arrest due to anesthesia. JAMA 1985; 253:2373.
13. Caplan RA, Posner KL, Ward RJ, et al: Adverse respiratory events in anesthesia: A closed claim analysis. Anesthesiology 1990; 72:828.
14. Eichhorn JH: Are there standards for intraoperative monitoring? Adv Anesth 1988; 5:1.
15. Eichhorn JH: The role of standard of care. Probl Anesth 1991; 5:188.
16. Eichhorn JH: Risk reduction in anesthesia. Probl Anesth 1992; 6:278.
17. Schwender D, Daunderer M, Kunze Kronawitter H, et al: Awareness during general anesthesia: Incidence, clinical relevance and monitoring. Acta Anaesthesiol Scand Suppl 1997; 111:313–314.
18. Eichhorn JH: Influence of practice standards on anaesthesia outcome. Baillière's Clin Anaesthesiol 1992; 6:663.
19. Eichhorn JH: Effect of monitoring standards on anesthesia outcome. Int Anesthesiol Clin 1993; 31:181.
20. Tinker JH, Dull DL, Caplan RA, et al: Role of monitoring devices in prevention of anesthetic mishaps: A closed claim analysis. Anesthesiology 1989; 71:541.
21. Ross AF, Tinker JH: Anesthesia risk. In Rogers MC, Tinker JH, Covino BG, Longnecker DE (eds): Principles and Practice of Anesthesiology. St Louis, Mosby–Year Book, 1993, p 625.

22. Lunn JN, Devlin HB: Lessons from the confidential inquiry into perioperative deaths in three NHS regions. Lancet 1987; 2:1384.

23. Zeitlin GL: Possible decrease in mortality associated with anaesthesia: A comparison of two time periods in Massachusetts, USA. Anaesthesia 1989; 44:432.

24. Keenan RS, Boyan CP: Decreasing frequency of anesthetic cardiac arrests. J Clin Anesth 1991; 3:354.

25. Taylor G, Larson CP, Prestwich R: Unexpected cardiac arrest during anesthesia and surgery: An environmental study. JAMA 1976; 236:2758.

26. Eichhorn JH: Documenting improved anesthesia outcome. J Clin Anesth 1991; 3:351.

27. Duncan PG, Cohen MM: Pulse oximetry and capnography in anaesthetic practice: An epidemiological appraisal. Can J Anaesth 1991; 38:619.

28. Tiret L, Desmonts JM, Hatton F, et al: Complications associated with anaesthesia: A prospective survey in France. Can Anaesth Soc J 1986; 33:336.

29. Moller JT, Pedersen T, Rasmussen LS, et al: Randomized evaluation of pulse oximetry in 20,802 patients. 11. Perioperative events and postoperative complications. Anesthesiology 1993; 79:445.

30. Eichhorn JH: Pulse oximetry as a standard of practice in anesthesia. Anesthesiology 1993; 78:423.

31. Hoker JF: Liability insurance issues in anesthesiology. Int Anesthesiol Clin 1989; 27:205.

32. Orkin FK. Practice standards: The Midas touch or the emperor's new clothes? Anesthesiology 1989; 70:567.

33. Keats AS: Anesthesia mortality in perspective. Anesth Analg 1990; 71:113.

34. International Task Force on Anaesthesiology: Recommended minimal standards for anaesthesia care. Eur J Anaesthesiol 1993; 10 (7 suppl):1–44.

5 Electrical Safety*

Jeffrey J. Schwartz, M.D.
Jan Ehrenwerth, M.D.

While the importance of a finger on the pulse and an eye on the patient cannot be denied, monitoring of the anesthetized patient in the next millennium requires a multitude of electronic devices. This equipment is often intentionally connected to the patient and is being used in an environment in which saline solutions can spill and catheters may enter the heart. Certainly no one would feel perfectly comfortable adjusting a radio while standing in a bathtub—the operating room can present similar hazards. In one study, 40% of electrical accidents in hospitals occurred in the operating room (OR).[1] Fortunately, electrocution is a rare event in the OR. This is due, in part, to various safeguards incorporated into both the electrical supply and the monitoring equipment. It is the responsibility of anesthesiologists to be familiar with electrical safety matters so that they may protect the patient and the operating room personnel.

Principles of Electricity

It is impossible to understand the principles of electrical safety without a basic understanding of electricity and its biologic effects. Electric current (I), the flow of electrons through a resistance (R) in a complete circuit, is measured in amperes. The drive that moves the electrons is the voltage or the electromotive force (E), measured in volts. The relationship between the applied voltage and the resulting current is given by Ohm's law.

$$E = I \times R$$

Practitioners may find that the relationship between the driving force of the circulation and the flow of blood, MAP = CO × SVR, where MAP is mean arterial pressure, CO is cardiac output, and SVR is systemic vascular resistance, makes Ohm's law more intuitive. Electric power is measured in watts and can be calculated by the formula W = E × I, where W is the power dissipated. The energy or work performed by electricity is equal to the power multiplied by the duration of the current flow. Some numerical examples may clarify these relationships.

Consider a 1200-W hair dryer that is powered by a conventional 120-V household outlet. The current flow through the dryer is 1200 W / 120 V = 10 A (W = E × I). The resistance of the hair dryer is 120 V / 10 A = 12 ohms (Ω) (E = I × R). If the dryer is used for 6 minutes, one-tenth of an hour, the energy dissipated is 1200 W × 1/10 hour = 120 watt-hours or, more conventionally, 0.12 kilowatt-hour.

Dry intact skin has a resistance of approximately 100,000 Ω. If a person with this skin resistance accidentally becomes part of a 120-V electric circuit, then a current of 120/100,000 = 1.2 milliamperes (mA) would flow through that person. As discussed later, this is not dangerous and is, in fact, barely perceptible. However, wet skin may have a resistance as low as 1000 Ω. If a person then contacts the same 120-V, a current of 120/1000 = 120 mA will flow, which would likely be fatal.

Alternating Current

When electron flow is always in one direction, it is termed direct current (DC). Batteries generate DC. When the flow of current periodically reverses itself, it is referred to as alternating current (AC).[2] Commercial utility companies in the United States generate electricity as AC to allow for easier distribution. The physics of AC is somewhat more complicated than that of DC. Surprisingly, a coiled piece of wire that would offer virtually no resistance to direct current will impede alternating current.[3] Conversely, a circuit that contains a gap or no physical connection may allow alternating current to pass. The sum of the forces that oppose current flow in an AC circuit is termed impedance and is designated by the letter Z.

A capacitor is defined as any two conductors separated by an insulator. A capacitor can store a charge on its conductors when a voltage is applied; the quantity of that charge, in proportion to the voltage, is the capacitance (C). When a DC voltage is initially applied to a capacitor, current flows briefly through the wires but not across the capacitor, and charges accumulate on the conductors.[4] If an AC voltage is applied, the capacitor will alternately charge and discharge and there will be a constant AC current in the wires. The opposition to electron flow in a capacitor is called the *capacitive impedance* and is inversely proportional to the frequency of the applied voltage. Direct current is blocked by a capacitor, while high-frequency alternating currents pass easily.

A capacitor need not be a fixed, constructed device. Any two conductors separated by an insulator will have some capacitance, known as "stray capacitance".[5] The patient or the anesthesiologist may be one of the conductors. This

*Adapted in part with permission from Ehrenwerth J: Electrical Safety. *In* Barash PG, Cullen BF, Stoelting RK, editors: Clinical Anesthesia, ed 3. Philadelphia, J.B. Lippincott, 1997.

57

situation implies that despite being apparently physically disconnected and apart from electric sources, small and possibly dangerous currents may still flow.

Any wire with a current flowing through it is associated with a magnetic field. The ability to store energy in the magnetic field is the wire's inductance (L). If the current is changing, as in AC, the magnetic field will be changing; this changing magnetic field actually opposes electron flow. This opposition is inductive impedance and is directly proportional to frequency. Inductance is less relevant than capacitance to electrical safety.

Physiology of Electric Shock

What exactly is the risk from electric shock and how does it come about? Electric shocks occur when a person becomes part of or completes an electric circuit. Thus, to receive a shock, one must contact the electric circuit at two different points at different voltages. By Ohm's law a current will then flow that is proportional to the voltage difference and inversely proportional to the impedance. Birds can sit happily on high-voltage wires because they are contacting only one part of a circuit.

The physiologic effects of electric shock depend on the current (which, by Ohm's law, is determined by the voltage and impedance), the duration of contact, the frequency at which the current changes direction, and the area through which the current flows. Electric shock may be divided into two categories, essentially depending on the path of current flow. Macroshock refers to large amounts of current flowing through intact skin, which can cause injury. Microshock refers to very small amounts of current that are dangerous because they are applied directly to the myocardium.[6, 7] This can occur in the electrically susceptible patient, that is, one who has an external conductor in direct contact with the heart. This may be a pacemaker wire or a saline-filled central venous catheter. Currents as low as 80 microamperes, when delivered through such a catheter, may cause ventricular fibrillation because all the current is concentrated over a small area.[8] This is 1/1000th the current that could cause fibrillation if applied externally.

Table 5-1 lists the effects of progressively increasing currents applied to the skin. Note that, as discussed in the numerical examples above, widely different currents may flow depending on the skin resistance. The longer the duration of contact, the more energy will be dissipated in the victim. Significant thermal burns are uncommon with household current but are a feature of lightning injuries and high-tension wire accidents. Ventricular fibrillation is more likely to develop with prolonged contact because of stimulation during the relative refractory period of the heart.

Electric shock does most of its damage by interfering with electrically excitable tissue: brain, nerve, and heart and skeletal muscle. Nerve stimulation leads to pain, while muscle stimulation leads to sustained contraction. Indeed, a current of 10 to 20 mA leads to sustained contractions and the inability of a conscious victim to release an energized wire. This is the "let-go" current, more properly termed the "can't-let-go" current.[9, 10] Stimulation of the heart can lead to ventricular fibrillation and cardiac tetany. Of course, DC applied to the chest wall can also treat fibrillation. Current through the brain can lead to unconsciousness and respiratory paralysis.

The electrosurgical unit (ESU) illustrates the influence of frequency on the danger of electric current. Surgeons regularly "electrocute" their patients with high-amperage, high-frequency current. The only ill effect is a thermal burn at the

Table 5-1 Effects of 60-Hz AC on a Normal Person for a 1-Second Duration of Contact

Current	Effect
MACROSHOCK	
1 mA (0.001 A)	Threshold of perception
5 mA (0.005 A)	Accepted as maximum harmless current intensity
10-20 mA (0.01-0.02 A)	"Let-go" current before sustained muscle contraction
50 mA (0.05 A)	Pain, possible fainting, mechanical injury, heart and respiratory functions continue
100-300 mA (0.1-0.3 A)	Ventricular fibrillation will start but respiratory center remains intact
6000 mA (6 A)	Sustained myocardial contractions, followed by normal heart rhythm; temporary respiratory paralysis; burns if current density is high
MICROSHOCK	
10 μA (0.01 mA)	Recommended maximum allowable 60-Hz leakage current
100 μA (0.1 mA)	Ventricular fibrillation

mA = milliampere   μA = microampere   A = Ampere

tip of the ESU pencil because the operating frequency of the ESU is so high that cardiac and neural tissues are not excited. Interestingly, the frequency of commercial electricity in the US—60 Hz—is probably the most dangerous one in terms of electrical shock hazard.[11]

Grounded Power

The electric company supplies electric current via two wires. The voltage between these wires is well maintained at about 120 volts. An uncommon mechanism of injury is simultaneous contact with both wires, thus completing a circuit. Pets and toddlers may lick or chew electrical outlets or wires. Electrical safety in the home certainly includes monitoring for this.

The electric company, to increase safety in the distribution and delivery of electric power, has connected one of the two wires to earth ground. Generally, this is via a large conducting rod buried deep in the earth. This wire is the neutral wire; the other is called the hot wire. The electric power is considered grounded.

This, unfortunately, leads to a much easier way to electrocute oneself (Fig. 5-1). To reiterate, in order for a person to sustain an electric shock, the person must become part of an electric circuit. If a person is in electric contact with the earth, one of the contacts in the circuit has been made. Only one additional contact point is necessary to complete the circuit and for the person to receive an electric shock. The reasoning behind the classic admonition not to touch a bathroom light switch while standing in a puddle of water is now apparent. In this situation, current could flow from a faulty switch through the bather, out the feet, through the puddle. The puddle might be in contact with a water pipe connected to the earth, which is where the electric company has connected its neutral wire.

The situation could be similar in the OR. There is a 120-V potential difference between the hot wire and the neutral wire as well as the hot wire and earth ground. Over time, the insulation covering wires may deteriorate and the bare

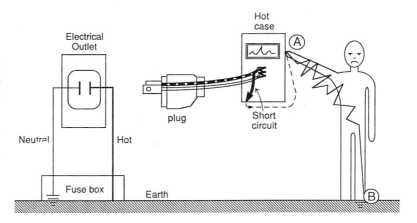

Figure 5-1. When a faulty piece of equipment without an equipment ground wire is plugged into an electric outlet not incorporating a ground wire, the case of the instrument will become hot. If a person touches the hot case (Point A), he or she will receive a shock, because standing on the earth (Point B) completes the circuit. The current (*dotted line*) will flow from the instrument through the person touching the hot case. (From Ehrenwerth J: Electrical safety. *In* Barash PG, Cullen BF, Stoelting RK (eds): *Clinical Anesthesia,* ed 3. Philadelphia, J.B. Lippincott, 1997.)

hot wire may internally come into contact with the case of an electrical instrument and constitute a shock hazard. When a person touches the equipment while also contacting earth ground, an electric shock will result, because the person is contacting the circuit at two points.

Modern electric wiring and equipment provide a safety feature to decrease the risk when a person comes into contact with an energized chassis. In addition to the hot and neutral wires, a third equipment ground wire is part of the electrical distribution system to all electrical outlets. This is the part of the electrical outlet that is round rather than flat. This wire is also connected to the earth ground. Most modern electric equipment connects the chassis to the ground wire via the third prong. When the chassis is connected to the equipment ground wire, the equipment is said to be grounded. Normally, no current would be expected to flow through the ground wire. However, if the chassis were to become energized, the bulk of the electric current would be shunted to earth ground via the equipment ground wire (Fig. 5-2). If the current were large enough, the circuit breaker would trip. (It should be noted that fuses or circuit breakers interrupt current to a circuit when it exceeds a designated amount. They are intended to prevent electrical fires due to overheating of wires. They do rather little to protect against electric shock because they generally do not trigger until the current is well above lethal levels.) If a person were to contact an energized but grounded chassis, the person may receive a shock but it would be unlikely to be fatal. This safety feature requires the consistent use of grounded equipment and the utter avoidance of "cheater plugs" that allow a three-pronged piece of equipment to plug into a two-

pronged outlet without connection of the third prong to earth ground.

Isolated Power

Because most of the potential risk for electric shock appears to be due to the grounding of the electric power supply and the ubiquitous connections of people to earth ground, it seems reasonable to utilize an ungrounded, or isolated, power supply to decrease this risk. In this case, neither of the two wires supplying current is connected to earth ground.

Grounded electric power can be converted to isolated power by means of an isolation transformer. This device uses electromagnetic induction to induce current in the ungrounded secondary winding of the transformer from energy supplied to the grounded primary winding. There is no electrical connection between the electric power supplied by the utility company and the power delivered to the electrical outlets. Thus, for safety reasons, in the isolated power system the equipment ground wire is still connected to earth ground; however, the power supply to the electrical outlets has no earth ground connection. The two secondary wires have a 120-V potential difference between them and no relationship to ground. The terms hot and neutral no longer make sense, so the wires are designated as line 1 and line 2 (Fig. 5-3).

Let's consider our potential victim standing in a puddle of water, connected to earth ground. If this person contacts one part of the isolated power circuit through a faulty chas-

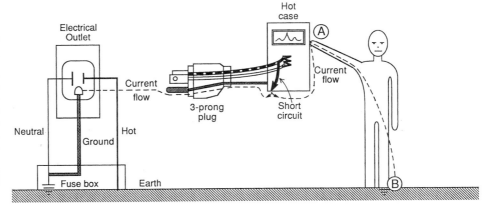

Figure 5-2. When a faulty piece of equipment that incorporates an equipment ground wire is properly connected to an electrical outlet with a grounding connection, the current (*dotted line*) will preferentially flow through the low-resistance ground wire. A person touching the case (Point A) and standing on the ground (Point B) will still complete the circuit; however, only a small part of the current will flow through the person. (From Ehrenwerth J: *Electrical Safety. In* Barash PG, Cullen BF, Stoelting RK (eds): *Clinical Anesthesia,* ed 3. Philadelphia, J.B. Lippincott; 1997.)

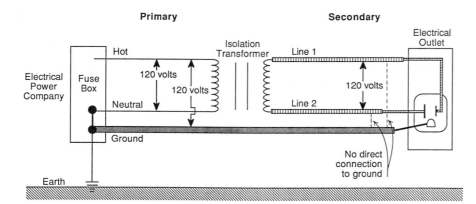

Figure 5–3. In the operating room, the isolation transformer converts the grounded power on the primary side to an ungrounded power system on the secondary side of the transformer. A 120-volt potential difference exists only between lines 1 and 2. There is no direct connection between the power on the secondary side and ground. The equipment ground wire is, however, still present. (From Ehrenwerth J: *Electrical Safety. In* Barash PG, Cullen BF, Stoelting RK (eds): *Clinical Anesthesia,* ed 3. Philadelphia, J.B. Lippincott, 1997.)

sis, he or she does *not* complete any circuit and will not receive a shock. That person has contacted one point of one circuit (isolated) and another point in an electrically distinct circuit (grounded). Because the person does not contact either the isolated or grounded circuit at two points, there is no current flow (Fig. 5–4).

The use of an equipment ground wire and connection of the chassis of the instrument to earth ground is still important in the isolated power system. Should one of the wires fray and come into contact with the chassis, no current will flow to ground and there is no shock hazard. The system, however, will no longer be isolated from ground and will, in fact, be identical to the original grounded power electrical system. It will require a second factor, such as another piece of faulty equipment, to pose an electrical hazard. In that unlikely event, the ground wire will still shunt most of the current to earth ground. It is a distinct advantage of the isolated power system that the first faulty piece of equipment will continue to function safely, as it may be life-supporting equipment.

It was somewhat incorrect to state that there was no electrical connection between the earth ground and the secondary circuit of the isolation transformer. As discussed earlier, stray capacitance exists between any two conductors and, when AC is involved, small leakage currents may flow from the isolated power lines to ground, thus degrading the isolation. These currents are generally small, 1 to 2 mA in total, and may be perceptible but not dangerous.

The integrity of the isolation is key to its acting as a safety feature. Because a malfunctioning device will continue to work normally in an isolated power supply, there must be some means for detecting the problem before a second fault can occur. This is the function of the line isolation monitor (LIM). The LIM continually checks the impedance between each of the isolated power lines and ground (Fig. 5–5). Rather than display the impedance, the LIM calculates how much current would flow to ground in the event of a first fault. Normally and ideally, the impedance would be infinite and the current would be zero. The inevitable stray capacitance and leakage currents make the impedance somewhat less. Modern LIMs are set to trigger an audible and visual alarm when the current exceeds 5 mA.[12] By Ohm's law this represents an impedance of 24,000 Ω (120 v/0.005 ampere.) Older LIMs triggered at 2 mA (60,000 Ω).

The LIM will trigger an alarm when a faulty piece of equipment is connected to the isolated power circuit. This will be a true fault to ground with a small impedance from one line to ground. The system is now equivalent to a grounded power supply but is still perfectly safe. It would

require another fault, in the same or different device, to pose a true risk of shock. The device that triggered the LIM should be removed from operation and serviced as soon as possible, but, because there is no immediate threat, the device may continue to be used if it is essential to the care of the patient.

The LIM may also trigger an alarm if many pieces of normally functioning equipment are all connected to the same isolated power supply. Although each piece may have a small leakage current, the sum may exceed the 5 mA threshold. For instance, if 30 devices each with a 200-microampere leakage current are connected to the same power supply, the total leakage current would be 6 milliamperes and the LIM would trigger. The change in threshold from 2 mA to 5 mA was prompted by an attempt to prevent this false alarm.

When the LIM alarms, the anesthesiologist should unplug each device in the room, one at a time—generally the most recently plugged items first—until the alarm disappears. This device should be removed for servicing unless essential at the time. If no faulty device is found, it may be that too many normally functioning devices are causing a total leakage current that triggers the LIM.

The equipment ground wire takes on added importance in the isolated power system. If this wire is broken or defeated with a cheater plug, a faulty piece of equipment that is plugged into an outlet will operate normally but the LIM will not alarm. The LIM can only sense the reduced impedance to ground and lack of isolation if the device's equipment ground wire is connected to ground.

Ground Fault Circuit Interrupters

A ground fault circuit interrupter (GFCI) can provide an inexpensive alternative method of decreasing the risk of shock when isolated power is not utilized. In a working electric circuit, the current in the hot wire must be equal to the current in the neutral wire; what goes in must come out. If a person becomes part of the circuit, some of the current will pass through that person to ground. Therefore, there will be a difference in current between the two limbs of the circuit. The GFCI monitors both sides of the circuit for equality of current flowing. If the difference between the currents exceeds a threshold, typically 5 mA, the GFCI will interrupt the power to the circuit. GFCIs are reliable devices. Modern building codes actually require them in "wet locations" such as bathrooms, kitchens, and outdoor outlets. Curiously, ORs are not always considered wet locations in

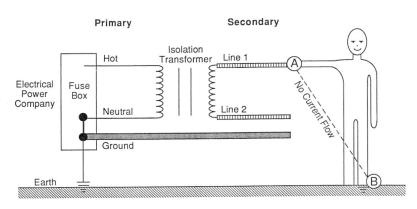

Figure 5–4. A safety feature of the isolated power system is illustrated. A person contacting one side of the isolated power system (Point A) and standing on the ground (Point B) will not receive a shock. In this instance, the person is not contacting the circuit at two points and thus is not completing the circuit. Point A (*cross-hatched lines*) is part of the isolated power system, and Point B is part of the primary or grounded side of the circuit (*solid lines*). (From Ehrenwerth J: *Electrical Safety. In* Barash PG, Cullen BF, Stoelting RK (eds): *Clinical Anesthesia,* ed 3. Philadelphia, J.B. Lippincott, 1997.)

the building codes. The main disadvantage of the GFCI in the OR is that the first warning of a piece of equipment becoming defective is that it turns off. A GFCI may be monitoring several devices, all of which will lose power if one of them is faulty. In addition, before the power can be restored, the faulty device must be identified and unplugged. This can be a serious problem if the equipment is life-supporting, such as a ventilator or cardiopulmonary bypass pump.

Operating Room Construction

The anesthesiologist is frequently called upon to help design new ORs. In 1984, the National Fire Protection Association (NFPA) revised its standards regarding isolated power systems in ORs. Currently, only ORs in which flammable agents are used are required to have isolated power systems. Operating rooms in which nonflammable agents are used may have isolated power systems, GFCIs, or maybe even no protection at all. If the area is considered a wet location, isolated power systems or GFCIs are required.

Anesthesiologists need to be aware of these changes and to insist that some form of protection be installed for patients and OR personnel. It is best to have isolated power because this system is safe *by design* and will limit fault

current to less than 5 mA. Although GFCIs are acceptable, they are an active system and require a fault current to be flowing before they interrupt the circuit. As already noted, if many outlets are protected by one GFCI, serious problems could result from patient monitors or life support equipment being shut off. If GFCIs are used, the best system is to have each electrical outlet in the room be its own branch circuit and be protected by an individual GFCI. It would be foolhardy to eliminate these important safety systems in order to obtain a small reduction in the cost of constructing the OR.[13, 14]

Microshock

Neither isolated power nor GFCIs can protect an electrically susceptible patient from the minuscule currents that represent a microshock hazard. When applied directly to the myocardium, currents as low as 80 μA may cause ventricular fibrillation.[15, 16] This is well below the threshold of perception (1000 μA) and well below the 5000-μA current that would trigger an LIM or a GFCI.

The stray capacitance that is part of any AC-powered circuit can cause a significant charge to build up on the chassis of a piece of equipment. The anesthesiologist who touches this chassis and then contacts the electrically suscep-

Figure 5–5. When a faulty piece of equipment is plugged into the isolated power system, it will markedly decrease the impedance from line 1 or line 2 to ground. This change will be detected by the LIM, which will sound an alarm. (From Ehrenwerth J: *Electrical Safety. In* Barash PG, Cullen BF, Stoelting RK (eds): *Clinical Anesthesia,* ed 3. Philadelphia, J.B. Lippincott, 1997.)

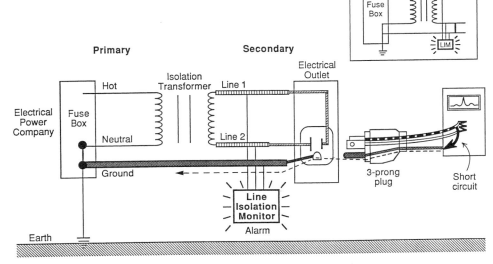

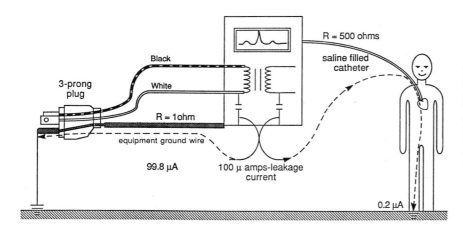

Figure 5–6. The electrically susceptible patient is protected from microshock by the presence of an intact equipment ground wire. The equipment ground wire provides a low-impedance path in which the majority of the leakage current (*dotted lines*) can flow. (From Ehrenwerth J: *Electrical Safety. In* Barash PG, Cullen BF, Stoelting RK (eds): *Clinical Anesthesia,* ed 3. Philadelphia, J.B. Lippincott, 1997.)

tible patient may cause a lethal, although imperceptible, current to flow directly into the heart. Radiofrequency output from an electrosurgical unit (ESU) may be redirected to the heart through the reference electrode in a right ventricular ejection fraction pulmonary artery catheter.[17] The principal protection against microshock is the presence of an intact functional equipment ground wire in all OR devices. Just as it provides a low resistance path to ground for large currents that may flow in the event of a fault, it also provides a low resistance path for pervasive leakage currents. Figure 5–6 illustrates a situation involving a patient who has a saline-filled catheter in the heart, with a resistance of approximately 500 Ω. The equipment ground wire has a resistance of 1 Ω. A leakage current of 100 μA due to stray capacitance will only cause 0.2 μA to flow into the patient while 99.8 μA take the lower resistance path to ground. If the ground wire were broken, all 100 μA would flow into the patient. Extra care must be taken when managing the electrically susceptible patient. Gloves should be worn when touching intracardiac catheters or pacemaker wires. Medical personnel should not simultaneously touch these catheters and other electrical devices.

Additional protection against microshock is obtained by attempting to isolate any electrical connection to the patient, such as electrocardiogram leads, from the power supply of the monitor. The original OR electrocardiogram actually intentionally connected the patient to the power supply to reduce the noise in the signal.[18] This is now recognized as being foolhardy. Optical isolators, transformers, and high-impedance amplifiers ensure that there is minimal leakage current between the monitor and the patient while allowing easy passage of the physiologic signal.

Electrosurgery

The ESU operates by generating very high-frequency currents (500,000 to 2,000,000 Hz). Heat is produced whenever a current flows through a resistance. The amount of heat produced is the product of the resistance and the square of the current and is inversely proportional to the area through which the current passes.[19] By concentrating the current at the tip of the ESU pencil, very localized cutting and coagulation can be achieved. As discussed, these high-frequency currents do not represent an electrical shock hazard. The risk is thermal burns at unintended sites.[20-25] The ESU current must return to the ESU generally through a dispersive or return electrode (often mistakenly given the misnomer "ground plate") of large surface area. The large surface en-

sures that the area of contact is extensive and the current density is small when it exits the patient. If the plate is improperly applied or becomes dislodged so that it covers only a small area, the patient may sustain a burn where the current exits as well as where it enters. The plate usually is the path of least resistance for the return current. If it is improperly applied or the cord connecting it to the unit is malfunctioning, the current will seek an alternative return pathway of lower resistance. If the return pathway is of a small area, such as an electrocardiography pad, a similar burn can result. While modern ESUs use a power supply isolated from ground that is not unlike the isolated power to the OR, it is impossible to totally isolate the energy. Capacitive impedance decreases as frequency increases; therefore, high-frequency current may travel easily through stray capacitance.

All OR personnel must be vigilant for proper application of the dispersive plate. The plate should be as far removed from electrocardiographic leads, pacemaker units, and metal implants as possible. If a surgeon requests a higher power because a proper cut is not being made, this should arouse suspicion that the plate is poorly applied.

Electromagnetic Interference (EMI)

Modern communication technology has increased the number of physicians and hospital personnel who have cellular phones. The number of wireless devices will undoubtedly increase dramatically in the near future. Reports have suggested that cellular devices may interfere with monitoring equipment, pacemakers, and automatic implantable cardioverter-defibrillators (AICDs). Many hospitals have developed policies that prohibit the use of cellular phones in critical care environments, and sometimes throughout the hospital, because of these concerns. Most studies show that electromagnetic interference (EMI) from cellular phones can cause temporary changes in pacemaker function such as pacing inhibition or erroneous sensing, but only when the phone is in close proximity to the pacemaker.[26, 27] In fact, the current FDA recommendation is that cellular phones be kept at least 6″ from the generator. One study found no clinically significant interference with cellular phones at ear level.[28] No permanent problems, such as reprogramming, have been noted. Similar studies show that AICDs are not susceptible to EMI from current cellular phones.[29]

A group at Hadassah Hospital in Jerusalem, Israel measured the electric field strength around various EMI-producing devices.[30] They concluded that the field strength from cellular phones was within the safe limits for medical devices. However, they instituted a policy banning cellular phones from their ORs, postanesthesia care units, emergency and trauma rooms, intensive care units, intermediate care areas, and the cardiac surgery department. With the lack of any reproducible data that demonstrate a patient safety problem with cellular phones, it seems unreasonable to ban these devices outright. The Emergency Care Research Institute (ECRI) has concluded that the risk to patients from cellular phones is minimal and that restrictive policies can be relaxed to allow the use of cellular phones in certain situations.[31] They further recommend maintaining a distance of 1 meter from medical devices if possible.

Unlike wired phones, cellular phones transmit an intermittent signal to the cellular tower whenever they are turned on, even when no actual call has been placed. Therefore, any policy that bans the use of cellular phones should also require that they be turned off. As pacemaker technology and cellular technology advance, the possibility of a new interaction in the future must be kept in mind. Using common sense, in combination with regular maintenance, and being aware of potential hazards along with the various safety devices, will markedly reduce the risk of electric shock to patients and OR personnel.[32, 33]

REFERENCES

1. Bruner JMR, Aronow S, Cavicchi RV: Electrical incidents in a large hospital: A 42 month register. JAAMI 1972; 6:222–230.
2. Bruner JMR: Hazards of electrical apparatus. Anesthesiology 1967; 28:396–425.
3. Miller F: College Physics, ed 2. New York; Harcourt Brace and World, 1967:457–459.
4. Leonard PF, Gould AB: Dynamics of electrical hazards of particular concern to operating-room personnel. Surg Clin North Am 1965; 45:817–828.
5. Leonard PF: Characteristics of electrical hazards. Anesth Analg 1972; 51:797–809.
6. Weinberg DI, Artley JL, Whalen RE, McIntosh HD: Electric shock hazards in cardiac catheterization. Circ Res 1962; 11:1004–1009.
7. Starmer CF, Whalen RE: Current density and electrically induced ventricular fibrillation. Med Instrum 1973; 7:158–161.
8. Raftery EB, Green HL, Yacoub MH: Disturbances of heart rhythm produced by 50-Hz leakage currents in human subjects. Cardiovasc Res 1975; 9:263–265.
9. Harpell TR: Electrical shock hazards in the hospital environment: Their causes and cures. Can Hosp 1970; 47:48–53.
10. Wald A: Electrical safety in medicine. In Skalak R, Chien S, (eds): Handbook of Bioengineering. New York, McGraw-Hill, 1987: 34.1.
11. Buczko GB, McKay WPS: Electrical safety in the operating room. Can J Anaesth 1987; 34:315–322.
12. Bernstein MS: Isolated power and line isolation monitors. BioMed-Instrum-Technol 1990; 24:221–223.
13. Pashayan AG, Ehrenwerth J: Lasers and electrical safety in the operating room. In Ehrenwerth J, Eisenkraft JB (eds): Anesthesia Equipment: Principles and Applications. St. Louis; Mosby-Yearbook, 1993, pp 436–469.
14. Matjasko MJ, Ashman MN: All you need to know about electrical safety in the operating room. In Barash PG, Deutsch S, Tinker J (eds): ASA Refresher Courses in Anesthesiology, vol 18. Philadelphia; JB Lippincott, 1990, p 251.
15. Hull CJ: Electrocution hazards in the operating theatre. Br J Anaesth 1978; 50:647–657.
16. Watson AB, Wright JS, Loughman J: Electrical thresholds for ventricular fibrillation in man. Med J Aust 1973; 1:1179–1182.
17. McNulty SE, Cooper M, Staudt S: Transmitted radiofrequency current through a flow directed pulmonary artery catheter. Anesth Analg 1994; 78:587–589.
18. Bruner JMR, Leonard PF: Electricity, Safety and the Patient. Chicago, Year Book Medical Publishers, 1989, p 43.
19. Dornette WHL: An electrically safe surgical environment. Arch Surg 1973; 107:567–573.
20. Meathe EA: Electrical safety for patients and anesthetists. In Saidman LJ, Smith NT (eds): Monitoring in Anesthesia, ed 2. Boston; Butterworths, 1984, p 497.
21. Rolly G: Two cases of burns caused by misuse of coagulation unit and monitoring. Acta Anaesthesiol Belg 1978; 29:313–316.
22. Parker EO: Electrosurgical burn at the site of an esophageal temperature probe. Anesthesiology 1984; 61:93–95.
23. Schneider AJL, Apple HP, Braun RT: Electrosurgical burns at skin temperature probes. Anesthesiology 1977; 47:72–74.
24. Bloch EC, Burton LW: Electrosurgical burn while using a battery-operated doppler monitor. Anesth Analg 1979; 58:339–342.
25. Becker CM, Malhotra IV, Hedley-Whyte J: The distribution of radiofrequency current and burns. Anesthesiology 1973; 38:106–122.
26. Schlegel RE, Grant FH, Raman S, Reynolds D: Electromagnetic compatibility study of the in-vitro interaction of wireless phones with cardiac pacemakers. Biomed Instrum Technol 1998; 32:645–655.
27. Chen WH, Lau CP, Leung SK, et al: Interference of cellular phones with implanted permanent pacemakers. Clin Cardiol 1996; 19:881–886.
28. Hayes DL, Wang PJ, Reynolds DW, et al: Interference with cardiac pacemakers by cellular telephones. N Engl J Med 1997; 336:1473–1479.
29. Fetter JG, Ivans V, Benditt DG, Collins J: Digital cellular telephone interaction with implantable cardioverter-defibrillators. J Am Coll Cardiol 1998; 21:623–628.
30. Adler D, Margulies L, Mahler Y, Israeli A: Measurements of electromagnetic fields radiated from communication equipment and of environmental electromagnetic noise: Impact on the use of communication equipment within the hospital. Biomed Instrum Technol 1998;32(6):581–590.
31. Emergency Care Research Institute: Cell phones and walkie-talkies: Is it time to relax your restrictive policies? Health Devices 1999; 28:409–413.
32. Nixon MC, Ghurye M: Electrical failure in theatre—a consequence of complacency? Anaesthesia 1997; 52(1):88–89.
33. Litt L, Ehrenwerth J: Electrical safety in the operating room: Important old wine, disguised new bottles. Anesth Analg 1994; 78:417–419.

6 Principles of Pressure Monitoring

Robert G. Loeb, M.D.
Jerry McCoy, Ph.D., M.D.

Arterial blood pressure monitoring, along with pulse rate, is historically and currently one of the most frequently monitored physiologic parameters during anesthesia. Invasive monitoring of arterial blood pressure in anesthesia and critical care is common. Invasive monitoring is more advantageous than noninvasive monitoring because continuous observation of the waveform is possible and arterial blood samples can be readily obtained. It is the gold standard. Invasive blood pressure monitoring is deceptively simple, as exemplified by the misnomer "direct pressure monitoring." As explained in this chapter, clinical monitoring of intravascular pressure is indirect rather than direct through transducers, filters, amplifiers, and displays. Attention to detail and an understanding of the frailties of such systems are necessary to avoid inaccuracy and misinterpretation.

Components of a Pressure Measurement System

Common clinical pressure measurement systems consist of four main subsystems (Fig. 6-1): the mechanical coupling system, the transducer, the electronic components, and the display. The mechanical coupling system transmits the pressure from the source to the transducer. The transducer converts the pressure into an electrical analog (usually voltage). The electronic components change the electrical analog into a form suitable for display and extract features of the waveform. The display converts the electrical signal and features into a visible form. The mechanical coupling system consists of an intravascular catheter, tubing, and stopcocks. The electronic components include amplifiers, filters, and circuits for peak detection and averaging.

Calibration and Performance

Static Calibration

The most important factor for ensuring the accuracy of a pressure measurement is the calibration of the system. Static calibration refers to the calibration of the system against a known static pressure. Clinical pressure monitoring systems are assumed to be linear; that is, a straight line describes the pressure input versus the system output. Therefore, a two-point calibration is sufficient.

Two-Point Calibration

Static calibration is performed by first exposing the mechanical coupling system to atmospheric pressure (this is usually done by opening a stopcock to air). On digital systems, a "zero" button is then pressed. This balances the preamplification circuitry to produce a zero voltage. Second, a known pressure is presented to the mechanical coupling system at the same site and level that the zero reading was taken. The known pressure is usually generated with a mercury manometer, but a water manometer (1.35 cm H_2O = 1 mmHg) or any calibrated manometer is acceptable. With the system exposed to a known pressure, the electrical "gain" control is adjusted to bring the displayed pressure to the calibrated value. This adjusts the gain of the preamplifier circuits to match the sensitivity of the transducer.

Two-point calibration should be performed before the system is attached to a patient. Because pressure transducers have a standard sensitivity of 5.0 μV, per volt excitation per millimeters of mercury input pressure, it can be argued that one-point calibration is sufficient. However, the only way to verify accuracy is by two-point calibration of the entire system. Disposable transducers are calibrated at the factory but may be damaged during shipping. Although the quality control of these devices seems to be good, two-point calibration before use identifies the rare defective unit.[1] Transducer cable malfunction can also result in artifactual hypotension if two-point calibration is not performed before use.[2, 3] Two-point calibration should be repeated during use if it is suspected that the transducer has malfunctioned.[4]

Reference Points. The pressure reference point varies with the pressure being measured and the position of the patient. Central venous pressure is measured at the level of the middle of the right atrium. Intracranial pressure is measured at the tragus of the ear. The pressure reference point for arterial blood pressure may be the middle of the right atrium when the patient is in the supine position or the level of the brain in neurosurgical procedures performed with the patient in a sitting position (Fig. 6-2). Recently it has been proposed that intracardiac pressure should be zero-referenced at the top of the heart rather than at the midchest level, since the midchest position may result in overestimates of pressure measurements due to hydrostatic effects.[5]

The column of fluid between the transducer and the pressure reference point represents a static pressure.[6] This static pressure can be zeroed mechanically or electrically. Mechanical zeroing is achieved by ensuring that the transducer is at the level of the pressure reference point. Electrical zeroing is achieved by rezeroing the system with a stopcock open at the pressure reference point, disregarding the level of the transducer. Either procedure needs to be repeated whenever the level of the transducer changes with respect to the pressure reference point.

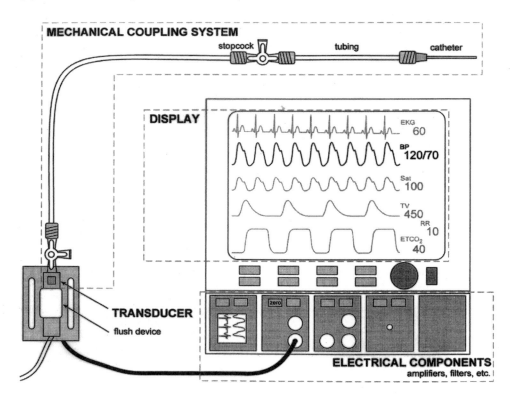

Figure 6-1. The four subsystems of a clinical pressure measurement system: mechanical coupling system, transducer, display, and electronic components.

Drift. The system should be rezeroed, without changing the gain, periodically during use. Usually the zero point drifts, with little change in sensitivity.[1] However, the output signal/voltage may change because of instability of transducer sensitivity, excitation voltage, or monitor amplification gain. Drift may lead to inaccuracy, especially when low pressures (e.g., venous or intracranial) are being measured. The main cause of drift is thermal effects on the transducer.[1]

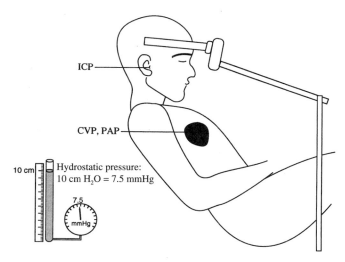

Figure 6-2. Zero reference points in the sitting position for intracranial pressure (ICP), central venous pressure (CVP), and pulmonary artery pressure (PAP). Arterial pressure is zeroed at the base of the skull to measure cerebral perfusion pressure (ICP = 0 when the dura is open). To calculate cardiovascular indices, such as systemic vascular resistance, 7.5 mmHg must be added to the arterial pressure for each 10 cm that the base of the skull is above the heart.

Temperature changes of 10°C usually change the measured pressure by less than 1 mmHg.[1] Transducer offset may also occur during electrocautery.[7] Therefore, pressure values obtained while electrosurgical units are active may not be accurate.

Daily calibration against a mercury manometer has been recommended.[8] To reduce the risk of air embolism, this should be done before the transducer is connected to the patient.[9] More recently, the accuracy of all disposable blood pressure transducers has been shown to be greater than required by the American National Standards Institute. Daily manometer calibrations may, therefore, be unnecessary.[10, 11]

Dynamic Calibration

Measuring static pressure is relatively straightforward. Accurately measuring dynamic pressures is more difficult by an order of magnitude. Fundamental to understanding the potential distortion is a conceptual knowledge of the behavior of oscillating systems. (For a mathematical description of the behavior of oscillating systems, see this chapter's appendix.)

There are many examples of oscillating systems: vibrating strings, pendulums, and waves on a pool of water. The vascular tree, the mechanical coupling subsystem, the pressure transducer, and electrical amplifier circuitry are also oscillating systems.

All oscillating systems have two energy storage compartments between which energy is transferred. In mechanical systems, the energy storage compartments are mass (which stores kinetic energy as inertia when in motion) and elasticity (which stores potential energy when distorted). Oscillations decrease with time, owing to friction, when no energy is added to the system (there are no perpetual motion machines). Damping or viscosity is a measure of the friction

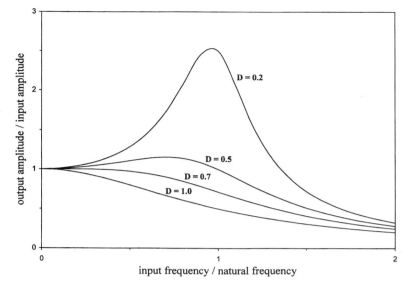

Figure 6-3. The effect of damping on the frequency response. Increasing the damping coefficient (D) results in less overshoot from oscillations near the natural frequency of the system. It also decreases the oscillating frequency. A damping coefficient around 0.7 is optimal because it yields an output-to-input amplitude ratio close to unity over the widest frequency range.

that counteracts the kinetic energy of the mass. To summarize, an oscillating system can be described by the coefficients of mass, stiffness (the inverse of elasticity), and damping.

Natural Frequency

All oscillating systems have a natural frequency. The natural frequency is the oscillating frequency of the *undamped* system. Oscillations at the natural frequency generate the largest displacement for a given input energy. The qualitative effects of changes in mass and stiffness on natural frequency are demonstrated by observations of piano strings. The low notes (slow oscillations) are generated by long, heavy, thick strings that are loosely stretched to be less stiff; high notes are generated by short, thin, light strings that are tightly stretched to be more stiff. Natural frequency decreases with increased mass and decreased stiffness.

Damping

Damping can be understood qualitatively by imagining a vibrating string immersed in honey. Two things would be noticed when comparing oscillations in honey with those in air: the oscillations in honey extinguish more quickly and the string oscillates at a lower frequency. That the oscillating frequency increases as damping decreases can also be demonstrated by the increasing pitch of the voice after inhaling a low-density gas such as helium. The resonant frequency is the oscillating frequency of a *damped* system. It is a function of the natural frequency and the damping coefficient (Fig. 6-3).

Figure 6-4 illustrates the effect of increasing the coefficient of damping on the response of an oscillating system to a sudden input of energy. Increasing the coefficient of damping decreases the overshoot but increases the response time of the system (response time is the time required to reach some fraction of the final value).

Mechanical Coupling Subsystem

The mechanical coupling subsystem (catheter, stopcock, and tubing) contains the elements of an oscillating system. The mass is represented by the mass of fluid within the system.

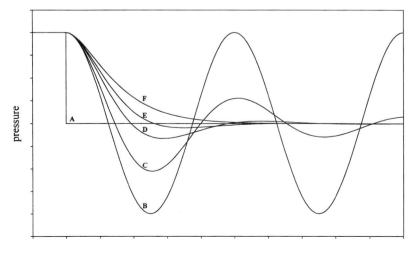

Figure 6-4. The effect of damping on the system response to a step change in pressure: *A,* The input signal. *B,* Response of a system with zero damping. *C,* Response of a system with a damping coefficient of 0.2. *D,* Response of a system with a damping coefficient of 0.5. *E,* Response of a system with an optimal damping coefficient of 0.7. *F,* Response of a system with a critical damping coefficient of 1.0. Note that a damping coefficient around 0.7 yields the best compromise between fast response time and small overshoot.

The distensibility of the plastics from which the components are made gives the system its elasticity. Damping is a function of the frictional resistance to movement of the fluid and distortion of the plastics.

Natural Frequency

Numerous studies have described the natural frequency and damping coefficient of commercial pressure monitoring systems. Bare transducers have resonant frequencies of 100 to 500 Hz.[12, 13] Transducer-tubing systems have much lower natural frequencies of 5 to 50 Hz.[14-17] The length of the tubing has a profound influence on the natural frequency.[16] Five feet of low-compliance tubing results in a natural frequency of 6.5 Hz compared with 33 Hz for 6 in. of tubing. This may be especially important when disposable systems with an option of patient- vs. pole-mounted transducers are used. In one study, the natural frequencies of seven brands of pole-mounted disposable units ranged from 19 to 28 Hz; mounting the same transducers on the patient resulted in increased natural frequencies in a range from 41 to 73 Hz.[18]

A major factor influencing the natural frequency of the mechanical coupling systems—and a factor that is too frequently ignored by clinicians—is the presence of air bubbles. Air bubbles are compressible and increase the elasticity of the system. Most clinicians know only that air bubbles increase the damping coefficient of the mechanical coupling system. However, air bubbles also cause a significant decrease in the natural frequency. The addition of 0.03 mL of air to pole-mounted disposable pressure transducer systems decreases the natural frequency from a range of 18 to 28 Hz to a range of 8 to 13 Hz.[18]

Damping Coefficient

The length of tubing and the presence of air bubbles also affect the damping coefficient. Five feet of low-compliance tubing results in a damping coefficient of 0.1 compared with 0.3 for 6 in. of tubing.[16] The addition of 0.3 mL of air to pole-mounted disposable pressure transducer systems increases the damping coefficient from a range of 0.14 to 0.22 to a range of 0.16 to 0.28.[18]

Frequency Content

To predict the effect of any combination of resonant frequency and damping coefficient on the accuracy of reproduction of a pressure waveform, one first needs to know the frequency content of the pressure waveform. Fourier analysis is a mathematical method of extracting the simple sine and cosine waves that sum to form a complex wave. Fourier analysis of blood pressure waveforms is demonstrated in Figure 6-5. Multiple studies have concluded that the original blood pressure waveform can be accurately reproduced by summing the first 5 to 10 harmonics.[13, 19] Because heart rate normally is in the range of 60 to 180 bpm (1 to 3 Hz), the 5th to 10th harmonics encompass a range of 5 to 30 Hz. Reexamination of Figure 6-3 reveals the amplitude distortion occurs around the natural frequency of the system. Small damping factors allow amplitude overshoot, whereas large damping coefficients result in low relative amplitudes below the natural frequency.

Two methods to preserve an accurate amplitude response are to increase the natural frequency of the system and to

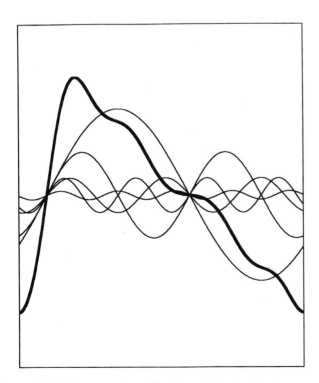
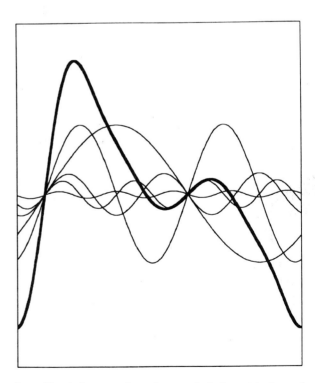

Figure 6-5. Two examples of Fourier analysis of a blood pressure waveform. The darker trace in each example is the original waveform. The fainter traces in each example are the sine wave harmonics which sum to yield the original waveform. The period of each sine wave is an integral multiple of the period of the original waveform. The only difference between the examples is the relative amplitude of each sine wave harmonic.

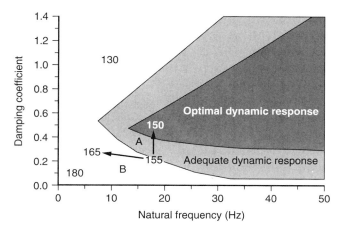

Figure 6-6. The adequate and optimal dynamic response ranges for invasive blood pressure measurement systems. The numbers are examples of output systolic pressures for a systolic input pressure of 150 mmHg. Increasing the damping coefficient decreases the systolic pressure. Systems with a high natural frequency have a wider range of acceptable damping coefficients. Systems with a natural frequency below 7.5 Hz are never adequate. *Arrow A* shows the effect of changing the damping coefficient of the mechanical coupling system with a commercial device for that purpose. *Arrow B* shows the effect of introducing an air bubble into the mechanical coupling system. (Modified from Gardner RM: Direct blood pressure measurement: Dynamic response requirements. Anesthesiology 1981; 54: 227-236.)

optimize the damping coefficient. Gardner[14] published a study that experimentally derived the adequate dynamic response range of invasive blood pressure measurement systems used for monitoring in intensive care units and operating rooms. His results indicate the combinations of natural frequency and damping coefficient that accurately reproduce arterial blood pressure waveforms (Fig. 6-6). Two ranges are depicted. Systems with adequate response accurately reproduce pressures at slow heart rates. Systems with optimal response may be necessary to accurately reproduce blood

pressure waveforms at fast heart rates or when fast upstrokes are present in the pressure waveform.[18]

The largest error introduced by inadequate dynamic response is an inaccurate systolic pressure. Because the systolic upstroke of the pressure waveform contains the highest-frequency components, these components are the most difficult to reproduce accurately. Figure 6-6 demonstrates the effect of dynamic response on the measured systolic pressure. Systolic pressure is underestimated by an overdamped system and overestimated by an underdamped system. Diastolic pressure is less sensitive to suboptimal dynamic response, but it is underestimated by underdamped systems and overestimated by overdamped systems. Mean pressure is least affected by the dynamic response of the measuring system.

Clinical Determination of Dynamic Response

There are two methods of determining the natural frequency and damping coefficient of a blood pressure measurement system. In the clinical laboratory, a pressure generator can be used to produce a constant amplitude sine wave pressure at progressively increasing frequency (sine wave method). Natural frequency and damping coefficient can be determined by comparing the pressure tracing recorded by the system under investigation with the pressure tracing recorded by a reference transducer (Fig. 6-7). In the operating room or intensive care unit, the natural frequency and damping coefficient of a pressure measurement system can be determined by the response of the system to a square wave pressure input. A square wave pressure can be generated by opening, then quickly closing, the fast-flush valve of a continuous flush mechanism (square wave method). Figure 6-8 demonstrates this method of determining the dynamic response of the system from the measured pressure waveform. Figure 6-9 provides a graph and table for determining the damping coefficient from the amplitude ratio.[14] The fast-flush test has proved to be an accurate method for determining dynamic response during normal pulsatile flow, cardio-

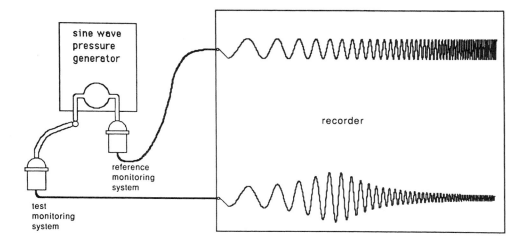

Figure 6-7. The sine wave method of determining dynamic response. A sine wave pressure of increasing frequency is simultaneously measured by a reference and test system. The reference system should have a flat response; the test system will have an output defined by the natural frequency and damping coefficient. Two measurements are made: the frequency at which there is peak amplitude from the test system (oscillating frequency), and the ratio of test system amplitude to reference system amplitude at the oscillating frequency. The damping coefficient and natural frequency can be calculated from these numbers (see the Appendix for formulas).

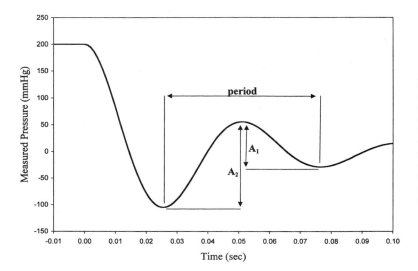

Figure 6–8. The square wave method of determining dynamic response. A square wave is generated by opening, then quickly closing the fast-flush valve of a continuous flush mechanism. Two measurements are then made from the recorded output: the oscillating frequency, which is the inverse of the period, and the amplitude ratio of two successive peaks, A_1/A_2. In this example the oscillating frequency is 19 Hz (1/0.052 second) and the amplitude ratio is 0.51. The damping coefficient and natural frequency can be derived from these numbers (see the Appendix and Fig. 6–9).

pulmonary bypass, and circulatory arrest.[20] It is generally accepted that the sine wave and square wave methods of determining dynamic response yield identical results.[18] However, differences in results obtained with these two methods have been documented. Differences in damping coefficients obtained with the two techniques have been attributed to damping effects of the catheter within the artery or the presence of air in the system when the flush method is used in vivo.[21-23]

Methods to Improve Dynamic Response

Most commercial blood pressure measurement systems are underdamped, with a borderline natural frequency for arterial blood pressure measurement.[17] What can the clinician do if the measured dynamic response of his or her system is outside the acceptable range? To optimize the dynamic response, the natural frequency should be as high as possible; a natural frequency below 7.5 Hz is never acceptable.[14] This is accomplished by using the shortest practical tubing (definitely less than 4 ft) and the fewest number of stopcocks (not more than one) between the transducer and the patient.[16] Tubing should be noncompliant; compliant devices such as T-connectors with injection ports should not be used.

Air bubbles should be meticulously removed from the mechanical coupling system.[24] Bubbles are often hidden in stopcocks and in the transducer housing. Air and other emboli injected through arterial and venous catheters can cause significant patient morbidity, especially in children.[25-27] To reduce the incidence of invisible bubbles, air should be removed from the intravenous bag before it is pressurized, the intravenous solution may be warmed or exposed to ultrasonic waves prior to use, and a filter may be used to trap air distal to the fast-flush mechanism.[25, 28]

After all measures have been taken to increase the natural frequency of the system, the dynamic response may still be inadequate owing to suboptimal damping. Two hydraulic devices are commercially available to increase the damping coefficient of the system without decreasing the natural frequency.[22, 29] The ROSE (Resonance OverShoot Eliminator, Gould Instruments Inc., Cleveland, OH) is a nonadjustable device that increases the damping coefficient by adding a second resonating element in parallel with the pressure measurement system. The Accudynamic (Sorenson, Salt Lake City, UT) is an adjustable device which operates on the same principle. The effect of using either device is illustrated in Figure 6–6.[14, 15] Schwid[29] has developed a semiautomatic electronic method for improving the dynamic response of a catheter-manometer system. With that method, a computer automatically determines the natural frequency and damping coefficient of the monitoring system after the clinician performs a fast flush. The computer then adapts calculations to the specific system to remove resonance artifacts and display an undistorted pressure waveform.

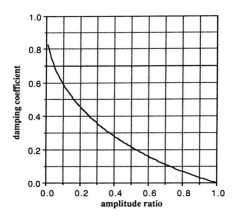

	0.00	**0.01**	**0.02**	**0.03**	**0.04**	**0.05**	**0.06**	**0.07**	**0.08**	**0.09**
.0	1.000	0.826	0.780	0.745	0.716	0.690	0.667	0.646	0.627	0.608
.1	0.591	0.575	0.559	0.545	0.531	0.517	0.504	0.491	0.479	0.467
.2	0.456	0.445	0.434	0.424	0.414	0.404	0.394	0.385	0.376	0.367
.3	0.358	0.349	0.341	0.333	0.325	0.317	0.309	0.302	0.294	0.287
.4	0.280	0.273	0.266	0.259	0.253	0.246	0.240	0.234	0.228	0.221
.5	0.215	0.210	0.204	0.198	0.192	0.187	0.181	0.176	0.171	0.166
.6	0.160	0.155	0.150	0.146	0.141	0.136	0.131	0.126	0.122	0.117
.7	0.113	0.108	0.104	0.100	0.095	0.091	0.087	0.083	0.079	0.075
.8	0.071	0.067	0.063	0.059	0.055	0.052	0.048	0.044	0.041	0.037
.9	0.034	0.030	0.027	0.023	0.020	0.016	0.013	0.010	0.006	0.003
1.0	0.000									

Figure 6–9. Two methods of determining the damping coefficient from the square wave method amplitude ratio. The conversion can be read from the graph, or, if greater accuracy is desired, from the table. For example, an amplitude ratio of 0.51 yields a damping coefficient of 0.210.

Transducers

A transducer is a device that converts one form of energy into another. All pressure transducers first convert pressure into movement. An elastic device, such as a Bourdon tube or a diaphragm, is exposed to the pressure, and its deflection is measured.

Historical Development

Geddes[13] has written a fascinating summary of the historical development of blood pressure transducers. Early transducers measured the deflection of a Bourdon tube using mechanical linkages, a method still used today in blood pressure manometers. However, purely mechanical manometers have a very low frequency response owing to the need for a large sensing element with a large displacement volume. This requirement is inherent because the energy to move the mechanical parts must come from the event being measured. A significant advance was made in the fidelity of blood pressure measurement with the development of mechano-optical transducers. These devices, developed between 1903 and 1945, further transduced the movement of the sensing element to the deflection of a beam of light. Ultimately, high fidelity was achieved using miniature low-elasticity glass membrane sensing elements to deflect the light beam. These devices, although useful in the physiology laboratory, were never used clinically because pressure recordings required a darkened room and photographic techniques. However, optical transducers that attach to standard monitors have been developed.[30] These optical transducers share several important features, such as minimal drift, high accuracy, and minimal interference or signal degradation along the optic fiber length.[31] They may be especially useful for measurement of pressure during magnetic resonance scanning.[32]

Given the advanced state of electrical technology, it is not surprising that modern blood pressure transducers convert movement of the sensing element into current or voltage. This conversion is usually accomplished by inducing a change in capacitance, inductance, or resistance. High-frequency response is achieved using small sensing elements with low fluid displacement.

Types

Capacitance Transducers

In a capacitance transducer, the sensing element is one plate of the capacitor (Fig. 6-10). As pressure is applied, the two plates of the capacitor move closer together and capacitance increases. An oscillating voltage is applied across the plates of the capacitor, and an alternating current that varies with the pressure on the sensing element results. This alternating current is then demodulated (converted to direct current) for further processing. Capacitance transducers have a number of practical problems.[13, 33, 34] They have poor temperature stability and require separate temperature-compensating circuitry. Electrical cables are themselves capacitors; therefore, the oscillator and demodulator must be built into the transducer housing to avoid interference. This feature increases the size of the unit. Further, in order to be used with biologic amplifiers, the current produced must first be converted to voltage.

Inductance Transducers

Inductance is an electrical property of coils produced by the forces of an induced magnetic field that causes the coil to resist changes in current flow. The inductance of a coil is affected by the position of an iron core within the coil. Inductance transducers have a core attached to the sensing element (see Fig. 6-10). As pressure is applied, the core is displaced into the coil and inductance increases. Like capacitance, inductance is measured with an oscillating current. Therefore, the transducer housing usually contains oscillators and demodulators. Inductance transducers have a number of advantages. They are stable over a useful temperature range and can be designed to have a large electrical output for a

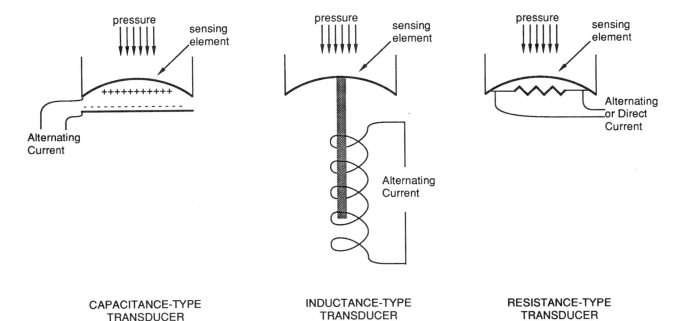

CAPACITANCE-TYPE TRANSDUCER   INDUCTANCE-TYPE TRANSDUCER   RESISTANCE-TYPE TRANSDUCER

Figure 6-10. The three common types of electronic pressure transducers.

small mechanical displacement. The most sensitive transducers based on the property of inductance use a miniature linear variable differential transformer. These units use a core and four coils to produce a multivolt output for 0.001-in. deflection of the sensing element.

Resistance Transducers

Change in resistance is the most common way of measuring displacement of the sensing element. The principle of measurement is based on the fact that the resistance of a wire increases as it is stretched (see Fig. 6–10). Nondisposable pressure transducers are usually bonded strain gauges. In these, a resistor or a group of resistors is bonded to the back of the diaphragm. As pressure is applied to the diaphragm, the resistors are distorted and their resistance changes. Resistive-type transducers have a major advantage over capacitance- and inductance-type transducers. A change in resistance is easily converted to change in voltage by use of a Wheatstone bridge. Therefore, bulky circuits for modulation-demodulation are not necessary. Strain gauges are temperature and light sensitive. This led to treatment of artifactual hypotension when warming lights were used.[35] The Wheatstone bridge can be designed to compensate for temperature sensitivity of the strain gauge. Certain transducer manufacturers use dyes designed to decrease light sensitivity. Other manufacturers provide information concerning photosensitivity in their respective transducers.[35] The popular disposable pressure transducers are resistive-type transducers. The diaphragm is a piece of silicon with the resistive elements etched onto it.

Intravascular Transducers

Most clinical pressure transducers are for external use, but intravascular transducers can be of the inductive, capacitance, or resistive type. The advantage of intravascular transducers is that there is no mechanical coupling system to distort the pressure waveform. The frequency response of an intravascular transducer system can be flat to over 100 Hz.

Unfortunately, intravascular transducers have a number of drawbacks. They are expensive and fragile, a bad combination for clinical devices. Although they are miniature compared with external transducers, they are too large to be passed through a catheter smaller than 18 gauge. Finally, they cannot be recalibrated during use. The result is that intravascular transducers are not widely used for clinical measurement of intravascular pressures.

Standardization

Manufacturers have adopted a standard blood pressure transducer output of 5 μV/V/mmHg. This standardization means that transducers from different manufacturers are functionally interchangeable. Because the interface plug between the transducer and the preamplifier has not been standardized, a conversion unit may still be required to connect any particular combination of transducer and monitor.

Amplifiers and Filters

Electrical amplification and filtering occur between the generation of the electrical analog at the transducer and the display of the pressure waveform. Many modern monitors also perform analog-to-digital conversion of the signal at this point. The actual mechanism of this "electronic massage" for any given monitor is unimportant and proprietary, but the specifications of the amplifiers, filters, and analog-to-digital converters are important since they influence the waveform and derived values. Amplifiers are used to increase the voltage and power of the signal. They contain oscillating electronic circuits but have a frequency response 100 times better than that of the mechanical coupling system.

Low-pass filters are included for three reasons: to remove high-frequency noise due to electrocautery; to smooth the waveform, which is often reconstructed from discretely sampled points; and to give the waveform a more pleasant appearance. Removal of electrocautery noise is clinically necessary. However, filtering to yield a more rounded appearance of the waveform is unwarranted. It is a serious problem because it is not standardized and the filters affect the frequencies of interest. For example, Hewlett-Packard monitor models 78353/4 and 78833/4 (Hewlett-Packard Co., Waltham, MA) have a bandwidth of 0 to 12 Hz, whereas the Tektronix model 414 monitor (Tektronix, Inc., Beaverton, OR) has a bandwidth of 0 to 20 Hz. (Bandwidth is the frequency range over which the output has between 70% and 140% the power of the input.) Nonstandardization may cause discrepancies, especially in systolic values and derived cardiovascular parameters, whenever a patient is moved from one monitor to another.

There are two reasons that a waveform may be sampled as discrete points and then reconstructed. Some monitors electronically disconnect the transducer hundreds of times per second (chop the signal) and subtract any baseline voltage during that time to maintain baseline stability of the internal electronic components. More important, most modern monitors convert the analog voltage to a digital value. This process, known as analog-to-digital conversion, occurs 60 to a few hundred times per second. The advantages of having the information in a digital form are that it can be stored and manipulated. Stored values allow display of frozen waveforms and trends. Digital computer manipulation of the values allows feature detection, automatic calculation of derived variables, and other sophisticated algorithms discussed later.

Electronic Signal Analysis

The shape of the pressure waveform is important to detect artifact, to judge the effect of arrhythmias on blood pressure (see Chapter 13), and perhaps to estimate the inotropic and volume status of the cardiovascular system. In addition to displaying the waveform, clinical monitors extract and digitally display four features: rate, systolic pressure, diastolic pressure, and mean pressure. These values are used, either directly or in derived parameters, to guide diagnostic and therapeutic decisions. These values are affected by dynamic and static calibration and electronic filtering as well as by the method of signal analysis.

What information is important from a physiologic viewpoint? Heart rate is one description of cardiovascular status. Cardiac output is affected by heart rate, especially in children. Heart rate also affects the oxygen supply-to-demand ratio of the heart. Heart rate variability with respiration indicates active autonomic control, and variability with surgical stimulus is helpful to evaluate depth of anesthesia. Therefore, the absolute value of heart rate and some measure of heart rate variability are clinically useful parameters.

The systolic blood pressure, that is, the average aortic pressure during systole, estimates left ventricular afterload. The mean blood pressure indicates tissue perfusion pressure. Perfusion pressure of the coronary arteries is influenced by the diastolic pressure, that is, the average aortic pressure during diastole. Normally these systemic pressures are relatively uniform, beat to beat, over the respiratory cycle. However, hypovolemia is associated with increased variability with respiration. For systemic pressures, the clinically useful values are the average systolic pressure, the average diastolic pressure, the average mean pressure, and some measure of blood pressure variability.

Central vascular pressures (central venous pressure, pulmonary artery pressure, and pulmonary capillary wedge pressure) are used as correlates of atrial filling pressure and end-diastolic volume. These pressures are dramatically affected by respiration, especially in critically ill patients. The physiologically important values occur at end-expiration when the intrathoracic pressure is closest to atmospheric pressure. Therefore, for central vascular pressure the average end-expiratory mean pressure is the most desirable measurement.

Digital Processing Algorithms

Digital signal processing is also used in most of the new blood pressure monitors. It is performed by one or more internal microprocessors. Digital processing algorithms are proprietary, and manufacturers rarely reveal the details of their methods. In general, algorithms are used to determine the beginning and end of a cardiac cycle. The maximum and minimum pressures during that cycle are then selected as systolic and diastolic values. These values, averaged over a constant period of time, are displayed. Mean pressures are also calculated beat to beat. Digital algorithms do perform better than analog algorithms found in older monitors. Maloy and Gardner[36] found that the numeric values displayed by monitors using digital technology agreed more closely with clinicians' readings than did monitors using analog technology. Even using current digital algorithms, systolic values are less reliable than diastolic values, and machine-generated values are sensitive to artifacts in the waveform.

Fluctuations in intrathoracic pressure during the respiratory cycle introduce a respiratory artifact in central venous and pulmonary artery occlusion pressures. Currently, it is recommended that the clinician determine these pressures from a calibrated paper-strip recording at end-exhalation.[37, 38] Simultaneous measurement of airway pressure accurately identifies end-expiration.[39] Alternatively, stable digital values can be obtained during a prolonged expiratory pause in the paralyzed and anesthetized patient.[4] However, this procedure has the risk of morbidity from failure to reinitiate mechanical ventilation. With current algorithms, the displayed mean value of central vascular pressures during mechanical ventilation is completely inaccurate and should not be used as either an absolute value or a trend.[38, 40]

A number of methods have been described in an attempt to automatically determine end-expiratory values of pulmonary artery pressures. The goal of each of these algorithms is to detect end-expiration. Measuring the pressure, temperature, flow, or CO_2 concentration in the respiratory gas does this most accurately.[39, 41] Unfortunately, these techniques require additional measuring equipment.

An alternative method is described by Ellis.[42] He noted that the beat-to-beat mean pressure fluctuates least during end-expiration whenever expiratory time exceeds or equals inspiratory time. He used this observation to develop an algorithm that identifies end-expiration from information present in the pressure waveform itself.[42]

After end-expiration is identified, end-expiratory pressures can be estimated in a number of ways. One way is to average all values but to give greater weight to the values with less beat-to-beat variability.[42] This method is currently used in some monitors. Another way is to average only the end-expiratory values.[41] These methods are slightly more accurate than simple averaging techniques but become inaccurate at high respiratory rates. They also have the disadvantage that they do not display the pressure waveform with the respiratory artifact removed.

Mitchell and coworkers have reported a microprocessor-based method of removing the respiratory artifact from the pressure waveform.[43] To separate the cardiac and respiratory components, they used an adaptive filter that changes its characteristics based on the measured heart rate. They then determined the mean intravascular pressure using Ellis's algorithm and added this offset to the cardiac component. The result is a continuous pulmonary artery pressure waveform with the respiratory artifact removed. The method is equally applicable to central venous pressure and pulmonary capillary wedge pressures. Hoeksel et al.[44] have developed a similar algorithm that removes both respiratory and extraneous artifacts.

Digital processing algorithms have also been developed to remove other types of artifacts, derive related physiologic variables, and improve alarm performance. For instance, Elghazzawi et al.[45] described a method to automatically identify arterial blood pressure features during use of an intra-aortic balloon pump, based on timing obtained from the electrocardiogram tracing.[45] Takazawa et al.[46] described the application of a generalized transfer function to estimate aortic root pressure from the radial artery pressure. Derrick and coworkers[47] described the use of a proportional-differential control algorithm to generate blood pressure alarms. Other, equally promising, algorithms have been developed.[48, 49]

Commercially available monitors use simple digital methods to determine average systolic, mean, and diastolic pressures. Algorithms are being developed to remove or identify artifact in invasive pressure waveforms. It is hoped that future commercial monitors will use more sophisticated electronic signal analysis.

Displays

Most clinicians are familiar with the variety of displays available on commercial monitors. Early blood pressure monitors used a simple oscilloscope to display the waveform. Systolic, diastolic, and mean values were displayed on separate analog or digital meters. Today, monitor displays have increased in complexity and sophistication. Waveforms and numbers are displayed simultaneously on a cathode ray tube. Display format can be partially defined by the user and can automatically change as different combinations of transducers are connected to the monitor. Remote displays are available; these are classified as "smart" or "dumb." Dumb terminals simply echo the monitor's integrated display. They are usually large screens used in operating rooms so that all members of the surgical team can observe cardiovascular parameters. Smart terminals allow various levels of display control from a remote location. These are most frequently used in intensive care units to display information from multiple monitors in a central location.

Two major improvements in displays have become available: color and trend displays. Color displays help the user to find and focus her or his attention on a particular waveform or value. This is important since displays often contain multiple waveforms and values from a number of sources. Many commercial monitors now have the ability to store a few hours of information and display it on a compressed time scale. The immediate advantages are twofold: (1) A clinician who has not been in constant attendance has access to an accurate record of the patient's physiologic status during the clinician's absence. (2) The clinician can view physiologic parameters on a compressed time scale to detect trends that may not be apparent in real time. Trend displays are underutilized by clinicians. Most clinicians are accustomed to the standard monitor display of real-time waveforms; this is the most frequently selected display for continual observation in the operating room and intensive care unit.

No studies have been done to determine whether physiologic stability can be better maintained by a clinician using real-time waveforms or trend displays as feedback, but trend displays may be the better choice under many circumstances. We humans are very effective in detecting patterns, but our memory limits our ability to detect patterns occurring over a span of time. By allowing the clinician to focus on the changes in relevant physiologic variables over a relevant period of time, trend displays aid in the detection and treatment of undesirable conditions.

Effects of Catheters

Superficial arteries are commonly cannulated for arterial pressure measurement. Barr[50] first described the over-the-needle catheter that is inserted percutaneously for indwelling use. Central arteries and veins are commonly cannulated using the method first described by Seldinger[51] (see Chapters 13 and 14).

Catheter Size and Type

The size of the catheter influences the rate of complications and the dynamic response of the system. Bedford[52] studied the incidence of temporary radial artery occlusion as a function of catheter size. He found a 34% incidence of occlusion 24 hours after insertion with 18-gauge catheters compared to 8% with 20-gauge catheters.[52] The incidence of arterial occlusion is directly related to the percentage of the vessel lumen that is occupied by the catheter. Wrist circumference is a noninvasive measurement that is well correlated with the risk of radial arterial occlusion; a wrist circumference less than 18 cm is associated with a greater than 25% incidence of occlusion, using an 18-gauge catheter.[53] In a more recent study, approximately 25% of radial artery catheters were associated with abnormal artery flows. However, there were no indications of resultant hand ischemia.[54] Although radial artery occlusion is usually temporary, persistent occlusion can result.[55] The lower incidence of thrombosis with smaller catheters is an advantage to the clinician. Infection and bleeding are also risks associated with arterial cannulation. The incidence of either is relatively low and not influenced by insertion site or patient condition (i.e., medical versus surgical).[56-59] Risk of catheter-related infection is correlated with advanced age, duration of catheterization and hospital stay, and concurrent infection with *Staphylococcus aureus*.[56, 61] Distal occlusion of the radial artery causes overshoot of the measured systolic pressure owing to increased wave reflection, whereas proximal occlusion causes a reduction in measured pulse pressure owing to overdamping[62] Small catheters have an additional effect of increasing the dynamic accuracy of the system. Although small catheters have a slightly lower resonant frequency than do large catheters, they have a significantly larger damping coefficient.[63, 64] Because most blood pressure monitoring systems are under-

damped, this results in increased accuracy of the system. The major clinical disadvantage of smaller catheters is that they kink more easily.

In neonates, radial artery cannulation with 24-gauge catheters yields accurate pressures and has a low complication rate.[65, 66] Femoral artery cannulation, even with relatively large catheters (3F), also has a low complication rate and can be considered an alternative site for invasive blood pressure monitoring in infants.[58]

Catheter Composition

The material from which the catheter is made also influences the rate of complications. Intravascular catheters are commonly manufactured from polyethylene, polypropylene, polyvinylchloride, or polytef (Teflon). Numerous studies have documented the increased thrombogenicity of polypropylene and polyethylene over Teflon.[62, 67-70] Polyvinylchloride is comparable to Teflon in its incidence of thrombus formation.[69, 71] Thrombogenicity is also affected by the smoothness of the catheter surface; roughened Teflon catheters are more thrombogenic than polyethylene catheters.[68] This factor may be clinically important, since pulmonary artery catheters have a higher incidence of thrombus formation when they are passed through introducers or protective sleeves.[72] Heparin impregnation of catheters reduces the incidence of thrombus formation initially, especially in larger vessels, but the effect is lost after 48 hours, probably because the heparin leaches out of the catheter.[69, 73] However, improved methods to attach heparin to surfaces are being developed.[73] In heparin-bonded catheters, the decrease in thrombus formation, is correlated with a decrease in catheter-related positive blood cultures.[74] Significant catheter-induced thrombus formation can occur without evidence of catheter malformation.[75] Therefore, the potential for complications associated with catheter thrombus can occur without forewarning. Fortunately, the incidence of thrombus in normally functioning catheters is low. Polyethylene catheters also cause injuries to the vessel, which can serve as a nidus for atherosclerotic plaques.[76]

A notable exception to the findings presented here are the data from Slogoff and coworkers.[77] In their study of 1699 patients after radial artery cannulation, they were unable to find any correlation between the risk of thrombus and catheter size (18 or 20 gauge) or catheter composition (Teflon or polypropylene).[77] They did report a statistically higher incidence of thrombosis in women (who tend to have a smaller wrist circumference).[77]

Maintenance of Catheter Patency

Catheters for pressure monitoring are kept patent by one of three methods: intermittent bolus of heparin-containing solution, continuous flush of heparin-containing solution, or continuous flush of non-heparin-containing solution.

Intermittent Bolus Technique

Historically, intermittent boluses of heparin-containing solution was the only method available. There are two major problems with the intermittent bolus technique. The first is that it is not particularly effective in preventing catheter thrombosis, leading to waveform damping.[69] Wesseling and Smith[78] reported that the duration of waveform loss owing to damping with the intermittent bolus technique is 2 to 10 times that of the continuous flush technique. More important, significant patient morbidity can result from a manual bolus when thrombotic or air emboli are forced retrograde into the central or cerebral circulation.[26] The volume of the bolus necessary to reach the central circulation correlates with the height of the patient. Therefore, extreme care is necessary during bolus injection in pediatric patients.

Continuous Flush Technique

In 1970, Gardner and colleagues[79] published a report of the first commercial continuous flush device for clinical use. Such devices, which infuse fluid through the catheter at a nominal rate of 3 to 6 mL/hour, are now widely used. Advantages of continuous flush include effectiveness, ease of use, and the ability to maintain a closed sterile system. An additional advantage is that constantly wedged pulmonary artery catheters may be identified by a steady rise in the measured pulmonary artery pressure with loss of the waveform.[80]

There are, of course, some disadvantages with continuous flush. A static error is introduced in the pressure measurement. The magnitude of the error depends on the infusion rate and the resistance to flow through the catheter. Static errors between 0.1 and 2.5 mmHg have been reported.[28, 79] For arterial pressure monitoring this error is clinically insignificant. A more important disadvantage is the potential for inadvertent excess fluid administration. This event can occur if the flush mechanism is defective[81] However, in neonates and children, even a flow of 3 to 6 mL/hour through multiple pressure monitoring lines may exceed the fluid requirements for that patient. In such cases the standard system can be modified so that the fluid for the flush device is dispensed from a syringe pump or volumetric infusion pump.[82] A final potential problem of continuous flush is the introduction of air into the pressure monitoring system. If the fluid source for the flush device is a pressurized bag of fluid that contains air, an air embolism may occur when the bag empties. This may be avoided if all the air is removed from the bag prior to applying pressure. Smaller amounts of air can also be introduced during a fast flush. This occurs owing to the vortex created when a stream of fluid enters the drip chamber. The best solution is to inspect the system for air after a fast flush or to use an appropriate filter.

The final issue in maintaining catheter patency is whether to use heparin in a continuous flush solution. Most practitioners use 1 or 2 U of heparin per milliliter of flush solution.[83] However, heparin administration carries the risk of heparin-induced thrombocytopenia or accidental heparin overdose.[84] Two early studies investigated whether heparin was necessary in a continuous flush solution to maintain arterial catheter patency. Heparin at a concentration of 2.5 U/mL did not maintain catheter patency better than lactated Ringer's solution in a nonrandomized unblinded study of 50 adult patients.[85] But catheter occlusion *was* more frequent when heparin (4 U/mL) was omitted from the continuous saline flush in a blinded and randomized study of 30 medical intensive care patients.[86] Similar results have been obtained with 24-gauge catheters in neonates.[87] A meta-analysis of 13 studies revealed no significant difference in duration of catheter patency between heparin and saline flush.[88] However, a more recent meta-analysis of 26 randomized controlled trials revealed a significantly longer duration of patency in radial artery catheters and when a low-dose heparin infusion was used instead of saline.[89] Other studies indicate that catheter patency may not only depend on the presence or absence of heparin but also on the type of catheter involved. The failure

rate of pulmonary artery catheters may not be influenced by the use of heparinized flush.[90] Thus, the use of heparin in arterial flush solutions is still controversial.

Pressure Alteration in Vasculature

The preceding discussions imply that systems with an optimal dynamic response accurately measure blood pressure. However, although the pressure at the site of measurement is accurately reproduced, the pressure may already be distorted at the site where it is measured. The vascular tree is a complex oscillating system that acts to change the blood pressure in different areas of the body. Parry et al.[91] demonstrated significantly higher pressure measured from the dorsalis pedis artery than from the radial artery. This difference was not affected by position of the patient.[91] Usually the pressures in peripheral arteries contain more high-frequency components than do central arteries; the systolic pressure is usually higher in peripheral arteries.[92, 93] However, there are exceptions. Multiple studies have demonstrated that the systolic pressure is often lower in peripheral arteries than it is in central arteries immediately after cardiopulmonary bypass.[92, 94-96] Iatrogenic compression of an upstream artery can also cause a falsely low peripheral blood pressure, for example, during sternal retraction.[97, 98] In neonates the peripheral pressure correlates well with the central umbilical artery pressure.[99]

Three major factors cause the vascular tree to change peripheral blood pressure: oscillations, wave reflections, and phase shift. The effects of oscillation on pressure measurements have been discussed previously. The vascular tree acts like many oscillating segments connected in series.[100] The damping coefficient and resonant frequency of each segment are functions of the vascular tone and blood volume. Computer modeling demonstrates how changes in vascular compliance and resistance alter the radial artery pressure independent of central aortic pressure. Not only are the systolic, diastolic, and mean pressures affected, but the entire shape of the pressure waveform is changed.[100] The dicrotic notch of the radial artery pressure waveform is an artifact[93, 100]; there is no correlation between it and the dicrotic notch of the central aortic pressure waveform.

The influence of wave reflection and phase shift on the resultant peripheral pressure is probably less than that of oscillations. Wave reflections occur when the pressure wave reaches the resistance arterioles.[101] At the arterioles, some of the energy of the pressure wave forces blood past the resistance, some of the energy is absorbed by the vessel, and the remainder is reflected. The tone of the arterioles influences the amount of energy reflected. Normal femoral vascular beds reflect 80% of the incident wave; reflections are decreased to almost zero after intra-arterial vasodilator injections.[101] The location of the pressure measurement site with respect to the wave reflection site and the elasticity of the arterial tree influence the effect of reflected waves on the measured pressure. Reflected waves coincident with the systolic part of the incident waveform cause an increased systolic pressure; those transmitted slower or detected farther away contribute to a diastolic peak.[101]

Wave reflection is easily demonstrated. When pressure is applied with the finger over the intravascular portion of an arterial catheter, an increase in systolic pressure is observed.[62] This is because a situation is created in which there is 100% energy reflection coincident with the systolic pressure. A similar situation occurs when there is thrombosis obstructing the artery distal to the site of measurement.[62]

Phase shift occurs because higher frequencies are transmitted at different rates than lower frequencies.[102] This distorts the peripheral pressure, causing the leading edge of the systolic pressure to be exaggerated.[19]

Because the pressure waveform in peripheral vessels is so different from that in the central aorta, care should be used in interpreting peripheral invasive blood pressures. The pressures in peripheral arteries differ from the aortic pressures to which the heart is exposed. Derived values that are meaningful when calculated from aortic pressures are meaningless when calculated from peripheral pressures. For example, the ratio of the area under the diastolic portion of the aortic pressure to the area under the systolic aortic pressure (diastolic pressure–time index-to-systolic pressure–time index ratio, DPTI/SPTI) has been used to predict the myocardial oxygen supply-to-demand ratio. This ratio is magnified by 25% when peripheral instead of aortic pressures are used.[103] Similarly, derivations of myocardial contractility and stroke volume from the peripheral blood pressure are inaccurate.[100]

Invasive blood pressure measurements are used clinically to judge the cardiovascular status of the patient. Extrapolations are made from arterial blood pressure to flow conditions in the brain, heart, kidney, and other organs, to the work of the heart, and even to cardiovascular volume status. The vascular tree and measurement devices modulate the pressure waveform in complex and dynamic ways. It is appropriate to use blood pressure trends to direct therapy; however, one should avoid placing too much confidence in the absolute value displayed on the blood pressure monitor.

REFERENCES

1. Disposable pressure transducers—Evaluation. Health Devices 1984; 13:268–290.
2. Navedo AT, Wald A: Erroneous measurement with invasive monitoring of blood pressure (letter). Anesth Analg 1991; 73: 96–97.
3. Raines DE, Hogue CJ, Wickens C, et al: Artifactual hypertension due to transducer cable malfunction. Anesthesiology 1991; 74: 1149–1151.
4. Barbieri LT, Kaplan JA: Artifactual hypotension secondary to intraoperative transducer failure. Anesth Analg 1983; 62:112–113.
5. Courtois M, Fattal PG, Kovacs SJ Jr, et al: Anatomically and physiologically based reference level for measurement of intracardiac pressures. Circulation. 1995; 92:1994–2000.
6. Fernandez-Cano F: A simple accurate technique for establishing zero reference levels for pressure measurements (letter). Anesthesiology 1984; 61:478.
7. Milne B, Cervenko FW, Henderson MB, et al: Transducer offset by electrocautery resulting in erroneous blood pressure measurement. Can J Anaesth 1986; 33:234–236.
8. Bailey RH, Bauer JH, Yanos J: Accuracy of disposable blood pressure transducers used in the critical care setting. Crit Care Med 1995; 23:187–192.
9. Disposable blood pressure transducers: Calibration methods. Health Devices 1993; 22:97.
10. Ahrens T, Penick JC, Tucker MK: Frequency requirements for zeroing transducers in hemodynamic monitoring. Am J Crit Care 1995; 4:466–471.
11. Gardner RM: Accuracy and reliability of disposable pressure transducers coupled with modern pressure monitors. Crit Care Med 1996; 24:879–882.
12. Fox F, Morrow DH, Kacher EJ, et al: Laboratory evaluation of pressure transducer domes containing a diaphragm. Anesth Analg 1978; 57:67–76.
13. Geddes LA: The Direct and Indirect Measurement of Blood Pressure. St. Louis, Mosby–Year Book, 1970, pp 1–69.
14. Gardner RM: Direct blood pressure measurement—dynamic response requirements. Anesthesiology 1981; 54:227–236.
15. Abrams JH, Olson ML, Marino JA, et al: Use of a needle valve variable resistor to improve invasive blood pressure monitoring. Crit Care Med 1984; 12:978–982.
16. Boutros A, Albert S: Effect of the dynamic response of transducer-tubing system on accuracy of direct blood pressure measurement in patients. Crit Care Med 1983; 11:124–127.
17. Shinozaki T, Deane RS, Mazuzan JE: The dynamic responses of liquid-filled catheter systems for direct measurements of blood pressure. Anesthesiology 1980; 53:498–504.
18. Hunziker P: Accuracy and dynamic response of disposable pressure transducer-tubing systems. Can J Anaesth 1987; 34:409–414.
19. Geddes LA, Baker LE: Principles of Applied Biomedical Instrumentation. New York, John Wiley & Sons, 1968, pp 446–467.
20. Kleinman K, Frey K, Stevens R: The fast flush test—is the clinical comparison equivalent to its *in vitro* simulation? J Clin Monit Comput 1988; 14:485–489.
21. Schwid HA: Frequency response evaluation of radial artery catheter-manometer systems: Sinusoidal frequency analysis versus flush method. J Clin Monit Comput 1988; 4:181–185.
22. Hipkins SF, Rutten AJ, Runciman WB: Experimental analysis of catheter-manometer systems *in vitro* and *in vivo*. Anesthesiology 1989; 71:893–906.
23. Kleinman B, Powell S, Gardner RM: Equivalence of fast flush and square wave testing of blood pressure monitoring systems. J Clin Monit Comput 1996; 12:149–154.
24. Wade LD, Krejcie TC: The effect of air bubbles on the dynamic response of invasive pressure monitoring systems (abstract). Anesth Analg 1983; 62:S289.
25. Soule DT, Powner DJ: Air entrapment in pressure monitoring lines. Crit Care Med 1984; 12:520–522.
26. Lowenstein E, Little JW, Lo HH: Prevention of cerebral embolization from flushing radial-artery cannulas. N Engl J Med 1971; 285:1414–1415.
27. Hayes A, Doherty P: Defective arterial monitoring kits. Anaesthesia 1998; 53:410.
28. Gardner RM, Bond EL, Clark JS: Safety and efficacy of continuous flush systems for arterial and pulmonary artery catheters. Ann Thorac Surg 1977; 23:534–538.
29. Schwid HA: Semiautomatic algorithm to remove resonance artifacts from the direct radial artery pressure. Biomed Instrum Technol 1989; 23:40–43.
30. Roos CF, Carroll FE Jr: Fiber-optic pressure transducer for use near MR magnetic fields. Radiology 1985; 156:548.
31. Narendran N, Corbo MA, Smith W: Fiber optic pressure sensor for biomedical applications. ASAIO J 1996; 42:M500–506.
32. Hackman CH, Tan PS, Chakrabarti MK, et al: A new optical transducer for arterial pressure measurement. Br J Anaesth 1991; 67:346–352.
33. Rushmer RF: Cardiovascular Dynamics. Philadelphia, WB Saunders, 1976, pp 36–75.
34. Lee APB: Biotechnological principles of monitoring. Int Anesthesiol Clin 1981; 19:197–207.
35. Garrett JS, Vernon DD, Xanos N, et al: Spurious hemodynamic alterations resulting from light sensitive pressure transducers. Crit Care Med. 1993; 21:1401–1402.
36. Maloy L, Gardner RM: Monitoring systemic arterial blood pressure: Strip chart recording versus digital display. Heart Lung 1986; 15:627–635.
37. Schmitt EA, Brantigan CO: Common artifacts of pulmonary artery and pulmonary artery wedge pressures: Recognition and interpretation. J Clin Monit Comput 1986; 2:44–52.
38. Maran AG: Variables in pulmonary capillary wedge pressure: Variation with intrathoracic pressure, graphic and digital recorders. Crit Care Med 1980; 8:102–105.
39. Berryhill RE, Benumof JL, Rauscher LA: Pulmonary vascular pressure reading at the end of exhalation. Anesthesiology 1978; 49:365–368.
40. Riedinger MS, Shellock FG, Swan HJC: Reading pulmonary artery and pulmonary capillary wedge pressure waveforms with respiratory variations. Heart Lung 1981; 10:675–678.
41. Oden R, Mitchell MM, Benumof J: Detection of end-exhalation period by airway thermistor: An approach to automated pulmonary artery pressure measurement. Anesthesiology 1983; 58: 467–471.

42. Ellis DM: Interpretation of beat-to-beat blood pressure values in the presence of ventilatory changes. J Clin Monit Comput 1985; 1:65–70.

43. Mitchell MM, Meathe EA, Jones BR, et al: Accurate, automated, continuously displayed pulmonary artery pressure measurement. Anesthesiology 1987; 67:294–300.

44. Hoeksel SA, Blom JA, Jansen JR, et al: Correction for respiration artifact in pulmonary blood pressure signals of ventilated patients. J Clin Monit Comput 1996; 12:397–403.

45. Elghazzawi ZF, Welch JP, Ladin Z, et al: Algorithm to identify components of arterial blood pressure signals during use of an intra-aortic balloon pump. J Clin Monit Comput 1993; 9:297–308.

46. Takazawa K, O'Rourke MF, Fujita M, et al: Estimation of ascending aortic pressure from radial arterial pressure using a generalised transfer function. Z Kardiol 1996; 85(suppl 3): 137–139.

47. Derrick JL, Thompson CL, Short TG: The application of a modified proportional-derivative control algorithm to arterial pressure alarms in anesthesiology. J Clin Monit Comput 1998; 14: 41–47.

48. Panerai RB, Rennie JM, Kelsall AW, et al: Frequency-domain analysis of cerebral autoregulation from spontaneous fluctuations in arterial blood pressure. Med Biol Eng Comput 1998; 36:315–322.

49. Hoeksel SAAP, Jansen JRC, Blom JA, et al: Detection of dicrotic notch in arterial pressure signals. J Clin Monit Comput 1997; 13:309–316.

50. Barr PO: Percutaneous puncture of the radial artery with a multi-purpose Teflon catheter for indwelling use. Acta Physiol Scand 1961; 51:343–347.

51. Seldinger SI: Catheter replacement of the needle in percutaneous arteriography. Acta Radiol 1953; 39:368–376.

52. Bedford RF: Radial arterial function following percutaneous cannulation with 18- and 20-gauge catheters. Anesthesiology 1977; 47:37–39.

53. Bedford RF: Wrist circumference predicts the risk of arterial occlusion after cannulation. Anesthesiology 1978; 48:377–378.

54. Sfeir R, Khoury S, Khoury G, et al: Ischaemia of the hand after radial artery monitoring. Cardiovas Surg 1996; 4:456–458.

55. Weiss BM, Gattiker RI: Complications during and following radial artery cannulation: A prospective study. Intensive Care Med 1986; 12:424–428.

56. Falk PS, Scuderi PE, Sheretz RJ, et al: Infected radial artery pseudoaneurysms occurring after percutaneous cannulation. Chest 1992; 101:490–495.

57. Frezza EE, Mezghebe H: Indications and complications of arterial catheter use in surgical or medical intensive care units: Analysis of 4932 patients. Am Surg 1998; 64:127–131.

58. Graves PW, Davis AL, Maggi JC, et al: Femoral artery cannulation for monitoring in critically ill children: Prospective study. Crit Care Med 1990; 18:1363–1366.

59. Leroy O, Billiau V, Beuscart C, et al: Nosocomial infections associated with long-term radial artery cannulation. Intensive Care Med 1989; 15:241–246.

60. Myles PS, Buckland MR, Burnett WJ: Single versus double occlusive dressing technique to minimize infusion thrombophlebitis: Vialon and Teflon cannulae reassessed. Anaesth Intensive Care 1991; 19:525–529.

61. Raad I, Umphrey J, Khan A, et al: The duration of placement as a predictor of peripheral and pulmonary arterial catheter infections. J Hosp Infect 1993; 23:17–26.

62. Kim JM, Arakawa K, Bliss J: Arterial cannulation: Factors in the development of occlusion. Anesth Analg 1975; 54:836–841.

63. Browning DH, Graves SA, van der Aa J: Catheters for arterial pressure monitoring in pediatrics (abstract). Anesthesiology 1981; 55:A131.

64. Goodwing SR, Graves SA, van der Aa J: Umbilical catheters and arterial blood pressure monitoring. J Clin Monit Comput 1985; 1:227–231.

65. Gevers M, van Genderingen HR, Lafeber HN, et al: Radial artery blood pressure measurement in neonates: An accurate and convenient technique in clinical practice. J Perinat Med 1995; 23: 467–475.

66. Gevers M, Hack MWM, van Genderingen HR, et al: Calculated mean arterial pressure in the posterior tibial and radial artery pressure wave in newborn infants. Basic Res Cardiol 1995; 90: 247–1251.

67. Davis FM, Stewart JM: Radial artery cannulation. Br J Anaesth 1980; 52:41–47.

68. Mortensen JD, Schaap RN: Further experience with an acute intra-arterial implantation screening test for thrombogenicity of intravascular catheters. Trans Am Soc Artif Intern Organs 1980; 26:284–288.

69. Downs JB, Chapman RL Jr, Hawkins IF Jr: Prolonged radial-artery catheterization. Arch Surg 1974; 108:671–673.

70. Bedford RF: Percutaneous radial-artery cannulation—increased safety using Teflon catheters. Anesthesiology 1975; 42:219–222.

71. Brown AE, Sweeney DB, Lumley J: Percutaneous radial artery cannulation. Anaesthesia 1969; 24:532–536.

72. Youngberg JA, Texidor M, Cantrell C, et al: Introducers and protective sleeves increase thrombogenicity of pulmonary artery catheters (abstract). Anesthesiology 1985; 63:A181.

73. Eberhart RC, Clagett CP: Catheter coatings, blood flow, and biocompatibility. Semin Hematol 1991; 28:42–48.

74. Krafte-Jacobs B, Sivit CJ, Mejia R, et al: Catheter-related thrombosis in critically ill children: Comparison of catheters with and without heparin bonding. J Pediatr 1995; 126:50–54.

75. Bolz KD, Fjermeros G, Wideroe TE, et al: Catheter malfunction and thrombus formation on double-lumen hemodialysis catheters: An intravascular ultrasonographic study. Am J Kidney Dis 1995; 25:597–602.

76. Madsen JK, Garbarasch C, Nielsen PE: Endothelial injury of arteries following catheterization with polyethylene tubes: Experimental studies on rabbit aorta using the Seldinger technique. Cardiovasc Res 1979; 13:541–546.

77. Slogoff S, Keats AS, Arlund C: On the safety of radial artery cannulation. Anesthesiology 1983; 59:42–47.

78. Wesseling KH, Smith NT: Availability of intraarterial pressure waveform from catheter-manometer systems during surgery. J Clin Monit Comput 1985; 1:11–16.

79. Gardner RM, Warner HR, Toronto AF, et al: Catheter-flush system for continuous monitoring of central arterial pulse waveform. J Appl Physiol 1970; 29:911–913.

80. Shin B, Ayella RJ, McAslan C: Pitfalls of Swan-Ganz catheterization. Crit Care Med 1977; 5:125–127.

81. Morray J, Todd S: A hazard of continuous flush systems for vascular pressure monitoring in infants. Anesthesiology 1983; 58:187–189.

82. Johnson DL: Invasive pressure monitoring: A modified system for pediatrics. Dimens Crit Care Nurs 1986; 5:93–96.

83. Ledbetter C, Ahrens T, Brown B, et al: Comparison of normal saline and heparin solutions for maintenance of arterial catheter patency (letter). Heart Lung 1991; 20:316.

84. Silver D, Kapsch DN, Tsoi EKM: Heparin-induced thrombocytopenia, thrombosis, and hemorrhage. Ann Surg 1983; 198:301–305.

85. Hook ML, Reuling J, Luettgen ML, et al: Comparison of the patency of arterial lines maintained with heparinized and non-heparinized infusions. Heart Lung 1987; 16:693–699.

86. Clifton GD, Branson P, Kelly HJ, et al: Comparison of normal saline and heparin solutions for maintenance of arterial catheter patency. Heart Lung 1991; 20:115–118.

87. Mudge B, Forcier D, Slattery MJ: Patency of 24-gauge peripheral intermittent infusion devices: A comparison of heparin and saline flush solutions. Pediatr Nurs 1998; 24:142–145, 149.

88. Peterson FY, Kirchhoff KT: Analysis of the research about heparinized versus nonheparinized intravascular lines. Heart Lung 1991; 20:631–640.

89. Randolph AG, Cook DJ, Gonzales CA, et al: Benefit of heparin in peripheral venous and arterial catheters: Systematic review and meta-analysis of randomised controlled trials. BMJ 1998; 316:969–975.

90. Zevola DR, Dioso J, Moggio R: Comparison of heparinized and nonheparinized solutions for maintaining patency of arterial and pulmonary artery catheters. Am J Crit Care. 1997; 6:52–55.

91. Parry T, Hirsch N, Fauvel N: Comparison of direct blood pressure measurement at the radial and dorsalis pedis arteries during surgery in the horizontal and reverse Trendelenburg positions. Anaesthesia 1995; 50:553–555.

92. Gallagher JD, Moore RA, McNicholas KW, et al: Comparison of radial and femoral arterial blood pressures in children after cardiopulmonary bypass. J Clin Monit Comput 1985; 1:169–171.

93. Bruner JMR: Handbook of Blood Pressure Monitoring. Littleton, MA: PSG, 1978.

94. Mohr R, Lavee J, Goor DA: Inaccuracy of radial artery pressure measurement after cardiac operations. J Thorac Cardiovasc Surg 1987; 94:286–290.

95. Rulf EN, Mitchell MM, Prakash O, et al: Measurement of arterial pressure after cardiopulmonary bypass with long radial artery catheters. J Cardiothorac Anesth 1990; 4:19–24.

96. Stern DH, Gerson JI, Allen FB, et al: Can we trust the direct radial artery pressure immediately following cardiopulmonary bypass? Anesthesiology 1985; 62:557–561.

97. Saka D, Lin TY, Oka Y: An unusual cause of false radial-artery blood-pressure readings during cardiopulmonary bypass. Anesthesiology 1975; 43:487–489.

98. Diamant M, Arkin DB: False radial-artery blood-pressure readings (letter). Anesthesiology 1976; 44:273.

99. Butt WW, Whyte H: Blood pressure monitoring in neonates: Comparison of umbilical and peripheral artery catheter measurements. J Pediatr 1984; 105:630–632.

100. Schwid HA, Taylor LA, Smith NT: Computer model analysis of the radial artery pressure waveform. J Clin Monit Comput 1987; 3:220–228.

101. O'Rourke MF, Yaginuma T: Wave reflections and the arterial pulse. Arch Intern Med 1984; 144:366–371.

102. Remington JW: Contour changes of the aortic pulse during propagation. Am J Physiol 1960; 199:331–334.

103. Reitan JA, Martucci RW, Levine NA: A computer evaluation of the ratio of the diastolic pressure-time index to the time-tension index from three arterial sites in dogs. J Clin Monit Comput 1986; 2:95–99.

Appendix

The oscillating behavior of the mechanical coupling system can be described by this differential equation,

$$M\frac{d^2x}{dt^2} + R\frac{dx}{dt} + Ex = P(t), \tag{6.1}$$

which describes the displacement of the fluid (x) for a given pressure waveform, P(t). M is the kinetic fluid mass of the system, R is the viscous damping, and E is the effective modulus of volume elasticity.

With zero damping the system oscillates at the natural frequency (f_n) in response to a sudden input pressure:

$$f_n = \frac{1}{2\pi}\sqrt{\frac{E}{M}} \tag{6.2}$$

E can be calculated from the physical characteristics of the transducer:

$$E = A^2\frac{\Delta P}{\Delta V} \tag{6.3}$$

where A is the exposed area of the transducer sensing element and $\Delta P/\Delta V$ is the change in pressure required to cause a volume of fluid to enter the transducer.

M can also be related to the physical characteristics of the system:

$$M = \frac{4}{3}\left(\frac{A}{a}\right)^2 l a\rho + LA\rho \tag{6.4}$$

where a is the cross-sectional area of the tubing, ρ is the densitiy of the fluid, and L and l are the lengths of the columns of fluid in the transducer and tubing, respectively. Of course, the cross-sectional area is related to the diameter of the tubing, d, by

$$a = \frac{\pi d^2}{4} \tag{6.5}$$

Thus the natural frequency is increased by decreasing the elasticity and surface area of the transducer sensing element, by using short wide-bore tubing, and by using a fluid of low density.

The damping coefficient (D) is the viscous damping of the system expressed as a fraction of the critical damping. The damping coefficient can be calculated from the physical characteristics of the system:

$$D = \frac{16\eta}{d^3}\sqrt{\frac{3L}{\pi\rho E}} \tag{6.6}$$

where η is the fluid viscosity. Note that damping is inversely related to the cube of the diameter of the tubing.

The natural frequency and damping coefficient can be calculated by measuring the output of the system for a step pressure input or an increasing frequency sine wave input. In either case the damped resonant frequency (f_d) of the system is measured. The damped resonant frequency is related to the natural frequency as follows:

$$f_d = f_n\sqrt{1 - D^2} \tag{6.7}$$

Using the step pressure method, the damping coefficient is calculated by measuring the amplitude ratio of two successive peaks (A_s) (see Fig. 6–8):

$$D = -\ln\left[\frac{A_s}{\sqrt{\pi^2 + (\ln A_s)^2}}\right] \tag{6.8}$$

Using the sine wave method, the damping coefficient is calculated by measuring the amplitude ratio of the test system to the reference system at the frequency of test system peak amplitude (Ar_{fd}):

$$D = \sqrt{\frac{1 - \sqrt{1 - \frac{1}{(Ar_{fd})^2}}}{2}} \tag{6.9}$$

Once the damping coefficient and natural frequency have been determined, the response of the system to a step pressure input and an increasing frequency sine input can be predicted. The output of the system over time to a step pressure input is

$$P(t) = P_o + \frac{P_o}{\sqrt{1 - D^2}} \, e^{-D2\pi f_n t} \sin (2\pi f_n t \sqrt{1 - D^2} + \\ \sin^{-1}\sqrt{1 - D^2}) \quad (6.10)$$

for $0 < D \leq 1$. The output-to-input ratio amplitude ratio (A_r) for any sine wave input frequency (f) (see Fig. 3-2) is

$$A_r = \frac{1}{\sqrt{\left(\dfrac{f}{f_n}\right)^4 + 2\left(\dfrac{f}{f_n}\right)^2 (2D^2 - 1) + 1}} \quad (6.11)$$

PART TWO

Central and Peripheral Nervous Systems

7 Evoked Potentials

S. S. Moorthy, M.D.
R. V. Reddy, M.D.

Evoked potential (EP) recording is a useful diagnostic tool in the evaluation of certain neurologic disorders. It is also a useful technique in monitoring the functional integrity of the sensory and motor pathways during many surgical procedures and preventing potential injury to the vital neural structures. EPs are extremely small-amplitude (microvolts) electrical potentials generated by nervous tissue in response to stimulation. In this chapter the focus is on the practical applications of this technology as it applies to intraoperative monitoring. The basic methods and standard recording parameters are described. There are excellent books and reviews on the technology and usefulness of EPs.[1-8]

The Source of Evoked Potentials

Application of a stimulus to the nervous system is followed by the development of a neural signal, which is transmitted along a specific pathway, for example, sensory stimuli through the spinothalamic tract or auditory stimuli through auditory and visual stimuli through visual pathways. The EPs are represented as waveforms, voltage over time, and are described in terms of amplitude, latency, and morphology (Fig. 7–1). *Amplitude* is peak to peak or baseline to peak voltage difference. *Latency* can be described as absolute, measured from the stimulus to the response, or interpeak, the interval between the two peaks of interest. *Morphology* is described as the overall shape or series of positive and negative waves. These waves can be monophasic, biphasic, or polyphasic. Recording of these waves is complicated by their small potentials and the presence of background noise. Fat and bone attenuate the signals. Cerebrospinal fluid, hematomas, hygromas, or other fluid cavities are good conductors. Metal plates and rods (Harrington rods) can distort the potentials.

Near-Field and Far-Field Evoked Potentials

In the near-field recordings the neuronal potentials created by depolarization are immediately below the recording electrode. The near-field recordings have relatively large amplitude. They exhibit marked changes in size and waveform with even small alterations in the position of the recording electrode. This is the case with the scalp recordings of many of the potentials generated in the cortex and the potentials recorded over an activated nerve. In the near-field potentials, there is an initial positive wave due to the outward current flow in advance of the active region of depolarization, a negative wave due to inward current flow in the actively depolarized area, and a final positive wave due to outward current flow as depolarization passes and repolarization occurs.

In the far field, a depolarizing volley (action potential front) within the central nervous system white matter tracts travels toward the cortical mantle and produces a positive-going activity. These far-field potentials are produced by the deeper nuclei and tracts and are widely distributed, and their amplitude and morphology remain relatively constant despite changes in the electrode position.

Latencies

The latencies are described as short latency (up to 10 ms), middle latency (10 to 50 ms), and long latency (over 50 ms). The visual latency is a long-latency response and the somatosensory EPs and auditory EP are short-latency potentials.

Method of Stimulation and Recording

Stimulation

The stimulus type, intensity, duration, rates, number of stimuli, and size and location of the stimulated area are important for obtaining the EPs consistently. The types of stimuli and recording parameters are described in detail under the individual EPs.

Recording Methods

The electrical activity at the surface of the skull and body are best recorded using cup-type pure silver electrodes coated with silver chloride, commonly used for electroencephalogram (EEG) recording. A conducting medium, usually an isotonic gel (electrolyte), forms the interface between the scalp or skin and the electrodes. This forms the first and in many ways vital link needed to act as a transmission bridge.

The scalp electrode placement is done using the 10–20 electrode placement system as recommended by the International Federation of Societies for EEG and Clinical Neurophysiology[9] (Fig. 7–2). The skin electrode placement is done using bony landmarks as a guide. The electrodes are attached to the scalp or skin, after preparation of the scalp or skin with alcohol or acetone, using collodion. The electrolyte is injected into the cup of the electrode using a blunt-tipped

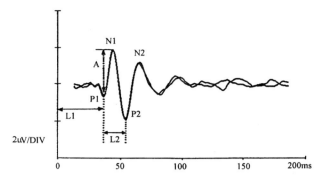

2uV/DIV

Figure 7-1. A cortical somatosensory evoked potential showing peak P1 (first positive peak) and N1 (first negative peak). Note that upward deflections are negative. A indicates the peak-to-peak (P1 to N1) amplitude. L1 indicates the (absolute) latency between the onset of the stimulus and the P1. L2 is the interpeak latency between P1 and P2.

needle. The electrodes can also be applied using a conductive paste. Clip, stick-on type silver and silver chloride, or needle electrodes can also be used. Special diagnostic electrodes for cochleograms and electroretinograms are not used in intraoperative recording on a routine basis. Electrode impedance should be checked at the start of every recording and should be repeated during the recording if there is a need to suspect bad electrode contact. The impedance of an electrode should be between 1000 and 5000 Ω. The skin-electrolyte-electrode interface forms the most important link for faithful acquisition of potentials. A poor interface leads to the most common recording problems.

The recording machines are computers with averagers, amplifiers, input selector switches, calibration units, and filters. The EP equipment averages the responses that are time-locked to the stimulus and the signal appears as an amplified wave at a fixed latency. The background activity that is not time-locked to the stimulus produces nearly a flat line by the equipment averaging effect on random noise.

Artifacts should be recognized and appropriate measures should be taken to eliminate or minimize them. Artifacts can be of environmental, stimulus, or physiologic origin. The sources of environmental interference in the operating room include electrical current from the operating tables, warming blankets, fluid warmers, fluorescent lights, and electrosurgical instruments (cautery and the like). Crossed cables, improper grounding, improperly attached electrodes, patient grounding, and movement of wires that link the electrodes and preamplifier also contribute to the noise.

The effective ways of dealing with electrostatic and magnetic interference are to (1) ensure good electrical contact for all electrodes and ground, (2) shield the main supply leads, (3) keep good distance, preferably 2 m or more, between the patient and all forms of electrical equipment, (4) change the orientation of the equipment with respect to the offending sources, and (5) entwine the pairs of input electrode leads to make a twisted pair or simply bunch together all the electrode leads to reduce magnetic pickup. The stimulus artifacts are usually due to current flow in stimulators and their output leads that can induce currents in recording electrodes. Such artifacts are especially conspicuous in somatosensory and auditory stimulation. These artifacts overlap and distort the early parts of the EPs and also prolong the averaging process if artifact rejection controls are used. Placing the ground electrode between stimulating and recording electrodes can reduce somatosensory stimulus artifacts. Artifacts in the auditory stimuli can be reduced by using ear inserts instead of earphones to administer click stimuli. The

physiologic artifacts are due to generation of large voltage changes by many structures within the head and body. The most troublesome sources of interference are the eyes, heart, and skeletal muscle. When monitoring is done in the operating room, eye movements and muscle artifacts are not usually a problem, although electrocardiogram artifacts can be troublesome. Use of appropriate filters can minimize these artifacts.

Somatosensory Evoked Potentials

Somatosensory pathways for touch, pressure vibration, and proprioception from the trunk and lower extremities are shown in Figure 7-3. The somatosensory evoked potential (SSEP) testing basically examines the integrity of the proprioceptive sensory pathways. The axons of the proprioceptive peripheral neurons enter the spinal cord through the dorsal roots, where some branch, sending collateral axons to the anterior horn, and some continue posteriorly in the dorsal column of the spinal cord. The axons from the lower body ascend in the fasciculus gracilis and axons from the upper body ascend in the fasciculus cuneatus. Fasciculi gracilis and cuneatus terminate at the medulla in their respective nuclei. The second-order neurons, after their origin, decussate to

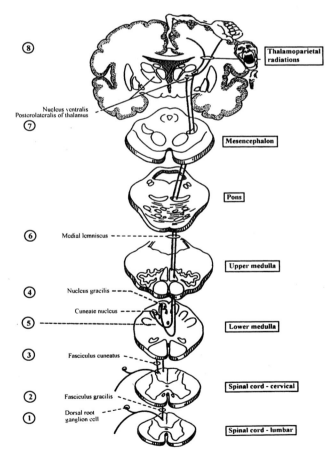

Figure 7-2. The international 10-20 system of scalp electrode positions. Electrodes are placed either 10% or 20% of the distance between landmarks on the skull. (From Harner P, Sannit T: A Review of the International Ten-Twenty System of Electrode Placement. Grass Instruments, Quincy, MA, 1974; and Aminoff MJ: Electrodiagnosis in Clinical Neurology, ed 3. New York, Churchill Livingstone, 1992.)

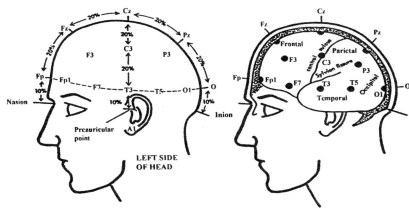

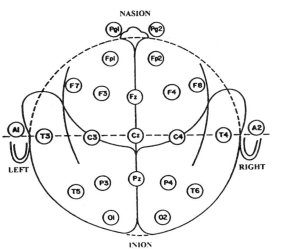

Figure 7-3. The somatosensory pathway for touch, proprioception, pressure, and vibratory stimuli. (Modified from DeJong RN: The Neurological Examination, ed 5. Philadelphia, JB Lippincott, 1992.)

the opposite side, forming the medial lemniscus in the brainstem, and ascend to synapse in the ventral posterior limb of the internal capsule, and synapse in the postcentral gyrus of the parietal lobe, the primary somatosensory cortex. Somatotopic organization is represented according to the homunculus as shown in the cortex (see Fig. 7-3).

SSEPs are electrical responses of brain or spinal cord to electrical stimulation of peripheral nerves. The most commonly studied nerves are median, ulnar, peroneal, and tibial. The stimulus for SSEPs is a brief electric pulse delivered to the distal portion of the nerve. The intensity of the stimulus is adjusted so there is a small muscle twitch. The intensity is sufficient to activate low-threshold myelinated nerve fibers. The compound nerve action potential enters the spinal cord through the dorsal root and is conducted through the spinal column to reach the gracile and cuneate nuclei. The second-order neurons in turn conduct these impulses through the brainstem to the thalamus and then make extensive projections to the cortex. The SSEPs are useful in the diagnosis of spinal cord diseases and are routinely used for intraoperative monitoring of some surgical procedures, such as Harrington rod placement for scoliosis.

Median Nerve Somatosensory Evoked Potentials

Median nerve SSEPs are useful in assessing the conduction in the upper cervical cord and brain. Median nerve SSEPs, when used in conjunction with lower extremity SSEPs, may help to recognize the lesions between cauda equina and

cervical spinal cord. The parameters are described in Table 7-1.

The electrodes are placed in the following locations for median nerve SSEPs: (1) Erb's points on the left (EP-1) and right (EP-2); (2) over the seventh or second cervical spine (C7 or C2); (3) at C3′ and C4′; and (4) Fz (frontal midline region). Erb's point is 2 to 3 cm above the clavicle, just

Table 7-1. Median and Tibial Nerve Recording Parameters for Somatosensory Evoked Potentials*

	Median Nerve	**Tibial Nerve**
Stimulation rate	4–7/s	4–7/s
Duration	200–300 μs	200–300 μs
Low-frequency filter	5–30 Hz	5–30 Hz
High-frequency filter	2500–4000 Hz	2500–4000 Hz
No. of trials	500–2000	1000–4000
Stimulating electrodes	Wrist	Behind medial malleolus
Montages		
Channel 1	Cc–Fz	Fz–Cz
Channel 2	C2/C7–Fz	L1–T12/IIC
Channel 3	EP-1–EP-2	PF–REF

Cc, contralateral central cortex; Fz, frontal midline region; Cz, central midline region; IIC, ipsilateral iliac crest; EP-1, Erb's point 1 (left) or ipsilateral Erb's point; EP-2, Erb's point 2 (right) or contralateral Erb's point; PF, popliteal fossa; REF, reference electrode.

*It is recommended that each laboratory establish its own normative data for these parameters.

lateral to the attachment of the sternocleidomastoid muscle. The C2 is the prominent spinous process at the base of the neck and can be identified by counting up from the most prominent C7 spinous process. C3′ and C4′ are 2 cm posterior to electrode positions C3 and C4, respectively, of the 10–20 electrode placement system. These electrodes are over the sensory cortex. The Fz is identical to the Fz of the 10–20 system. The recommended channels are contralateral central cortex (Cc) to Fz, cervical (C2 or C7) to Fz, and EP-1 (ipsilateral Erb's point) to EP-2 (contralateral Erb's point). With stimulation of the median nerve at the wrist, the potentials recorded at the Erb's point, neck, and contralateral scalp are N9, N14, and N20, respectively. The Erb's potential (N9) arises from the afferent volley in the brachial plexus at a latency of about 9 to 12 ms, the cervical potential (N14) arises from dorsal column nuclei at about 14 ms, and the cortical potential (N20) arises from thalamocortical projections at about 20 ms. The upper and lower extremity recordings of SSEPs are shown in Figure 7–4.

Tibial Somatosensory Evoked Potentials

SSEPs from the lower extremity are obtained by stimulation of either the tibial or peroneal nerve. For posterior tibial nerve stimulation at the ankle, the recording electrodes are placed over the tibial nerve in the popliteal fossa (PF), usually at the middle of the popliteal crease, and the reference electrode (REF) on the medial surface of the knee about 5

cm medial to the PF; over the first lumbar spinous process (L1) and 3 cm rostral to L1 (T12) or to the ipsilateral iliac crest (IIC); and over the cortex, Fz, and Cz (central midline region), using the 10–20 electrode placement system. The lumbar response sometimes can be better visualized if the ipsilateral iliac crest is used as a reference. The montage includes channel 1, Cz–Fz; channel 2; L2–T12; and channel 3; PF–REF. The recorded waveforms include the potential recorded from the afferent volley in the PF at about 13 ms; the potential recorded over the L1 spinous process at about 22 ms; and two potentials recorded over the cortex: N30 and P40 at about 30 and 40 ms, respectively. The stimulus intensity is just enough to produce a visual twitch. SSEPs can also be recorded from the spinal cord at different levels depending upon the clinical needs.

Conditions Producing Changes in Somatosensory Evoked Potentials

Anesthetic agents have variable and complex effects on SSEPs and central conduction time (CCT).[10–12] Surgical anesthesia is associated with prolonged latency and diminished amplitude of the SSEP component. Premedication with atropine, morphine, and diazepam has little effect on SSEPs. However, increasing doses of morphine and diazepam can attenuate SSEPs. Induction with thiopental does not affect SSEP, but barbiturate coma reduces the amplitude of N20 and increases latency and CCT. Halogenated anesthetic

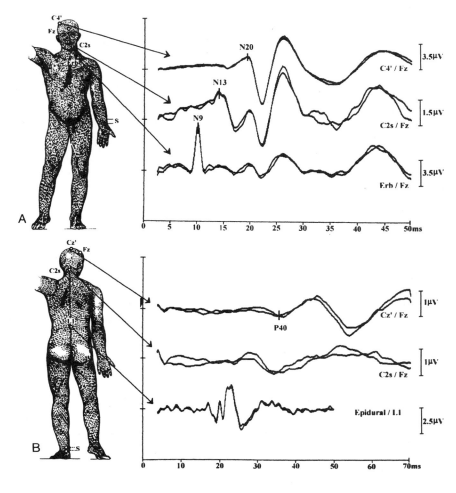

Figure 7–4. *A,* Somatosensory evoked potentials (SSEPs) following stimulation to the left median nerve(s), recorded transcutaneously from points along the somatosensory pathway, from Erbs point (Erb/Fz), and over the somatosensory cortex (C4′/Fz). The difference between N13 and N20 represents the central somatosensory conduction time. *B,* SSEPs following stimulation to the left tibial nerve (S), recorded from points along the somatosensory pathway, from the L1 epidural space (Epidural/L1), from the skin overlying the C2 spinous process (C2s/Fz), and from the scalp overlying the somatosensory cortex (Cz′/Fz).

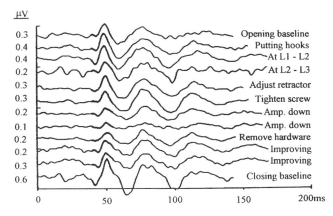

Figure 7-5. Cortical sensory evoked potentials (CSEPs) recorded in a patient with idiopathic scoliosis undergoing Cotrel-Dubousset instrumentation following bilateral tibial nerve stimulation. After spinal distraction, the CSEP amplitude decreased to 0.1 V. The surgeon was warned of the evoked potential change, and he removed the instrumentation. The CSEPs fully recovered, and the patient had no postoperative neurologic deficits. (The number on the left refers to the amplitude of the first negative peak.) (From Deletis V: The Sentinel-4 Evoked Potential/Electroencephalographic Analyzer. Anesth Rev 1991;16:27-31.)

agents reduce the amplitude and increase the latencies of the SSEP in a dose-dependent manner. CCT is also prolonged with the use of halogenated agents. Nitrous oxide (50% or greater) following fentanyl administration is associated with reduction in amplitude and increase in latency. SSEPs recorded from the spinal column are markedly attenuated with the use of halogenated agents. These agents should be avoided during spinal surgery. Etomidate increases the amplitude of cortical SSEPs and prolongs CCT and the latency of SSEP. Adjunct drugs, antibiotics, and other cardiovascular drugs do not have any significant effects on SSEPs. Hypotension and hypothermia increase the latencies and reduce the amplitude of the SSEPs. The anesthetic regimens with successful monitoring of SSEPs include narcotic technique or narcotic and low concentrations of inhalation agents such as isoflurane, halothane, enflurane, sevoflurane, and desflurane.

Somatosensory Evoked Potentials and Spinal Cord Function

Somatosensory Evoked Potentials During Spinal Surgery

SSEP monitoring during spinal surgery has been found to be very useful in preventing potential damage to the spinal cord[13-19] (Fig. 7-5). Before the introduction of SSEPs the only method of evaluation during spinal surgery was to wake the patient during surgery and ask the patient to move the lower limbs (wake-up test).

SSEPs are also useful in evaluating spinal cord function during thoracic aortic surgery. The incidence of paraplegia following repair of aortic coarctation is between 0.4% and 1.5%. The incidence is higher following repair of thoracic aortic aneurysm (up to 15%). SSEP monitoring is useful and sensitive for spinal cord ischemia.[20] Spinal arteriography and therapeutic transvascular embolization are associated with SSEP changes (Fig. 7-6). Recovery takes place in 2 to 4 minutes unless the patient has neurologic deficit. In patients undergoing thoracic aortic surgery, if the SSEP changes are

detected, a shunt procedure or femoral-femoral bypass may be needed.

Somatosensory Evoked Potentials in Other Surgeries

SSEPs can be used for monitoring during extracranial carotid reconstruction, carotid endarterectomy, cerebrovascular surgery with induced hypotension, and clipping and intraoperative localization of sensorimotor cortex[21-24] (Fig. 7-7). Carotid endarterectomy is highly beneficial to patients with high-grade (>70%) stenosis with or without symptoms. The complication rate in this group of patients is variable, death occurring in 0% to 5%, and stroke in 1.5% to 16%. Carotid cross-clamping is associated with risk of ipsilateral cerebral ischemia unless satisfactory collateral circulation is present. In patients undergoing carotid endarterectomy, SSEPs are recorded with stimulation of the median nerve at the wrist on both sides. After obtaining baseline or control SSEPs before anesthetic induction, recordings are obtained before the use of neuromuscular blocking drugs and then continuously during surgery. Particular attention is paid to the SSEPs before cross-clamping of the carotid artery, during cross-clamping and repair, and following release of the cross clamp. The evoked responses are continuously displayed on an oscilloscope and later printed. The morphology, latencies, and amplitudes of the waves are continuously compared. The waveforms N14 and N19 and CCT (interval between N14 and N19) are evaluated for changes. SSEP changes on the side of the carotid endarterectomy compared with the opposite side indicate cerebral ischemia. There are a number of reports confirming the usefulness of monitoring SSEPs during carotid endarterectomy. One disadvantage is the difficulty in detecting only motor tract ischemia during surgery as SSEP monitors only the sensory tracts.

Intracranial vascular surgeries can be done with the use

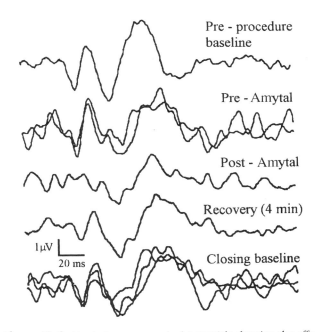

Figure 7-6. Cortical sensory evoked potentials showing the effect of an injection of amobarbital (Amytal) into a high thoracic feeding vessel in a patient undergoing embolization of vessels feeding a spinal cord tumor. (From Young W, Mollin D: Intraoperative somatosensory evoked potential monitoring of spinal surgery. *In* Desmedt JE [ed]: Neuromonitoring in Surgery. Amsterdam, Elsevier, 1989, pp 165-173.)

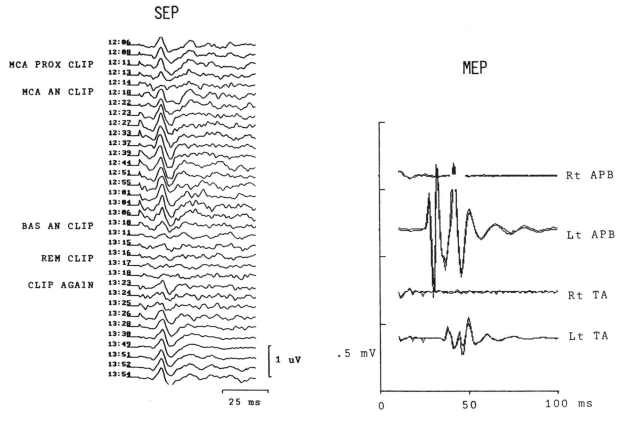

Figure 7–7. Cortical sensory evoked potentials (SEPs) recorded from a patient undergoing surgical repair of a middle cerebral artery (MCA) aneurysm and a basilar artery aneurysm, after stimulation of the right median nerve. The SEP disappeared temporarily after clipping the proximal middle cerebral artery (MCA PROX CLIP) and basilar aneurysm (BAS AN CLIP), but recovered fully by the end of the surgery. The patient woke with intact sensation, but with right-sided hemiplegia. Motor evoked potentials (MEPs) recorded postoperatively after transcranial magnetic stimulation showed the absence of a motor response from the right extremities (abductor pollicis brevis [APB] and tibialis anterior [TA] muscles). (From Deletis V: Intraoperative monitoring of the functional integrity of the motor pathways. *In* Devinski O, Beric A, Dogali M [eds]: Electrical and Magnetic Stimulation of the Brain and Spinal Cord. New York, Raven Press, 1993.)

of SSEPs. Stimulation of the median nerves at the wrist for middle cerebral artery surgery and stimulation of the posterior tibial nerve at the ankle for anterior cerebral artery surgery are appropriate. It has been found that monitoring SSEPs or auditory evoked potentials (AEPs) may not be useful during basilar artery surgery and the duration of ischemia should be limited to less than 10 minutes. Brain retraction during induced hypotension may have greater effect on the SSEPs, and the retractor may have to be adjusted for better outcome. False-negative SSEPs can occur in 2% to 22% of patients undergoing neurologic surgery. However, the number of false-positive SSEPs is low (2%). If there are changes in SSEPs, they indicate central nervous system (CNS) ischemia. Small areas of injury, motor area injury, or lenticulostriate area injury may not be associated with changes in SSEPs.

Auditory Evoked Potentials

The clinical application of AEPs includes the assessment of peripheral auditory function and the integrity of the central auditory pathways. They can be classified according to the relative latency of the components (short, middle, and long). The short-latency potentials can be identified in the first 10 ms following a click stimulus and have peaks that are positive at the vertex with reference to the ear. The waves are labeled with roman numerals I to V (Fig. 7–8). Waves I, III,

and V are constant, while waves II and IV may not always be identifiable in some normal tracings. The middle-latency potentials comprise the domain from 10 to 50 ms following the click stimulus and are labeled by their polarity at the vertex (positive [P] or negative [N]) and approximate latency in milliseconds, N20, P30, and N40, and sometimes called Na, Pa, and Nb, respectively. They are usually of the largest amplitude at the vertex. The long-latency potentials comprise the time domain from 50 to 500 ms following the click stimulus and are labeled by convention with the polarity and mean normal latency, N100 and P200. They are of maximal amplitude over the midline at the end and frontal regions.

Important short-latency potentials are generated by the eighth cranial nerve external to the brainstem (wave I), superior olivary nucleus and lateral lemniscus (wave III), and midbrain (wave V). The middle-latency peaks are probably generated from early cortical potentials, and long-latency potentials from later cortical excitation.

The most commonly used stimulus consists of clicks generated by applying a brief square wave to a calibrated earphone. Tone pips, which are brief tone bursts, have been employed to activate restricted portions of the basilar membrane of the cochlea for defining frequency-specific AEPs.

The most important measurements are wave I latency and interpeak I–III and III–V latencies. The usual rate of clicks for middle latency is the same as for short-latency potentials (8 to 10/second) and it is 1/second for long-latency potentials.

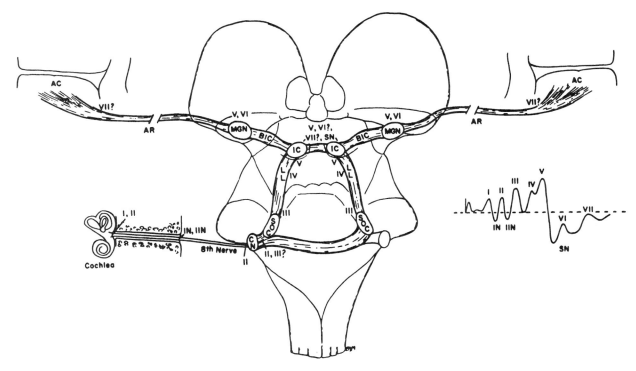

Figure 7–8. Schematic drawing of the auditory system and possible generators of different waves of the brainstem auditory evoked potential. See text for details. (From Legatt AD, Arezzo JC, Vaughan HG: Neurologic Clinics: Evoked Potentials. Philadelphia, WB Saunders, 1988.)

For recording, the electrodes are placed at the vertex and on the ear lobes. The ear electrode may be placed on the left (A1) and right ear lobe (A2) or on the left and right mastoid bone (M1, M2). All the AEPs, short-latency (SAEPs), middle-latency (MLAEPs), and late-latency potentials (LLAEPs) can be recorded with the same electrode placements. The parameters for obtaining AEPs are described in Table 7–2.

Age, sex, body temperature, and hearing can alter AEPs. Control AEPs can be recorded before monitoring during anesthesia and surgery. Abnormal AEPs can be seen in a number of conditions, for example, acoustic nerve lesions, cochlear lesions, pontomedullary lesions, lower brainstem lesions, upper brainstem lesions, and conditions with hearing loss. Some of the common conditions include multiple sclerosis, intramedullary and extramedullary brainstem tumors, coma from metabolic and structural causes, and some heredofamilial neurologic disorders.

Surgical Monitoring

Anesthetic agents have dose-dependent effects on AEPs.[25,26] Absolute latencies of waves III and V and I–III and I–V interpeak latencies increase with increasing inhaled concentrations of halothane, enflurane, and isoflurane. Intravenous induction agents like thiopental and propofol also may have an effect on AEPs. Middle-latency AEPs can be used for monitoring the depth of anesthesia.

Usefulness of Auditory Evoked Potentials During Surgical Procedures

AEPs are useful in monitoring during surgeries of cerebellopontine angle tumors, microvascular decompressions in the posterior fossa, and surgeries on the cavernous sinus with manipulation of the brainstem.[27–33] Usually, latency of peak V is affected. Interpeak latencies of I and III are preserved. By stimulation of the ear opposite to the side of surgery, as in acoustic neuroma, changes in latencies of peak V without changes of peak III indicated brainstem ischemia with surgical manipulation.[28] Hypotension during surgery may produce similar changes. Hypothermia may also produce changes in latencies of the waves.

Visual Evoked Potentials

The visual evoked potentials (VEPs) commonly used for monitoring are obtained using checkerboard pattern reversals at 2/second, recorded as midline occipital potentials. They are characterized by a major positive peak at a latency of 90 to 110 ms and amplitude of 10 mV, and this peak is referred to as P100. This large positive wave is preceded by a small negative peak at 60 to 80 ms (N75 or N1) and a negative peak following P100 (N145) (Fig. 7–9). Stroboscopic goggles are used for intraoperative monitoring.

Electrode placement for recording is midline occipital

Table 7–2. Parameters for Brainstem Auditory Evoked Potentials

Rate	8–10/s
Intensity	65 db SL
No. of trials	1000–4000
Low-frequency filter	10–30 Hz
High-frequency filter	2500–3000 Hz
Analysis time	15 ms
Montages	
Channel 1	Ai–Cz (vertex)
Channel 2	Ac–Cz (vertex)

SL, sensory level; Ai, ipsilateral ear; Ac, contralateral ear; Cz, central midline region.

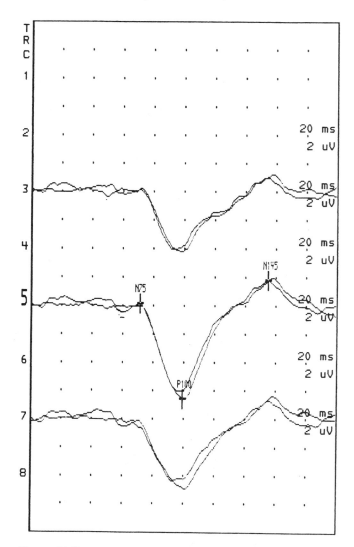

Figure 7–9. Normal visual evoked potentials using checkerboard pattern reversal at 2/second. The potentials include an initial small negative peak (N75) and a large positive peak (N100) followed by a negative peak (N145).

Table 7-3. Parameters for Visual Evoked Potentials Using Pattern Reversal Method

Pattern reversal rate	2/s
Check size	28–32 min of arc
No. of trials	100–200
Montages	
Channel 1	O1–Fz
Channel 2	O1–Fz
Channel 3	O2–Fz
Analysis period	250 s

O1, left occipital; O2, right occipital; Fz, frontal midline region.

Motor Evoked Potentials

Motor evoked potentials (MEPs) can be used to detect damage to motor cortex or motor pathway from motor cortex to the muscle. Because of the use of neuromuscular blocking drugs and the difficulty in monitoring the muscles, recording from spinal epidural space has been recommended. Stimulation of the motor cortex can be done by transcranial electric stimulation, stimulation of exposed motor cortex, or transcranial magnetic stimulation of motor cortex to the spinal cord. Although these methods are not commonly used, the details are described in textbooks on EPs.[1-3] The principle of magnetic stimulation is based on varying time or changing the magnetic field, thereby inducing an electric field that impedes the original magnetic field. A stationary magnetic field does not induce an electric field, whereas changing the magnetic field induces an electric field in a conductive medium. A typical magnetic stimulator consists of a power supply, a storage capacitor, and solid-state switching elements and a magnetic stimulating cord. A high-voltage power source is needed for stimulation. The magnetic stimulation is still not extensively used. The side effects include seizures, hormonal changes, and cognitive or memory changes.[38-40]

Monitoring EPs can give important and useful information during surgery involving the nervous system. This method of monitoring has not become popular because of the complexity and time involved in setting up the monitors, and interpretation of the evoked responses. Specially trained technicians, an anesthesiologist, or a neurologist should be available for monitoring and interpretation.

(Oz), at 5 cm above the inion; Fz, placed at 12 cm above the nasion; right occipital (O2), placed at 5 cm to the right of the Oz; and left occipital (O1), placed at 5 cm to the left of Oz. The parameters for recording VEPs are given in Table 7-3.

Abnormal VEPs may be due to technical problems; prechiasmal, chiasmal, or postchiasmal lesions; bilateral optical nerve lesions; or ocular lesions. A number of neurologic diseases involve the optic nerve or optic pathway.

Monitoring of VEPs under anesthesia is associated with some difficulties. Inhaled anesthetic drugs have dose-dependent effects on VEPs. Although VEPs are found to be extremely useful outside the operating room in the diagnosis of disease involving the optic nerve and its pathways, VEP monitoring is associated with difficulties in the operating room, giving a greater number of false-positive and false-negative results. VEP monitoring has been used in surgery involving the optic chiasm, pituitary gland, transsphenoidal surgeries, and frontotemporal and parieto-occipital areas.[34-37] The results of these studies have not clearly demonstrated the usefulness of VEPs for monitoring. In addition, anesthetic agents and temperature changes affect the VEPs markedly.

REFERENCES

1. Linden RD, Zapulla R, Shields CB: Intraoperative Evoked Potential Monitoring. Philadelphia, Lippincott-Raven, 1997, pp 601–689.
2. Misulis KE: Spehlomann's Evoked Potential Primer. Boston, Butterworth-Heinemann, 1994.
3. Nuwer MR: Evoked Potential Monitoring in the Operating Room. New York, Raven Press, 1986.
4. Loftus CM, Traynelis VC: Intraoperative Monitoring Techniques in Neurosurgery. New York, McGraw-Hill, 1994.
5. Deletis V: Evoked potentials. In Lake CL (ed): Clinical Monitoring for Anesthesia and Critical Care. Philadelphia, WB Saunders, 1994, pp 288–314.
6. Jones SJ: Evoked potentials in intraoperative monitoring. In Halliday JD (ed): Evoked Potentials in Clinical Testing. New York, Churchill Livingstone, 1986, pp 565–599.
7. Møller AR: Evoked Potentials in Intraoperative Monitoring. Baltimore, Williams & Wilkins, 1988.
8. Raudzens PA: Intraoperative monitoring of evoked potentials. Ann N Y Acad Sci 1982; 388:308–326.
9. American Electroencephalographic Society guidelines for clinical evoked potential studies. J Clin Neurophysiol 1986; 3(suppl 1): 43–92.

10. Sloan TB, Koht A: Depression of cortical somatosensory evoked potentials by nitrous oxide. Br J Anaesth 1985; 57:849–852.
11. Sebel PS, Erwin CW, Neville WK: Effects of halothane and enflurane on far and near field somatosensory evoked potentials. Br J Anaesth 1987; 59:1492–1496.
12. Pathak KS, Brown RH, Cascorbi HF, et al: Effects of fentanyl and morphine on intraoperative somatosensory cortical-evoked potentials. Anesth Analg 1984; 63:833–837.
13. Jones SJ, Howard L, Shawkak F: Criteria for detection and pathological significance of response decrement during spinal cord monitoring. *In* Ducker TB, Brown RH (eds): Neurophysiology and Standard of Spinal Cord Monitoring. New York, Springer-Verlag, 1988.
14. Mostegl A, Bauer R, Eichenauer M: Intraoperative somatosensory potential monitoring. A clinical analysis of 127 surgical procedures. Spine 1988; 13:396–400.
15. Ginsburg HH, Shetter AG, Raudzens PA: Postoperative paraplegia with preserved intraoperative somatosensory evoked potentials. J Neurosurg 1985; 63:296–300.
16. Lesser RP, Raudzens P, Lüders H, et al: Postoperative neurological deficits may occur despite unchanged intraoperative somatosensory evoked potentials. Ann Neurol 1986; 19:22–25.
17. Machida M, Weinstein SL, Yamada T, et al: Spinal cord monitoring: Electrophysiological measures of sensory and motor function during spinal surgery. Spine 1985; 10:407–413.
18. Ryan TP, Britt RH: Spinal and cortical somatosensory evoked potential monitoring during corrective spinal surgery with 108 patients. Spine 1986; 11:352–361.
19. Whittle IR, Johnston IH, Besser M: Recording of spinal somatosensory evoked potentials for intraoperative spinal cord monitoring. J Neurosurg 1986; 64:601–612.
20. Kaplan BJ, Friedman WA, Alexander JA, et al: Somatosensory evoked potentials monitoring of spinal cord ischemia during aortic operations. Neurosurgery 1986; 19:82–90.
21. Amantini A, Bartelli M, de Scisciolo G, et al: Monitoring of somatosensory evoked potentials during carotid endarterectomy. J Neurol 1992; 239:241–247.
22. Nargadine JR, Branston NM, Symon L: Central conduction time in primate brain ischemia—A study in baboons. Stroke 1980; 11:637–642.
23. Haupt WF, Horsch S: Evoked potentials monitoring in carotid surgery—A review of 994 cases. J Neurol 1992; 42:835–838.
24. Moorthy SS, Markand ON, Dilley R, et al: Somatosensory evoked response during carotid endarterectomy. Anesth Analg 1982; 61:879–883.
25. Samra SK, Lilly DJ, Rush NL, et al: Fentanyl anesthesia and human brainstem auditory evoked potentials. Anesthesiology 1984; 61:261–265.
26. Levine RA: Short latency auditory evoked potentials: Intraoperative application. Int Anesthesiol Clin 1990; 28:147–153.
27. Levine RA, Ojemann RG, Montgomery WW, et al: Monitoring auditory evoked potentials during acoustic neuroma surgery: Insights into the mechanism of hearing loss. Ann Otol Rhinol Laryngol 1984; 93:116.
28. Grundy BL, Lima A, Procopio PT, et al: Reversible evoked potential changes with retraction of 8th cranial nerve. Anesth Analg 1981; 60:835–838.
29. Radtke RA, Erwin W, Wilkins RH: Intraoperative brainstem auditory evoked potentials: Significant decrease in postoperative morbidity. J Neurol 1989; 39:187–191.
30. Daspit CP, Raudzens PA, Shetter AG: Monitoring of intraoperative auditory brainstem responses. Otolaryngol Head Neck Surg 1982; 90:108–116.
31. Schramm J, Mokrusch T, Fahlbusch R, et al: Detailed analysis of intraoperative changes monitoring brainstem acoustic evoked potentials. J Neurosurg 1988; 22:694–702.
32. Møller AR, Jannetta PJ, Møller MB: Neural generators of brainstem evoked potentials. Results from human intracranial recordings. Ann Otol 1981; 90:591–596.
33. Grundy BL, Jannetta PJ, Procopio PT, et al: Intraoperative monitoring of brainstem auditory evoked potentials. J Neurosurg 1982; 57:674–681.
34. Cedzich C, Schramm J, Mengedoht CF, et al: Factors that limit the use of flash visual evoked potentials for surgical monitoring. Electroencephalogr Clin Neurophysiol 1988; 71:142–145.
35. Wilson WB, Kirsch WM, Neville H, et al: Monitoring of visual function during parasellar surgery. Surg Neurol 1976; 5:323–329.
36. Jones SJ: The value of evoked potentials in surgical monitoring. *In* Cracco RQ, Bodis-Wollmer J (eds): Evoked Potentials. New York, ARL Press, 1986.
37. Costa e Silva J, Wang AD, Symon L: The application of visual evoked potentials during operations of the anterior visual pathway. Neurol Res 1985; 7:11–16.
38. Kandler R: Safety of transcranial magnetic stimulation. Lancet 1990; 335:469–470.
39. Homberg V, Netz J: Generalized seizures induced by transcranial magnetic stimulation of motor cortex. Lancet 1989; 2:1223.
40. Fauth C, Meyer BU, Prosiegel M, et al: Seizures induction and magnetic brain stimulation after stroke. Lancet 1992; 339:362.

8 Electroencephalography and Monitoring of Anesthetic Depth

Marc J. Bloom, M.D., Ph.D.

Although the main site of action of anesthesia is the brain, it is not routinely monitored in the operating room. It is generally assumed that without prior cerebral pathologic findings, maintaining adequate mean arterial blood pressure and oxygen saturation will assure that no harm will come to the brain.[1] Despite adequate blood pressure, cerebral ischemia can occur secondary to increases in intracranial pressure or changes in cerebrovascular resistances.[2] Since these cannot be routinely measured in the operating room, electroencephalography (EEG) offers a noninvasive way to monitor cerebral well-being. Monitoring for adequate cerebral perfusion is not the only application for intraoperative EEG monitoring. EEG can be used to monitor for the occurrence of seizures, and the degree of barbiturate burst suppression, and most recently the level of sedation produced by drugs.

Advances in technology have made intraoperative EEG monitoring easier and less costly, but interpretation and recognition of spurious results still requires a basic understanding of the recording methods and physiology of EEG.[3, 4]

Physiology of the Electroencephalogram

Although the electrical energy to produce EEG is generated by the separation of ions across the semipermeable membrane of the neuronal cell, EEG is not the product of propagated action potentials. Mylenization of axons tends to limit the spread of ionic current to a few hundred micrometers, making it impossible to record axon potentials on the scalp. Instead, EEG is derived from the summation of nearly synchronous depolarization of cell bodies and dentrites, secondary to neurotransmitter release (Fig. 8-1). The scalp tends to act as an averager of the positive and negative voltages from many cells and much of the signal is canceled out unless the activity is synchronous.[5]

Methods

Standard Multilead Electroencephalography

Standard raw EEG recording is done by placing as many as 21 electrodes on the scalp at locations standardized by the international 10-20 system[6] (Fig. 8-2). These electrodes can be used in pairs for bipolar recording or individually using a common reference (frequently, linked earlobes).[7] Referential montages have the advantage of allowing each electrode to produce its own channel of EEG. This reduces the number of electrodes that must be placed for multichannel recordings. Bipolar montages require two electrodes for each chan-

nel, but have the advantages of better regional selectivity and lower noise because signals common to both inputs of the differential amplifiers are rejected.[8] Various montages can be configured to examine particular regions or conditions of the brain.[9] Complex pattern recognition is required to derive diagnostic information from the analog waveforms, and this requires extensive training, usually in an apprenticeship.

Many types of electrodes are used for intraoperative EEG monitoring. The lowest-impedance and highest-quality signals can be obtained by using metallic cups attached to the scalp with collodion and filled with conductive gel. Although cups attached with collodion also have the advantage of secure attachment even in hair, the process is time-consuming, requiring at least 1 to 2 minutes for each electrode. All of the electrodes used must be made of the same metal to prevent bimetallic battery effects. Needle electrodes can be applied much more quickly and can be secured during anesthesia with a surgical skin staple, but the low surface area of these electrodes tends to produce higher impedances and may be prone to DC (direct current)-offset voltage secondary to polarization when used for extended periods.

While advances have been made in self-adhesive electrodes,[10] they cannot be applied to hair, thereby limiting the available montages. Several designs have recently been produced which have an entire montage of electrodes embedded in a cap[11] or meshwork which can be quickly pulled down over the head, but these cannot be used during surgery of the head or upper neck. No matter what kind of electrode is used, extreme care must be taken to carefully apply and secure the electrodes to minimize artifacts during the monitoring (Fig. 8-3).

Problems During Electroencephalographic Monitoring

The EEG is measured in microvolts, and is extremely susceptible to noise. Contamination of the EEG signal can lead to misinterpretation and failures in monitoring. Great care must be taken to identify and eliminate all sources of artifact.[12]

The most common source of noise in the EEG is from high electrode impedances. This may be due to improper site preparation, poor adhesion, mechanical disruption, desiccation, oxidation, or broken contacts. Fastidious attention must be paid to proper electrode application (Fig. 8-4). While accurate placement using the international 10-20 system is important for diagnostic testing, minor deviations in electrode placement rarely have significant impact on perioperative monitoring. Maintaining symmetry, however, is important for making comparisons between channels.

Impedance mismatch between electrodes is another po-

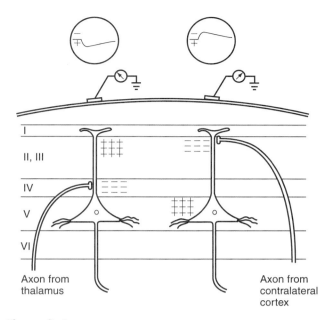

Figure 8–1. Underlying synaptic mechanisms produce positive or negative scalp potentials. Ascending thalamic input usually terminates in layer IV (left neuron), producing a positive surface potential. Intercortical connections typically terminate in superficial layers (right neuron), producing negative scalp potentials. Actual scalp potentials are the summation of the synchronous activity of many such neurons often sharing common input.

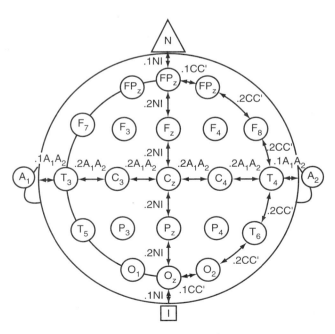

Figure 8–2. International 10–20 system for scalp electrode placement. Positions are determined by multiplying the distances from nasion to inion (NI), auditory canals ($A_1 A_2$) and hemicircumference (CC′) by 10% or 20%. Regions are named frontal pole (FP), frontal (F), central (C), parietal (P), occipital (O), and temporal (T), with odd numbers on the left and even numbers on the right.

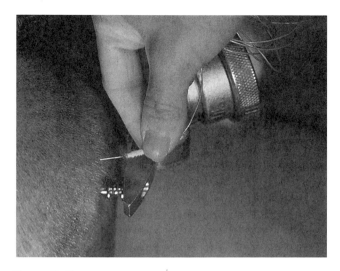

Figure 8–3. Photograph of needle electrode about to be inserted into the scalp.

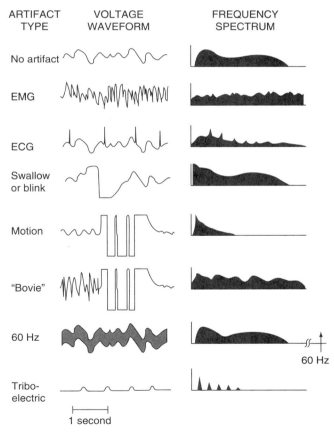

Figure 8–4. Stylized artifacts illustrated in both the time and frequency domains. Electromyogram adds wide-band noise, Electrocardiographic complexes appear in the frequency spectrum as blips at multiples of the heart rate. Blinks and motion add low-frequency artifacts. Electrocautery is wide-band, but usually just saturates the amplifiers. Power-line interference can be filtered out if not too large. (From Rampil IJ: A primer for EEG signal processing in anesthesia. Anesthesiology 1998; 89:980–1002.)

Table 8-1. Frequency Bands of the Electroencephalogram

Band	Frequency Range
Delta	<3.5 or 4 Hz
Theta	3.5–7.5 or 8 Hz
Alpha	7.5–13 Hz
Beta	>13 Hz (to 25–40 Hz)

tential source of artifact in EEG monitoring. All electrode impedances should be within 2000 Ω of each other to avoid decreasing the effectiveness of the differential amplifiers used to record the EEG.

The bane of every encephalographer's efforts is power-line noise. In the United States, AC (alternating current) power is supplied at 60 Hz. Although slightly above the usual range of frequencies of interest in EEG, this contaminant can be so large that it masks the actual EEG or appears as phantom signals at lower frequencies due to inadequate filtering before digitization. While "notch" filters around 60 Hz may help to lessen the problem, it is best to keep power lines and sources as far from the EEG electrodes as possible.

Another possible source of external noise is the ground line. Most EEG equipment uses an optically isolated amplifier to connect to the patient. This minimizes the risks of ground-line noise, but it can still cause problems in systems that have nonisolated circuits before the signal is digitized. Vibration and other forms of motion can create artifacts. Common sources of motion artifacts are pumps, ventilators, air-powered tools, and some suction devices.[13] Electrocautery uses kilovolts of electricity and it is not possible to record EEG while it is in use. The best systems are those that quickly reject signals contaminated with electrocautery and recover within a few seconds when it is discontinued.

Electroencephalographic Waveforms

Conventional EEG is recorded on a strip chart recorder at a rate of 30 mm/second. This generates about 360 pages per hour of recording. While such recordings are regarded as the gold standard for diagnostic purposes, there are significant problems with their use in the operating room. Interpretation requires specialized training.[8] The recording must be watched continuously, since looking back through the paper records while the paper is still moving is very challenging, and monitoring is only active while the paper is moving and must not be stopped. Quantitative analysis or comparison is impossible while the recording is being made, and annotation for later interpretation is limited. While newer digital instruments have begun to address these concerns, this methodology is not commonly used in the operating room. However, even in the computer-processed EEG monitors in use today, it is important to be able to constantly examine the raw analog EEG signal to recognize common artifacts and physiologic patterns such as slowing and burst suppression.

The clinically observed frequency range of EEG is 0.2 to 40 Hz. This frequency range is classically divided into bands describing various physiologic rhythms. The ranges are detailed in Table 8-1. The most common normal rhythm seen in awake EEG is the *alpha* rhythm, a steady wave in the 8- to 13-Hz range. This is typically seen in a resting subject with eyes closed. When this alpha rhythm is disrupted, particularly by excitation, a less synchronous, higher-frequency

beta rhythm is seen. With cortical depression or some other pathologic conditions, lower-frequency *theta* waves can be recorded, and at the most severe depressions, such as cerebral ischemia, very-low-frequency *delta* waves may be manifested. Particular pathologic morphologies of waveforms may also be present, the most common of these being various spikes and waves of epileptic conditions.

Compressed Spectral Arrays

The detailed examination of individual waveforms across many channels is usually not done in the setting of acute monitoring. Most of what is important in acute monitoring can be seen in a simplified display of amplitudes and frequencies.[14]

The initial method of compressing EEG spectral data into a more compact display was to compute the power spectrum from fast fourier transformation (FFT)[15] which converts the EEG signal from amplitude as a function of time to amplitude as a function of frequency. This is sometimes called shifting from the "time domain" to the "frequency domain," making it easier to see effects like "slowing" of dominant frequencies, and the loss of high-frequency components. It also helps the user to better assess the increase in low-frequency power often associated with EEG abnormalities. The individual spectra are computed every few seconds and then stacked or "compressed" into an array (compressed spectral array, CSA) for easy comparison of successive periods.[16]

Density-Modulated Spectral Arrays

There are problems with the CSA format. In order to keep the individual traces from crossing back and forth over each other, the separation of the traces much be kept fairly wide, thereby limiting the amount of time that can be displayed on a screen (Fig. 8-5). When the EEG is highly variable, this spacing must be increased even further, sometimes limiting the screen to only a few minutes of CSA. If, instead of encoding the amplitude as the height of a trace, it is represented by the intensity or color of a dot, then the spectral

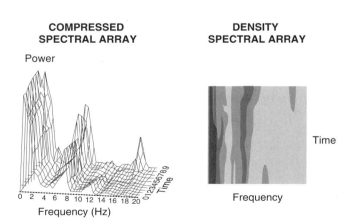

Figure 8-5. Compressed spectral array (CSA) and density spectral array (DSA) of the same data. Rapid changes and subtle shifts are easier to assess in the DSA and can display more time in the same amount of space.

array can be further compressed without confusion or lack of interpretability. This is the density spectral array (DSA).[17]

One problem with the DSA is that when the amplitudes of the EEG get very low, the dots on the display are very few and pale. By having the dots represent the percent of total power during that period, one can create a spectral percent power array (SPPA) which makes seeing shifts in frequency distribution easier, but total power must then be presented separately on the display.

Indications for Electroencephalographic Monitoring

The most obvious reason for EEG monitoring is to assure cerebral well-being when a full neurologic examination cannot be done.[18, 19] In particular, EEG monitoring has been used to detect the need for shunt placement during carotid endarterectomy.[20-22] Although insertion of a shunt can provide some blood flow around a cross-clamped carotid artery, insertion of a shunt carries risks of embolization and malfunction.[23] Presence of a shunt also limits the exposure of the artery, making a clean intimal repair more difficult. EEG monitoring allows the avoidance of the risks of shunting in the 85% or more of patients who have adequate collateral flow without it. EEG changes associated with carotid cross-clamping are usually not subtle. The temporal association of any perceptible change that persists for more than half a minute after the clamp is applied can be considered indicative of the need for a shunt.[24] This conservative approach will only increase the incidence of shunting by a few percent over the more stringent criteria used by experts.[25]

Another application where EEG monitoring for cerebral ischemia appears to be of value is during cardiac surgery. Various studies have found that neuropsychiatric deficits may be present in 40% to 70% of patients after cardiac surgery,[26-28] but that rate can be lowered to less than 4% by aggressive intervention when EEG monitoring indicates cerebral ischemia.[29-31]

The number of channels that should be monitored depends on the degree to which injury may be limited to a small region rather than occurring globally.[25] Highest regional sensitivity is achieved by using 16 to 32 channels of EEG, which can be used to create an interpolated map of the cortical surface.[32] For acute monitoring of perioperative changes, eight or even four channels may be sufficient to see changes caused by sudden hemodynamic shifts.[33] Monitoring of two channels will allow only the detection of hemispheric differences.

A second indication for EEG monitoring is when the brain is believed to be at risk for ischemia and cerebral protection measures are applied such as barbiturate therapy.[34] While the optimal dose of barbiturate is not known, the usual endpoint used is the production of periods of suppression in the EEG.[35, 36] The dose necessary to produce this suppression may vary 10-fold from patient to patient and cannot be chosen without monitoring the EEG.[37]

Perioperative seizure activity may not be easy to detect, especially if the seizures do not involve the motor areas or muscle relaxants are being used. EEG monitoring allows immediate seizure detection and can help to guide effective therapy.[38-41] EEG monitoring can help to assess the progress and prognosis of patients in coma.[39] One of the worst prognostic signs in comatose patients is a monotonous unreactive EEG.[42, 43]

EEG monitoring must be applied with caution because, while sensitivity is high, specificity can be significantly affected by anesthetic technique and analysis methods. EEG changes occur at variable times and in varying severity. Quantitative measures of EEG are imperfect and should not be used as an isolated guide to therapy.[44]

One of the most recent and increasingly prominent applications of EEG is to measure the effects of anesthetics.

Monitoring of Anesthetic Depth: The Bispectral Monitor

Indications

The use of an EEG-derived pharmadynamic index to guide dosing of sedative drugs requires a major shift in the clinician's approach to applied pharmacodynamics. This new approach can be used in several circumstances.

In the intraoperative setting, monitoring of anesthetic or sedative effects allows a differentiation between the need for deeper hypnosis, more analgesia, or direct autonomic control. Instead of relying on predictions from population statistics (such as minimum alveolar concentration, MAC), the direct measurement of the functional effects of the drugs on the brain allows individualized pharmacologic management.

In the intensive care unit, monitoring of sedation is made more difficult because the patient is not under the constant assessment of an anesthesiologist.[45] Instead, nurses are given vague guidelines for sedation and these are applied in an inconsistent manner according to the priorities and judgments of a nurse who may not completely understand the pharmacology. This is particularly problematic in patients receiving muscle relaxants, because it is nearly impossible to assess the level of sedation in patients who cannot move.

Another application for an EEG monitor is to guide the dosing of barbiturates for cerebral "protection" therapy. Reliable control of barbiturate coma is not possible without a constant measure of the degree of EEG suppression.[37, 46, 47] Continuous recording of raw EEG data is cumbersome and impractical, but the BIS monitor is easy to apply and maintain without the constant attendance of a technician. It provides a continuous and trended value of the suppression ratio (SR), reflecting the percent of time the EEG is nearly isoelectric over the past minute.

Individualized Dosing

Drug dosing schemes in most clinical practice are anything but optimized for individual patients. Clinicians choose a standard effective dose (e.g., ED_{50} or ED_{95}), guess the degree to which a patient is tolerant or sensitive to the drug, and then adjust the dose by trial and error. The major goal is to avoid toxicity while achieving some therapeutic endpoint that is poorly defined. The drugs are most commonly given as a bolus, for convenience of administration, or by continuous infusion in cases where infusion pumps are available and appropriate.

In an effort to move one step closer to a physiologic control point, target-controlled infusion systems that employ pharmacokinetic models derived from population statistics have been recently introduced in Europe, but these systems cannot adjust for interpatient variability.[48] Efforts at quantifying the "depth of anesthesia" from EEG have met with limited success because the metric of anesthesia is not uniquely defined.

Anesthesia is NOT Just One Thing. While the concept of MAC has been stretched to indicate the level of a particular anesthetic, even the definitions of MAC vary. Furthermore, there are different anesthetic goals for different patients, different anesthetic approaches by different clinicians, and different goals at different times in the individual case.

Components of Anesthetic Depth

There are at least four components to what is commonly referred to as "anesthetic depth":

1. Sedation or hypnosis produces unconsciousness or a state of oblivion.
2. Analgesia reduces the somatic responses to painful stimuli.
3. Amnesia is either achieved by direct pharmacologic therapy or indirectly by achieving unconsciousness.
4. The blockade of autonomic reflexes may be a byproduct of the previous conditions or addressed directly.

In an effort to characterize the effects of anesthetic agents, many monometric parameters from the EEG have been investigated. Among them are median frequency, an indication of the overall frequency content of the EEG; the spectral edge frequency, an indication of the highest frequencies present in the EEG; and various power bands, to describe the redistribution of power across frequencies of the EEG. None has been found to have universal acceptability. The reason is that there are many confounding problems in the application of quantitative analysis to EEG. Pharmacologic effects on the EEG are time-varying. EEG differs from region to region in the brain and the locus of anesthetic effect is unknown. Most drugs have unique effects on EEG, making a universal descriptor difficult to find. Despite investigation for over 30 years, the "magic number" to describe anesthetic effects on the EEG has eluded definition. No single number was found to describe the complex signal, but when two or three descriptors were chosen post hoc, they could be 85% to 90% correct. Even this, however, was insufficient to be of practical clinical use.

Statistically Derived Indices

To overcome the problems discussed above, statistically derived multiparametric indices have been developed:

- The Bispectral Index (BIS index)[49] has been the most commercially successful so far.
- The Midlatency Auditory Evoked Response Index has shown some success in Great Britain.[50, 51]
- Autoregressive models of MAC have been incorporated into a machine called the Narcograph.[52]

Although unproven at this time, neural network models appear to hold promise of an alternative method to classify the EEG.[53, 54]

The Bispectral Index

The BIS index was designed to reflect the common sedative effects of anesthetic drugs in a reliable monotonic fashion. The BIS index was derived statistically and optimized to classify EEG of observed sedation states, which were defined behaviorally. It has been validated for many drugs (Fig. 8–6A and B). To understand the BIS index one must first understand the *bispectrum,* which is included as a component in the index. The bispectrum (B) is defined as

$$B(f_1 \cdot f_2) = X(f_1) \cdot X(f_2) \cdot X^*(f_1 + f_2)$$

where X^* is the complex conjugate. The bicoherence is the bispectrum normalized for differences in power at various frequencies by dividing by the real triple product. A term is then derived from the bicoherence that describes the relative synchrony of fast and slow regions of the bispectrum.

Once the component parameters were selected to characterize the features of the EEG, a discriminant function was derived to classify segments into states defined by the Modified Observer's Assessment of Alertness/Sedation Scale. The scale is shown in Table 8–2. The performance of the derived index is shown in Table 8–3. Several results are of particular note in the table. For propofol, the correlation coefficients are higher for the BIS index than even the measured arterial blood concentrations. This is due to the fact that the pharmacodynamics (the response of the brain to a given drug concentration) are significantly different between individuals.

Enhancements

Subsequent versions of the BIS index have included several enhancements. Early versions used prediction of movement as the endpoint. The performance of this index was inconsistent and prompted a shift to better-defined sedation levels. This greatly improved the performance of the index. The BIS index has been further improved by eliminating artifacts and other errors in the data used to define the discriminant function, by improved artifact detection and rejection, by revised components for burst suppression, and by recognizing and eliminating electrocardiographic (ECG) contamination.

Electromyographic (EMG) contamination can be particularly problematic. Electrodes placed over the temporalis and frontalis muscles can pick up large broad-band signals that extend down into the range of beta rhythm EEG (16 to 40 Hz). While the amplitudes of higher frequencies, up to 300 Hz, can be displayed and act to alert the user to possible artifactual elevation of the BIS index, current versions of the software do not try to compensate for this contamination.

A BIS index value above 80 indicates a high probability of the patient responding to a command. The probability then falls sharply (for all sedative agents), reaching a very low probability of response below a BIS index of 50. Since the BIS index was statistically derived to correlate with response to command and *not* specifically to recall, the variance between drugs is wider for recall but nonetheless falls to very low probabilities below 80, long before the usual endpoint for unconsciousness (Figs. 8–7 and 8–8).

Use of the BIS Index in Practice

To make optimal use of the BIS index, one must not only understand what it is, but also what it is NOT. In particular, the BIS index is not a "MAC-meter." That is, it does not predict the likelihood of movement in response to an incision, or to any other noxious stimulus, for that matter. Furthermore, it is not a *predictor* of any future behavior, but rather an indicator of the level of sedation over the past minute. It is still the task of the clinician, now armed with information about where the patient's level of consciousness was over the past minute, the sequence and timing of drugs given, and the impending level of noxious stimuli, to predict what the patient's response will be.

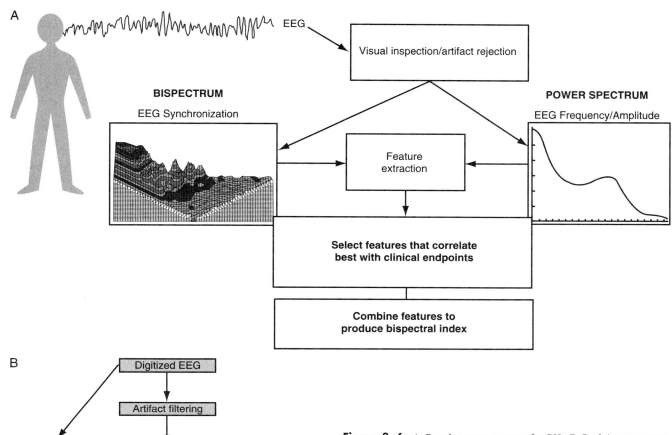

Figure 8-6. *A*, Development process for BIS. *B*, Real-time computation used in monitoring. Analog electroencephalography is first digitized and then processed to detect and remove artifacts. The signal is then analyzed for suppression detection and also fast Fourier transformed (FFT). The suppression information is used to compute the burst suppression ratio (BSR) and to quantify quasi-suppression (QUASI). The FFT is used to compute a beta power ratio and also used to compute the bispectrum, from which the relative synchrony of fast and slow wave is derived (Synch Fast Slow). All of these components are combined using multipliers derived from discriminant analysis, with the result scaled to 0 to 100.

While it is true that cerebral ischemia can cause a loss of consciousness, and that the BIS index may consequently decrease, significant cerebral ischemia can occur without a notable decrease in the BIS index. Thus the BIS index cannot be considered a reliable detector of cerebral ischemia. Lastly, as with any monitor used in patient care, failures and dysfunction can occur which require clinical judgment as to whether the displayed BIS index value is consistent with the entire clinical state (Figs. 8-9 and 8-10).

Table 8-2. Modified Observer's Assessment of Alertness/
Sedation Scale

Response	Score
Responds readily to name spoken in normal tone	5
Lethargic response to name spoken in normal tone	4
Responds only after name is called loudly or repeatedly	3
Responds only after mild prodding or shaking	2
Does not respond to mild prodding or shaking	1
Does not respond to noxious stimulus	0

Anesthetic Management Using Bispectral Monitoring

To effectively apply BIS monitoring to anesthetic management, the clinician should use a systematic approach to the individual components of the anesthetic. Using whatever drug is chosen for the sedative-hypnotic component, the delivery should be adjusted until an average BIS index value of 50 is obtained. Then, to minimize the capability of noxious stimuli to produce an arousal response, the dose of analgesic should be adjusted to decrease the maximum-to-

Table 8-3. Correlation Coefficients to Sedation Score

Drug (n)	Bispectral Index	Target [ ]	Actual [ ]	Log [ ]
Propofol (399)	.88	−.81	−.78	−.77
Isoflurane (70)	.85	−.89	−.89	−.85
Midazolam (50)	.76	−.77	−.75	−.65
Alfentanil (50)	.44	−.17	−.25	−.24

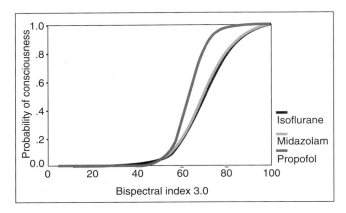

Figure 8-7. Actual logistic regression curves show nearly identical steep response for sedative drugs. Propofol difference was not statistically significant. Consciousness was defined as response to command.

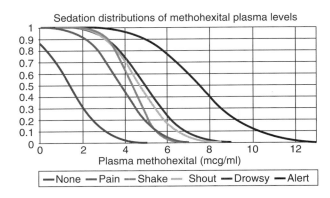

Figure 8-9. All intermediate levels of sedation fall in the same range of methohexital plasma level, making it impossible to predict the level of sedation even if the pharmacokinetic models could produce a precise targeted plasma concentration.

minimum variation over a few minutes to less than 10. If otherwise unexplained sympathetic activity produces tachycardia or hypertension, a trial of additional analgesic may be appropriate before directly treating the autonomic responses.

Conversely, if hypotension occurs, it may be appropriate to decrease dose of analgesic, while assessing the volume status of the patient and treating with sympathetic agonists. To optimize the emergence benefits of BIS monitoring, the sedative dosing should be decreased to bring the BIS index up toward 65 during closure. If the BIS index rises above 70 too soon, a short-acting sedative (inhalation agent, lidocaine, propofol, etc.) can be used to avoid premature emergence.

As long as the patient does not have complete blockade of the neuromuscular junction, respiratory effort may be observed as the PCO_2 is allowed to rise toward 40 mm Hg. If the respiratory rate is above normal, this can be used as a guide to supplementation of analgesia during emergence. The continued rise in the BIS index will assure a rapid emergence without the need to withhold narcotics in an effort to arouse the patient with pain.

Once sedation and analgesia have been controlled at ap-

propriate levels, any remaining hemodynamic responses can be directly controlled using vasoactive or direct autonomic drugs, thus minimizing cardiovascular instability during emergence.

Pitfalls and Caveats

When using BIS monitoring, one must be aware that as with any other instrument, spurious readings are possible. In the case of the BIS monitor, in order to minimize the chance of a patient being conscious with a low BIS index reading, it is designed to "fail upward." Therefore, if other clinical signs make the anesthesia provider suspicious that the level of unconsciousness is significantly lower than the BIS index indicates, one should look for possible sources of spuriously high BIS index values.

The most common cause of spurious BIS index values is noise contaminating the EEG signal. High impedance or poor contact of the electrodes frequently causes this. The electrode impedances should be tested immediately and should be less than 2000 Ω for highest reliability of the BIS index. If the impedances are higher than this, each contact

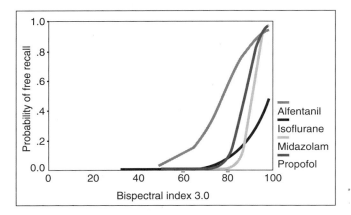

Figure 8-8. Logistic regression curves for free recall are not as drug-independent since that was not the endpoint the discriminant function was optimized for. Free recall was defined as the ability to remember, without a cue, words or images previously presented.

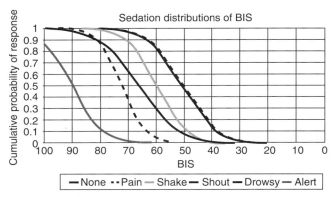

Figure 8-10. Data from the same methohexital study as in Figure 8-9. Each level of sedation falls in a separate Bispectral Index range of (BIS) values, making it possible to choose a specific range of values for a desired level of sedation.

CHOOSING AN APPROPRIATE BIS LEVEL

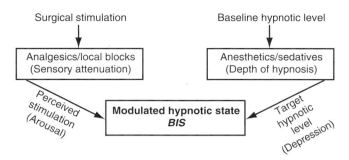

- The balance between stimulation and sensory suppression is critical
- Patient arousal can occur at any hypnotic level if stimulation is not blocked
- Patients can be maintained at light hypnotic levels (BIS 55–65) if the perceived levels of stimulation are minimal
- Changes in BIS in response to stimulation can provide an alternative real-time measure of patient reactiveness under anesthesia

Figure 8–11. Choosing an appropriate Bispectral Index level.

point should be pressed firmly until a small amount of conductive jelly is extruded. It is important to examine the raw EEG waveform for obvious forms of artifact such as ECG and 60 Hz power contamination. These sources should be sought out and eliminated if possible.

Another source of contamination causing spuriously elevated BIS index values is EMG activity from the frontalis muscle directly beneath the BIS electrodes. Because this EMG activity occurs in frequencies all the way down into the beta rhythm EEG range, it may be erroneously interpreted as an arousal response. In the event that EMG activity is recorded, a small dose of neuromuscular relaxant can be used, if not otherwise contraindicated, to see if BIS index values return to expected values. In earlier versions of the BIS software, there was a problem of brief periods of burst suppression causing artificial elevations in the BIS index, but this has been eliminated in the newer version of the calculation.

If none of the above reasons can be found for a suspiciously high BIS index value, a small dose of drug with strong sedative properties (e.g., propofol, thiopental, or halogenated gas) should be given and the BIS index watched for a prompt decrease. If this occurs, then the patient likely needed more sedation than was initially suspected.

Paradoxical Arousal Response

Although almost all erroneous BIS index values are too high, there is one condition that will cause the BIS index to suddenly drop to low values even though the patient's level of sedation is actually decreasing. Since the condition produces a pattern of intense slow-wave activity characteristic of a deep level of sedation, it has been referred to as a "paradoxical arousal" response. It is usually seen at a light anesthetic level, and usually in the setting of minimal analgesia. It can possibly be provoked by a strong noxious stimulus, and typically has a very sudden onset and resolution. It is best treated by a bolus of narcotics, which will "paradoxically"

return the BIS index to the elevated value it usually began with. Unless a sudden and immediate arousal to consciousness is desired, one should NOT decrease sedation further, and additional sedative may be indicated if imminent emergence is not planned.

Control of the Opiate Dosing

BIS index values are not directly influenced by opiates. Therefore, choosing appropriate doses of opiates for intraoperative analgesia requires other strategies. Most commonly, the clinician chooses a dose based on population ranges scaled to body weight. This is usually done without any direct measurement of a response variable. A loading bolus is often followed by either intermittent incremental doses or a continuous infusion. Recently, pharmacokinetic models have been available to predict the expected plasma concentration of an average patient, but adjustment is not made for an individual patient's deviation from the average.

Recently it has been reported that the variance in BIS index readings appears to have useful information for adjusting the opiate infusion.[55] Large swings in BIS (>10) over 1 to 2 minutes suggest the need for increased analgesia.

Summary

Clinical utility studies have found that BIS monitoring–managed anesthetics offer significant advantages over standard practice without BIS index measurement.[56] Where BIS index values have been continuously recorded, there has never been a case of awareness without values above 75 near the time of awareness, and only one anecdotal case has been verified of potential awareness with a BIS index less than 70. This patient had an unusual and abnormal EEG at baseline.[57] Knowing how much sedative is required to keep an individual patient unconscious avoids the need to use a much higher dose (e.g., ED$_{95}$) to allow for interpatient variability. By avoiding higher maintenance doses and monitoring the speed of emergence, more reliable times of emergence are obtained,[58] and the phenomenon of the patient who unexpectedly fails to emerge is all but eliminated.

Observation of the BIS index response to doses of sedative drugs allows the detection of patients with unusual tolerance or oversensitivity to these and other drugs. This greatly enhances the clinician's ability to tailor the dose of drugs to the individual, using a more objective measure than guessing by stereotype or medical history.[59] In the case of critically ill and unstable patients, the ability to determine a sufficient anesthetic dose helps to avoid hypotension while guiding the need for further amnestic therapy.

Finally, in the course of using BIS monitoring routinely, the clinician may be struck by the magnitude of the interpatient variability in pharmacodynamics. The potency, onset, and duration of a drug may vary more than an order of magnitude from patient to patient, making one wonder how we have seen such remarkable safety and reliability in routine anesthetic management.

REFERENCES

1. Stockard JJ, Bickford RG, Schauble JF: Pressure-dependent cerebral ischemia during cardiopulmonary bypass. Neurology 1973; 23:521–529.

2. Sundt TM, Sharbrough FW, Piepgras DG: Correlation of cerebral blood flow and electroencephalographic changes during carotid endarterectomy with results of surgery and hemodynamics of cerebral ischemia. Mayo Clin Proc 1981; 56:533–543.

3. Levy WJ, Shapiro HM, Maruchak G, et al: Automated EEG processing for intraoperative monitoring: A comparison of techniques. Anesthesiology 1980; 53:223–236.

4. Nuwer MR: Intraoperative electroencephalography [review]. J Clin Neurophysiol 1993; 10:437–444.

5. Delucchi M, Garoutte B, Aird R: The scalp as an electroencephalographic averager. Electroencephalogr Clin Neurophysiol 1962; 14:191–196.

6. Jasper H: The ten-twenty electrode system of the International Federation. Electroencephalogr Clin Neurophysiol 1958; 10:371–375.

7. American Electroencephalographic Society: Guideline one: Minimum technical requirements for performing clinical electroencephalography. J Clin Neurophysiol 1994; 11:2–5.

8. Nuwer MR, Daube J, Fischer C, et al: Neuromonitoring during surgery. Report of an IFCN Committee [see comments]. Electroencephalogr Clin Neurophysiol 1993; 87:263–276.

9. Rampil IJ: What every neuroanesthesiologist should know about electroencephalograms and computerized monitors. In Bissonnette B (ed): Cerebral Protection, Resuscitation, and Monitoring: A Look in the Future of Neuroanesthesia. Philadelphia, WB Saunders, 1996, pp 683–718.

10. Jopling M, Lang E, Embree P, et al: An evaluation of the aspect "ZIPprep" surface electrode. Anesth Analg 1995; 80:SCA90.

11. Blom J, Annevelt M: An electrode cap tested. Electroencephalogr Clin Neurophysiol 1982; 54:591–594.

12. Barlow JS: Artifact processing (rejection and minimization) in EEG data processing. In Lopes da Silva FH, Storm van Leeuwen W, Remond A (eds): Clinical Applications of Computer Analysis of EEG and other Neurophysiological Signals. Amsterdam, Elsevier, 1986, pp 15–62.

13. Levy WJ, Shapiro HM, Meathe E: The identification of rhythmic EEG artifacts by power-spectrum analysis. Anesthesiology 1980; 53:505–507.

14. Pichlmayr I, Lehmkuhl P, Lips U: EEG Atlas for Anesthesiologists. New York, Springer-Verlag, 1987.

15. Blackman R, Tukey J: The Measurement of Power Spectra. New York, Dover, 1958.

16. Bickford RG, Fleming N, Billinger T: Compression of EEG data. Trans Am Neurol Assoc 1971; 96:118–122.

17. Fleming RA, Smith NT: An inexpensive device for analyzing and monitoring the electroencephalogram. Anesthesiology 1979; 50: 456–460.

18. Sharbrough FW, Messick JM Jr, Sundt TM Jr: Correlation of continuous electroencephalograms with cerebral blood flow measurements during carotid endarterectomy. Stroke 1973; 4: 674–683.

19. Sundt TM Jr: The ischemic tolerance of neural tissue and the need for monitoring and selective shunting during carotid endarterectomy. Stroke 1983; 14:93–98.

20. Grady RE, Weglinski MR, Sharbrough FW, et al: Correlation of regional cerebral blood flow with ischemic electroencephalographic changes during sevoflurane–nitrous oxide anesthesia for carotid endarterectomy. Anesthesiology 1998; 88:892–897.

21. Plestis KA, Loubser P, Mizrahi EM, et al: Continuous electroencephalographic monitoring and selective shunting reduces neurologic morbidity rates in carotid endarterectomy. J Vasc Surg 1997; 25:620–628.

22. Ballotta E, Dagiau G, Saladini M, et al: Results of electroencephalographic monitoring during 369 consecutive carotid artery revascularizations. Eur Neurol 1997; 37:43–47.

23. Jansen C, Moll FL, Vermeulen FE, et al: Continuous transcranial Doppler ultrasonography and electroencephalography during carotid endarterectomy: A multimodal monitoring system to detect intraoperative ischemia. Ann Vasc Surg 1993; 7:95–101.

24. Facco E, Deriu GP, Dona B, et al: EEG monitoring of carotid endarterectomy with routine patch-graft angioplasty: An experience in a large series. Neurophysiol Clin 1992; 22:437–446.

25. Chiappa KH, Burke SR, Young RR: Results of electroencephalographic monitoring during 367 carotid endarterectomies. Use of a dedicated minicomputer. Stroke 1979; 10:381–388.

26. Sotaniemi K: Prediction of cerebral outcome after extracorporeal circulation. Acta Neurol Scand 1982; 66:697–704.

27. Sotaniemi K: Five-year neurological and EEG outcome after open-heart surgery. J Neurol Neurosurg Psychiatry 1985; 48: 569–575.

28. Sotaniemi KA, Juolasmaa A, Hokkanen ET: Neuropsychologic outcome after open-heart surgery. Arch Neurol 1981; 38:2–8.

29. Arom KV, Cohen DE, Strobl FT: Effect of intraoperative intervention on neurological outcome based on electroencephalographic monitoring during cardiopulmonary bypass. Ann Thorac Surg 1989; 48:476–483.

30. Edmonds HL Jr, Rodriguez RA, Audenaert SM, et al: The role of neuromonitoring in cardiovascular surgery [review]. Cardiothorac Vasc Anesth 1996; 10:15–23.

31. Edmonds HL Jr, Griffiths LK, van der Laken J, et al: Quantitative electroencephalographic monitoring during myocardial revascularization predicts postoperative disorientation and improves outcome [see comments]. J Thorac Cardiovasc Surg 1992; 103:555–563.

32. Duffy FH: Topographic Mapping of Brain Electrical Activity. Boston, Butterworth, 1986.

33. Craft RM, Losasso TJ, Perkins WJ, et al: EEG monitoring for cerebral ischemia during carotid endarterectomy (CEA): How much is enough? (abstract). Anesthesiology 1994; 81:A214.

34. Nussmeier NA, Arlund C, Slogoff S: Neuropsychiatric complications after cardiopulmonary bypass: Cerebral protection by a barbiturate. Anesthesiology 1986; 64:165–170.

35. Nehls DG, Todd MM, Spetzler RF, et al: A comparison of the cerebral protective effects of isoflurane and barbiturates during temporary focal ischemia in primates. Anesthesiology 1987; 66: 453–464.

36. Hicks RG, Kerr DR, Horton DA: Thiopentone cerebral protection under EEG control during carotid endarterectomy. Anaesth Intensive Care 1986; 14:22–28.

37. Winer JW, Rosenwasser RH, Jimenez F: Electroencephalographic activity and serum and cerebrospinal fluid pentobarbital levels in determining the therapeutic end point during barbiturate coma. Neurosurgery 1991; 29:739–741; discussion 741–742.

38. Marino R Jr, Radvany J, Huck FR, et al: Selective electroencephalograph-guided microsurgical callosotomy for refractory generalized epilepsy. Surg Neurol 1990; 34:219–228.

39. Nuwer MR: Electroencephalograms and evoked potentials. Monitoring cerebral function in the neurosurgical intensive care unit. Neurosurg Clin North Am 1994; 5:647–659.

40. Tasker RC, Boyd SG, Harden A, et al: EEG monitoring of prolonged thiopentone administration for intractable seizures and status epilepticus in infants and young children. Neuropediatrics 1989; 20:147–153.

41. Fiol ME, Gates JR, Mireles R, et al: Value of intraoperative EEG changes during corpus callosotomy in predicting surgical results. Epilepsia 1993; 34:74–78.

42. Bricolo A, Faccioli F, Grosslercher JC, et al: Electrophysiological monitoring in the intensive care unit. Electroencephalogr Clin Neurophysiol Suppl 1987; 39:255–263.

43. Bricolo A, Turazzi S, Faccioli F, et al: Clinical application of compressed spectral array in long-term EEG monitoring of comatose patients. Electroencephalogr Clin Neurophysiol 1978; 45: 211–225.

44. Adams DC, Heyer EJ, Emerson RG, et al: The reliability of quantitative electroencephalography as an indicator of cerebral ischemia [see comments]. Anesth Analg 1995; 81:80–83.

45. De Deyne C, Struys M, Decruyenaere J, et al: Use of continuous bispectral EEG monitoring to assess depth of sedation in ICU patients. Intensive Care Med 1998; 24:1294–1298.

46. Turcant A, Delhumeau A, Premel-Cabic A, et al: Thiopental pharmacokinetics under conditions of long-term infusion. Anesthesiology 1985; 63:50–54.

47. Kim JH, Kim SH, Yoo SK, et al: The effects of mild hypothermia on thiopental-induced electroencephalogram burst suppression. J Neurosurg Anesthesiol 1998; 10:137–141.

48. Kenny GN, White M: A portable target controlled propofol infusion system. Int J Clin Monit Comput 1992; 9:179–182.

49. Rampil IJ: A primer for EEG signal processing in anesthesia [see comments]. Anesthesiology 1998; 89:980–1002.

50. Jordan C, Weller C, Thornton C, et al: Monitoring evoked poten-

tials during surgery to assess the level of anaesthesia. J Med Eng Technol 1995; 19:77–79.

51. Mantzaridis H, Kenny GN: Auditory evoked potential index: A quantitative measure of changes in auditory evoked potentials during general anaesthesia. Anaesthesia 1997; 52:1030–1036.

52. Bender R, Schultz B, Schultz A, et al: I: Identification of EEG patterns occurring in anesthesia by means of autoregressive parameters. Biomed Tech (Berl) 1991; 36:236–240.

53. Muthuswamy J, Roy RJ: The use of fuzzy integrals and bispectral analysis of the electroencephalogram to predict movement under anesthesia. IEEE Trans Biomed Eng 1999; 46:291–299.

54. Sharma A, Roy RJ: Design of a recognition system to predict movement during anesthesia. IEEE Trans Biomed Eng 1997; 44:505–511.

55. Iselin-Chaves IA, Flaishon R, Sebel PS, et al: The effect of the interaction of propofol and alfentanil on recall, loss of con-sciousness, and the Bispectral Index. Anesth Analg 1998; 87:949–955.

56. Gan TJ, Glass PS, Windsor A, et al: Bispectral case monitoring allows faster emergence and improved recovery from propofol, alfentanil, and nitrous oxide anesthesia. BIS Utility Study Group. Anesthesiology 1997; 87:808–815.

57. Schnider TW, Luginbuhl M, Petersen-Felix S, et al: Unreasonably low bispectral index values in a volunteer with genetically determined low-voltage electroencephalographic signal (letter). Anesthesiology 1998; 89:1607–1608.

58. Song D, Joshi GP, White PF: Titration of volatile anesthetics using bispectral index facilitates recovery after ambulatory anesthesia. Anesthesiology 1997; 87:842–848.

59. Sebel PS, Lang E, Rampil IJ, et al: A multicenter study of bispectral electroencephalogram analysis for monitoring anesthetic effect. Anesth Analg 1997; 84:891–899.

9 Monitoring Intracranial Pressure

Wayne K. Marshall, M.D.
Carlos U. Arancibia, M.D.
Charles L. Williams, M.D.

The goal of any anesthetic technique for neurologic surgery is to create the best environment for surgery while preserving neurologic function. Although preoperative brain function can be determined with a routine neurologic examination that includes memory, cognition, sensation, motor strength, cranial nerve integrity, cerebellar tests, and level of consciousness, the patient's cooperation is generally required. Except during certain forms of regional anesthesia, such tests are impossible intraoperatively and in the early portions of the recovery period, so alternative methods of monitoring brain function have evolved.

Brain function directly depends on cerebral blood flow (CBF) and the delivery of oxygen and nutrients to support metabolism and cellular electrical activity. Anesthetic agents, intracranial pressure (ICP), hydrogen ion concentrations, and the partial pressures of oxygen and carbon dioxide may affect CBF. Intraoperative neurologic monitoring can therefore be based on evaluation of the brain's electrical activity or on evaluation of the physiologic parameters affecting the delivery of CBF. Cellular electrical activity can be monitored using electroencephalography (EEG) (see Chapter 8) or evoked potentials (see Chapter 7), and regional CBF can be monitored directly using techniques such as xenon 133 washout. This latter technique, however, is limited to only a few medical centers because it is invasive (inhalation, intravenous or intracarotid administration of radioactive tracer is required), requires radiation exposure, and provides only an intermittent measurement of blood flow. ICP, however, is more easily evaluated.

This chapter discusses the origin and importance of normal cerebrospinal fluid (CSF) pressure and intracranial hypertension, the effects of commonly used drugs and anesthetics on ICP, the rationale for clinical measurement of ICP, and the common devices used for measurement of ICP.

Physiology of Normal Cerebral Blood Flow

Normal CBF in awake humans averages $50 \ mL \cdot 100 \ g^{-1} \cdot minute^{-1}$ for whole brain.[1, 2] Blood flow to the brain provides nutrients (glucose) and oxygen, and removes the waste products of cellular metabolism (CO_2, lactic acid, and so on). Brain cells acutely depend on adequate blood flow to accomplish these tasks. As CBF decreases, both the delivery of glucose and oxygen and the removal of waste products decrease.

At levels of CBF under $25 \ mL \cdot 100 \ g^{-1} \cdot minute^{-1}$, early changes in cerebral electrical activity become apparent, so this point is called the "critical CBF."[3] These EEG changes represent ischemia of brain cells. CBF of $25 \ mL \cdot 100 \ g^{-1} \cdot minute^{-1}$ corresponds to a cerebral perfusion pressure (CPP) of approximately 45 mmHg[4] (Fig. 9-1). This correlation of CPP to level of CBF provides a readily available, objective clinical indication of adequacy of cerebral perfusion.

In normal individuals, CBF is regulated by three factors, categorized as metabolic activity, neurogenic factors (pressure), and viscosity.[5] These various factors interact to produce an effect known as autoregulation. Cerebral autoregulation is the maintenance of CBF over a range of blood pressures, blood viscosity, and metabolic activity. All these effects are ultimately mediated through changes in cerebral vessel size and therefore changes in the relative resistance to blood flow.

Metabolic Control

Four metabolic mechanisms affect CBF: H^+ concentration, oxygen, CO_2, and basic cerebral metabolic rate.

pH Effect

The concentration of H^+ in the tissues surrounding the vessels in the brain affects blood flow. This is known as the pH effect. An increased extracellular fluid H^+ concentration decreases pH, and the resulting acidosis produces vasodilation with increased blood flow.[6] Likewise, decreased extracellular fluid H^+ concentration increases pH, and this alkalosis produces vasoconstriction and a decrease in blood flow.[7] Substances that affect pH by changing the H^+ concentration are given in Table 9-1. The pH effect, although functional, usually plays a secondary role in regulation of CBF when compared with other factors.[8]

Oxygen and Carbon Dioxide Effects

The effects of the respiratory gases O_2 and CO_2 are usually considered in relation to the arterial partial pressure of each gas (PaO_2 and $PaCO_2$).

PaO_2 Effect. Insufficient oxygen supply to the brain, whether due to inadequate volume of blood or to inadequate oxygen tension in the blood, increases CBF through vasodilation of the cerebral vessels. This occurs when the PaO_2 falls

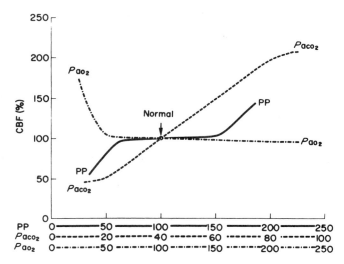

Figure 9-1. The effects on cerebral blood flow (CBF) of arterial oxygen tension (Pao$_2$ [mm Hg]), arterial carbon dioxide tension (Pao$_2$ [mm Hg]), as a percentage of control, and cerebral perfusion pressure (PP [mm Hg]). CBF is little affected by Po$_2$ except during hypoxia. Autoregulation of CBF occurs between perfusion pressures of about 60 to 150 mm Hg. CBF is quite sensitive to changes in Paco$_2$. (From Michenfelder, JD: The cerebral circulation. *In* Prys-Roberts C [ed]. The Circulation in Anaesthesia. London, Blackwell, 1980, p 212).

below 60 mmHg[9] (see Fig. 9-1). High arterial oxygen tensions only minimally affect the cerebral vessels by vasoconstriction[10] (see Fig. 9-1).

Paco$_2$ Effect. The Paco$_2$ exerts a vasoactive effect through two mechanisms. The direct effects of Paco$_2$ are progressive vasoconstriction and decreased blood flow in response to a decreased Paco$_2$, and progressive vasodilation and increased blood flow in response to an increased Paco$_2$[11, 12] (see Fig. 9-1). Both of these responses affect CBF in a nearly linear manner, and are independent of changes in H$^+$ concentration.[13-15]

The indirect effect of Paco$_2$ operates through the pH effect. Both arterial and tissue CO$_2$ combine with water to produce carbonic acid, which in turn dissociates to increase H$^+$ concentration.[7] Therefore, increased Paco$_2$ produces increased H$^+$ concentration, decreased pH, and resultant vasodilation and increased CBF.[7, 9] Decreased Paco$_2$ produces decreased H$^+$ concentration, increased pH, and resultant vasoconstriction and decreased CBF.[16]

The duration of the vasoconstrictive effect of decreased Paco$_2$, however, may be limited. Sustained hyperventilation to reduce ICP is no longer effective beyond 24 hours due to

Table 9-1. Substances Affecting Cerebral Vasculature

Substance Affecting [H$^+$]	Effect on pH	Effect on Cerebral Vessels
Increased Paco$_2$	Acidosis	Vasodilation
Decreased Paco$_2$	Alkalosis	Vasoconstriction
Increased HCO$_3^-$	Alkalosis	Vasoconstriction
Decreased HCO$_3^-$	Acidosis	Vasodilation
Increased metabolic acid (lactic, pyruvic)	Acidosis	Vasodilation
Decreased metabolic acid	Alkalosis	Vasoconstriction

buffering of the induced pH changes by the CSF.[17] In fact, it has been suggested that hyperventilation beyond this time may even be detrimental, because the depletion of the CSF bicarbonate buffer makes the cerebral vessels more sensitive to even the subtlest CO$_2$ changes. Intubated patients may no longer tolerate brief suctioning without large increases in ICP.[18]

Metabolic Rate Effect

Finally, the overall basic rate of metabolism of brain cells also affects blood flow.[19] An increase in cerebral metabolic rate results in vasodilation and increased blood flow as CBF tries to supply adequate oxygen and nutrients to satisfy the brain's increased demand.[20, 21] Similarly, a decrease in cerebral metabolic rate results in vasoconstriction and decreased blood flow.[21] This relationship is called flow-metabolism coupling, and it can be dysfunctional in a wide range of pathologic states. Cerebral metabolic rate can be influenced by general anesthetics, temperature, and seizure activity.

Neurogenic Control

The effects of neurogenic influences on CBF are usually masked by the powerful metabolic mechanisms previously described,[7] but cerebral vessels are also under the control of the autonomic nervous system. The intracranial vessels are innervated by both sympathetic and parasympathetic fibers, and under certain circumstances (e.g., severe exercise, intracranial hemorrhage, stroke), strong sympathetic outflow produces cerebral vasoconstriction and decreased CBF.[19, 22, 23]

Pressure Autoregulation

The multiple mechanisms previously described interact through control of cerebral vessel size to produce CBF levels that closely match the metabolic needs of the brain. Normally, this system of autoregulation operates over a range of mean CPPs from 60 to 150 mmHg[4] (see Fig. 9-1) *Cerebral perfusion pressure* is defined as the mean arterial pressure minus the ICP (or central venous pressure [CVP] if it is higher than ICP), and represents the ability of blood to circulate through the head. Below a CPP of 60 mmHg, cerebral vessels are maximally dilated in an effort to preserve CBF, and with any further reduction of CPP, CBF becomes dependent directly on mean arterial pressure (see Fig. 9-1). Conversely, at CPPs above 150 mmHg, blood flow is again pressure-dependent because of maximal vessel constriction, and flow increases with pressure[4] (see Fig. 9-1).

The effects of the respiratory gases O$_2$ and CO$_2$ can defeat normal autoregulation.[10, 24] Thus, at any given perfusion pressure, Pao$_2$ less than 60 mmHg or an increase in Paco$_2$ produces vasodilation and increases CBF; a decrease in Paco$_2$ produces vasoconstriction and decreases blood flow.[4]

Viscosity Autoregulation

Changes in blood viscosity are paralleled by intracranial vessel size, and appear to be closely associated with pressure autoregulation.[25, 26] Mannitol, with its ability to reduce intravascular viscosity by hemodilution, may exert a significant portion of its therapeutic value of ICP reduction by this mechanism.

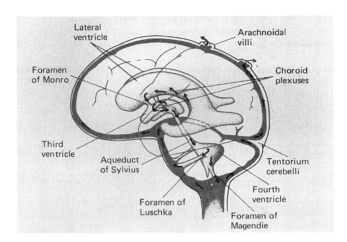

Figure 9-2. In the normal brain, cerebrospinal fluid flows from the lateral ventricles through the foramen of Monro to the third ventricle, through the aqueduct of Sylvius to the fourth ventricle, through the foramina of Magendie and Luschka to the cisterna magna, and finally to the cerebral and spinal subarachnoid spaces. (From Guyton AC: Textbook of Medical Physiology, ed. 7. Philadelphia, WB Saunders, 1986, p 374.)

Physiology of Intracranial Pressure

Cerebrospinal Fluid Physiology

CSF is the body's shock absorber for the central nervous system (CNS). It bathes and surrounds the entire brain and spinal cord to act as a natural cushion for delicate neural structures.

The normal intracranial-intraspinal volume of the CNS is approximately 1650 mL, of which 150 mL is CSF.[7] The normal rate of CSF production is approximately 500 mL/day.[27]

CSF is mainly produced by the choroid plexus in all four ventricles of the brain, with the major portion coming from the lateral ventricles.[7, 27, 28] It flows from the lateral ventricles through the foramen of Monro to the third ventricle, through the aqueduct of Sylvius to the fourth ventricle, through the foramen of Luschka and foramen of Magendie to the cisterna magna, and then into the subarachnoid space surrounding the brain and spinal cord (Fig. 9-2). Absorption (into the venous blood) occurs through the arachnoid villi in the sagittal venous sinus. In the absence of a pathologic condition, the rate of absorption back into the blood is equal to the rate of production.[7] The fact that production is largely active (pressure-independent) and absorption is largely passive (pressure-dependent) produces a measurable CSF pressure (ICP) that is normally less than 15 mmHg.[7, 24]

Determinants of Intracranial Pressure

The intracranial cavity is bordered by the cranium, a rigid structure of bone with only one real outlet for the intracranial contents, the foramen magnum. CSF is only one of the substances contained in this cavity, the normal contents of which are listed in Figure 9-3.[29]

An increase in the volume of one or more of the normal constituents of the intracranial cavity produces a concomitant and compensating decrease in the volume of other intracranial contents to partially maintain volume and pressure at a constant level.[29] Glial cells, neurons, and extracellular fluid are minimally compressible, have no ready avenue to exit

the cranial vault, and are usually not part of this compensatory mechanism. Thus, volume compensation results from the decrease of either intracranial intravascular blood volume, CSF volume, or both. An overwhelming pathologic increase in intracranial volume exhausts this mechanism for compensation, and ICP increases. Any further increase in intracranial volume produces a concomitant increase in ICP.[29]

This pressure-volume (intracranial compliance) relationship can be examined by injecting very small increments (0.1 mL, 0.5 mL, and 1.0 mL) of sterile preservative-free saline into the CSF space and measuring the concomitant change in CSF pressure produced. An intracranial pressure-volume curve can then be produced for individual patients (Fig. 9-4). The higher on the sharp limb of the curve, the tighter the brain is, and the more dramatic the increase in ICP becomes with each increment of increasing intracranial volume.

This relationship can also be expressed by the pressure-volume index (PVI), a measure of brain compliance. It is the calculated volume (in milliliters) required to be added to the CSF to raise the ICP by a factor of 10.[30] If autoregulation is intact, the PVI remains about 20 mL throughout the CPP range of 60 to 150 mmHg, but when autoregulation is pathologically absent, the PVI falls dramatically with higher CPPs.

The effect of intracranial volume on ICP also depends on the rate of volume increase. Compensatory mechanisms respond more readily to slower increases in intracranial volume, so slower changes in volume produce less acute changes in ICP.[31] A very rapid increase in volume rapidly increases ICP. However, there is an absolute limit to the volume compensatory mechanisms, and when that limit is exceeded, the rate of volume expansion becomes irrelevant.[32]

Causes of Intracranial Hypertension

Abnormal increases in ICP are produced by many different pathologic conditions. The mechanisms of production of in-

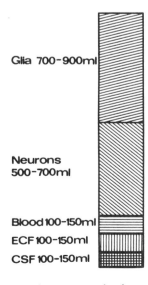

Figure 9-3. Intracranial contents and volume in an average adult human. Total intracranial volume is 1500 to 2050 mL. ECF, extracellular fluid; CSF, cerebrospinal fluid. (From Jennett B, Teasdale G: Management of Head Injuries. Philadelphia, FA Davis, 1981, p 60.)

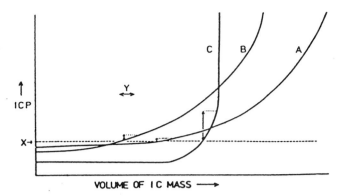

Figure 9-4. Three possible intracranial pressure-volume curves. The most widely accepted is curve C. As the volume of intracranial (IC) mass increases, the intracranial pressure (ICP) increases. In curve C, the flat portion represents the volume compensation of normal brain. Once this compensation is exhausted, further increases in volume produce greater and greater increases in ICP. A patient with an elevation of ICP to point X is on the steep portion of the curve. Any further increase in volume (Y) produces a large increase in ICP in curve C, but smaller increases in curves A and B. The relative position of any patient on the curve (intracranial compliance) can be determined by injecting small increments of volume into the CSF (*arrows*) and observing the concomitant change in pressure (see text). (From Leech P, Miller JD: Intracranial volume-pressure relationships during experimental brain compression in primates. Pressure responses to changes in ventricular volume. J Neurol Neurosurg Psychiatry 1974; 37:1093–1098.)

creased ICP include an expanding intracranial mass, cerebral edema formation, increased intracranial CSF volume, and increased intracranial blood volume.[7] Some conditions are caused by more than one mechanism.

Intracranial Masses

Expanding intracranial masses include tumors and hematomas. These are conditions in which a normal or abnormal constituent of the intracranial vault increases in size and adds to intracranial volume.

Cerebral Edema

Cerebral edema represents an increase in intracellular volume (cytoxic edema) or an increase in extracellular fluid volume (vasogenic edema). Cerebral edema may be classified as either global or regional. Conditions producing global edema include closed head injury with contusions, cerebral anoxic damage, Reye's syndrome,[33] and severe systemic hypertension. Some examples of conditions producing regional cerebral edema are edema surrounding an intracranial tumor,[34] localized cerebral trauma, and stroke.

Increased Cerebrospinal Fluid Volume

Intracranial CSF volume increases because of decreased absorption of CSF, obstruction of venous outflow from the head, or pathologic overproduction of CSF that exceeds normal reabsorption. Decreased absorption of CSF produces hydrocephalus. Communicating hydrocephalus occurs when the CSF is not normally absorbed through the arachnoid villi. Noncommunicating hydrocephalus is produced by an obstruction to CSF flow through the ventricles to the subarachnoid space. Usually, this obstruction occurs in the aqueduct of Sylvius between the third and fourth ventricles.

Venous outflow obstruction decreases CSF absorption, probably by increasing the passive filtration pressure across the arachnoid villi via an increase in sagittal sinus venous pressure. Venous outflow obstruction can occur intracranially secondary to traumatic disruption of the venous sinus tract or extracranially from jugular venous compression. It may even occur with the assumption of the supine position, removing the negative venous hydrostatic pressure gradient present in the upright position.

Increased Intracranial Blood Volume

Increased circulating intracranial blood volume is a consequence of cerebral vasodilation or venous outflow obstruction. Cerebral vasodilation in turn can be caused by severe systemic hypertension, direct vasodilator drugs, and acute respiratory failure. It is also produced by a decrease in PaO_2 (hypoxia), an increase in $PaCO_2$ (hypercarbia), and a decrease in arterial pH (acidosis).[7, 9, 11, 15]

Intracranial Pressure Waveforms

When measured and displayed on an oscilloscope, the CSF pressure normally exhibits a characteristic pulsatile waveform.[32] The amplitude varies with the cardiac cycle, owing to transient changes in blood volume, and with respiration, probably owing to transient changes in intrathoracic pressure that are transmitted via the venous system to the venous sinus in the cranium. These pulsatile variations are superimposed on a steady-state volume level of CSF (Fig. 9-5).

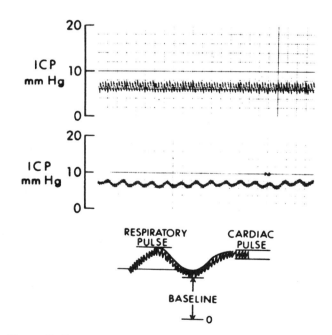

Figure 9-5. Normal intracranial pressure (ICP) is a pulsatile waveform with pressures of 5 to 7 mm Hg. On this pressure are superimposed the effects of the cardiac and respiratory cycles. The top graph is at high paper speed to illustrate the cardiac effect; the middle graph represents the respiratory effect; the bottom graph illustrates the basic components of an ICP waveform during one respiratory cycle. (From Marmarou A, Tabaddor K: Intracranial pressure: Physiology and Pathophysiology. *In* Cooper PR [ed]: Head Injury. Baltimore: Williams & Wilkins, 1982, pp 115–127.)

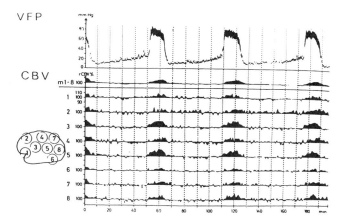

VFP

CBV

Figure 9-6. Simultaneous recordings of intracranial pressure (ICP; ventricular fluid pressure, VFP) and cerebral blood volume (CBV) regionally in eight separate areas of the left hemisphere in a single patient. The y-axis represents time in minutes during the measurement. The top graph illustrates VFP (ICP) A waves or plateau waves. The second graph represents average CBV from the eight areas. Note the similar course of VFP (ICP) and CBV; the A waves are accompanied by increases in CBV. (From Risberg J, Lundberg N, Ingvar DH: Regional cerebral blood volume during acute transient rises of the intracranial pressure [plateau waves]. J Neurosurg 1969; 31:303-310.)

Normal CSF pressures are less than 15 mmHg. In cases of abnormally increased ICP, the amplitude of the pulsatile component increases. Abnormal waveforms seen in cases of pathologically increased ICP are usually intermittent and of two basic types: A waves (Fig. 9-6), or plateau waves, last for several minutes and acutely exhibit an ICP of 50 to 100 mmHg; B waves are of lower amplitude with shorter duration than A waves and are not associated with the very poor neurologic outcome that A waves denote.[35] Normal-appearing pressure tracings typically surround these pathologic waves, so continuous ICP monitoring is recommended.

Anesthetic Effects on Intracranial Pressure

The effects of various drugs on the ICP are summarized in Table 9-2. The potent anesthetic agents desflurane, enflurane, halothane, isoflurane, and sevoflurane increase ICP primarily by direct cerebral vasodilation and resultant increased cerebral blood volume.[36, 37] Uncompensated respiratory depression from these agents may also cause cerebral vasodilation secondary to an increase in $PaCO_2$.[12]

The influence that nitrous oxide (N_2O) exerts upon CBF and ICP has been difficult to study in humans, because it is an incomplete anesthetic and must be used with other drugs, most of which have their own effects. However, it is generally accepted that N_2O will increase CBF and ICP through an increase in regional metabolic activity.[38-41] Stronger influences, such as mannitol, hyperventilation, or hypothermia, tend to easily dominate and lower ICP, so the effects of N_2O are rarely seen clinically. Concerns of increasing the size of a pneumocephalus from exposure to N_2O are warranted, so its use in craniotomies remains controversial.

The barbiturate drugs, of which thiopental sodium is commonly used in anesthesia, decrease ICP by decreasing cerebral metabolism in normal brain, which results in direct

cerebral vasoconstriction and decreased cerebral blood volume.[42, 43] Narcotic agents such as morphine and fentanyl either do not affect CSF pressure or may even decrease ICP by primarily decreasing the cerebral metabolic rate and CBF.[44, 45] However, like the potent anesthetic agents, narcotics also depress respiration; unless ventilation is supported when necessary, increased $PaCO_2$ may increase ICP.[12] The newer synthetic narcotics sufentanil and alfentanil, however, have demonstrated variable effects on ICP in different studies.[45, 46] These drugs should be used with care and the knowledge that some question of their efficacy may yet exist in patients with increased ICP.

Ketamine produces an increase in ICP owing to an increase in CBF from sympathomimetic effects and cerebral vasodilation.[47-49] The benzodiazepines (diazepam, lorazepam, midazolam) decrease ICP by cerebral vasoconstriction.[50-52] Etomidate decreases ICP by decreasing CBF.[99]

A more recent drug used in neuroanesthesia and neurologic intensive care is propofol, an intravenous anesthetic agent. Propofol decreases ICP secondary to a decrease in the

Table 9-2. Drug Effects on Intracranial Pressure

Drug	Primary	Secondary	References
Potent Anesthetic Agents			
Halothane	++		36
Enflurane	++		96
Isoflurane	++		97
Desflurane	++		98
Sevoflurane	++		37
Barbiturates			
Thiopental sodium	−−		42, 43
Propofol			53-54
Narcotics			
Morphine	0	+	44
Fentanyl citrate	0	+	45
Alfentanil	±	+	45
Sufentanil	±	+	46
Ketamine Hydrochloride	+		47-49
Benzodiazepines			
Diazepam	−		50-52
Lorazepam	−		50-52
Midazolam	−		50-52
Neuromuscular Blocking Drugs			
Succinylcholine chloride	+	0	61-63
d-Tubocurarine	0	+	55
Pancuronium bromide	0		55, 56
Vecuronium bromide	0		57, 58
Atracurium besylate	0		59, 60
Etomidate	−		99
Diuretics			
Mannitol	−		65, 66
Furosemide	−		64
Vasodilators			
Sodium nitroprusside	+		67
Hydralazine hydrochloride	+		68
Nitroglycerin	+		69
Trimethaphan camsylate	0	+	67, 70
Calcium Channel Blocking Drugs			
Nimodipine	0		74
Nicardipine	++		75
β-Adrenergic Blocking Drugs			
Propranolol	0		71
Labetalol	0		72
Esmolol	0		73
Nitrous Oxide	0	+	38-41

++, major increase; +, moderate increase; 0, no effect; −−, major decrease; −, moderate decrease; ±, positive or negative change may occur.

cerebral metabolic rate for oxygen, a decrease in CBF, and an increase in cerebral vascular resistance.[53] Although there is agreement on the effect of propofol on ICP, there is some evidence that propofol may decrease CBF and CPP because of a decrease in arterial blood pressure.[54]

The muscle relaxants commonly used in anesthesia vary in their effects on ICP. Pancuronium, vecuronium, and atracurium have all been shown to have no effect on ICP,[55-60] but d-tubocurarine may increase ICP secondary to histamine release and cerebral vasodilation.[55] Succinylcholine is the most controversial member of this group because evidence shows that, although the drug causes increases in ICP, this effect may be attenuated by pretreatment with a nondepolarizing relaxant drug.[61-63]

Diuretic agents, including furosemide and mannitol, are commonly used to treat intracranial hypertension. Furosemide is a loop diuretic that decreases ICP by producing a fluid diuresis through the kidney.[64] The resultant fluid shifts effectively reduce cerebral edema. Mannitol, an osmotic diuretic, also produces this effect through diuresis, although it may also increase ICP transiently through an osmotic effect on brain water.[65, 66] Both drugs ultimately depend on normal renal function for their effect.

Hypotensive agents, such as primary vasodilators, trimethaphan, and β-adrenergic blockers, are occasionally needed to control systemic hypertension or to produce deliberate hypotension (e.g., in cerebral aneurysm surgery). The primary vasodilator agents nitroprusside, hydralazine, and nitroglycerin produce dose-related increases in ICP by dilating cerebral vessels and increasing CBF and cerebral blood volume.[67-69] Trimethaphan, a ganglionic blocking agent, may also increase ICP through vasodilation secondary to histamine release, although this effect is still debated.[67, 70] The β-adrenergic blocking drugs propranolol, labetalol, and esmolol do not primarily affect ICP.[71-73]

Calcium channel blocking drugs, specifically nimodipine, are useful in the treatment of vasospasm secondary to subarachnoid blood. Nimodipine reduces vasospasm, increases CBF, and decreases cerebral vascular resistance without increasing ICP.[74] However, care should be used with this drug because decreases in arterial blood pressure may result in deterioration of CPP. Nicardipine has been shown to increase ICP, decrease CPP, and decrease arterial pressure in normal subjects and therefore is not a drug of choice in craniotomy patients.[75]

Pathophysiology of Intracranial Hypertension

Cerebral Perfusion Pressure

To understand why increased ICP is a problem, it is necessary to understand the concept of CPP.[29] As discussed earlier, CPP is defined as the pressure gradient across the cerebral capillary bed, which perfuses blood through the brain. The CPP is calculated according to the following formula:

$$CPP = MAP - ICP$$

where:

> MAP = mean arterial inflow pressure
> ICP = intracranial pressure.

For accuracy, MAP should be measured at the level of the external auditory meatus. If CVP is higher than ICP, CVP measured at the level of the external auditory meatus may be used in place of ICP. When ICP increases (intracranial hypertension) or MAP decreases substantially, CPP and the effective perfusion of blood through the brain are compromised.

Intracranial hypertension produces pathologic insults through two basic mechanisms: ischemia of brain tissue and mechanical damage due to bulk shifts of brain tissue.

Cerebral Ischemia

The final common pathway leading to cell damage from intracranial hypertension is ischemia of the cells in the brain.[76] As stated previously, CBF delivers oxygen and glucose and removes CO_2 and waste products from metabolizing brain cells. Ischemia of these cells produces hypoxia and acidosis of brain tissue. When CPP decreases below approximately 45 mmHg, CBF decreases to ischemic levels[3] (see Fig. 9-1).

From the preceding formula, it can be seen that CPP decreases as MAP decreases or ICP increases. Normal CPP is between 60 and 150 mmHg. This corresponds to a CBF of 50 mL · 100 g^{-1} · $minute^{-1}$ (see Fig. 9-1). As the CPP decreases below 60 mmHg, autoregulation is defeated and CBF decreases with systemic mean arterial pressure. At a CPP of 45 mmHg, CBF is approximately 50% of normal, that is, 25 mL · 100 g^{-1} · $minute^{-1}$ (see Fig. 9-1). At this point, the first electrical evidence of ischemia appears,[3] and further reduction in CBF produces more profound changes. In addition to the level of CBF achieved, the duration of time spent at that level plays an important role in determining the survival of cells. The absolute safe level of CBF during low-flow states that does not produce permanent cell damage is not known, but preexisting abnormal cerebral vessels reduce the margin for decreased CBF (as in chronic hypertension).[77] Therefore, when possible, every attempt should be made to maintain CPP at or near normal levels.

Herniation

Bulk shifts of brain tissue can produce mechanical damage to brain cells through the process known as herniation.[29, 32] Although herniation through a craniotomy is possible, brain herniation in the intact cranium occurs through the foramen magnum (cerebellum), the tentorium (temporal lobe or uncus), and under the falx (cingulate gyrus and cerebral hemisphere). The tentorium and the falx are dividing structures within the intracranial vault that create smaller compartments. Herniation occurs when a pressure differential develops between these different compartments, usually due to mass effects from tumors, edema, or hematomas. The type of herniation that occurs depends on the location of the mass. Supratentorial masses include temporal masses, which produce severe midbrain herniation, and frontal or occipital masses, which affect the brainstem less severely for the same size of mass and same ICP level. In addition to location, rapidly increasing masses produce a greater effect on the ICP and herniation than do more slowly growing masses.[32]

Intracranial Pressure Monitoring Devices

General Considerations

Historically, many different devices have been used to measure ICP, some of which are presently in common clinical

Table 9-3. Manufacturing of Intracranial Pressure Monitoring Devices

Manufacturer	Address	Telephone
Camino Laboratories Inc.	5955 Pacific Center Blvd., San Diego, CA 92121	619-455-1115
Cordis Corporation	PO Box 025700, Miami, FL 33102	800-327-2490
Fiber Optic Sensor Technologies	501 Avis Drive, Ann Arbor, MI 48108	313-665-6707
InnerSpace Medical	1923 South East Main Street, Irvine, CA 92714	800-447-0304
Ladd Research Industries Inc.	PO Box 1005, Burlington, VT 05402	800-451-3406
Medical Measurements Inc.	53 Main Street, Hackensack, NJ 07601	800-833-8031
Pudenz-Schulte Medical	125 B Cremona Drive, Goleta, CA 93117	805-968-1546

use. Several aspects should be considered when deciding which device to use in a given clinical situation. First, the ICP monitor should be reliable and stable during long-term use. In general, the simpler the device, the more reliable it is. Second, the placement procedure should be as innocuous to the patient's CNS as possible, and the risks of bleeding and infection should be minimal. Third, the monitor should allow for continuous measurement and recording of ICP while allowing adequate comfort and nursing care for the patient. Fourth, it may be advantageous to choose a monitor that is both informative and potentially therapeutic, and finally, the monitor chosen should be within the realm of expertise of the operator and as inexpensive as possible.[78] Tables 9-3 and 9-4 list available products and manufacturers.

Monitoring Indications

After an initial insult to the brain, severe secondary injuries can occur, usually by producing ischemia from a decrease in CPP and a concomitant decrease in CBF.[76] Prevention of this secondary injury is where ICP monitoring and therapy may help, because no therapy can reverse the damage already produced by the primary insult. Therefore, ICP monitoring should be considered whenever secondary injury is of concern. These conditions include the following:

1. Patients with head injuries with a Glasgow Coma Scale score of 7 or less.[69]

2. Patients with Reye's syndrome, because uncontrolled increases in ICP are a major factor in mortality.[33]

3. Patients with intracranial tumors, especially during induction of anesthesia when peritumoral edema is present.[34]

4. Any patient with an intracranial abnormality when the clinical neurologic examination cannot be followed (a) intraoperatively (this becomes ineffective once the dura is opened), (b) during barbiturate-induced coma, and (c) when neuromuscular blocking agents are used in neurosurgical patients in the intensive care unit.

5. Whenever therapeutic maneuvers adversely affect CPP and ICP.[76]

Classification of Devices

The devices and techniques now available for monitoring ICP can be classified into groups by location of the device in the CNS, inherent invasiveness of the device, and method of measuring ICP. All of the devices outlined in this chapter require placement through surgical entry into the skull; therefore, they should be inserted only by an experienced operator.

Insertion sites of the device can vary among the lumbar spine, the cervical spine, the posterior fossa, and the supratentorial area of the cranium. Supratentorial placement is almost always preferred because of pathologically decreased flow of CSF around the tentorium in the subarachnoid space and subsequent intracranial herniation.[78] In patients with increased ICP, invasion of the subarachnoid space in the spinal canal and subsequent loss of CSF below the tentorium or foramen magnum may even produce downward herniation.

ICP monitoring devices also can be described by method of measurement. Devices that place the pressure-measuring transducer at a site remote from the patient utilize a column of fluid in tubing to transmit the pressure wave from the CSF to the transducer. These devices are said to be fluid-coupled. The fluid and fluid path must be sterile, nonirritating to tissues, and free of leaks and air bubbles. The transducer should usually be placed at the level of the external auditory meatus for accuracy. Care must be taken to prevent any inadvertent injection of drugs or volume into this system. This has been a problem and is a continuing risk owing to the close resemblance of this system to other physiologic pressure monitoring equipment, for example, an arterial pressure apparatus.

Another necessary precaution is preventing the use of continuous flush systems in this setting. Nursing personnel and physicians caring for patients with fluid-coupled monitoring devices must know the differences between other physiologic monitoring equipment and ICP monitors. Experienced operators, however, can safely perform clinical intracranial pressure-volume determinations on patients with this apparatus.

Table 9-4. Types of Intracranial Pressure Monitoring Devices and Their Manufacturers*

Device Type	Manufacturer
Intraventricular Devices	
Catheter	Cordis Corporation; Pudenz-Schulte Medical
Fiberoptic transducer	Camino Laboratories Inc.; Inner-Space Medical
Intraparenchymal Devices	
Fiberoptic transducer	Camino Laboratories Inc.; Inner-Space Medical
Subarachnoid Devices	
Bolt	Pudenz-Schulte Medical
Cup catheter	Cordis Corporation
Fiberoptic transducer	Camino Laboratories Inc.; Inner-Space Medical
Epidural Devices	
Strain-gauge transducer	Medical Measurements Inc.
Fiberoptic transducer	Camino Laboratories Inc.; Inner-Space Medical
Pneumatic transducer	Ladd Research Industries Inc.

*For address and telephone numbers, see Table 9-3.

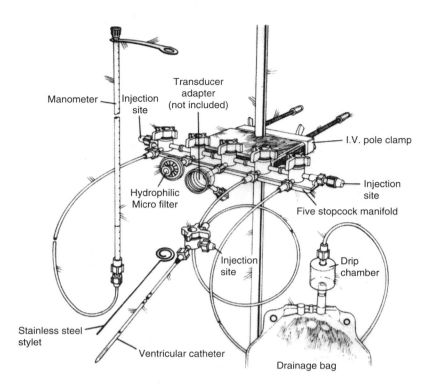

Figure 9-7. One arrangement of tubing, transducer, and drainage bag originally proposed by Becker. Note the transducer dome in the center, the absence of a continuous flush system, and ports for injection and drainage of cerebrospinal fluid. The transducer should be positioned at the level of the external auditory meatus. This apparatus may be used for measurement of either intraventricular or subarachnoid pressures. (From Wilkinson HA: Intracranial pressure monitoring: Techniques and pitfalls. *In* Cooper PR [ed]: Head Injury. Philadelphia: Williams & Wilkins, 1982, p 155.)

Newer devices utilize light transmission (fiberoptics) or a column of gas (pneumatics) instead of fluid-coupling to transmit the CSF pressure wave to the pressure-measuring electronic device. At least one device places the transducer directly in contact with the dura. There are also several experimental devices that attempt to implant the pressure transducer directly into the CSF. The major problems with newer devices are reliability and miniaturization of the electronics or power supplies. Another development in ICP measurement is the implantation of devices into brain parenchyma. Pressures obtained in this way are reliable and compare well with conventionally measured pressures.[79] Intraparenchymal placement precludes therapeutic CSF drainage or flushing of the device.

Intraventricular Devices

Classification according to the invasive nature of the device distinguishes among intraventricular devices, subarachnoid devices, epidural devices, and surface devices.

The intraventricular catheter is one of the oldest and simplest devices used to measure ICP.[80-82] It is classified as a fluid-coupled device; ICP waves are transmitted via an uninterrupted fluid path to a pressure sensor, usually a strain-gauge transducer outside of the cranium. This is accomplished by directly placing a hollow fluid-filled catheter into one of the lateral ventricles through a cranial bur hole and intact brain tissue. A typical arrangement of the tubing and transducer is shown in Figures 9-7 and 9-8. With this device, although it is very invasive, long-term ICP measurements can be made, pressure-volume determinations can be

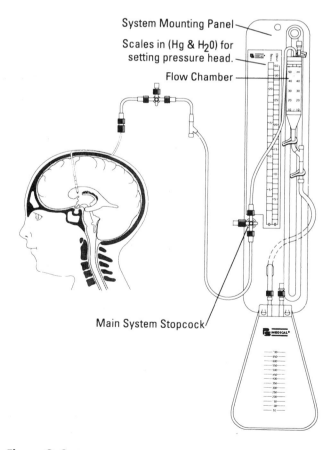

Figure 9-8. A new ICP measurement and drainage system. (Courtesy of Pudenz-Schulte Medical, Goleta, CA.)

performed, intrathecal drugs (antibiotics) can be injected, and CSF can be withdrawn for both diagnostic studies and therapeutic needs (e.g., to decrease ICP). To achieve accurate ICP measurements with this device, the external transducer should be located at the level of the external auditory meatus.

Because the tubing arrangement for this device closely resembles that of other intravascular pressure monitoring devices, care must be taken to remove any continuous flush system from the apparatus. Flushing of the tubing and catheter is occasionally necessary but should be done carefully, only with preservative-free saline, and only by an experienced operator. Because this technique requires invasion of tissue and violation of the dura, infection is possible and carries an estimated incidence of less than 6.3%.[83-85] Likewise, if the ventricular system is collapsed or relatively small, the operator may be unable to accurately place a catheter into the lateral ventricle (Fig. 9-9). Computed tomography (CT) or fiberoptic ventriculoscopy can facilitate intraventricular catheter placement by locating the lateral ventricles.

Subarachnoid Devices

Subarachnoid Bolt

In an effort to circumvent brain tissue perforation (as with a ventricular catheter) and still directly interface with CSF, the subarachnoid bolt was developed (Fig. 9-10). Sometimes referred to as the Richmond bolt because of pioneering work done by Becker, Vires, Young, and others at the Medical College of Virginia, this device is also placed via a bur hole in the supratentorial area of the skull, with the tip placed

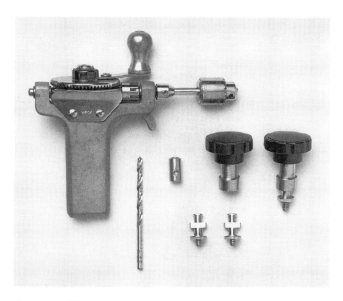

Figure 9-10. A subarachnoid bolt and the equipment for its insertion. The twist drill has a movable collar that produces a well in the outer table of the skull to allow accurate depth of placement. The black handles are for insertion of the bolt itself.

below the arachnoid membrane.[78, 80, 86] Figure 9-11 compares optimal insertion sites with undesirable locations. Like the intraventricular catheter, the bolt is fluid-coupled to an external pressure transducer, which should be placed at the level of the external meatus. Continuous flushing systems should be excluded from the fluid path (see Fig. 9-7). Regular flushing of the bolt should be performed manually but only with very small amounts of preservative-free saline. Be-

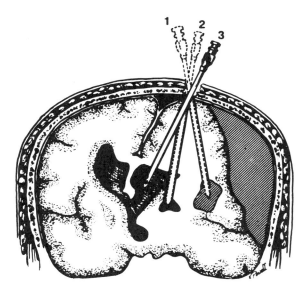

Figure 9-9. Potential problems encountered in placing an intraventricular catheter. The subdural hematoma has shifted the brain to the contralateral side and compressed the ipsilateral ventricle. Needle position 3 is the appropriate placement in this case and was achieved after blind passage, as in 1 and 2. With the ready availability of computed tomography, needle placement is much more precise. (From Wilkinson HA: intracranial pressure monitoring: Techniques and pitfalls. *In* Cooper PR [ed]: Head Injury. Baltimore: Williams & Wilkins, 1982, p 158.)

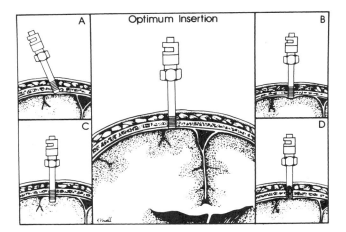

Figure 9-11. Optimum placement of the subarachnoid bolt is seen in the center of the figure. Potential problems with bolt placement: *A*, Oblique placement does not allow full approximation to the subarachnoid space. *B*, A thin cranium allows movement of the bolt and occlusion; *C*, Bolt placed too deep damages brain tissue; *D*, Herniation of brain tissue into the bolt and subsequent occlusion. (From Wilkinson HA: Intracranial pressure monitoring: Techniques and pitfalls. *In* Cooper PR [ed]: Head Injury. Philadelphia: Williams & Wilkins, 1982, p 161.)

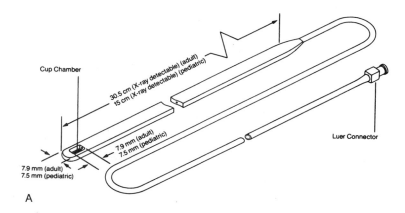

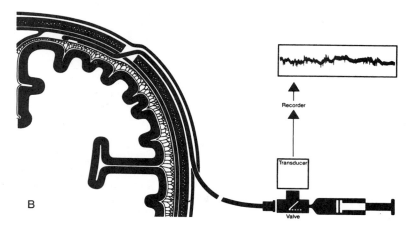

Figure 9-12. The cup catheter *(A)* is ribbon-shaped, and has a cup formed in its end. It is designed as a surface-monitoring device to be placed so that the open cup rests on the brain surface *(B)*. This device is also fluid-coupled and must be flushed periodically. (Courtesy of Cordis Corporation.)

cause the tip of the bolt actually rests close to or on the brain surface, withdrawal of CSF is impossible. Pressure-volume determinations are possible, but drugs cannot be reliably injected. Potential for infection does exist but is considered to be less likely than with a ventricular catheter.[85, 86] Despite the relative ease of placement and the relative accuracy of the pressure measurement, the subarachnoid bolt is no longer widely used for measuring ICP because of its lack of therapeutic flexibility.

Cup Catheter

Another available subarachnoid device is the cup catheter, which operates similarly to the subarachnoid bolt (Fig. 9-12). This device is a ribbon-shaped catheter passed into the cerebral subarachnoid space through a bur hole, with the skin incision remote from the craniotomy site, thus possibly decreasing the incidence of infection.[87] The cup catheter is also fluid-coupled to ensure filling of the cup. This catheter is somewhat more difficult to place than the bolt and is even less widely used.

Epidural Devices

Three devices are currently available for epidural ICP measurement: the epidural transducer, fiberoptic transducer, and pneumatic transducer. All three devices measure ICP through the intact dura, avoiding the use of a fluid path (i.e., they are not fluid-coupled), and because the dura is not opened, the

risk of infection is thought to be less than with intraventricular or subarachnoid devices.

Epidural Transducer

The epidural transducer is produced and marketed by NV Philips, the Netherlands. It is designed to be threaded into a bur hole in the skull far enough to stretch the intact dura

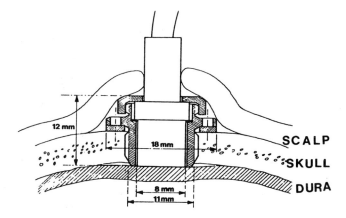

Figure 9-13. A schematic diagram of the epidural transducer. The clear layer overlapping the top edge of the device is scalp. The transducer is threaded into a burr hole in the skull, and the transducer surface adheres directly to the dura. (From Koster WG, Kuypers MH: Intracranial pressure and its epidural measurement. Med Prog Technol 1980; 7:21-27.)

across the flat sensor at the tip[88] (Fig. 9-13). The measurement of ICP with this device depends on the principle of coplanarity; that is, the flat sensor must be exactly parallel to the plane of the dura and in intimate contact with it.[89] The CSF pressure waves are transmitted across the intact dura to the transducer surface. Therefore, accuracy of placement is crucial. When properly placed, however, the pressure measurements correspond well with those obtained from an intraventricular catheter.[88] Because there is no fluid-coupling, injection of drugs and intracranial pressure-volume measurement are impossible, and the device does not need to be flushed periodically, as do fluid-coupled devices. Unfortunately, the transducer is nondisposable and relatively expensive.[88, 89]

Epidural Catheter Tip Pressure Transducer

This catheter differs from other catheters in that the pressure transducer is located at the catheter tip and is covered by a thin membrane[90, 91] (Figs. 9-14 and 9-15). No fluid-couple is needed because the thin membrane rests directly on the strain-gauge pressure measuring device during measurement. The entire apparatus then connects to an existing pressure measuring module via an adapter.

Usually used as an epidural sensor (Fig. 9-16), this device has been used in the subdural space and even intraventricularly. Manufactured by Gaeltec (Hackensack, NJ) and marketed by Medical Measurements Inc., the catheter is designed to allow in vivo calibration and zero checks.

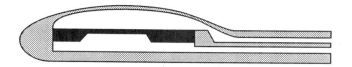
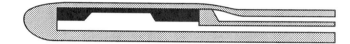

Figure 9-15. The Gaeltec dual-channel catheter allows for in vivo zero calibration of the device. One channel allows atmospheric pressure to the reverse side of the transducer during measurement; the membrane is in contact with the transducer during this phase *(bottom)*. To calibrate the unit in vivo, equal pressure is applied to both sides of the transducer via the first and second channels *(top)*. (Courtesy of Medical Measurements Inc., Hackensack, N.J.)

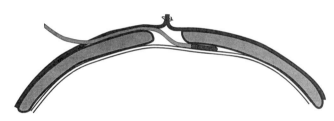

Figure 9-16. Gaeltec catheter placed epidurally. (Courtesy of Medical Measurements Inc., Hackensack, NJ.)

Gaeltec Model ICT/b
Intracranial epidural pressure sensor

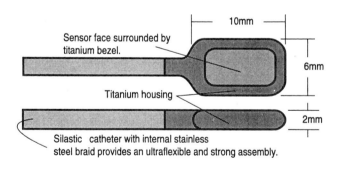

10mm

Sensor face surrounded by titanium bezel.

6mm

Titanium housing

2mm

Silastic catheter with internal stainless steel braid provides an ultraflexible and strong assembly.

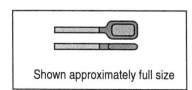

Shown approximately full size

Figure 9-14. The Gaeltec catheter is made up of a dual-channel catheter with an electronic strain gauge pressure measuring device at the tip. A thin membrane covers the pressure sensor and lies in contact with it during measurement. (Courtesy of Medical Measurements Inc., Hackensack, NJ.)

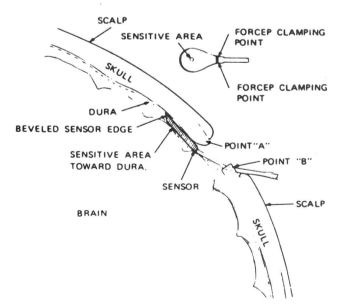

Figure 9-17. Placement of the Ladd sensor. The membrane surface is placed against the dura through a bur hole in the skull. (From Levin AB: The use of a fiberoptic intracranial pressure monitor in clinical practice. Neurosurgery 1977; 1:266-271.)

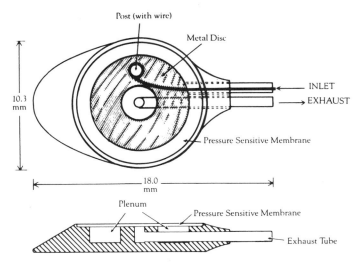

Figure 9–18. The disposable sensor for the Ladd-Steritek intracranial pressure monitoring system. The pressure-sensitive membrane is a thin metal disk that can occlude the exhaust gas port. Gas enters the sensor through the inlet port at 40 mL/minute. (Courtesy of Ladd Research Industries, Burlington, VT.)

Designed to act as a pneumatic flow switch, pressure will build up within the plenum of the sensor to overcome any outside pressure (ICP) against the membrane and reestablish air flow.

Pneumatic Epidural Monitor

The Ladd-Steritek (Ladd Research Industries, Burlington, VT) ICP monitoring system utilizes a disposable pneumatic sensor, which is placed in either the epidural or subdural space through a bur hole in the skull (Figs. 9–17, 9–18, and 9–19). The sensor membrane is placed toward the dura or brain surface. The sensor is designed to self-calibrate in vivo.

The Ladd-Steritek base unit (containing an air pump, transducer, and microprocessor) provides a constant flow of air at 40 mL/minute into a sensor chamber (see Figs. 9–18 and 9–19) where the pressure inside the chamber is measured constantly by a transducer. A metal disk membrane occludes the air exhaust port when acted on by pressure outside the sensor ICP, so air is pumped into the chamber until the pressure inside is sufficient to lift the membrane and open the exhaust port. This internal pressure now reflects the ICP outside the catheter. Advantages of the Ladd-Steritek unit are disposability, lower cost, and less fragile sensors, but it is a dedicated monitor that can be used on only one patient at a time, and has no other uses.

All of the epidural devices presented here eliminate the need for fluid-coupling with the inherent problems of fluid systems (e.g., leakage and sterility). However, they are generally more expensive and more difficult to place, and are dedicated instruments with only one use.

Fiberoptic Monitor

The most recent advance in ICP monitoring devices is the use of fiberoptics, one of which is manufactured by Camino Laboratories (San Diego, CA) (Fig. 9–20). This device requires the use of only the manufacturer's monitor and recorder (Fig. 9–21), but the system may be used as an epidural, subdural, intraventricular, or intraparenchymal monitor[92-95] (Fig. 9–22).

The device measures ICP by the use of fiberoptic light paths in the catheter. One light path transmits light generated in the monitor itself to the tip of the catheter, which then reflects off a flat reflecting surface, the other side of which is in contact with CSF or brain tissue. The second fiberoptic pathway transmits reflected light back to the monitor unit, where it is quantitatively measured and compared to the level of generated light. As pressure in the CSF in-

creases, the reflecting surface is displaced at an ever-increasing angle, resulting in less and less of the reflected light being captured by the return fiberoptic pathway. The difference in the generated light and returned light gives a measure of the pressure at the catheter tip and therefore ICP. This fiberoptic catheter compares favorably with other methods of measuring ICP but cannot be zeroed or recalibrated in vivo. The only major fault with the catheter appears to be breakage of the fiber bundles with prolonged use, but this can be remedied by inserting the catheter into the patient through a device that remains in situ (see Fig. 9–22).

Another similar fiberoptic device is the OPX catheter marketed by Innerspace Medical (Irvine, CA) (Fig. 9–23). This device again requires the use of only the manufacturer's monitoring technology (Fig. 9–24), but does allow drainage of CSF when used in the intraventricular mode.

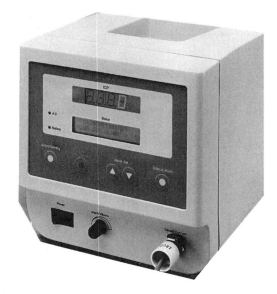

Figure 9–19. The microprocessor-based Ladd-Steritek intracranial pressure monitor base unit. The unit houses the microprocessor, transducer, and pneumatic pump. This device can be used for only one patient at a time. (Courtesy of Ladd Research Industries, Burlington, VT.)

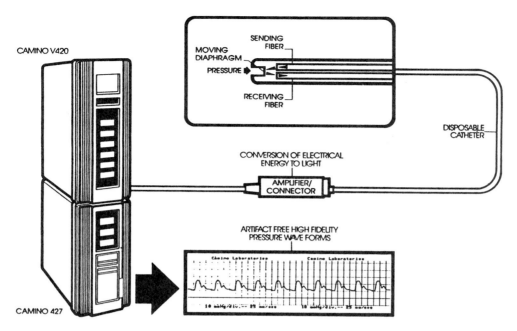

Figure 9-20. The Camino fiberoptic catheter utilizes dual fiberoptic light fibers and a moving diaphragm. As the diaphragm moves, light transmitted from the unit is deflected so that a smaller proportion is returned to the unit from the sensor. This differential is used to calculate the pressure needed to deflect the diaphragm and displayed as intracranial pressure on the unit. Waveforms generated from this device compare very favorably with direct intraventricular waves. (Courtesy of Camino Laboratories, San Diego.)

Therapy of Increased Intracranial Pressure

The therapy of increased ICP is based on the contents of the intracranial cavity. In a rigid, enclosed container such as the cranial vault, a decrease in pressure is best achieved by a decrease in the volume of the intracranial contents. Simply venting the interior to atmospheric pressure would create dangerous pressure differentials that could lead to outward herniation of brain tissue. Therefore, a therapeutic decrease in ICP can best be achieved by (1) decreasing the volume of CSF through ventriculostomy drainage; (2) decreasing intracranial blood volume through hyperventilation, barbiturate therapy, prevention of hypoxia, improving venous drainage (head-up position), avoiding jugular venous compression,

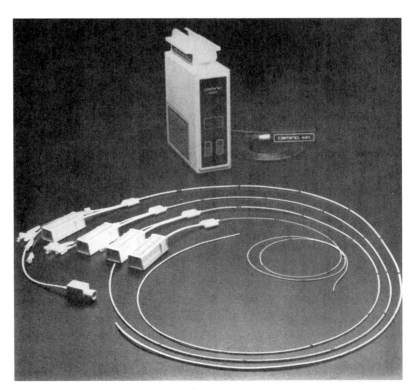

Figure 9-21. The Camino Laboratories intracranial pressure fiberoptic system.

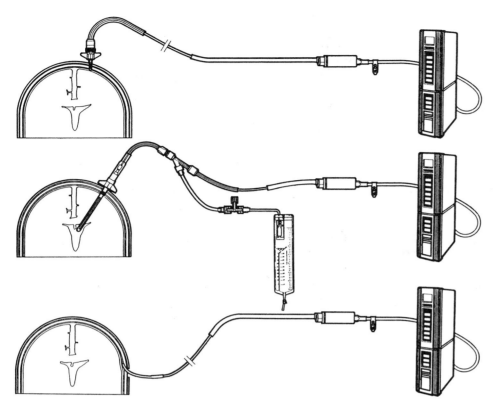

Figure 9-22. The fiberoptic system from Camino Laboratories can be used epidurally, subdurally, intraventricularly, and intraparenchymally. In most applications, the sensor is placed via a stable cranial bolt and can be replaced as needed without removing the bolt.

maintaining normal CPP by avoiding hypotension, and avoiding cerebral vasodilator drugs; (3) decreasing cerebral edema and extracellular fluid with diuretics and avoidance of fluid overload; or (4) surgical removal of any existing intracranial mass such as a hematoma or tumor.[29, 76]

The need to measure ICP to guide therapy in pathologic conditions and the significance of elevated ICP in those circumstances stem from a sound knowledge of cerebral circulation physiology and the dynamics of the CSF. All clinical monitoring techniques available today require surgical procedures for placement, and of the various systems currently available, the older techniques of intraventricular and subarachnoid fluid-coupled devices are still the simplest, most reliable, and most cost-effective.

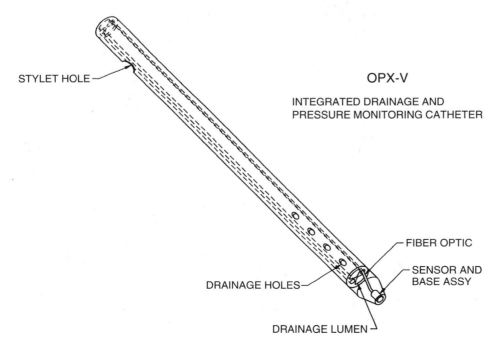

STYLET HOLE —

OPX-V

INTEGRATED DRAINAGE AND
PRESSURE MONITORING CATHETER

— FIBER OPTIC

DRAINAGE HOLES —

— SENSOR AND
BASE ASSY

DRAINAGE LUMEN —

Figure 9-23. The OPX-V catheter from InnerSpace Medical. The integration of catheter and miniature sensor allows for cerebrospinal fluid (CSF) drainage when placed intraventricularly. The sensor is a fiberoptic unit. (Courtesy of InnerSpace Medical, Irvine, CA.)

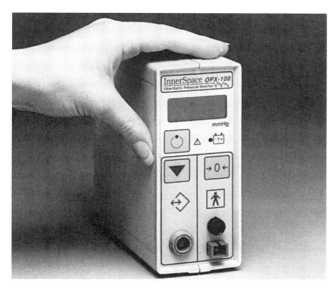

Figure 19–24. The OPX base unit. (Courtesy of InnerSpace Medical, Irvine, CA.)

REFERENCES

1. Lassen NA, Ingavar DH: Radioisotopic assessment of regional cerebral blood flow. Prog Nucl Med 1972; 1:376–409.
2. Obrist WD, Thompson HK, Wang HS, et al: Regional cerebral blood flow estimated by 133-xenon inhalation. Stroke 1975; 6: 245–256.
3. McKay RD, Sundt TM, Michenfelder JD: Internal carotid artery stump pressure and cerebral blood flow during carotid endarterectomy: Modification by halothane, enflurane, and innovar. Anesthesiology 1976; 45:390–399.
4. Michenfelder JD: The cerebral circulation. In Prys-Roberts C (ed): The Circulation in Anesthesia. London, Blackwell Scientific, 1980, p 212.
5. Halsey JH, McFarland S: Oxygen cycles and metabolic autoregulation. Stroke 1974; 5:219–225.
6. Shapiro BA, Harrison RD, Walton JR: Clinical Application of Blood Gases, ed 3. St Louis, Mosby-Year Book, 1982, 14.
7. Guyton AC: Textbook of Medical Physiology, ed 7. Philadelphia, WB Saunders, 1986, p 339.
8. Siesjo BK: Cerebral circulation and metabolism. J Neurosurg 1984; 60:883–908.
9. Seymour SS, Kety S, Schmidt CF: The effects of altered arterial tensions of carbon dioxide and oxygen on cerebral blood flow and cerebral oxygen consumption of normal young men. J Clin Invest 1948; 27:484–492.
10. Turner J, Lambertsen CJ, Owen SG, et al: Effects of .08 and .8 atmospheres of inspired PO_2 of 43 mmHg (abstract). Fed Proc 1967; 16:130.
11. Raichle ME, Posner JB, Plum F: Cerebral blood flow during and after hyperventilation. Arch Neurol 1970; 23:394–403.
12. Raichle ME, Stone HL: Cerebral blood flow during and after hypercapnia. Eur Neurol 1971–72; 6:1–5.
13. Lambertsen CJ, Smyth SM, Gelfand R: H^+ and PCO_2 as chemical factors in respiratory and cerebral circulatory control. J Appl Physiol 1961; 16:473–484.
14. Harper AM, Bell RA: The effect of metabolic acidosis and alkalosis on the blood flow through the cerebral cortex. J Neurol Neurosurg Psychiatry 1963; 26:341–344.
15. Sokoloff L: The effect of carbon dioxide on the cerebral circulation. Anesthesiology 1960; 21:664–673.
16. Reivich M: Arterial PCO_2 and cerebral hemodynamics. Am J Physiol 1964; 206:25–35.
17. Muizelaar P, van der Poel H, Li Z, et al: Pial arteriolar vessel diameter and CO_2 reactivity during prolonged hyperventilation in the rabbit. J Neurosurg 1988; 69:923–927.
18. Bouma GJ, Muizelaar JP: Cerebral blood flow, cerebral blood volume, and cerebrovascular reactivity after severe head injury. J Neurotrauma 1992; 9:S333–S348.
19. Lassen NA: Control of cerebral circulation in health and disease. Circ Res 1974; 34:749–760.
20. Olesen J: Contralateral focal increase of cerebral blood flow in man during arm work. Brain 1971; 94:635–646.
21. Lassen NA, Christensen MS: Physiology of cerebral blood flow. Br J Anaesth 1976; 48:719–734.
22. Wolfgang K, Wahl M: Local, chemical and neurogenic regulation of cerebral vascular resistance. Physiol Rev 1978; 58:656–689.
23. Bevegard BS, Shepherd JT: Regulation of the circulation during exercise in man. Physiol Rev 1967; 47:178–213.
24. Michenfelder JD, Gronert GA, Rehder K: Neuroanesthesia. Anesthesiology 1969; 30:65–100.
25. Muizelaar JP, Wei EP, Kontos HA: Mannitol causes compensatory vasoconstriction and vasodilation in response to blood viscosity changes. J Neurosurg 1983; 59:822–828.
26. Hudak AL, Jones MD, Popel AS, et al: Hemodilution causes size-dependent constriction of pial arterioles in the cat. Am J Physiol 1989; 257:H912–H917.
27. Cutler RWP, Page L, Galicich J, et al: Formation and absorption of cerebrospinal fluid in man. Brain 1968; 91:707–720.
28. Cserr HF: Physiology of the choroid plexus. Physiol Rev 1971; 51:273–311.
29. Jennett B, Teasdale G: Management of Head Injuries. Philadelphia, FA Davis, 1981.
30. Mamarou A, Shulman K, Rosende R: A nonlinear analysis of the cerebrospinal fluid system and intracranial pressure dynamics. J Neurosurg 1978; 48:332–344.
31. Leech P, Miller JD: Intracranial volume-pressure relationships during experimental brain compression in primates. Pressure responses to changes in ventricular volume. J Neurol Neurosurg Psychiatry 1974; 37:1093–1098.
32. Marmarou A, Tabaddor K: Intracranial pressure: Physiology and pathophysiology. In Cooper PR (ed): Head Injury. Baltimore, Williams & Wilkins, 1982, pp 115–127.
33. Venes JL, Shaywitz BA, Spender DD: Management of severe cerebral edema in the metabolic encephalopathy of Reye-Johnson syndrome. J Neurosurg 1978; 48:903–915.
34. Bedford RF, Morris L, Jane JA: Intracranial hypertension during surgery for supratentorial tumor: Correlation with preoperative computed tomography scans. Anesth Analg 1982; 61:430–433.
35. Risberg J, Lundberg, N, Ingvar DH: Regional cerebral blood volume during acute transient rises of the intracranial pressure (plateau waves). J Neurosurg 1969; 31:303–310.
36. McDowall DG: The effects of clinical concentrations of halothane on the blood flow and oxygen uptake of the cerebral cortex. Br J Anaesth 1967; 39:186–196.
37. Scheller MS, Tateishi A, Drummond JC, et al: The effects of sevoflurane on cerebral blood flow, cerebral metabolic rate for oxygen, intracranial pressure, and the electroencephalogram are similar to those of isoflurane in the rabbit. Anesthesiology 1988; 68:548–551.
38. Henriksen HT, Jorgensen PB: The effect of nitrous oxide on intracranial pressure in patients with intracranial disorders. Br J Anaesth 1973; 45:486–492.
39. Laitinen LV, Johansson GG, Tarkkanen L: The effect of nitrous oxide on pulsatile cerebral impedance and cerebral blood flow. Br J Anaesth 1967; 39:781–785.
40. Sokoloff L: The action of drugs on the cerebral circulation. Pharmacol Rev 1959; 11:1–85.
41. Smith AI, Wollman H: Cerebral blood flow and metabolism: Effects of anesthetic drugs and techniques. Anesthesiology 1972; 36:378–400.
42. Pierce ED, Lambertsen CJ, Deutsch S, et al: Cerebral circulation and metabolism during thiopental anesthesia and hyperventilation in man. J Clin Invest 1962; 41:1664–1671.
43. Shapiro HM, Galindo A, Wyte SR, et al: Rapid intraoperative reduction of intracranial pressure with thiopentone. Br J Anaesth 1973; 45:1057–1062.
44. Jobes DR, Kennell E, Bitner R, et al: Effects of morphine–nitrous oxide anesthesia on cerebral autoregulation. Anesthesiology 1975; 42:30–34.
45. Jung R, Shah N, Reinsel R, et al: Cerebrospinal fluid pressure in patients with brain tumors: Impact of fentanyl versus alfentanil during nitrous oxide–oxygen anesthesia. Anesth Analg 1990; 71: 419–422.

46. Milde LN, Milde JH, Gallagher WJ: Effects of sufentanil on cerebral circulation and metabolism in dogs. Anesth Analg 1990; 70: 138–146.
47. Gibbs JM: The effect of intravenous ketamine on cerebrospinal fluid pressure. Br J Anaesth 1971; 44:1298–1302.
48. Shapiro HM, Wyte SR, Harris AB: Ketamine anaesthesia in patients with intracranial pathology. Br J Anaesth 1972; 44:1200–1204.
49. Sari A, Okida Y, Takeshita H: The effect of ketamine on cerebrospinal fluid pressure. Anesth Analg 1972; 51:560–565.
50. Carlsson C, Chapman AG: The effect of diazepam on the cerebral metabolic state in rats and its interaction with nitrous oxide. Anesthesiology 1981; 54:488–495.
51. Foster A, Juge O, Morel D: Effects of midazolam on cerebral blood flow in human volunteers. Anesthesiology 1982; 56:453–455.
52. Rockoff MA, Naughton KVH, Shapiro HM, et al: Cerebral circulatory and metabolic responses to intravenously administered lorazepam. Anesthesiology 1980; 53:215–218.
53. Sebel PS, Lowden JD: Propofol: A new intravenous anesthetic. Anesthesiology 1989; 71:260–277.
54. Pinaud M, Lelausque JN, Chetanneau A, et al: Effects of propofol on cerebral hemodynamics and metabolism in patients with brain trauma. Anesthesiology 1990; 73:404–409.
55. Varma YS, Sharma PL, Minocha KB: Comparative evaluation of cerebral and hepatic blood flow under d-tubocurarine and pancuronium in dogs. Indian J Med Res 1977; 66:317–322.
56. Belik J, Wagerle LC, Delivoria-Papadopoulos M: Cerebral blood flow and metabolism following pancuronium bromide in newborn lambs. Pediatr Res 1984; 18:1305–1308.
57. Griffin JP, Hartung J, Cottrell JE, et al: Effect of vecuronium on intracranial pressure, mean arterial pressure and heart rate in cats. Br J Anaesth 1986; 58:441–443.
58. Rosa G, Sanfilippo M, Vilardi M, et al: Effects of vecuronium bromide on intracranial pressure and cerebral perfusion pressure. Br J Anaesth 1986; 58:437–440.
59. Minton MD, Stirt JA, Bedford RF, Haworth C: Intracranial pressure after atracurium in neurosurgical patients. Anesth Analg 1985; 64:1113–1116.
60. Lanier WL, Milde JH, Michenfelder JD: The cerebral effects of pancuronium and atracurium in halothane-anesthetized dogs. Anesthesiology 1985; 63:589–597.
61. Lanier WL, Milde JM, Michenfelder JD: Cerebral stimulation following succinylcholine in dogs. Anesthesiology 1986; 64:551–559.
62. Minton MD, Grosslight K, Stirt JA, Bedford RF: Increases in intracranial pressure from succinylcholine: Prevention by prior nondepolarizing blockade. Anesthesiology 1986; 65:165–169.
63. Stirt JA, Grosslight KR, Bedford RF, Vollmer D: "Defasciculation" with metocurine prevents succinylcholine-induced increases in intracranial pressure. Anesthesiology 1987; 67:50–53.
64. Cottrell JE, Robustelli A, Post K, Turndorf H: Furosemide- and mannitol-induced changes in intracranial pressure and serum osmolality and electrolytes. Anesthesiology 1977; 47:28–30.
65. Leech P, Miller JD: Intracranial volume-pressure relationships during experimental brain compression in primates. J Neurol Neurosurg Psychiatry 1974; 37:1105–1111.
66. Johnston IH, Harper AM: The effect of mannitol on cerebral blood flow: An experimental study. J Neurosurg 1973; 38:461–471.
67. Turner JM, Powell D, Gibson RM, et al: Intracranial pressure changes in neurosurgical patients during hypotension induced with sodium nitroprusside or trimetaphan. Br J Anaesth 1977; 49:419–424.
68. James DJ, Bedford RF: Hydralazine for controlled hypotension during neurosurgical operations. Anesth Analg 1982; 61:1016–1019.
69. Ghani GA, Sung YF, Weinstein MA, et al: Effects of intravenous nitroglycerin on the intracranial pressure and volume pressure response. J Neurosurg 1983; 58:562–565.
70. Fahmy NR, Soter NA: Effects of trimethaphan on arterial blood histamine and systemic hemodynamics in humans. Anesthesiology 1985; 62:562–566.
71. Berntman L, Carlsson C, Siesjo BK: Influence of propranolol on cerebral metabolism and blood flow in the rat brain. Brain Res 1978; 151:220–224.
72. Aken HV, Puchstein C, Schweppe ML, et al: Effect of labetalol on intracranial pressure in dogs with and without intracranial hypertension. Acta Anaesthesiol Scand 1982; 26:615–619.
73. Benfield P, Sorkin EM: Esmolol. A preliminary review of pharmacodynamic and pharmacokinetic properties, and therapeutic efficacy. Drugs 1987; 33:392–412.
74. Hadley MN, Spetzler RF, Fifield MS, et al: The effect of nimodipine on intracranial pressure. J Neurosurg 1987; 66:387–393.
75. Nishikawa T, Omote K, Namiki A, et al: The effects of nicardipine on cerebrospinal fluid pressure in humans. Anesth Analg 1986; 65:507–510.
76. Marshall LF, Bowers SA: Medical management of intracranial pressure. In Cooper PR (ed): Head Injury. Baltimore: Williams & Wilkins, 1982, pp 129–146.
77. Strandgaard S: Autoregulation of cerebral blood flow in hypertensive patients. Circulation 1975; 53:720–727.
78. Wilkinson HA: Intracranial pressure monitoring: Techniques and pitfalls. In Cooper PR (ed): Head Injury. Baltimore: Williams & Wilkins, 1982, pp 147–184.
79. Sundbarg G, Nordstrom CH, Messeter K, et al: A comparison of intraparenchymatous and intraventricular pressure recording in clinical practice. J Neurosurg 1987; 67:841–845.
80. Mendelow AD, Rowan JO, Murray L, Kerr AE: A clinical comparison of subdural screw pressure measurements with ventricular pressure. J Neurosurg 1983; 58:45–50.
81. Jorgensen PB, Riishede J: Comparative clinical studies of epidural and ventricular pressure. In Brock M, Dietz H (eds): Intracranial Pressure: Experimental and Clinical Aspects. Berlin, Springer-Verlag, 1972, pp 41–45.
82. Friedman WA, Vries JK: Percutaneous tunnel ventriculostomy. J Neurosurg 1980; 53:662–665.
83. Narayan RK, Kishore PR, Becker DP, et al: Intracranial pressure: To Monitor or not to monitor? J Neurosurg 1982; 56:650–659.
84. Langfitt TW: Clinical methods for monitoring intracranial pressure and measuring cerebral blood flow. Clin Neurosurg 1976; 23:302–320.
85. Rosner MJ, Becker DP: ICP monitoring: Complications and associated factors. Clin Neurosurg 1976; 23:494–519.
86. Vries JK, Becker DP, Young HF: A subarachnoid screw for monitoring intracranial pressure. J Neurosurg 1973; 39:416–419.
87. Wilkinson HA: The intracranial pressure-monitoring cup catheter: Technical note. Neurosurgery 1977; 1:139–141.
88. Koster WG, Kuypers MH: Intracranial pressure and its epidural measurement. Med Prog Technol 1980; 7:21–27.
89. Kleiber M: Physical instruments for the biologist. Rev Sci Instr 1945; 15:79–81.
90. Barlow P, Mendelow AD, Lawrence AE, et al: Clinical evaluation of two methods of subdural pressure monitoring. J Neurosurg 1985; 63:578–582.
91. Allen R: Intracranial pressure: A review of clinical problems, measurement techniques and monitoring methods. J Med Eng Tech 1986; 10:299–320.
92. Crutchfield JS, Narayan RK, Robertson CS, et al: Evaluation of a fiberoptic intracranial pressure monitor. J Neurosurg 1990; 72: 482–487.
93. Ostrup RC, Luerssen TG, Marshall LF, et al: Continuous monitoring of intracranial pressure with a miniaturized fiberoptic device. J Neurosurg 1987; 67:206–209.
94. Rabow L, Bergenheim T, Balfors E: Intraparenchymal and conventional monitoring of intracranial pressure. J Clin Monit Comput 1990; 6:163.
95. Chambers IR, Menelow AD, Sinar EJ, et al: A clinical evaluation of the Camino subdural screw and ventricular monitoring kits. Neurosurgery 1990; 26:421–423.
96. Artru AA: Relationship between cerebral blood volume and CSF pressure during anesthesia with halothane or enflurane in dogs. Anesthesiology 1983; 58:533–539.
97. Cucchiara RF, Theye RA, Michenfelder JD: The effects of isoflurane on canine cerebral metabolism and blood flow. Anesthesiology 1974; 40:571–574.
98. Muzzi DA, Losasso TH, Dietz NM, et al: The effect of desflurane and isoflurane on cerebrospinal fluid pressure in humans with supratentorial mass lesions. Anesthesiology 1992; 76:720–724.
99. Milde LN, Milde JH, Michenfelder JD: Cerebral functional, metabolic and hemodynamic effects of etomidate in dogs. Anesthesiology 1985; 63:371–377.

10 Monitoring the Neuromuscular Junction

Michael H. Wall, M.D.
Richard C. Prielipp, M.D.

Neuromuscular blocking (NMB) drugs have been used extensively in the operating room (OR) for over 55 years, whereas their widespread use in the intensive care unit (ICU) is more recent. All NMB drugs not only interrupt normal neuromuscular transmission but also produce potent autonomic, hemodynamic, respiratory, and immunologic effects. Appropriate clinical utilization of these drugs relies on a thorough understanding of normal neuromuscular transmission, the pharmacology and monitoring of NMB drug actions, and potential complications of their use.

The Neuromuscular Junction in Health and Disease

The neuromuscular junction, which is the triad of a motor nerve terminus, the neurotransmitter acetylcholine (ACh), and the postsynaptic muscle endplate, controls voluntary muscle contraction. An action potential reaching the motor nerve terminus causes release of ACh from synaptic vesicles, each one containing about 10,000 molecules of the neurotransmitter. This concentrated release of ACh rapidly diffuses across the 20-nm gap to the postsynaptic endplate (Fig. 10-1). The motor endplate contains specialized ligand-gated, nicotinic ACh receptors (nAChRs), which convert the chemical signal (i.e., binding of two ACh molecules) into electrical signals (i.e., a transient permeability change and depolarization in the postsynaptic membrane of striated muscle).[1] Voluntary muscle contraction follows.

nAChRs are clustered at the muscle endplate, concentrated on the crests of the postjunctional membrane folds. Each nAChR is a pentameric glycoprotein complex (total molecular weight of 250 kD) composed of four subunits—alpha, beta, epsilon, and delta—in a ratio of 2:1:1:1.[1, 2] Each of the two alpha subunits acts as an ACh binding site (Fig. 10-2). When stimulated simultaneously by two ACh molecules, the channel undergoes conformational change and opens for 1 ms, allowing nonselective passage of small positively charged ions, mainly sodium (Na^+, peak rate of $\geq 30,000$ ions per channel per millisecond), potassium, and calcium. This Na^+ influx depolarizes the nearby muscle membrane, triggering local voltage-gated Na^+ channels, and thereby creates a self-propagating depolarization (i.e., a muscle action potential). Excitation-contraction coupling results in voluntary muscle contraction. Under most circumstances, a "safety margin" for neuromuscular transmission exists whereby excess ACh is released to ensure effective signal transduction. The action of ACh is terminated by dissociation and passive diffusion away from the endplate, along with

enzymatic degradation by acetylcholinesterase. Subsequently, the nAChR channel makes a transition rapidly through desensitized and closed states to recycle itself for the next nerve impulse.

One of the striking features of the neuromuscular junction is the concentration of nAChR on the postsynaptic membrane (each endplate has 1 to 10 million receptors). Normal *neural* activity and stimulation of the motor endplate regulates the translation and membrane integration of the nAChR. Before synapse formation, ACh receptors (AChRs) are evenly distributed across the muscle membrane, but within hours after interaction with the nerve, receptor density increases 1000-fold to a concentration of greater than 10,000 receptors per microgram.[2] Figure 10-3 shows a schematic model of the organization and structure of this postsynaptic region. Agrin is the nerve-derived extracellular protein that is instrumental in triggering receptor clustering during synapse formation.[3] However, receptor aggregation appears to occur in distinct steps, with small clusters followed by formation of larger ones, and then final stabilization of mature receptor domains. Initial nAChR clusters probably form around the protein rapsyn, whereas utrophin may be principally involved in the enlargement of these early AChR clusters into larger ones. Meanwhile, ∂-dystroglycan, the extracellular component of dystrophin-associated glycoprotein complex (DGC), appears to be the agrin receptor which transduces final AChR clustering. Lastly, utrophin bridges the maturing clusters to underlying strands of F-actin in the internal muscle cytoskeleton, thus forming immobile, mature, functional receptor domains.

Adult skeletal muscle retains an ability to synthesize both the mature, adult AChR, as well as an immature nAChR variant (see Fig. 10-2), in which a gamma subunit is substituted for the normal epsilon subunit.[2] In diseases such as Guillain-Barré syndrome, stroke, poliomyelitis, spinal cord injury, burns, severe muscle trauma, enforced immobilization, or other conditions producing loss of nerve function, synthesis of immature (fetal) receptors may be triggered (see Fig. 10-2). These immature nAChRs are distinguished by three features. First, immature receptors are not localized to the muscle endplate, but migrate across the entire membrane surface.[1, 2] Second, the immature receptors are metabolically short-lived (<24 hours) and more ionically active, having a 2- to 10-fold longer channel "open time." Lastly, these immature receptors are more sensitive to the depolarizing effects of drugs such as succinylcholine or decamethonium, and more resistant to the effects of competitive antagonists such as *d*-tubocurarine. The clinical consequences of upregulation of these abnormal receptors are profound and prob-

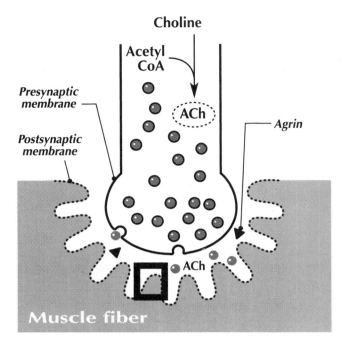

Figure 10-1. Schematic diagram of a motor nerve terminus, where the neurotransmitter acetylcholine (ACh) is synthesized and stored in vesicles. A neuronal action potential induces release of ACh from these synaptic vesicles, where it diffuses the 20-nm gap to the postsynaptic endplate. The junctional folds of the motor endplate concentrate several million specialized nicotinic acetylcholine receptors (nAChR), which induce a transient membrane depolarization resulting in striated muscle contraction. The area within the black box (at the junctional fold of the motor endplate) is enlarged in Figures 10-2 and 10-3 to illustrate the molecular details of the nAChR complex.

lematic.[2, 4-6] For example, in acute spinal cord injury and burn patients, denervation-induced proliferation of immature (gamma subunit) nAChR may explain the observed sensitivity and potentially lethal hyperkalemic response to depolarizing agonists such as succinylcholine.[5, 6] In addition, this same phenomenon may explain NMB drug resistance and tachyphylaxis to nondepolarizing NMB drugs such as *d*-tubocurarine, vecuronium, and atracurium in these same ICUs of patients.

Neuromuscular Blocking Drugs

Relationship of Structure to Activity

The neurotransmitter ACh has a positively charged quaternary ammonium ($[N-C_4]^+$) group which binds with the negatively charged alpha subunit of the nAChR at the neuromuscular junction.[1, 2] All clinically available NMB drugs also contain one or more quaternary ammonium groups that promote molecular binding. The structure of the ACh molecule is functionally duplicated in the chemical structure of NMB drugs and helps impart receptor specificity. All NMB drugs interact at the postjunctional alpha-subunit receptor sites, but they vary in their associated autonomic effects. Muscarinic "contamination" may result in bradycardia or tachycardia, while blockade of nicotinic autonomic ganglia may produce significant hypotension. Endogenous release of vasoactive amines such as histamine leads to hypotension and flushing.

Drug structure is also related to NMB drug potency. The greater potency of certain NMB drugs, used in relatively smaller doses, has two clinical implications. Increased potency allows the administration of fewer drug molecules, generally resulting in fewer unwanted side effects. Thus, drugs such as doxacurium and pipecuronium are noteworthy for their lack of hemodynamic or autonomic interactions. However, administration of less drug also means fewer molecules to antagonize neuromuscular junctional receptors and a slower onset of action. This phenomenon is explained by

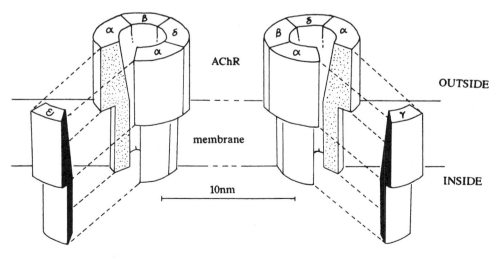

Figure 10-2. The mature nicotinic acetylcholine receptor (nAChR) (left) with its glycoprotein subunits arranged around the central cation core. Two molecules of acetylcholine bind simultaneously to the two alpha subunits to convert the channel to an open state. The immature, or fetal-variant receptor, is shown on the right with a single subunit substitution, which follows major stress (e.g., burns or denervation). These immature receptors are characterized by 10-fold greater ionic activity, rapid metabolic turnover, and extrajunctional proliferation. Use of a depolarizing muscle relaxant (succinylcholine) in patients with proliferating, immature nAChRs will lead to severe, acute hyperkalemia. (From Martyn JAJ, White DA, Gronert GA, et al: Up-and-down regulation of skeletal muscle acetylcholine receptors. Anesthesiology 1992; 76: 822-843.)

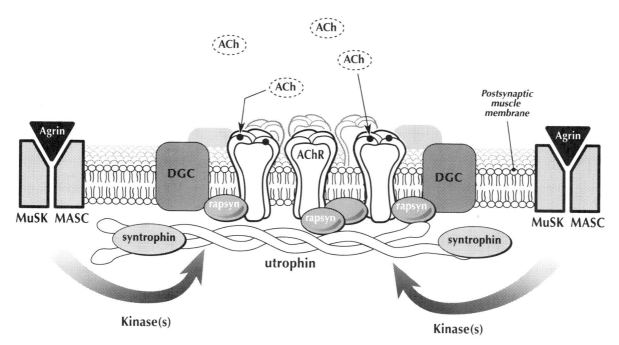

Figure 10-3. Schematic drawing of the molecular organization of the nicotinic acetylcholine receptors (nAChR) in the postsynaptic muscle membrane. Agrin is the *nerve-derived* ~200-kD protein that triggers clustering of receptor proteins during synapse formation, as well as concentrating other synaptic proteins such as acetylcholinesterase, rapsyn, and utrophin. Evidence suggests that MuSK (muscle-specific kinase), along with a cofactor MASC (myotube-associated specificity component) activates certain kinase activity which initiates clustering of synaptic proteins. Receptor aggregation occurs in distinct steps, however, initiated with nAChR localization by rapsyn. Meanwhile, ∂-dystroglycan (not shown), the extracellular component of dystrophin-associated glycoprotein complex (DGC), may also function as an agrin receptor, and promotes further nAChR clustering. The final process utilizes the structural organization of additional proteins like utrophin, which stabilize the mature, immobile domains by interaction with the underlying cytoskeleton (F-actin). When completed, this process concentrates nAChR density 1000-fold compared to unmodified muscle membrane. The agrin signaling mechanism must remain active throughout the life of the synapse in order to maintain stability. (Drawn from Apel ED, Merlie JP: Assembly of the postsynaptic apparatus. Curr Opin Neurobiol 1995; 5: 62–67; Burden SJ: The formation of neuromuscular synapses. Genes Dev 1998; 12:133–148; and Wells DG, Fallon JR: Neuromuscular junctions: The state of the union. Curr Biol 1996; 6:1073–1075.)

the large proportion (≥75% to 80%) of receptors which must be occupied for the clinical onset of neuromuscular blockade to occur. Thus, low-potency drugs deliver a larger number of drug molecules at higher concentration more quickly to the nAChR of the neuromuscular junction. In addition, there are intrinsic drug differences based on the equilibrium dissociation constants of various NMB drugs that dictate the speed of drug-nAChR interaction.

Drug Action

NMB drugs produce muscle relaxation by either sustained activation of the nAChR or blocking of the activation of the nAChR. Succinylcholine is the depolarizing NMB drug that initially activates nAChR and opens the receptor channel. However, unlike ACh, succinylcholine is not metabolized by acetylcholinesterase in the neuromuscular junction, and repeatedly binds with the nAChR, leading to prolonged endplate depolarization and subsequent flaccid paralysis. Nondepolarizing NMB drugs competitively bind to the nAChR, preventing binding of ACh and depolarization. The nondepolarizing drugs can be further categorized by their chemical structure (aminosteroid versus benzylisoquinolinium) or by the duration of action of neuromuscular blockade.

Depolarizing Neuromuscular Blockade

Succinylcholine is the only depolarizing NMB agent in common use today. Succinylcholine is synthesized by binding

two molecules of ACh together. Succinylcholine is very rapidly metabolized to choline and succinylmonocholine by plasma cholinesterase (also known as pseudo- or butyryl cholinesterase), while a minority of succinylcholine actually reaches the neuromuscular junction. Succinylcholine binds to the ACh receptors located pre- and postsynaptically, as well as to extrajunctional AChRs. (Succinylcholine binding to presynaptic nAChR may be responsible for the commonly observed muscle fasciculations.) Succinylcholine repeatedly binds alpha subunits of the nAChR, producing a motor endplate that is electrically refractory and functionally unexcitable. The prolonged depolarization of the neuromuscular junction also inactivates perijunctional, voltage-sensitive sodium channels, which also prevents propagation of an action potential.[5] The neuromuscular junction remains depolarized, and the muscle flaccid, until the succinylcholine diffuses away from the neuromuscular junction.[5, 6]

The administration of 1.0 mg/kg of succinylcholine intravenously (IV) (twice the dose that produces the desired effect on 95% of a population, or ED_{95}) causes fasciculations, followed by flaccid paralysis within 30 to 60 seconds, with full recovery occurring after 7 to 12 minutes. This is termed phase I block and is characterized by decreased single-twitch height and no fade with sustained tetanus, train-of-four (TOF), or double-burst stimulation (DBS); no post-tetanic facilitation; and potentiation by anticholinesterase inhibitors[5] (Fig. 10–4). Activation of the nAChR by succinylcholine may also cause prolonged muscular contraction of the masseter and adductor pollicis muscles: the mechanism is unclear, but this effect can be blocked by the administration of a paralyz-

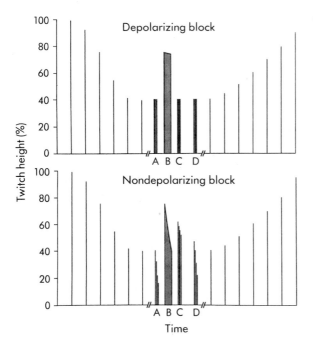

Figure 10–4. Phase I depolarizing block (upper panel) showing decreased single twitch height, no fade with train-of-four (TOF) stimulation (A) or tetany (B) and no post-tetanic facilitation (C and D). The lower panel shows the characteristics of nondepolarizing block with fade to TOF (A) and tetanus (B) and post-tetanic facilitation (C and D). (From Brull SJ, Silverman DG: Neuromuscular block monitoring. *In* Ehrenwerth J, Eisenkraft JE (eds): Anesthesia Equipment: Principles and Applications. St Louis, Mosby–Year Book, 1993, pp 297–318.)

ing dose of a nondepolarizing NMB drug (atracurium) prior to the administration of succinylcholine.[7] Thus, this effect is probably mediated by postsynaptic receptors.[7]

When succinylcholine is used as an infusion or with repeated boluses, a block resembling a nondepolarizing block, with tetanic fade, post-tetanic potentiation, and reversal with anticholinesterase drugs (called phase II block) may occur. The mechanism is unclear; however, phase II block may be due to desensitization, actual blockade of the AChR ion channel by succinylcholine, or interference with production and release of ACh.[8]

Nondepolarizing Neuromuscular Blockade

The nondepolarizing NMB drugs are categorized on the basis of their chemical structure, that is, aminosteroids (pancuronium, vecuronium, pipecuronium, rocuronium) or benzylisoquinoliniums (*d*-tubocurarine, dimethyltubocurarine, atracurium, cisatracurium, doxacurium, mivacurium, gallamine). They may also be differentiated by their duration of action as short (<30 minutes after an "intubating dose" of twice the ED_{95}—mivacurium), intermediate (30 to 60 minutes after an "intubating dose" of twice the ED_{95}—vecuronium, rocuronium and atracurium, or cisatracurium) or long-acting (>60 minutes after an "intubating dose" of twice the ED_{95}—*d*-tubocurarine, dimethyltubocurarine, pancuronium, pipecuronium, gallamine, or doxacurium). These drugs also bind to the prejunctional AChR, preventing the rapid reaccumulation of ACh within the nerve axon, which may account for "fade" seen with repetitive stimulation.[6] Nondepolarizing

neuromuscular block is characterized by decreased single-twitch height, fade with tetanus, TOF and DBS, and post-tetanic facilitation (see Fig. 10–4).

Indications for Monitoring

In the OR, the degree of neuromuscular blockade is routinely monitored by qualitative grading of a motor response to transcutaneous peripheral nerve stimulation.[9, 10] Monitoring depth of neuromuscular blockade should be routine in the ICU to prevent excess administration of NMB drugs and to maintain the least degree of neuromuscular block necessary to provide optimal patient care. The use of peripheral nerve stimulation also allows neuromuscular function to be assessed.[11, 12] Traditionally, the ulnar nerve at the wrist is stimulated while the motor response of the adductor pollicis brevis muscle of the thumb is evaluated. Other peripheral nerve sites (such as facial nerve stimulation while grading the orbicularis oculi muscle, or stimulating the peroneal nerve of the upper leg and grading foot dorsiflexion) are also available, but exhibit slightly different neuromuscular blockade profiles.[11, 12] Patients with stroke, paraplegia, or dense peripheral neuropathies should be monitored on unaffected limbs, because affected extremities exhibit resistance to neuromuscular blockade.

The TOF is the most reliable and convenient method for clinical monitoring of neuromuscular blockade, particularly in awake patients when the more vigorous tetanic stimulation is both uncomfortable and stressful. The TOF response delivers four supramaximal stimuli (50- to 80-mA current) at 2 Hz (one stimulus every 0.5 second), while the motor twitch response of the fourth twitch (T4) is compared to the twitch response of the first stimulus (T1). Visual or tactile evaluation of the TOF response is adequate for most clinical applications. More precise characterization of the motor response is possible with commercially available force-displacement transducer recorders, mechanomyography (MMG), electromyography (EMG), or accelerography (ACG). In addition, new patterns of nerve stimulation, such as DBS (two train-of-three stimulations separated by 750 ms), are designed to detect residual neuromuscular blockade in awake patients without causing excessive discomfort. The following sections describe the types of nerve stimulators, stimulating patterns, and muscles commonly used for monitoring patients in the OR and ICU.

Monitor Stimulators

Nerve stimulators pass an electrical current across peripheral nerves. If enough current is applied to depolarize an axon, an action potential is generated and transmitted to the nerve terminal, where ACh is released. When 5% to 20% of AChRs are activated by ACh, the endplate reaches a threshold potential of 45 mV, and a motor action potential is generated. Sodium receptors along the entire muscle fiber are then activated, leading to mechanical contraction.[8, 13]

Because peripheral nerves are made up of a large number of axons of different sizes and depolarizing thresholds, not all nerves will depolarize at equal currents. As higher currents are applied, more axons are depolarized, leading to a stronger muscular contraction. Eventually a point is reached where further increases in current do not cause further significant increases in the force of contraction. This relationship between current applied and force generated is sigmoidal[14] (Fig. 10–5).

The amount of current needed for neuromuscular moni-

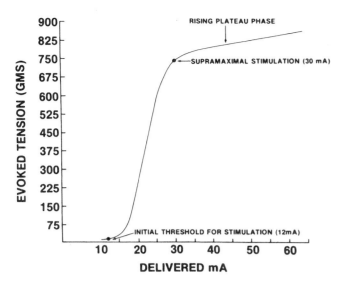

Figure 10–5. Increases in delivered transcutaneous current produce no response until a threshold is reached (the initial threshold for stimulation). Beyond a point of supramaximal stimulation, further increases in current cause minimal additional increases in contractile force. (From Kopman AF, Lawson D: Milliamperage requirements for supramaximal stimulation of the ulnar nerve with surface electrodes. Anesthesiology 1984; 61:83–85.)

toring depends on the nerve being stimulated, the type of electrodes used, and the impedance present. The lowest current needed to generate muscular activity is the initial threshold for stimulation (ITS) current.[14] With surface electrodes on properly prepared skin the ITS is usually less than 15 mA.[15] The current required to depolarize all fibers of a nerve bundle is called the *maximal current,* and when single-twitch height is being monitored, a supramaximal current (10% to 20% more than the maximal current) should be used. The supramaximal current at the wrist for ulnar nerve stimulation is 2.75 to 3 times the ITS.[14]

Surface electrodes using pregelled sodium and sodium chloride, silver and silver chloride, or conductive rubber are commonly used. The skin should be prepared by removing excess hair, followed by light abrasion to remove cornified skin, and then cleansing with alcohol. This will produce an ITS of less than 15 mA. If the ITS cannot be obtained below this threshold, the impedance may be too high, and consideration should be given to using percutaneous needle electrodes. Needle electrodes may also be considered in obese patients, edematous patients, and patients who are very hypothermic. Needle electrode systems usually have a low impedance of 500 to 2000 ωms, allowing for currents of less than 10 mA for supramaximal stimulation. However, caution is warranted because needle electrodes are invasive and painful, may be a site for skin infection, and can cause localized burn.[15]

If possible, the negative (black or stimulating) electrode should be placed distally over the nerve, while the positive (red) electrode should be placed more proximally (not over any other nerves). This electrode orientation allows for a lower supramaximal stimulation threshold, and is more important the greater the distance between the stimulating electrodes.[16]

The ideal nerve stimulator would be small, durable, and battery-powered. It should produce a constant current, square wave impulse of 0.1 to 0.2 ms, because shorter stimulus times may not depolarize all axons in the nerve and longer times may cause direct muscle stimulation or exceed

the refractory period of the nerve.[17] The current setting needs to be adjustable from 0 to 5 mA for subcutaneous nerve localization, 5 to 10 mA for subcutaneous nerve stimulation, and 30 to 100 mA for transcutaneous electrode stimulation. Ideally there should be two separate outputs for low and high currents. There should be an audible and visual signal with each stimulus, as well as alarms for excessive impedance, lead disconnection, or low battery condition. The stimulator should have several patterns of stimulation, including single twitch, TOF, tetanus, DBS, and post-tetanic count. The ideal stimulator would also have a simple, easy-to-use recording of the results of stimulation[15, 18, 19] (Fig. 10–6).

Patterns of Stimulation

Both depolarizing and nondepolarizing NMB drugs decrease single-twitch height—but nondepolarizing block (and phase II depolarizing block) also cause fade with sustained tetanus, TOF stimulation, and DBS. These modalities are commonly used to monitor nondepolarizing neuromuscular blockade, and are explained later (Table 10–1, Fig. 10–7).

Single Twitch

A supramaximal stimulus current is applied at intervals of 10 seconds or more and the twitch height is compared to a pre-NMB drug baseline. Limitations of this form of monitoring include the need for a baseline measurement and the lack of sensitivity with very deep levels of blockade. In addition, twitch height is normal until more than 70% of receptors are occupied and twitch height is zero when 90% to 95% of the receptors are blocked.

Tetanus

There is sustained muscle tetanus without fade when a frequency of 50 Hz is applied for 5 seconds, even when up to 75% of nAChRs are occupied by nondepolarizing NMB drugs. Use of frequencies of 50 Hz for 5 seconds will cause fade when more than 75% of receptors are occupied by nondepolarizing NMB drugs. Tetanus stimulation of greater than 100 Hz for 5 seconds may cause fade in patients anesthetized only with isoflurane or enflurane at 1.25 minimum anesthetic concentration (MAC) (i.e., without NMB drugs).[20]

Tetanus at 50 Hz for 5 seconds is a useful modality clinically because there is no need for a baseline measurement. The presence of fade means more than 75% of receptors are blocked—and the absence of fade means fewer than 75% of receptors are blocked. Absence of fade usually correlates with the ability to protect the airway after tracheal extubation. The main disadvantage of tetanus stimulation is that it is painful in awake patients and may cause post-tetanic facilitation (PTF). PTF will cause an exaggerated response to single twitch and TOF monitoring if single twitch or TOF stimulation is performed within 1 to 2 minutes of tetanus (see below).[5, 21]

Train-of-Four

TOF is the most commonly used mode of nerve stimulation, wherein four stimuli are delivered at 2 Hz.[22] The response can be recorded as the TOF count (TOFc) or the TOF ratio (TOFr). The TOFc is the easiest to perform and is used most commonly in clinical anesthesia and in ICUs. The TOFr is

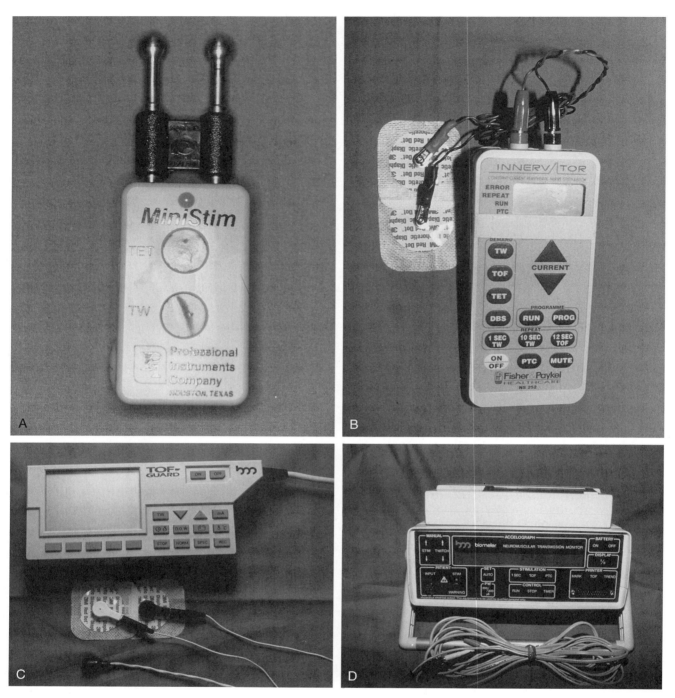

Figure 10–6. *A–D,* Four models of commercially available peripheral nerve stimulators are pictured. All units deliver variable voltage, constant current nerve stimulation for monitoring the depth of neuromuscular block. The more complex (and expensive) models provide improved accuracy, greater operator control of current selection, and a wider array of available stimulation patterns. *A,* The MiniStim (Professional Instruments Company, Houston, TX). *B,* The Innervator Model NS 252 (Fisher & Paykel Healthcare, Auckland, New Zealand). *C,* The TOF-Guard (Biometer, Turnhout, Belgium). *D,* The Accelograph Model US 1 (Biometer International A/S, DK-5210 Odense NV, Denmark). The first two stimulators (*A* and *B*) rely on visual or tactile response of the adductor pollicis brevis muscle to ulnar nerve stimulation. The latter two (*C* and *D*) stimulators utilize an acceleration transducer attached to the thumb to automatically record the muscle twitch response to stimulation. Skeletal muscle acceleration is linearly related to traditional force-displacement measurements usually recorded in scientific or research studies.

most commonly used experimentally; however, unless monitored with a transducer and recording system, visual or tactile assessment of the TOFr is not reliable.[23] The advantage of TOF stimulation is there is no need for a prerelaxant baseline, because comparing T1 with T4 serves as its own comparator. The TOFr and TOFc of the adductor pollicis have been extensively studied with a variety of nondepolarizing NMB drugs. The TOFr is equal to 1 in the absence of

Table 10–1. Relationship of Receptor Occupancy, Neuromuscular Monitoring, and Clinical Signs at Adductor Pollicis With Nondepolarizing Neuromuscular Blockade

NMJ Receptions Blocked (%)	T1 Twitch % Baseline	T4 Twitch % Baseline	TOFr	TOFc	Tetanus	Comments*
100	0	0	0	0		
95	5	0	0	0		Adequate for tracheal intubation
90	10	0	0	1		PTC ≥ 10
	20	0	0	2		
80	25	0	0	3	Onset of fade at 30 Hz	
80	80–90	55–65	0.6–0.7	4		VC ≥ 15 mL/kg, MIP ≥ −22 cm H_2O, V_T ≥ 8 mL/kg, sustained eye opening, hand grip
	95	65–70	0.7–0.75	4		
75	100	75–100	0.75–1.0	4		Diplopia common
	100	90–100	0.8–1.0	4	Sustained at 50 Hz	5-s leg lift, 5-s head lift, MIP ≥ −42 cm H_2O, effective swallowing, masseter strength normal
			0.9–1.0	4		Normal UES tone, pharyngeal function
50	100	100	1.0	4	Onset of fade at 100 Hz	
35	100	100	1.0	4	Onset of fade at 200 Hz	

NMJ, neuromuscular junction; T1, first twitch; T4, fourth twitch; TOFr, train-of-four ratio (T4/T1); TOFc, train-of-four count; PTC, post-tetanic count; VC, vital capacity; V_T, tidal volume; MIP, maximum inspired pressure; UES, upper esophageal sphincter.
*Clinical signs: tests do not always correlate with TOFr and TOFc and do not always ensure normal NMJ function, adequacy of ventilatory function, or the ability to protect the airway.
Modified from Silverman DG, Brull SJ: Patterns of stimulation. *In* Silverman DG (ed.): Neuromuscular Block in Perioperative and Intensive Care. Philadelphia, JB Lippincott, 1994, pp 37–50.

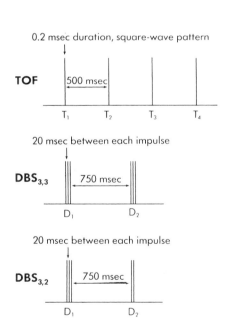

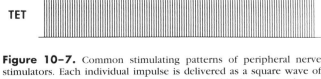

Figure 10–7. Common stimulating patterns of peripheral nerve stimulators. Each individual impulse is delivered as a square wave of 200-μs duration. TOF, train-of-four; DBS, double burst stimulation; TET, tetanic stimulation. (From Brull SJ, Silverman DG: Neuromuscular block monitoring. *In* Ehrenwerth J, Eisenkraft JE (eds): Anesthesia Equipment: Principles and Applications. St. Louis, Mosby–Year Book, 1993, pp 297–318.)

neuromuscular blockade. When the TOFr is greater than 70%, there is sustained tetanus at 50 Hz, and single twitch has reached control height, all of which correlates to less than 75% receptor blockade.[24]

When more than 70% of the neuromuscular junction receptors are blocked by nondepolarizing NMB drugs, there is fade at 50 Hz, T4 is less than T1, and the TOFr is less than 1.[25] The degree of fade of T4 is similar to the degree of fade after 5 seconds of tetanus at 50 Hz.[26] With progressive increases in receptor occupancy, the TOFr continues to decrease. At greater than 80% receptor occupancy T1 is 25% of baseline, and T4 is no longer present (TOFr = 0, TOFc = 3). At 90% receptor occupancy T1 is 10% of baseline and T2 and T3 are lost (TOFc = 1), and at greater than 90% occupancy there are no twitches (TOFc = 0).[5, 27] TOF monitoring is valid when repeated as often as every 10 to 15 seconds.

Double Burst Stimulation

DBS is two bursts of two to four impulses. The impulses are of 0.2-ms duration at 50 Hz. The bursts are separated by 0.75 second. Many patterns have been evaluated, but the most common pattern used clinically is two bursts of three impulses at 50 Hz (DBS$_{3,3}$). The first burst is called D$_1$ and the second burst D$_2$.[28–30] The D2/D1 ratio of DBS$_{3,3}$ correlates with T4/T1, and DBS fade is easier to detect manually than T4/T1 fade.[30] Also, DBS can be used at deeper levels of blockade because D$_1$ can be detected when T1 is absent.[31]

Post-tetanic Count

With deep levels of neuromuscular blockade there may be no response to single twitch, tetanus, TOF, or DBS. However, the application of 5 seconds of 50 Hz, with a 3-second pause, followed by single twitches at 1 Hz, should be evaluated (Fig. 10–8). The number of visible twitches correlates

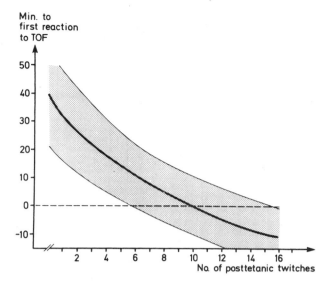

Figure 10-8. Relationship between the number of post-tetanic twitches and the time to the first response to train-of-four stimulation. (The mean curve and 95% confidence limits are shown.) (From Viby-Mogensen J, Howardy-Hansen P, Chraemmer-Jorgensen B, et al: Posttetanic count (PTC): A new method of evaluating an intense nondepolarizing neuromuscular blockade. Anesthesiology 1981; 55: 458-461.)

inversely with the time required for return of neuromuscular function. The number of twitches is called the post-tetanic count (PTC). This mode of stimulation can be done every 2 to 6 minutes.[32, 33] A PTC of 1 or less is a very deep level of neuromuscular blockade, with near total paralysis of the diaphragm. A PTC of greater than 9 usually means T1 will be detected on TOF stimulation, and T1 will be decreased to greater than 90% of control.[15]

Methods of Recording Responses of Neuromuscular Junction

Following depolarization of a muscle fiber, there is an electrical event followed shortly by a mechanical event. Both of these events can be measured.

Visual and Tactile

The simplest, cheapest, and most commonly used method to evaluate muscle contraction is to look or feel for a response. However, multiple studies have shown that TOF fade or tetanic fade is not detected by visual or tactile means when the T4/T1 is as low as 0.3. DBS is more easily perceived by most practitioners but still may not be detected with D1/D2 of 0.5. to 0.6.[29, 30] Despite these limitations, visual or tactile TOF is by far the most common method of neuromuscular monitoring because of ease of use and clinical utility.

Electromyogram

The EMG records the electrical response generated by the muscle action potentials following a stimulus. The recording electrode is placed over the middle of the tendinous insertion of the stimulated muscle. The EMG response may be measured by the peak amplitude or by finding the area under the EMG response curve. The integrated area is the most commonly used.

Mechanomyography and Accelerography

The MMG measures the contractive response of a stimulated muscle by measuring force translation or angular acceleration. Force translation is measured by placing a fixed preload on a muscle, aligning a force transducer with the direction of movement, and recording the force. ACG is similar to force translation monitoring except that the acceleration of muscle contraction (rather than force of contraction) is measured by a piezoelectric transducer. The responses of force translation and ACG have similar T4/T1 ratios in response to nondepolarizing relaxants.[34]

Muscle Monitoring Locations

Different muscles have different onset and offset times and sensitivities to NMB drugs.[15] The muscles of the larynx and diaphragm cannot be easily monitored but have predictable correlations with muscle groups that are more conventionally monitored. The ulnar nerve is the most commonly monitored site. The negative (black) electrode is placed proximal to the wrist on the vertical side of the flexor carpi ulnaris. The proximal (red) electrode can be placed more than 2 cm proximal or over the olecranon groove. The adductor pollicis brevis is the most commonly monitored skeletal muscle, both clinically and in research applications. Several studies have shown that the adductor pollicis takes longer to reach maximal paralysis and takes longer to recover than the larynx, orbicularis oculi, or the diaphragm[35] (Fig. 10-9). The adductor pollicis can be used to assess recovery or reversal of neuromuscular blockade. Because the adductor pollicis is more sensitive and recovers later than the larynx and diaphragm, there is additional safety when monitoring this muscle for reversal of NMB drug effects.

The adductor digiti minimi can also be monitored. However, it is 15% to 20% more resistant to NMB drugs than the adductor pollicis (i.e., when the TOF at the adductor pollicis is 70%, the TOF at the adductor digiti minimi will be 90%).[36] This muscle has been used for EMG recordings because it gives good EMG signals and may be less sensitive to movement artifact.[36] The first dorsal interosseous has sensitivities to nondepolarizing NMB drugs that are similar to the adductor pollicis. EMG electrodes are easy to place and there is little movement artifact.[37] EMG of the first dorsal interosseous also correlates well with adductor pollicis force.[38]

The facial nerve can be stimulated 2 to 3 cm posterior to the lateral borders of the orbit, causing contraction of the orbicularis oculi. Onset and recovery of blockade are similar to those of the diaphragm and larynx, with both occurring before that of the adductor pollicis. This is an ideal muscle to monitor for the *onset* of neuromuscular blockade of the larynx and because it is more resistant to NMB drags. It is also appropriate to monitor if deeper levels of paralysis are needed.[39]

The posterior tibial nerve (posterior to the medial malleolus) can stimulate the flexor hallucis brevis, causing plantar flexion of the great toe. This has a similar response to the adductor pollicis when both are monitored.[40] However, ability to detect fade in response to TOF or DBS by tactile

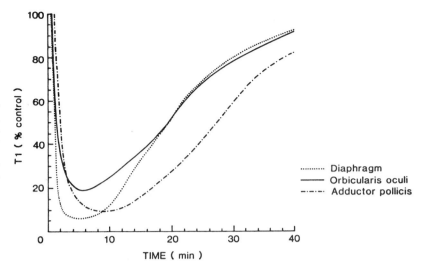

Figure 10-9. First stimulus (T1) in the train-of-four (TOF) obtained in three different muscles following a dose of vecuronium 0.07 mg/kg showing that paralysis and recovery of the diaphragm occurs before the adductor pollicis. (From Donati F, Meistelman C, Plaud B: Vecuronium neuromuscular blockade at the diaphragm, the orbicularis oculi, and adductor pollicis muscles. Anesthesiology 1990;73:870–875.)

means is not as reliable.[41] Finally, stimulation of the common peroneal (fibular) nerve, placing electrodes above and below the head of the fibula, causes dorsiflexion of the foot; however, these have not been correlated with other motor responses.

Monitoring Return of Normal Neuromuscular Function

NMB drug studies that assess the return of "normal" neuromuscular function commonly use healthy surgical patients who are paralyzed for a short period of time and have neuromuscular blockade reversed with anticholinesterase drugs. Even acknowledging these "ideal" study conditions, recent information has highlighted important limitations regarding NMB drug reversal[42]:

1. A TOFc of 4 means that there may still be up to 70% of nAChR blockade, and a TOFr may be as low as 0.6 (see Table 10–1).

2. 100% of awake, healthy normal volunteers exhibited pharyngeal dysfunction when the TOFr is 90.[43]

3. Patients who receive long-acting NMB drugs (pancuronium) are more likely to have a postoperative TOFr of less than 70% in the postanesthesia care unit (PACU), and are more likely to have postoperative pulmonary complications.[44]

4. A negative inspiratory force of -42 cm H_2O (or greater) is needed to control airway secretions in awake, healthy volunteers, and a negative inspiratory force of -53 cm H_2O is necessary to perform a 5-second head lift or leg raise.[45]

5. Tests of clinical recovery such as negative inspiratory force (NIF), head lift, vital capacity, tidal volume, and so forth *do not* always correlate with TOFr greater than 90 or receptor blockade of less than 30%.[46-48]

Because of these limitations inherent with current monitoring modalities, vigilance is still required in the PACU to observe patients for recurarization or silent aspiration. Indeed, some authors suggest that intermediate-acting NMB drugs (compared to long-acting NMB drugs) provide a greater safety margin for patients when extubation, spontaneous ventilation, and airway protection are required after paralysis.[42]

Use and Complications of Neuromuscular Blocking Drugs in the Intensive Care Unit

The main shortcoming of peripheral nerve stimulation is that global muscle function is inferred from the response of a single peripheral muscle group. As already noted, the diaphragm and laryngeal muscles are more resistant to neuromuscular blockade than the adductor pollicis brevis muscle and also recover more quickly after cessation of NMB drugs. In some patients, a TOF count of 0 at the adductor pollicis muscle may not correlate with a level of neuromuscular block sufficient to adequately manage clinical endpoints such as elimination of coughing during suctioning, elimination of peripheral motor movements, or dyssynchrony ("triggering") of the ventilator. Thus, a TOF count of 0 does not necessarily represent a failure of monitoring or drug titration, but may reflect both the difficulty of administering NMB drugs in the ICU and the need for clinical endpoints discrepant with the monitored twitch at the adductor pollicis brevis muscle. It is important, therefore, to utilize a combination of both peripheral nerve stimulation and clinical assessment to evaluate neuromuscular function and degree of neuromuscular blockade. Critically ill patients rarely require dense, 100% receptor blockade.[49] NMB drugs should be titrated to the minimally effective dose, maintaining the least degree of neuromuscular block that provides optimal patient care. Regardless, a fixed level of neuromuscular block is difficult to maintain in ICU patients owing to factors such as changing body temperature, alterations of muscle blood flow, altered electrolytes, and use of concomitant medications such as aminoglycosides, magnesium, calcium channel blockers, and so forth.

Prolonged recovery (defined as neuromuscular recovery that is significantly longer than predicted by recognized pharmacokinetic and pharmacodynamic parameters) and myopathy (defined as the clinical triad of persistent clinical paresis, increased creatine phosphokinase (CK) concentrations, and abnormal EMG and nerve conduction studies after ICU administration of NMB drugs) are the most feared com-

Table 10-2. Neuromuscular Blocking (NMB) Drug–Drug
Interactions

Drugs that Potentiate the Action of Nondepolarizing NMB Drugs

Local anesthetics
Lidocaine
Antibiotics
Aminoglycosides (gentamicin, tobramycin, amikacin)
Polypeptides (polymyxin B)
Other antibiotics (clindamycin, tetracycline)
Antiarrhythmics
Procainamide
Quinidine
Magnesium
Calcium channel blockers
β-Adrenergic blockers
Chemotherapeutic agents
Cyclophosphamide
Dantrolene
Diuretics
Furosemide (biphasic response)
Thiazides
Lithium carbonate
Cyclosporine

Drugs that Antagonize the Actions of Nondepolarizing NMB Drugs

Phenytoin
Carbamazepine
Theophylline
Ranitidine
Chronic exposure to nondepolarizing NMB drugs

plications after NMB drug use in the ICU.[50-52] These adverse effects may be divided into pharmacologic, physiologic, and toxic categories.

Pharmacologic

The steroid-based NMB drugs (e.g., pancuronium and vecuronium) have been associated with the majority of past case reports of prolonged weakness or myopathy in ICU patients.[53] For instance, vecuronium undergoes hepatic hydrolysis to three metabolites: 3-des, 17-des, and 3,17-desacetylvecuronium.[54, 55] The 3-desacetyl metabolite is estimated to be 80% as potent as the parent compound, while the 17- and 3,17- metabolites are far less potent. The hepatic elimination of 3-desacetylvecuronium is decreased in patients who are uremic for longer than 36 hours. The accumulation of both 3-desacetylvecuronium and vecuronium in renal failure likely contributes to prolonged weakness in this subset of ICU patients. In patients with renal failure, the combination of decreased clearance, increased volume of distribution, and accumulation of active 3-OH metabolites may be the pharmacologic explanation for prolonged weakness in some ICU patients.

There is a wide range of drugs with complex interactions with NMB drugs. These drug-drug interactions may either antagonize or potentiate the effect of NMB drug motor block (Table 10-2). Great concern is focused on patients who receive both NMB drugs and exogenous corticosteroids.[53] However, the long-term effect and potential toxicity of some of these interactions have yet to be defined.

Physiologic

Pathophysiologic changes occur at the nerve, neuromuscular junction, and muscle in critically ill patients.[56] Physiologic changes are enhanced when patients are immobilized or denervated secondary to spinal cord injury, as well as during NMB drug-induced paralysis. The nAChR may be triggered to revert to a fetal variant structure, characterized by an increase in total number, frequent extrajunctional proliferation, and "resistance" to nondepolarizing NMB drugs (see Fig. 10-2). This may account for the observations of some ICU patients developing tachyphylaxis to NMB drugs. The proliferation and distribution of these altered receptors across the myomembrane may, however, simultaneously sensitize patients to depolarizing drugs such as succinylcholine. Succinylcholine stimulation of the immature, fetal receptors allows increased cation transport, which may clinically manifest as life-threatening hyperkalemia in these patients.

Additional investigation and evaluation of the effect of prolonged NMB exposure to nerves, neuromuscular junctions, and muscle are ongoing. For instance, there is increasing recognition of an entity termed *critical illness polyneuropathy* (CIP). The sensorimotor polyneuropathy of CIP differentiates this process from other neurologic and myopathic processes encountered in the critically ill (Table 10-3). CIP occurs most commonly in elderly, septic patients who are severely ill for prolonged periods.[57-59] Up to 70% of septic ICU patients are reported to develop some elements of CIP. CIP is a diagnosis of exclusion, after examination of the clinical setting, determination of a diffuse sensorimotor deficit, and EMG and nerve conduction studies.[56]

Toxic

The incidence of prolonged weakness after NMB drugs remains unknown. Murray et al.[60] prospectively monitored patients in the ICU at the Mayo Clinic and estimated the risk of clinically significant prolonged neuromuscular block was 5%. The actual incidence probably depends on numerous factors, perhaps including the administration of various antibiotics (aminoglycosides), corticosteroids, anticonvulsants, magnesium, calcium channel blocking drugs, and other medications which may interact with NMB drugs. The incidence of true myopathy is certainly less than the occurrence of prolonged weakness in the ICU.

The acute myopathy, often referred to as postparalytic "quadriparesis" or "tetraparesis," is an infrequent but major complication after prolonged NMB drug administration in the critically ill. This entity must be differentiated from other neuromuscular disorders noted earlier (see Table 10-3). Afflicted patients demonstrate diffuse weakness that persists long after the NMB drug administration is discontinued. Neurologic examination reveals primarily a global motor deficit,

Table 10-3. Causes of Weakness in Intensive Care Unit Patients

Residual neuromuscular blocking drug effects: secondary to parent drug, drug metabolite, or drug-drug interaction
Myasthenia gravis
Eaton-Lambert syndrome
Muscular dystrophies
Guillain-Barré syndrome
Central nervous system injury or lesion
Spinal cord injury
Steroid myopathy
Critical illness polyneuropathy
Disuse atrophy
Severe electrolyte toxicity (e.g., magnesium)
Severe electrolyte deficiency (e.g., hypophosphatemia)

Table 10-4. Characteristics of Various Causes of Weakness After Prolonged Use of Neuromuscular Blocking Drugs

Diagnosis	History	Physical Examination and Laboratory Tests	Muscle/Nerve Biopsy	EMG/NCS	Course
Postparalysis syndrome	NMB use (aminosteroid more common) May occur with NMB alone Consider drug interactions (esp. concurrent steroids)	Diffuse weakness Sparing of sensory function Potential for elevation in CK	Early change: selective thick filament degeneration on EM or local loss of ATPase activity on LM Late change: muscle fiber necrosis	Small CMAP SNAP Nl NCV Nl or near Nl Myopathic change (only in patient with steroids and NMBs) NMB alone; see type II atrophy (disuse)	Favorable for the most part, but patient may have prolonged recovery period
Critical polyneuropathy	Commonly occurs with sepsis More frequent in elderly, severely ill patients	Sensorimotor involvement	Predominantly axonal degeneration	Consistent with distal axonal sensorimotor polyneuropathy	May have protracted process with unfavorable outcome Outcome mainly related to underlying pathologic condition
Steroid-induced myopathy	Acute or chronic process Occurs more commonly in proximal muscles	Systemic sequelae of steroid use (skin and body habitus changes, diabetes, hypertension)	Type II muscle fiber atrophy	Nl or if severe—mild myopathic change	Tends to be favorable
Deconditioning syndrome	Occurs with immobile, highly catabolic patients in ICU May be exacerbated by deafferentation associated with dense neuromuscular blockade	Diffuse weakness and loss of muscle mass and skin	Muscle biopsy not indicated but if done shows type II fiber atrophy	Essentially Nl	Dependent on underlying pathologic condition
Guillain-Barré syndrome	Associated with underlying viral infection and ascending polyneuropathy	Diffuse motor weakness Potential involvement of cranial nerves Possible autonomic lability	Not indicated	Compatible with demyelinating sensorimotor polyneuropathy	Favorable, appears to improve with immunoglobulin or plasmapheresis
Myasthenia gravis	Variable but frequent progressive fatigue and bulbar signs	Muscle fatiguability	Not indicated	Decremental response on repetitive stimulation at 2 Hz MUP variability on EMG	Dependent on aggressiveness of disease, favorable with cholinesterase inhibitors, steroids, and thymectomy as needed
Acute rhabdomyolysis	Associated with crush injuries, drug overdose, or toxic ingestions	Increased CK; check HPO$_4$, urine myoglobin	Diffuse muscle fiber necrosis	Spontaneous activity with myopathic changes	Favorable, depends on associated pathologic condition and injury
Central pontine myelinolysis	Rapid electrolyte alterations	Locked-in syndrome	Not indicated	Nl	Poor

ICU, intensive care unit; ATPase, adenosinetriphosphatase; CK, creatine kinase; CMAP, compound motor action potential; EM, electron microscopy; EMG, electromyography; LM, light microscopy; MUP, motor unit potential; NCS, nerve conduction study; NCV, nerve conduction velocities; Nl, normal; NMB, neuromuscular blocking drug; SNAP, sensory action potential. (From Prielipp RC, Coursin DB, Wood KE, et al: Complications associated with sedative and neuromuscular blocking drugs in critically ill patients. Crit Care Clin 1995; 11:983–1003.)

which tends to affect proximal and distal muscles equally. Barohn et al.[61] described three patients with myopathy, characterized by low-amplitude compound motor action potentials, normal sensory studies, and fibrillations. Muscle biopsy showed loss of thick myosin filaments. Variable increases in CK may be detected, depending on the timing of laboratory determinations and the initiation of the myopathic process. Thus, there may be some justification for routine screening of high-risk patients with serial CK determinations during the infusion of NMB drugs. It is unclear whether drug combinations such as aminosteroid NMB drugs and concurrent ad-

ministration of exogenous corticosteroids confer any specific increased risk; however, this practice is probably best avoided.

There are now a small number of well-documented reports of myopathy developing after ICU administration of benzylisoquinolinium drugs (i.e., doxacurium, atracurium, cisatracurium) as well.[62-64] We and others have diagnosed myopathy (clinical weakness or paresis, increased CK concentrations, and abnormal EMG studies) without sensory deficits in patients after ICU administration of atracurium or cisatracurium for 3 to 10 days. However, these reports are complicated by patients receiving concurrent administration of corticosteroids, aminoglycosides, or other drugs noted in Table 10-2.

The diagnosis of the patient with prolonged weakness, paresis, and possible myopathy after discontinuation of NMB drugs requires a systematic approach. This includes a thorough history and physical examination combined with review of recent medications and identification of related nerve or muscle abnormalities. First, potential residual neuromuscular blockade should be investigated with a peripheral nerve stimulator. In addition, early neurologic consultation with appropriate diagnostic examination including EMG and nerve conduction velocity, CK analysis, and muscle biopsy should be undertaken when indicated (Table 10-4).

Summary

NMB drugs are an integral part of current anesthesia practice in the OR and the ICU. However, there are numerous potential complications and limitations that clinicians must recognize. Monitoring the neuromuscular junction with a peripheral nerve stimulator remains the mainstay of safe administration and reversal of these drugs. Current practitioners must also recognize the large number of drug-drug interactions, as well as interactions with concurrent illness, which may confound interpretation of the actions of the common monitoring modalities.

In theory, NMB drugs should be carefully selected and titrated for each patient and anesthetic, and discontinued as soon as is clinically possible. The evaluation of neuromuscular recovery must correlate both clinical and monitoring endpoints to ensure the adequacy of neuromuscular recovery. When used appropriately, NMB drugs should optimize patient care in the OR and ICU without increasing morbidity or mortality.

REFERENCES

1. Rama Sastry BV: Nicotinic receptor. Anaesth Pharmacol Rev 1993; 1:6-19.
2. Martyn JAJ, White DA, Gronert GA, et al: Up-and-down regulation of skeletal muscle acetylcholine receptors. Anesthesiology 1992; 76:822-843.
3. Apel ED, Merlie JP: Assembly of the postsynaptic apparatus. Curr Opin Neurobiol 1995; 5:62-67.
4. Hogue CW Jr, Ward JM, Itani MS, et al: Tolerance and upregulation of acetylcholine receptors follows chronic infusion of d-tubocurarine. J Appl Physiol 1992; 72:1326-1331.
5. Bevan DR, Donati F: Muscle relaxants. In Barash PG (ed): Clinical Anesthesia, ed 3. Philadephia, Lippincott-Raven, 1996, pp 385-412.
6. Silverman DG, Standaert FG: Mechanisms of neuromuscular block. In Silverman DG (ed): Neuromuscular Block in Perioperative and Intensive Care. Philadelphia, JB Lippincott, 1994, pp 11-22.
7. Smith CE, Saddler JM, Bevan JC, et al: Pretreatment with nondepolarizing neuromuscular blocking agents and suxamethonium-induced increases in resting jaw tension in children. Br J Anaesth 1990; 64:577-581.
8. Haspel KL, Ali HH, Kitz RJ: Physiology of neuromuscular transmission and mechanism of action of neuromuscular blocking agents. In Rogers MC, Tinker JH, Covino BG, et al (eds): Principles and Practice of Anesthesiology. St Louis, Mosby-Year Book, 1993, pp 1507-1517.
9. Hudes E, Lee KC: Clinical use of peripheral nerve stimulators in anaesthesia. Can J Anaesth 1987; 34:525-534.
10. Brull SJ: An update on monitoring of neuromuscular function. Curr Opin Anaesthiol 1992; 5:577-583.
11. Donati F, Bevan DR: Not all muscles are the same (editorial). Br J Anaesth 1992; 68:235-236.
12. Donati F, Antzaka C, Bevan DR: Potency of pancuronium at the diaphragm and the adductor pollicis muscle in humans. Anesthesiology 1986; 65:1-5.
13. Silverman DG, Standaert FG: Anatomy and physiology of neuromuscular transmission. In Silverman DG (ed): Neuromuscular Block in Perioperative and Intensive Care. Philadelphia, JB Lippincott 1994 pp 1-10.
14. Kopman AF, Lawson D: Milliamperage requirements for supramaximal stimulation of the ulnar nerve with surface electrodes. Anesthesiology 1984; 61:83-85.
15. Beemer GH, Reeves JH, Bjorksten AR: Accurate monitoring of neuromuscular blockade using a peripheral nerve stimulator—a review. Anaesth Intensive Care 1990; 18:490-496.
16. Brull SJ, Silverman DG: Pulse width, stimulus intensity, electrode placement and polarity during assessment of neuromuscular block. Anesthesiology 1995; 83:702-709.
17. Epstein RA, Jackson SH: Repetitive muscle depolarization from single indirect stimulation in anesthetized man. J Appl Physiol 1970; 28:407-410.
18. Silverman DG, Brull SJ. Features of neurostimulation. In Silverman DG (ed): Neuromuscular Block in Perioperative and Intensive Care. Philadelphia, JB Lippincott, 1994, pp 23-36.
19. Beemer GH, Reeves JH: An evaluation of eight peripheral nerve stimulators for monitoring neuromuscular blockade. Anaesth Intensive Care 1988; 16:464-477.
20. Fogdall RP, Miller RD: Neuromuscular effects of enflurane, alone and combined with d-tubocurarine, pancuronium, and succinylcholine in man. Anesthesiology 1975; 42:173-178.
21. Brull SJ, Connelly NR, O'Connor TZ, et al. Effect of tetanus on subsequent neuromuscular monitoring in patients receiving vecuronium. Anesthesiology 1991; 74:64-70.
22. Ali HH, Utting JE, Gray C: Stimulus frequency in the detection of neuromuscular block in humans. Br J Anaesth 1970; 42:967-978.
23. Viby-Mogensen J, Jensen NH, Engbaek J, et al. Tactile and visual evaluation of the response to train-of-four nerve stimulation. Anesthesiology 1985; 63:440-443.
24. Ali HH, Savarese JJ, Lebowitz PW, et al. Twitch, tetanus and train-of-four as indices of recovery from nondepolarizing neuromusclar blockade. Anesthesiology 1981; 54:294-297.
25. Waud BE, Waud DR: The relation between response to "train-of-four" stimulation and receptor occlusion during competitive neuromuscular block. Anesthesiology 1972; 37:413-416.
26. Lee C, Katz RL: Fade of neurally evoked compound electromyogram during neuromuscular block by d tubocurarine. Anesth Analg 1977; 56:271-275.
27. Lee CM: Train-of-4 quantitation of competitive neuromuscular block. Anesth Analg 1975; 54:649-653.
28. Engbaek J, Ostergaard D, Viby-Mogensen J: Double burst stimulation (DBS): A new pattern of nerve stimulation to identify residual neuromuscular block. Br J Anaesth 1989; 62:274-278.
29. Gill SS, Donati F, Bevan DR: Clinical evaluation of double-burst stimulation. Its relationship to train-of-four stimulation. Anaesthesia 1989; 45:543-548.
30. Drenck NE, Ueda N, Olsen NV, et al: Manual evaluation of residual curarization using double burst stimulation: A comparison with train-of-four. Anesthesiology 1989; 70:578-581.
31. Braude N, Vyvyan HA, Jordan MJ: Intraoperative assessment of atracurium-induced neuromuscular block using double burst stimulation. Br J Anaesth 1991; 67:574-578.
32. Viby-Mogensen J, Howardy-Hansen P, Chraemmer-Jorgensen B, et al: Posttetanic count (PTC): A new method of evaluating an intense nondepolarizing neuromuscular blockade. Anesthesiology 1981; 55:458-461.
33. Muchhal KK, Viby-Mogensen J, Fernando PU, et al: Evaluation of intense neuromuscular blockade caused by vecuronium using posttetanic count (PTC). Anesthesiology 1987; 66:846-849.
34. Werner MU, Kirkegaard Nielson H, May O, et al: Assessment of neuromuscular transmission by the evoked acceleration response. An evaluation of the accuracy of the acceleration transducer in comparison with a force displacement transducer. Acta Anaesthesiol Scand 1988; 32:395-400.

35. Donati F, Meistelman C, Plaud B: Vecuronium neuromuscular blockade at the adductor muscles of the larynx and adductor pollicis. Anesthesiology 1991; 74:833–837.

36. Kopman AF: The relationship of evoked electromyographic and mechanical responses following atracurium in humans. Anesthesiology 1985; 63:208–211.

37. Kalli I: Effect of surface electrode position on the compared action potential evoked by ulnar nerve stimulation during isoflurane anaesthesia. Br J Anaesth 1990; 65:494–499.

38. Kopman AF: The dose-effect relationship of metocurine: The integrated electromyogram of the first dorsal interosseous muscle and the mechanomyogram of the adductor pollicis compared. Anesthesiology 1988; 68:604–607.

39. Donati F, Meistelman C, Plaud B: Vecuronium neuromuscular blockade of the diaphragm, the orbicularis oculi and adductor pollicis muscles. Anesthesiology 1990; 73:870–875.

40. Sopher MJ, Sears DH, Walts LF: Neuromuscular function monitoring comparing the flexor hallucis brevis and the adductor pollicis muscles. Anesthesiology 1988; 69:129–131.

41. Saitoh Y, Koitabashi Y, Makita K, et al: Train-of-four and double burst stimulation fade at the great toe and thumb. Can J Anaesth 1997; 44:390–395.

42. Savarese JJ: Some considerations on the new muscle relaxants. Anesth Analg 1998; (suppl): 119–127.

43. Eriksson LI, Sundman E, Olsson R, et al: Functional assessment of the pharynx at rest and during swallowing in partially paralyzed humans: Simultaneous videomanometry and mechanomyography of awake human volunteers. Anesthesiology 1997; 87:1035–1043.

44. Berg H: Is residual neuromuscular block following pancuronium a risk factor for postoperative pulmonary complications? Acta Anaesthesiol Scand Suppl 1997; 110:156–158.

45. Pavlin EG, Holle RH, Schoene RB: Recovery of airway protection compared with ventilation in humans after paralysis with curare. Anesthesiology 1989; 70:381–385.

46. Beemer GH, Rozental P: Postoperative neuromuscular function. Anaesth Intensive Care 1986; 14:41–45.

47. Hutton P, Burchett KR, Madden AP: Comparison of recovery after neuromuscular blockade by atracurium or pancuronium. Br J Anaesth 1988; 60:36–42.

48. Kopman AF, Yee PS, Neuman GG: Relationship of the train-of-four fade ratio to clinical signs and symptoms of residual paralysis in awake volunteers. Anesthesiology 1997; 86:765–771.

49. Sharpe MD: The use of muscle relaxants in the intensive care unit. Can J Anaesth 1992; 39:949–962.

50. Danon MJ, Carpenter S: Myopathy with thick filament (myosin) loss following prolonged paralysis with vecuronium during steroid treatment. Muscle Nerve 1991; 14:1131–1139.

51. Margolis BD, Khachikian D, Friedman Y, et al: Prolonged reversible quadriparesis in mechanically ventilated patients who received long-term infusions of vecuronium. Chest 1991; 100:877–878.

52. Partridge BL, Abrams JH, Bazemore C, et al: Prolonged neuromuscular blockade after long-term infusion of vecuronium bromide in the intensive care unit. Crit Care Med 1990; 18:1177–1179.

53. Watling SM, Dasta JF. Prolonged paralysis in intensive care unit patients after the use of neuromuscular blocking agents: a review of the literature. Crit Care Med 1994; 22:884–893.

54. Segredo V, Caldwell JE, Matthay MA, et al: Persistent paralysis in critically ill patients after long-term administration of vecuronium. N Engl J Med 1992; 327:524–528.

55. Caldwell JE, Szenohradszky J, Segredo V, et al: The pharmacodynamics and pharmacokinetics of the metabolite 3-desacetylvecuronium (ORG 7268) and its parent compound, vecuronium, in human volunteers. J Pharmacol Exp Ther 1994; 270:1216–1222.

56. Coakley JH, Nagendran K, Yarwood GD, et al: Patterns of neurophysiological abnormality in prolonged critical illness. Intensive Care Med 1998; 24:801–807.

57. Bolton CF, Young GB, Zochodne DW: The neurologic complications of sepsis. Ann Neurol 1993; 33:94–100.

58. Bolton CF: Muscle weakness and difficulty in weaning from the ventilator in the critical care unit. Chest 1994; 106:1–2.

59. Witt NJ, Zochodne DW, Bolton CF, et al: Peripheral nerve function in sepsis and multiple organ failure. Chest 1991; 99:176–184.

60. Murray MJ, Strickland RA, Weiler C: The use of neuromuscular blocking drugs in the intensive care unit: A US perspective. Intensive Care Med 1993; 19(suppl 2):S40–44.

61. Barohn RJ, Jackson CE, Rogers SJ, et al: Prolonged paralysis due to nondepolarizing neuromuscular blocking agents and corticosteroids. Muscle Nerve 1994; 17:647–654.

62. Marik PE: Doxacurium-corticosteroid acute myopathy: Another piece to the puzzle. Crit Care Med 1996; 24:1266–1267.

63. Davis NA, Rodgers JE, Gonzalez ER, et al: Prolonged weakness after cisatracurium infusion: A case report. Crit Care Med 1998; 26:1290–1292.

64. Meyer KC, Prielipp RC, Grossman JE, et al: Prolonged weakness after infusion of atracurium in two intensive care unit patients. Anesth Analg 1994; 78:772–774.

11 Specialized Neurophysiologic Monitoring

Timothy McCulloch, M.B.B.S., FANZCA
Arthur M. Lam, M.D., F.R.C.P.C.

Cerebral ischemia is a major cause of morbidity following such insults as traumatic brain injury, subarachnoid hemorrhage, neurovascular surgery, and cardiopulmonary bypass (CPB). Routine management of patients at risk of cerebral ischemia usually focuses on treatment of raised intracranial pressure (ICP) and maintenance of adequate cerebral perfusion pressure (CPP). The aim of specialized monitoring is to provide information beyond these hemodynamic variables to give the clinician more direct information regarding the adequacy of oxygen delivery to the brain.

The monitors discussed in this chapter are primarily aimed at detecting ischemia and monitoring the efficacy of therapies aimed at prevention or treatment of ischemia. In some situations, monitoring may also provide diagnostic information as to the cause of cerebral ischemia. Other causes of brain damage such as hyperperfusion and cerebral emboli can also be detected by specialized monitoring.

Transcranial Doppler Ultrasonography

Since the introduction of transcranial Doppler (TCD) ultrasound in 1982[1] it has been possible to noninvasively assess blood flow in the major intracranial arteries. Doppler ultrasound can be performed at the bedside or in the operating room and may be used continuously over many hours. In contrast, other techniques for measuring cerebral blood flow (CBF) such as nitrous oxide washin, xenon–computed tomography (CT), and single-photon emission computed tomography (SPECT) are not suited to frequently repeated or continuous monitoring.

The proximal segments of the middle, anterior, and posterior cerebral arteries, as well as the vertebral, basilar, ophthalmic, and terminal internal carotid arteries, can be accessed with the TCD. This technique allows monitoring of a variety of pathologic states and also enables investigation of cerebrovascular physiology in a wide range of clinical and experimental situations.

Principles

High-frequency sound waves penetrate biologic tissues and are reflected when they encounter boundaries between tissues of differing acoustic impedance. According to the Doppler principle, the reflected sound waves are "compressed," and therefore have a shorter wavelength and higher frequency if the reflector (such as a red blood cell) is moving toward the source. Conversely, the ultrasound frequency is lowered when reflected from an object moving away from the source. This frequency (f) change is called the Doppler shift and its magnitude is related to the velocity (v) of the reflector according to the formula

$$v = \frac{c}{2\cos\theta} \times \frac{f}{f_0}$$

where f_0 is the frequency of the emitted ultrasound and c is the ultrasound propagation velocity. The angle (θ) between the direction of movement and the direction of the ultrasound is termed the angle of insonation.

Flow Velocity as a Measure of Cerebral Blood Flow

Flow velocity (FV) is only indirectly related to the actual blood flow in the vessel. TCD measurements of FV in the middle cerebral artery (MCA) of normal subjects range from 35 to 90 cm · s^{-1}.[1] This wide range is due largely to variation in MCA diameter among individuals. Although FV correlates poorly with absolute CBF, *changes* in CBF can be accurately detected with TCD. The measured FV bears a constant relation to the actual rate of blood flow in the insonated vessel provided the following two criteria are met:

1. *Constant angle of insonation.* It is important to note that the Doppler technique only measures the component of velocity in the direction of the ultrasound beam. Any angulation with respect to the direction of flow causes an underestimate of the FV. Inspection of the preceding formula shows that measured FV is reduced in proportion to the cosine of the angle of insonation. In the worst case, blood flow is perpendicular to the ultrasound beam so there is no velocity vector in the direction of the sound wave, no Doppler shift, and no measured flow. In practice, it is not usually possible to be certain that the angle of insonation is near to zero, but provided that the ultrasound can be directed to within ±30 degrees of the direction of flow, the error will be less than 15% (cos 30° = 0.87). As long as the angle remains constant, changes in measured FV are proportional to changes in blood flow.

2. *Constant vessel diameter.* The vessels investigated by TCD are conductance vessels and, as such, their diameter is thought to remain constant. Physiologic changes in cerebrovascular resistance (CVR) are due to adjustments in the diameter of the smaller resistance vessels. The assumption of constant vessel diameter underlies the usefulness of TCD as a monitor of CBF. Validation of this assumption is required in each new situation investigated because different patho-

physiologic and pharmacologic circumstances could potentially alter the diameter of the basal cerebral arteries.

Alterations in $PaCO_2$ and blood pressure profoundly influence cerebrovascular resistance but have been found not to appreciably affect measurements of MCA diameter.[2, 3] Studies of CO_2 reactivity using TCD have reported good correlation with the results of direct measurement of CBF,[4-6] providing further evidence that basal cerebral artery diameter is not responsive to CO_2. Furthermore, basal cerebral artery diameter appears to remain constant despite alterations in arterial blood pressure. Changes in MCA flow velocity (V_{mca}) have been shown to accurately reflect changes in internal carotid artery (ICA) blood flow occurring in response to incidental[7] or induced[8] falls in blood pressure under anesthesia.

Phenylephrine and nitroprusside, when used to produce mild changes in blood pressure, do not appreciably alter MCA diameter.[3] On the other hand, nitroglycerin has been reported to cause a 25% fall in V_{mca} with no associated change in CBF,[9] implying significant dilation of the MCA. Direct evidence regarding the effects of anesthetic drugs on human basal cerebral artery diameter is lacking. Intravenous anesthetics probably do not alter MCA diameter.[10] There is indirect evidence that volatile anesthetics at low doses do not affect MCA diameter as well,[11] although other authors suggest that MCA dilation may occur at doses greater than 1 MAC (minimal alveolar concentration).[10, 12] Even if anesthetic agents are found to alter MCA diameter, if anesthetic concentration remains steady, then changes in TCD velocity measurements can be assumed to represent changes in blood flow.

Cerebral vasospasm represents a special situation in which there is a profound change in the diameter of major cerebral arteries. With severe vasospasm, TCD demonstrates a dramatic increase in FV, while actual flow may fall to the point of causing ischemia or infarction. Paradoxically, although vasospasm invalidates the use of TCD as a monitor of CBF, the noninvasive diagnosis and monitoring of vasospasm are major clinical applications of TCD.

Maximum Velocity

When ultrasound reflected from a blood vessel is analyzed there is never a single, pure frequency shift. Rather, there is a spectrum of frequency shifts representing a range of velocities due to the parabolic profile of flow such that cells in the center of the stream move faster than those at the edges. Furthermore, the sample volume may contain a curving or branching vessel with blood flowing over a range of angles with respect to the ultrasound.

Although it is difficult to extract a reliable estimate of the mean FV within the insonated vessel, it has been found that the maximum velocity (V_{max}) is directly proportional to the mean velocity.[13] V_{max} is relatively simple to determine from the Doppler spectrum and TCD monitors incorporate software to continuously outline the peak velocity of the waveform. V_{max} varies throughout the cardiac cycle, following the arterial pressure waveform. A time-mean of the maximum flow velocity (V_m) can be automatically derived by the monitor or can be estimated by the formula $V_m = V_d + (V_s - V_d)/3$ where V_d represents the lowest V_{max} during diastole and V_s the highest V_{max} during systole.

Pulsatility

The difference between the systolic and diastolic flow velocity is called the pulsatility. Various indices have been used to quantify pulsatility, the one most commonly employed being the Gosling pulsatility index (PI): $PI = (V_s - V_d)/V_m$. The normal PI for the MCA is 0.9 ± 0.5. Changes in CVR affect pulsatility. If the cerebral arterioles constrict, then the compliance of the cerebrovascular system is reduced and flow becomes more pulsatile. However, the PI cannot be taken as a simple indicator of CVR because multiple other factors influence pulsatility. Pulsatility varies inversely with CPP, regardless of any autoregulatory change in CVR. For example, if CPP falls due to an increase in ICP, there is a proportionately greater fall in perfusion pressure during diastole compared to systole, so pulsatility increases. Pulsatility can also be influenced by stenosis upstream from the insonated vessel and by changes in systemic arterial pulsatility.

Equipment and Technique

TCD requires specialized ultrasound equipment, including probes designed specifically for transcranial use. To enable adequate penetration of the skull, TCD utilizes ultrasound at a lower frequency (e.g., 2 MHz) than usually employed for cardiovascular ultrasound. The most commonly employed probes are for freehand use but probes designed for attachment to fixation devices are also available. Equipment is available that permits simultaneous monitoring with two or more probes.

Signal Presentation

The Doppler ultrasound shift is presented as an audio signal with volume representing the intensity of the signal and pitch representing the velocity. The signal is also displayed on a video monitor as a Fourier transform with the height of the waveform representing velocity while signal intensity at each range of velocity is represented on either a gray or color scale. The video display also allows differentiation between flow toward or away from the probe.

Sample Volume

Only the signal from a circumscribed volume is processed. This sample volume is defined laterally by the width of the ultrasound beam, but the depth of the sample volume is determined by a technique called range-gating. Range-gating utilizes pulsed ultrasound and only the reflected signal arriving within a certain time period after each pulse is analyzed. The propagation speed in tissue is known so signals that make the round trip in a predetermined time represent flow at a known depth from the probe. The depth of the sample volume can be adjusted by the operator.

To compensate for signal attenuation by bone, the sample volume used for TCD is larger than for other Doppler ultrasound equipment. This means that it is not uncommon for the sample volume to include both the vessel of interest and a nearby vessel or branch.

Technique

For most monitoring purposes, it is sufficient to obtain TCD signals from the MCA that is the largest branch of the circle of Willis and normally carries 75% to 80% of the ipsilateral ICA blood flow. Fortunately, the MCA is relatively easy to locate and identify in most subjects, although it is still necessary to spend some time gaining skill in locating and optimizing the signal.

A complete TCD examination of all accessible arteries is complex and requires both skill and training. Locating and identifying signals can be difficult and requires a knowledge of the multiple variations of flow in the circle of Willis that occur due to anatomic anomalies and disease processes. Such examinations are usually performed by technicians with specific training in TCD.

Cranial Windows

The technique of TCD depends on locating areas of the skull known as cranial windows in which attenuation of the ultrasound is low enough to allow adequate signal transmission. There are three primary cranial windows: (1) the temporal window, which lies immediately superior to the zygomatic arch and allows insonation of the MCA, the proximal anterior cerebral artery, the terminal ICA, and the posterior cerebral artery; (2) the orbital window, which allows insonation of the ophthalmic artery and the carotid siphon; and (3) the suboccipital window, which allows insonation via the foramen magnum of the vertebral arteries and the basilar artery.

Clinical Application

Carotid Endarterectomy

Use of the TCD for monitoring during carotid endarterectomy (CEA) is now standard in a growing number of institutions. A TCD probe can be fixed over the temporal window for MCA monitoring without interfering with the surgical field. TCD monitoring provides information relevant to all the major causes of perioperative cerebrovascular morbidity; that is, intraoperative and postoperative emboli, hypoperfusion during cross-clamping, hypoperfusion due to thrombosis or intimal flaps, and postoperative hyperperfusion syndrome.

Decision to Shunt

There is continuing controversy regarding the use of an intraluminal shunt during CEA. Ideally, shunts should be placed in only those few patients who have critically reduced CBF on carotid artery cross-clamping. V_{mca} monitoring is proving useful in determining which patients may benefit from shunt placement. At the time of cross-clamping there is normally a fall in V_{mca} followed by a rise over the next few seconds due to autoregulatory vasodilation. The V_{mca} then plateaus at a flow rate that is usually lower than it was prior to cross-clamping. The reduction in blood flow can be quantified in a standardized way by expressing the V_{mca} 10 seconds after cross-clamping as a percentage of the V_{mca} immediately prior to clamping. A typical tracing is shown in Figure 11–1.

Halsey[14] published results from 1495 CEAs in an attempt to define the relationship between intraoperative measurements of V_{mca} and the indication for shunting. The data were collected retrospectively and there was no standardization of surgical or anesthetic technique and no standardization of criteria for shunt placement. Despite these drawbacks, this study provides strong evidence that patients with a 85% or greater fall in V_{mca} who are not shunted have a very high risk of perioperative stroke. In over 75% of patients, V_{mca} fell by less than 60% and within that group there was a better outcome in those who were *not* shunted. In the intermediate group (V_{mca} fall between 60% and 85%) there was no difference in outcome between the shunted and nonshunted patients. Based on these data, if V_{mca} stabilizes at 40% or greater of the preclamp value, it is unlikely the patient would benefit from a shunt.

TCD compares favorably with other methods of identifying patients likely to benefit from an intraluminal shunt. There appears to be excellent correlation between TCD and electroencephalographic (EEG) criteria of ischemia,[15-17] although it is possible to have severe reduction in V_{mca} and subsequent stroke without EEG evidence of ischemia.[18] Cerebral symptoms in awake patients having CEA under local

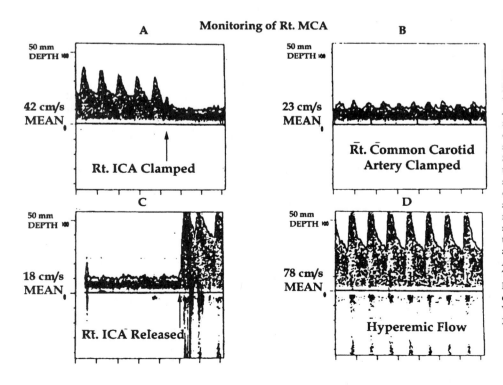

Monitoring of Rt. MCA

A
50 mm DEPTH 100
42 cm/s MEAN
Rt. ICA Clamped

B
50 mm DEPTH 100
23 cm/s MEAN
Rt. Common Carotid Artery Clamped

C
50 mm DEPTH 100
18 cm/s MEAN
Rt. ICA Released

D
50 mm DEPTH 100
78 cm/s MEAN
Hyperemic Flow

Figure 11–1. Characteristic changes in middle cerebral artery (MCA) flow velocity during carotid endarterectomy. *A*, Cross-clamp of the internal carotid artery (ICA) leads to an abrupt decrease in flow velocity and loss of pulsatility from maximal vasodilation. *B*, Slight increase in pulsatility with continuous cross-clamp, most likely a result of increased flow with collaterals. *C*, Release of clamp is followed by reactive hyperemia. The vertical streaks represent air emboli whose acoustic signatures overwhelmed the range of the instrument. *D*, Persistent hyperemia after release in this patient. (From Lam AM, Matta BF: Cerebral blood flow: Transcranial Doppler and microvascular Doppler. *In* Andrews RJ (ed): Intraoperative Neuroprotection. Baltimore, Williams & Wilkins, 1996, pp 217–247.)

anesthesia are usually, but not always, accompanied by a significant fall in V_{mca}[19] (conversely, it cannot be assumed that all awake patients who develop ischemic symptoms would have suffered a stroke had they been operated on under general anesthesia without being shunted). In a careful comparison of V_{mca} and stump pressure, Spencer et al.[20] reported a good correlation, but they found stump pressure to be sensitive to zeroing errors, and a small error in stump pressure estimation may represent a crucial difference in cerebral perfusion.

Some patients with severe ischemia on TCD criteria do not suffer stroke.[14, 17] This could be due to perfusion via cortical (leptomeningeal) collaterals, which may be better developed in patients with severe carotid stenosis. Also, a false diagnosis of critically reduced V_{mca} can arise from technical problems such as probe dislodgment or inadvertent monitoring of the distal ICA rather than the MCA.

When a shunt is used, TCD confirms restoration of MCA flow and provides a continuous monitor of shunt function. An obstructed shunt causes an immediate reduction in FV that precedes any change in cerebral function or EEG.

In summary, as with other monitors employed under general anesthesia, TCD criteria for cerebral hypoperfusion will be liable to false positives and possibly false negatives. The combination of intraoperative TCD and EEG to detect cross-clamp ischemia and aid in the decision to shunt should theoretically improve patient safety.

Detection of Emboli

Cerebral emboli are the major cause of perioperative stroke from CEA.[21] Microemboli can easily be recognized by the characteristic "chirping," "clicking," or "whistling" sounds on the TCD monitor. The TCD features of particulate and gas emboli have been characterized,[22] and software is available for automatic emboli detection and counting.

TCD monitoring has provided unique information about the prevalence and timing of perioperative cerebral emboli associated with CEA. Cerebral microemboli are noted during the majority of CEAs (97% in one recent report[23]). Emboli are sometimes noted during dissection of the carotid artery, stump pressure measurement, and during insertion of shunts. Most emboli are detected on restoration of ICA perfusion but these are predominately air, which is believed to be less harmful than particulate emboli. Ongoing embolization is sometimes detected immediately postoperatively and this may necessitate therapy such as heparin, dextrans, or other antiplatelet drugs.[24, 25]

It has become clear from TCD studies that most microemboli do not result in stroke. However, there is a strong correlation between the number of perioperative emboli detected and the incidence of embolic stroke,[21] cognitive deterioration,[26] and asymptomatic cerebral infarctions.[18, 27] A consistently reported benefit of the introduction of TCD monitoring is that the audible feedback to the surgeon provokes adjustments in technique that then reduce the frequency of emboli in subsequent patients.[17, 21]

Postoperative Hyperperfusion

Postoperative hyperperfusion syndrome occurs in about 1% of patients following CEA, and when cerebral hemorrhage occurs the prognosis is very poor. The syndrome is thought to occur when abnormally high blood flow develops in vascular beds that have been habituated to a low perfusion pressure and are suddenly exposed to normal arterial pressure.[28, 29] These vascular beds have apparently lost the ability to autoregulate at normal blood pressure.[30] Hyperperfusion can be diagnosed by TCD before clinical signs develop. Elevated ipsilateral V_{mca} on the order of 30% to 230% is found in 10% to 20% of patients after CEA, only some of whom develop headaches or more serious sequelae. Early diagnosis with TCD allows strict control of blood pressure to restore flow velocities to the normal range and perhaps prevent serious complications.

Postoperative Occlusion

Immediate postoperative cerebral ischemia may be due to problems at the site of endarterectomy such as thrombosis or intimal flap. Neurologic deterioration in the recovery room should prompt immediate TCD evaluation, and if ipsilateral flow is poor, rapid reexploration may be indicated to prevent stroke. An advantage of TCD is that carotid occlusion can be diagnosed even before emergence from anesthesia.[14]

Cardiac Surgery

Stroke and more subtle neuropsychological changes are a complication of cardiac surgical procedures. As with CEA, the mechanism may be either cerebral hypoperfusion or cerebral emboli. Theoretically, TCD can aid in the diagnosis of both. It has been demonstrated that increase in embolic count is associated with increase in postoperative cognitive deficits.[31, 32] The relationship between V_{mca} and CBF after institution of hypothermic CPB for coronary bypass remains controversial. While Trivedi et al.[33] and Endoh et al.[34] demonstrated that there is good correlation between CBF and relative V_{mca} changes, other investigators failed to observe this relationship.[35-37] Clearly, this is an area in which more investigation is required.

Subarachnoid Hemorrhage

TCD provides a very useful clinical tool for the management of patients at risk of vasospasm from ruptured cerebral aneurysm[38, 39] or traumatic brain injury.[40-42] Abnormal accelerated increases in FV can be detected noninvasively prior to the development of clinical signs of ischemia.[43] Repeated measurements are practical and reduce the need for multiple angiograms. The efficacy of angioplasty can also be monitored serially.[44] Despite the wide range of FVs in normal individuals, it is possible to define criteria for diagnosis of vasospasm. FVs in excess of 200 cm · s^{-1} are highly suggestive of vasospasm. Global reduction in CBF, for example due to coma, may cause normalization of FV even in the presence of significant vasospasm. To increase the sensitivity of TCD diagnosis, the cerebral artery FV can be compared with the flow in the extracranial ICA; a ratio of greater than 3 is generally considered to be consistent with vasospasm rather than hyperemia. However, TCD for diagnosis of vasospasm does not replace angiography because it does not have comparable sensitivity and specificity.[45]

Head Injury

Autoregulation

Severe, and even mild, head injury is frequently associated with loss of cerebral autoregulation.[46] CBF then becomes passively dependent on perfusion pressure, and such patients may be at increased risk of cerebral ischemia or hemorrhage if CPP fluctuates outside the normal range. TCD allows bedside testing of cerebral autoregulation and, in contrast to previously available methods, permits beat-to-beat observation of the autoregulatory response. With TCD, it is possible to measure the dynamic autoregulatory response to a rapid, transient change in blood pressure produced by deflation of thigh cuffs.[46] Another simple method for assessing autoregulation is to measure the response to a static change in blood pressure produced by infusion of a vasopressor such as phenylephrine. Using this technique, we have observed impaired cerebral autoregulation in head-injured patients having general anesthesia for peripheral injuries, and this can occur even after mild head injury (unpublished data).

Vasospasm

Similar to vasospasm from aneurysmal rupture, 20% to 40% of patients with traumatic subarachnoid hemorrhage may develop secondary ischemia from vasospasm, with a similar time course. TCD facilitates the diagnosis and management of these patients.[40-42]

Brain Death

The TCD features of critically reduced CBF and cerebral circulatory arrest have been described.[47, 48] As ICP approaches arterial pressure, diastolic blood flow falls, then ceases. When CBF reaches zero, it is often possible to detect forward flow during systole and reverse flow in diastole (to-and-fro or oscillatory flow) (Fig. 11-2). At this time, TCD evidence of cerebral circulatory arrest is gaining acceptance as an ancillary criterion or confirmatory test for diagnosis of brain death.[49, 50] The usefulness of the technique lies in its ability to rapidly assess blood flow and the response to therapeutic interventions. For example, we have used TCD intraoperatively in patients with acute polytrauma requiring urgent surgery to control blood loss and identified those with evidence of critically reduced CPP. Prognosis is generally dismal if TCD identifies cerebral circulatory arrest that does not respond to therapeutic interventions such as elevation of systemic blood pressure or administration of hyperosmolar fluids.

Limitations

A major frustration within the application of TCD as a routine monitor is that insonation via the temporal region is not possible in up to 10% of adults. A temporal window cannot be found if the bone is too thick to transmit the ultrasound signal adequately, this being more likely with advancing age, female sex, and some racial groups.[51] Patients with bony or soft tissue injuries over the temporal window may also be unsuitable for monitoring. TCD instruments are designed primarily as diagnostic devices and their use as a monitor requires a method for fixation of the probe. In patients with a poor temporal window, very small movements of the probe may result in loss of signal. The fixation device must be robust enough to hold the probe steady and, if intraoperative monitoring is required, it must not interfere with the surgical field.[52] Issues relating to possible variation in vessel diameter invalidating the use of TCD as a monitor of flow have already been discussed.

Jugular Bulb Oximetry

Jugular bulb catheterization permits monitoring of various metabolic parameters in the venous drainage of the brain. The unique physiologic information obtained is potentially useful in the management of patients at risk of cerebral ischemia.

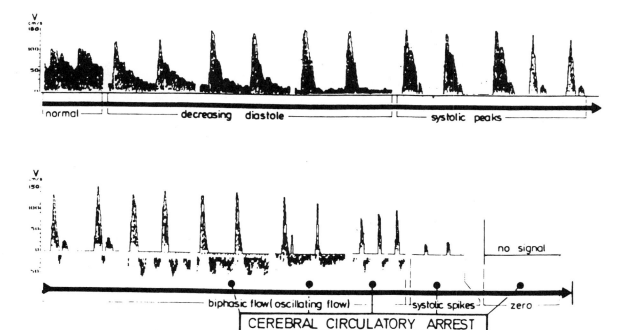

Figure 11-2. Changes in flow velocity profile with increasing intracranial pressure. Progressive decrease in diastolic flow velocity is followed by the appearance of the oscillating flow pattern, which signifies the onset of intracranial circulatory arrest. (From Hassler W, Steinmetz H, Pirschel J: Transcranial Doppler study of intracranial circulatory arrest. J. Neurosurg 1989; 71:195-201.)

Table 11–1. Reference Values for Cerebral Blood Flow and Metabolic Rate of Oxygen

$CMRO_2$: 3.3 ± 0.4 mL · 100 g⁻¹ · min⁻¹	$(1.5 \pm 0.18$ mmol · g⁻¹ · min⁻¹)*
CBF: 54 ± 12 mL · 100 g⁻¹ · min⁻¹	
$C(a-v)O_2$: 6.3 (5.0–7.5) vol%	$(2.8$ (2.2–3.3) mmol · mL⁻¹)*
$SjvO_2$: 55%–70%	

$CMRO_2$, cerebral metabolic rate of oxygen; CBF, cerebral blood flow; $C(a-v)O_2$, arteriovenous oxygen content difference; $SjvO_2$, jugular venous oxygen saturation.
*1 mL gas = 45 mmol.

Physiologic Principles

Arteriovenous Oxygen Difference

The difference between the arterial oxygen content (CaO_2) and the venous oxygen content (CvO_2) is termed the cerebral arteriovenous oxygen content difference [$C(a-v)O_2$].

$$C(a-v)O_2 = CaO_2 - CjvO_2 \qquad (1)$$
$$= 1.39 \times Hb \times [SaO_2 - SjvO_2] - 0.003 \times [PaO_2 - PjvO_2] \qquad (2)$$

Some authors use the affinity constant of 1.34 instead of 1.39.

This formula gives the $C(a-v)O_2$ (vol%) as determined by the arterial and jugular venous hemoglobin (Hb) saturations (SaO_2 and $SjvO_2$, respectively), Hb concentration (in g/dL), and oxygen tensions in arterial (PaO_2) and jugular venous ($PjvO_2$) blood (mmHg). The normal values are shown in Table 11–1.

Arteriovenous Oxygen Content Difference as an Indicator of Cerebral Blood Flow

By rearranging the Fick equation, the relationship between $C(a-v)O_2$ CBF, and the cerebral metabolic rate of oxygen ($CMRO_2$) can be expressed thus:

$$C(a-v)O_2 = \frac{CMRO_2}{CBF} \qquad (3)$$

From this equation it can be seen that as long as the relationship between cerebral metabolism and blood flow remains constant, the $C(a-v)O_2$ remains unchanged. In the normal brain, flow-metabolism coupling ensures a tight match between metabolic requirements and blood flow and the $C(a-v)O_2$ indeed remains constant despite fluctuations in oxygen consumption.

Changes in $C(a-v)O_2$ can be used to monitor deviations from the normal ratio of flow to metabolism. Excess blood flow for the metabolic rate (i.e., hyperemia or luxury perfusion) results in a fall in the $C(a-v)O_2$ and hence an abnormally high $SjvO_2$. This may be due to an absolute rise in blood flow in excess of metabolic requirements or it may be due to a fall in cerebral metabolism not accompanied by an appropriate fall in CBF. The reverse situation, that is, inadequate CBF for the metabolic rate (ischemia), results in a widened $C(a-v)O_2$ and a low $SjvO_2$.

In some circumstances $CMRO_2$ can be assumed to remain constant while CBF may be subject to change. For example, changes in $PaCO_2$ alter CBF independently of $CMRO_2$. Also, severe head injury sometimes impairs cerebral autoregulation so that CBF changes passively with changes in CPP. From

Equation (3), it can be seen that if $CMRO_2$ is constant, then the $C(a-v)O_2$ serves as an indicator of CBF.[53] The relationship is hyperbolic: if CBF is low, then further small decreases in CBF cause progressively larger rises in $C(a-v)O_2$ (Fig. 11–3).

One important caveat should be given. If CBF falls to the point of causing ischemia, $C(a-v)O_2$ can no longer be expected to represent CBF. This is because $CMRO_2$ can no longer be constant but will become flow-dependent as oxygen delivery itself limits metabolism. In this situation, further falls in CBF will not cause a corresponding rise in $C(a-v)O_2$.

Factors Determining Jugular Venous Hemoglobin Saturations

If dissolved oxygen is ignored, Equation (2) may be simplified thus:

$$C(a-v)O_2 \approx 1.39 \times Hb \times [SaO_2 - SjvO_2] \qquad (4)$$

Substituting this equation for Equation (3) allows us to derive an equation that summarizes all the important factors determining $SjvO_2$:

$$SjvO_2 \approx SaO_2 - \frac{CMRO_2}{CBF \times Hb \times 1.39} \qquad (5)$$

Arterial Oxygen Content

Oxygen delivery to the brain is the product of CBF and CaO_2. If oxygen delivery falls due to a change in one or both of these parameters, the brain must increase oxygen extraction to maintain the cerebral metabolic rate. Therefore, ane-

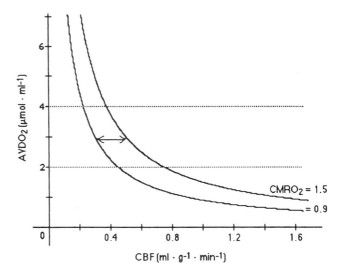

Figure 11–3. Relationship between cerebral blood flow (CBF) and arteriovenous oxygen content difference ($AVDO_2$). Shown are two curves representing two different cerebral metabolic rates for oxygen (1.5 and 0.9 mmol · g⁻¹ · min⁻¹). If CBF changes while the cerebral metabolic rate of oxygen ($CMRO_2$) remains constant, then the arteriovenous oxygen content difference changes according to the hyperbolic relationship shown. A metabolically coupled change in CBF and $CMRO_2$ is represented by a shift to a new curve and the arteriovenous oxygen content difference remains unchanged (*arrow*). (Adapted from Robertson CS, Narayan RK, Gokaslan ZL, et al: Cerebral arteriovenous oxygen difference as an estimate of cerebral blood flow in comatose patients. J Neurosurg 1989; 70:223.)

mia or hypoxemia leads to a lower $SjvO_2$ unless CBF increases to preserve cerebral oxygen delivery. Increasing CBF lowers the $C(a-v)O_2$, tending to maintain the $SjvO_2$ within the normal range. However, if blood flow does not rise enough to maintain oxygen delivery, $SjvO_2$ falls, indicating impending ischemia.

Arteriovenous Lactate Difference

In the presence of adequate oxygen transport to the brain there is no anaerobic metabolism and the brain does not produce lactate. In fact, a small consumption of lactate is normal. Therefore, while the absolute value of jugular bulb lactate varies with the arterial lactate, the difference between the two concentrations is usually small. Detection of cerebral lactate production by determining the arteriovenous lactate difference (AVDL) is a potential method of diagnosing cerebral ischemia. The AVDL (arterial lactate concentration minus jugular bulb lactate concentration) is normally 0.17 (0.17 to 0.37) $mmol \cdot L^{-1}$.[53] A value less than 0.17 is indicative of ischemia.

In coma, although overall cerebral metabolism is reduced, patients are sometimes hyperemic. The increased CBF reduces both the $C(a-v)O_2$ and AVDL and this may reduce the ability to diagnose ischemia. It has been proposed that an index of lactate production versus oxygen consumption, the lactate-oxygen index (LOI), should give a more sensitive guide to the presence of ischemia.[53] $LOI = -AVDL/C(a-v)O_2$ (AVDL and $C(a-v)O_2$ are both converted to $\mu mol \cdot mL^{-1}$). The LOI is normally less than 0.03 and a threshold of 0.08 or greater appears to be diagnostic of cerebral ischemia or infarction.[53]

Anatomic Considerations

Blood in the jugular bulb is representative of the venous drainage of the whole brain. This fact underlies the usefulness of measuring metabolic parameters at this site. Based on cadaver studies in the 1930s, it is often stated that blood from the cortex drains preferentially into the dominant lateral sinus (usually the right) and hence into the jugular bulb on that side. Conversely, blood from deeper brain structures is said to drain to the contralateral side. The significance of these findings has been disputed,[54] and it is now generally accepted that blood from both cortical and subcortical structures drains bilaterally. It is worth noting that the classic Kety-Schmidt method of measuring CBF relies on simultaneous sampling of arterial and jugular bulb blood. The validity of that technique as a measurement of global CBF depends on the assumption that unilateral jugular bulb measurements are representative of the brain as a whole. In normal human subjects, estimations of oxygen saturation, lactate production, CBF, and $CMRO_2$ are nearly equal when measured simultaneously from both jugular bulbs.[55]

Usually, one lateral sinus and internal jugular vein (IJV) are dominant, draining a larger proportion of the total CBF. Most commonly the right side is dominant. Occasionally, the IJV is vestigial or absent on one side. There is cross-drainage of venous blood such that, on average, two thirds of blood in the jugular bulb originates from the ipsilateral ICA and one third from the contralateral ICA.[54] This incomplete mixing across the midline means that a unilateral lesion sometimes causes changes in the ipsilateral jugular bulb only.

Excessive contamination with extracranial venous blood can invalidate jugular bulb measurements. The extraction of oxygen in the facial circulation is much lower than in the brain, so contamination will artifactually raise the measured venous saturation. Normally, blood in the jugular bulb is only 0% to 6% extracranial in origin (mean, 2.7%),[54] but care must be taken because facial veins enter the IJV only a few centimeters downstream from the jugular bulb. Malpositioning of catheters, either inadvertently up the facial veins or too low in the IJV, leads to artifactual measurements.[56] Rapid aspiration from the jugular bulb could draw contaminated blood retrogradely from the IJV so blood should be drawn no faster than about 1 mL/30 seconds.[57]

Choice of Side

A common problem with the clinical application of jugular bulb monitoring is the choice of side for placement of the catheter. Typically, only one jugular bulb is catheterized and various strategies have been used to determine the appropriate side. If monitoring is for global effects (e.g., hyperventilation), it is probably unimportant which side is chosen and an acceptable strategy is to always cannulate the right, the right being more frequently dominant. In patients with head injury, it is common to cannulate the side of dominant venous drainage. The dominant side may be determined by compressing each IJV in turn; the side on which compression causes the greater rise in ICP is taken to be the dominant.[58, 59] Alternatively, CT scans can be examined to determine which jugular foramen is larger. Lastly, if there is a unilateral lesion, it is reasonable to cannulate on the ipsilateral side.[60] Analysis of bilateral measurements in head-injured patients suggests that the best strategy for unilateral monitoring is to choose the side of the lesion or, when the injury is diffuse, the side of the larger jugular foramen.[61] Even so, a significant number of the episodes of desaturation and raised LOI detected in that study would have been missed with any unilateral strategy.

Equipment and Technique

For many years jugular bulb sampling has been safely performed by placement of a needle percutaneously anterior to the mastoid process. This technique is unsuitable for long-term monitoring, and today jugular bulb monitoring is easily performed by passage of a catheter retrogradely up the IJV. Jugular bulb saturation can be assayed intermittently or continuously. For intermittent sampling, a catheter is placed and blood samples are drawn as required. A 4F fiberoptic oximetric catheter (originally designed for umbilical artery placement) is inserted for continuous monitoring.

For intermittent sampling, we insert a 16-gauge, 13.3-cm Angiocath catheter (Becton Dickinson, Sandy, UT) using the catheter-over-needle technique. Anatomic considerations are comparable to those for routine anterograde central venous catheterization via the IJV. Briefly, the operator stands at the supine patient's side and identifies the apex of the triangle between the two heads of the sternocleidomastoid muscle. With a syringe attached, the needle is angled about 30 degrees from the horizontal and directed toward the ipsilateral mastoid process. After skin puncture, the needle is advanced 1 to 2 cm until blood is freely aspirated. If blood is not aspirated, the needle is slowly withdrawn while maintaining gentle negative pressure and observing again for free flow of blood. As with anterograde catheterization of the IJV, it is common for the advancing needle to compress the vein and then "pop" through both walls simultaneously so that the needle will then reenter the lumen during withdrawal. Once the lumen is identified, the catheter is advanced off the needle and should pass without resistance up the vein. The jugular bulb is entered at approximately the same distance from the puncture site as the mastoid process. The catheter may impinge on the wall of the bulb, in which case a slight elastic resistance may be felt and the catheter is withdrawn 1 cm. If the catheter does not freely advance to the depth of the mastoid, it may be passing up a facial branch. In this case the catheter is partially withdrawn and then readvanced. Occasionally, a J-tipped guidewire is useful to help guide the catheter.

Catheterization can usually be performed with the patient in the supine position without head-down tilt or turning of the head. These positioning considerations may be important in trauma patients with possible cervical fractures and in patients with raised ICP. A bedside ultrasound image (e.g., Site-Rite) may be useful in localizing the IJV and confirming that the vein is "full" in this patient position.

For continuous monitoring of $SjvO_2$, a fiberoptic oximetric catheter is inserted in a manner similar to that described above. An appropriately-sized introducer (4F) is placed using the Seldinger technique. The catheter is advanced up the IJV until a slight elastic resistance is felt and then withdrawn 1 cm. Calibration is checked against a blood sample drawn via the fiberoptic catheter and the monitor is then recalibrated if necessary. Fiberoptic catheters are flexible and hence prone to misplacement due to coiling within the vessel or placement up a branch vein. Radiographic confirmation of placement is required for fiberoptic catheters but is usually unnecessary for uncomplicated insertion of stiffer intermittent sampling catheters.[62]

With either type of catheter, a slow infusion of a heparin-containing solution (1 to 2 U/mL) is commenced to reduce the risk of clot formation.

Complications and Contraindications

Inability to catheterize the jugular bulb is unusual (1% to 3%).[60, 62] Malpositioning may be a problem as outlined earlier, and correct position can be confirmed on a plain anteroposterior (AP) radiograph in which the catheter should be medial to the mastoid process and curve slightly medially.[56] Because indwelling catheters can coil within the vessel after initial correct positioning,[58] it has been recommended that position be confirmed by daily radiographs.

The local complications of and contraindications to regular central venous catheter placement via the IJV apply equally to the retrograde catheter. Local trauma or infection may preclude placement. Accidental carotid artery puncture is the commonest reported complication, although there are no reports of subsequent patient morbidity.[56, 60, 62, 63]

Of theoretical concern is exacerbation of raised ICP due to impaired venous drainage. This could occur due to patient manipulation and positioning during insertion, venous obstruction by the catheter itself, or venous thrombosis. Studies in infants and children documenting ICP during insertion report no clinically significant rise.[60, 63] Testing of venous patency has not documented any instance of impaired venous drainage attributed to a jugular bulb catheter.[60] However, subclinical nonobstructive venous thrombosis has been reported to occur in up to 40% of patients monitored with indwelling fiberoptic oximetric catheters.[64]

Clinical Applications

Traumatic Brain Injury

The greatest interest in jugular bulb monitoring is in the intensive care management of traumatic brain injury (TBI).

This monitoring has become standard care in many institutions. The aim of early hospital care of TBI is prevention of secondary injury; that is, ischemic brain damage. Jugular bulb oximetry provides a minimally invasive method of continuous monitoring for inadequate CBF.

When CBF has been measured in head-injured patients it has confirmed that a widened $C(a-v)O_2$ correlates well with globally reduced CBF.[65, 66] Episodes of jugular bulb desaturation[67, 68] and raised $C(a-v)O_2$[69] are associated with poor outcome after TBI. Robertson et al.[70] observed that multiple episodes of desaturation in patients with severe head injury are associated with a significantly higher mortality compared with that in patients without any desaturation episodes (Fig. 11–4). Increased lactate production, as evidenced by a high LOI, is strongly associated with a poor outcome.[71] In some patients with raised LOI, the $SjvO_2$ is normal or raised.[53, 59] It is unclear why these patients with critically reduced blood flow and raised lactate production should have a high $SjvO_2$. Possibly, these patients have large areas of ischemia or infarction while some blood continues to flow through other pathologic areas with little or no metabolism of oxygen. This is supported by the observation that regional decrease in brain tissue PO_2 and increase in lactate can occur with an unchanged $SjvO_2$.[72]

One of the problematic issues in management of TBI is the use of hyperventilation. The benefits of hyperventilation-induced vasoconstriction in reducing cerebral blood volume and ICP, raising the CPP, and averting brain herniation are well known. However, as the indiscriminate use of hyperventilation in TBI has been shown to be harmful[73] and as hyperventilation can itself induce cerebral ischemia,[65, 74] the use of jugular bulb oximetry has been recommended as a method of detecting ischemia and optimizing hyperventila-

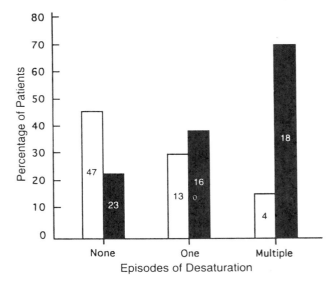

Figure 11–4. The association of cerebral venous desaturation episodes with outcome of patients with severe traumatic brain injury. The numbers in bars represent the actual number of patients. White bar = good recovery/moderate disability, black bar = dead patients. The difference in outcome between the groups (no desaturation, one episode, multiple episodes) is statistically significant ($P < .001$). (From Lam AM, Mayberg TS: Jugular bulb venous oximetry monitoring. Anesth Clin North Am 1997; 15:533–549; adapted from Robertson CS, Gopinath SP, Goodman JC, et al: $SjvO_2$ monitoring in head-injured patients. J Neurotrauma 1995; 12:891–896.)

tion.[75] Excessive hyperventilation is frequently identified as a cause of jugular bulb desaturation.[67]

Interpretation of Jugular Bulb Oxygen Saturation

Normal. A normal $SjvO_2$ can be taken as reassuring that there is no global cerebral ischemia. The most important provison is that areas of regional ischemia may be missed by any global monitor.[72] Calculating the AVDL and the LOI may increase the sensitivity for detection of ischemia, but lactate is not measured continuously and requires intermittent blood sampling.

Raised. A high $SjvO_2$, and therefore low $C(a-v)O_2$, is indicative of hyperemia, otherwise known as "luxury perfusion." In the setting of coma following TBI, a significant proportion of patients have increased CBF relative to their reduced $CMRO_2$. Compared with coma patients with a normal $C(a-v)O_2$, these patients with hyperemia are more likely to have intracranial hypertension.[65] Observation of increased $SjvO_2$ associated with spontaneous increases in blood pressure is suggestive of impaired cerebral autoregulation.[76] Other causes of raised $SjvO_2$ include hypercapnia, arteriovenous admixture via atrioventricular (A-V) malformations, and hypothermic CPB. A high $SjvO_2$ estimation can also be artifactual due to contamination by facial venous blood or calibration drift of indwelling catheters.

Low. An $SjvO_2$ less than 50% is considered pathologic and indicates that there is reduced oxygen delivery relative to the metabolic requirements of the brain. If desaturation is indicated by an indwelling fiberoptic catheter, it is first necessary to confirm the reading by checking for reduced light intensity and drawing a blood sample for in vitro analysis. Causes of desaturation to be considered and treated are summarized in Table 11-2.

Other Applications

Neurosurgical Anesthesia. Jugular bulb catheterization can be safely performed in patients undergoing anesthesia for neurosurgery. An inexpensive catheter for intermittent sampling allows monitoring of the effects of hyperventilation on $SjvO_2$ and AVDL. The level of $PaCO_2$ at which jugular venous desaturation occurs is highly variable. Monitoring the $SjvO_2$ permits detection of hypoperfusion in some pa-

tients[62, 77] while allowing the safe use of more aggressive hyperventilation in others. Blood pressure management during cerebral aneurysm surgery can also be optimized.[78] With experience, it is possible to place jugular bulb catheters in patients undergoing emergency evacuation of space-occupying lesions without delaying surgery or compromising optimal patient positioning. This may allow optimization of hyperventilation and CPP at an early phase when there is a high risk of ischemic brain injury.

Cardiopulmonary Bypass. Neurologic and neuropsychological deficits after CPB continue to be a problem; methods of monitoring cerebral perfusion during bypass could provide an obvious advantage. Although $SjvO_2$ is usually high during hypothermic CPB, this may not represent excessive CBF. During rewarming, jugular venous desaturation is common and occurs in about 20% of the patients.[79] Patients who undergo normothermic CPB may develop desaturation during early bypass.[80] Although the significance of cerebral venous desaturation as an important contributor to postoperative neurologic deficit remains unproved, one report suggests that it is associated with impaired postoperative cognitive test performance.[79]

Limitations of Jugular Bulb Monitoring

Calibration of indwelling fiberoptic catheters is subject to drift, and routine recalibration is required between 4 and 12 hours.[58, 67, 76] Reports consistently indicate that the catheter will require recalibration on about 50% of the instances that blood saturation is checked in vitro.[76, 81] For this reason, whenever the monitor indicates desaturation it is necessary to check the result with a blood sample, and about half of these instances will turn out to be false alarms.[67, 68] A major source of artifactually low saturation readings is loss of reflected light intensity. This is due to impingement of the fiberoptic catheter tip against the vessel wall or formation of clot on the tip. The monitor warns of reduced light intensity and the signal can often be improved by manipulation or flushing of the catheter. Suggested design improvements with potential to improve reliability include a stiffer catheter (less liable to malpositioning), a mechanism for centering the catheter within the vessel lumen, and central placement of the light fibers.[76]

A major limitation of monitoring for CBF with jugular bulb oximetry is that the measurement is global. In some situations global effects are likely and jugular bulb monitoring is particularly useful. For example, $SjvO_2$ monitoring is useful for detecting hypoperfusion due to hyperventilation in the intensive care unit or the operating room. Discrete regions of ischemia may be disguised because the desaturated blood draining from such areas mixes with normal venous blood from the rest of the brain.[72] Therefore, while jugular bulb desaturation is specific for hypoperfusion, it is unfortunately not a sensitive indicator of ischemia.

Near-Infrared Spectroscopy

Principles

Near-infrared spectroscopy (NIRS) is a technique that aims to provide continuous, noninvasive monitoring of regional cerebral oxygenation. Near-infrared light (wavelength 700 to 1000 nm) penetrates biologic tissues, including the scalp, skull, and brain. Light in this wavelength is absorbed by the biologic chromophores which include Hb, oxygenated Hb

Table 11-2. Causes of and Treatments for Jugular Bulb Desaturation

Causes	Treatment Strategies
Reduced Arterial Oxygen Content	
Anemia	Blood transfusion
Hypoxemia	Correct hypoxemia
Reduced Cerebral Blood Flow	
Arterial hypotension	IV fluid, vasopressors/inotropic agents
Intracranial hypertension	CSF drainage, hyperosmolar fluids, hyperventilation, surgery
Excessive hyperventilation	Increase arterial CO_2
Vasospasm	Hypertension, hypervolemia, hemodilution, nimodipine
Increased Cerebral Metabolism	
Fever	Antipyretics, physical cooling
Seizures	Anticonvulsants, barbiturates, propofol

(HbO₂), and oxygenated cytochrome-*c* oxidase. Simultaneous measurement of the absorption of several wavelengths of near-infrared light allows calculation of the relative concentrations of these chromophores.[82] This is similar to the principle used in pulse oximetry with the exception that it is based on reflectance oximetry rather than transmission oximetry.

When a near-infrared light source is applied to the scalp the light penetrates to a depth of several centimeters. The light is scattered in the tissues and some returns to the surrounding scalp where it can be detected and the absorbance measured. The average path of photons scattering back to the scalp is parabolic so the depth of the tissue penetrated is related to the distance between the light source and the detector (Fig. 11–5).

Commercially available monitors utilizing two wavelengths can solve for only two chromophores, Hb and HbO₂. Cytochrome-*c* oxidase may be ignored as its contribution to changes in absorbance is small compared to Hb. Monitors such as the INVOS (Somanetics Corp., Troy, MI) estimate the ratio of oxygenated and deoxygenated Hb to calculate the regional Hb saturation (rSO₂): rSO₂ = [HbO₂]/([Hb] + [HbO₂]). The familiar technique of pulse oximetry utilizes a similar method for estimating the relative concentrations of Hb and HbO₂ in arterial blood. Alternatively, monitors such as the NIRO (Hamamatsu Photonics, Mamamatsu City, Japan) convert changes in absorbance to a change in the concentration of Hb and HbO₂ in the light path (expressed in mmol · L⁻¹). In addition, the sum of the changes in Hb and HbO₂ gives an indication of alteration in tissue blood volume, as might occur with changes in arterial carbon dioxide.

Cerebral blood is 75% to 80% venous so the absorbance measured by NIRS is assumed to be predominately influenced by regional venous blood. The INVOS algorithm assumes an arbitrary partition of arterial and venous blood volume to derive the regional saturation. Therefore, NIRS provides a monitor of the adequacy of O₂ delivery similar to jugular bulb saturation. The former technique is a regional measurement whereas the latter is global. Average saturations of 70% to 75% are found in normal subjects.

Perhaps the greatest difficulty in applying NIRS is the confounding effect of absorbance from the scalp and skull. The INVOS monitor attempts to account for this by having two detectors, one closer to the light source than the other. The absorbance measured at the closer detector represents the superficial tissues, and this is used to correct measurements from the more distant detector. The corrected reading is an attempt at estimating the Hb saturation in the area of interest: the cortex deep to the probe. There is some clinical evidence that this system is effective in reducing the contribution of extracranial blood to the saturation reading.[83] The other problem is the variable length of optical path among individuals. Thus there is a close correlation between SjvO₂ and rSO₂ within individuals but not between individuals.[84]

Equipment and Technique

NIRS equipment incorporates a system for applying light-emitting and -detecting probes to the patient. The probes must be placed on skin free of hair so the usual place to monitor is over the forehead, close to the hairline. The midline is avoided to prevent sampling the sagittal sinus while the temporalis muscle is avoided laterally. Adequate distance between the light source and the detector, for example, 40 to 60 mm, is required to enable sampling of cortical tissue.

The three probes in the INVOS monitor (one light source and two detectors) are incorporated into a single adhesive pad for application to the scalp. Other monitors, such as the NIRO, require separate fixation of two probes. A method of excluding extraneous light is required and application of constant pressure may improve reliability by reducing scalp blood flow.

Clinical Applications

The first clinical application of NIRS was in the field of neonatal intensive care.[85] In neonates it is possible to transilluminate across the entire skull, allowing monitoring of transmitted rather than reflected light.

NIRS monitoring for cerebral ischemia in adults has been studied in most situations where cerebral perfusion is threatened. These include CEA,[83, 86] carotid occlusion tests,[87] CPB,[88] circulatory arrest,[89] and severe head injury.[86]

Initial experience in intensive care monitoring of head-injured patients suggests that NIRS has a greater sensitivity than jugular bulb oximetry in detecting episodes of impaired cerebral oxygenation.[90] Another study reported opposite results, with NIRS monitoring failing to detect any of 14 episodes of cerebral hypoxia diagnosed by jugular bulb oximetry[91] (this study utilized a version of the INVOS monitor that has since been superseded).

Limitations

The various technical and clinical problems to be overcome in the application of this technology have been reviewed.[92] The extent to which the signal is contaminated by extracerebral blood remains a subject of debate.[93] In a study examining cerebral oximetry values in dead subjects, a considerable overlap in values was observed between the control group and the study group in whom circulation had ceased for many hours before the study.[94] This is of particular concern in situations where extracranial blood flow cannot be assumed to remain constant; for example, during cross-clamping of the common or external carotid arteries.

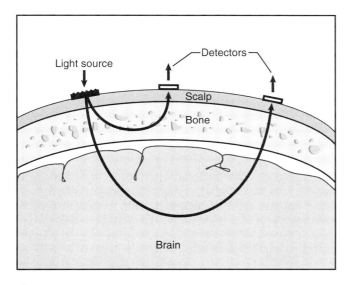

Figure 11–5. Diagrammatic illustration of the principles of the INVOS cerebral oximeter (Somanetics, Troy, MI). The light reflected from superficial and deep tissues is measured by respective electrodes positioned at strategic positions from the source.

A minimum threshold of rSO_2, or a maximum acceptable decrease, is required for clinical application of NIRS, but such values are yet to be established. A decrease in rSO_2 value is generally observed during cross-clamping of the ipsilateral carotid artery. However, correlation of rSO_2 with neurologic changes during awake CEA,[95] and EEG[96] or somatosensory evoked potential (SSEP)[97, 98] changes during the same procedure under general anesthesia have failed to establish NIRS criteria for the diagnosis of ischemia.

NIRS allows focal monitoring of only a few cubic centimeters of brain. If an ischemic insult is localized to areas distant from the monitored cortex, then the NIRS monitor is not useful. In carotid surgery, for example, monitoring of the frontal lobe may be falsely reassuring if the patient happens to have both anterior cerebral arteries supplied by the contralateral ICA.[99]

The accuracy of NIRS is also limited if blood accumulates between the brain and the probe. For example, subdural or extradural hematoma and even scalp hematoma will cause the monitor to measure the saturation of the pooled blood rather than cerebral blood.

The INVOS system for estimating rSO_2 assumes that the optical path length is identical for the two wavelengths utilized. This assumption is not valid for a significant proportion of subjects. The monitor is able to detect variation in path length and displays a "signal quality index" to warn of unreliable absolute saturation readings (trends in regional saturation remain valid). Clearly, significant improvement in technology and design is required before this monitor can become a clinically useful device.

Brain Parenchymal Oxygen Tension

Principles

Microcatheters incorporating miniature Clark electrodes for continuous in vivo measurement of PaO_2 are now commercially available. The physical principles of these monitors are described in Chapter 19. These probes (Licox, GMS, Kiel-Mielkendorf, Germany; Paratrend 7, Biomedical Sensors, Malvern, PA) have been inserted directly into brain parenchyma and are being evaluated as a monitor of cerebral oxygenation.[81, 100] In addition to PO_2, they can also measure pH and PCO_2.

The monitor provides continuous measurement of tissue oxygen partial pressure ($PtiO_2$) with a response time of around 2 to 3 minutes. This technology offers the potential for directly monitoring the availability of a vital substrate for brain metabolism, oxygen, at the site of the tissue at risk. The actual area of brain monitored is limited to the few cubic millimeters surrounding the probe.

Equipment and Technique

Insertion of parenchymal catheters requires a surgical procedure for drilling a bur hole, placing the catheter through the dura into cortex or white matter and fixation of the catheter. One of the commercially available catheters has the oxygen electrode 35 mm from the catheter tip so it is important to ensure that the catheter is inserted to an adequate depth. The catheter is calibrated in vivo prior to insertion and a period of about half an hour is required for $PtiO_2$ to stabilize following the local microtrauma of insertion. Once the probe is inserted, no recalibration is possible and drift cannot be detected.

Clinical Applications

Although interest is growing, measurement of parenchymal oxygen tension must still be regarded as experimental. The technique has been tried in patients at risk of cerebral ischemia who are having invasive procedures performed as part of routine management. These include patients having ICP monitors inserted for management of head injury and patients having craniotomy for hematoma or cerebrovascular surgery.[101] Because of the invasive nature of the monitor, it has not been studied in other patients at risk of ischemia such as those undergoing CEA.

There is debate over how low the $PtiO_2$ can fall before endangering neurons (see below). A value of 20 mmHg has been suggested, but lower values have also been advanced and the difference may relate to differences between the performance of the two commercially available probes at low oxygen tensions.[102]

A comparison between indwelling fiberoptic probes for jugular bulb saturation monitoring and parenchymal oxygen probes found $PtiO_2$ monitoring to be more robust with fewer artifacts.[81] Possible complications are similar to other invasive techniques such as parenchymal pressure transducers and ventriculostomy catheters. These include hematoma and infection.

Limitations

As with NIRS, but to an even greater degree, ischemia is detected only in a limited area of cortex. This would be acceptable if the ischemic insult could be assumed to be uniformly global. Alternatively, if it is known which area is most at risk for ischemia, then highly localized monitoring may be appropriate, assuming that the area is suitable for probe insertion. With heterogeneous pathologic changes, a localized area of ischemia more than a few millimeters away from the probe would not be detected by this technology, a concern that is borne out by reports of patients with normal $PtiO_2$ despite lactate production detected with jugular bulb monitoring.[103] Conversely, the probe might be placed in a pathologic area that is beyond salvage and data from such a region may be misleading if used to guide therapy for the remainder of the brain.[104]

A major difficulty in the clinical application of this technology is that threshold $PtiO_2$ values predictive of ischemic brain damage have not yet been determined. A recent study of severely head-injured patients reported increasing chance of death with increasing cumulative time at which $PtiO_2$ is below 15 mmHg, and any episode of $PtiO_2$ below 6 mmHg was highly predictive of death.[105] While such data help confirm the validity of the monitor as a measure of brain oxygenation, death is a crude outcome variable; it will be more useful if thresholds can be determined above which optimal recovery is ensured. There may turn out to be considerable overlap between $PtiO_2$ values measured in patients with adequate oxygen delivery compared with those measured in patients who would benefit from improved CBF or CaO_2.

Interpatient variability in $PtiO_2$ may be partly artifactual. A study in normal rat brains reported that microhemorrhage sometimes occurs around the catheter tip and is associated with reduced $PtiO_2$ readings.[106] Brain $PtiO_2$ can fall below 10 mmHg during ischemic insults and the accuracy of the miniaturized Clark electrodes in this range has been questioned. Once the probe is inserted it cannot be recalibrated and calibration drift may be significant at low PO_2.[105]

Summary

The ideal monitor for cerebral ischemia would be noninvasive and simple to use at the bedside or in the operating room. It would provide continuous detection of local, regional, and global ischemia, allowing corrective therapy before neuronal damage occurs. Unfortunately, such an ideal monitor is yet to be realized.

Of the monitors discussed in this chapter, jugular bulb oximetry suffers from being a global measure and may fail to detect regional ischemia. Conversely, NIRS and parenchymal oxygen probes are localized and may fail to detect ischemia outside the monitored region. TCD ultrasonography is capable of monitoring a large proportion of the CBF but is not possible in some situations and in some patients.

Despite their limitations, jugular bulb oximetry and TCD are assuming an important role in clinical practice. Jugular bulb oximetry monitoring now has an established role in the management of head injury and has also been found to be useful as an intraoperative monitor. TCD has an established role in the management of vasospasm and a growing place in CEA. Besides its role as a monitor for cerebral ischemia, TCD gives other diagnostic information such as emboli detection and detection of hyperemia and can be used for bedside assessment of cerebral autoregulation. As with almost all forms of monitoring, there are no outcome studies demonstrating a benefit from monitoring for cerebral ischemia.

Regarding NIRS, a monitor that is noninvasive, reliable, simple to apply, and gives continuous and rapidly responsive information regarding adequacy of oxygenation has obvious appeal. Pulse oximetry has been rapidly adopted as a monitor of arterial oxygenation, but SaO_2 is only one aspect of oxygen delivery. A noninvasive monitor of tissue oxygenation within a critical organ such as the brain would be advantageous. If the limitations regarding signal contamination with extracranial blood could be overcome, then NIRS might even find a place in routine anesthetic and critical care monitoring. However, the usefulness of NIRS in adults at high risk of cerebral ischemia may be limited by the fact that it monitors a very localized area of cortex, and diagnostic criteria for ischemia have not yet been established.

Measurement of brain parenchymal oxygen tension has the attraction of directly monitoring availability to the neurons of a vital metabolic substrate. Other monitoring modalities such as CPP, TCD, and $SjvO_2$ provide only indirect information regarding oxygen delivery. However, the highly focal nature of the monitor, absence of a clearly defined ischemic threshold, and technical problems such as calibration drift, limit its clinical applicability at this time.

Because each monitor has advantages and limitations, it may be useful to monitor with two or more modalities simultaneously.[107] Multimodal monitoring may detect cerebral ischemia or altered cerebral function where any single monitor would be unreliable. Furthermore, analysis of trend data recorded simultaneously from multiple monitors may allow inference of causal relationships between physiologic variables.

REFERENCES

1. Aaslid R, Markwalder T, Nornes H: Noninvasive transcranial Doppler ultrasound recording of flow velocity in basal cerebral arteries. J Neurosurg 1982 57:769–774.
2. Huber P, Handa J: Effect of contrast material, hypercapnia, hyperventilation, hypertonic glucose and papaverine on the diameter of the cerebral arteries—angiographic determination in man. Investigative Radiology 1967; 2:17–32.
3. Giller CA, Bowman G, Dyer H, et al: Cerebral arterial diameters during changes in blood pressure and carbon dioxide during craniotomy. Neurosurgery 1993; 32:737–742.
4. Bishop CCR, Powell S, Rutt D, et al: Transcranial Doppler measurement of middle cerebral artery blood flow velocity: A validation study. Stroke 1986; 17:913–915.
5. Markwalder T, Grolimund P, Seiler RW, et al: Dependency of blood flow velocity in the middle cerebral artery on end-tidal carbon dioxide partial pressure—a transcranial ultrasound Doppler study. J Cereb Blood Flow Metab 1984; 4:368–372.
6. Kirkham FJ, Padayachee TS, Parsons S, et al: Transcranial measurement of blood velocities in the basal cerebral arteries using pulsed Doppler ultrasound: Velocity as an index of flow. Ultrasound Med Biol 1986; 12:15–21.
7. Lindegaard K, Lundar T, Wiberg J, et al: Variations in middle cerebral artery blood flow investigated with noninvasive transcranial blood velocity measurements. Stroke 1987; 18:1025–1030.
8. Newell DW, Aaslid R, Lam AM, et al: Comparison of flow and velocity during dynamic autoregulation testing in humans. Stroke 1994; 25:793–797.
9. Dahl A, Russell D, Nyberg-Hansen R, et al: Effect of nitroglycerin on cerebral circulation measured by Doppler and SPECT. Stroke 1989; 20:1733–1736.
10. Schregel W, Schafermeyer H, Muller C, et al: The effect of halothane, alfentanil and propofol on blood flow velocity, blood vessel cross section and blood volume flow in the middle cerebral artery. Anaesthetist 1992; 41:21–26.
11. Lam AM, Matta BF: Isoflurane does not dilate the middle cerebral artery appreciably. Anesth Analg 1995; 80:S262.
12. Schregel W, Schaefermeyer H, Sihle-Wissel M, et al: Transcranial Doppler sonography during isoflurane/N$_2$O anesthesia and surgery: Flow velocity, "vessel area" and "volume flow". Can J Anaesth 1994; 41:607–612.
13. Aaslid R: Developments and principles of transcranial Doppler: In Newell DW, Aaslid R (eds): Transcranial Doppler. New York, Raven Press, 1992, pp 1–8.
14. Halsey JH: Risks and benefits of shunting in carotid endarterectomy. Stroke 1992; 23:1583–1587.
15. Fiori L, Parenti G, Marconi F: Combined transcranial Doppler and electrophysiologic monitoring for carotid endarterectomy. J Neurosurg Anesthesiol 1997; 9:11–16.
16. Chiesa R, Minicucci F, Melissano G, et al: The role of transcranial Doppler in carotid artery surgery. Eur J Vasc Surg 1992; 6:211–216.
17. Jansen C, Vriens EM, Eikelboom BC, et al: Carotid endarterectomy with transcranial Doppler and electroencephalographic monitoring: A prospective study in 130 operations. Stroke 1993; 24:665–669.
18. Jansen C, Ramos LMP, van Heesewijk JPM, et al: Impact of microembolism and hemodynamic changes in the brain during carotid endarterectomy. Stroke 1994; 25:992–997.
19. Cao P, Giordano G, Zannetti S, et al: Transcranial Doppler monitoring during carotid endarterectomy: Is it appropriate for selecting patients in need of shunt? J Vasc Surg 1997; 26:973–980.
20. Spencer MP, Thomas GI, Moehring MA: Relation between cerebral artery blood flow velocity and stump pressure during carotid endarterectomy. Stroke 1992; 23:1439–1445.
21. Spencer MP: Transcranial Doppler monitoring and causes of stroke from carotid endarterectomy. Stroke 1997; 28:685–691.
22. Spencer MP. Detection of cerebral arterial emboli with transcranial Doppler. In Newell DW, Aaslid R (eds): Transcranial Doppler. New York, Raven Press, 1992, pp 215–230.
23. Smith JL, Evans DH, Gaunt ME, et al: Experience with transcranial Doppler monitoring reduces the incidence of particulate embolization during carotid endarterectomy. Br J Surg 1998; 85:56–59.
24. Lennard N, Smith JL, Hayes P, et al: Transcranial Doppler directed dextran therapy in the prevention of carotid thrombosis: Three-hour monitoring is as effective as six hours. Eur J Vasc Endovasc Surg 1999; 17:301–305.
25. Lennard N, Smith J, Dumville J, et al: Prevention of postoperative thrombotic stroke after carotid endarterectomy: The role of transcranial Doppler ultrasound. J Vasc Surg 1997; 26:579–584.

26. Gaunt ME, Martin PJ, Smith JL, et al: Clinical relevance of intraoperative embolization detected by transcranial Doppler ultrasonography during carotid endarterectomy: A prospective study of 100 patients. Br J Surg 1994; 81:1435–1439.

27. Cantelmo NL, Babiken VL, Samaraweera RN, et al: Cerebral microembolism and ischemic changes associated with carotid endarterectomy. J Vasc Surg 1998; 27:1024–1031.

28. Schroeder T, Sillesen H, Sørensen O, et al: Cerebral hyperperfusion following carotid endarterectomy. J Neurosurg 1987; 66:824–829.

29. Piepgras DG, Morgan MK, Sundt TM, et al: Intracerebral hemorrhage after carotid endarterectomy. J Neurosurg 1998; 68:532–536.

30. Jorgensen LG, Schroeder T: Defective cerebrovascular autoregulation after carotid endarterectomy. Eur J Vasc Surg 1993; 7:370–379.

31. Pugsley W, Klinger L, Paschalis C, et al: The impact of microemboli during cardiopulmonary bypass on neuropsychological functioning. Stroke 1994; 25:1393–1399.

32. Barbut D, Lo YW, Gold JP, et al: Impact of embolization during coronary artery bypass grafting on outcome and length of stay. Ann Thorac Surg 1997; 63:998–1002.

33. Trivedi UH, Patel RL, Turtle MR, et al: Relative changes in cerebral blood flow during cardiac operations using xenon-133 clearance versus transcranial Doppler sonography. Ann Thorac Surg 1997; 63:167–174.

34. Endoh H, Shimoji K: Changes in blood flow velocity in the middle cerebral artery during nonpulsatile hypothermic cardiopulmonary bypass. Stroke 1994; 25:403–407.

35. Weyland A, Stephan H, Kazmaier S, et al: Flow velocity measurements as an index of cerebral blood flow. Validity of transcranial Doppler sonographic monitoring during cardiac surgery. Anesthesiology 1994; 81:1401–1410.

36. Nuttall GA, Cook DJ, Fulgham JR, et al: The relationship between cerebral blood flow and transcranial Doppler blood flow velocity during hypothermic cardiopulmonary bypass in adults. Anesth Analg 1996; 82:1146–1151.

37. Grocott HP, Amory DW, Lowry E, et al: Transcranial Doppler blood flow velocity versus^{133} Xe clearance cerebral blood flow during mild hypothermic cardiopulmonary bypass. J Clin Monit Comput 1998; 14:35–39.

38. Aaslid R, Huber P, Nornes H: A transcranial Doppler method in the evaluation of cerebrovascular spasm. Neuroradiology 1986; 28:11–16.

39. Newell DW, Winn HR: Transcranial Doppler in cerebral vasospasm. Neurosurg Clin North Am 1990; 1:319–328.

40. Romner B, Bellner J, Kongstad P, et al: Elevated transcranial Doppler flow velocities after severe head injury: Cerebral vasospasm or hyperemia? J Neurosurg 1996; 85:90–97.

41. Martin NA, Doberstein C, Alexander M, et al: Posttraumatic cerebral arterial spasm. J Neurotrauma 1995; 12:897–901.

42. Weber M, Grolimund P, Seiler RW: Evaluation of posttraumatic cerebral blood flow velocities by transcranial Doppler ultrasonography. Neurosurgery 1990; 27:106–112.

43. Grosset DG, Straiton J, du Trevou M, et al: Prediction of symptomatic vasospasm after subarachnoid hemorrhage by rapidly increasing transcranial Doppler velocity and cerebral blood flow changes. Stroke 1992; 23:674–679.

44. Eskridge JM, McAuliffe W, Song JK, et al: Balloon angioplasty for the treatment of vasospasm: Results of first 50 cases. Neurosurgery 1998; 42:510–516.

45. Laumer R, Steinmeier R, Gonner F, et al: Cerebral hemodynamics in subarachnoid hemorrhage evaluated by transcranial Doppler sonography. Part 1. Reliability of flow velocities in clinical management. Neurosurgery 1993; 33:1–8.

46. Junger EC, Newell DW, Grant GA, et al: Cerebral autoregulation following minor head injury. J Neurosurg 1997; 86:425–432.

47. Hassler W, Steinmetz H, Pirschel J: Transcranial Doppler study of intracranial circulatory arrest. J Neurosurg 1989; 71:195–201.

48. Ducrocq X, Braun M, Debouverie M, et al: Brain death and transcranial Doppler: Experience in 130 cases of brain dead patients. J Neurol Sci 1998; 160:41–46.

49. Assessment: Transcranial Doppler. Report of the American Academy of Neurology, Therapeutics and Technology Assessment Subcommittee. Neurology 1990; 40:680–681.

50. Ducrocq X, Hassler W, Moritake K, et al: Consensus opinion on diagnosis of cerebral circulatory arrest using Doppler-sonography: Task Force Group on cerebral death of the Neurosonology Research Group of the World Federation of Neurology. J Neurol Sci 1998; 159:145–150.

51. Eden A: Transcranial Doppler ultrasonography and hyperostosis of the skull (letter). Stroke 1988; 19:1445–1446.

52. Lam AM: Intraoperative transcranial Doppler monitoring. Anesthesiology 1995; 82:1536–1537.

53. Robertson CS, Narayan RK, Gokaslan ZL, et al: Cerebral arteriovenous oxygen difference as an estimate of cerebral blood flow in comatose patients. J Neurosurg 1989; 70:222–230.

54. Shenkin HA, Harmel MH, Kety SS: Dynamic anatomy of the cerebral circulation. Arch Neurol Psychiatry 1948; 60:240–252.

55. Gibbs EL, Lennox WG, Gibbs FA: Bilateral internal jugular blood: comparison of A-V differences, oxygen-dextrose ratios and respiratory quotients. Am J Psychiatry 1945; 102:184–190.

56. Jakobsen M, Enevoldsen E: Retrograde catheterization of the right internal jugular vein for serial measurements of cerebral venous oxygen content. J Cereb Blood Flow Metab 1989; 9:717–720.

57. Matta BF, Lam AM: The speed of blood withdrawal affects the accuracy of jugular venous bulb oxygen saturation measurements. Anesthesiology 1997; 88:806–808.

58. Andrews PJD, Dearden NM, Miller JD: Jugular bulb cannulation: Description of a cannulation technique and validation of a new continuous monitor. Br J Anaesth 1991; 67:553–558.

59. Lam JMK, Chan MSY, Poon WS; Cerebral venous oxygen saturation monitoring: Is dominant jugular bulb cannulation good enough? Br J Neurosurg 1996; 10:357–364.

60. Goetting MG, Preston G: Jugular bulb catheterization: Experience with 123 patients. Crit Care Med 1990; 18:1220–1223.

61. Metz C, Holzschuh M, Bein T, et al: Monitoring of cerebral oxygen metabolism in the jugular bulb: Reliability of unilateral measurements in severe head injury. J Cereb Blood Flow Metab 1998;18:332–343.

62. Matta BF, Lam AM, Mayberg TS, et al: A critique of the intraoperative use of jugular venous bulb catheters during neurosurgical procedures. Anesth Analg 1994; 79:745–750.

63. Gayle MO, Frewen TC, Armstrong RF, et al: Jugular venous bulb catheterization in infants and children. Crit Care Med 1989; 17:385–388.

64. Coplin WM, O'Keefe GE, Grady MS, et al: Thrombotic, infectious, and procedural complications of the jugular bulb catheter in the intensive care unit. Neurosurgery 1997; 41:101–107.

65. Obrist WD, Langfitt TW, Jaggi JL, et al: Cerebral blood flow and metabolism in comatose patients with acute head injury: Relationship to intracranial hypertension. J Neurosurg 1984; 61:241–253.

66. Robertson CS, Contant CF, Gokaslan ZL, et al: Cerebral blood flow, arteriovenous difference, and outcome in head injured patients. J Neurol Neurosurg Psychiatry 1992; 55:594–603.

67. Sheinberg MS, Kanter MJ, Robertson CS, et al: Continuous monitoring of jugular venous oxygen saturation in head-injured patients. J Neurosurg 1992; 76:212–217.

68. Gopinath SP, Robertson CS, Contant CF, et al: Jugular venous desaturation and outcome after head injury. J Neurol Neurosurg Psychiatry 1994; 57:717–723.

69. Le Roux PD, Newell DW, Lam AM, et al: Cerebral arteriovenous oxygen difference: a predictor of cerebral infarction and outcome in patients with severe head injury. J Neurosurg 1997; 87:1–8.

70. Robertson CS, Gopinath SP, Goodman JC, et al: SjvO$_2$ monitoring in head-injured patients. J Neurotrauma 1995; 12:891–896.

71. Sahuquillo J, Poca MA, Garnacho A, et al: Early ischaemia after head injury: Preliminary results in patients with diffuse brain injuries. Acta Neurochir 1993; 122:204–214.

72. Robertson CS, Gopinath SP, Uzura M, et al: Metabolic changes in the brain during transient ischemia measured with microdialysis. Neurol Res 1998; 20 (suppl 1):S91–94.

73. Muizelaar JP, Marmarou A, Ward JD, et al: Adverse effects of prolonged hyperventilation in patients with severe head injury: A randomized clinical trial. J Neurosurg 1991; 75:731–739.

74. Cold G: Does acute hyperventilation provoke cerebral oligemia in comatose patients after acute head injury? Acta Neurochir (Wien) 1989; 96:100–106.
75. Cruz J: The first decade of continuous monitoring of jugular bulb oxyhemoglobin saturation: Management strategies and clinical outcome. Crit Care Med 1998; 26:344–351.
76. Fortune JB, Feustel PJ, Weigle CGM, et al: Continuous measurement of jugular venous oxygen saturation in response to transient elevations of blood pressure in head-injured patients. J Neurosurg 1994; 80:461–468.
77. Schaffranietz L, Heinke W: The effect of different ventilation regimes on jugular venous oxygen saturation in elective neurosurgical patients. Neurol Res 1998; 20:S66–S70.
78. Moss E, Dearden NM, Berridge JC: Effects of changes in mean arterial pressure on SjO$_2$ during cerebral aneurysm surgery. Br J Anaesth 1995; 75:527–530.
79. Croughwell ND, Newman MF, Blumenthal JA, et al: Jugular bulb saturation and cognitive dysfunction after cardiopulmonary bypass. Ann Thorac Surg 1994; 58:1702–1708.
80. Cook DJ, Oliver WC Jr, Orszulak TA, et al: A prospective, randomized comparison of cerebral venous oxygen saturation during normothermic and hypothermic cardiopulmonary bypass. J Thorac Cardiovasc Surg 1994; 107:1020–1028.
81. Kiening KL, Unterberg AW, Bardt TF, et al. Monitoring of cerebral oxygenation in patients with severe head injuries: Brain tissue PO$_2$ versus jugular vein oxygen saturation. J Neurosurg 1996; 85:751–757.
82. Jöbsis-Vandervliet FF, Fox E, Sugioka K: Monitoring of cerebral oxygenation and cytochrome aa3 redox state. Int Anesthesiol Clin 1987; 25:209–230.
83. Cho H, Nemoto EM, Yonas H, et al. Cerebral monitoring by means of oximetry and somatosensory evoked potentials during carotid endarterectomy. J Neurosurg 1998; 89:533–538.
84. Henson LC, Calalang C, Temp JA, et al. Accuracy of a cerebral oximeter in healthy volunteers under conditions of isocapnic hypoxia. Anesthesiology 1998; 88:58–65.
85. Osmond E, Reynolds, McCormick DC, et al. New non-invasive methods for the investigation of cerebral oxidative metabolism and haemodynamics in newborn infants. Ann Med 1991; 23:681–686.
86. Kirkpatrick PJ, Smielewski P, Whitfield PC, et al. An observational study of near-infrared spectroscopy during carotid endarterectomy. J Neurosurg 1995; 82:756–763.
87. Dujovny M, Misra M, Widman R: Cerebral oximetry—techniques. Neurol Res 1998; 20(suppl 1):S5–S12.
88. Daubeney PE, Smith DC, Pilkington SN, et al: Cerebral oxygenation during paediatric cardiac surgery: Identification of vulnerable periods using near infrared spectroscopy. Eur J Cardiothorac Surg 1998; 13:370–377.
89. Ausman JI, McCormick PW, Stewart M, et al: Cerebral oxygen metabolism during hypothermic circulatory arrest in humans. J Neurosurg 1993; 79:810–815.
90. Kirkpatrick PJ, Smielewski P, Czosnyka M, et al. Near-infrared spectroscopy in patients with head injury. J Neurosurg 1995; 83:963–970.

91. Lewis SB, Myburgh JA, Thornton EL, et al. Cerebral oxygenation monitoring by near-infrared spectroscopy is not clinically useful in patients with severe closed-head injury: A comparison with jugular venous bulb oximetry. Crit Care Med 1996; 24:1334–1338.
92. Wahr JA, Tremper KK, Samra S, et al. Near-infrared spectroscopy: Theory and applications. J Cardiothorac Vasc Anesth 1996; 10:406–418.
93. Kirkpatrick PJ, Smielewski P, Al-Rawi P, et al. Resolving extra- and intracranial changes during adult near infrared spectroscopy. Neurol Res 1998; 20(suppl 1):S19–S22.
94. Schwarz G, Litscher G, Kleinert R, et al: Cerebral oximetry in dead subjects. J Neurosurg Anesthesiol 1996; 8:189–193.
95. Samra SK, Dorje P, Zelenock GB, et al. Cerebral oximetry in patients undergoing carotid endarterectomy under regional anesthesia. Stroke 1996; 27:49–55.
96. de Letter JAM, Sie HT, Thomas BMJH, et al: Near-infrared spectroscopy and electroencephalography during carotid endarterectomy—in search of a new shunt criterion. Neurol Res 1998; 20(suppl 1):S23–S27.
97. Beese U, Langer H, Lang W, et al. Comparison of near-infrared spectroscopy and somatosensory evoked potentials for the detection of cerebral ischemia during carotid endarterectomy. Stroke 1998; 29:2032–2037.
98. Duffy CM, Manninen PH, Chan A, et al. Comparison of cerebral oximeter and evoked potential monitoring in carotid endarterectomy. Can J Anaesth 1997; 44:1077–1081.
99. Kirkpatrick PJ, Lam JL, Al-Rawi P, et al: Defining thresholds for critical ischemia by using near-infrared spectroscopy in the adult brain. J Neurosurg 1998; 89:389–394.
100. Hoffman WE, Charbel FT, Edelman G, et al: Brain tissue oxygen pressure, carbon dioxide pressure and pH during ischemia. Neurol Res 1996; 18:54–56.
101. Doppenberg EM, Watson JC, Broaddus WC, et al: Intraoperative monitoring of substrate delivery during aneurysm and hematoma surgery: Initial experience in 16 patients. J Neurosurg 1997; 87:809–816.
102. Doppenberg EM, Zauner A, Watson JC, et al: Determination of the ischemic threshold for brain oxygen tension. Acta Neurochir Suppl (Wien) 1998; 71:166–169.
103. Holzschuh M, Metz C, Woertgen C, et al. Brain ischemia detected by tissue-Po$_2$ measurement and the lactate-oxygen index in head injury. Acta Neurochir Suppl (Wien) 1998; 71:170–171.
104. Sarrafzadeh AS, Kiening KL, Bardt TF, et al. Cerebral oxygenation in contusioned vs. nonlesioned brain tissue: monitoring of PtiO$_2$ with Licox and Paratrend. Acta Neurochir Suppl (Wien) 1998; 71:186–189.
105. Valadka AB, Gopinath SP, Contant CF, et al. Relationship of brain tissue PO$_2$ to outcome after severe brain injury. Crit Care Med 1998; 26:1576–1581.
106. Van Der Brink WA, Haitsma IK, Avezaat CJJ, et al: Brain parenchyma/pO$_2$ catheter interface: A histopathological study in the rat. J Neurotrauma 1998; 15:813–824.
107. Czosnyka M, Kirkpatrick PJ, Pickard JD: Multimodal monitoring and assessment of cerebral haemodynamic reserve after severe head injury. Cerebrovasc Brain Metab Rev 1996; 8:273–295.

PART THREE

Cardiac Monitoring

12 Electrocardiographic Monitoring for Ischemia and Arrhythmias

Peter C. Brath, M.D.
Daniel J. Kennedy, M.D.
Roger L. Royster, M.D.

Electrocardiographic (ECG) monitoring of patients in the operating room (OR) and intensive care unit (ICU) setting has become standard practice. Myocardial ischemia and cardiac arrhythmias occur frequently in patients undergoing surgery and in patients with serious illness in the ICU. The many arrhythmogenic influences in this setting and the high prevalence of cardiac disease in these patients put them at substantial risk for developing cardiac arrhythmias and myocardial ischemia. Arrhythmias may be innocuous or may have profound hemodynamic consequences, while ischemia may lead to arrhythmias or myocardial infarction. A thorough understanding of the incidence, genesis, and diagnosis of myocardial ischemia and specific cardiac arrhythmias is crucial for individuals caring for patients in the OR or ICU.

Electrocardiographic Lead Systems

The selection of which lead system to use depends on the clinical situation and monitor capabilities. The American Heart Association Task Force on continuous ECG monitoring recommends that monitors display two and preferably three or more leads to maximize facilitation of P wave recognition, distinction between supraventricular and ventricular rhythms, axis shifts, ST segment detection, and artifact detection.[1]

Surface Leads

The standard lead system consists of three bipolar limb leads of Einthoven (leads I, II, III), which measure potential differences between two points, and three unipolar limb leads (aVR, aVL, and aVF), also known as augmented leads, which measure the potential between the positive electrode on the limb and a common negative pole. The electrical axes of the unipolar limb leads are perpendicular to the axes of standard limb leads (Fig. 12-1). There are also six standard chest leads, designated leads V_1 to V_6, which are unipolar leads measured against a common value (Wilson's central terminal) created by electrically joining all three limb leads (Fig. 12-2). Leads placed on the right chest at locations corresponding to V_1 to V_6 are labeled V_{1R} to V_{6R}, and are useful for the detection of right ventricular ischemia. In addition to these standard leads, many modifications have been made, including moving the limb leads to the torso to minimize movement artifact (the Mason-Likar modification).[2]

Modified chest leads (MCLs) have the negative electrode just below the left clavicle at the midclavicular line, the ground electrode below the right clavicle, and the positive electrode placed in the precordial position corresponding to V_1 to V_6. MCL leads are bipolar leads that simulate unipolar chest leads and offer similar ECG information (Fig. 12-3). MCR leads are similar to MCL leads, but the negative electrode is below the right clavicle and the ground electrode is below the left clavicle. Central back leads (CBLs), such as CBL_5, a bipolar lead with the negative electrode over the right scapula posteriorly and the positive electrode at the usual V_5 site, offer good P wave morphology and ischemia detection.[3] Central manubrial (CM) leads, such as CM_5 where the negative electrode is over the manubrium and the positive electrode is at the V_5 site, have excellent ischemia detection.[4]

Leads I, II, and aVF offer excellent P wave detection and morphology, as do MCL_1, MCL_2, MCP_1, and CBL_5. Lead II, frequently monitored in the OR and ICU, is inadequate for detecting bundle branch blocks or aberrancy, and is not helpful in evaluating wide-complex tachycardia. Leads V_1, V_6, MCL_1, and MCL_6 are the best leads for detecting bundle branch block, aberrancy or evaluating wide-complex tachycardia.[5] With a dual channel monitor and a four-lead system, it is possible to simultaneously monitor MCL_1 and MCL_6 (Fig. 12-4). This lead montage allows easy P wave recognition and is very effective for arrhythmia diagnosis.

Esophageal Leads

Often the P wave is not detected or the relationship of the P wave to the QRS complex is unclear on surface leads and an esophageal electrode is used. The P waves are much larger in this lead owing to the proximity of the esophagus to the left atrium[6] (Fig. 12-5). Posterior myocardial ischemia can be detected and cardiac pacing via the esophagus is feasible.[7] One commercially available esophageal stethoscope has external electrodes 7 and 20 cm from the distal end, which are connected to standard ECG lead wires. A 3F balloon-tipped temporary transvenous pacing electrode, used as an esophageal electrode, correctly identified the rhythm in 10 of 12 patients when the surface ECG was nondiagnostic.[8] A J guidewire inserted through an 8F red Robinson catheter taped to an esophageal stethoscope can be used.[9] Care must be taken to avoid esophageal burns when electrocautery units are in use.[10]

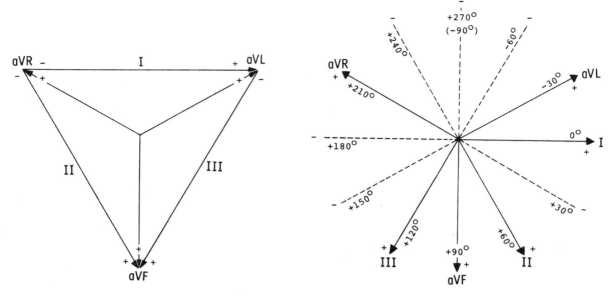

Figure 12-1. Einthoven's triangle, composed of the standard bipolar limb leads and the augmented limb leads. The Hexaxial Reference System is a modified Einthoven's triangle, and is more useful for rhetorical axis determinations. (From Chung EK. Electrocardiography: Practical Applications With Vectoral Principles, ed 3. Norwalk, CT, Appleton-Century-Crofts, 1985.)

Epicardial Leads

Many patients have temporary transcutaneous pacer wires sutured to the atrium and ventricle during cardiac surgery to overcome transient postoperative bradycardia or atrioventricular (AV) block. These leads allow monitoring of electrical activity directly from the surface of the heart in the OR or

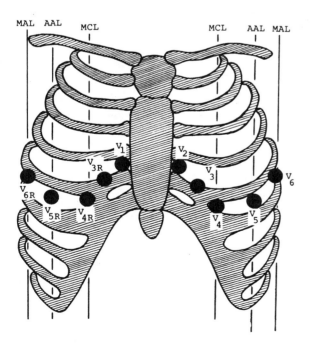

Figure 12-2. Precordial lead system showing standard V and right-sided VR chest lead positions. MAL, midaxillary line; AAL, arterial axillary line; MCL, midclavicular line. (From Chung EK: Electrocardiography: Practical Applications with Vectorial Principles, ed 3. Norwalk, CT, Appleton-Century-Crofts, 1985.)

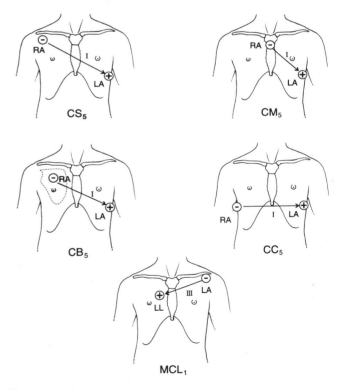

Figure 12-3. The modified bipolar limb leads. These alternatives to lead V_5 are recorded by selecting lead I on the monitor. The positive (exploring) electrode (LA) is placed in the V_5 position, and the negative (RA) electrode in either central subclavian (CS_5), central manubrium (CM_5), central back (CB_5) or central chest (CC_5). The MCL_1 lead is recorded by choosing lead III on the monitor and placing the electrodes as shown. (From Mark JB: Atlas of Cardiovascular Monitoring. New York, Churchill Livingstone, 1998.)

Figure 12–4. Electrode placement for simultaneous monitoring of MCL₁ and MCL₆ with a four-lead system. With selector dial for channel 1 placed on lead I, left arm (LA) is the positive and right arm (RA) is the negative electrode. Bipolar precordial lead MCL₁ is displayed. With selector dial for channel 2 placed on lead II, left leg (LL) is the positive and RA remains the negative electrode. The resultant lead on channel 2 is bipolar chest lead MCL₆. The right leg (RL) electrode is a reference or ground electrode, and may be placed anywhere on the body. (From Drew BJ: Bedside electrocardiographic monitoring: State of the art for the 1990s. Heart Lung 1991; 20: 610.)

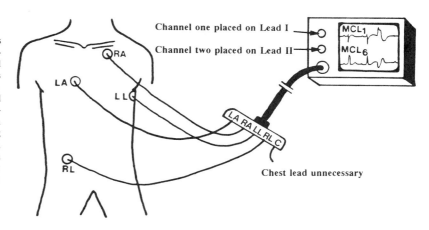

cardiac surgical ICU. Atrial electrograms (AEGs) are unsurpassed in detecting atrial activity in situations in which the surface ECG fails to detect P waves or establish their relationship with the QRS complex.[11] Ventricular epicardial electrograms are of little value because the QRS complex is usually readily detected on standard surface ECG.[12]

Unipolar and bipolar AEGs can be obtained. Unipolar AEGs best establish the relationship between atrial and ventricular activity and are obtained by attaching one atrial epicardial lead to one of the limb leads[13] (Fig. 12–6). A bipolar AEG is obtained when both atrial epicardial wires are connected, using alligator clips, to the positive and negative leads of a standard bipolar lead, such as lead I (Fig. 12–7). Bipolar AEGs enhance while avoiding masking atrial activity within simultaneously occurring ventricular complexes. Attaching both epicardial wires to the right and left arm leads allows monitoring of the bipolar AEG by selecting lead I, while selection of lead II or III displays a unipolar AEG.

Appropriate electrical grounding and insulation must be used to prevent electrical injury when recording AEGs. The direct contact of the leads with the heart places the patient at risk for microshock, which can lead to atrial extrasystoles, atrial flutter, or atrial fibrillation. Extreme caution is advised to avoid microshock, which can precipitate ventricular fibrillation when ventricular pacing leads are in use. Rubber gloves should be worn when the epicardial leads are handled; when not in use, these should be kept dry and coiled inside a rubber glove to insulate the exposed wires when not in use.[14]

Intracardiac Leads

Recording of intracardiac electrical potentials via temporary transvenous pacemaker leads yields information similar to that obtained with epicardial leads.[15] Intra-atrial electrograms may be recorded through a saline-filled central venous[16] or a pulmonary artery catheter,[17] or by inserting a flexible pacing wire through the catheter.[18] Concerns about electrical safety and microshock are the same as for epicardial leads.

Diagnostic Versus Monitoring Mode

Many monitors are equipped with a bandwidth filter which removes signals above or below a certain frequency. The high-frequency filter removes 60 cps (Hz) and other electrical interference, such as from electrocautery units (1 × 10⁶ Hz).[19] In the diagnostic mode, the lower-frequency re-

sponse of most monitors is 0.14 Hz, below which signals are attenuated by the low-frequency filter.[19] Monitor mode involves an additional low-frequency filter which removes all signals below 0.5 Hz.[19] Low-frequency signals are often associated with respiratory movements or the movement of ECG lead wires and can lead to wandering baselines and difficulty in interpretation of the cardiac rhythm. However, distortion of the ST segment and T waves, mimicking ischemic ECG changes, often occurs when the low-frequency filter is used (Fig. 12–8). Thus, when monitoring for myocardial ischemia, either the diagnostic mode must be used or the monitor must be calibrated in the monitoring mode. The amplitude and morphology of the P wave may be altered by the low-frequency filter, leading to difficulty in interpretation of arrhythmias.

Risks of Electrocardiographic Monitoring

The risks of ECG monitoring include electrical shock injury, burns, and institution of inappropriate therapy as a result of misdiagnosis of arrhythmias.

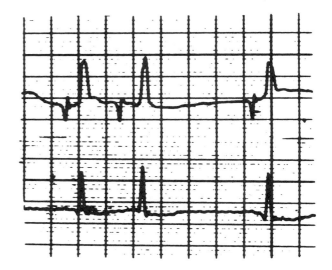

Figure 12–5. Esophageal electrode recording showing prominent atrial activity (downward deflections), which is not seen on the simultaneous surface ECG. (Adapted from Kaplan JA, Thys DM: Electrocardiography. *In* Miller RD (ed): Anesthesiology, ed 3. New York, Churchill Livingstone, 1990.)

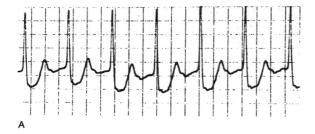

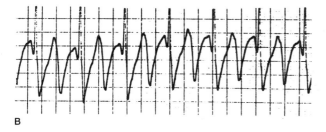

Figure 12–6. Simultaneous recording of an ECG surface lead (top tracing) and unipolar atrial electrogram (AEG) in patient with new-onset tachycardia and hypotension following cardiopulmonary bypass surgery. Surface ECG suggests sinus tachycardia, but AEG (bottom tracing) clearly shows atrial activity at a rate of 270 bpm (downward deflections) with 2:1 ventricular response (upward deflections), thus establishing atrial flutter as the diagnosis.

Electrical Hazards

A basic appreciation of the principles of electricity is essential to understanding the risks of ECG monitoring. Ohm's law ($V = I \times R$) describes the relationship between current (I), resistance to current flow (R), and the voltage potential (V). For a given voltage, the current will vary inversely with the resistance. In order for current to flow, a circuit must be completed from the voltage source, through the resistance(s), and back to the voltage source. Current flows from the potential source through a hot wire to the resistance and returns via a neutral wire.[19] A ground wire connects the neutral side of the circuit to an object with zero voltage potential, such as the earth. Current (units are amperes) divided by the cross-sectional area of flow is the current density. Power (units are watts) is the product of volts and current, and energy (units are joules or watt-seconds) is the product of energy and time. If a person contacts a nonisolated circuit at two points, current can flow though the individual and lead to injury or death. Since the earth is the usual ground source for electrical circuits, contact with the circuit at only one point will complete the circuit.

A line-isolation transformer is a device that isolates the power source from the ground, such that connecting one of the two power contacts to the ground does not complete the circuit (Fig. 12–9). In an isolated system, because there is no contact between the power supply and the ground, contact at one point does not complete the circuit, and no current flows.[19] A line-isolation monitor (LIM) measures current flow between the isolated circuit and the ground, allowing for detection of abnormal ground connections (short circuits), indicating that the circuit has become nonisolated.[20] When the LIM alarm indicates a current flow greater than 2 mA, each electrical device attached to the circuit must be investigated to determine where the short circuit is located.[19] Each monitor should be sequentially unplugged until the LIM alarm ceases, starting with the device plugged

in most recently. The LIM ceases alarming when the device unplugged contains the short circuit, and this device or monitor should not be used until thoroughly evaluated by the biomedical engineering department.

Electricity applied to the surface of the body travels by the path of least resistance, namely via the great vessels, muscles, nerves, and connective tissues. This is termed *macroshock* and, if greater than 100 to 200 mA, may result in ventricular fibrillation.[21, 22] Smaller currents applied directly to the heart via pacemaker wires, fluid-filled intracardiac catheters, or directly during surgery are termed *microshock*, and the fibrillatory threshold is approximately 50 to 100 µA (0.05 to 0.1 mA).[21] Extreme care must be taken to ensure that all instruments are safely grounded and isolated, as this microshock current is below the threshold for perception (approximately 1 mA) by most personnel working in the OR or ICU.

Burns

Heat is generated whenever current passes through a resistor and is proportional to the resistance and the current density. Electrocautery units utilize a large surface area dispersive plate, which decreases the current density as the electrocautery current exits the body.[23] If the grounding pad is poorly applied, the current may exit the patient via an ECG lead with a significantly smaller surface area, in which case the heat generation will be greater, and cutaneous burns can result.[23] Nuclear magnetic resonance (NMR) units employ shifting magnetic fields that can generate electrical currents in metallic items such as ECG monitor leads.[24, 25] The current density exiting via these leads, if significantly large, can generate sufficient heat to cause burns. The use of nonferromagnetic ECG leads eliminates this hazard.[26]

Artifacts

The ECG is subject to many external influences that may generate false signals or interfere with rhythm interpretation. Electrocautery units may completely distort ECG tracings,

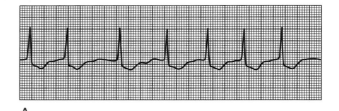

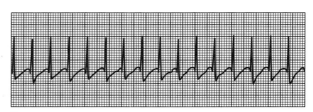

Figure 12–7. Simultaneous recording of surface ECG (top tracing) suggesting atrial fibrillation at approximately 100 bpm, but a bipolar AEG (bottom tracing), demonstrating atrial tachycardia at 200 bpm with variable atrioventricular conduction.

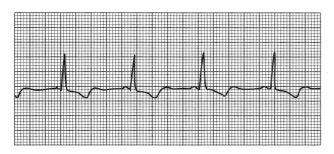

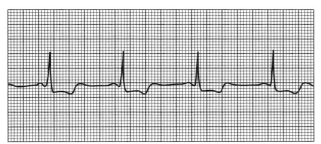

Figure 12–8. Apparent ST segment depression in a patient with T-wave inversion produced by switching from diagnostic mode (*A*) to monitor mode (*B*). (Adapted from Kaplan JA, Thys DM: Electrocardiography. *In* Miller RD (ed): Anesthesiology, ed 3. New York, Churchill Livingstone, 1990.)

and patient movements such as shivering or hiccupping may create artifacts resembling P waves, atrial fibrillation, or even ventricular tachycardia. The arterial pump roller head during cardiopulmonary bypass often mimics myocardial electrical activity (Fig. 12–10).

Electrocardiographic Monitoring for Myocardial Ischemia

Myocardial ischemia is the result of an imbalance of myocardial oxygen supply and demand leading to anaerobic metabolism, and, if continued, eventually to cell death. It is brought about either by an increase in myocardial oxygen demand (e.g., tachycardia, increased afterload) or a decrease in oxygen supply (e.g., coronary artery spasm, plaque rupture or thrombus, angioplasty, hypotension). Ischemia produces a predictable and consistent derangement in myocardial function. With as little as a 20% to 50% reduction in coronary flow, early thinning of the ventricular wall occurs during isovolumic relaxation,[27-29] and with increasing reductions in coronary artery blood flow, the morphologic pattern pro-

ceeds to a reduction in myocyte shortening (hypokinesis), no shortening (akinesis), and then expansion during ventricular systole (dyskinesis).[28] Concomitant with this change are metabolic signs of increased anaerobic metabolism such as decreases in adenosine triphosphate (ATP),[30] increases in regional lactate production,[29, 31, 32] decreases in coronary sinus oxygen saturation,[33] and elevated coronary sinus plasma potassium levels.[32]

It is now well known that up to 90% of ischemic episodes are symptomatically silent in both the perioperative[34-37] and nonperioperative periods.[38-45] Silent myocardial ischemia produces deficits in myocardial function similar to ischemic episodes that are symptomatic.[46, 47] Episodes of asymptomatic ischemia appear to have a cumulative effect,[37, 44, 48-50] which has led to the term "total ischemic burden."[51] These asymptomatic ischemic events have been shown to have an adverse effect on cardiac outcome in both nonperioperative[43, 44, 52-61] and perioperative patients,[35-37, 50, 62-69] and also may be associated with a failure to wean from the ventilator in ICU patients.[70, 71] Therapy directed at reducing this burden has recently been shown to improve outcome in perioperative patients in whom the survival benefit of prophylactic β-blockade seemed to be related to the reduction of ischemic events.[72]

Electrocardiographic Changes During Myocardial Ischemia

The ECG hallmark of myocardial ischemia is ST segment displacement. The amplitude and direction of the displacement depend on the location of recording and the extent of injury. Ischemia causes membrane dysfunction leading to an efflux of potassium.[73] This leads to a partial diastolic depolarization and creates a potential difference between the injured tissue and nearby normal tissue. This produces a current of injury that shifts the electrical baseline.[74] Electrocardiographically, this shift is seen as elevation in the ST segment on the surface ECG during transmural ischemia. When the ischemic area is separated from the exploring electrode by an area of healthy tissue (as in subendocardial ischemia with a surface ECG), the ST segment is depressed because the vector of the current of injury is directed away from the electrode (Fig. 12–11). With a progressive reduction in coronary blood flow, endocardial electrodes consistently show ST elevation, while epicardial electrodes show ST depression until a critical reduction in coronary flow occurs and the injury becomes transmural, leading to epicardial ST elevation.[75] Other less specific ECG markers of ischemia include intraventricular conduction delays, U wave inversions,[76] and J-point depression.[32] Most investigators define

Figure 12–9. This diagram illustrates a safety feature of the isolated power system. An individual contacting one side of the isolated power system (point A) and standing on the ground (point B) will not receive a shock. The individual is not contacting the isolated circuit at two points and thus not completing the circuit. Point A is part of the isolated circuit, while the ground (point B) is part of the primary or grounded side of the circuit. (From Ehrenwerth J: Electrical Safety. *In* Barash PG, Cullen BF, Stoelting RK (eds): Clinical Anesthesia. Philadelphia, JB Lippincott, 1989, p 625.)

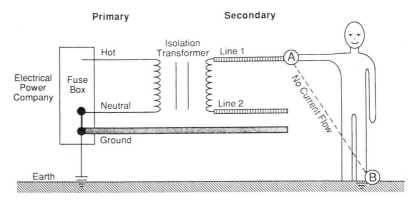

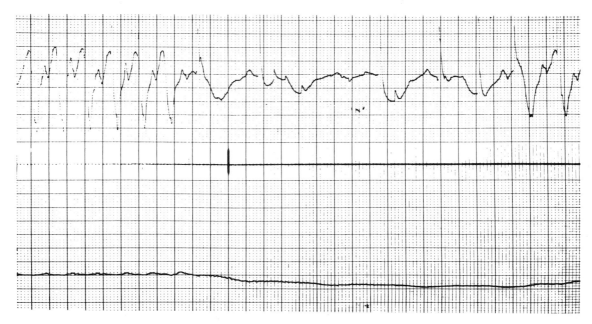

Figure 12-10. Artifact produced by the arterial roller pump head during cardiopulmonary bypass, mimicking ventricular tachycardia. The pump was briefly turned off, revealing an underlying slower cardiac rhythm.

ECG evidence of myocardial ischemia as ST segment depression that is horizontal or downsloping, 1.0 mm (0.1mV) or greater in magnitude (measured 60 to 80 ms after the J point) lasting for at least 1 minute.

Lead Selection for Ischemic Detection and Monitoring

ECG determination of myocardial ischemia is affected by many factors, not the least of which is location and number of ECG leads. In patients undergoing exercise treadmill testing, it was determined that 85% of ST segment depression was localized to leads II and V_5.[77] Data obtained during stress testing, however, may not be entirely applicable to perioperative monitoring. Stress testing induces ischemia through an increase in myocardial oxygen demand, while most perioperative ischemic events are not precipitated by changes in hemodynamic variables and are thought to be primarily a result of decreased myocardial oxygen supply.[34, 65, 67, 68, 78] This finding has also been noted in nonoperative patients with silent ischemia.[39-41, 45, 79, 80] Despite this, the value of the V_5 lead has been demonstrated by Kaplan and King[81] and Roy et al.,[82] who showed improvement in the intraoperative recognition of ST segment depression in patients undergoing both cardiac and noncardiac surgery, compared with monitoring lead II. London et al.[83] monitored all 12 standard leads in 105 patients undergoing noncardiac operations and found that lead V_5 had the most sensitivity of any single lead (75%). Leads II and V_5 had an 80% sensitivity; leads V_4 and V_5 had a 90% sensitivity; and leads II, V_4 and V_5 had a combined 96% sensitivity (Fig. 12-12). In 120 patients undergoing cardiac surgery, Jain[84] found that leads III and V_5 recorded 15 out of 16 ischemic ST segment elevations and all 8 ischemic ST segment depressions, but V_5 alone missed one half of the ischemic ST segment elevations and 1 of 8 ischemic ST segment depressions. Other authors have found that the modified bipolar leads CS_5 and CB_5 are reasonable alternatives to lead V_5.[3, 85] One shortcoming of these leads is their difficulty in detecting posterior and right-sided ischemia.

Right-sided ischemia can be detected by application of the right-sided precordial leads. De Hert et al.[86] demonstrated that application of a V_{4R} lead in patients with angiographically documented disease of the right coronary artery al-

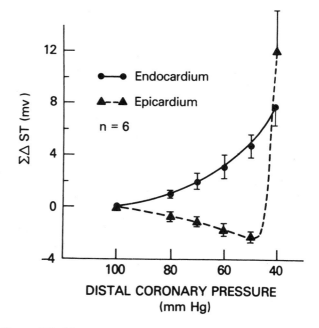

Figure 12-11. ST segment changes measured by endocardial and epicardial electrodes, during graded coronary artery occlusion with constant aortic pressure, heart rate, and cardiac output. Endocardial ST segment elevation is uniformly present (injury current directed toward the electrode) while epicardial ST segments are depressed (injury current directed away from electrode) until a critical point of flow reduction creates transmural ischemia and epicardial ST segment elevation. (From Guyton RA, McClenathan JH, Newman GE, et al: Significance of subendocardial S-T segment elevation caused by coronary stenosis in the dog. Epicardial S-T segment depression, local ischemia and subsequent necrosis. Am J Cardiol 1977; 40:377.)

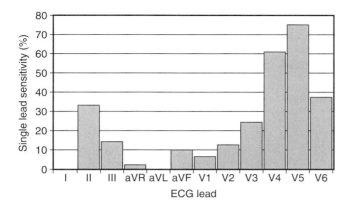

Figure 12–12. Distribution of ischemic ST segment changes in each lead in high-risk patients undergoing noncardiac surgery. (From London MJ, Hollenberg M, Wong MG, et al: Intraoperative myocardial ischemia: Localization by continuous 12-lead electrocardiography. Anesthesiology 1988; 69:237.)

lowed detection of 20% of ischemic events that would have been undetected by monitoring leads I, II, and CB$_5$.[86] Right-sided precordial leads have also been shown to demonstrate right ventricular infarcts in patients without any changes in the standard 12-lead ECG. Posterior ischemia can be detected with an esophageal electrode,[6, 87–90] although the baseline may be subject to more drift and can require extra filtering. Other monitoring sites include the endotracheal tube[91] and intracardiac electrodes.[92]

Trend Analysis

Trend analysis of the ST segment, either with dedicated components in bedside monitors or ambulatory monitors, has become more important recently. This is due to the high incidence of silent ischemia, the low probability of the routine 12-lead ECG in recording an ischemic event,[93] and the inability of routine observation of a bedside monitor to accurately detect episodes of ischemia.[94]

Ambulatory Ischemic Monitoring

Ambulatory ECG was originally designed for arrhythmia monitoring because of its capability for detailed analysis of signals recorded over a longer period of time than the standard ECG. Original ambulatory monitors were battery-powered analog tape recorders. The recordings were made either by amplitude-modulated (AM) or frequency-modulated (FM) techniques. Problems arose with trying to accurately record the low-frequency response of the ST segment (Fig. 12–13). Artifactual ST segment changes were possible due to inadequate low-frequency response or phase distortion (inherent in any system that employs filters) in the AM recorders. FM recorders have good low-frequency response but are subject to phase distortions and recorder speed variation (wow and flutter) which are enhanced by the slow recording speeds of tape-based systems. These fluctuations may be augmented by a weakening battery which further slows tape speed (generally toward the end of a recording session).[95–99]

Recent advances in ambulatory monitoring include the development of a programmable digital device for long-term ambulatory monitoring.[100] The device (Monitor One, Q-Med, Laurence Harbor, NJ) digitized the input signal, which is then analyzed by the microprocessor that uses variations in a

time-averaged ST segment amplitude as an indicator of ischemia. Abnormal events can be stored in random access memory. The device is powered by a lithium battery that allows up to 8 days of continuous recording, extending the monitoring period well into the postoperative period when ischemia is still highly prevalent.[101] This device also has a tone generator and a liquid-crystal display. The microprocessor determines and constantly updates the baseline through a programmable algorithm, allowing the level of significant ST depression to be input, and the ST segment to be averaged and stored every 8 seconds. When ST segment depression remains below the preset threshold value for more than 40 seconds, the event is validated and the timing begins (Fig. 12–14).

Subsequent studies have validated this device, the sensitivity ranging from 81% to 100% and the specificity ranging from 92% to 100%,[102, 103] with one of the studies[102] showing that the audible tone allowed guided therapy with nitroglycerin, reducing the total ischemic time. Other studies have shown its usefulness or potential usefulness in the perioperative period. Dunn et al.[104] showed that directed therapy was easily applied in a patient undergoing a carotid bypass procedure because of the audible alarm. Clements et al.[105] presented a case report of a patient who, after resection of an abdominal aortic aneurysm, had prolonged ischemia detected by the Monitor One. However, the audible alarm had been turned off as part of a study protocol, and the ischemia went unnoticed by the staff during continuous bedside monitoring; ventricular fibrillation eventually resulted.

Many ORs and ICUs use monitors that have been outfitted with ST segment trending capabilities. These generally require the user to obtain a stable baseline of the patient's ECG, and then the measuring points (isoelectric and J points) can be modified for each patient. The monitors display a graphic trend of the ST segment amplitude, allowing for prompt recognition and therapy. These trend monitors have been validated[106, 107] and have been found to be reasonably sensitive and specific[108, 109] and potentially to be of benefit. In a 2-year study of ischemia detected by ST segment trend monitoring in patients undergoing cardiac surgery, Kotter et al.[110] demonstrated a decrease in ischemia from 17% in the first 6 months to 6% in the last 6 months. The authors thought that, along with the uncontrollable vari-

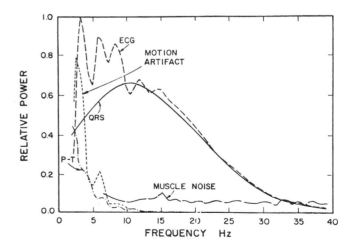

Figure 12–13. Power spectrum analysis of ECG showing low frequency of the ST segment, and the influence of muscle noise and motion artifact. (From Thakor NV: From Holter monitors to automatic defibrillators: Developments in ambulatory arrhythmia monitoring. IEEE Trans Biomed Eng 1984; 31:772. © 1984 IEEE.)

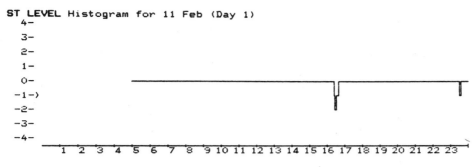

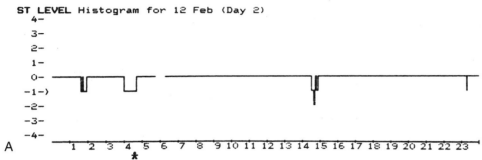

A

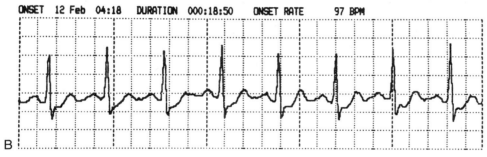

B

Figure 12-14. Recording of the ST amplitude on the Q-Med Monitor One over a 2-day period showing several episodes of ST segment depression. *A,* The small character under the event at 4:00 on the second day is the patient-generated event marker signifying an episode of anginal pain that was present for at least 15 minutes prior to symptoms. *B,* The ECG tracing generated at that time clearly shows significant ST segment depression. (From Levin RI: Quantitation of transient myocardial ischemia by digital, ambulatory electrocardiography. Am J Cardiol 1988; 61:15B.)

ables of preoperative management and anesthetic and surgical techniques, the addition of the trend monitor heightened awareness and earlier intervention.

Another recent development is the ELI 100 (Mortara Instruments, Milwaukee, WI), which is a programmable, portable microprocessor-based device that can acquire, analyze, and store standard 12-lead ECGs at programmable intervals or automatically in the presence of ST segment changes. The device has already proved useful in the emergency room.[111-114] This monitor has also been used for identification of reocclusion after revascularization (either by angioplasty or thrombolytics) of coronary arteries. The ST segment trend (either during balloon occlusion or before thrombolytics) can be downloaded and displayed three-dimensionally on a graph, creating an "ischemic fingerprint"[115] (Fig. 12-15). Plotted over time, this allows for temporal and spatial analysis of ST segment trends and has been validated clinically.[115-118]

Limitations of Electrocardiographic Monitoring for Ischemia

Despite all the advances made in ECG, the ECG does have many limitations involving diagnosis of ischemia. Baseline ECG abnormalities can interfere with ST segment evalua-

tion.[119] These include bundle branch blocks, intraventricular conduction delays, and left ventricular hypertrophy. Many drugs, especially digoxin, can also affect the ST segment, even in healthy patients.[120] Other factors affecting the ST segment include aging,[121] sex of the patient,[122] hyperventilation,[123-125] and body position.[126-129] Additional artifacts can arise from the filtering modality used (diagnostic versus monitoring),[130, 131] inaccurate setting of ST segment trend monitoring parameters,[132] electrode placement,[133] and interference from medical devices such as cardiopulmonary bypass machines.[134-136] Design of the ECG monitor itself can interfere with accurate monitoring. The filters incorporated in the monitor to minimize artifact from muscle noise, motion, 60-Hz line interference, and electrocautery can interfere with ECG processing. Inherent in any filtering system is phase distortion, which can produce ECG changes similar to those seen in ischemia.[95, 99] Artifact can be minimized by using properly designed monitors, decreasing skin impedance by proper site preparation, correctly placing leads to minimize motion artifact, and using quality electrodes and cables.[1, 137]

Even with optimization, the ECG can be relatively insensitive and nonspecific. There can be significant discordance between ECG changes and the site of exercise-induced perfusion deficit or anatomic site of coronary artery disease.[104, 138-141] Also, surface ECG recordings have failed to show injury patterns in ischemia induced experimentally by alterations in supply[142] and demand.[143] In addition, postoper-

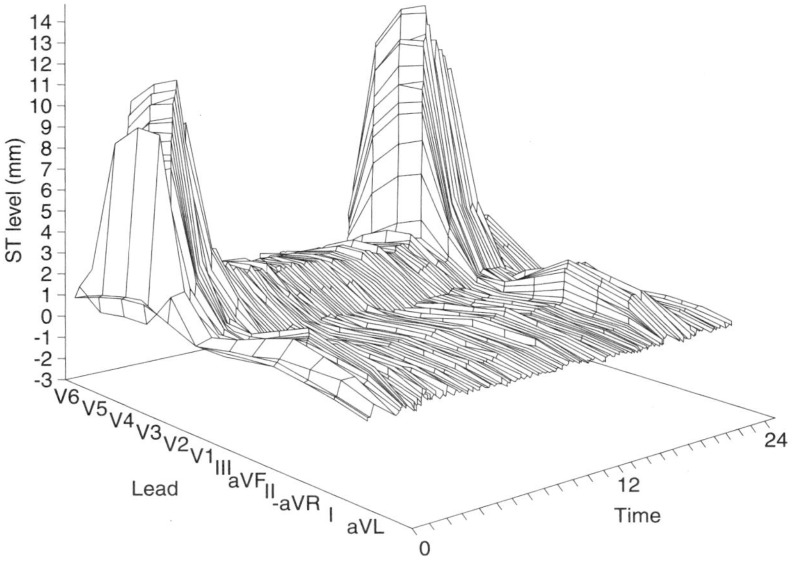

Figure 12–15. Twelve-lead ST segment monitoring processed to show spatial and temporal relations. The initial rise in the ST segments is due to balloon occlusion during angioplasty of the patient's left anterior descending coronary artery. The ST segment elevation normalizes after deflation of the balloon and remains stable for 16 hours. Reappearance of ST segment elevation signifies acute artery reocclusion. (From Drew BJ, Adams MG, Pelter MM, et al: Comparison of standard and derived 12-lead electrocardiograms for diagnosis of coronary angioplasty–induced myocardial ischemia. Am J Cardiol 1997; 79:643.)

ative T wave changes[44] and even ST segment changes intraoperatively[145] have been demonstrated but shown not to have any immediate clinical significance.

Alternatives to Electrocardiographic Ischemia Monitoring

The shortcomings in ECG monitoring for myocardial ischemia have led to the use of other monitors for the identification of myocardial ischemia, such as the hemodynamic indices of the rate-pressure product (RPP) or pressure/rate quotient (PRQ), the pulmonary artery (PA) catheter, and transesophageal echocardiography. The RPP is calculated by multiplying the peak systolic pressure by the heart rate. The PRQ is calculated from the mean arterial pressure divided by the heart rate. Several studies, however, have shown that an RPP greater than 12,000 or a PRQ less than 1 are insensitive predictors of myocardial ischemia.[146–148] Many factors may play a part in this apparent discrepancy, but the most likely explanation relates to the fact that most ischemic events are precipitated by decreased oxygen supply, not by acute changes in myocardial demand.[34, 39–41, 45, 65, 67, 68, 78, 79]

Another device that has been used for many years to monitor myocardial ischemia is the PA catheter. The pulmonary artery occlusion pressure (PAOP) is used as an estimate of left ventricular end-diastolic pressure (LVEDP), which is then used as a correlate of left ventricular end-diastolic volume (LVEDV). Myocardial ischemia may produce an increase in both LVEDV and LVEDP through its effect on systolic and diastolic function.[149–151] This may be manifest by either an increase in mean PAOP or the production of abnormal waveforms (such as large a or v waves) signifying decreased left ventricular compliance or mitral regurgitation (either from papillary muscle ischemia or mitral annular dilatation). Notwithstanding the problems inherent in correlating pressures and volumes in the face of changing compliance, investigators have had varying success in using the PA catheter as an ischemia monitor. Kaplan and Wells,[152] in a study of 40 patients undergoing elective coronary artery bypass surgery, showed that an elevation in the PAOP was the only sign of ischemia in 55% of the patients. Other studies have demonstrated that alterations in PAOP occur quicker and are more sensitive than ECG changes.[153, 154] Still other studies have

demonstrated that changes in the PAOP waveform are less predictive of ischemia than the more sensitive indicator of regional wall motion abnormalities (RWMAs) seen by transesophageal echocardiography,[155–157] myocardial lactate production,[158] and postoperative perfusion deficits.[159] Development of significant changes in ventricular function may be required to produce abnormal waves.[160]

Transesophageal echocardiography (TEE) has gained in appeal as a monitor of ischemia with the developing knowledge of the physiologic derangements of myocardial ischemia. In both graded reductions in coronary flow[27, 29–31, 161] and acute coronary obstruction,[162–168] RWMAs occur prior to the development of ECG changes. These RWMA changes develop within 8 to 30 seconds of occlusion, while ST segment changes may require 20 to 90 seconds or more. Wall motion abnormalities occur more frequently than ECG changes in high-risk operations (cardiac and major vascular), are not precipitated by acute changes in hemodynamics, and when they persist are more predictive of adverse cardiac outcome.[169–172] The TEE can be an important monitor for the guidance of anti-ischemic theraphy,[173, 174] although Eisenberg et al.[175] did not find in their study of patients at high preoperative risk for ischemia that routine TEE monitoring showed any added benefit in detection of intraoperative ischemia over monitoring a standard two-lead ECG. TEE is also used for the detection of coronary artery disease in stress testing with favorable results as compared with other modalities.[176, 177]

The standard view for intraoperative detection of ischemia is the transgastric short-axis view at the midpapillary level. This allows for monitoring of all three major coronary artery distributions in the same field of view[178] (Fig. 12–16). However, this view may pick up as little as 17% of RWMAs in patients undergoing cardiac or major vascular surgery, and additional transverse and longitudinal views are needed to detect other segmental abnormalities.[179] Semiquantitative scoring of the wall motion can be made (Table 12–1) and myocardial ischemia can be diagnosed by a *change* of 2 points or more in the semiquantitative score.[180] As with all other monitors, TEE determination of ischemia has limitations, including difficulty in accurately assessing ischemic changes in the presence of changing preload and afterload, left bundle branch block, and cardiac pacing. The effect of rotational and translational motion of the ventricle on the

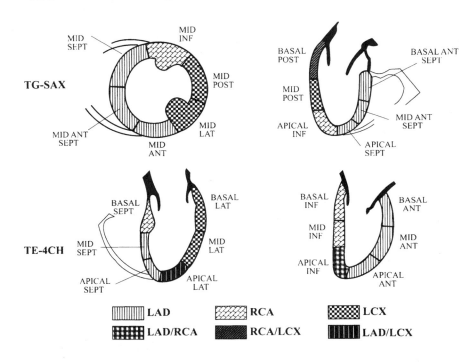

Figure 12–16. Assignment of myocardial segments to coronary artery distribution. Note that the transgastric short-axis view allows monitoring of all three major arteries simultaneously. (From Siostrzonek P, Mundigler G, Hassan A, et al: Echocardiographic diagnosis of segmental wall motion abnormalities. Acta Anaesthesiol Scand Suppl 1997; 111:272.)

TEE image must also be considered. Another difficulty is the need for diagnostic interpretation in real time. Bergquist et al.[181] showed that among five full-time cardiac anesthesiologists, real-time detection of ischemia by TEE had a sensitivity and specificity of 76% when compared with off-line examination, but there was variability in quantifying the severity of regional dysfunction. An additional problem is that the incidence of intraoperative ischemia is low relative to the incidence in the preoperative and postoperative periods.[34, 65, 67, 68] Half of all ischemic events occurred before induction[68] and therefore before a TEE probe would be placed. Continuous TEE monitoring is also not possible postoperatively.

Because of the overlap of all of these monitors, it may be desirable to use more than one in high-risk patients to confirm ischemia and guide therapy.[174, 182, 183] One solution might be ambulatory ST segment monitoring preoperatively in high-risk patients to identify those with frequent ischemic episodes, giving time for potential intervention. Intraoperatively, monitoring would include multiple-lead ECG monitoring with ST segment trending and the possible addition of more invasive monitors such as TEE or the PA catheter, or both, in operations with a high inherent risk of cardiac morbidity. Postoperative ambulatory ST segment monitoring with alarms should be done during the first postoperative week for identification and rapid treatment of ischemic events to minimize adverse cardiac outcome.

Monitoring for Cardiac Arrhythmias

Incidence of Arrhythmias

The true incidence of arrhythmias is difficult to know. Studies often assign arbitrary classifications, evaluate certain arrhythmias while excluding others, or do not use continuous beat-by-beat monitoring. Other studies have looked only at patients undergoing cardiac surgery, patients with cardiac disease undergoing noncardiac surgery, and patients with respiratory failure. The first large series of ECG monitoring in operative patients undergoing surgery was reported by Kurtz

et al. in 1936.[184] This study revealed a high incidence of sinus arrhythmias, premature ventricular contractions (PVCs), and junctional rhythms.[184] In 1968, Vanik and Davis[185] reported a 34% incidence of intraoperative arrhythmias in patients with cardiac disease undergoing halothane anesthesia, and, interestingly, found arrhythmias in 16% of otherwise healthy patients. Kuner et al.[186] reported a 62% incidence of arrhythmias in relatively healthy patients, with sinus tachycardia being most common, while junctional rhythms were seen in 20% and PVCs in 15% of patients.

Certain subgroups have repeatedly been found to be at increased risk for arrhythmias during surgery (Table 12–2). Bertrand et al.[187] reported a 60% incidence of ventricular arrhythmias in patients with known cardiac disease, compared with an incidence of 37% in patients without known heart disease. Furthermore, 92% of patients with cardiac disease developed either a supraventricular or ventricular arrhythmia during surgery and anesthesia.[187] Arrhythmias were most common at times of endotracheal intubation and extubation. In a study of patients undergoing cardiac surgery, Angelini et al.[188] reported that 58% of patients undergoing valvular surgery and 45% of patients undergoing coronary artery bypass surgery developed significant postoperative arrhythmias. More important, the arrhythmias tended to correlate with the severity of the heart disease, led to a prolonged

Table 12–1. Semiquantitative (Subjective) Segmental Wall Motion Scoring

	Meaning	Score
Normal	No evidence of dysfunction	0
Mild hypokinesis	Minimal diminution in function	1
Severe hypokinesis	Barely perceptible movement	2
Akinesis	Total lack of movement or thickening	3
Dyskinesis	Paradoxical outward movement or wall thinning	4

Modified from Huemer G, Weber T, Tschernich H, et al: Intraoperative myocardial ischemia and transesophageal echocardiography. Acta Anaesthesiol Scand Suppl 1997;111:274–276.

Table 12-2. Incidence of Arrhythmias During Anesthesia and Surgery

Study (yr)	N	Arrhythmia (%)	Monitoring	Highest Incidence Related to
Vanik and Davis (1968)[185]	5013	17.9	Intermittent	Age Intubation Heart disease
Kuner et al. (1967)[186]	154	61.7	Holter	Neurologic, head and neck, thoracic surgery Intubation Surgery >3 hr
Bertrand et al. (1971)[187]	100	84.0	Holter	Intubation Extubation Heart disease
Angelini et al. (1974)[188]	128	50.0	Holter	Severity of heart disease

Modified from Royster RL: Causes and consequences of arrhythmias. *In* Benumof JL, Saidman LJ (eds): Anesthesia and Perioperative Complications. St Louis, Mosby–Year Book, 1992, p 228.

hospital stay, and were responsible for up to 80% of the surgical mortality in the series.

Arrhythmias are relatively common in otherwise healthy people as well. Fifty male medical students without heart disease were followed with 24-hour continuous ECG monitoring. Sinus arrhythmia occurred in 50%, sinus pauses in 28%, atrial extrasystoles in 56%, and ventricular premature beats in 50% of students.[189] In a more recent study, arrhythmias were seen in greater than 60% of patients undergoing anesthesia and surgery when continuous methods of monitoring were used.[190]

Atrial contraction contributes only 15% to 20% of left ventricular end-diastolic volume in patients with a normally functioning heart[191] but may account for as much as 30% to 40% of left ventricular end-diastolic volume in patients with a dilated left ventricle, left ventricular hypertrophy, or other abnormalities of myocardial performance.[192] Loss of AV synchrony due to an arrhythmia may be associated with a significant decrease in cardiac output, systemic blood pressure, and organ perfusion, and is tolerated very poorly by many patients. Tachyarrhythmias increase myocardial oxygen consumption, decrease diastolic coronary perfusion duration, and may precipitate myocardial ischemia, further exacerbating the arrhythmogenic potential of the myocardium.

Therefore, during ECG monitoring, the physician must be aware of the incidence and significance of arrhythmias in healthy people as well as those with cardiac disease. The individual must be familiar with situations in which arrhythmias are most common. Most important, the physician must realize that a change in cardiac rate or rhythm may be a warning signal that something extracardiac is abnormal, such as hypoxemia or hypercarbia.

Electrophysiology

Normal Action Potentials

An electrical potential difference exists across the cell membrane in excitable tissue and is maintained by the active pumping of Na^+ out of, and K^+ into, the cell, against their concentration gradients (Table 12-3). As a result, the resting cellular transmembrane potential is maintained at -60 to -90 mV. The time course of the cell membrane potential actively changing during depolarization and repolarization is called the action potential[193] (Fig. 12-17). As the cardiac cell membrane slowly depolarizes to its threshold potential (-45 to -65 mV), a conformational change in membrane Na^+ channels allows for a rapid, massive increase in Na^+ permeability. Phase 0 of the action potential begins as

Na^+ rushes into the cell and the transmembrane potential quickly becomes less negative. Phase 1 (early repolarization) begins as the Na^+ channels quickly inactivate and an increased K^+ permeability allows an outward flow of K^+. An inward Cl^- flux may also occur during phase 1. Slower Ca^{2+} currents entering the cell inhibit repolarization and are responsible for the sustained depolarization known as phase 2 (plateau phase) of the action potential. During phase 3 (rapid repolarization), the inward Ca^{2+} current diminishes, while K^+ continues to flow rapidly out of the cell, thus restoring the electrical gradient across the cell membrane (see Table 12-3). Phase 4 of the action potential represents resting membrane potential in nonpacemaking cells. In cells with pacemaker potential, phase 4 represents slow diastolic depolarization due to an inward movement of Na^+ and possibly Ca^{2+}, allowing resting membrane potential to slowly approach threshold potential.

This ability to spontaneously generate action potentials is known as automaticity.[193] The rate of depolarization of a pacemaker cell depends on the slope of phase 4 depolarization, the resting membrane potential, and the threshold potential (Fig. 12-18). Normally, cells in the sinoatrial (SA) node have the steepest slope of phase 4 depolarization, and the least negative resting membrane potential (-60 mV) and threshold potential (-40 mV). They are capable of the most rapid rate of depolarization, allowing them to act as the predominant pacemaker cells controlling the heart rate. Other potential pacemaker cells, including cells near the AV node, Purkinje cells, and certain ventricular myocytes, exhibit slower rates of spontaneous phase 4 depolarization. These cells can function as secondary pacemakers if the rate of depolarization from the SA node decreases or their own rate of depolarization increases. Sympathetic stimulation in-

Table 12-3. Major Ion Movement During Phases of the Cardiac Action Potential

Phase	Ion	Movement Across Cell Membrane
0	Na^+	In
1	K^+	Out
	Cl^-	In
2	Ca^{2+}	In
	K^+	Out
3	K^+	Out
4	Na^+	In

From Stoelting RK: Heart. *In* Pharmacology and Physiology in Anesthetic Practice, ed 2. Philadelphia, JB Lippincott 1991, p 692.

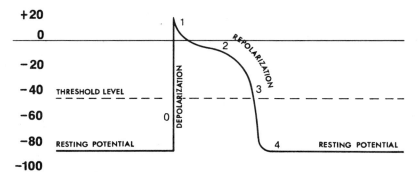

Figure 12-17. Cardiac action potential from a non-pacemaking cell. The resting potential, threshold potential, and phases of depolarization and repolarization are illustrated. (Adapted from Mangiola S, Ritota J: Basic Principles: Cardiac Arrhythmias. Philadelphia, JB Lippincott, 1974.)

creases the rate of phase 4 depolarization. Vagal stimulation slows the rate of pacemaker depolarization by making the resting membrane potential more negative (hyperpolarizing the cell) and slowing the rate of phase 4 depolarization.

The Na⁺ channels, which are activated during the upstroke, are rapidly inactivated and remain so until the membrane potential has been restored to threshold potential (−60 mV). During this time—the absolute refractory period—the membrane is completely unexcitable.[193] The Na⁺ channels are gradually reactivated by the increasingly negative membrane potential. As the action potential voltage falls below threshold potential, an action potential can be generated only by a greater-than-normal electrical stimulus. This is known as the relative refractory period.[193] Cell membrane refractoriness to depolarization prevents rapid repetitive stimulation and allows for completion of mechanical contraction prior to the onset of the next action potential.

The action potential generated in the SA node spreads through adjacent conducting tissues in the atria to the AV node, and then through the His-Purkinje system to the ventricular myocardium. The P wave and QRS complexes of the surface ECG are generated by phase 0 depolarization of millions of atrial and ventricular muscle cells respectively, while the T wave is generated by phase 3 repolarization of the ventricular cells. Repolarization of the atria occurs in a similar manner and direction as depolarization. However, repolarization of the human His-Purkinje system occurs last in the first cells to depolarize (the proximal bundle branches) and vice versa. This phenomenon explains aberrant ventricular conduction with premature atrial beats and the positive deflection of the ventricular T wave.

Mechanisms of Arrhythmias

Arrhythmias occur when there is disruption of the normal sequence of depolarization of the SA node, atrial tissue, AV node, His-Purkinje system, and ventricular muscle. Arrhythmias may result from normal physiologic mechanisms that enhance or depress the normal automaticity of pacemaking cells (sinus tachycardia, sinus arrhythmia, etc.). If the rate of impulse generation from a secondary pacemaker such as an AV nodal cell becomes more rapid than the depolarization rate of the SA node, the secondary pacemaker will assume primary control of the heart rate and rhythm (escape rhythm, AV dissociation), and so forth. An arrhythmia arises from one of many possible clinical scenarios involving reentry, as with accessory AV pathways. Specific therapy for arrhythmias may depend on deciding which of the following mechanisms is its cause: abnormal automaticity, triggered automaticity, or reentry.

Abnormal Automaticity

Abnormalities in the action potential, such as a decrease in the resting membrane potential, an increase in threshold potential, or an increase in the slope of phase 4 diastolic depolarization, will increase the depolarization rate for any cell with pacemaker potential.[194] Abnormal automaticity is usually the result of a movement of the resting membrane potential toward the threshold potential (less negative) which makes the cell more likely to depolarize. Less negative membrane potentials occur most frequently in areas of ischemia and infarction.[195] Abnormal automaticity with spontaneous depolarization of nonpacemaker cells may occur when the resting membrane potential is −60 mV.

Triggered Automaticity

Depolarization of the cell membrane that is triggered by the preceding action potential during or after repolarization is termed *afterdepolarization*. Early afterdepolarizations occur during phase 3 of repolarization, whereas late afterdepolarizations occur during phase 4, after repolarization is complete. Early afterdepolarizations develop because of a change in movement of K⁺ out of the cell or an abnormal increased movement of Na⁺ or Ca²⁺ into the cell. Conditions which cause early afterdepolarizations include hypokalemia, excess catecholamines, acidosis, hypoxia, delayed repolarization, and slow heart rates.[195] Delayed afterdepolarizations are primarily due to enhanced Ca²⁺ entry into the cell. Digitalis toxicity, hypomagnesemia, myocardial ischemia, catecholamine excess, and Ca²⁺ administration all can precipitate delayed afterdepolarizations.[195] Triggered activity may be initiated by premature stimuli or rapid pacing and may terminate spontaneously with rapid pacing or with spontaneous or programmed premature stimuli.

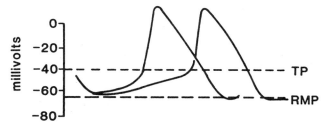

Figure 12-18. The rate of pacemaker discharge is dependent upon the slope of spontaneous phase 4 depolarization, negativity of the resting membrane potential (RMP), and the threshold potential (TP). (From Stoelting RK: Heart. *In* Pharmacology and Physiology in Anesthetic Practice, ed 2. Philadelphia, JB Lippincott, 1991, p 692.)

Reentry

The classic mechanism for arrhythmia generation involves reentry of a stimulus into the conducting system.[196] Anatomically contiguous but functionally diverse myocardial tissue is required for reentry to occur. Three conditions must exist: (1) an area of unidirectional block of impulse propagation, (2) a pathway with slow conduction velocity, and (3) distal recovery of excitability in the area formerly blocked (Fig. 12–19).

Reentry has been found to be involved in the generation of many arrhythmias. Supraventricular tachycardia can be caused by reentry occurring in the sinus node, the atrium, the AV node, or via an accessory pathway.[197] Reentrant arrhythmias tend to start and stop abruptly, are frequently precipitated by premature beats, and can be terminated with programmed insertion of premature stimuli.[198] Elongation of conducting pathways, as seen with dilation of the heart (especially left atrial dilatation associated with mitral stenosis) and decreased conduction velocity from myocardial ischemia, create a situation in which reentry via the Purkinje fibers can occur.

Arrhythmogenic Influences in the Intensive Care Unit and Operating Room

Critically ill patients are constantly exposed to a number of factors which can precipitate arrhythmias in the emergency department, OR, and ICU. Failure to maintain temperature during trauma surgery, anesthesia, and exposure to cold hospital environments may lead to hypothermia. Electrolyte disturbances such as hypokalemia, hypomagnesemia, and metabolic alkalosis may result from diuretic use,[199] intravenous fluid administration, or acid-base shifts. Hypocalcemia can result from rapid administration of albumin or blood products that contain citrate as an anticoagulant.[200] The presence of an indwelling central venous or PA catheter may increase risk of arrhythmias in certain patients.[201] Transient right bundle branch block, frequent ventricular ectopy, or nonsustained ventricular tachycardia are common with insertion of a PA catheter.[202] Medications such as digitalis, theophylline,[203] tricyclic antidepressants,[204] anesthetic agents, and antiarrhythmic agents may generate or enhance arrhythmias. Sympathetic stimulation occurs with hypoxia, hypercarbia, endotracheal intubation, surgical incision, pain, sepsis, or catecholamine infusions. This may lead to tachycardia, increased myocardial oxygen consumption, myocardial ischemia, and ventricular ectopy in patients with preexisting coronary artery disease. Parasympathetic stimulation occurs with pain, distention of a hollow viscus such as the bladder, and certain medications. Electrical microshock hazards exist due to the myriad of monitoring devices used in the critical care setting and may also precipitate arrhythmias.

Common Arrhythmias

Normal Sinus Rhythm

Normal sinus rhythm is characterized by (1) regular atrial activity originating in the SA node with a rate between 60 and 100 bpm; (2) upright P waves in leads I, II, and aVF and V_2 through V_6; (3) a P-R interval between 120 and 200 ms; (4) a P wave preceding each QRS complex; and (5) a QRS complex following each P wave. The rate of sinus node discharge depends on the balance between sympathetic and parasympathetic tone.

Sinus Tachycardia

Sinus tachycardia is essentially sinus rhythm occurring at a rate greater than 100 bpm in adults or 140 bpm in children.[205] Sinus tachycardia may be caused by many medications, including aminophylline, caffeine, isoflurane, ketamine, and quinidine.[205] Increases in sympathetic tone may result in rates of up to 160 to 200 bpm in adults, and greater than 220 bpm in children. Hypermetabolic states such as exercise, fever, sepsis, thyrotoxicosis, and malignant hyperthermia are associated with increased oxygen consumption and tachycardia. Inhibition of vagal tone occurs with anticholinergic medications such as atropine or glycopyrrolate. Sinus tachycardia is a physiologic sign of systemic perturbations, and one should attempt to identify and correct the underlying causes. Sinus tachycardia per se does not usually result in hemodynamic compromise but may lead to myocardial ischemia in patients with coronary artery disease or, if it is sustained, ischemia may develop in otherwise healthy individuals. Shortened diastolic time, a consequence of sinus tachycardia, leads to impaired ventricular filling in patients with decreased ventricular compliance or mitral stenosis. This causes a reduction in stroke volume, and may significantly decrease cardiac output.

Sinus Bradycardia

Sinus bradycardia is a sinus rhythm with a rate below 60 bpm in adults, or below 100 bpm in infants.[206] It is commonly seen in healthy young adults and well-trained athletes.

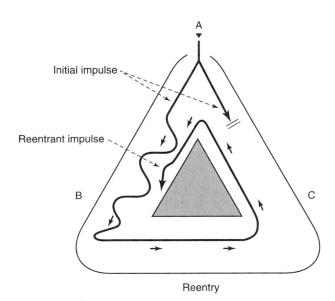

Figure 12–19. The essential requirement for initiation of a reentry circuit is a unidirectional block preventing anterograde propagation of the cardiac impulse. A premature impulse arriving at A finds pathway C refractory. Conduction in pathway B is slowed because of incomplete repolarization. The impulse travels retrograde via pathway C which has repolarized during the time required for the impulse to traverse pathway B, thus setting up the reentry circuit. (From Akhtar M: Management of ventricular tachyarrhythmias. JAMA 1982; 247:671–674.)

Sinus bradycardia may be due to inhibition of sympathetic activity with drugs such as β blockers, narcotics, and other anesthetic agents. Augmentation of parasympathetic tone with cholinergic agents such as pilocarpine, succinylcholine, or the anticholinesterases edrophonium or neostigmine reduces heart rate. Intraoperative traction on the peritoneum or mesentery, manipulation of the carotid sinus, or distention of a hollow viscus can cause vagally mediated bradycardia. Traction on the extraocular muscles or compression of the globe triggers the oculocardiac reflex, with pronounced bradycardia, or occasionally asystole. Increased intracranial pressure leads to systemic hypertension, reflex bradycardia, and respiratory irregularities, a trait known as Cushing's reflex. Hypoxia and hypothermia may lead to sinus bradycardia.

Inferior wall myocardial ischemia or infarction is frequently associated with sinus bradycardia. The blood supply to the SA node most commonly arises from the right coronary artery, and may be compromised during inferior ventricular wall ischemia. Chest pain may initiate a vagally mediated bradycardia. Cardiac sensory fibers may cause a systemic vagotonia resulting in nausea, hypotension, bradycardia, and occasionally varying degrees of heart block (Bezold-Jarisch reflex).

Excessively slow heart rates compromise cardiac output, which can lead to hypotension and shock. Heart rates less than 35 to 40 bpm increase the risk of cardiac escape rhythms. Withdrawal of the inciting stimulus, such as relief of traction on the mesentery, is often all that is necessary to correct this reflex sinus bradycardia. If clinically significant, bradycardia can be treated with atropine or catecholamines and, if refractory to medical therapy, with cardiac pacing.

Sinus Node Exit Block, Sinus Arrest

Occasionally, the SA node generates impulses that cannot escape the node to trigger the atrium. This is designated an SA node exit block and is occasionally a cause of bradycardia. Characteristics of SA exit block (Fig. 12-20) include the absence of a P wave in any lead, with the next P wave occurring at the anticipated time. This is different from a sinus arrest, in which the SA node fails to form an impulse and the subsequent P wave usually occurs earlier than anticipated.

Sinus Arrhythmia

Sinus arrhythmia is a benign, rhythmic variation in the sinus rate occurring usually as a result of changes in vagal tone associated with respiration (Fig. 12-21). The heart rate slowly increases during inspiration and slowly decreases during exhalation. A nonrespiratory variant of sinus arrhythmia may be seen with digitalis toxicity, hypothyroidism, calcium channel blocking medications, and with myocardial infarction,[207] or may occur in young, healthy individuals. In sinus arrhythmia, the P-R interval and P wave and QRS morphologies do not vary.

Wandering Atrial Pacemaker

The term *wandering atrial pacemaker* is applied when two or more supraventricular pacemaker foci are competing for control of the heart rhythm (Fig 12-22). The cycle length is regular, while P wave morphology and P-R intervals change with each pacemaker focus. This rhythm rarely requires treatment or deteriorates into a more significant arrhythmia. It must not be confused with an AV node reentrant tachycardia with a retrograde P wave occurring immediately before the QRS complex.

Premature Atrial Contraction

When the atrial impulse originates from a focus other than the SA node, the P wave has a different morphology than the sinus-generated P wave. If this occurs before the next sinus P wave, it is called a premature atrial complex (PAC) (Fig. 12-23). An ectopic focus located high in the atrium will generate an ectopic P wave closely resembling the normal sinus P wave. The ectopic P wave will be inverted in leads I, II, and aVF if the focus is low in the atrium. Often, the ectopic P wave is hidden in the T wave of the preceding complex. The ectopic P-R interval may be shorter than normal with a low atrial focus or may be prolonged due to partial refractoriness of the AV node. The pause following the PAC is equal to or slightly longer than the sinus cycle length, if the sinus node is depolarized by the PAC and reset, causing a noncompensatory pause. However, the SA node may depolarize in a normal sequence without interference from the PAC, but not conduct due to atrial refractoriness. The next sinus node beat occurs at the normal interval and the resulting pause between complexes is fully compensated.

PACs occurring very early in diastole may find the AV node refractory, and depolarization will not spread to the ventricles. This is known as a blocked PAC (Fig. 12-24). Alternatively, the AV conduction system may be only partially repolarized, and the PAC is conducted aberrantly[208] (Fig. 12-25). This usually results in a right bundle branch block pattern since the right bundle frequently has a longer refractory period than the left bundle. Aberrant conduction of a PAC combined with the absence of a noncompensatory pause can lead to the erroneous diagnosis of a ventricular premature beat. (See Premature Ventricular Contractions.)

Electrolyte disturbances, especially hypokalemia, hypoxemia, hypercarbia, acidosis, digitalis toxicity, and mechanical irritation of the atrium by indwelling catheters or pacemaker leads, can cause atrial ectopy. PACs do not usually require treatment unless they become so frequent as to impair cardiac output. A PAC may trigger other supraventricular arrhythmias, such as supraventricular tachycardias and atrial flutter or fibrillation, and is the most frequent reason for treating PACs in the OR or critical care setting.[209]

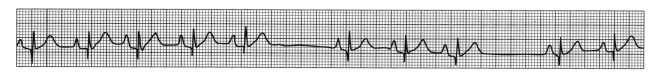

Figure 12-20. Sinus node exit block. Note the absence of a P wave (following the fifth and eighth QRS complexes), and subsequent P waves occurring at the anticipated time. (From Zipes DP: Specific arrhythmias: Diagnosis and treatment. *In* Braunwald E (ed): Heart Disease: A Textbook of Cardiovascular Disease, ed 3. Philadelphia, WB Saunders, 1988, p 660.)

Inspiration   Expiration   Inspiration

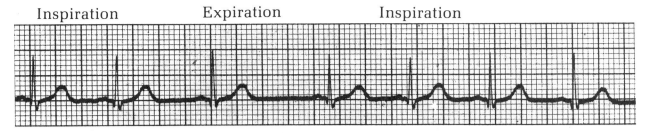

Figure 12-21. Sinus arrhythmia associated with respiration in a young, healthy adult. Note the constant P-R interval and P wave and QRS complex morphology, with varying R-R intervals. (From Conover MB: Understanding Electrocardiography, ed 6. St Louis: Mosby–Year Book, 1992.)

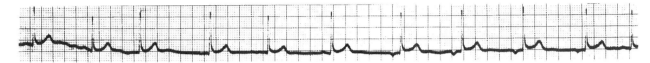

Figure 12-22. Wandering atrial pacemaker. The first three beats are sinus, then the pacemaking shifts to another pacemaker focus. Note the different P wave morphology, but no significant change in the rate. The sinus node regains control in the bottom tracing. (From Zipes DP: Specific arrhythmias: Diagnosis and treatment. *In* Braunwald E (ed): Heart Disease: A Textbook of Cardiovascular Disease, ed 3. Philadelphia, WB Saunders, 1988, p 666.)

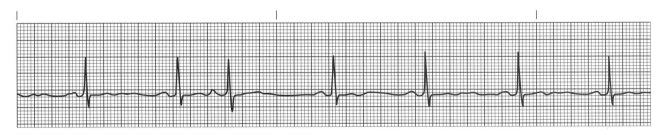

Figure 12-23. The third beat arrives early and has a different P wave morphology than the preceding beats, identifying it as a premature atrial contraction (PAC).

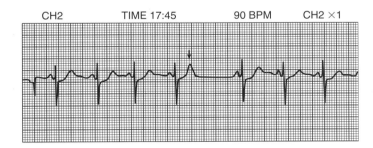

Figure 12-24. Sinus rhythm with a nonconducted premature atrial contraction (PAC). The blocked PAC marked by the *arrow* distorts the T wave morphology compared with the other T waves.

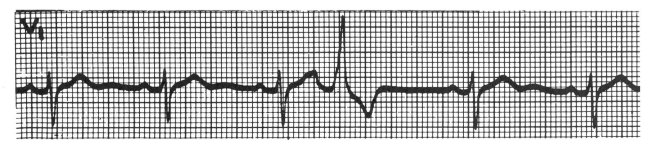

Figure 12-25. After three normally conducted beats a premature atrial contraction arises and is conducted aberrantly with a right bundle branch block pattern. A P wave identifiable in the preceding T wave distinguishes this from a ventricular premature beat. (From Marriott HJK: Practical Electrocardiography, ed 7. Baltimore, Williams & Wilkins, 1983.)

Premature Nodal Complexes

The AV node consists of three regions according to cell types: transitional, midnodal, and lower nodal. The transitional zone, also known as the atrionodal (AN) region, is the gradual merging of atrial and nodal fibers. The midnodal, or N region, accounts for most of the physiologic delay in AV conduction. The lower nodal or nodal-His (NH) zone, where nodal and His-Purkinje fibers merge, is the usual focus for nodal pacemaker activity.

The AV node normally acts as an escape pacemaker whenever the atrial rate slows below the intrinsic nodal rate. However, early depolarization of this tissue leads to premature nodal complexes (PNCs). Retrograde conduction to the atrium is possible and is evident by an inverted P wave in leads I, II, and aVF. The retrograde P wave may precede, follow, or be buried within the QRS complex (Fig. 12-26).

The AV node may become the primary cardiac pacemaker if the nodal rate exceeds the sinus rate. Nodal rhythm is regular at the intrinsic rate of 45 to 60 bpm. The term *accelerated nodal rhythm* is used when a nodal rhythm occurs at a rate between 60 and 100 bpm, and nodal tachycardia when the rate exceeds 100 bpm. PNCs and nodal rhythms may result from the same causes as PACs.

Paroxysmal Supraventricular Tachycardia

Paroxysmal supraventricular tachycardia (PSVT) is a generic term encompassing all tachycardias originating in cardiac tissue other than ventricular tissue. The common characteristic is the sudden onset of this arrhythmia. PSVT includes SA node and AV nodal reentry, atrial tachycardias, and AV reentry tachycardias using an accessory pathway. AV nodal reentrant tachycardia (AVNRT) is the most common PSVT in adults, representing greater than 50% of all PSVTs.[197] AVNRT is often precipitated and terminated physiologically by a PAC or retrograde conduction of a PVC. The AV node consists of

two separate pathways, conventionally named alpha (slow conduction velocity and short refractory period) and beta (fast conduction velocity and long refractory period). Reentry is possible when a PAC is blocked in the beta pathway with the longer refractory period and travels slowly through the alpha pathway. ECG diagnosis reveals a rate of 140 to 200 bpm, and a regular rhythm with a narrow QRS complex without visible P waves (Fig. 12-27). Retrograde P waves may be seen preceding or following the QRS complex but most commonly are obscured in the QRS complex owing to almost simultaneous activation of the atria and ventricles. An atrial or esophageal electrogram may document atrial activity in a 1:1 relationship to ventricular activity. At faster rates, widening of the QRS complex due to rate-related bundle branch block may make differentiation from ventricular tachycardia difficult. Adenosine or calcium channel blockers are very effective in converting AVNRT to sinus rhythm (>90% of patients).

Paroxysmal atrial tachycardia (PAT) may result either from an automatic or reentry focus.[210] ECG diagnosis reveals a narrow-complex tachycardia with a rate of 150 to 200 bpm. P waves usually precede the QRS complexes, but with a morphology different from normal sinus P waves. Depending on heart rate, the P waves may be hidden in the T wave of the preceding QRS complex (Fig. 12-28). When an automatic focus is responsible for PAT, carotid sinus massage and calcium channel blockers may slow the rate but usually fail to terminate the arrhythmia. Therapy aims to correct the underlying process, be it myocardial ischemia, chronic obstructive pulmonary disease with hypoxia and hypercarbia, or electrolyte disturbance.

Atrial tachycardia, which may be associated with varying degrees of AV block, is seen with digitalis toxicity, catecholamine excess, and critical illness involving hypoxia, acidosis, and electrolyte disturbances (Fig. 12-29). This rhythm may reflect underlying sinus node dysfunction and may be seen as part of the sick sinus syndrome (SSS). This clinical syndrome of abnormal sinus node function is caused by abnormalities in SA node automaticity, SA conduction, and occasionally AV node dysfunction.[211] Sinus node ischemia, mitral valve prolapse, inflammatory and infiltrative diseases, and atrial trauma may all be associated with SSS. Although it usually manifests as bradycardia, it is often associated with recurrent episodes of tachycardia alternating with bradyarrhythmias (Fig. 12-30). In this context, it is known as tachycardia-bradycardia syndrome. Insertion of a permanent pacemaker may be required for control of prolonged sinus pauses or symptomatic bradycardia in addition to medical control of the tachycardia.

Multifocal atrial tachycardia, also known as chaotic atrial tachycardia, is characterized by three or more morphologically distinct P waves at a rate greater than 100 bpm, with varying P-P and P-R intervals (Fig. 12-31). It is most commonly seen in critically ill patients with underlying pulmonary disease,[212] and theophylline has been implicated as the inciting factor in this arrhythmia.[213]

Accessory AV connections are the second most common cause of PSVT (25 to 30%) of patients.[214] Wolff-Parkinson-White (WPW) syndrome is associated with an accessory pathway (bundle of Kent). This abnormal connection between the atrial and ventricular myocardium bypasses the normal delay imposed by the AV node. ECG diagnosis reveals a short P-R interval and delta wave when the patient is in sinus rhythm (Fig. 12-32). The accessory pathway (James fibers) in the Lown-Ganong-Levine syndrome connects the atrium to the AV node or bundle of His. A shortened P-R interval without a delta wave is seen on surface ECG. Reen-

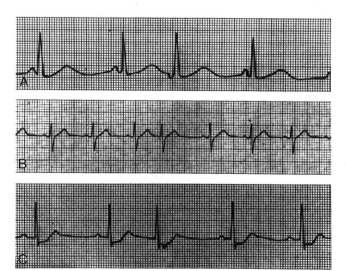

Figure 12-26. Junctional premature complexes. In tracing A, the retrograde P wave precedes the QRS complex; in strip B it is buried within the QRS; in strip C, the retrograde P wave follows the QRS complex. (From Conover MB: Understanding Electrocardiography, ed 6. St Louis: Mosby-Year Book, 1992.)

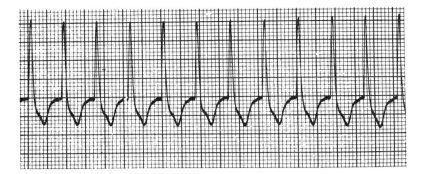

Figure 12-27. Paroxysmal supraventricular tachycardia. The retrograde P waves are lost within the Q-T complex and are not definitely discernible. This is typical of atrioventricular nodal reentry tachycardia.

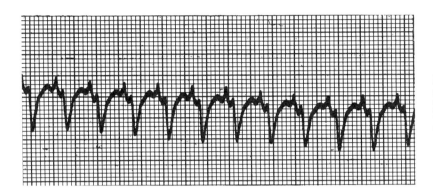

Figure 12-28. Paroxysmal atrial tachycardia at a rate of 188 bpm. The P waves have a different morphology than do sinus P waves. (From Mangiola S, Ritota J: Basic Principles: Cardiac Arrhythmias. Philadelphia, JB Lippincott, 1974, p 1.)

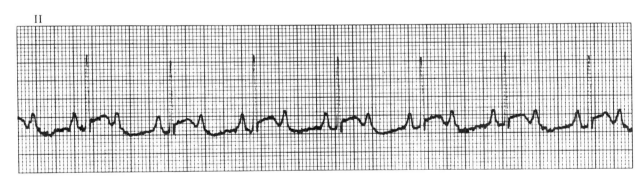

Figure 12-29. Atrial tachycardia with 2:1 atrioventricular block, in a patient with digoxin toxicity. (From Conover MB: Understanding Electrocardiography, ed 6. St Louis, Mosby-Year Book, 1992.)

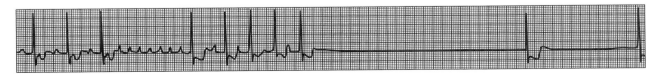

Figure 12-30. Sick sinus syndrome manifesting as the tachycardia-bradycardia syndrome. Irregular atrial tachycardia is followed by prolonged sinus pause. A junctional escape rhythm begins after 4.8 seconds. (From Zipes DP: Specific arrhythmias: Diagnosis and treatment. *In* Braunwald E (ed): Heart Disease: A Textbook of Cardiovascular Disease, ed 3. Philadelphia, WB. Saunders, 1988, p 667.)

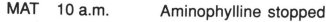

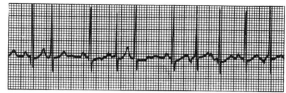

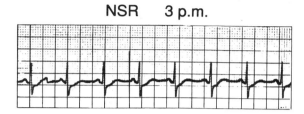

Figure 12-31. Multifocal atrial tachycardia (chaotic atrial tachycardia) with several different P wave morphologies evident in a patient with chronic obstructive pulmonary disease. Normal sinus rhythm (NSR) is restored after aminophylline is discontinued. (From Royster RL: Causes and consequences of arrhythmias. *In* Benumof JL, Saidman JL (eds): Anesthesia and Perioperative Complications. St. Louis, Mosby–Year Book, 1992, p 228.)

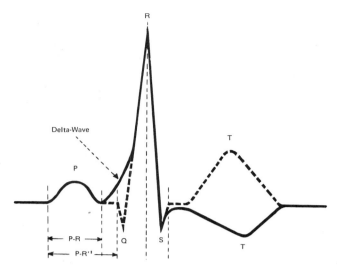

Figure 12-32. The solid line indicates the anomalous conduction in the Wolff-Parkinson-White syndrome, and the dotted line indicates normal conduction. The P-R interval is shortened because of the delta wave. The T wave is inverted because of secondary T wave changes. (From Chung EK: Electrocardiography: Practical Applications With Vectoral Principles, ed 3. Norwalk, CT Appleton Century-Crofts, 1985.)

try occurs with anterograde (atria to ventricle) AV nodal conduction and retrograde (ventricle to atria) conduction through the accessory pathway. This results in a narrow-complex tachycardia with QRS morphology similar to normally conducted beats. The inverted P wave usually follows closely or is hidden within the preceding QRS complex (Fig. 12-33). Occasionally, anterograde conduction is via the accessory pathway with retrograde conduction through the AV node, resulting in a wide QRS complex due to the delta wave of preexcitation.[215] The morphology and QRS–P interval will depend upon the location of the accessory pathway.[216] PSVT, atrial flutter, or atrial fibrillation may result in extremely rapid ventricular rates (>300 bpm) because of the very fast conduction velocity and short refractory period of the accessory pathway. Significant hemodynamic compromise can occur. Carotid sinus massage, adenosine, or calcium channel blockers may convert narrow-complex tachycardia to sinus rhythm by primarily slowing AV node conduction. Class Ia antiarrhythmic agents (e.g., procainamide) may convert wide-complex tachycardias through slowing of conduction in the accessory pathway. If hemodynamically unstable, immediate cardioversion is indicated.

Sinus node reentry is an uncommon form of PSVT, and is characterized by abrupt onset of a narrow-complex tachycardia, with P waves identical to normal sinus P waves. As with most reentrant tachycardias, sinus node reentry may be terminated by carotid sinus massage, calcium channel blockers, or programmed insertion of a premature beat.

Atrial Fibrillation

Atrial fibrillation is characterized by a rapid, irregular, disorganized atrial activity representing multiple foci firing simultaneously. Microreentry is likely the predominant mechanism. On surface ECG, no discernible P waves are seen, but the baseline may show very fine or coarse fibrillatory activity (Fig. 12-34). The AEG reveals complexes having a myriad of shapes, sizes, polarities, and amplitudes.[13] Ventricular activity is irregular, reflecting the constant bombardment of the AV node with impulses which traverse the AV node in a variable manner. The ventricular rate in untreated, healthy patients may vary between 120 and 200 bpm. Aberrant conduction, often with a right bundle branch block pattern, is common in atrial fibrillation. Accessory AV pathways allow very rapid conduction of impulses to the ventricles and may lead to ventricular tachycardia or fibrillation. Atrial fibrillation is common in patients with ischemic cardiac disease, valvular heart disease, thyroid disease, and in critically ill patients. Therapy is aimed at control of the ventricular rate to allow adequate time for ventricular filling in the absence of an atrial contraction. The ventricular response is slowed with digitalis, β blockers, or calcium channel blockers, singly or in combination.[217] Conversion of acute atrial fibrillation to sinus rhythm is often successful with procainamide,[218] esmolol,[217] and intravenous amiodarone. Cardioversion is indicated for hemodynamically unstable patients with acute atrial fibril-

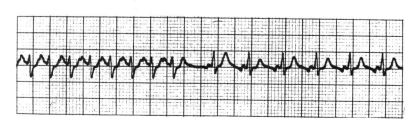

Figure 12-33. Narrow complex reentrant tachycardia in a child with Wolff-Parkinson-White syndrome. The tachycardia terminates abruptly with the ensuing normal sinus rhythm characterized by a short P-R interval and a nondistinct delta wave.

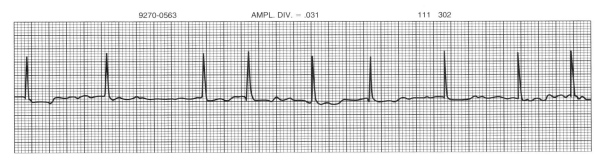

Figure 12-34. Atrial fibrillation with a slow ventricular response. Note the total irregularity of QRS complexes with a fine fibrillatory baseline.

lation or if the arrhythmia persists for several days. Cardioversion of acute atrial fibrillation after 5 to 7 days requires anticoagulation.[219]

Atrial Flutter

Atrial flutter is commonly seen with many cardiac diseases, especially mitral valve disease. Atrial flutter is categorized into two types on the basis of atrial rate and susceptibility to overdrive pacing.[220] Type I (classic) atrial flutter occurs at a rate of 300 bpm, with typical sawtooth or biphasic flutter waves (F waves) seen in the inferior leads (Fig. 12-35). Rapid overdrive pacing is usually successful in terminating type I atrial flutter.[221] Type II atrial flutter is characterized by a flatter baseline with positive flutter waves in the inferior leads, at a rate of 350 to 400 bpm (Fig. 12-36). Overdrive pacing usually fails to capture the atria in the presence of type II flutter, although conversion to type I flutter may occur with pharmacologic therapy. Ventricular rate depends upon the state of the AV node, with conduction ranging from 2:1 to 8:1. The ventricular response is frequently 150 bpm due to 2:1 AV block. Carotid sinus massage will increase the block, and the flutter waves will become more readily discerned. AEGs are useful for defining atrial activity when clear flutter waves are not present on the surface ECG (see Fig. 12-6). Control of ventricular response is obtained by increasing the AV block with digitalis, β blockers, calcium channel blockers, or a combination of these. Esmolol is effective in rate control and appears to convert acute atrial fibrillation or flutter to sinus rhythm in a high percentage of patients[222] (Table 12-4). Cardioversion with very low energy levels (10 to 25 J) may be required if the patient is hemodynamically unstable or atrial flutter persists despite adequate medical therapy.

Arrhythmias Due to Atrioventricular Block

Delayed or blocked impulse propagation between the atria and ventricles may occur in the atrium, AV node, or His-Purkinje system. First-degree AV block is a delay in AV conduction, almost invariably occurring in the AV node. The P-R interval is greater than 200 ms, with normal P wave and QRS complexes, and with each P wave resulting in a QRS complex. First-degree AV block is usually benign and occurs in children, well-conditioned athletes, patients on digoxin or β blockers, and in patients with enhanced vagal tone.

Second-degree AV block is defined as failure of some but not all P waves to be transmitted to the ventricles and occurs in two types. Mobitz type I AV block, also known as Wenckebach block, is characterized by progressive lengthening of the P-R interval followed by a blocked beat (Fig. 12-37). The site of this block is usually in the AV node, so it is sometimes referred to as a "proximal block." This rhythm is usually temporary, and does not progress to complete heart block. It is a result of reflex slowing of AV conduction as occurs with carotid sinus massage, oculocardiac reflex, Bezold-Jarisch reflex with inferior myocardial infarction, and in well-conditioned athletes. Proximal AV block is usually responsive to atropine. Mobitz type II second-degree AV block, or "distal block," is less common but more severe than type I. The ECG shows fixed P-R intervals and intermittent nonconducted P waves (Fig. 12-38). This type of AV block is frequently associated with intraventricular conduction delays such as bundle branch blocks, and often progresses to complete heart block. Seen more commonly with anterior myocardial infarctions, it is less responsive to atropine than proximal block and may necessitate permanent pacemaker insertion. When the P/R ratio is 2:1 (every other P wave blocked), it is difficult to differentiate type I from type II AV block. If the P-R interval of the conducted beats is pro-

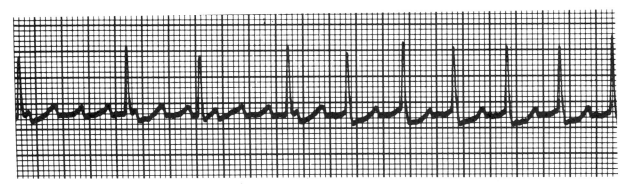

Figure 12-35. Type I atrial flutter at a rate of 300 bpm, with classic sawtooth flutter waves and variable atrioventricular block.

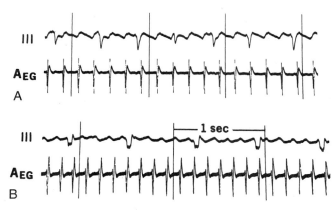

Figure 12–36. Simultaneous surface ECG (lead III) and atrial electrogram (A$_{EG}$) demonstrating type I atrial flutter (patient A) with classic sawtooth flutter waves at a rate of 300 bpm, and type II atrial flutter (patient B) with atrial activity at a rate of 400 bpm, and absence of discrete sawtooth flutter waves. (From Waldo AL, Kaiser GA: Electrophysiologic consideration for the cardiac surgical patient. *In* Litwak RS, Jurado RA, (eds): Care of the Cardiac Surgical Patient. Norwalk, CT: Appleton-Century-Crofts, 1982, p 241.)

Table 12–4. Results of Pharmacologic Therapy vs. Placebo 1 Hour After Initiation of Therapy in Patients With Recent-Onset Atrial Fibrillation or Flutter

Drug†	Converted to Normal Sinus Rhythm	Ventricular Response (bpm mean ± SEM)
Esmolol (n = 21)	10/21*	151 ± 6 → 104 ± 3**
Verapamil (n = 20)	4/20	147 ± 6 → 94 ± 3**
Digoxin (n = 20)	3/20	139 ± 5 → 135 ± 4
Placebo (n = 18)	2/18	137 ± 4 → 135 ± 4

*$P < .05$ vs. verapamil, digoxin, placebo.
**$P < .05$ vs. digoxin, placebo.
†Drugs were administered as follows: esmolol 10–20 mg bolus followed by infusion 2–16 mg/hr; verapamil 10–20 mg bolus in two titration steps; digoxin 0.5 mg single bolus; placebo = saline.
Data from Platia EV, Michelson EL, Porterfield JK, et al: Esmolol versus verapamil in the acute treatment of atrial fibrillation or atrial flutter. Am J Cardiol 1989; 63:925; and Platia EV, Waclawski SH, Pluth TA, et al: Management of acute-onset atrial fibrillation/flutter: Esmolol vs verapamil vs digoxin vs placebo. Circulation 1987; 76(suppl 4):IV–520.

longed and there is no bundle branch block, it is more likely a type I or Wenckebach block.

Third-degree AV block, or complete heart block, occurs when no P waves are transmitted to the ventricles. The atria and ventricles each are beating independently (Fig. 12–39). The ventricular rate is determined by the site of the escape pacemaker. An AV nodal focus results in narrow QRS complexes (junctional escape rhythm), while a focus within the ventricular myocardium generates wide QRS complexes (idioventricular escape rhythm). Common causes of complete heart block include myocardial ischemia and infarction, infiltrative cardiomyopathies, and excessive vagal tone.

Arrhythmias Due to Intraventricular Conduction Abnormalities

Electrical impulse transmission through the ventricular conduction system may also be disturbed, leading to abnormalities in the morphology of the QRS complex. The bundle of His separates into right and left bundle branches, with the left bundle branch giving rise to anterior and posterior divisions or fascicles. The fascicles terminate in an extensive branching network of small Purkinje fibers which interdigitate with cardiac myocytes. The left anterior fascicle is responsible for depolarization of the anterior and anterolateral portions of the left ventricle, the posterior fascicle depolarizes the posterior and inferior left ventricle, and the right bundle branch controls depolarization of the right ventricle. Septal depolarization occurs due to small branches arising from the main left bundle branch. Myocardial ischemia, in-

farction, electrolyte disturbances, or mechanical trauma may lead to delayed or interrupted impulse propagation. In the absence of coordinated transmission of activation from the His-Purkinje system, electrical activation must spread from myocyte to myocyte, resulting in a prolonged time course of ventricular activation. In addition, the magnitude and direction of the ECG electrical vectors are altered. Detection of many arrhythmias resulting from interventricular conduction defects is often very difficult utilizing single-channel or two-lead systems. Isolated right or left fascicular block may be manifest only by changes in the mean electrical QRS axis in the precordial plane.

Complete bundle branch blocks are characterized by prolongation of the QRS complex (>120 ms) and delayed activation of the affected ventricle. The right bundle branch is relatively long and thin, running just under the endocardial surface of the right side of the interventricular septum and right ventricular outflow tract, terminating at about the level of the anterior papillary muscle. With complete right bundle branch block the QRS width is prolonged, the initial portion of the QRS complex is normal, and delayed right ventricular depolarization creates a widened, slurred S wave in leftward-directed ECG leads, such as I, II, aV$_L$, V$_5$, and V$_6$[223] (Fig. 12–40). Transient right bundle branch block may be seen during insertion of a flow-directed PA catheter as the balloon traverses the right ventricular outflow tract, but rarely progresses to complete heart block, even in the presence of preexisting left bundle branch block.[224, 225] When conduction through the left bundle branch is blocked, the initial portion of the QRS complex is abnormal because depolarization of the interventricular septum occurs from right to left. Depo-

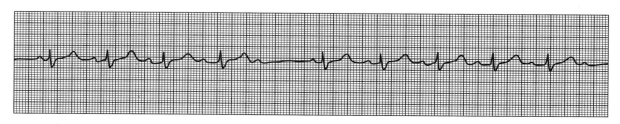

Figure 12–37. Second-degree Mobitz type I (Wenckebach) atrioventricular block. Note progressive P-R prolongation, and nonconduction of the P wave before each pause.

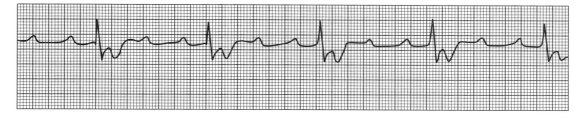

Figure 12-38. Second-degree Mobitz type II atrioventricular block. The P-R interval remains constant.

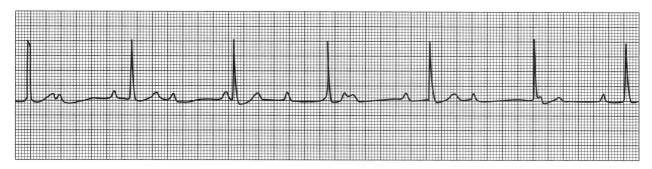

Figure 12-39. Third-degree or complete heart block, with junctional escape focus at a rate of 45 bpm. Note complete dissociation of atrial and ventricular activity.

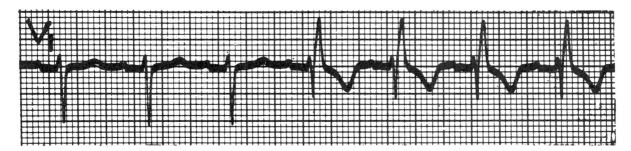

Figure 12-40. ECG tracing showing intermittent right bundle branch block (RBBB). The first three beats are conducted normally, then RBBB morphology becomes evident. The initial part of the QRS complex is normal, the QRS duration is widened, and the T wave is opposite the direction of the QRS. (From Marriott HJK: Practical Electrocardiography, ed 7. Baltimore, Williams & Wilkins, 1983, p 79.)

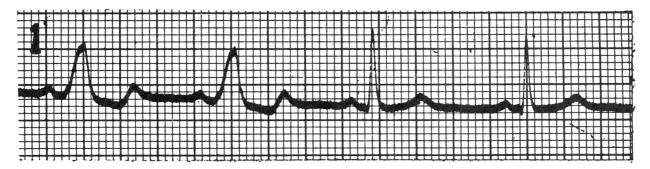

Figure 12-41. ECG tracing showing left bundle branch block (LBBB). The first two beats have a classic LBBB pattern followed by resumption of normal conduction in the following two beats. Note that the initial portion of the QRS differs from the initial part of the normal QRS complexes. Also note the widened QRS with the T wave directed opposite the QRS in the beats with LBBB morphology. (From Marriott HJK: Practical Electrocardiography, ed 7. Baltimore, Williams & Wilkins, 1983, p 68.)

larization of the left ventricle is prolonged as the wave of activation must pass from cell to cell, resulting in a widened QRS complex. As a result of the depolarization-repolarization disturbance produced by the block,[223] the T wave is generally directed opposite to the main QRS complex (Fig. 12–41). These changes are usually evident in all leads but most pronounced in lateral leads such as I, aV_L, V_5, and V_6. Bundle branch blocks can be found in healthy, asymptomatic individuals with apparently normal hearts, with right bundle branch block seen more frequently (5.0 to 18.9/100,000) than left bundle branch block (1.0 to 5.0/100,000).[226-232]

Although ischemic heart disease is the most worrisome cause, other common causes of cardiac conduction disturbances include electrolyte imbalances, rheumatic heart disease, tertiary syphilis, Chagas' disease, congenital rubella, calcific degeneration of the conducting system, and infiltrative cardiac diseases such as sarcoidosis or amyloidosis. Bundle branch blocks may also be entirely rate-dependent, becoming manifest during faster, or, occasionally, slower heart rates. Rate-related conduction defects are frequently associated with subclinical or overt ischemic coronary artery disease. The new onset of any conduction abnormality should always raise concern over myocardial ischemia or infarction, until proven otherwise.

Premature Ventricular Contractions

PVCs, also known as ventricular premature beats, originate from the ventricular myocardium. Conduction through the myocardium occurs without the specialized His-Purkinje conduction system, and thus the QRS duration is widened (>0.12 second), and the QRS morphology is significantly altered. The QRS is wide and slurred, with ST segments sloping in the opposite direction to the main QRS deflection (Fig. 12–42).

Differentiation between PVCs and PACs with aberrant conduction can be difficult.[208] Obviously, the presence of P waves before the QRS complexes favors PACs, although their absence does not rule them out. Retrograde P waves may be seen following a PVC when conduction through the AV node is slowed significantly. PVCs tend to have a fixed coupling interval—that is, the time between the normal QRS and the PVC tends to be constant (Fig. 12–43). The coupling interval is more variable with PACs. Fusion beats, in

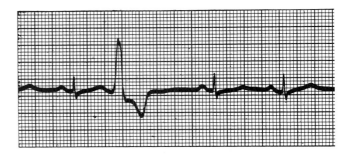

Figure 12-42. Premature ventricular contraction, demonstrating a fully compensatory pause. (From Mangiola S, Ritota J: Basic Principles: Cardiac Arrhythmias. Philadelphia, JB Lippincott, 1974.)

which the QRS complex is a blend of normal and PVC morphologies, favor a ventricular origin (Fig. 12–44). PVCs usually do not penetrate the SA node and reset its rate, so the pause following a PVC will be longer than expected. The next normal QRS complex will occur at two cycle lengths after the previous normal QRS complex. The pause is said to be fully compensatory (Fig. 12–42), in contrast to a PAC, which resets the SA node and results in a less than fully compensated pause. A PVC may, however, reset the SA node, so a noncompensatory pause does not totally rule out a ventricular origin.

PVCs are commonly seen in otherwise healthy patients.[189] PVCs are also seen in patients with myocardial ischemia, catecholamine excess, hypokalemia, hypomagnesemia, hypoxemia, and ventricular irritation from indwelling catheters. They may be harbingers of more threatening arrhythmias, such as ventricular tachycardia or fibrillation in certain patients. Multifocal PVCs are associated with a higher risk of degeneration into ventricular tachycardia or fibrillation (Fig. 12–45). A PVC occurring on the peak of the T wave, the vulnerable period of the ECG, may trigger sustained ventricular tachycardia or fibrillation. In bigeminy, every other beat is a PVC, usually with a fixed coupling interval (see Fig. 12–43). This may be from slow reentry or triggered activity. Medical therapy for isolated PVCs remains controversial, but frequent, multiform, or "R on T" beats may trigger sustained ventricular tachycardia or fibrillation, and probably should be suppressed.

V_1

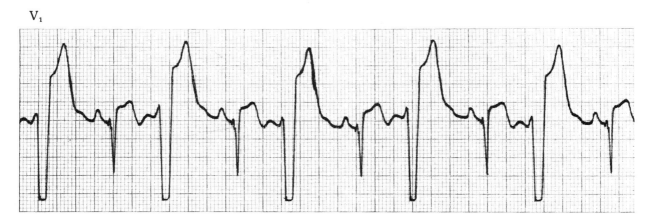

Figure 12-43. Ventricular bigeminy with a fixed coupling interval. Note that the interval between the sinus beat and the PVC is constant. (From Conover MB: Understanding Electrocardiography, ed 6. St Louis, Mosby–Year Book, 1992.)

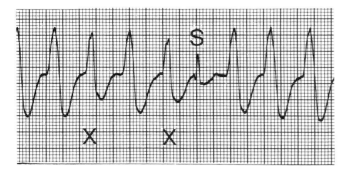

Figure 12-44. Fusion beats. Ventricular tachycardia is interrupted by two fusion beats (X) with sinus depolarization of the ventricles fusing with the ventricular ectopic activity. Complete capture of the ventricles by the sinus occurs (S). (From Royster RL, Robertie PG: Recognition and treatment of ectopic beats. Anesthesiol Clin North Am 1989; 7:315.)

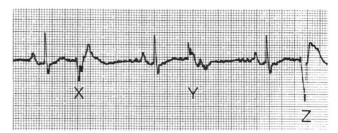

Figure 12-45. Multifocal premature ventricular contractions (PVCs). Note the different morphologies of the three PVCs (X,Y,Z). (From Royster RL, Robertie PG: Recognition and treatment of ectopic beats. Anesthesiol Clin North Am 1989; 7:315.)

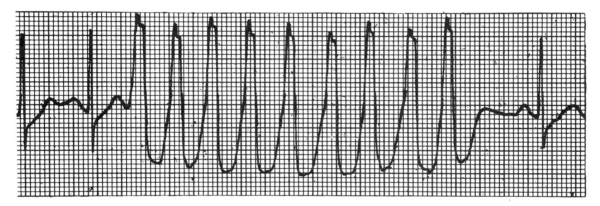

Figure 12-46. Ventricular tachycardia during sinus rhythm. (From Mangiola S, Ritota J: Basic Principles: Cardiac Arrhythmias. Philadelphia, JB Lippincott, 1974, p 1.)

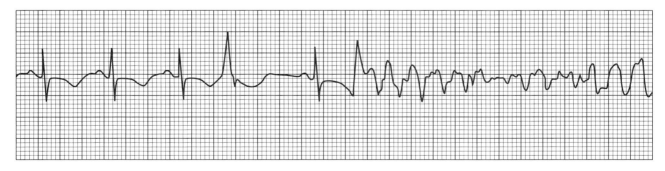

Figure 12-47. Polymorphic ventricular tachycardia, or torsades de pointes, in a patient with prolonged Q-T interval.

Table 12-5. Factors in the Electrocardiographic Diagnosis of Ventricular Tachycardia (VT) or Supraventricular Tachycardia (SVT) With Aberration

	VT	SVT With Aberration
AV dissociation	+	−
Fusion beats	+	−
QRS width	>140 ms	<140 ms
QRS morphology		
RBBB	Monophasic, LAD	Triphasic, normal axis
LBBB	Wide R in lead V₁	−
	RAD	−
Onset	PVC	PAC with ↑ QRS
CSM effective	−(<2%)	+(30%)

AV, atrioventricular; PAC, premature atrial concentration; CSM, carotid sinus massage; LAD, left axis deviation; LBBB, left bundle branch block; RAD, right axis deviation; RBBB, right bundle branch block; PVC, premature ventricular contraction.

Ventricular Tachycardia

Three or more consecutive PVCs at a rate greater than 100 bpm constitutes ventricular tachycardia (Fig. 12-46). If the rate is less than 100 bpm, the term *accelerated idioventricular rhythm* is used. As with PVCs, differentiating ventricular tachycardia from supraventricular tachycardia with aberrancy is often quite difficult.[233] Criteria that suggest ventricular tachycardia include wide QRS complex (>0.14 second), left axis deviation (> −60 degrees), fusion beats, certain QRS morphologies, and AV dissociation (Table 12-5). Establishing ventricular tachycardia as the diagnosis is of extreme importance because many therapeutic options for supraventricular tachycardia will not affect ventricular tachycardia. Ventricular tachycardia is often poorly tolerated for extended periods and may deteriorate into ventricular fibrillation. An AEG or esophageal lead may show evidence of AV dissociation, establishing the diagnosis of ventricular tachycardia. Immediate treatment with antiarrhythmic drugs or electrical countershock is almost always indicated. Correc-

tion of any underlying condition such as electrolyte disturbances, hypoxemia, myocardial ischemia, or intracardiac catheter malposition is necessary.

Polymorphic ventricular tachycardia, also known as torsades de pointes, is associated with prolongation of the Q-T interval on the surface ECG (Fig. 12-47). Acquired prolongation of the Q-T interval is seen with myocardial ischemia, myocarditis, intracranial disorders, hypothermia, and electrolyte abnormalities.[234] A number of drugs, most notably the class Ia antiarrhythmic agents such as procainamide, quinidine, and disopyramide, can also cause torsades de pointes.[235] Treatment is aimed at shortening the Q-T interval, and includes rapid overdrive pacing, isoproterenol infusion, and intravenous magnesium.[236] In contrast, the congenital prolonged Q-T syndromes are treated with β-adrenergic blockers or surgical sympathectomy.[237] Cardiac arrest during anesthesia is a distinct possibility in this syndrome and preoperative institution of β-blockers is critical.[238]

Ventricular Fibrillation

Ventricular fibrillation is chaotic, asynchronous electrical activity of the ventricular myocardium, associated with minimal to no cardiac output. Factors associated with an increased risk for ventricular fibrillation include myocardial ischemia or infarction, electrolyte disturbances such as hypokalemia or hypomagnesemia, hypoxemia, hypothermia, and catecholamine excess. Direct mechanical irritation of the heart during surgery or central venous catheter insertion can precipitate ventricular fibrillation in patients at risk. ECG tracings in ventricular fibrillation may show high-amplitude (coarse) or low-amplitude (fine) fibrillatory activity. Low-amplitude fibrillation may be confused with asystole depending on the leads used for monitoring. Ventricular fibrillation requires immediate recognition and initiation of cardiopulmonary resuscitation, including electrical defibrillation.

Asystole

Asystole is the absence of ventricular electrical activity, also known as cardiac standstill. No ventricular complexes are

Table 12-6. The NASPE/BPEG Generic Pacemaker Code

	Position				
	I	II	III	IV	V
	CHAMBER(S) PACED	CHAMBER(S) SENSED	RESPONSE TO SENSING	PROGRAMMABILITY RATE MODULATION	ANTITACHYARRHYTHMIA FUNCTION(S)
Letter codes	O = None	O = None	O = None	O = None	O = None
	A = Atrium	A = Atrium	T = Triggered	P = Simple programmable	P = Pacing (antitachyarrhythmia)
	V = Ventricle	V = Ventricle	I = Inhibited	M = Multiprogrammable	S = Shock
	D = Dual (A + V)	D = Dual (A + V)	D = Dual (T + I)	C = Communicating	D = Dual (P + S)
				R = Rate modulation	
Manufacturers designation only	S = Single (A or V)	S = Single (A or V)			

NASPE, North American Society of Pacing and Electrophysiology; BPEG, British Pacing and Electrophysiology Group. Modified from Bernstein AD, Camm AJ, Fletcher RD, et al: The NASPE/BPEG generic pacemaker codes for antibradyarrhythmia and adaptive-rate pacing and antitachyarrhythmia devices. Pacing Clin Electrophysiol 1987; 10:794.

Table 12–7. Rate-Responsive Pacemakers and Possible Interference Sources

Pacemaker Sensor	Physiologic Basis	Algorithm of the Pacemaker	Pacemaker Name	Manufacturer	Approval	Anesthetic Hazard
Activity	Muscle movement	Piezoelectric crystal activation	Activitrax Sensolog	Medtronic Siemens	Clinical Clinical	Vibration of patient or pacemaker
Q–T interval	Q–T decreases as heart rate increases	Onset of paced QRS to end of T wave	Quintech TX	Vitatron	Clinical	Drugs interfering with intracardiac conduction time
Respiratory	Respiratory rate	Thorax impedance changes	Biorate	Biotec	Clinical	Ventilation rate
Respiratory	Minute ventilation	Thorax impedance changes	META	Telectronics	Clinical	Hyperventilation
Temperature	Central venous blood temperature	Measurement of temperature changes	Kelvin 500 Nova MR Thermos	Cook Intermedics Biotronik	Clinical Clinical Clinical	Changes in blood temperature
pH	Central venous pH	pH measurement changes			Preclinical	pH changes
dP/dt	Right ventricular pressure	Piezoelectric crystal in the pacing lead	Deltatrax	Medtronic	Clinical	Factors affecting right ventricular pressure
O₂ saturation	Central venous blood saturation	Hemoreflectorimetry	Oxytrax	Medtronic	Clinical	Oxygen treatment
RVSV		Intraventricular impedance			Preclinical	
Ventricular depolarization gradient		Integration of paced evoked QRS complex	Prism CL	Telectronics	Clinical	

RVSV, right ventricular stroke volume.
From Anderson C, Madsen GM. Rate-responsive pacemakers and anaesthesia: A consideration of possible implications. Anaesthesia 1990; 45:474.

seen on ECG, although continued atrial activity may be seen. Immediate institution of cardiopulmonary resuscitation (CPR) is required, with atropine, isoproterenol, epinephrine, or temporary pacing. Care must be taken when a flat ECG tracing is seen not to assume ECG lead disconnection, and delay the diagnosis of asystole. Presence of an arterial pulse rules out asystole.

Electrocardiographic Monitoring of Pacemakers

Approximately 2 million persons worldwide have a permanent, implanted pacemaker, including many patients undergoing surgery or those admitted to the ICU. Indications for permanent pacing include symptomatic bradycardia, SSS, high-grade conduction block such as bifascicular or complete heart block, as well as some cases of unexplained syncope. Malfunction of a pacemaker can lead to AV dyssynchrony, decreased cardiac output, hypotension, and malignant cardiac arrhythmias. Many factors can interfere with pacemaker function, and an understanding of basic pacemaker technology is crucial to diagnosis and management of patients with implanted pacemakers. Pacemakers may be classified according to which cardiac chambers are paced (unipolar vs. bipolar), the capability of sensing intrinsic electrical activity (demand pacemakers), as well as other higher-level functions.

A three-letter code designation was developed in 1974 by the Inter-Society Commission for Heart Disease Resources[239] and has been revised several times, reflecting advances in pacemaker capabilities. The North American Society of Pacing and Electrophysiology (NASPE), in conjunction with the British Pacing and Electrophysiology Group (BPEG) established the NASPE/BPEG generic pacemaker code in 1987,[240] the most widely used and accepted code system used today (Table 12–6). The first letter designates the cardiac chamber

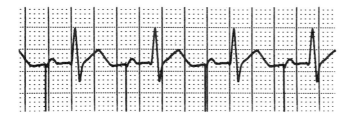

Figure 12–48. Appropriate capture during atrial pacing. Each pacemaker spike is followed by a P wave. (From Morton PG: The pacemaker and defibrillator codes: Implications for critical care nursing. Crit Care Nurs 1997; 17:56.)

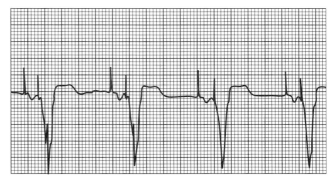

Figure 12–49. ECG of a patient with a dual chamber pacemaker. A pacing stimulus precedes each P wave and QRS complex. (From Morton PG: The pacemaker and defibrillator codes: Implications for critical care nursing. Crit Care Nurse 1997; 17:56.)

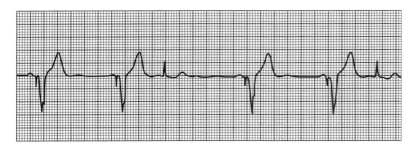

Figure 12–50. Following two paced ventricular complexes, a P wave is conducted normally to the ventricle, and the VVI pacemaker senses the QRS complex and inhibits the pacemaker. (From Zipes DP, Duffin EG: Cardiac pacemakers. *In* Braunwald E (ed): Heart Disease: A Textbook of Cardiovascular Disease, ed 3. Philadelphia, WB Saunders, 1988, p 725.)

paced, the second letter represents the chamber sensed, and the third letter reflects the pacemaker's response to sensing electrical activity. The letter *I* in position III means that the pacemaker *i*nhibits further firing when electrical activity is sensed. The letter *T* in the III position denotes a pacemaker that *t*riggers pacing activity in response to sensed electrical activity. A "triggering" pacemaker will pace the ventricle in response to sensing atrial activity, for example. A pacemaker with the letter *D* (for *d*ual) in the III position combines both inhibition and triggering activity. Positions IV and V relate to programmability and antitachyarrhythmia functions. The letter *R* in the IV position represents a pacemaker with the ability to alter its pacing *r*ate in *r*esponse to sensed changes in some physiologic parameter.[240-242] These "rate-responsive" pacemakers allow for increased cardiac output and oxygen delivery in response to increased demand, as seen with exercise, metabolic stress, and so forth. Table 12–7 lists some rate-responsive pacemakers, the physiologic parameter that is monitored to alter the pacing rate, and some possible hazards that can adversely affect the pacemaker.

ECG assessment of pacemaker function involves evaluation of "capture" or pacing capacity, sensing of intrinsic electrical activity, and response to the sensed signals. Appropriate capture is noted whenever the pacemaker-generated electrical spike is followed by an appropriate P wave or QRS complex (Figs. 12–48 and 12–49). Appropriate inhibitory function of the pacemaker can be demonstrated by the absence of pacemaker stimuli after sensed intrinsic electrical activity (Figure 12–50). Loss of sensing ability usually precedes loss of pacing activity in most pacemakers, with pacemaker stimuli noted at inappropriate times during the ECG cycle (Fig. 12–51). Pacemakers can also sense and be inappropriately inhibited by noncardiac events such as lithotripsy,[243-247] electrocautery,[248-253] muscular activity, or nearby electromagnetic interference.[254, 255] Applying an external magnet or preemptively resetting the pacemaker into a nonsensing mode such as atrial asynchronous (AOO), ventricular asynchronous, (VOO), or dual-chamber asynchronous (DOO) will prevent inadvertent suppression due to external stimuli. In addition, strong electromagnetic interference such as surgical electrocautery may reprogram the pacemaker generator, potentially creating an unstable rhythm (i.e., runaway pacemaker).[252, 255] Careful interrogation of the pacemaker generator should be immediately undertaken following any potential reprogramming.

REFERENCES

1. Mirvis DM, Berson AS, Goldberger AL, et al: Instrumentation and practice standards for electrocardiographic monitoring in special care units. A report for health professionals by a Task Force of the Council on Clinical Cardiology. Circulation 1989; 79:464–471.
2. Mason RE, Likar I: A new system of multiple-lead exercise electrocardiography. Am Heart J 1966; 71:196–205.
3. Bazaral MG, Norfleet EA: Comparison of CB₅ and V₅ leads for intraoperative electrocardiographic monitoring. Anesth Analg 1981; 60:849–853.
4. Blackburn H, Katigbak R: What electrocardiographic leads to take after exercise? Am Heart J 1964; 67:184–185.
5. Drew BJ: Bedside electrocardiographic monitoring: State of the art for the 1990s. Heart Lung 1991; 20:610–623.
6. Kates RA, Zaidan JR, Kaplan JA: Esophageal lead for intraoperative electrocardiographic monitoring. Anesth Analg 1982; 61: 781–785.
7. Fletcher RD, Saunders RC: Technique of esophageal electrocardiography. *In* Hurst JW (ed): The Heart, ed 6. New York, McGraw-Hill, 1986, pp 1690–1703.
8. Katz A, Guetta V, Ovsyshcher IA: Transesophageal electrocardiography using a temporary pacing balloon-tipped electrode in acute cardiac care. Ann Emerg Med 1991; 20:961–963.
9. Rice MJ, Atlee JL III: Electrocardiography: Monitoring for arrhythmias. *In* Lake CL (ed): Clinical Monitoring. Philadelphia, WB Saunders, 1990, pp 53–84.
10. Parker EO III: Electrosurgical burn at the site of an esophageal temperature probe. Anesthesiology 1984; 61:93–95.
11. Waldo AL, Henthorn RW, Plumb VJ: Temporary epicardial wire electrodes in the diagnosis and treatment of arrhythmias after open heart surgery. Am J Surg 1984; 148:275–283.
12. Lombness PM: Taking the mystery out of rhythm interpretation: Atrial electrograms. Heart Lung 1992; 21:415–426.
13. Waldo AL, Kaiser GA: Electrophysiologic consideration for the cardiac surgical patient. *In* Litwak RS, Jurado RA (eds): Care of the Cardiac Surgical Patient. Norwalk, CT, Appleton-Century-Crofts, 1982, pp 241–280.
14. Schultz CK, Woodall CE: Using epicardial pacing electrodes. J Cardiovasc Nurs 1989; 3:25–33.
15. Donovan KD, Power BM, Hockings BE, et al: Usefulness of atrial electrocardiograms recorded via central venous catheters in the diagnosis of complex cardiac arrhythmias. Crit Care Med 1993; 21:532–537.
16. Martin JT: Neuroanesthetic adjuncts for patients in the sitting position. III. Intravascular electrocardiography. Anesth Analg 1970; 49:793–808.

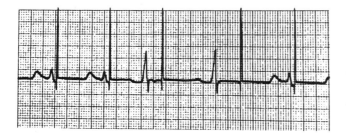

Figure 12–51. Loss of pacemaker sensing function, with pacer stimuli following, during, and immediately following native QRS complexes. (From Hayes DL: Pacemaker electrocardiography. *In* Furman S, Hayes D, Holmes D Jr. (eds): A Practice of Cardiac Pacing, ed 3. Mount Kisco, NY, Futura, 1993, pp 30–359.)

17. Kint PP, Spaa W, van den Berg A, et al: Recording the right atrial electrogram through the fluid column of a pulmonary artery catheter. Crit Care Med 1985; 13:982–984.
18. Vincent J-L: New developments in pulmonary artery catheterization. Int Care World 1986; 3:42–43.
19. Ehrenwerth J: Electrical safety. *In* Barash PG, Cullen BF, Stoelting RK (eds): Clinical Anesthesia. Philadelphia, JB Lippincott, 1989, pp 625–644.
20. Barker SJ, Tremper KK: Physics applied to anesthesia. *In* Barash PG, Cullen BF, Stoelting RK (eds): Clinical Anesthesia. Philadelphia, JB Lippincott, 1989, pp 91–133.
21. Geddes LA, Tacker WA, Rosborough J, et al: The electrical doses for ventricular defibrillation with electrodes applied directly to the heart. J Thorac Cardiovasc Surg 1974; 68:593–602.
22. Watson AB, Wright JS, Loughman J: Electrical thresholds for ventricular fibrillation in man. Med J Aust 1973; 1:1179–1182.
23. Becker CM, Malhotra IV, Hedley-Whyte J: The distribution of radiofrequency current and burns. Anesthesiology 1973; 38:106–122.
24. Menon DK, Peden CJ, Hall AS, et al: Magnetic resonance for the anesthetist. Part I: Physical principles, applications, safety aspects. Anaesthesia 1992; 47:240–255.
25. Tobin JR, Spurrier EA, Wetzel RC: Anaesthesia for critically ill children during magnetic resonance imaging. Br J Anaesth 1992; 69:482–486.
26. Roth JL, Nugent M, Gray JE, et al: Patient monitoring during magnetic resonance imaging. Anesthesiology 1985; 62:80–83.
27. Sabbah HN, Stein PD: Early segmental thinning of the left ventricular wall following regional ischemia. Cathet Cardiovasc Diagn 1983; 9:473–482.
28. Forrester JS, Wyatt HL, Da Luz PL, et al: Functional significance of regional ischemic contraction abnormalities. Circulation 1976; 54:64–70.
29. Watanabe S, Buffington CW: Speed and sensitivity of mechanical versus electrographic indicators to mild or moderate myocardial ischemia in the pig. Anesthesiology 1994; 80:582–594.
30. Mori H, Ogawa S, Hayashi J, et al: Electrophysiologic and myocardial metabolic changes in the acute phase of partial coronary occlusion. Am Heart J 1983; 106:624–630.
31. Waters DD, Da Luz P, Wyatt HL, et al: Early changes in regional and global left ventricular function induced by graded reductions in regional coronary perfusion. Am J Cardiol 1977; 39:537–543.
32. Case RB, Nasser MG, Crampton RS: Biochemical aspects of early myocardial ischemia. Am J Cardiol 1969; 24:766–775.
33. Chierchia S, Brunelli C, Simonetti I, et al: Sequence of events in angina at rest: Primary reduction in coronary flow. Circulation 1980; 61:759–768.
34. Knight AA, Hollenberg M, London MJ, et al: Perioperative myocardial ischemia: Importance of the preoperative ischemic pattern. Anesthesiology 1988; 68:681–688.
35. Raby KE, Goldman L, Cook EF, et al: Long-term prognosis of myocardial ischemia detected by Holter monitoring in peripheral vascular disease. Am J Cardiol 1990; 66:1309–1313.
36. McCann RL, Clements FM: Silent myocardial ischemia in patients undergoing peripheral vascular surgery: Incidence and association with perioperative cardiac morbidity and mortality. J Vasc Surg 1989; 9:583–587.
37. Pasternack PF, Grossi EA, Baumann FG, et al: The value of silent myocardial ischemia monitoring in the prediction of perioperative myocardial infarction in patients undergoing peripheral vascular surgery. J Vasc Surg 1989; 10:617–625.
38. Gunther H, Osterspey A, Treis-Muller I, et al: The sensitivity of 24 h Holter monitoring and exercise testing for the recognition of myocardial ischaemia: A comparative study. Eur Heart J 1988; 9(suppl N):46–49.
39. Selwyn AP, Shea M, Deanfield JE, et al: Character of transient ischemia in angina pectoris. Am J Cardiol 1986; 58:21B–25B.
40. Nademanee K, Intarachot V, Singh PN, et al: Characteristics and clinical significance of silent myocardial ischemia in unstable angina. Am J Cardiol 1986; 58:26B–33B.
41. Schang SJ Jr, Pepine CJ: Transient asymptomatic S-T segment depression during daily activity. Am J Cardiol 1977; 39:396–402.
42. Cecchi AC, Dovellini EV, Marchi F, et al: Silent myocardial ischemia during ambulatory electrocardiographic monitoring in patients with effort angina. J Am Coll Cardiol 1983; 1:934–939.
43. Rocco MB, Nabel EG, Campbell S, et al: Prognostic importance of myocardial ischemia detected by ambulatory monitoring in patients with stable coronary artery disease. Circulation 1988; 78:877–884.
44. Gottlieb SO, Weisfeldt ML, Ouyang P, et al: Silent ischemia as a marker for early unfavorable outcomes in patients with unstable angina. N Engl J Med 1986; 314:1214–1219.
45. Biagini A, Mazzei MG, Carpeggiani C, et al: Vasospastic ischemic mechanism of frequent asymptomatic transient ST-T changes during continuous electrocardiographic monitoring in selected unstable angina patients. Am Heart J 1982; 103:13–20.
46. Deanfield JE, Ribiero P, Oakley K, et al: Analysis of ST-segment changes in normal subjects: Implications for ambulatory monitoring in angina pectoris. Am J Cardiol 1984; 54:1321–1325.
47. Wohlgelernter D, Jafe CC, Cabin HS, et al: Silent ischemia during coronary occlusion produced by balloon inflation: Relation to regional myocardial dysfunction. J Am Coll Cardiol 1987; 10:491–498.
48. Parthenakis F, Kochiadakis G, Simantirakis E, et al: Incidence of ventricular arrhythmias during silent myocardial ischaemia in coronary artery disease. Int J Cardiol 1996; 57:61–67.
49. Geft IL, Fishbein MC, Ninomiya K, et al: Intermittent brief periods of ischemia have a cumulative effect and may cause myocardial necrosis. Circulation 1982; 66:1150–1153.
50. Landesberg G, Einav S, Christopherson R, et al: Perioperative ischemia and cardiac complications in major vascular surgery: Importance of the preoperative twelve-lead electrocardiogram. J Vasc Surg 1997; 26:570–578.
51. Cohn PF: Total ischemic burden: Pathophysiology and prognosis. Am J Cardiol 1987; 59:3C–6C.
52. Amsterdam EA: Relation of silent myocardial ischemia to ventricular arrhythmias and sudden death. Am J Cardiol 1988; 62:24I–27I.
53. Aronow WS, Epstein S: Usefulness of silent myocardial ischemia detected by ambulatory electrocardiographic monitoring in predicting new coronary events in elderly patients. Am J Cardiol 1988; 62:1295–1296.
54. Weiner DA, Ryan JT, Parsons L, et al: Significance of silent myocardial ischemia during exercise testing in patients with diabetes mellitus: A report from the Coronary Artery Surgery Study (CASS) Registry. Am J Cardiol 1991; 68:729–734.
55. Aronow WS, Mercando AD, Epstein S: Prevalence of silent myocardial ischemia detected by 24-hour ambulatory electrocardiography, and its association with new coronary events at 40-month follow-up in elderly diabetic and nondiabetic patients with coronary artery disease. Am J Cardiol 1992; 69:555–556.
56. Stone PH, Chaitman BR, Forman S, et al: Prognostic significance of myocardial ischemia detected by ambulatory electrocardiography, exercise treadmill testing, and electrocardiogram at rest to predict cardiac events by one year (the Asymptomatic Cardiac Ischemia Pilot [ACIP] study). Am J Cardiol 1997; 80:1395–1401.
57. Bridges SL Jr, Hollowell JS, Stagg SW, et al: Is silent ischemia on the routine admission ECG an important finding? J Electrocardiol 1993; 26:131–136.
58. Gottlieb SO, Weisfeldt ML, Ouyang P, et al: Silent ischemia predicts infarction and death during 2 year follow-up of unstable angina. J Am Coll Cardiol 1987; 10:756–760.
59. Mark DB, Hlatky MA, Califf RM, et al: Painless exercise ST deviation on the treadmill: Long-term prognosis. J Am Coll Cardiol 1989; 14:885–892.
60. Quintana M, Lindvall K, Brolund F: Assessment and significance of ST-segment changes detected by ambulatory electrocardiography after acute myocardial infarction. Am J Cardiol 1995; 76:6–13.
61. Hohnloser SH, Kasper W, Zehender M, et al: Silent myocardial ischemia as a predisposing factor for ventricular fibrillation. Am J Cardiol 1988; 61:461–463.
62. Landesberg G, Luria MH, Cotev S, et al: Importance of long-duration postoperative ST-segment depression in cardiac morbidity after vascular surgery. Lancet 1993; 341:715–719.
63. Pasternack PF, Grossi EA, Baumann FG, et al: Silent myocardial

ischemia monitoring predicts late as well as perioperative cardiac events in patients undergoing vascular surgery. J Vasc Surg 1992; 16:171–180.

64. Weiner DA, Ryan TJ, Parsons L, et al: Prevalence and prognostic significance of silent and symptomatic ischemia after coronary bypass surgery: A report from the Coronary Artery Surgery Study (CASS) randomized population. J Am Coll Cardiol 1991; 18:343–348.

65. Slogoff S, Keats AS: Further observations on perioperative myocardial ischemia. Anesthesiology 1986; 65:539–542.

66. Ganz LI, Andrews TC, Barry J, et al: Silent ischemia preceding sudden cardiac death in a patient after vascular surgery. Am Heart J 1994; 127:1652–1654.

67. Raby KE, Barry J, Creager MA, et al: Detection and significance of intraoperative and postoperative myocardial ischemia in peripheral vascular surgery. JAMA 1992; 268:222–227.

68. Slogoff S, Keats AS: Does perioperative myocardial ischemia lead to postoperative myocardial infarction? Anesthesiology 1985; 62:107–114.

69. Raby KE, Goldman L, Creager MA, et al: Correlation between preoperative ischemia and major cardiac events after peripheral vascular surgery. N Engl J Med 1989; 321:1296–1300.

70. Hurford WE, Favorito F: Association of myocardial ischemia with failure to wean from mechanical ventilation. Crit Care Med 1995; 23:1475–1480.

71. Chatila W, Ani S, Guaglianone D, et al: Cardiac ischemia during weaning from mechanical ventilation. Chest 1996; 109:1577–1583.

72. Wallace A, Layug B, Tateo I, et al: Prophylactic atenolol reduces postoperative myocardial ischemia. Anesthesiology 1998; 88:7–17.

73. Waters DD, Forrester JS: Myocardial ischemia: detection and quantitation. Ann Intern Med 1978; 88:239–250.

74. Kleber AG, Janse MJ, van Capelle FJ, et al: Mechanism and time course of S-T and T-Q segment changes during acute regional myocardial ischemia in the pig heart determined by extracellular and intracellular recordings. Circ Res 1978; 42:603–613.

75. Guyton RA, McClenathan JH, Newman GE, et al: Significance of subendocardial S-T segment elevation caused by coronary stenosis in the dog. Epicardial S-T segment depression, local ischemia and subsequent necrosis. Am J Cardiol 1977; 40:373–380.

76. Belic N, Gardin JM: ECG manifestations of myocardial ischemia. Arch Intern Med 1980; 140:1162–1165.

77. Blackburn H, Katigbak R: What electrocardiographic leads to take after exercise? Am Heart J 1964; 67:184–185.

78. Smith H, Nathan H, Harrison M: Failure to predict intraoperative myocardial ischaemia in patients with coronary artery disease. Can J Anaesth 1989; 36:539–544.

79. Chierchia S, Lazzari M, Freedman B, et al: Impairment of myocardial perfusion and function during painless myocardial ischemia. J Am Coll Cardiol 1983; 1:924–930.

80. Singh BN, Nademanee K, Figueras J, et al: Hemodynamic and electrocardiographic correlates of symptomatic and silent myocardial ischemia: Pathophysiologic and therapeutic implications. Am J Cardiol 1986; 58:3B–10B.

81. Kaplan JA, King SB III: The precordial electrocardiographic lead (V5) in patients who have coronary-artery disease. Anesthesiology 1976; 45:570–574.

82. Roy WL, Edelist G, Gilbert B: Myocardial ischemia during noncardiac surgical procedures in patients with coronary-artery disease. Anesthesiology 1979; 51:393–397.

83. London MJ, Hollenberg M, Wong MG, et al: Intraoperative myocardial ischemia: Localization by continuous 12-lead electrocardiography. Anesthesiology 1988; 69:232–241.

84. Jain U: An electrocardiographic lead system for coronary artery bypass surgery. J Clin Anesth 1996; 8:19–24.

85. Griffin RM, Kaplan JA: Myocardial ischaemia during non-cardiac surgery. A comparison of different lead systems using computerised ST segment analysis. Anaesthesia 1987; 42:155–159.

86. De Hert SG, Moens MM, Vermeyen KM, et al: Use of the right-sided precordial lead V4R in the detection of intraoperative myocardial ischemia. J Cardiothorac Vasc Anesth 1993; 7:659–667.

87. Machler HE, Lueger A, Rehak P, et al: A new high-resolution esophageal electrocardiography recording technique: An experimental approach for the detection of myocardial ischemia. Anesth Analg 1998; 86:34–39.

88. Jadvar H, Jenkins JM, Arzbaecher RC: A system for simultaneous esophageal atrial pacing and ventricular recording in computer analysis of posterior ischemia. J Electrocardiol 1989; 22(suppl):248–252.

89. Trager MA, Feinberg BI, Kaplan JA: Right ventricular ischemia diagnosed by an esophageal electrocardiogram and right atrial pressure tracing. J Cardiothorac Anesth 1987; 1:123–125.

90. Jain U: Wave recognition and use of the intraoperative unipolar esophageal electrocardiogram. J Clin Anesth 1997; 9:487–492.

91. Hayes JK, Peters JL, Smith KW, et al.: Monitoring normal and aberrant electrocardiographic activity from an endotracheal tube: Comparison of the surface, esophageal, and tracheal electrocardiograms. J Clin Monit Comput 1994; 10:81–90.

92. Siegel S, Brodman R, Fisher J, et al: Intracardiac electrode detection of early or subendocardial ischemia. Pacing Clin Electrophysiol 1982; 5:892–902.

93. Triposkiadis F, Papadopoulos P, Masdrakis G, et al: Continuous electrocardiographic monitoring in patients with unstable angina pectoris: Evaluation of medical treatment. Acta Cardiol 1987; 42:263–271.

94. Arbeit SR, Rubin IL, Gross H: Dangers in interpreting the electrocardiogram from the oscilloscope monitor. JAMA 1970; 211:453–456.

95. Bragg-Remschel DA, Anderson CM, Winkle RA: Frequency response characteristics of ambulatory ECG monitoring systems and their implications for ST segment analysis. Am Heart J 1982; 103:20–31.

96. Hinderliter AL, Bragdon E, Herbst M, et al: A comparison of amplitude-modulated and frequency-modulated ambulatory monitoring systems. Am J Cardiol 1989; 64:76–80.

97. Schluter P: Magnetic tape recording and playback for ST-segment analysis. J Electrocardiol 1988; 21(suppl):S20–26.

98. Shook TL, Balke CW, Kotilainen PW, et al: Comparison of amplitude-modulated (direct) and frequency-modulated ambulatory techniques for recording ischemic electrocardiographic changes. Am J Cardiol 1987; 60:895–900.

99. Tayler DI, Vincent R: Artefactual ST segment abnormalities due to electrocardiograph design. Br Heart J 1985; 54:121–128.

100. Levin RI: Quantitation of transient myocardial ischemia by digital, ambulatory electrocardiography. Am J Cardiol 1988; 61:13B–17B.

101. Mangano DT, Wong MG, London MJ, et al: Perioperative myocardial ischemia in patients undergoing noncardiac surgery—II: Incidence and severity during the 1st week after surgery. The Study of Perioperative Ischemia (SPI) Research Group. J Am Coll Cardiol 1991; 17:851–857.

102. Barry J, Campbell S, Nabel EG, et al: Ambulatory monitoring of the digitized electrocardiogram for detection and early warning of transient myocardial ischemia in angina pectoris. Am J Cardiol 1987; 60:483–488.

103. Jamal SM, Mitra-Duncan L, Kelly DT, et al: Validation of a real-time electrocardiographic monitor for detection of myocardial ischemia secondary to coronary artery disease. Am J Cardiol 1987; 60:525–527.

104. Dunn RF, Freedman B, Bailey IK, et al: Localization of coronary artery disease with exercise electrocardiography: Correlation with thallium-201 myocardial perfusion scanning. Am J Cardiol 1981; 48:837–843.

105. Clements FM, McCann RL, Levin RI: Continuous ST segment analysis for the detection of perioperative myocardial ischemia. Crit Care Med 1988; 16:710–711.

106. London MJ, Ahlstrom LD: Validation testing of the spacelabs PC2 ST-segment analyzer. J Cardiothorac Vasc Anesth 1995; 9:684–693.

107. London MJ: Validation testing of the SEER real-time digital holter monitor. J Cardiothorac Vasc Anesth 1996; 10:497–501.

108. Ansley DM, O'Connor JP, Merrick PM, et al: On line ST-segment analysis for detection of myocardial ischaemia during and after coronary revascularization. Can J Anaesth 1996; 43:995–1000.

109. Leung JM, Voskanian A, Bellows WH, et al: Automated electrocardiograph ST segment trending monitors: Accuracy in detecting myocardial ischemia. Anesth Analg 1998; 87:4–10.

110. Kotter GS, Kotrly KJ, Kalbfleisch JH, et al: Myocardial ischemia during cardiovascular surgery as detected by an ST segment trend monitoring system. J Cardiothorac Anesth 1987; 1:190–199.

111. Fesmire FM, Smith EE: Continuous 12-lead electrocardiograph monitoring in the emergency department. Am J Emerg Med 1993; 11:54–60.

112. Fesmire FM, Percy RF, Bardoner JB, et al: Usefulness of automated serial 12-lead ECG monitoring during the initial emergency department evaluation of patients with chest pain. Ann Emerg Med 1998; 31:3–11.

113. Finefrock SC: Continuous 12-lead ST segment monitoring: an adjunct to identifying silent ischemia and infarct in the emergency department. J Emerg Nurs 1995; 21:413–416.

114. Fu GY, Joseph AJ, Antalis G: Application of continuous ST-segment monitoring in the detection of silent myocardial ischemia. Ann Emerg Med 1994; 23:1113–1115.

115. Krucoff MW, Wagner NB, Pope JE, et al: The portable programmable microprocessor-driven real-time 12-lead electrocardiographic monitor: A preliminary report of a new device for the noninvasive detection of successful reperfusion or silent coronary reocclusion. Am J Cardiol 1990; 65:143–148.

116. Drew BJ, Adams MG, Pelter MM, et al: Comparison of standard and derived 12-lead electrocardiograms for diagnosis of coronary angioplasty-induced myocardial ischemia. Am J Cardiol 1997; 79:639–644.

117. Krucoff M: Identification of high-risk patients with silent myocardial ischemia after percutaneous transluminal coronary angioplasty by multilead monitoring. Am J Cardiol 1988; 61:29F–35F.

118. Krucoff MW, Jackson YR, Kehoe MK, et al: Quantitative and qualitative ST segment monitoring during and after percutaneous transluminal coronary angioplasty. Circulation 1990; 81(suppl 3):IV20–26.

119. Meyers DG, Bendon KA, Hankins JH, et al: The effect of baseline electrocardiographic abnormalities on the diagnostic accuracy of exercise-induced ST segment changes. Am Heart J 1990; 119:272–276.

120. Sundqvist K, Atterhog JH, Jogestrand T: Effect of digoxin on the electrocardiogram at rest and during exercise in healthy subjects. Am J Cardiol 1986; 57:661–665.

121. Jones J, Srodulski ZM, Romisher S: The aging electrocardiogram. Am J Emerg Med 1990; 8:240–245.

122. Dellborg M, Herlitz J, Emanuelsson H, et al: ECG changes during myocardial ischemia. Differences between men and women. J Electrocardiol 1994; 27(suppl):42–45.

123. Ardissino D, De Servi S, Barberis P, et al: Significance of hyperventilation-induced ST segment depression in patients with coronary artery disease. J Am Coll Cardiol 1989; 13:804–810.

124. Lary D, Goldschlager N: Electrocardiographic changes during hyperventilation resembling myocardial ischemia in patients with normal coronary arteriograms. Am Heart J 1974; 87:383–390.

125. Magarian GJ, Jones S, Calverley T: Hyperventilation testing for coronary vasospasm: Induction of spontaneous ventricular tachycardia in association with transmural ischemia without obstructive coronary disease. Am Heart J 1990; 120:1447–1449.

126. Adams MG, Drew BJ: Body position effects on the ECG: Implication for ischemia monitoring. J Electrocardiol 1997; 30:285–291.

127. Gavrielides S, Kaski JC, Tousoulis D, et al: Duration of ST segment depression after exercise-induced myocardial ischemia is influenced by body position during recovery but not by type of exercise. Am Heart J 1991; 121:1665–1670.

128. Mangar D, Lightly GW Jr, Camporesi EM: Electrocardiographic changes associated with the prone position (letter). J Clin Monit Comput 1992; 8:92–93.

129. Wetherbee JN, Bamrah VS, Ptacin MJ, et al: Comparison of ST segment depression in upright treadmill and supine bicycle exercise testing. J Am Coll Cardiol 1988; 11:330–337.

130. Slogoff S, Keats AS, David Y, et al: Incidence of perioperative myocardial ischemia detected by different electrocardiographic systems. Anesthesiology 1990; 73:1074–1081.

131. Camann W, Trunfio GV, Kluger R, et al: Automated ST-segment analysis during cesarean delivery: Effects of ECG filtering modality. J Clin Anesth 1996; 8:564–567.

132. Brooker S, Lowenstein E: Spurious ST segment depression by automated ST segment analysis. J Clin Monit Comput 1995; 11:186–188.

133. Wenger W, Kligfield P: Variability of precordial electrode placement during routine electrocardiography. J Electrocardiol 1996; 29:179–184.

134. Khambatta HJ, Stone JG, Wald A, et al: Electrocardiographic artifacts during cardiopulmonary bypass. Anesth Analg 1990; 71:88–91.

135. Kleinman B, Shah K, Belusko R, et al: Electrocardiographic artifact caused by extracorporeal roller pump (letter). J Clin Monit Comput 1990; 6:258–259.

136. Metz S: ECG artifacts during cardiopulmonary bypass—an alternative method. Anesth Analg 1991; 72:715–716.

137. Gardner RM, Hollingsworth KW: Optimizing the electrocardiogram and pressure monitoring. Crit Care Med 1986; 14:651–658.

138. Dwyer EM Jr: The predictive accuracy of the electrocardiogram in identifying the presence and location of myocardial infarction and coronary artery disease. Ann N Y Acad Sci 1990; 601:67–76.

139. Fox RM, Hakki AH, Iskandrian AS: Relation between electrocardiographic and scintigraphic location of myocardial ischemia during exercise in one-vessel coronary artery disease. Am J Cardiol 1984; 53:1529–1531.

140. Freedman SB, Dunn RF: Relation between electrocardiographic and scintigraphic location of myocardial ischemia in 1-vessel coronary artery disease (letter). Am J Cardiol 1985; 56:704.

141. Fuchs RM, Achuff SC, Grunwald L, et al: Electrocardiographic localization of coronary artery narrowings: Studies during myocardial ischemia and infarction in patients with one-vessel disease. Circulation 1982; 66:1168–1176.

142. Lamberti JJ, Silver H, Howell J, et al: Transmural gradients of experimental myocardial ischemia: Limited correlation of ultrastructure with epicardial S-T segment elevation. Am Heart J 1978; 96:496–506.

143. Barnard RJ, Buckberg GD, Duncan HW: Limitations of the standard transthoracic electrocardiogram in detecting subendocardial ischemia. Am Heart J 1980; 99:476–482.

144. Breslow MJ, Miller CF, Parker SD, et al: Changes in T-wave morphology following anesthesia and surgery: A common recovery-room phenomenon. Anesthesiology 1986; 64:398–402.

145. Jakobsson J, Rehnqvist N, Davidson S: Computerised evaluation of the electrocardiogram during and for a short period after gall bladder surgery. Acta Anaesthesiol Scand 1989; 3:474–477.

146. Gordon MA, Urban MK, O'Connor T, et al: Is the pressure rate quotient a predictor or indicator of myocardial ischemia as measured by ST-segment changes in patients undergoing coronary artery bypass surgery? Anesthesiology 1991; 74:848–853.

147. Harris SN, Gordon MA, Urban MK, et al: The pressure rate quotient is not an indicator of myocardial ischemia in humans. An echocardiographic evaluation. Anesthesiology 1993; 78:242–250.

148. Leung JM, O'Kelly BF, Mangano DT: Relationship of regional wall motion abnormalities to hemodynamic indices of myocardial oxygen supply and demand in patients undergoing CABG surgery. Anesthesiology 1990; 73:802–814.

149. Bourdillon PD, Lorell BH, Mirsky I, et al: Increased regional myocardial stiffness of the left ventricle during pacing-induced angina in man. Circulation 1983; 67:316–323.

150. McCans JL, Parker JO: Left ventricular pressure-volume relationships during myocardial ischemia in man. Circulation 1973; 48:775–785.

151. McLaurin LP, Rolett EL, Grossman W: Impaired left ventricular relaxation during pacing-induced ischemia. Am J Cardiol 1973; 32:751–757.

152. Kaplan JA, Wells PH: Early diagnosis of myocardial ischemia using the pulmonary arterial catheter. Anesth Analg 1981; 60:789–793.

153. Sanchez R, Wee M: Perioperative myocardial ischemia: Early diagnosis using the pulmonary artery catheter. J Cardiothorac Vasc Anesth 1991; 5:604–607.

154. Sharkey SW, Aberg NB: Hemodynamic evidence of painless myocardial ischemia with acute pulmonary edema in coronary disease. Am Heart J 1995; 129:188–191.

155. Haggmark S, Hohner P, Ostman M, et al: Comparison of hemo-dynamic, electrocardiographic, mechanical, and metabolic indi-cators of intraoperative myocardial ischemia in vascular surgical patients with coronary artery disease. Anesthesiology 1989; 70:19-25.

156. Hogue CW Jr, Davila-Roman VG: Detection of myocardial ische-mia by transesophageal echocardiographically determined changes in left ventricular area in patients undergoing coronary artery bypass surgery. J Clin Anesth 1997; 9:388-393.

157. van Daele ME, Sutherland GR, Mitchell MM, et al: Do changes in pulmonary capillary wedge pressure adequately reflect myo-cardial ischemia during anesthesia? A correlative preoperative hemodynamic, electrocardiographic, and transesophageal echo-cardiographic study. Circulation 1990; 81:865-871.

158. Hall RI, O'Regan N, Gardner M: Detection of intraoperative myocardial ischaemia—a comparison among electrocardio-graphic, myocardial metabolic, and haemodynamic measure-ments in patients with reduced ventricular function. Can J Anaesth 1995; 42:487-494.

159. Cheng DC, Chung F, Burns RJ, et al: Postoperative myocardial infarction documented by technetium pyrophosphate scan us-ing single-photon emission computed tomography: Significance of intraoperative myocardial ischemia and hemodynamic con-trol. Anesthesiology 1989; 71:818-826.

160. Konstadt S, Goldman M, Thys D, et al: Intraoperative diagnosis of myocardial ischemia. Mt Sinai J Med 1985; 52:521-525.

161. Battler A, Froelicher VF, Gallagher KP, et al: Dissociation be-tween regional myocardial dysfunction and ECG changes dur-ing ischemia in the conscious dog. Circulation 1980; 62:735-744.

162. Alam M, Khaja F, Brymer J, et al: Echocardiographic evaluation of left ventricular function during coronary artery angioplasty. Am J Cardiol 1986; 57:20-25.

163. Distante A, Rovai D, Picano E, et al: Transient changes in left ventricular mechanics during attacks of Prinzmetal's angina: An M-mode echocardiographic study. Am Heart J 1984; 107:465-474.

164. Hauser AM, Gangadharan V, Ramos RG, et al: Sequence of mechanical, electrocardiographic and clinical effects of re-peated coronary artery occlusion in human beings: Echocardio-graphic observations during coronary angioplasty. J Am Coll Cardiol 1985; 5:193-197.

165. Sugishita Y, Koseki S, Matsuda M, et al: Dissociation between regional myocardial dysfunction and ECG changes during myo-cardial ischemia induced by exercise in patients with angina pectoris. Am Heart J 1983; 106:1-8.

166. Tzivoni D, Diamond G, Pichler M, et al: Analysis of regional ischemic left ventricular dysfunction by quantitative cineangio-graphy. Circulation 1979; 60:1278-1283.

167. Visser CA, David GK, Kan G, et al: Two-dimensional echocardi-ography during percutaneous transluminal coronary angio-plasty. Am Heart J 1986; 111:1035-1041.

168. Wohlgelernter D, Cleman M, Highman HA, et al: Regional myo-cardial dysfunction during coronary angioplasty: Evaluation by two-dimensional echocardiography and 12 lead electrocardiog-raphy. J Am Coll Cardiol 1986; 7:1245-1254.

169. Koolen JJ, Visser CA, Reichert SL, et al: Improved monitoring of myocardial ischaemia during major vascular surgery using transoesophageal echocardiography. Eur Heart J 1992; 13:1028-1033.

170. Leung JM, O'Kelly B, Browner WS, et al: Prognostic importance of postbypass regional wall-motion abnormalities in patients undergoing coronary artery bypass graft surgery. Anesthesiol-ogy 1989; 71:16-25.

171. London MJ, Tubau JF, Wong MG, et al: The "natural history" of segmental wall motion abnormalities in patients undergoing noncardiac surgery. Anesthesiology 1990; 73:644-655.

172. Smith JS, Cahalan MK, Benefiel DJ, et al: Intraoperative detec-tion of myocardial ischemia in high-risk patients: Electrocardi-ography versus two-dimensional transesophageal echocardiogra-phy. Circulation 1985; 72:1015-1021.

173. Bergquist BD, Bellows WH, Leung JM: Transesophageal echo-cardiography in myocardial revascularization: II. Influence on intraoperative decision making. Anesth Analg 1996; 82:1139-1145.

174. Kato M, Nakashima Y, Levine J, et al: Does transesophageal echocardiography improve postoperative outcome in patients undergoing coronary artery bypass surgery? J Cardiothorac Vasc Anesth 1993; 7:285-289.

175. Eisenberg MJ, London MJ, Leung JM, et al: Monitoring for myo-cardial ischemia during noncardiac surgery. A technology as-sessment of transesophageal echocardiography and 12-lead elec-trocardiography. JAMA 1992; 268:210-216.

176. Lambertz H, Kreis A, Trumper H, et al: Simultaneous trans-esophageal atrial pacing and transesophageal two-dimensional echocardiography: A new method of stress echocardiography. J Am Coll Cardiol 1990; 16:1143-1153.

177. Sheikh KH, Bengtson JR, Helmy S, et al: Relation of quantitative coronary lesion measurements to the development of exercise-induced ischemia assessed by exercise echocardiography. J Am Coll Cardiol 1990; 15:1043-1051.

178. Siostrzonek P, Mundigler G, Hassan A, et al: Echocardiographic diagnosis of segmental wall motion abnormalities. Acta Anaes-thesiol Scand Suppl 1997; 111:271-274.

179. Rouine-Rapp K, Ionescu P, Balea M, et al: Detection of intraop-erative segmental wall-motion abnormalities by transesophageal echocardiography: The incremental value of additional cross sections in the transverse and longitudinal planes. Anesth Analg 1996; 83:1141-1148.

180. Huemer G, Weber T, Tschernich H, et al: Intraoperative myo-cardial ischemia and transesophageal echocardiography. Acta Anaesthesiol Scand Suppl 1997; 111:274-276.

181. Bergquist BD, Leung JM, Bellows WH: Transesophageal echo-cardiography in myocardial revascularization: I. Accuracy of in-traoperative real-time interpretation. Anesth Analg 1996; 82:1132-1138.

182. Ellis JE, Shah MN, Briller JE, et al: A comparison of methods for the detection of myocardial ischemia during noncardiac sur-gery: Automated ST-segment analysis systems, electrocardiogra-phy, and transesophageal echocardiography. Anesth Analg 1992; 75:764-772.

183. Wickey GS, Larach DR, Keifer JC, et al: Combined interpreta-tion of transesophageal echocardiography, electrocardiography, and pulmonary artery wedge waveform to detect myocardial ischemia. J Cardiothorac Anesth 1990; 4:102-104.

184. Kurtz CM, Bennett JH, Shapiro HH: ECG studies during surgical anesthesia. JAMA 1936; 106:434-441.

185. Vanik PE, Davis HS: Cardiac arrhythmias during halothane anes-thesia. Anesth Analg 1968; 47:299-307.

186. Kuner J, Enescu V, Utsu F, et al: Cardiac arrhythmias during anesthesia. Dis Chest 1967; 52:580-587.

187. Bertrand CA, Steiner NV, Jameson AG, et al: Disturbances of cardiac rhythm during anesthesia and surgery. JAMA 1971; 216:1615-1617.

188. Angelini P, Feldman MI, Lufschanowski R, et al: Cardiac ar-rhythmias during and after heart surgery: Diagnosis and man-agement. Prog Cardiovasc Dis 1974; 16:469-495.

189. Brodsky M, Wu D, Denes P, et al: Arrhythmias documented by 24-hour continuous electrocardiographic monitoring in 50 male medical students without apparent heart disease. Am J Cardiol 1977; 39:390-395.

190. Atlee JL III, Bosnjak ZJ: Mechanisms for cardiac dysrhythmias during anesthesia. Anesthesiology 1990; 72:347-374.

191. Ruskin J, McHale PA, Harley A, et al: Pressure-flow studies in man: Effect of atrial systole on left ventricular function. J Clin Invest 1970; 49:472-478.

192. Rahimtoola SH, Ehsani A, Sinno MZ, et al: Left atrial transport function in myocardial infarction. Importance of its booster function. Am J Med 1975; 59:686-694.

193. Wojtczak JA: Basic cellular electrophysiology of the heart. In Thys DM, Kaplan JA, (eds): The ECG in Anesthesia and Critical Care. New York, Churchill Livingstone, 1987, pp 109-125.

194. Hoffman BF, Rosen MR: Cellular mechanisms for cardiac ar-rhythmias. Circ Res 1981; 49:1-15.

195. Gorgels APM, Vos MA, Brugada P, et al: The clinical relevance of abnormal automaticity and triggered activity. In Brugada P, Wellens HJJ, (eds): Cardiac Arrhythmias: Where to Go From Here? New York, Futura, 1987, pp 147-169.

196. Rosen MR: Mechanisms for arrhythmias. Am J Cardiol 1988; 61:2A-8A.

197. Manolis AS, Estes NA III: Supraventricular tachycardia. Mechanisms and therapy. Arch Intern Med 1987; 147:1706–1716.
198. Akhtar M: Management of ventricular tachyarrhythmias. Part I. JAMA 1982; 247:671–674.
199. Hollifield JW: Thiazide treatment of hypertension. Effects of thiazide diuretics on serum potassium, magnesium, and ventricular ectopy. Am J Med 1986; 80:8–12.
200. Denlinger JK, Kaplan JA, Lecky JH, et al: Cardiovascular responses to calcium administered intravenously to man during halothane anesthesia. Anesthesiology 1975; 42:390–397.
201. Royster RL, Johnston WE, Gravlee GP, et al: Arrythmias during venous cannulation prior to pulmonary artery catheter insertion. Anesth Analg 1985; 64:1214–1216.
202. Damen J, Bolton D: A prospective analysis of 1,400 pulmonary artery catheterizations in patients undergoing cardiac surgery. Acta Anaesthesiol Scand 1986; 30:386–392.
203. Weinberger M: Pharmacology and therapeutic use of theophylline. J Allergy Clin Immunol 1986; 77:525.
204. Frommer DA, Kulig KW, Marx JA, Rumack B: Tricyclic antidepressant overdose. A review. JAMA 1987; 257:521–526.
205. Brown RE, Galford RE: Sinus tachycardia. In Galford RE (ed): Problems in Anesthesiology: Approach to Diagnosis. Boston, Little, Brown, 1992, pp 67–70.
206. Kennedy DJ, Galford RE: Sinus bradycardia. In Galford RE (ed): Problems in Anesthesiology: Approach to Diagnosis. Boston: Little, Brown, 1992, pp 71–74.
207. Zaidan JR: Electrocardiography. In Barash PG, Cullen BF, Stoelting RK (eds): Clinical Anesthesia. Philadelphia, JB Lippincott, 1989, pp 587–623.
208. Singer DH, Ten Eick RE: Aberrancy: Electrophysiologic aspects. Am J Cardiol 1971; 28:381–401.
209. Josephson ME, Kastor JA: Supraventricular tachycardia: Mechanisms and management. Ann Intern Med 1977; 87:346–358.
210. Wu D: Supraventricular tachycardias. JAMA 1983; 249:3357–3360.
211. Scarpa WJ: The sick sinus syndrome. Am Heart J 1976; 92:648–660.
212. Shine KI, Kastor JA, Yurchak PM: Multifocal atrial tachycardia. Clinical and electrocardiographic features in 32 patients. N Engl J Med 1968; 279:344–349.
213. Levine JH, Michael JR, Guarnieri T: Multifocal atrial tachycardia: A toxic effect of theophylline. Lancet 1985; 1:12–14.
214. Josephson ME, Wellens HJ: Differential diagnosis of supraventricular tachycardia. Cardiol Clin 1990; 8:411–442.
215. Richardson JM: Ventricular preexcitation. Practical considerations. Arch Intern Med 1983; 143:760–764.
216. Mandel WJ, Laks MM, Obayashi K, et al: The Wolff-Parkinson-White syndrome: Pharmacologic effects of procainamide. Am Heart J 1975; 90:744–754.
217. Platia EV, Michelson EL, Porterfield JK, et al: Esmolol versus verapamil in the acute treatment of atrial fibrillation or atrial flutter. Am J Cardiol 1989; 63:925–929.
218. Fenster PE, Comess KA, Marsh R, et al: Conversion of atrial fibrillation to sinus rhythm by acute intravenous procainamide infusion. Am Heart J 1983; 106:501–504.
219. Dunn M, Alexander J, de Silva R, et al: Antithrombotic therapy in atrial fibrillation. Chest 1986; 89:68S–74S.
220. Wells JL Jr, MacLean WA, James TN, et al: Characterization of atrial flutter. Studies in man after open heart surgery using fixed atrial electrodes. Circulation 1979; 60:665–673.
221. Waldo AL, Wells JL Jr, Cooper TB, et al: Temporary cardiac pacing: Applications and techniques in the treatment of cardiac arrhythmias. Prog Cardiovasc Dis 1981; 23:451–474.
222. Platia EV, Waclawski SH, Pluth TA, et al: Management of acute-onset atrial fibrillation/flutter: Esmolol vs verapamil vs digoxin vs placebo. Circulation 1987; 76(suppl 4):IV-520.
223. Marriott HJL: Bundle branch blocks. In Marriott JHL (ed): Practical Electrocardiography, ed. 7. Baltimore, Williams & Wilkins, 1983, pp 62–83.
224. Sprung CL, Elser B, Schein RM, et al: Risk of right bundle-branch block and complete heart block during pulmonary artery catheterization. Crit Care Med 1989; 17:1–3.
225. Morris D, Mulvihill D, Lew WY: Risk of developing complete heart block during bedside pulmonary artery catheterization in patients with left bundle-branch block. Arch Intern Med 1987; 147:2005–2010.

226. Canaveris G: Intraventricular conduction disturbances in flying personnel: Right bundle branch block. Aviat Space Environ Med 1986; 57:591–596.
227. Hardarson T, Amason A, Eliasson GJ, et al: Left bundle branch block: Prevalence, incidence, and follow-up and outcome. Eur Heart J 1987; 8:1075–1079.
228. Thrainsdottir IS, Hardarson T, Thorgeirsson G, et al: The epidemiology of right bundle branch block and its association with cardiovascular morbidity—the Reykjavik Study. Eur Heart J 1993; 14:1590–1596.
229. Fahy GJ, Pinski SL, Miller DP, et al: Natural history of isolated bundle branch block. Am J Cardiol 1996; 77:1185–1190.
230. Lamb LE, Kable KD, Averill KH: Electrocardiographic findings in 67,375 asymptomatic subjects. V. Left bundle branch block. Am J Cardiol 1960; 6:130–142.
231. Johnson RL, Averill KH, Lamb LE: Electrocardiographic findings in 67,375 asymptomatic subjects. VI. Right bundle branch block. Am J Cardiol 1960; 6:143–152.
232. Hiss RG, Lamb LE: Electrocardiographic findings in 122,043 individuals. Circulation 1962; 25:947–961.
233. Wellens HJ, Bar FW, Lie KI: The value of the electrocardiogram in the differential diagnosis of a tachycardia with a widened QRS complex. Am J Med 1978; 64:27–33.
234. Galloway PA, Glass PS: Anesthetic implications of prolonged QT interval syndromes. Anesth Analg 1985; 64:612–620.
235. Roden DM, Woosley RL, Primm RK: Incidence and clinical features of the quinidine-associated long QT syndrome: Implications for patient care. Am Heart J 1986; 111:1088-1093.
236. Tzivoni D, Banai S, Schuger C, et al: Treatment of torsade de pointes with magnesium sulfate. Circulation 1988; 77:392–397.
237. Moss AJ, McDonald J. Unilateral cervicothoracic sympathetic ganglionectomy for the treatment of the long QT interval syndrome. N Engl J Med 1971; 285:903–904.
238. Medak R, Benumof JL: Perioperative management of the prolonged Q-T interval syndrome. Br J Anaesth 1983; 55:361–364.
239. Parsonnet V, Furman S, Smyth NP: Report of the Inter-Society Commission for Heart Disease Resources. Implantable cardiac pacemakers: status report and resource guideline. Am J Cardiol 1974; 34:487–500.
240. Bernstein AD, Camm AJ, Fletcher RD, et al: The NASPE/BPEG generic pacemaker code for antibradyarrhythmia and adaptive-rate pacing and antitachyarrhythmia devices. Pacing Clin Electrophysiol 1987; 10:794–799.
241. Andersen C, Madsen GM: Rate-responsive pacemakers and anaesthesia. A consideration of possible implications. Anaesthesia 1990; 45:472–476.
242. Zaiden JR: Perioperative considerations for rate-adaptive implantable pacemakers. In Lynch C III, (ed): Clinical Cardiac Electrophysiology: Perioperative Considerations. Philadelphia, JB Lippincott, 1994, pp 259–283.
243. Albers DD, Lybrand FE III, Axton JC, et al: Shockwave lithotripsy and pacemakers: Experience with 20 cases. J Endourol 1995; 9:310–313.
244. Celentano WJ, Jahr JS, Nossaman BD: Extracorporeal shock wave lithotripsy in a patient with a pacemaker. Anesth Analg 1992; 74:770–772.
245. Drach GW, Weber C, Donovan JM: Treatment of pacemaker patients with extracorporeal shock wave lithotripsy: Experience from 2 continents. J Urol 1990; 143:895–896.
246. Fetter J, Patterson D, Aram G, et al: Effects of extracorporeal shock wave lithotripsy on single chamber rate response and dual chamber pacemakers. Pacing Clin Electrophysiol 1989; 12:1494–1501.
247. Cooper D, Wilkoff B, Masterson M, et al: Effects of extracorporeal shock wave lithotripsy on cardiac pacemakers and its safety in patients with implanted cardiac pacemakers. Pacing Clin Electrophysiol 1988; 11:1607–1616.
248. Nercessian OA, Wu H, Nazarian D, Mahmud F: Intraoperative pacemaker dysfunction caused by the use of electrocautery during a total hip arthroplasty. J Arthroplasty 1998; 13:599–602.
249. Kellow NH: Pacemaker failure during transurethral resection of the prostate. Anaesthesia. 1993; 48:136–138.
250. Chauvin M, Crenner F, Brechenmacher C: Interaction between

permanent cardiac pacing and electrocautery: The significance of electrode position. Pacing Clin Electrophysiol 1992; 15: 2028–2033.

251. Mangar D, Atlas GM, Kane PB: Electrocautery-induced pacemaker malfunction during surgery. Can J Anaesth 1991; 38: 616–618.

252. Heller LI: Surgical electrocautery and the runaway pacemaker syndrome. Pacing Clin Electrophysiol 1990; 13:1084–1085.

253. Domino KB, Smith TC: Electrocautery-induced reprogramming of a pacemaker using a precordial magnet. Anesth Analg 1983; 62:609–612.

254. Belott PH, Sands S, Warren J: Resetting of DDD pacemakers due to EMI. Pacing Clin Electrophysiol 1984; 7:169–172.

255. Godin JF, Petitot JC: STIMAREC report. Pacemaker failures due to electrocautery and external electric shock. Pacing Clin Electrophysiol 1989; 12:1011.

13 Invasive and Noninvasive Blood Pressure Monitoring

Nitin Shah, M.D.
Robert F. Bedford, M.D.

Systemic Arterial Pressure

The arterial pulse-pressure wave results from the left ventricular stroke volume creating aortic distention within the closed vascular system. Peak aortic blood flow acceleration produces the initial rate of rise of the pressure pulse, whereas the ejection of ventricular volume fills out and sustains the pulse waveform.[1] The initial rapid upstroke of the aortic root pulse reaches a peak that can be viewed as the inotropic component of the pressure-pulse wave. The pressure and flow phenomena at this time expand primarily the upper aorta and produce a higher pressure than would occur if the entire aorta were to distend uniformly. The rounded, sustained portion of the aortic pulse-pressure wave represents a combined effect of (1) ventricular volume ejection, (2) distention of the entire aorta (capacitance), and (3) runoff into the branches of the aorta. The initial peak of the arterial waveform is followed by a more or less well-defined notch and subsequently by a second peak, the systolic pressure. The second peak falls away to the descending limb of the waveform, which often contains a dicrotic notch[2] (Fig. 13-1). The nadir of the pulse-pressure wave is defined as the diastolic pressure, occurring immediately before the subsequent systolic upstroke begins.

Ventricular ejection produces both a true pressure wave and a flow wave in the ascending aorta. The aortic blood flow is not transmitted to the periphery with the pulse-pressure wave. The left ventricular stroke volume is absorbed by the distensible elastic aortic arch, which serves as a "fixed-capacity, high-pressure reservoir."[2] While the blood flow wave moves out of the aorta at a relatively slow 0.5 m/second during aortic elastic recoil from the volume ejected from the left ventricle, the pulse-pressure wave moves at the rate of 10 m/second.[2] In fact, by the time ventricular systole is completed, the dorsalis pedis artery has already started to receive the arterial pulse-pressure wave.

As the pulse-pressure wave moves away from the aortic root, there is a delay in transmission, the initial upstroke becomes steeper, the high-frequency components (such as the anacrotic and dicrotic notches) disappear, and the systolic maximum becomes progressively more peaked (Fig. 13-2). The dicrotic notch starts out as an incisura and gradually gets lost in transmission, becoming a deep, drawn-out hump or anacrotic wave in the upper extremities, while virtually disappearing into the diastolic pressure in the femoral system. The tidal wave after the primary systolic peak appears in the axillary-brachial-radial system but does not appear in the femoral artery. Mean pressure must decrease peripherally for flow to continue, although mean pressure changes less than either systolic or diastolic pressure. In general, the farther into the periphery blood pressure (BP) is measured, the greater the increase in systolic and pulse pressure, the lower the diastolic and mean values, and the narrower the waveform appears.

The reasons for the changing pattern of the arterial pulse wave are extremely complex, and yet they are important for the clinician's understanding of BP monitoring techniques. Because BP is usually measured in peripheral arteries, probably the most important factor in modifying the pulse-pressure waveform obtained clinically—particularly the systolic component—is the reflection of waves from the periphery. Just as surface waves are produced by dropping an object into a pool of water, when the waves hit the edge of the pool they are reflected back, and those reflected waves produce a standing wave that adds to the incident wave (Fig. 13-3). In the arterial tree, the artery-arteriole junction is thought to be the principal site of reflection, and standing waves are produced that add or subtract from different portions of the pulse wave.[3, 4] It has been estimated that as much as 80% of the incident wave is reflected with normal arterial resistance. When peripheral vasodilation occurs (vasodilator therapy, systemic inflammatory response syndrome, exercise, arteriovenous fistula), the energy in the pressure pulse is passed on into the periphery and absorbed without reflection, resulting in marked changes in the pulse-pressure contour.[5, 6] Conversely, when a cannulated radial or dorsalis pedis artery is occluded by a catheter or thrombus, the site of wave reflection is at the catheter tip, and the summation of the reflected and incident waves results in augmentation of the systolic pressure value.[7, 8]

Reflection of the arterial waveform also is thought to occur at branching points of vessels. The changes in the shape of the dicrotic notch are thought to result from reflected waves from the lower aorta summating with the incident pulse-pressure wave, because there is no dicrotic notch visible in the femoral arterial tree, whereas it is clearly evident in the arteries of the upper extremities.

There are other causes of change in the configuration of the arterial pulse-pressure wave as it moves peripherally:

1. The decreasing content of elastic fibers (and lower compliance) as the more peripheral arteries become more muscular.
2. The tapering of vessel diameter, which acts to amplify arterial waves similar to the way an ear trumpet amplifies sound waves (see Fig. 13-3).
3. The fact that the high pressure levels of the arterial pulse travel faster than the low pressure levels so that the peak of the arterial pulse curve "catches up" and summates

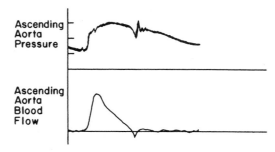

Figure 13–1. Aortic root pressure-pulse wave and the corresponding flow generated in the ascending aorta. See text for explanation. (From Bedford RF, Shah NK: Blood pressure monitoring: Invasive and noninvasive. In Blitt CD, Hines RL: Monitoring in Anesthesia and Critical Care Medicine. New York, Churchill Livingstone, 1995, p 95.)

with the earlier pressure components in the more peripheral arteries.[9]

The observation that older patients have less discrepancy between systolic pressures measured in the aorta and peripherally is thought to be due to less vessel wall pliability and a faster pulse-wave velocity with increasing age.[10] Conversely, the marked augmentation of the dicrotic notch (actually a wave) often observed in children's radial arteries is a function of greater vessel compliance and greater opportunity for wave reflection and amplification due to slower wave transmission time.

The changes in arterial waveform, particularly those of the systolic component, account in large part (although not entirely) for the disparities observed between cuff pressures measured in the brachial artery and invasive pressures measured at a more distal site such as the radial or dorsalis pedis arteries.

In summary, the arterial system functions as a damped, resonant transmission line, transmitting various frequencies with different degrees of attenuation. The reshaping of the aortic pulse-pressure wave as it travels into the peripheral

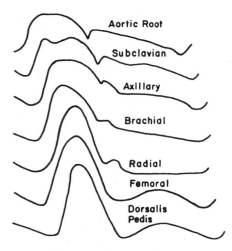

Figure 13–2. Configuration of the pressure-pulse wave at various sites in the arterial tree. See text for a more complete description of the changes as the arterial pulse wave travels to the periphery. (From Bedford RF, Shah NK: Blood pressure monitoring: Invasive and noninvasive. In Blitt CD, Hines RL: Monitoring in Anesthesia and Critical Care Medicine. New York, Churchill Livingstone, 1995, p 95.)

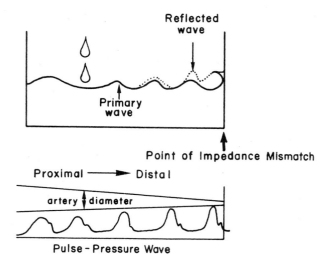

Figure 13–3. Some factors affecting the arterial pressure-pulse wave shape: Reflection at the artery-arteriole junction and progressive decrease in diameter of arterial lumen. See text for further description.

arterial pressure wave is the result of the attenuation of some frequencies and the augmentation of other frequencies. Although the mean pressure measured in the periphery will be only slightly lower than the value in the aortic arch, the clinician should not be fooled into believing that systolic and diastolic pressures measured in the periphery accurately reflect the same pressures as those at the takeoff of the coronary arteries.[11]

Noninvasive Methods for Blood Pressure Measurement

Considerable effort has been expended in refining the technology for noninvasive blood pressure (NIBP) measurement. Ever since 1903, when Cushing[12] first advocated clinical use of BP measurement, most arterial pressure monitoring has been done noninvasively, either with a manually operated sphygmomanometer or with an automated noninvasive device. Currently there are approximately 200,000 automated noninvasive BP devices in clinical use worldwide, both in operating rooms and critical care units.

One of the problems with NIBP measurement is the considerable variance in BP data, both within and between the different techniques available.[13] Common to nearly all the contemporary methods for noninvasive arterial pressure measurement is an inflatable circumferential cuff that is placed around an extremity and inflated to a pressure exceeding systolic pressure and that stops either blood flow or arterial wall motion. However, there is little standardization for the estimation of NIBP, and there are multiple techniques available for measuring changes in systolic, diastolic, mean arterial, and pulse pressures.

The lack of standardization is further complicated by the multiplicity of sites available for NIBP measurement. As discussed in the section on invasive BP monitoring, the intra-arterial pressure changes as it moves away from the aortic root, a consequence of changes in vessel diameter, vessel wall elasticity, and the state of arteriolar tone. It is because of these limitations and the observed inconsistencies in NIBP measurement that Brunner and colleagues concluded, "Blood pressure is a function of the way it is measured."[1]

Figure 13-4. The effect of cuff fit on blood pressure reading. Shaded areas indicate the magnitude of tissue pressure (= cuff pressure). 1) With a proper fit the pressure of the cuff is transmitted undiminished to the artery and compresses it. 2) A cuff that is too narrow requires greater pressure and results in a higher blood pressure reading. 3) A loose cuff also results in artifactual elevation of the blood pressure. A cuff that is too wide is merely bulky and does not distort readings. (From Rushmer RF: Cardiovascular Dynamics, 3rd ed. Philadelphia, WB Saunders, 1976, p 157.)

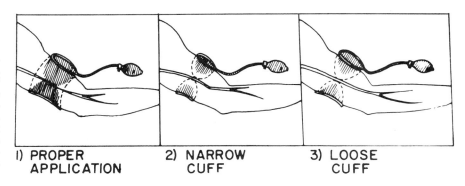

1) PROPER APPLICATION   2) NARROW CUFF   3) LOOSE CUFF

History

Although the circulation of blood in the human body had been known since first described in 1628 by William Harvey, it was not until 1876 that Von Basch developed a technique for occluding a peripheral artery using hydraulically applied pressure over a bone. The pressure was increased until pulsations in the artery disappeared; this point was taken as the systolic pressure. A variation of this technique of arterial occlusion was undertaken in 1876 by E. J. Marey, who inserted a subject's arm through a seal into a cylinder of water that could have its pressure recorded as well as changed. Marey also developed a somewhat less bulky method using a cylinder that fit tightly around one finger, but this method did not win clinical acceptance, perhaps because of the low amplitude of the oscillations in the manometer.[14]

The use of a pneumatic cuff around the arm was first described in 1896 by Riva-Rocci and in 1897 by Hill and Barnard.[15] Using palpation of the radial artery (the so-called palpatory method) the cuff was gradually inflated until the radial pulse first disappeared; the cuff was then deflated and the pressure at which the pulse then reappeared was recorded. These two readings were averaged to give the systolic pressure.

The auscultatory method of BP determination was first proposed in 1905 by Korotkoff.[15] He believed that the sounds that were heard through a stethoscope placed over the brachial artery distal to an occluding cuff were caused by the breakthrough of a pulse wave and that the subsequent lessening and then disappearance of the sounds were caused by the passage of an unobstructed pulse wave. He noted that the first sound occurred at a higher pressure than was obtained with palpation of the radial artery and concluded that more of the pulse waveform had to pass down the artery before the pulse was palpable.

Methods of Measurement

NIBP measurement is currently performed either manually or with a variety of automated electromechanical devices employing techniques such as auscultation, oscillometry, blood flow detection, and photometric pulse wave delay.[7] The following is a partial list of techniques and devices used in contemporary medical practice. Each will be discussed in some detail:

Auscultation
Oscillometry
Blood flow detection: palpation, ultrasonic, and photoelectric
Ultrasonic detection of arterial wall movement
Infrasonde (Puritan Bennett)
Finapres
Arterial tonometry
Photometric wave velocity

Auscultation

The auscultatory or Riva-Rocci method for NIBP monitoring has been, and continues to be, the most commonly used NIBP measurement technique.[16] It relies on Korotkoff sounds, a complex series of audible frequencies produced by turbulent flow, instability of the arterial wall, and shock wave formation that are created as external occluding cuff pressure on a major artery is reduced.[17] The pressure at which the first sound (phase I) is heard is usually taken as the systolic value. The sound character changes (phases II and III), then becomes muffled (phase IV), and finally absent (phase V). Diastolic pressure is recorded at phase IV or V, although phase V may never occur in certain pathophysiologic states, such as aortic regurgitation.[18]

As familiar as the standard BP cuff may be, a number of caveats should be considered in its use. It is of paramount importance to match the size of BP cuff to the size of the patient's arm. Too small a cuff, or one that is wrapped too loosely, will result in falsely elevated BP readings because of the excessive cuff pressure required to occlude a deep artery (Fig. 13-4). Other causes of falsely elevated BP include the extremity's being placed below heart level or uneven cuff compression transmitted to the underlying artery. Falsely low estimates result when cuffs are too large, when the extremity is above heart level, or if the cuff is deflated too rapidly to detect appropriate Korotkoff sounds.[19]

Geddes[14] stated that the width of the BP cuff should be 40% of the circumference of the arm. The pneumatic bladder should span at least one half of this circumference and should be centered over the artery. One of the cuffs shown in Table 13-1 will be accurate in most patients.

Table 13-1. Commonly Available Blood Pressure Cuff Sizes

Cuff	Arm Circumference (cm)	Bladder Size (cm)
Newborn	6-11	2.5 × 5
Infant	10-19	6 × 12
Child	18-26	9 × 18
Adult	25-35	12 × 23
Large arm	33-47	15 × 33
Thigh	46-66	18 × 36

Courtesy of WA Baum Co., Inc., Copiague, NY.

Consideration should also be given to placement of the stethoscope over the brachial artery. Loose-fitting diaphragm-type stethoscopes, a poor seal with a bell-type stethoscope, or motion of either stethoscope will result in attenuation of the Korotkoff sounds. The Diasyst stethoscope bell is particularly helpful for achieving good skin contact over the brachial artery.

The cuff deflation rate should be slow enough for the sensing process to detect appropriate Korotkoff sound changes and to assign them to the pressure of the cuff. Failure to do so will result in falsely low pressures. A deflation rate of 3 mmHg per second limits this source of error. Coupling of the deflation rate to heart rate (2 mmHg per beat) has been found to further improve accuracy.[20]

Oscillometry

The oscillometric method of NIBP monitoring senses variations in the pressure within a BP cuff during deflation. The cuff is pressurized until no oscillations are seen and is then allowed to deflate until sudden fluctuations in the pressure of the cuff are noted on a pressure gauge. At this point, the cuff pressure is at or near the systolic pressure. The inflation pressure is then allowed to fall further, until the oscillations are seen to reach a maximum and begin to decrease. This point has been shown to be near the *mean* arterial pressure, not the diastolic pressure as had been previously thought (Fig. 13-5). Two cardiac cycles are compared at each increment if "noise" conditions are low. With increased noise (patient or cuff movement), inflation is held until successive comparative beats occur. Under these conditions, measurement becomes time-dependent, although normally the entire sequence from measurement to display is 20 to 45 seconds. The averaged pairs of oscillations and the corresponding cuff pressures are stored and analyzed electronically to determine systolic, diastolic, and mean pressures. The heart rate is the median of rates obtained by analysis of all pressure pulses in a given determination.

The first commercially produced automatic oscillometric BP monitor, the Dinamap (Critikon, Tampa, FL), entered routine clinical use in 1976.[21] Initially, it determined only mean arterial pressure (MAP), primarily because a change in MAP is easier to interpret than changes in systolic or diastolic pressure, which can often move in opposite directions. Also, at the capillary bed level, most of the pulsation caused by the oscillations of systolic and diastolic pressure has been damped out by the resistance and compliance of the proximal vascular bed. In addition, MAP measurement is less affected by changes in vascular tone than systolic or diastolic pressure measurement because it is determined when the oscillations of cuff pressure reach the greatest amplitude. This property allows MAP to be measured reliably even in cases of hypotension with vasoconstriction and diminished pulse pressure.[22] In fact, oscillometry is the only noninvasive method that directly estimates mean BP.

The technique for ideal oscillometric NIBP measurement is illustrated in Figure 13-6. All three pressures are determined individually, and, in contrast to the manual auscultatory method, there is little effect on the accuracy of the measurement when venous engorgement from cuff inflation is not allowed to subside.

Difficulties in BP measurement by oscillometry may arise due to (1) incorrect cuff size, (2) incorrect cuff application, (3) undetected leaks in the cuff, hoses, or connectors, (4) failure to keep the cuff at heart level, (5) arm movement, and (6) inadequate pulse-pressure waves due to shock or vascular compression proximal to the cuff.[22]

In spite of these potential difficulties, numerous reports attest to the accuracy and reliability of the Dinamap monitor in both neonates and adults.[23-25] Most of these studies have shown that there is less than 5 mmHg mean error with a standard deviation of less than 8 mmHg when a Dinamap is compared with a centrally placed arterial catheter. The current models of the Dinamap display systolic, mean, and diastolic BP as well as heart rate (Fig. 13-7).

Blood Flow Detection

There are three commonly used techniques for measurement of systolic BP by detection of blood flow distal to an occlusive cuff. There is *no* way to measure the mean or the diastolic pressure using this technique.

Palpation. The first method utilizes palpation of the arterial pulse distal to a pneumatic cuff. In brief, an arm cuff of sufficient width is inflated to a point 30 mmHg higher than the point of disappearance of the pulse. The cuff is deflated at a rate of 2 to 3 mmHg per heartbeat. The point of return of the radial pulse denotes the systolic pressure. Patients with irregular heart rates such as those in atrial fibrillation will demonstrate a wide range of systolic pressures, particularly if the cuff is allowed to deflate rapidly. Whenever two systoles occur in close proximity, there is less time for filling of the left ventricle and both stroke volume and BP are lower during the second beat. It is thus possible to miss a beat or two and interpret the BP as lower than it actually is. If the palpated vessel is some distance from the cuff, flow transmission time will delay sensing of systolic pressure slightly (flow velocity is approximately 8 to 10 m/second).[26] Overall, systolic BP measurements by palpation are lower than those determined with Korotkoff systems. This technique has been found useful in neonates, infants, obese patients, and those in whom Korotkoff sounds are inconsistent.[27] (In infants, the "flush" method, a variation of the palpation method wherein the pressure at which limb color

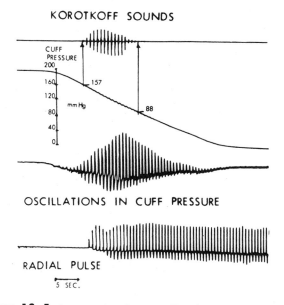

Figure 13-5. A comparison between Korotkoff sounds, cuff pressure oscillation, and radial pulse. There is a good correlation between the onset of the first Korotkoff sound, the onset of oscillations in the cuff pressure, and the radial pulse wave. By contrast, there is no correlation with the disappearance of the cuff oscillations. (From Reitan JA, Barash PG: Noninvasive monitoring. In Saidman LJ, Smith NT (eds): Monitoring in Anesthesia, 2nd ed. London, Butterworth, 1984.)

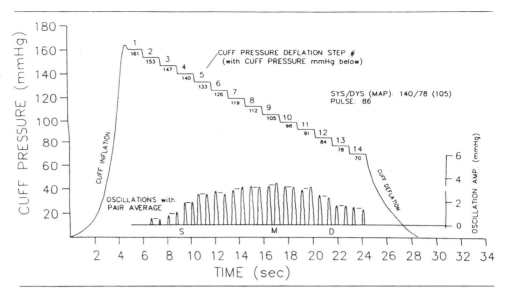

Figure 13-6. Blood pressure measurement technique illustrating the ideal measurement condition in the absence of artifact. The cuff pressure and oscillation amplitude (AMP) are plotted on the same axis, with the cuff pressure amplitude axis on the left and the oscillation amplitude axis on the right. Mean arterial pressure (MAP, M) is calculated from systolic (SYS, S) and diastolic (DYS, D) pressures. In this subject, cuff pressure is considerably above systolic pressure and no cuff pressure oscillations are visible either in the figure or the microprocessor. (From Ramsey M: Blood pressure monitoring: Automated oscillometric devices. J Clin Monit Comput 1991; 7:56.)

returns, is noted. The flush method depends highly on speed of cuff deflation, peripheral perfusion, and operator skill.)

Ultrasonic. More sensitive than the palpation method of measurement of blood flow, an ultrasonic blood flow detector employs an ultrasonic Doppler unit placed over a distal artery. The Doppler transceiver monitors blood flow in the artery by sensing the velocity of erythrocytes.[28] As the ipsilateral upper arm cuff is inflated above systolic BP, the audio output from the unit becomes silent as arterial erythrocyte movement ceases. Systolic pressure is signaled by the cuff pressure at which "chirps" from the Doppler unit indicate blood flow that rhythmically follows the heartbeat. Diastolic pressure is signified by the point at which full pulsatile flow occurs. This method is particularly useful when the peripheral pulse is faint or absent as in patients who are cold and in shock and in infants or obese patients whose Korotkoff sounds may be absorbed by fatty tissue.

A significant disadvantage of ultrasonic blood flow detectors is that electrosurgical equipment produces audible interference, which can be annoying or even render BP determination impossible. Newer Doppler flow detectors employ circuits to eliminate this problem by automatically shutting off the external speaker circuit when the electrosurgery unit is activated.

Photoelectric. This technique measures the absorption of light from a source placed against the skin, most conveniently on a finger. The pulsatile changes in blood volume associated with blood flow produce changes in absorption of infrared light. If a cuff is inflated above arterial pressure and then allowed to deflate, a sudden small oscillation in the output of the blood flow detector is seen that is equivalent to the systolic pressure. When the pulse volume amplitude no longer increases, diastolic pressure is reached.

The technique fails, however, if the blood vessels in the finger become constricted due to either hypothermia or hypotension. Furthermore, the constant light source produces a moderate amount of heat that, in combination with poor blood flow under the transducer, may lead to thermal injury.

Ultrasonic Detection of Arterial Wall Movement

In addition to detecting the flow of erythrocytes, the Doppler principle can be used to indirectly measure BP by detecting motion of an arterial wall distal to an occlusive pneumatic cuff (Arteriosonde 1216, Roche Medical Electronics Division, Cranbury, NJ). A dual piezoelectric crystal ultrasonic transducer is placed over the artery. One crystal acts as the transmitter of an ultrasonic signal (commonly 2 to 10 MHz), while the other receives the reflected sound wave. With no target (artery) movement, the receiver crystal senses a constant signal frequency. When the cuff pressure falls just below systolic pressure, the vessel opens and then quickly closes as the peak (systolic) pressure wave subsides. This sudden movement of the arterial wall causes a Doppler frequency shift, which is noted by the receiving crystal. The initial arterial opening is taken as the systolic pressure read-

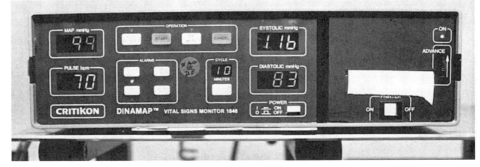

Figure 13-7. Dinamap. (Courtesy of Critikon, Tampa, FL.)

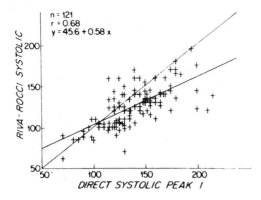

Figure 13-8. Comparison between systolic blood pressure determined by the Riva-Rocci method and blood pressures determined by direct intra-arterial monitoring. Note the large scatter in the data. (From Brunner JMR, et al: Comparison of direct and indirect methods of measuring arterial blood pressure. Part III. Med Instrum 1981; 15:182.)

ing. Diastolic pressure is determined when cuff pressure falls to the point where the artery is open throughout the pulse cycle so that the rhythmic arterial opening and closing is no longer present. Several studies comparing NIBP measured by ultrasound to direct intra-arterial pressures in both adults and infants found satisfactory results in most clinical applications.[29-31]

Infrasonde

The Infrasonde (Puritan Bennett Corp., Carlsbad, CA) uses the auscultatory method to automatically determine systolic and diastolic pressures. Like the Dinamap, the Infrasonde provides for automatic inflation of an arm cuff. Two crystal microphones are positioned over the brachial artery and are used to determine the point at which the Korotkoff sounds first appear. The cuff deflates at a rate selected by the operator; a determination is then made of the systolic, mean, and diastolic BPs. Accuracy is ensured by a display of the signal strength, a useful feature that aids the operator both in accurately positioning the cuff and for indicating the signal-to-noise ratio under which the machine is operating. As one might infer, the leading disadvantage of the Infrasonde is that it must have its sensors placed accurately over an artery. If the sensors shift away from the artery, the signal strength drops and the machine is unable to give a satisfactory NIBP reading. Unlike the Dinamap, the Infrasonde cannot be placed easily over any portion of an extremity. It thus trades convenience of cuff placement for rapidity of BP determination.[32]

Finapres

First described by Penaz in Czechoslovakia, the Finapres (*finger arterial pressure*) consists of a small cuff placed over a patient's finger. The cuff is connected to a very rapidly responding solenoid that inflates and deflates the cuff, keeping the volume of the finger constant as pulsatile blood flow increases or decreases. When the instrument senses that finger volume is expanding due to inflow of blood under the constricting cuff, the solenoid pressurizes the cuff just enough to prevent further blood flow. Thus, the device tends to track the mean arterial BP in digital arteries underlying the cuff by nulling the transmural pressure under the

cuff. A waveform that closely approximates arterial BP in the finger is displayed on the screen.[2]

The accuracy of the Finapres has been the subject of considerable study. Stokes and coworkers[33] compared Finapres values with invasive arterial pressures and concluded that, while providing useful beat-to-beat information on arterial pressure trends, the Finapres could not be recommended as a universal substitute for invasive arterial pressure monitoring. Kurki et al.[34] looked at the optimal measurement conditions and factors affecting reliability. They found that pressures measured in the thumb correlate with intra-arterial pressure better than do pressures measured in other digits. Changes in hemoglobin saturation affect the transmission of light to the device but not the pressure readings.[34] Gorback and associates[35] compared the Finapres with the Dinamap and found that readings by both correlated well for diastolic and mean arterial pressures, while the accuracy of the Finapres appeared to be slightly superior for systolic pressure. Epstein and coworkers[36] compared Finapres and Dinamap measurements with intra-arterial pressures. They found that the Finapres had a significantly higher bias than the Dinamap for diastolic and mean BP when compared to intra-arterial pressure. They concluded that the Finapres monitor could not be relied on to accurately measure BP (without a second method of BP measurement) in patients undergoing general anesthesia.

Additional studies comparing NIBP and invasive arterial pressure readings were performed by Brunner and colleagues[7] and are summarized in Figures 13-8, 13-9, and 13-10. In their series of patients, they found that the correlation between invasive and automated noninvasive measurements was not very good for systolic pressures and that the correlation with diastolic pressures was even worse. In contrast, the correlation between Riva-Rocci systolic pressure and intra-arterial catheter occlusion pressure was found to be quite good.

Arterial Tonometry

The technique of arterial tonometry utilizes a pressor sensor positioned over a superficial artery and records arterial wall displacement, which is then converted into an electrical signal.[37-39] It requires an adequately sized superficial artery that is supported by a bony structure. The sensor exerts pressure

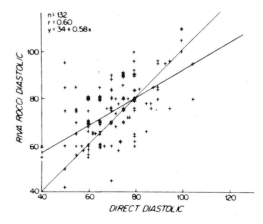

Figure 13-9. Comparison between diastolic blood pressures determined by the Riva-Rocci method and by direct intra-arterial monitoring. There is even more scatter in the data than that in Figure 13-8. (From Brunner JMR, et al: Comparison of direct and indirect methods of measuring arterial blood pressure. Part III. Med Instrum 1981; 15:182.)

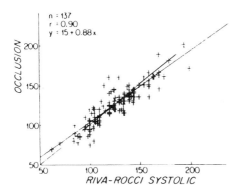

Figure 13-10. Comparison between systolic blood pressure determined by the Riva-Rocci method and by the occlusion method of observing an intra-arterial trace from a catheter in the radial artery while a proximal cuff is inflated above systolic pressure and then deflated. The point of appearance of the pulse wave is taken as the systolic pressure. These two methods show the best correlation. (From Brunner JMR, et al: Comparison of direct and indirect methods of measuring arterial blood pressure. Part III. Med Instrum 1981; 15:182.)

on the artery, partially flattening it against the underlying bone (Fig. 13-11). The force exerted by the blood vessel is then transmitted through the skin with near-perfect fidelity. The technique is based on the following assumptions: (1) the skin thickness is insignificant compared to the arterial diameter; (2) the arterial wall behaves essentially as an ideal membrane; and (3) the sensor is smaller than the flattened area of the artery and is centered above the flattened area. It has been shown that the electrical output signal of the generated force is directly proportional to the intra-arterial BP.

The CBM-3000 (Colin Medical Instruments Corp., San Antonio, TX) is a multiparameter monitor that employs the newly developed transducer array for tonometric BP monitoring. The transducer array is incorporated into a sensor that is placed over the radial artery just proximal to the wrist joint. The sensor assembly is formed to hold the wrist with the proper degree of extension. A microcomputer analyzes the signal from each transducer of the sensor array and selects the transducer that is properly positioned based on maximum pulse amplitude of the signal. Hold-down pressure is set via microprocessor control of a pneumatic bladder that is incorporated into the sensor assembly. The tonometric BP readings require calibration to oscillometer cuff measurements at user-selected intervals of either 5 or 10 minutes.

Several studies have compared tonometric BP measurements against invasive radial artery pressure tracings in anesthetized patients. A good correlation was found between the two techniques, with identical pressure waveforms found in both tonometric and intra-arterial BP recordings.[40-42]

Photometric Wave Velocity Technique

The refinement of pulse oximetry technology has led to advances in photometric sensor development and signal processing techniques that permit NIBP measurement without use of artery occlusion. Instead, systolic and diastolic BP values are determined by measuring arterial pulse wave velocity and changes in local blood volume. The ARTRAC 7000 monitor uses two photometric sensors similar to those used by pulse oximeters, one of which is placed on the ear and the other on a finger. The pulse oximeters sense each heartbeat, with the proximal (ear) pulse arriving before the distal (finger) pulse. The difference in arrival time is called the pulse transit time. The proximal sensor also senses changes in microvascular volume. The pulse wave velocity is a relative measure of diastolic pressure, so that an initial calibration with a traditional BP cuff is necessary to obtain absolute pressure values.

When compared with NIBP data obtained with a BP cuff, the ARTRAC has been found to be within the American Association of Medical Instrumentation (AAMI) and American National Standards Institute (ANSI) standards. When compared with invasive arterial pressures, the bias was within standards for systolic and mean pressures and within a mean value of 7 mmHg for diastolic pressures (D. H. Wong and D. R. Bogard, personal communication, 1999.)

Special Situations

NIBP Measurement at Rest and During Exercise

Accurate and reliable determination of BP is important for assessment and interpretation of exercise tests.[43] Unfortunately, both "gold standard" methods of BP measurement, intra-arterial and manual auscultatory sphygmomanometry, are problematic and unreliable.[44, 45] A new motion-tolerant BP monitor, the CardioDyne NBP 2000 unit (Luxtec, Worcester, MA), uses a proprietary differential sensor to detect the Korotkoff sounds produced during BP measurement. This machine was compared with standard manual sphygmomanometry at rest and during exercise in 19 healthy normotensive subjects. The automated device largely eliminated prob-

Figure 13-11. Diagram of the multisensor arterial tonometer in use. The tonometer is placed over the artery and secured with sufficient force to partially flatten the artery. The arterial waveform is then recorded with near-perfect fidelity. (From Eckerle JS: Arterial tonometry. *In* Webster JG (ed): Encyclopedia of Medical Devices and Instrumentation. New York, John Wiley & Sons, 1988, pp 2270-2288.)

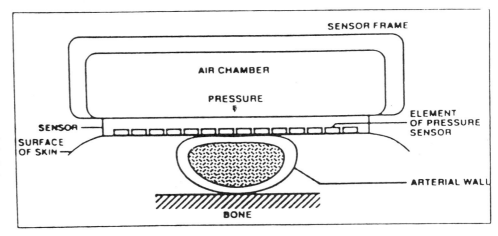

lems associated with manual measurement, such as variable hearing acuity among technicians, intertechnician variability, and technician terminal digit bias.[46] MacRae and Allen[47] found CardioDyne NBP 2000 to provide accurate and verifiable information.

Ambulatory Blood Pressure Monitor in Children

The importance of BP in early life has been highlighted by Barker et al.,[48] and 24-hour studies in children have been carried out by a number of groups.[49-51] If NIBP monitoring devices are to be used in children, they should be validated in the pediatric population, as BP measurement in children poses specific problems. The Takeda 2421 (A & D, Japan) is a monitor that uses both the oscillometric and auscultatory (Korotkoff) methods of BP measurement in normal school children. From a study in 529 school children, O'Sullivan et al.[52] found that the Korotkoff method gave more satisfactory readings as compared with oscillometric readings.[52]

Blood Pressure Measurement in Pregnancy

The indirect measurement of BP has an established place in antenatal care, although there is no universal agreement regarding the use of the fourth (K4, muffling prior to final disappearance) versus fifth (K5, final disappearance) Korotkoff sounds to identify the diastolic BP. The World Health Organization (WHO) and International Society for the Study of Hypertension in Pregnancy (ISSHP) favor the use of K4 to determine the diastolic BP in pregnant women, whereas K5 is favored in the United States.[53, 54] Duggan,[55] from a study of 132 pregnant women, found K5 to be more often and more reliably detected than K4.

Complications of Noninvasive Blood Pressure Devices

Skin and tissue compression from NIBP monitors, which can lead to skin irritation and bruising, are probably the most common complications. Prolonged use and frequent BP determinations can lead to venous pooling and congestion. Excessive venous pressures can lead to tissue ischemia and nerve damage; in fact, ulnar nerve damage has been reported when a cuff applied too distally on the arm caused direct compression of the ulnar nerve in the ulnar groove.[56, 57] Intravenous injection of irritating substances during cuff inflation may cause tissue damage owing to a locally increased concentration. Accidental injection of succinylcholine into a vein distal to the inflated cuff of an automated device during a rapid-sequence anesthetic induction may preclude timely intubation.

Invasive Blood Pressure Monitoring

Catheter Insertion Technique

By definition, invasive BP monitoring involves insertion of a hollow device into the lumen of the arterial tree so that it can be connected to an appropriate pressure transducer via a fluid-filled tube (Fig. 13–12). Whereas the radial artery is by far the most common cannulation site, there are a number of additional sites that may be indicated depending on the patient's size and physical limitations (Fig. 13–13). Since the early 1960s, the most widely used technique for percuta-

neous cannulation for direct arterial monitoring has been the "catheter-over-needle" approach first described for radial artery cannulation by Barr.[58] This approach requires meticulous antiseptic skin preparation, identification of the course of the artery by palpation, and advancing of the catheter-stylet device at a shallow angle relative to the vessel. When blood is observed in the flash chamber of the stylet, the catheter is advanced into the lumen of the vessel (Fig. 13–14).

Because peripheral arteries are frequently difficult to palpate in hypotensive or vasoconstricted patients, a variety of techniques have evolved to assist in successful cannulation. Among these are use of transillumination to help identify arteries in infants[59] and fine-tip Doppler ultrasound probes to identify weakly palpable arteries in adults (Fig. 13–15). A common clinical problem is that the tip of the needle may enter the vessel but the catheter, being larger, will not "thread" into the lumen. Miniature, flexible guidewire introducers for 20- and 22-gauge catheters have helped to obviate this problem, since the small guidewire usually can be introduced into the vessel lumen and inserted past intima, atheromas, or other obstructions that prevent successful catheter passage. Additional techniques to rescue cannulation from the "no thread" phenomenon include removing the needle from the catheter and alternately (1) withdrawing the catheter until a flash of blood indicates that the catheter tip is in the middle of the lumen, or (2) attaching an air- or fluid-filled plastic extension tube to the catheter and withdrawing the catheter until the air bubble pulsates maximally,[60] again indicating that the catheter tip is in a central location in the vessel lumen. With either of these techniques and a bit of good fortune, the catheter can then be advanced up the lumen of the vessel. A variant on these techniques is the "liquid stylet" approach, where a 10-mL syringe is applied to the cannula hub after a "no thread" is encountered. The cannula is withdrawn while suction is applied to the syringe until blood flows readily; the cannula is then advanced while 1 to 2 mL is injected with the syringe.[61] Because the "no thread" phenomenon usually results from the catheter impinging on the lateral or deep wall of the artery while only part of the needle tip is in the arterial lumen, meticulous identification of the vessel and stabilization of the extremity all seem to help to minimize this problem.

Physical Factors of Arterial Cannulas

Arterial catheters are manufactured from a variety of plastics, each with different structural properties and tissue reactivity. Most utilize polytex (Teflon), polypropylene, polyvinyl chloride, or polyethylene. Although polypropylene catheters were originally popular because they were stiff enough to avoid kinking and could be extruded into a very fine tip, several clinical studies found them to be more thrombogenic than Teflon catheters.[62, 63] While Teflon catheters are prone to kink, particularly at fine gauges (22 to 25), Teflon is currently the most widely used plastic catheter material because both in vivo animal testing and clinical use in humans have shown it to be less thrombogenic than polyethylene, polyvinyl chloride, or polypropylene.[62-65] Although heparin coating or impregnation has been shown to be of short-term value for arterial cannulation, the heparin leaches out of the plastic after a day or two and no further reduction in thrombogenicity is gained.[66]

The size of an arterial catheter is also an important consideration, both for the monitoring system to perform optimally and for minimizing vascular damage induced by the

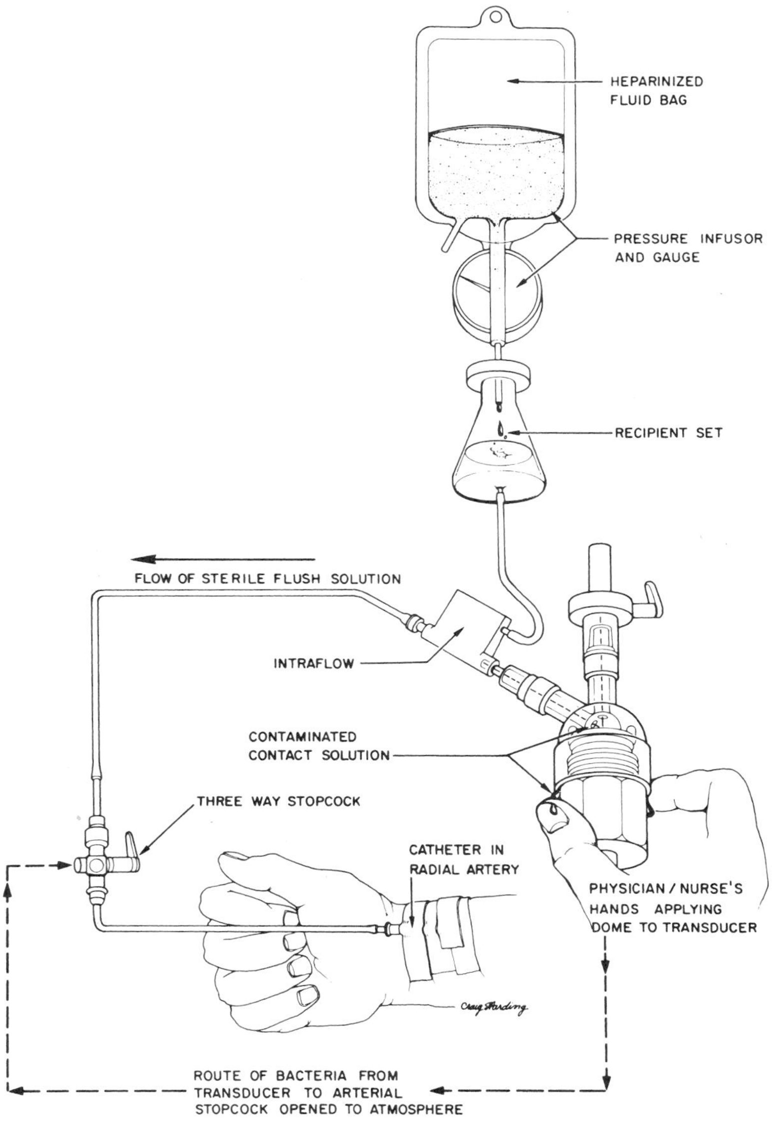

Figure 13–12. Diagram of arterial pressure monitoring system including arterial catheter, extension tubes, stopcocks, constant infusion device, disposable pressure dome, and transducer. Note the route of bacterial contamination in a sterile system: from the nonsterile transducer to the patient-access stopcock via a health professional's fingers. (From Bedford RF, Shah NK: Blood pressure monitoring: Invasive and noninvasive. In Blitt CD, Hines RL: Monitoring in Anesthesia and Critical Care Medicine. New York, Churchill Livingstone, 1995, p 95.)

catheter. In terms of minimizing vascular damage, it appears that the smaller an arterial catheter is relative to the size of the artery, the lower the incidence of vessel thrombosis[67] (Fig. 13–16). Conversely, however, smaller catheters are manufactured with thinner walls and are more prone to kink between the skin and the artery (Fig. 13–17). Within 24 hours of insertion, 20% of 20-gauge radial artery catheters kink, resulting in significant degradation of catheter performance. The BP pulse wave becomes damped, and difficulty is encountered in recovery of blood samples. Occasionally, a kinked catheter can be straightened by rotating the catheter through a 180-degree arc, or by applying distal traction and withdrawing it slightly. In the case of a kinked radial artery catheter, the temptation to hyperextend the wrist to straighten the kink and restore a pulse-pressure wave should be avoided, as this may lead to stretching of the median nerve with subsequent hand numbness.[68] As a last resort, a kinked catheter may be replaced by inserting a sterile, flexible guidewire into the catheter while it is straightened with distal traction; the old catheter is then removed, and a new one is introduced into the vessel over the guidewire.

General Hazards of Invasive Blood Pressure Monitoring

In general terms, the hazards of invasive arterial pressure monitoring can be summarized as (1) vascular compromise, (2) disconnection, (3) accidental injection, (4) infection, and (5) damage to nearby nerves. The problems of vascular compromise and nerve damage will be considered in the individual sections discussing the various sites suitable for arterial cannulation.

In a monitoring system exposed to systemic arterial pressures, it should go without saying that a disconnection could potentially result in a patient's rapid exsanguination. Accidental injection of noxious substances into a peripheral artery can be disastrous for an entire limb. The serious complications of intra-arterial thiopental and thiamylal injection are well known,[69] as are those of intravascular vasoconstrictors.[70] Ketamine injected via a dorsalis pedis artery catheter caused severe skin necrosis that extended proximally over the anterior and lateral portion of the leg and foot, and required 5

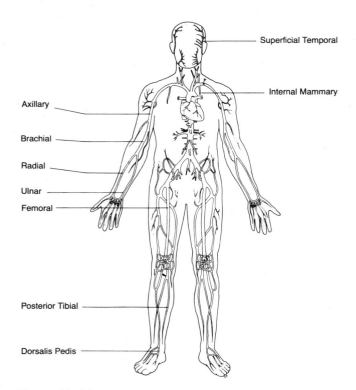

Axillary

Brachial

Radial

Ulnar

Femoral

Superficial Temporal

Internal Mammary

Posterior Tibial

Dorsalis Pedis

Figure 13–13. Sites for cannulation of the systemic arterial circulation. Although the most common location for catheterization is the radial artery, other sites (axillary, brachial, femoral, dorsalis pedis, superficial temporal) are used when radial collateral circulation is inadequate or radial pressures may be erroneous. Not demonstrated is the umbilical artery cannulation site. (From Lake C: Monitoring of arterial pressure. In Lake C: Clinical Monitoring for Anesthesia and Critical Care, 2nd ed. Philadelphia, WB Saunders, 1994.)

weeks for the patient to recover.[71] Similarly, retrograde injection of blood clots via a radial artery cannula have resulted in cerebrovascular ischemia,[72] as well as distal embolization and ischemia.[66, 73]

Arterial monitoring catheters may result in nosocomial infection due to either local or systemic sepsis. Local infections are thought to be caused by introduction of cutaneous bacteria at the time of cannulation and are usually of staphylococcal origin. The longer the cannula is in place, the greater the risk of local infection.[74-78] Unlike peripheral venous catheters, however, femoral arterial cannulas are not associated with a higher infection rate than other cannulation sites.[79] Ointments applied to intravascular catheter sites reduced the local infection rate from 6.5% in nontreated patients to 3.6% with iodophor and 2.2% with polymyxin, neomycin, or bacitracin ointment. However, these ointments have been associated with an increased incidence of *Candida* infections. Iodophor ointment is recommended for intravascular cannulation sites.[80] In addition, use of antibiotic-impregnated catheters has been advocated to reduce infectious complications from peripheral arterial catheters.[81]

Bacteremia is also associated with use of arterial monitoring systems. This may be the result of contamination of the tubing system,[82-84] or the catheter itself may become a nidus for infection due to seeding from septicemia. Stopcocks are often the route of access when bacteria are manually transferred to the tubing system (see Fig. 13–12), although the use of contemporary isolated disposable transducer systems (as opposed to the disposable dome shown in Fig. 13–12) has markedly reduced the risks of bacterial contamination[85]

and studies support the use of these systems for up to 4 days without replacement.[86] Arterial thrombi induced by monitoring catheters also may act as a septic nidus,[87, 88] occasionally requiring surgical removal of the thrombus to treat the infection.[89, 90]

Current Centers for Disease Control and Prevention (CDC) recommendations[91] for prevention of infections related to peripheral arterial cannulas include the following:

1. Use sterile technique, including gown, mask, and gloves and sterile drapes for catheter insertion.

2. Cleanse the skin site with appropriate antiseptic before catheter insertion and allow antiseptic to remain in the insertion site for an appropriate duration before insertion.

3. Replace dressings when damp, loosened, or soiled.

4. If local cutaneous infection is present at the skin puncture site, remove the catheter.

5. If catheter-related infection is suspected, replace the catheter using guidewire assistance. If catheter-related infection is documented, remove the catheter.

6. Use disposable, rather than reusable, transducer assemblies with closed, continuous flush systems whenever possible.

7. Sterilize and disinfect reusable transducers in a central processing area.

8. Treat stopcocks as a sterile field and keep covered with a cap or syringe when not in use. Do not use arterial catheters for routine blood sampling that does not require arterial blood.

9. In adults, replace catheters, transducers, and flush tubing at 96-hour intervals.

10. If persistent bacteremia occurs while an arterial catheter is in place, remove the catheter 24 to 48 hours from the time antimicrobial therapy has been started.

Sites for Invasive Blood Pressure Cannulation

Radial Artery Cannulation

Advantages and Disadvantages. Percutaneous radial artery cannulation rapidly achieved widespread popularity for invasive BP monitoring shortly after its initial description by Barr in 1961.[58] The reasons for this popularity are obvious: (1) the vessel is superficial and easy to identify; (2) the cannulation site is accessible; (3) the procedure is reasonably reliable and pain-free for the patient; and (4) collateral circulation to the hand is abundant and easy to document and the likelihood of inducing distal vascular ischemia is quite low.

On the other hand, the radial artery is not the ideal cannulation site for acquiring hemodynamic data. The radial pulse-pressure wave is subject to considerable systolic pressure augmentation because it is distal and close to the point of pulse wave reflection. Furthermore, the radial artery lumen diameter is relatively small (2 to 3 mm), and it frequently becomes occluded by either the catheter or catheter-induced thrombus.[92] Thus, the site of pulse wave reflection is right at the site of cannulation, and systolic pressure becomes augmented with high-frequency pressure wave transients that give a falsely elevated systolic pressure value.

Radial arterial pressures are also fraught with abnormal pressure gradients between the aortic and radial arteries associated with cardiothoracic operations[93] and separation

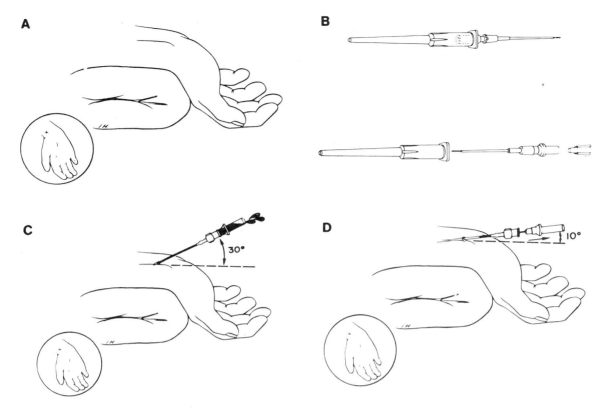

Figure 13–14. The technique of cannulation of a peripheral artery is similar for almost all arteries. The direct technique for the radial artery is demonstrated. *A,* Proper hand position with the hand dorsiflexed over a small roll. *B,* Technique of placing the catheter cover over the end of the catheter. This technique allows visualization of free flow of blood without environmental contamination. (K.R. Grosslight, M.D., personal communication, 1989.) *C,* The catheter is inserted at an angle of 30–40 degrees to the plane of the wrist until spurting blood flow is obtained. *D,* The angle of the catheter is reduced to 10 degrees while the plastic catheter is advanced into the artery. (From Lake CL: Cardiovascular Anesthesia. New York, Springer-Verlag, 1985, p 54.)

from cardiopulmonary bypass, particularly during and following rewarming.[94-96] It is thought that the latter differences (up to 32 mmHg) may be due to changes in vasomotor tone associated with the wide temperature fluctuations and endocrine responses to cardiopulmonary bypass.

A previous diagnostic catheterization performed in the brachial artery should probably preclude use of the ipsilateral radial artery, since pulse-pressure waves may be markedly damped and a low-flow state may tend to induce hand ischemia.[97] Other factors that might affect the site of radial artery cannulation include use of the right radial artery for thoracic aneurysm surgery, because the left subclavian is often occluded during surgery, or use of the right radial in premature infants with a patent ductus arteriosus, where the left side would receive desaturated blood from the ductus arteriosus. Finally, cannulation of the radial artery in a hand with inadequate ulnar artery collateral circulation may result in limb ischemia.[98]

There are probably as many techniques for cannulation of the radial artery as there are clinicians performing it. The radial artery is quite tortuous as it passes over the wrist joint (Fig. 13–18). Just palpating a pulse at one point near the wrist does not indicate where the vessel may be when the catheter reaches the depth of the artery, and it does not guarantee that the catheter will be aligned with the vessel lumen when it enters the vessel wall. Accordingly, dorsiflexion and immobilization of the wrist, and identification of the course of the vessel with palpating fingers or a skin-marking pencil may increase the likelihood of successful cannulation (see Fig. 13–14). Cannulation of the radial artery proximal to

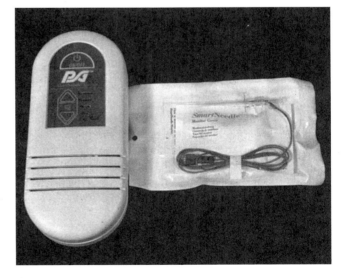

Figure 13–15. The Smart Needle Doppler device for cannulation of peripheral and central veins with ultrasound localization. Both 18- and 20-gauge cannulas may be inserted using this technique. (From Lake C: Monitoring of arterial pressure. In Lake C: Clinical Monitoring for Anesthesia and Critical Care, 2nd ed. Philadelphia, WB Saunders, 1994.)

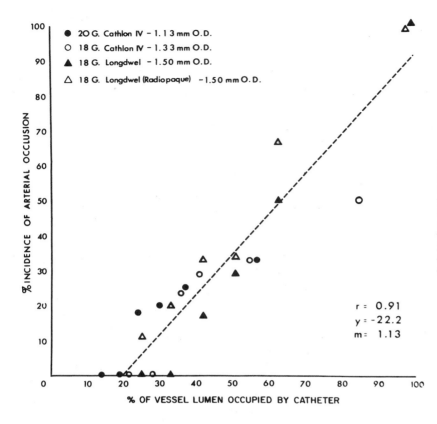

Legend:
● 20 G. Cathlon IV – 1.13 mm O.D.
○ 18 G. Cathlon IV – 1.33 mm O.D.
▲ 18 G. Longdwel – 1.50 mm O.D.
△ 18 G. Longdwel (Radiopaque) – 1.50 mm O.D.

r = 0.91
y = –22.2
m = 1.13

X-axis: % OF VESSEL LUMEN OCCUPIED BY CATHETER
Y-axis: % INCIDENCE OF ARTERIAL OCCLUSION

Figure 13-16. Radial artery thrombosis after 24 hours of cannulation. Incidence of radial artery occlusion plotted as a function of the percentage of the vessel lumen occupied by the arterial catheter. Small catheters in large vessels tended to induce thrombosis only rarely. Large catheters occupying the entire vessel lumen always induced thrombosis. (From Bedford RF: Radial arterial function following percutaneous cannulation with 18- and 20-gauge catheters. Anesthesiology 1977; 47:37.)

the wrist joint (where it is straighter) may also improve the success rate. Although its greater depth may make it more difficult to palpate, the catheter may slide into the vessel lumen more readily because the vessel is straighter at this location. The improved cannulation success rate of the Arrow radial artery catheterization set (Arrow International, Reading, PA), with its built-in flexible guidewire, is possibly due to the propensity of most clinicians to go where the artery is most superficial rather than where it is straightest.[98] Once the vessel lumen is entered, the flexible guidewire can negotiate turns that a straight needle and catheter assembly cannot manage.

The impact on vessel function of multiple arterial punctures during attempted cannulation is controversial. Some think that traumatic cannulation is responsible for most ischemic problems related to invasive BP monitoring,[99] whereas others have found no evidence for such a claim.[100] Transfixion of the radial artery during cannulation has not been found to cause a higher incidence of vascular occlusion than techniques where only the superficial wall of the vessel is punctured during cannulation.[101-103] Pseudoaneurysm formation, however, is a well-recognized complication of radial artery cannulation.[104] This is usually heralded by the presence of a pulsatile hematoma at the cannulation site as a result of a persistent hole in the vessel wall, often associated with anticoagulation. Conservative management, with Doppler-guided compression over the site of leakage, is thought to be the treatment of choice.[105]

Trauma during radial artery cannulation may, however, result in nerve damage or compartment syndrome, or both, at the wrist related to persistent bleeding from puncture sites.[106] Figure 13-19 shows extravasation of radiopaque contrast material outside of a radial artery that had just been cannulated by a transfixing technique. With multiple arterial punctures, particularly in anticoagulated patients, considera-

bly more extravasation probably occurs. While the radial nerve lies close to the radial artery, it is the median nerve that has been associated with evidence of neuropathy (pain, weakness, hand wasting) following multiple radial artery punctures, cutdown cannulation, or traumatic attempted percutaneous cannulation.[107, 108] Postmortem examination has shown hematoma from the radial artery extending over the flexor carpi radialis and compressing the median nerve proximal to the transverse carpal ligament. Presumably the median nerve is more susceptible because it is confined within the carpal tunnel and is subject to compression by spreading hematoma. Another possible cause of hand pain after radial artery cannulation is prolonged dorsiflexion of the wrist with stretching of the median nerve.[109] Thus, it is probably advisable to return the wrist to a more neutral position after cannulation.

Radial artery thrombosis occurs frequently after cannulation for BP monitoring and may contribute to catastrophic ischemic injury to the hand (see below). In general, a higher incidence of arterial occlusion results from progressively longer periods of cannulation,[74, 100, 110, 111] and the use of larger catheters made of non–Teflon-containing plastics. Data in adult patients suggest a 10% overall incidence of arterial occlusion in adults cannulated with 20-gauge Teflon catheters in place for a period of 1 to 3 days[110] (Fig. 13-20), whereas use of 22-gauge Teflon catheters for 24 hours reduces the risk of arterial occlusion to close to zero.[112]

The size of the radial artery lumen relative to the cross-sectional area of the cannula also affects the incidence of vessel thrombosis[67, 92] (see Fig. 13-16). Women have a higher incidence of radial arterial occlusion than men,[100, 113] and the incidence of radial arterial occlusion in neonates reaches as high as 72% when 22-gauge catheters are left in place for up to 10 days.[114] By contrast, adults sustain approximately a 30% incidence of occlusion when 20-gauge radial

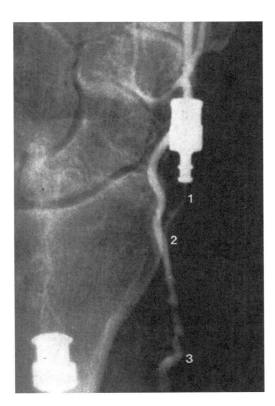

Figure 13–17. Radiograph of a nonfunctional, 20-gauge radial artery catheter showing three sites of kinking: 1, above the skin, 2, between the skin and the artery, and 3, within the artery lumen. (From Bedford RF, Shah NK: Blood pressure monitoring: Invasive and noninvasive. In Blitt CD, Hines RL: Monitoring in Anesthesia and Critical Care Medicine. New York, Churchill Livingstone, 1995, p 95.)

artery catheters remain in place for a similar length of time.[74, 115]

The pathophysiology of radial artery thrombosis is summarized in Figures 13–21 through 13–24. The presence of a catheter within the radial artery lumen first induces a thickening of the intimal lining which, in turn, is followed by loss of the intima and accumulation of platelet aggregates and fibrinous material. Radial arterial cannulation also causes scarring of the vessel media, and weakness of this layer may result in pseudoaneurysm formation after decannulation.

Thrombotic occlusion of the radial artery after cannulation appears to be a temporary phenomenon (Fig. 13–25), with studies showing a duration up to 75 days.[8, 100, 115] Smaller arteries remain thrombosed longer than larger arteries,[8] perhaps because they sustain greater anatomic damage while the cannula is in place. As recanalization of radial artery thrombi may take many days, it is not practical to rely on this process for alleviation of distal vascular ischemia should it develop while a cannula is in place. Some thrombi can be removed at the time of decannulation by aspirating vigorously through the catheter while it is being withdrawn from the radial artery[116] (Figs. 13–26 and 13–29). This technique has been used to successfully reinstate flow to patients' hands that have started to become ischemic during prolonged cannulation. Another approach to remove thrombi from radial arteries with an 18-gauge cannula in place is to perform a surgical cutdown onto the artery and to pass a small-diameter embolectomy catheter through the arteriotomy created by the 18-gauge cannula. Inflation of the balloon and withdrawal of the embolectomy catheter can re-

move clot from the artery and reestablish blood flow past the area of occlusion.[65]

The most common complication associated with radial artery cannulation that results in significant morbidity is *not* distal vascular insufficiency, but rather *ischemic necrosis* of the skin overlying the cannula (Fig. 13–27). This lesion requires several weeks to heal by secondary intention. Originally described as an incidental, isolated finding, this lesion is associated with 0.5% to 3.0% of all cannulations[117] and 10% of all thrombosed radial arteries regardless of the duration of cannulation or the size of the cannula.[74] Arteriography demonstrates occlusion of the small, cutaneous, perforating branches of the radial artery due to thrombosis around the cannula, and postmortem examination has found thrombus extending into the branches of the radial artery. The incidence of this problem has decreased with the use of smaller catheters, presumably because fewer thrombi are produced.[74]

Given that there is a high incidence of radial artery occlusion associated with percutaneous cannulation, the importance of collateral circulation to the hand should not be underestimated. Coleman and Anson[118] performed 650 anatomic dissections to identify the three arterial arches anastomosing between the radial and ulnar arteries: (1) a superficial volar arch (complete in 86% of specimens) formed primarily as a continuation of the ulnar artery; (2) a deep volar arch (complete in 50% of specimens) formed from the

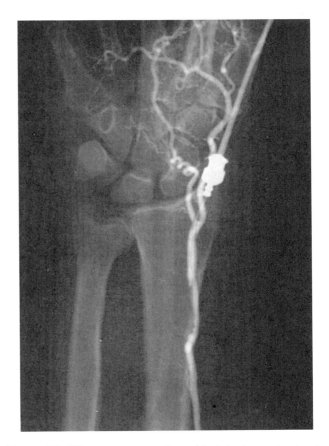

Figure 13–18. Arteriogram performed by injecting contrast material through a radial artery catheter. Note the tortuosity of the artery as it passes over the wrist joint. (From Bedford RF, Shah NK: Blood pressure monitoring: Invasive and noninvasive. In Blitt CD, Hines RL: Monitoring in Anesthesia and Critical Care Medicine. New York, Churchill Livingstone, 1995, p 95.)

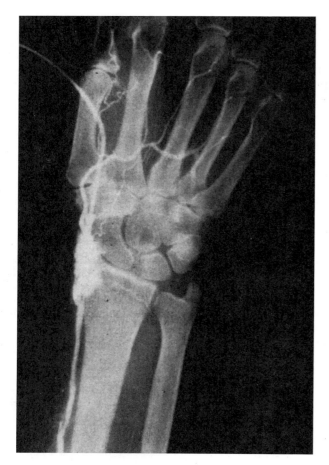

Figure 13-19. Contrast material extravasating from the deep wall of a radial artery recently cannulated with a transfixing technique. Such extravasation appears to play a role in median nerve dysfunction associated with radial artery cannulation. (From Bedford RF, Shah NK: Blood pressure monitoring: Invasive and noninvasive. In Blitt CD, Hines RL: Monitoring in Anesthesia and Critical Care Medicine. New York, Churchill Livingstone, 1995, p 95.)

continuation of the radial artery; and (3) a dorsal arch (complete in 85% of specimens) formed primarily as a continuation of the dorsal radial artery and anastomosing with either the interosseous or ulnar arteries. These findings have been verified by radiologic examinations, such as that seen in Figure 13-28, in which collateral flow from the ulnar artery supplies blood to the entire hand and radial artery distal to a cannula-induced, occlusive lesion. Digital blood flow in turn radiates from the palmar arches, such that if occlusion of the radial artery is caused by a monitoring cannula, it rarely results in distal vascular ischemia of the hand because of the abundant collateral circulation from the ulnar and median interosseous arteries.

Accurate assessment of ulnar collateral circulation seems warranted because anatomic studies predict that approximately 3% to 6% of patients have incomplete palmar arterial arches.[118] These findings have been verified clinically by Husum and Palm,[119] who found that 6% of 259 patients undergoing cardiovascular surgery had inadequate ulnar flow unilaterally (determined by a systolic BP of < 40 mmHg in the thumb during radial artery occlusion) and 4% had inadequate ulnar flow bilaterally. Furthermore, several studies have found markedly impaired radial artery flow soon after cannulation such that the hand is entirely perfused by collateral

flow.[97, 120] In patients with acromegaly, in which ulnar artery flow is often compromised by ligamentous hypertrophy at the wrist, it has been recommended either that radial artery cannulation be avoided or that particular attention be given to documenting adequate ulnar collateral circulation before the radial artery is cannulated.[121]

Allen's test, devised in 1929 as a method for diagnosing occlusive arterial lesions at the wrist caused by thromboangiitis obliterans,[122] is both popular and controversial as a technique for documenting adequate collateral circulation from the ulnar artery to the entire hand. Allen described having the patient alternately squeeze and relax his hand to exsanguinate it while the examiner occluded both the radial and ulnar arteries with fingertip pressure. Patency of the ulnar artery was indicated by a "prompt return to color" in the hand when pressure over the ulnar artery was released. Allen did not intend to document blood flow to the entire hand, but only to diagnose arterial occlusion at the wrist.[122]

When used to document collateral flow, Allen's test "return to color" has been a source of confusion. Some clinicians have mistaken a blush in the center of the palm as indicative of blood flow passing all the way from the ulnar artery to the thumb and thenar eminence. Others thought that a 15-second "return to color" indicated satisfactory collateral circulation.[100, 123] The result of these misinterpretations was a 10% incidence of cold, white thumbs associated with radial artery occlusion. More recent studies using a 5-second limit on complete "return to color" of the hand, particularly the thumb and thenar eminence, have found Allen's test to be a satisfactory technique for documenting patency of ulnar collateral circulation,[92] although Husum and Berthelson[123] found a 1% chance of inadequate thumb flow

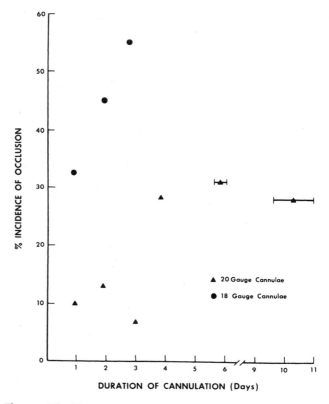

Figure 13-20. Incidence of radial artery thrombosis plotted against duration of cannulation for 18- and 20-gauge catheters. (From Bedford RF: Long-term radial artery cannulation: effects on subsequent vessel function. Crit Care Med 1978; 6:64.)

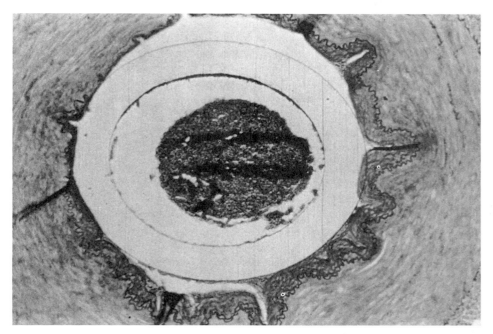

Figure 13–21. Microscopic section of a radial artery with catheter in situ. There is thickening of the intimal layer as a reaction to the introduction of the foreign body. (Elastic stain.) (From Bedford RF, Shah NK: Blood pressure monitoring: Invasive and noninvasive. In Blitt CD, Hines RL: Monitoring in Anesthesia and Critical Care Medicine. New York, Churchill Livingstone, 1995, p 95.)

with a 6-second "return to color" time from the ulnar artery while the radial artery was occluded.[123]

Additional problems with Allen's test are (1) the patient must be awake and cooperative; (2) it is difficult or impossible to interpret in patients who are burned, pale, or jaundiced; and (3) hyperextension of the digits may give a false pallor, resulting in misinterpretation of the test. Because of the problems in interpreting Allen's test, other techniques for documenting ulnar collateral circulation have been developed, including Doppler examination, pulse pressure measurement, or pulse oximetry distal to an occluding finger over the radial artery.[124-127] Slogoff et al.[113] concluded that Allen's test was not useful because they found no episodes of distal

vascular ischemia after cannulating the radial arteries of 16 patients with markedly impaired flow to the hand. Because they failed to document the duration of the cannulation, the size of the catheters used, and what proportion of the patients were men (with large radial arteries and a lower incidence of thrombosis), the results remain controversial.

Despite apparent evidence of satisfactory ulnar collateral circulation, many case reports of severe distal vascular ischemia and gangrene of the hand have been associated with radial artery cannulation[128-132] (see Figs. 13-27 and 13-29). To date, only one such case has been definitely associated with thromboembolic phenomena from the heart.[133] More commonly, however, hand gangrene is associated with low-

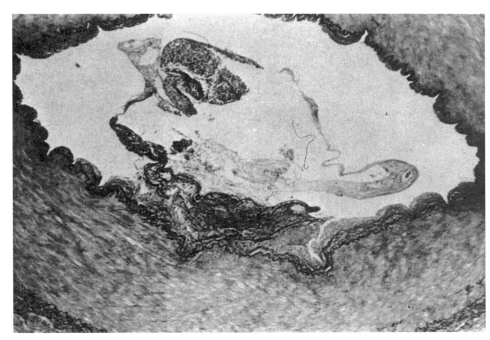

Figure 13–22. Continued presence of the catheter results in denuding of the intimal lining with accumulation of platelets and thrombotic material on the exposed internal elastic layer. (From Bedford RF, Shah NK: Blood pressure monitoring: Invasive and noninvasive. In Blitt CD, Hines RL: Monitoring in Anesthesia and Critical Care Medicine. New York, Churchill Livingstone, 1995, p 95.)

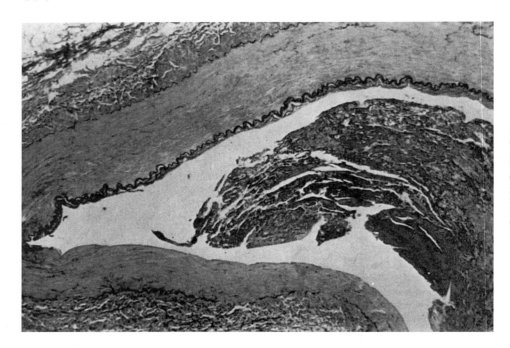

Figure 13-23. With prolonged cannulation there is complete denuding of the intimal lining and thrombotic occlusion of the vessel lumen. (From Bedford RF, Shah NK: Blood pressure monitoring: Invasive and noninvasive. In Blitt CD, Hines RL: Monitoring in Anesthesia and Critical Care Medicine. New York, Churchill Livingstone, 1995, p 95.)

flow states, high-dose vasopressor therapy, and no documentation of ulnar collateral flow.[63, 72, 76, 99, 134-137] Although distal vascular ischemia has been relieved in some of these cases by thrombectomy, sympathetic blockade, intra-arterial local anesthetic, or papaverine, the condition in many patients was totally refractory to therapy, and they ultimately required amputation of fingers, hands, or forearms. The overall incidence of severe vascular compromise has been estimated at 0.01% of all radial artery cannulations.[138] Because these catastrophes usually begin with radial arterial thrombosis, and thrombus around the catheter often causes catheter dysfunction in the form of damped pulse-pressure waves or difficulty in obtaining samples, it has been recommended that evidence of catheter dysfunction probably should be a signal for decannulation.[63] This should be performed preferably with vigorous aspiration on the catheter as it is withdrawn in an attempt to remove intra-arterial thrombus.[116] Attempts at relieving catheter dysfunction by vigorous flushing, however, may only result in cerebral ischemia due to retrograde flow of clot and flush solution to the carotid or vertebral circulation.[72] Such attempts have been shown to cause acute hypertension in neonates.[139]

Alternative Sites for Arterial Pressure Monitoring

Ulnar Artery. Ulnar artery cannulation is performed in a manner similar to cannulation of the radial artery, although it is somewhat more difficult because the vessel is not as superficial as the radial artery and it tends to be quite tortuous as it passes the wrist joint (see Fig. 13-28). Several studies have referred to the radial and ulnar arteries as interchangeable sites for peripheral arterial cannulation.[8, 97, 119] Because dominant collateral flow to the hand can be from either the radial or ulnar artery, it seems advisable to document collateral flow from the radial artery to the entire hand prior to attempting cannulation of the ulnar artery. Likewise, virtually every technical problem and clinical complication ascribed to radial artery cannulation can also occur in association with ulnar artery cannulation.

Brachial Artery. Cannulation of the brachial artery of-

fers several theoretical and practical advantages over radial and ulnar artery cannulation. It is a larger vessel than the radial or ulnar arteries and may be more amenable to cannulation in infants. In addition, it can accommodate a larger catheter with a higher natural frequency. Furthermore, it is more proximal and, therefore, less subject to systolic pressure augmentation due to reflection of the pulse-pressure wave from distal artery-arteriole junctions. As with other sites, however, the incidence of complications increases with duration of cannulation.[140-144]

In addition to vascular lesions, damage to the median nerve has also been reported with brachial artery cannulation, either associated with traumatic arterial puncture or hematoma formation.[145, 146] From a practical standpoint, brachial artery catheters work well when a patient is anesthetized but tend to be a problem in conscious patients in the intensive care unit in whom the elbow joint becomes more difficult to immobilize than the wrist.

Axillary Artery. There are several desirable aspects to cannulation of the axillary artery. The vessel is large, it can tolerate relatively large-bore catheters with a low incidence of thrombotic complications, and it leaves the patient's arms relatively unencumbered. The axillary artery is often palpable in critically ill infants[147] and adults, when more peripheral vessels are faint or absent. In addition, the axillary pulse-pressure trace closely represents that in the aortic arch.[148-153]

Because the axillary arterial catheter is close to the central circulation, meticulous attention must be directed at preventing the entry of air bubbles or clots into the cerebral circulation during catheter flushing or blood sampling. The left axillary artery is the preferred site, since the tip of a 6-in. catheter in the right axillary artery may lie in the innominate artery, with ready access to the cerebral circulation. Another disadvantage of the axillary artery is its location within a neurovascular sheath, where hematoma formation may result in neurologic consequences.[106, 107]

The approach to the axillary artery is similar to that for an axillary brachial plexus block. Once the vessel lumen is punctured, cannulation can be performed using either a 3-in.

catheter-over-needle device or a 6-in. pediatric central venous pressure catheter advanced into the vessel over a guidewire.

Dorsalis Pedis Artery. Cannulation of the dorsalis pedis artery is indicated in clinical situations in which the arteries of the upper extremities are inaccessible, as in extensive burns, trauma, or previous arterial catheterizations.[154] Due to its distal location, however, systolic and diastolic pressure readings are subject to considerable resonance and MAP is the only value that approximates aortic pressure values. Like other peripheral arteries, it is also subject to pseudoaneurysm formation following cannulation.[155] Because it is a small vessel, there is a high incidence of both unsuccessful cannulation and postcannulation arterial occlusion. Fortunately, there is an arterial arcade in the foot that usually supplies collateral circulation from the posterior tibial circulation in the event of occlusion of the dorsalis pedis artery. However, wedge-shaped distal infarcts and impaired toe perfusion have been reported.[156, 157] To assess collateral circulation, Kaplan[158] suggests occluding both the dorsalis pedis and posterior tibial pulses with digital pressure, then blanching the patient's great toe with direct compression. If the toe color does not promptly (< 5 seconds) return to normal when the posterior tibial artery pressure is released, another site should be selected for arterial cannulation.

Femoral Artery. When used for BP monitoring in adults, the femoral artery has been found to be no more risky than radial artery cannulation.[159-161] It is a large artery and should be relatively free from catheter-induced thrombosis. However, it is also subject to atheroma formation, which may lead to difficult cannulation, peripheral embolization, and possible distal vascular insufficiency. Several reports list an approximate incidence of 0.5% for ischemia requiring embolectomy after femoral artery cannulation, whereas transient self-limited vascular insufficiency occurs in approximately another 0.5%. In these studies, catheter sizes ranged from 14 to 20 gauge, with no obvious relationship between catheter diameter and the incidence of occlusive lesions. These data

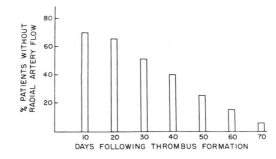

Figure 13-25. Duration of arterial occlusion in patients whose radial arteries had thrombosed after cannulation. (From Bedford RF, Wollman H: Complications of percutaneous radial artery cannulation: An objective prospective study in man. Anesthesiology 1973; 38: 228–236.)

suggest that atheromas may act as a prime cause of occlusion while femoral arterial catheters are in place.[162-164]

Hematoma and pseudoaneurysm formation are also prominent problems with femoral artery cannulation, with the former occurring in 8% to 13% of patients. Both are probably related to placement of catheters through larger needles or via a transfixing cannulation technique.[159, 162, 164-166] Noncompressible retroperitoneal hematomas have also been reported as a result of unsuccessful femoral artery catheterization,[167] occasionally leading to compartmental syndrome.[168]

As is the case with other intravascular catheters, the incidence of infection increases with the duration of femoral artery cannulation. A 1- to 3-day period appears to be safe, whereas longer periods (4 to 12 days) produce catheter-related infections at a rate of 8% to 17%.[149, 159, 162]

Indications for cannulation of the femoral artery include thoracic aortic surgery, in which the patency of a Gott shunt can be monitored by femoral artery pressure[169]; patients in shock whose other peripheral pulses may be nonpalpable; or those suffering from burns or multiple trauma in whom other sites are inaccessible.

In children, 18- or 20-gauge catheters are often more

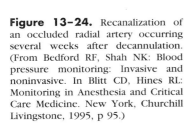

Figure 13-24. Recanalization of an occluded radial artery occurring several weeks after decannulation. (From Bedford RF, Shah NK: Blood pressure monitoring: Invasive and noninvasive. In Blitt CD, Hines RL: Monitoring in Anesthesia and Critical Care Medicine. New York, Churchill Livingstone, 1995, p 95.)

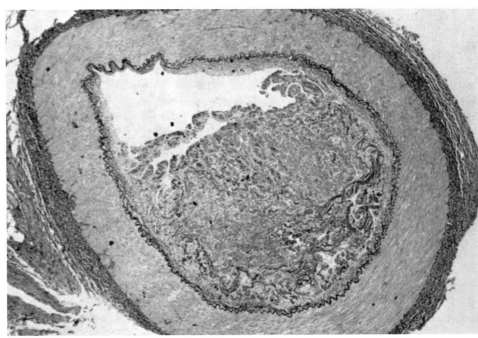

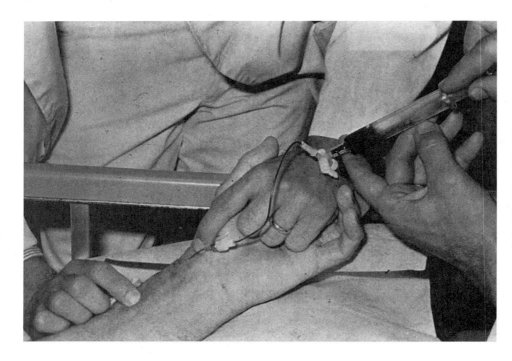

Figure 13-26. Attempted recovery of thrombus from a radial artery at decannulation. As the catheter is withdrawn, vigorous continuous suction is applied while digital pressure occludes the artery. Thrombus is aspirated into the syringe. (From Bedford RF: Removal of radial artery thrombi following percutaneous cannulation for monitoring. Anesthesiology 1977; 46:430.)

easily placed in the femoral than in the radial arteries. However, cannulation of the femoral artery is often avoided in children because of a high incidence of thrombosis in younger children with small vessels,[170] its proximity to the retroperitoneum,[171] the risk of hip capsule puncture with subsequent joint infection, and the potential for decreased limb growth if thrombotic occlusion should develop. In the series reported by Glenski and coworkers,[172] femoral catheterization was performed in 151 children undergoing cardiac surgery with only a 3.6% failure rate. Decreased limb perfusion occurred in 25% of neonates, but the overall rate of infectious complications was only 3.6% in 165 catheteriza-

tions and no permanent complications were noted.[172] Rosenthal and colleagues[173] noted no reduction in leg growth after femoral cannulation. In children under the age of 10 years, prophylactic administration of heparin 100 U/kg has been found to reduce the incidence of thromboembolic events significantly, from 40% to 8%.[174] In the event that thrombotic occlusion occurs in a child, thrombolytic therapy has been found to be successful in 85% of patients, with only 1% requiring surgical embolectomy.[175]

Superficial Temporal Artery. The temporal artery branches off the external carotid artery, which passes anterior to the tragus of the ear. Temporal cannulation may be useful on an emergent basis if there is no access to other sites, or as a primary cannulation site for BP monitoring during thoracic aortic procedures. The superficial temporal artery is often quite tortuous and difficult to cannulate. First delineating the arterial course with a Doppler probe may facilitate cannula passage by helping to align the vessel with the cannula assembly.[176] Arterial puncture is often performed at the superior edge of the helix of the ear,[177] either percutaneously or through a 3-mm to 2-cm incision (depending on patient size) with the catheter-needle device in a bevel-down position. The bevel-down position has been found to help prevent posterior arterial perforation, and the catheter can then be advanced centrally. Proper positioning of the catheter tip is crucial, with an optimal location in the external carotid artery at the junction with the external maxillary artery. Risks of superficial temporal cannulation include vessel thrombosis with resultant scalp ischemia and catheter malposition that permits embolic material to pass centrally to the cerebral circulation via the internal carotid artery. Because of the site, it is often difficult to secure the catheter so that it does not become dislodged.[176, 177]

Umbilical Artery. Cannulation of the umbilical artery is used in critically ill newborns, in whom access to more peripheral vessels may prove difficult or tenuous. The umbilical arteries originate from the internal iliac arteries, cross over the ureters, and pass inferiorly on either side of the

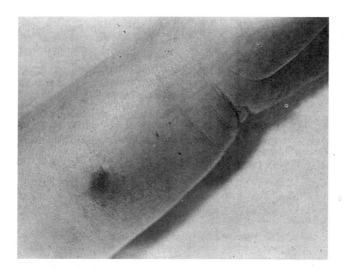

Figure 13-27. Skin necrosis overlying a segment of radial artery thrombus. The cannula puncture site is seen distal to the lesion. (From Bedford RF, Shah NK: Blood pressure monitoring: Invasive and noninvasive. In Blitt CD, Hines RL: Monitoring in Anesthesia and Critical Care Medicine. New York, Churchill Livingstone, 1995, p 95.)

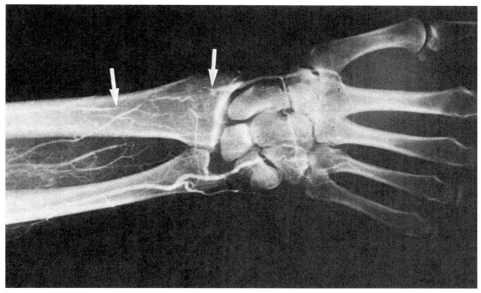

Figure 13–28. Brachial arteriogram of a patient with an occluded radial artery (*arrows*). Collateral circulation to the hand is supplied via the ulnar artery and two of the three palmar arterial arches described by Coleman and Anson.[118] (From Bedford RF, Shah NK: Blood pressure monitoring: Invasive and noninvasive. In Blitt CD, Hines RL: Monitoring in Anesthesia and Critical Care Medicine. New York, Churchill Livingstone, 1995, p 95.)

dome of the bladder and cephalad in the anterior abdominal wall to the umbilicus.[184] Either a percutaneous or a cutdown technique may be used. With the percutaneous method, a 16-gauge short catheter is initially placed as an introducer and then a longer 3.5F or 5F catheter is guided through the 16-gauge catheter into the aorta. The cutdown method requires placement of a suture at the base of the umbilicus prior to cutting the umbilical cord several millimeters above the skin. An umbilical artery is identified and a probe is inserted to dilate the vessel prior to passage of the catheter (a 3.5F or 5F catheter). After the catheter is successfully inserted, the suture at the umbilical base is tied around the catheter.[178]

Optimal locations for the catheter tip are just above the aortic bifurcation,[179] below the inferior mesenteric artery, or at the mid-dorsal aorta above the diaphragm. Undesirable locations include the celiac plexus and renal or superior mesenteric arteries.[180] Spasm at the junction of hypogastric and iliac arteries is the most common cause of failure to successfully catheterize the aorta via an umbilical artery.

Complications of umbilical arterial cannulation can be catastrophic, including abdominal organ ischemia if the catheter becomes dislodged into a specific intra-abdominal vessel, aortic thrombosis, lower extremity ischemia secondary to arterial vasospasm or embolism, vascular perforation causing hemorrhage and paradoxical central nervous system embolism via a patent foramen ovale.[180–182] Factors contributing to

complications include prolonged use and repeated manipulations. Prophylactic low-dose heparin administration has been shown to lower the incidence of thromboembolic complications.[183] Additional methods to avoid complications include radiographic confirmation of catheter tip location, avoidance of catheter manipulation, use of nonthrombogenic catheters, and timely removal of catheters when no longer indicated.

Conclusions

Will indirect measurement of BP ever replace direct intra-arterial BP monitoring? Probably not, because an arterial catheter also functions as a site for drawing multiple blood samples, when needed. On the other hand, the rapid development of noninvasive CO_2 and O_2 analysis, in combination with reliable NIBP measurements, has probably reduced the overall need for arterial catheterization.

It must always be remembered, however, that invasive arterial pressure monitoring and NIBP measurement reflect two different phenomena. When a catheter is placed in a patient's artery, the systolic, diastolic, and mean pressures can be obtained even when there is no blood flow in the vessel. In contrast, when an occluding cuff is wrapped around the patient's arm and inflated, detection of the systolic, diastolic, and mean pressure is possible only because of blood flow under the cuff. Thus, one technique measures

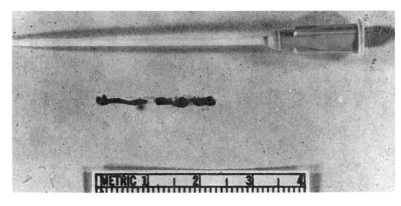

Figure 13–29. Thrombotic material recovered from a radial artery catheter during decannulation. (From Bedford RF: Removal of radial artery thrombi following percutaneous cannulation for monitoring. Anesthesiology 1977; 46:430.)

pressure directly, whereas the other detects flow and tries to infer pressure indirectly.

Should we resolve these differences? We believe probably not. Attempts to make the direct and indirect methods of BP measurements correspond can lower the accuracy and repeatability of both methods. One should be content with the fact that each method has its particular advantages, and comparisons, except in the most general terms, should be avoided. The important feature of BP monitoring is that the equipment gives a value, which, in turn, should cause the clinician to think about what is happening to the patient and to act accordingly.

REFERENCES

1. Brunner JMR: Handbook of Blood Pressure Monitoring. Littleton, MA, PSG, 1978.
2. Prys-Roberts C: Measurement of intravascular pressure. In Saidman LJ, Smith NT (eds): Monitoring in Anesthesia. New York, Churchill Livingstone, 1978, pp 64–83.
3. Brunner JMR, Krenis LJ, Kunsman JM, et al: Comparison of direct and indirect methods of measuring arterial blood pressure. Part I. Med Instrum 1981; 15:11–21.
4. O'Rourke MJF: Pressure and flow waves in systemic arteries and the anatomical design of the arterial system. J Appl Physiol 1967; 23:139–144.
5. Campbell B: Arterial waveforms: Monitoring changes in configuration. Heart Lung 1997; 26:204–214.
6. Shelley KH, Murray WB, Chang D: Arterial-pulse oximetry loops: A new method of monitoring vascular tone. J Clin Monit Comput 1997; 13:223–228.
7. Brunner JMR, Krenis LJ, Kunsman JM, et al: Comparison of direct and indirect methods of measuring arterial blood pressure. Part II. Med Instrum 1981; 15:97–102.
8. Kim JM, Arawaka K, Bliss J: Arterial cannulation: Factors in the development of occlusion. Anesth Analg 1977; 56:603–606.
9. Berne RM, Levy MN: Peripheral arterial pressure curves. In Cardiovascular Physiology. St Louis, Mosby–Year Book, 1977, pp 110–121.
10. O'Rourke MF, Taylor MG: Vascular impedance of the femoral bed. Circ Res 1966; 18:126–129.
11. Brunner JMR: Invasive pressure monitoring: Practical application and pitfalls. Presented at American Society of Anesthesiologists Annual Meeting, Refresher Course Lecture, Las Vegas, Oct. 1982.
12. Cushing H: On routine determinations of arterial tension in operating room and clinic. N Engl J Med 1903; 148:250–255.
13. Davis RF: Clinical comparison of automated auscultatory and oscillometric and catheter-transducer measurements of arterial pressure. J Clin Monit Comput 1985; 1:114–116.
14. Geddes LA: The Direct and Indirect Measurement of Blood Pressure. St Louis, Mosby–Year Book, 1970.
15. Hill L, Barnard H: A simple and accurate form of sphygmomanometer for arterial pressure gauge contrived for clinical use. BMJ 1897; 2:904–905.
16. Kirkendall WM, Feinleib M, Freis ED, Mark AL: American Heart Association: Recommendation for human blood pressure determination by sphygmomanometers. Circulation 1980; 62:1145A–1155A.
17. Gorback MS: Considerations in the interpretation of systemic pressure monitoring. In Lumb PD, Bryan-Brown CW (eds): Complications in Critical Care Medicine. St Louis, Mosby–Year Book, 1988.
18. Goldstein S, Killip T: Comparison of direct and indirect arterial pressures in aortic regurgitation. N Engl J Med 1962; 267:1121–1123.
19. Simpson JA, Jamieson G, Dickhaus DW, et al: Effect of size of cuff bladder on accuracy of measurement of indirect blood pressure. Am Heart J 1965; 70:206–208.
20. Young PG, Geddes LA: The effect of cuff pressure deflation rate on accuracy in indirect measurement of blood pressure with the auscultatory method. J Clin Monit Comput 1987; 3:155–157.
21. Ramsey M: Non-invasive automatic determination of mean arterial pressure. Med Biol Eng Comput 1979; 17:11–14.
22. Ramsey M: Blood pressure monitoring: Automated oscillometric devices. J Clin Monit Comput 1991; 7:56–58.
23. Cullen PM, Dye J, Huges DG: Clinical assessment of the neonatal Dinamap 847 during anesthesia in neonates and infants. J Clin Monit Comput 1987; 3:229–331.
24. Borow KM, Newburger JW: Noninvasive estimation of central aortic pressure during the oscillometric method: A comparative study of brachial artery pressure with simultaneous central aortic pressure measurements. Am Heart J 1982; 103:879–883.
25. Nystrom E, Keid KH, Bennett R, et al: A comparison of two automated indirect arterial blood pressure meters: With recordings from a radial arterial catheter in anesthetized surgical patients. Anesthesiology 1985; 62:526–527.
26. Eliakim M, Sapoznikov D, Weinman J: Pulse wave velocity in healthy subjects and in patients with various disease states. Am Heart J 1971; 82:448–451.
27. Ghanassia MD, Huynh KH, Rosenberg S, et al: Blood pressure during pediatric anesthesia: Four methods of preoperative indirect measurement. Anesth Analg (Paris) 1980; 37:399–403.
28. Lowry RL, Lichti EL, Eggers GWN: The Doppler: An aid in monitoring blood pressure during anesthesia. Anesth Analg 1973; 52:531–533.
29. Poppers PJ: Controlled evaluation of ultrasonic measurement of systolic and diastolic blood pressure in pediatric patients. Anesthesiology 1973; 38:187–189.
30. Gordon LS, Johnson PE, Penido JRF, et al: Systolic and diastolic blood pressure measurements by transcutaneous Doppler ultrasound in premature infants in critical care nurseries and at closed-heart surgery. Anesth Analg 1974; 53:914–916.
31. George DF, Lewis PJ, Petrie A: Clinical experience with use of ultrasound sphygmomanometer. Br Heart J 1975; 37:804–807.
32. Reitan JA: Noninvasive monitoring. In Saidman LJ, Smith NT (eds): Monitoring in Anesthesia. New York, John Wiley & Sons, 1978, pp 85–98.
33. Stokes DN, Clutton-Brock, Patil C, et al: Comparison of invasive and non-invasive measurement of continuous arterial pressure using the Finapres. Br J Anesth 1991; 67:26–29.
34. Kurki T, Smith NT, Head N, et al: Noninvasive continuous blood pressure measurement from the finger: Optimal measurement conditions and factors affecting reliability. J Clin Monit Comput 1987; 3:6–13.
35. Gorback MS, Quill TJ, Lavine ML: The relative accuracies of two automated noninvasive arterial pressure measurement devices. J Clin Monit Comput 1991; 7:13–16.
36. Epstein RH, Huffnagle S, Bartkowski RR: Comparative accuracies of a finger blood pressure monitor and an oscillometric blood pressure monitor. J Clin Monit Comput 1991; 7:161–167.
37. Pressman GL, Newgard PM: A transducer for the continuous external measurement of arterial blood pressure. IEEE Trans Biomed Eng 1963; 10:73–76.
38. Drzewiecki GM, Melbin J, Noodergraaf A: Arterial tonometry: Review and analysis. J Biomech 1983; 116:141–148.
39. Eckerle JS: Arterial tonometry. In Webster JG (ed): Encyclopedia of Medical Devices and Instrumentation. New York, John Wiley & Sons, 1988, pp 2770–2788.
40. Kemmotsu O, Ueda M, Otsuka K, et al: Evaluation of arterial tonometry for noninvasive, continuous blood pressure monitoring during anesthesia (abstract). Anesthesiology 1989; 71:A406.
41. Kemmotsu O, Ueda M, Otsuka K, et al: Blood pressure measurement by arterial tonometry in controlled hypotension (abstract). Anesthesiology 1989; 71:A407.
42. Kemmotsu O, Yokota S, Yamamura T, et al: A noninvasive blood pressure monitor based on arterial tonometry. Anesth Analg 1989; 68:S145.
43. American College of Sports Medicine: Guidelines for Exercise Testing and Prescription, ed 5. Baltimore, Williams & Wilkins, 1995, pp 94–96.
44. Ellestad MH: Reliability of blood pressure recordings. Am J Cardiol 1989; 63:983–985.
45. Rasmussen PH, Staats DJ, Driscoll K, et al: Direct and indirect blood pressure measurement during exercise. Chest 1985; 87:743–748.

46. Pannarle G, Bebb A, Sullivan C, et al: Bias and variability in blood pressure measurement with ambulatory recorders. Hypertension 1993; 22:591–598.
47. MacRae HS, Allen PJ: Automated blood pressure measurement at rest and during exercise: Evaluation of the motion tolerant CardioDyne NBP 2000. Med Sci Sports Exerc 1998; 30(2):328–331.
48. Barker DJP, Osmond C, Golding J, et al: Growth in utero, blood pressure in childhood and adult life. BMJ 1989; 298:564–567.
49. Harshfield G, Alpert B, Pulliam D, et al: Ambulatory blood pressure recordings in children and adolescents. Pediatrics 1994; 2:180–184.
50. Reusz GS, Hobor M, Tulassay T, et al: 24-hour blood pressure monitoring in healthy and hypertensive children. Arch Dis Child 1994; 70:90–94.
51. Reichert H, Lindinger A, Frey O, et al: Ambulatory blood pressure monitoring in healthy schoolchildren. Pediatr Nephrol 1995; 9:282–286.
52. O'Sullivan JJ, Derrick G, Griggs PE, et al: Validation of the Takeda 2421 ambulatory blood pressure monitor in children. J Med Eng Technol 1998; 22:101–105.
53. World Health Organization Study Group: The hypertensive disorders of pregnancy. World Health Organ Tech Rep Ser 1987; 758.
54. Davey DA, MacGillivray I: The classification and definition of the hypertensive disorders of pregnancy. Am J Obstet Gynecol 1988; 158:892–898.
55. Duggan PM: Which Korotkoff sound should be used for the diastolic blood pressure in pregnancy? Aust N Z J Obstet Gynaecol 1998; 38:194–197.
56. Sy WP: Ulnar nerve palsy possibly related to use of automatically cycled blood pressure cuff. Anesth Analg 1981; 60:687–688.
57. Ramsey M: Blood pressure monitoring: Automated oscillometric devices. J Clin Monit Comput 1991; 7:56–67.
58. Barr PO: Percutaneous puncture of the radial artery with a multipurpose Teflon catheter for indwelling use. Acta Physiol Scand 1961; 51:343–345.
59. Pearse RG: Percutaneous catheterization of the radial artery in newborn babies using transillumination. Arch Dis Child 1978; 53:549–550.
60. Brodsky JB, Wong AL, Meyer JA: Percutaneous cannulation of weakly palpable arteries. Anesth Analg 1977; 56:448–450.
61. Stirt JA: Liquid stylet for percutaneous radial artery cannulation. Can Anaesth Soc J 1982; 29:492–493.
62. Bedford RF: Percutaneous radial-artery cannulation: Increased safety using Teflon catheters. Anesthesiology 1977; 42:219–222.
63. Davis FM, Stewart JM: Radial artery cannulation: A prospective study in patients undergoing cardiothoracic surgery. Br J Anaesth 1980; 52:41–44.
64. Downs JB, Rackstein AD, Klein EF, et al: Hazards of radial-artery catheterization. Anesthesiology 1973; 38:283–286.
65. Feeley TW: Reestablishment of radial artery patency for arterial monitoring. Anesthesiology 1975; 46:73–75.
66. Downs JB, Chapman WL, Hawkins IF: Prolonged radial-artery catheterization: An evaluation of heparinized catheters and continuous irrigation. Arch Surg 1974; 108:671–675.
67. Bedford RF: Wrist circumference predicts the risk of radial-arterial occlusion after cannulation. Anesthesiology 1978; 48:377.
68. Kaplan JA: Hemodynamic monitoring. *In* Kaplan JA (ed): Cardiac Anesthesia, ed 2. Orlando, FL, Grune & Stratton, 1987, p 183.
69. Dotii S, Naito H: Intraarterial injection of 2.5 percent thiamylal does cause gangrene. Anesthesiology 1983; 59:154–155.
70. Young RJ, Lipman J, Freebairn RC: Accidental intra-arterial adrenaline administration. Anaesth Intensive Care 1995; 23:488–489.
71. Zweibel FR, Monies-Chas I: Accidental intraarterial injection of ketamine. Anaesthesia 1976; 31:1084.
72. Lowenstein E, Little JW III, Lo HH: Prevention of cerebral embolization from flushing radial-artery cannulas. N Engl J Med 1971; 285:1414–1415.
73. Andrew M, David M, deVeber G, et al: Arterial thromboembolic complications in paediatric patients. Thromb Haemost 1997; 78:715–725.
74. Bedford RF: Long-term radial artery cannulation: Effects on subsequent vessel function. Crit Care Med 1978; 6:64–65.
75. Pinella JC, Ross DF, Martin T, et al: Study of the incidence of intravascular catheter infection and associated septicemia in critically ill patients. Crit Care Med 1983; 11:21–25.
76. Gardner RM, Schwartz R, Wong HC, et al: Percutaneous indwelling radial artery catheters for monitoring cardiovascular function. N Engl J Med 1974; 290:1227–1231.
77. Norwood SH, Cormier B, McMahon NG, et al: Prospective study of catheter-related infection during prolonged arterial catheterization. Crit Care Med 1988; 16:836–839.
78. Read I, Umphewy J, Khan A, et al: The duration of placement as a predictor of peripheral and pulmonary arterial catheter infections. J Hosp Infect 1993; 23:17–23.
79. Thomas F, Burke JP, Parker J, et al: The risk of infection related to radial vs femoral sites for arterial catheterization. Crit Care Med 1983; 11:807–812.
80. Maki DG, Band JD: A comparative study of polyantibiotic and iodophore ointments in prevention of vascular catheter-related infections. Am J Med 1981; 70:739–744.
81. Kamal GD, Pfaller MA, Rempe LE, et al: Reduced intravascular catheter infection by antibiotic bonding. A prospective, randomized, controlled trial. JAMA 1991; 265:2364–2368.
82. Donowitz LG, Marsik FJ, Hoyt JW, et al: *Serratia marcescens* bacteremia from contaminated pressure transducers. JAMA 1979; 242:1749–1751.
83. Shinozaki T, Deane RS, Mazuzan JE, et al: Bacterial contamination of arterial lines: A prospective study. JAMA 1983; 249:223–225.
84. Stamm WE, Colella JJ, Anderson RL, et al: Indwelling arterial catheters as a source of nosocomial bacteremia: An outbreak caused by *Flavobacterium* species. N Engl J Med 1975; 292:1099–1102.
85. Luskin RL, Weinstein RA, Nathan C, et al: Extended use of disposable pressure transducers: A bacteriologic evaluation. JAMA 1986; 255:916–920.
86. O'Mally MK, Rhame FS, Cerra FB, et al: Value of routine pressure monitoring system changes after 72 hours of use. Crit Care Med 1994; 22:1424–1430.
87. Rose HD: Gas gangrene and *Clostridium perfringens* septicemia associated with the use of an indwelling radial arterial catheter. Can Med Assoc J 1979; 121:1595–1597.
88. Michaelson ED, Walsh RE: Osler's node: A complication of prolonged arterial cannulation. N Engl J Med 1970; 283:472.
89. Fanning WL, Aronson M: Osler node, Janeway lesions and splinter hemorrhages: Occurrence with an infected arterial catheter. Arch Dermatol 1977; 113:648–650.
90. Cohen A, Reyes R, Kirk M, et al: Osler's nodes, pseudoaneurysm formation and sepsis complicating percutaneous radial artery cannulation. Crit Care Med 1984; 12:1078–1079.
91. Pearson ML: Guidelines for prevention of intravascular device-related infections, parts I and II. Am J Infect Control 1996; 24:262–293.
92. Bedford RF: Radial arterial function following percutaneous cannulation with 18 and 20 gauge catheters. Anesthesiology 1977; 47:37–39.
93. Turnage WS, Laborde RJ: Loss of a right radial arterial pressure tracing during thoracic aortic aneurysm repair. J Cardiothorac Vasc Anesth 1995; 9:431–434.
94. Stern D, Gershon J, Allen F, et al: Can we trust the direct radial artery pressure immediately following cardiopulmonary bypass? Anesthesiology 1985; 62:557–561.
95. Pauca A, Hudspeth A, Wallenhaupt S, et al: Radial artery to aorta pressure difference after discontinuation of cardiopulmonary bypass. Anesthesiology 1989; 70:935–938.
96. Mohr R, Lavee J, Goor D: Inaccuracy of radial artery pressure measurements after cardiac operations. J Thorac Cardiovasc Surg 1987; 94:286–290.
97. Ryan JF, Raines J, Dalton BC, et al: Arterial dynamics of radial artery cannulation. Anesth Analg 1973; 52:1017–1020.
98. Mangar D, Thrush DN, Connell GR, et al: Direct or modified

Seldinger guide wire-directed technique for arterial catheter insertion. Anesth Analg 1993; 76:714-715.

99. Schwander D, Schwander A: Arterial trauma in anesthesia and in the intensive care unit: Surgical treatment. Z Gefasskr 1973; 2:330-340.

100. Bedford RF, Wollman H: Complications of percutaneous radial artery cannulation: An objective prospective study in man. Anesthesiology 1973; 38:228-236.

101. Cronin KD, Davies MJ, Domaingue CM, et al: Radial artery cannulation: The influence of method on blood flow after decannulation. Anaesth Intensive Care 1986; 14:400-405.

102. Davis FM: Methods of radial artery cannulation and subsequent arterial occlusion (letter). Anesthesiology 1982; 56:331.

103. Jones RM, Hill AB, Nahrwold ML, et al: The effect of method of radial artery cannulation on postcannulation blood flow and thrombus formation. Anesthesiology 1981; 55:76-77.

104. Wolf S, Mangano DT: Pseudoaneurysm, a late complication of radial-artery cannulation. Anesthesiology 1980; 52:80-81.

105. Fields JM, Saluja S, Schwartz DS, et al: Hemophilia presenting in an infant as a radial artery pseudoaneurysm following arterial puncture. Pediatr Radiol 1997; 27:763-764.

106. Qvist J, Peterfreund RA, Perlmutter GS: Transient compartment syndrome of the forearm after attempted radial artery cannulation. Anesth Analg 1996; 83:183-185.

107. Koenigsberger MR, Moessinger AC: Iatrogenic carpal tunnel syndrome in the newborn infant. J Pediatr 1977; 91:443-444.

108. Marshall G, Edelstein G, Hirschman CA: Median nerve compression following radial arterial puncture. Anesth Analg 1980; 59:953-954.

109. Ward RJ, Green HD: Arterial puncture as a safe diagnostic aid. Surgery 1963; 57:672-675.

110. Palm T: Evaluation of peripheral arterial pressure in the thumb following radial artery cannulation. Br J Anaesth 1977; 49:819-824.

111. Shenoy PNF, Leaman DM, Field JM: Safety of short-term percutaneous arterial cannulation. Anesth Analg 1979; 58:256-258.

112. Abadir AR, Ung K-A, Chaudhry MR: Complications following radial artery cannulation with 22 gauge cannula. Presented at American Society of Anesthesiologists Annual Meeting, Chicago, Oct. 1978, 523.

113. Slogoff S, Keats AS, Arlund C: On the safety of radial artery cannulation. Anesthesiology 1983; 59:42-47.

114. Barne PA, Summers J, Wirtschafter E, et al: Percutaneous peripheral arterial cannulation in the neonate. Pediatrics 1977; 57:1058-1061.

115. Cederholm I, Sorensen J, Carlson C: Thrombosis following percutaneous radial artery cannulation. Acta Anaesth Scand 1986; 30:277-279.

116. Bedford RF: Removal of radial artery thrombi following percutaneous cannulation for monitoring. Anesthesiology 1977; 46:430-432.

117. Wyatt R, Glaves I, Cooper DJ: Proximal skin necrosis after radial-artery cannulation. Lancet 1974; 2:1135-1136.

118. Coleman SS, Anson BJ: Arterial patterns in the hand based upon a study of 650 specimens. Surg Gynecol Obstet 1961; 113:409-419.

119. Husum B, Palm T: Arterial dominance in the hand. Br J Anaesth 1978; 50:913-916.

120. Kurki TS, Sanford TJ Jr, Smith NT, et al: Changes in distal blood flow during radial artery cannulation (abstract). Anesthesiology 1986; 65:A121.

121. Campkin TV: Radial artery cannulation: Potential hazard in patients with acromegaly. Anaesthesia 1980; 35:1008-1009.

122. Allen EV: Thromboangiitis obliterans: Methods of diagnosis of chronic occlusive arterial lesions distal to the wrist with illustrative cases. Am J Med Sci 1929; 178:237-244.

123. Husum B, Berthelson P: Allen's test and systolic arterial pressure in the thumb. Br J Anaesth 1981; 53:635.

124. McSwain GR, Ameriks JA: Doppler-improved Allen's test. South Med J 1979; 72:1620-1621.

125. Ramanathan S, Chalon J, Turndorf H: Determining patency of palmar arches by retrograde radial pulsation. Anesthesiology 1975; 42:756-758.

126. Brodsky JB: A simple method to determine patency of the ulnar artery intraoperatively prior to radial artery cannulation. Anesthesiology 1975; 42:626-627.

127. Raju R: The pulse oximeter and the collateral circulation. Anaesthesia 1986; 41:784-785.

128. Cartwright GW, Schreimer RL: Major complications secondary to percutaneous radial artery catheterization in the neonate. Pediatrics 1980; 65:139-143.

129. Johnson FE, Summer DS, Shandness DE Jr: Extremity necrosis caused by indwelling arterial catheters. Am J Surg 1976; 131:375-377.

130. Mangano DT, Hickey RF: Ischemic injury following uncomplicated radial artery catheterization. Anesth Analg 1979; 58:55-56.

131. Mayer T, Matlak ME, Thompson JA: Necrosis of the forearm following radial artery catheterization in a patient with Reye's syndrome. Pediatrics 1980; 65:141-143.

132. Lee KL, Miller JG, Laitung G: Hand ischaemia following radial artery cannulation. J Hand Surg [Br] 1995; 20:493-495.

133. Vender JS, Watts DR: Differential diagnosis of hand ischemia in the presence of an arterial cannula. Anesth Analg 1982; 61:465-466.

134. Hayes MF, Morello DC, Rosenbaum RW, et al: Radial artery cannulation by cutdown technique. Crit Care Med 1973; 1:151-153.

135. Dalton B, Laver MB: Vasospasm with an indwelling radial artery cannula. Anesthesiology 1971; 34:194-197.

136. Cannon BW, Meshier TW: Extremity amputation following radial artery cannulation in a patient with hyperlipoproteinemia Type V. Anesthesiology 1982; 56:222-223.

137. Baker RJ, Chunpraph B, Nybrus LN: Severe ischemia of the hand following radial artery catheterization. Surgery 1976; 80:449-450.

138. Wilkins RG: Radial artery cannulation and ischaemic damage: A review. Anaesthesia 1985; 40:896-900.

139. Butt WW, Gow R, Whyte H, et al: Complications resulting from use of arterial catheters: Retrograde flow and rapid elevation in blood pressure. Pediatrics 1986; 76:250-252.

140. Barnes RW, Foster EJ, Janssen GA, et al: Safety of brachial arterial catheters as monitors in the intensive care unit: Prospective evaluation with the Doppler ultrasonic velocity detector. Anesthesiology 1976; 44:260-264.

141. Moran F, Lorimer AR, Boyd G: Percutaneous arterial catheterization for multiple sampling. Thorax 1967; 22:253-254.

142. Bell JW: Treatment of post-catheterization arterial injuries: Use of survey plethysmography. Ann Surg 1962; 155:591-595.

143. Bjork L, Enghoff E, Grenvik A, et al: Local circulatory changes following brachial artery catheterization. Vasc Dis 1965; 2:283-285.

144. Comstock MK, Ellis T, Carter JG, et al: Safety of brachial vs. radial arterial catheters (abstract). Anesthesiology 1979; 51:A158.

145. Littler WA: Median nerve palsy: A complication of brachial artery cannulation. Postgrad Med J 1974; 52:110.

146. Luce EA, Futrell JW, Wilgris EFS: Compression neuropathy following brachial arterial puncture in anticoagulated patients. J Trauma 1976; 16:717-719.

147. Piotrowski A, Kawczynski P: Cannulation of the axillary artery in critically ill newborn infants. Euro J Pediatr 1995; 154:57-59.

148. Adler DC, Bryan-Brown CW: Use of the axillary artery for intravascular monitoring. Crit Care Med 1973; 1:148-150.

149. Brown M, Gordon LH, Brown OW, et al: Intravascular monitoring via the axillary artery. Anaesth Intensive Care 1984; 13:38-40.

150. De Angelis J: Axillary arterial monitoring. Crit Care Med 1976; 4:205-206.

151. Gurman GM, Kriemerman S: Cannulation of big arteries in critically ill patients. Crit Care Med 1985; 13:217-220.

152. Gordon LH, Brown M, Brown OW, et al: Alternative sites for continuous arterial monitoring. South Med J 1984; 77:1498-1500.

153. Brown M, Gordon LH, Brown OW, et al: Intravascular monitoring via the axillary artery. Anaesth Intensive Care 1984; 13:38-40.

154. Johnstone RE, Greenhow DEF: Catheterization of the dorsalis pedis artery. Anesthesiology 1973; 39:654-655.

155. Vasudevan A, Patel D, Brodrick P: Pseudoaneurysm of the dorsalis pedis artery (letter). Anaesthesia 1997; 52:926–927.
156. Husum B, Palm T, Eriksen J: Percutaneous cannulation of the dorsalis pedis artery. Br J Anaesth 1979; 51:1055–1058.
157. Youngberg JA, Miller ED Jr: Evaluation of percutaneous cannulation of the dorsalis pedis artery. Anesthesiology 1976; 44:80–83.
158. Kaplan JA: Hemodynamic monitoring. *In* Kaplan JA (ed): Cardiac Anesthesia, ed 2. Orlando, FL, Grune & Stratton, 1987, p 183.
159. Ersoz CJ, Hedden M, Lain L: Prolonged femoral arterial catheterization for intensive care. Anesth Analg 1970; 49:160–164.
160. Soderstrom CA, Wasserman DH, Denham CM, et al: Superiority of the femoral artery for monitoring: A prospective study. Am J Surg 1982; 144:309–314.
161. Frezza EE, Mezghebe H: Indications and complications of arterial catheter use in surgical and medical intensive care units: Analysis of 4932 patients. Am Surg 1998; 64:127–131.
162. Colvin MP, Curran JP, Jarvis D, et al: Femoral artery pressure monitoring. Anaesthesia 1977; 32:451–454.
163. Russell RA, Joel M, Hudson RJ, et al: A prospective evaluation of radial and femoral catheterization sites in critically ill patients. Crit Care Med 1981; 9:144.
164. Puri VK, Carlson RW, Bander JJ, et al: Complications of vascular cannulation in the critically ill: A prospective study. Crit Care Med 1980; 8:495–497.
165. Kazmers A, Meeker C, Nofz K, et al: Nonoperative therapy for postcatheterization femoral artery pseudoaneurysms. Am Surg 1997; 63:199–204.
166. Kronzon I: Diagnosis and treatment of iatrogenic femoral artery pseudoaneurysm: A review. J Am Soc Echocardiogr 1997; 10:236–245.
167. Christian CM, Naraghi M: A complication of femoral arterial cannulation in a patient undergoing cardiopulmonary bypass. Anesthesiology 1978; 49:436–437.
168. Selby IR, Darowski MJ: Compartment syndrome in a child occurring after femoral artery cannulation. Paediatr Anaesth 1995; 393–395.
169. Kopman E, Ferguson TB: Intraoperative monitoring of femoral artery pressure during replacement of aneurysm of descending thoracic aorta. Anesth Analg 1977; 56:603–606.
170. Mortensson W, Hallbook T, Lungstrom N: Percutaneous catheterization of the femoral vessels in children. II. Thrombotic occlusion of the catheterized artery: Frequency and causes. Pediatr Radiol 1975; 4:1–9.
171. Moran KM, Finkbeiner AA: Iliopsoas abscess following catheterization of the femoral artery: Diagnostic and treatment strategies. Am J Orthop 1997; 26:446–448.
172. Glenski JA, Beynen FM, Brady J: A prospective evaluation of femoral artery monitoring in pediatric patients. Anesthesiology 1987; 66:227–229.
173. Rosenthal A, Anderson M, Thomson SJ, et al: Superficial femoral artery catheterization in infants and small children. Circulation 1977; 56:102–105.
174. Freed M, Rosenthal A, Fyler D: Attempts to reduce arterial thrombosis after cardiac catheterization in children: Use of percutaneous technique and aspirin. Am Heart J 1974; 87:283–286.
175. Ino T, Benson LN, Freedom RM, et al: Thrombolytic therapy for femoral artery thrombosis after pediatric cardiac catheterization. Am Heart J 1988; 115:633–639.
176. Prian GW: New proximal approach works well in temporal artery catheterization. JAMA 1976; 235:2693–2694.
177. Hegemann CO, Rappaport I, Berger WJ: Superficial temporal artery cannulation. Arch Surg 1969; 99:619–624.
178. Cole AFD, Rolbin SH: A technique for rapid catheterization of the umbilical artery. Anesthesiology 1980; 53:254–255.
179. Vidyasagar D, Downes JJ, Boggs TR: Respiratory distress syndrome of newborn infants: II—Technic of catheterization of umbilical artery and clinical results of treatment. Clin Pediatr 1970; 9:332–336.
180. Paster SB, Middleton P: Roentgenographic evaluation of umbilical artery and vein catheters. JAMA 1975; 231:742–746.
181. McFadden PM, Ochsner JL: Neonatal aortic thrombosis: Complication of umbilical artery cannulation. J Cardiovasc Surg 1983; 24:1–4.
182. Marsh JL, Fonkalsrud EW: Serious complications after umbilical artery catheterization for neonatal monitoring. Arch Surg 1975; 110:1203–1208.
183. Rajani K, Goetzman B, Wennberg R, et al: Effect of heparinization of fluids infused through an umbilical artery catheter on catheter patency and frequency of complications. Pediatrics 1979; 63:552–556.
184. Cole AFD, Rolbin SH: A technique for rapid catheterization of the umbilical artery. Anesthesiology 1980; 53:254–255.

14 Pulmonary Artery Catheterization

Roberta Hines, M.D.
Michael Griffin, M.B., M.R.C.P.I., F.F.A.R.C.S.I.

Since its development more than 20 years ago as a research tool for the study of myocardial infarction (MI), the balloon-tipped pulmonary artery (PA) flotation catheter (Swan-Ganz catheter) has become one of the most important and valuable clinical tools for monitoring the critically ill patient. Recently, the indications for and clinical application of this monitoring modality have been reexamined; it remains an extremely useful tool for use in the perioperative period. In 1929, Werner Forssman, a German surgical resident, used a mirror to catheterize his own right atrium via the left antecubital vein.[1] Skill in cardiac catheterization increased markedly over the next several decades, until this procedure became common in the cardiac catheterization laboratory. However, the technique required fluoroscopic guidance and was time-consuming, often requiring 20 to 30 minutes for catheter passage. In addition, approximately 30% of all attempts at catheter placement were unsuccessful. Fortunately, in 1953, in conjunction with their experiments isolating each lung, Lategola and Rahn[2] developed a catheter with an inflatable balloon at the tip. They reported that the catheter consistently and easily slipped into the PA without extensive manipulation. However, no clinical notice was taken of the accomplishment and it remained for the "rediscovery" of the principle 2 decades later by Jeremy Swan, William Ganz, and colleagues.[3, 4] Bedside monitoring of the critically ill became a reality because fluoroscopy was no longer needed and rapid passage to the PA was easily achieved. As originally designed, the catheter measured PA and pulmonary capillary wedge pressures. Subsequently, the catheter was modified to perform a wide variety of functions, including measurement of cardiac output by thermodilution, performance of angiography, intracavitary electrography and atrial or ventricular pacing, calculation of ejection fraction, and detection of venous air embolism.[5-14]

Catheter Design

The standard 7F thermodilution (TD) pulmonary artery catheter (PAC) consists of a single catheter 110 cm in length containing four lumina.[15] It is constructed of flexible radiopaque polyvinyl chloride (PVC) (Fig. 14-1). Ten-centimeter increments are marked in black on the catheter beginning at the distal end. At the distal end of the catheter is a latex rubber balloon of 1.5 mL capacity. When inflated, the balloon extends slightly beyond the tip of the catheter but does not obstruct it. This feature prevents the tip of the catheter from contacting the right ventricular (RV) wall during passage and is responsible for the reduced incidence of arrhyth-

mias during insertion. Not only does the balloon reduce the force of contact against the RV wall but it also acts to float the catheter into the PA. Balloon flotation in blood strongly influences PAC tip location, and this assists in preferentially directing its placement.[16] Finally, inflation of the balloon allows measurement of the pulmonary capillary wedge pressure (PCWP). During inflation, the development of high intraballoon pressure may cause disruption of the PA[19, 20]; therefore, the duration of balloon inflation should be kept to a minimum.

Studies have implicated high peak intraballoon pressures, which are transmitted to the PA, as the main cause of this problem.[17-21] Early studies evaluated the pressure-volume relationship of the balloon in four different PACs.[22] A study by Ikedo et al.[22] demonstrated that a slower rate of balloon inflation (over 2.5 to 6.0 seconds) resulted in a lower peak pressure and a lower balloon volume. Therefore, these authors suggested that to minimize the potential for excessive intraballoon pressure (and secondary increases in volume), air should be injected slowly, preferably over at least 3 seconds. In addition, initial reports suggested that the composition of the PAC balloon (particularly PVC) may also increase the risk of PA perforation.[23] As a result, polyurethane has been suggested as an alternative material for balloon manufacture.[24] A potential advantage of polyurethane is that the material softens at body temperature and does not stiffen over time (a trait of PVC catheters). Although theoretically attractive, the clinical advantage of polyurethane balloons remains to be elucidated.

Information Obtained With the Pulmonary Artery Catheter

Information provided by the PAC includes (1) right- and left-sided intracardiac pressures; (2) cardiac output by the TD method; and (3) mixed venous blood for gas and chemical analysis. In addition, modifications of the "traditional" PAC provide data necessary for calculation of derived hemodynamic variables, facilitate diagnosis of complex arrhythmias, provide continuous measurement of mixed venous oxygen saturation, and allow for pacing of atrium or ventricle.

Intracardiac Pressure Measurements

PCWP is an indirect measurement of left ventricular end-diastolic pressure (LVEDP) (Fig. 14-2). Traditionally, LVEDP measurement has been employed to access left ventricular

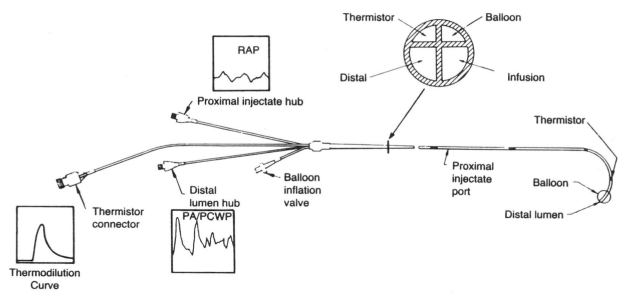

Figure 14-1. A 7F thermodilution Swan-Ganz catheter. *Inset:* Cross-section detailing lumen design. (Courtesy of Baxter Healthcare Corp., Edwards Division, Irvine, CA.)

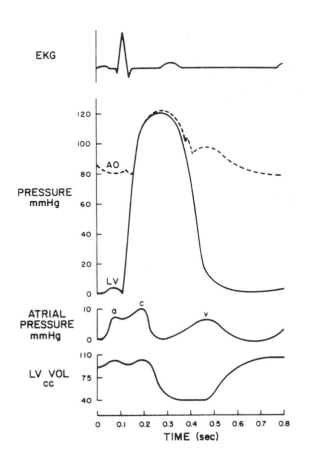

Figure 14-2. Simultaneous measurement of electrocardiogram, systemic blood pressure (BP), left ventricular pressure (LVP), left atrial pressure (LAP), left ventricular volume (LV).

(LV), function. However, a normal LVEDP (6 to 12 mmHg) does not ensure normal ventricular function. Conversely, an abnormal LVEDP (>15 mmHg) cannot directly measure the degree of LV impairment. LVEDP has also been used to assess preload.

Preload is classically derived from measurement of end-diastolic fiber length (or end-diastolic volume). However, due to logistic problems of routinely obtaining ventricular volume, a pressure measurement has been employed. Depending on the state of ventricular compliance, LVEDP may or may not have a linear relationship to LVEDV. In the absence of mitral valve disease, PCWP approximates left atrial pressure (LAP). Therefore, a more clinically available measurement of preload is the PCWP (normal, 8 to 12 mmHg).

PCWP correlates with LVEDP (LAP) over a wide range of filling pressures (5 to 25 mmHg).[25-29] To avoid complications with PAC balloon inflation, pulmonary artery end-diastolic pressure (PAEDP) is frequently used as an estimate of PCWP.[30-35] In the absence of increased pulmonary vascular resistance (PVR) (e.g., chronic mitral stenosis, chronic LV failure, pulmonary disease) the gradient between PAEDP and PCWP is approximately 1 to 4 mmHg.[36-39] PAEDP may be greater than PCWP in a patient with tachycardia because diastolic filling time is decreased.[28] The anatomic site of the PAC also influences the PCWP-LAP relationship. The ideal position for obtaining a PCWP is in a large branch of the PA. This will result in a good PCWP-LAP correlation. However, wedging in a small artery yields a PCWP higher than LAP.[40, 41] Occasionally the transition from PA to PCWP may not be evident by changes in the waveform. In these situations aspiration of pulmonary capillary blood will confirm the PAC location.[42]

A number of additional factors alter the correlation between PCWP and LAP, including incorrect catheter placement, transducer-related artifacts, eccentric balloon occlusion, non-zone III PCWP, pulmonary venous occlusive disease, valvular heart disease, pericardial tamponade, and altered LV compliance and the presence of mitral regurgitation (v waves).[43-45] In addition, depending on the state of ventricular compliance, LVEDP may or may not have a linear relationship to LVEDV.[46-50] An elegant study by Pichard et

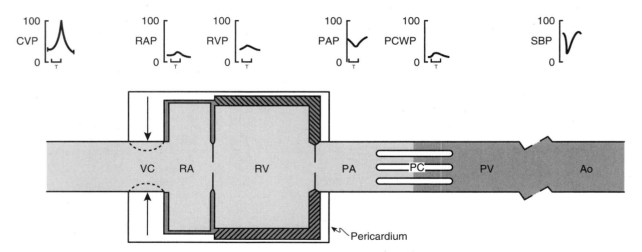

Figure 14–3. Schematic representation of cardiac tamponade in a canine model using saline infusion into the intact pericardial sac. Owing to anatomic relationships of the pericardium, the central venous pressure will give the first indications of tamponade.

al.[35] has clearly demonstrated how the left atrial (LA) waveforms are affected by compliance changes. They showed that the patient would develop a large v wave without ischemia or mitral regurgitation when the preload was acutely increased; a large cardiac filling volume makes the pulmonary venous and atrial systems noncompliant where a small stroke volume can create a significant v wave. In contrast, if the pulmonary artery opening pressure (PAOP) is low and the pulmonary veins and the atrium are compliant, severe mitral regurgitation may be associated with a normal-sized v wave. This study demonstrated a poor correlation between the severity of mitral regurgitation and the height of the v wave.

Right atrial pressure (RAP) (normal, 0 to 8 mmHg), obtained from the proximal port of the standard TD catheter, yields valuable information regarding RV performance.[10, 51-53] Studies show that RV ischemia has been detected by continuous monitoring of RAP combined with electrocardiography (ECG).[54] RAP is also critical to the early diagnosis of cardiac tamponade (Fig. 14-3). However, by itself RAP has been shown to be a poor predictor of LV filling pressure.[55-58]

When used in combination with a measurement of flow (i.e., cardiac output) the information gained from the PCWP measurement will be maximized. This is especially applicable when making a diagnosis or instituting a new therapy. For example, a patient may have a reduced blood pressure (BP) and decreased PCWP (e.g., BP = 70/50, PCWP = 4 mmHg). Clinically, this may be interpreted as hypovolemia. This would be true if the patient had a low cardiac output (<3 L/minute). However, the same patient had a high cardiac output state (8 L/minute); septic shock may lead the differential diagnosis list. Therefore, a cardiac output determination should accompany the measurement of PCWP when any clinically important diagnostic, therapeutic, or prognostic decision is to be made. Left-sided cardiac output measurement with a Swan-Ganz catheter and estimation of mitral valve area (MVA) by the Gorlin formula has been reported.[59] The use of right-sided cardiac output after balloon mitral valvotomy can give an inaccurate estimation of MVA with the Gorlin formula because of the atrial septal defect (ASD) created during the procedure.

Thermodilution Cardiac Output

The ability to obtain accurate, rapid, and repetitive measurements of cardiac output is one of the principal advantages of the PAC.[60-62] The information gained from serial measurements of cardiac output can be vital to diagnosis, evaluation of therapeutic interventions, and assessing prognosis.[63-66] Estimation of cardiac output from physical diagnosis has been shown to be unreliable[67-69]; therefore, direct measurement is essential.

The TD method of measuring cardiac output was first described in 1954 by Fegler.[70] Subsequent incorporation of a thermistor into the PAC greatly enhanced the usefulness of the technique in clinical medicine.[1, 71, 72] An excellent correlation has been reported between TD cardiac output and other techniques, including dye dilution techniques, the Fick method, Doppler method, and radionuclear and electromagnetic flowmeters.[73-84] The noninvasive Doppler, Fick, and carbon dioxide rebreathing techniques tend to overestimate cardiac output compared to TD and the poor agreement has to be taken into consideration, especially in measurement of low cardiac output.[85]

TD cardiac output is a variant of the indicator dilution technique, with "cold" used as the trace indicator. Cooling of the blood is accomplished by injection of 5% dextrose and noting that the change in temperature at the downstream sampling site is proportional to cardiac output.

The TD principle is described by the Stewart-Hamilton equation:

$$Q = \frac{V_I(T_B - T_I)K_1K_2}{T_B(t)dt}$$

where

Q = cardiac output
V_I = injectate volume
T_B = blood temperature
T_I = injectate temperature
K_1 = density factor

$$\frac{(\text{specific heat})(\text{specific gravity}) \text{ injectate}}{(\text{specific heat})(\text{specific gravity}) \text{ blood}}$$

K_2 = a computation constant that includes heat change in transit, dead space of the catheter, and injection rate, and adjusts the units to liters per minute
$T_B(t)dt$ = change in blood temperature as a function of time

Solution of this equation is accomplished by the cardiac

output computer, which integrates the area under the TD curve and displays a digital readout of cardiac output in liters per minute.[83] Cardiac output is inversely proportional to the area under the curve $[T_B(t)dt]$.

Volume of Injectate

Standard cardiac output measurements are performed with 2.5, 5.0, or 10 mL of injectate (D5W). The volume of injectate must be accurately measured as it will affect the total amount of thermal indicator injected. If careful attention is paid to filling syringes, the error introduced by variations in volume is small, amounting to 1%. If a separate injectate catheter is used, it should have the same volume as the proximal port of the PAC,[86, 87] or the computation constant (K_2) should be changed.

Blood Temperature

A stable baseline blood temperature is essential for computing an accurate TD curve. Currently available cardiac output computers utilize a thermistor to measure PA temperature. Even so, baseline temperatures can be seen to vary in phase with the respiratory cycle. These variations are small with normal respiration, amounting to 0.01° to 0.02°C, but are accentuated in dyspneic patients or patients being mechanically ventilated. To obviate or minimize the effect of these variations, each injection of the thermal indicator should be performed at the same time in the respiratory cycle.[55]

Injectate Temperature

Of equal importance is the accurate measurement of injectate temperature. Temperatures ranging from 0°C to room temperature (19° to 24°C) can be used. However, warm solutions require larger injectate volumes and higher thermistor sensitivities than do iced solutions.[88] The use of iced solutions increases the signal-to-noise ratio by a factor of 2 to 3. In theory, this may lead to greater reproducibility of results. Commercial systems are now available for maintaining cold injectate syringes and accurately measuring injectate temperature at the proximal port. However, studies using an in vitro model failed to show any difference in accuracy or reproducibility between iced injectate and room temperature injectate. A potential hazard of cold injectate has been recently reported by Nishikawa and Dohi,[89] who observed a transient bradycardia following injection of 10 mL of iced D5W.

The time between withdrawal of the injectate and injection should be as short as possible. Significant warming of the iced injectate can occur in handling and during prolonged injection phases. Little warming of room temperature injectate occurs between filling the syringe and injection. As a result, newer methods using in-line temperature probes have been developed that allow for measurement of injectate temperature as the injection proceeds. A 1°C increase in the temperature of the injectate will cause an error of 3% in cardiac output. Therefore, to create a smooth TD curve, injection should be made as rapidly and smoothly as possible and at the same point in the respiratory cycle. Most computation constants assume injection to have been made in less than 4 seconds. Rapid continuous infusion of fluid through the venous infusion port of the PAC significantly limits the accuracy of simultaneous intermittent bolus TD (BTD) measurement.[90] Optimally, measurements should be avoided during rapid volume infusion.

Density Factor

D5W and normal saline (NS) are the two most commonly used injectates. The choice of solutions *does not* significantly affect the computation of K_1 because both yield nearly identical results (NS/blood K_1 = 1.08; D5W/blood K_1 = 1.10). Although the specific gravity of blood changes with hematocrit, K_1 shows little variation, decreasing only slightly from 1.13 to 1.07 as hematocrit is significantly changed from 52% to 30%.

Computation Constant

The computation constant combines several components of the Stewart-Hamilton equation. Calculation is based on the volume of injectate, temperature change of injectate, and the capacity of the injectate port of the cardiac output catheter.

Correction is required to allow for the warming of injectate as it passes through the intravascular portion of the catheter.[91, 92] The magnitude of this change may be appreciated by the fact that a 4°C injectate yields an effective temperature of 12°C at the point of entry into the circulation. It should be noted that each computer manufacturer determines K_2 in a different manner. Therefore, the user should be aware of particular assumptions made by the manufacturer of a particular cardiac output computer.

Change in Blood Temperature With Time

When a bolus of thermal indicator is injected, a time-temperature plot is constructed. The computer then integrates the area under this curve $[T_B(t)dt]$. Methods that employ this technique to calculate cardiac output include integrating to a point on the downslope equal to 10% of the peak, integrating the entire curve, extrapolating the downslope to zero, or the use of a constant to multiply a certain portion of the curve.[93, 94] The thermistor of the PAC is balanced through use of a whetstone bridge. As a result, variations in temperature will alter resistance and current flow. To ensure correct calculations, it is important that a smooth TD curve be obtained. Low-amplitude curves may be caused by small injectate volumes, a high cardiac output, or an inadequate blood-to-injectate temperature differential. Irregular curves may result from poor mixing, changes in BP or heart rate, or contact between the thermistor and vessel wall.

Other Factors

The location of the thermistor is also important for the determination of an accurate cardiac output. A thermistor located at the catheter tip is likely to impinge upon the vessel wall, giving rise to irregular TD curves. Such curves are characterized by a prolonged upslope, a reduced peak deflection, and an increased downslope. Early models of the TD catheters had the thermistor located in this position and were plagued by this problem. New modifications in PAC design locate the thermistor 4 cm from the catheter tip. With this change, abnormalities in cardiac output results from contact with the vessel wall have been minimized.[15] Room temperature TD cardiac output determinations from the venous infusion port can be used in place of the central venous port if the central port becomes nonfunctional.[95, 96]

Technique

The clinical determination of cardiac output by the TD method is a simple technique, well suited to use during the perioperative period. However, to optimize accuracy and reproducibility, measurements should be obtained paying careful attention to technique.[44, 92] The following is a summary of key features that influence both the accuracy and reproducibility of TD measurements.

1. The correct computation constant (K_2) must be entered into the computer. This may vary with manufacturer and size of catheter, as well as with injectate volume and temperature.

2. The volume of injectate must be accurately measured. For example, an error or 0.5 mL in a 5-mL injection will cause a 10% error in the measurement.

3. The time between withdrawal of the sample and injection should be as short as possible, certainly less than 30 seconds, if possible. As previously described, a 1°C increase in the temperature of the injectate will cause an error of 3% in cardiac output.

4. Each injection should be timed to occur at the same point in the respiratory cycle to ensure comparability of measurements. However, an average of multiple determinations with injections equally dispersed throughout the respiratory cycle has been shown to provide the best estimate of mean cardiac output.[97] The results of this study suggest that the manual technique of determining cardiac output at end-exhalation may not accurately reflect the average cardiac output.

In summary, to create a smooth TD curve, injection should be made as rapidly and smoothly as possible and at the same point in the respiratory cycle[81, 98] (Table 14-1).

Complications of Thermodilution Cardiac Output

In general, complications of cardiac output measurement are few. The most frequently encountered errors result from inaccurate measurements or misinterpretation of results. Either of these may lead to the initiation of inappropriate therapeutic maneuvers.[21, 99] Although there are no published reports documenting the development of septic complications that can be specifically traced to cardiac output de-

Table 14-1. Guidelines for Best Results in Hemodynamic Monitoring

---

Acquisition of Pressure Data

Completely eliminate any air or blood clots from the system

Discard catheters or tubes with kinks or bends

Do not depend on internal calibration alone; use a mercury manometer for external calibration

Check calibration routinely (3 or 4 times a day) or any time that unexpected pressures are recorded

Always recheck the zero reference and calibration before measuring pressures

Measure pressures at end-expiration, regardless of whether the patient is breathing spontaneously or is on mechanical ventilation

Derive pressures manually off hard copy when tracing artifact is present

Cardiac Output Measurements

Ensure proper positioning of the distal thermistor and right atrial lumen

Use 5 or 10 mL of cold injectate or 10 mL of room temperature injectate

Injection should be rapid and smooth, with minimal time wasted between picking up the injectate syringe, turning on the computer switch, and actually injecting the fluid

Adjust the computer constant according to the type, volume, and temperature of the injectate and the type of catheter used (predetermined constants are available)

terminations, the potential for such contamination does exist.[36, 100-103] Inadvertent injection through a catheter containing potent cardiovascular drugs can occur. Fluid overload (due to repeated determinations) or hypothermia (if ice injectate is used) are additional possibilities for complications in pediatric patients. Bradycardia and atrial fibrillation have been reported following use of iced injectate.[89, 104] An occupational disease of caregivers ("Swan-Ganz elbow") has been described as the result of obtaining repetitive cardiac output injections.[105]

Mixed Venous Oxygen Tension

Serial measurements of mixed venous oxygen tension ($P\bar{v}O_2$) can provide valuable diagnostic and prognostic information.[106-111] $P\bar{v}O_2$ is also necessary for the calculation of several important derived respiratory and hemodynamic parameters such as arteriovenous oxygen content difference [$C(a-v)O_2$], intrapulmonary shunt (Qs/Qt), and oxygen consumption (VO_2).[112] Mixed venous carbon dioxide tension ($P\bar{v}CO_2$) is used for calculating carbon dioxide production and respiratory quotient, and can be used for estimating changes in cardiac output. Continuous mixed venous oximetry is presently being used to supplement traditional hemodynamic monitoring in critically ill patents.[106, 107, 113-116]

The technology which measures mixed venous oxygen saturation (by PAC) is based on the use of reflectance spectrophotometry. Using this technique, the determination of SvO_2 is based on the differential capacity of oxyhemoglobin and desaturated hemoglobin to absorb light. Of note, desaturated hemoglobin absorbs more light than saturated (oxy) hemoglobin. When SvO_2 monitoring was initially developed, the systems transmitted the different wavelengths of light along fiberoptic wires, which were incorporated into one of the lumina of the PAC. These fiberoptic components are used to measure hemoglobin oxygen saturation by the process of reflectance spectrophotometry.[117] One of these wavelengths, identified as the *indicator* wavelength, is sensitive to changes in oxygen saturation. The second wavelength, or *isosbestic* wavelength, is relatively insensitive to changes in oxygen saturation but is quite sensitive to potential sources of interference such as temperature, pH, velocity blood flow, and hematocrit. Light from either of these two wavelengths is reflected back along the catheter and then sensed by a photodetector connected to a microprocessor located within the monitor. The microprocessor then computes the ratio of the light reflection from wavelength 1 and wavelength 2 (in an attempt to minimize any effect of the interferences previously described). By doing this, the microprocessor theoretically determines the changes in light intensity due solely to changes in oxygenation. In practice, however, the relationship of light intensity to oxygenation is a nonlinear function. As a result, early prototypes of SvO_2 monitors often produced values that intermittently or variably correlated with in vitro data obtained by co-oximetry measurement. More recently, a third wavelength was incorporated into the SvO_2 monitoring system, which allows for the nonlinear computation of the relationship between light intensity and oxygen saturation and appears to have increased the clinical utility of this technology.[115, 117]

Clinical studies comparing three wavelength systems in vivo with in vitro (transmission spectrophotometry) techniques demonstrated an excellent correlation between these two techniques ($r = .912$ to $.99$).[117, 118] Hecker et al.[117] demonstrated that a two-wavelength determination differed significantly from co-oximetry values ($r = .762$), but a three-wavelength system correlated more closely with co-oximetry values ($r = .92$) in patients undergoing cardiac surgery.[117] Two other studies in cardiac surgery and intensive care unit (ICU) patients demonstrated acceptable agreement between two- and three-wavelength SvO_2 systems using reflectance spectrophotometry (SAT2 and OX3 respectively) and SvO_2 measured by co-oximetry using transmission spectrophotometry.[119, 120] The latter study demonstrated a tendency for catheter venous oximetry to underestimate oxygen saturation at lower SvO_2 levels. The latter group used a dual ejection fraction and oximetry catheter and had previously demonstrated an acceptable estimation of right ventricular-ejection fraction (RVEF).[121] A relatively high coefficient of variation of 16% for the estimation of RVEF is due to a number of factors such as nonhomogeneous mixing, respiratory artifact, and small changes in injectate temperature.[120]

Nelson[122] reported a correlation between SvO_2 and the oxygen utilization coefficient reflecting the overall balance between VO_2 and delivery. Subsequently, decreases in SvO_2 have been shown to directly correlate with decreases in cardiac output in a variety of clinical settings.[106, 112, 123-125] When arterial oxygen content and VO_2 are held constant, mixed venous oxygen varies directly with cardiac output. Consequently, this value can be used to directly assess the adequacy of cardiac output in relation to tissue oxygen requirements.[106] In a study assessing clinical usefulness, SvO_2 PAC monitoring was deemed useful in 57% of patients.[126] Usefulness was defined as a change in therapy triggered solely by continuous SvO_2 data that would not have been obtained from other routine data or earlier recognition of significant adverse events. This study also defined independent preoperative factors associated with SvO_2 PAC monitoring and proposed a cutoff point above which SvO_2 may be useful.

The oxygen tension of venous blood varies according to the location from which the sample is obtained. Due to the large nonmetabolic blood flow (shunt) from the kidneys, blood from the inferior vena cava (IVC) usually has a higher oxygen tension than superior vena cava (SVC) blood. The high oxygen extraction ratio of the myocardium results in the low oxygen tension of the coronary sinus (CS). Use of blood from the right atrium (RA) for determination of oxygen tension may yield an inaccurate measurement, since streaming is present from the IVC, SVC, and CS. Numerous empiric formulas have been developed in an attempt to relate RA oxygen tension to true $P\bar{v}O_2$.[43, 127] However, in critically ill patients, measurements of central venous oxygen tension correlate poorly with true $P\bar{v}O_2$ obtained from the PA.[128] It has been shown that mixing of the three streams of venous blood occurs in the RV; however, the risk of arrhythmias does not allow a catheter to be placed in the RV. A sample from the SVC is useful when a "true" mixed venous blood cannot be obtained, for example, in children with an intracardiac left-to-right shunt (ASD).

$P\bar{v}O_2$ represents the final balance between total body oxygen supply and demand. The normal $P\bar{v}O_2$ is 40 mmHg (SvO_2 = 75%). Due to regional differences in blood flow, a normal $P\bar{v}O_2$ does not necessarily indicate adequate perfusion in each organ system. Factors that reduce $P\bar{v}O_2$ include:

1. Decreased O_2 delivery
   Decreased arterial oxygen content (CaO_2)
   Decreased PaO_2
   Decreased hemoglobin
2. Increased tissue requirements
   Hypermetabolic states
   Fever
   Endocrinopathies

An elevated $P\bar{v}O_2$ may be seen in patients who have a left-to-right shunt, for example, a ventricular septal defect (VSD) complicating an acute myocardial infarction (AMI).[129, 130] Impairment of cellular respiration as seen with sepsis or cyanide poisoning also results in an elevated $P\bar{v}O_2$. The latter is of particular importance to the anesthesiologist. Cyanide ion resulting from sodium nitroprusside administration may poison the cytochrome oxidase system.

Significant errors can result from contamination of mixed venous blood by pulmonary capillary blood. This may occur with distal migration of the catheter to a wedge position or blood withdrawal with the balloon inflated. In these circumstances retrograde flow from pulmonary capillaries is the only possible source of blood. When the catheter tip is positioned more proximally, experimental results have been conflicting. Several studies demonstrate contamination accompanying rapid blood withdrawal, while several investigators could not support this observation.[41, 131] Therefore, in light of current evidence, it is recommended that mixed venous blood samples be obtained only from properly positioned catheters and that a slow rate of withdrawal be used. Proponents of continuous mixed venous saturation monitoring claim it is associated with minimal risk and is cost-effective.

Pacing Catheter

A multipurpose PAC composed of five pacing electrodes may be used for atrial, ventricular, or atrioventricular (A-V) sequential pacing. An additional advantage provided by this catheter is its ability to record an intracardiac ECG.[132, 133] Roth and Zaidan[134] evaluated the ability of the pacing PAC to detect atrial and ventricular endocardial electrical activity during hypothermic cardioplegia arrest and compared it with the activity found on the standard ECG.[134] These results demonstrated that the atrial electrodes detected activity that was noted also by visual inspection. However, the ventricular electrodes detected receiving electrical activity in 7 of 18 patients. Three of these 7 patients did not have simultaneous ECG activity, indicating that, in the usual monitoring circumstance, this ventricular electrical activity would have gone untreated. As a result of the ventricular activity seen with the pacing catheter, additional cardioplegia was administered. The authors therefore recommend that when a pacing Swan-Ganz catheter is used for clinical care, it can also be used to monitor myocardial electrical activity during cardioplegia arrest.[134]

The multipurpose PAC that is presently available has two intraventricular electrodes situated 18.5 and 19.5 cm from the distal end and three intra-atrial electrodes situated 28.5, 31.0, and 33.5 cm further distal (Swan-Ganz flow-directing pacing catheter, Model 93-200H-7F, Baxter Healthcare Corp., Irvine, CA). Incorporation of a third intra-atrial electrode enables proper positioning in hearts of varying chamber sizes. The ability of the catheter to provide successful pacing was evaluated in a series of 30 patients undergoing cardiac surgery.[133] Atrial pacing was possible in 80% of patients, ventricular pacing in 93% and A-V sequential pacing in 73%. Transmyocardial pacing is feasible using one temporary epicardial pacing lead and one endocardial lead of a pacing PAC.[135]

In addition to the multipurpose PAC, a new modification of the PAC with an additional RV port placed 19 cm from the catheter tip has been introduced (Paceport, Baxter Healthcare Corp.). This additional lumen allows for the introduction of a pacer wire for emergency RV pacing (Fig. 14–4). With the Paceport system, the pacing wire is packaged separately from the PAC. This allows the flexibility of having

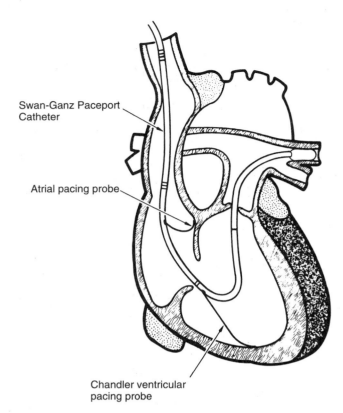

Swan-Ganz Paceport
Catheter

Atrial pacing probe

Chandler ventricular
pacing probe

Figure 14–4. Paceport catheter with a right ventricular port which allows for passage of a ventricular pacing wire. (Chandler Ventricular Pacing Probe.)

ventricular pacing compatibility available (i.e., the pacing wire with the additional lumen in the RV) but not having to use the technology unless it becomes indicated. The present Paceport system allows for rapid and accurate placement of the pacing wire into the RV. To ensure the wire is in contact with the RV and to minimize the risk of RV injury, the manufacturer recommends using either an intracavity ECG (looking for injury current, or verifying capture by the pacing wire in the conventional manner; see Fig. 14–4). A recent modification of the Paceport catheter provides an additional RA port (in addition to the RV port) that allows for A-V sequential pacing (AV Paceport Catheter Model 93A-991H-7.5F, Baxter Healthcare Corp.). Seltzer et al.[136] have reported a high degree of successful placement and A-V pacing ability with this new Paceport modification. Lumb[137] evaluated the ability of A-V sequelae pacing with transluminal atrial and ventricular pacing probes inserted via the PAC with results obtained using epicardial pacing wires. In this study, there was no statistically significant difference between the electrical currents delivered either through epicardial wires or transluminal pacing probes in the PAC. A subsequent study by Trankina and White[138] revealed a 98% rate for atrial capture and a 100% rate of ventricular capture using an A-V pacing PAC in 40 cardiac surgical patients. The ability to provide atrial pacing following cardiopulmonary bypass (CPB) decreased slightly to 95%.[138] The pacing PAC has proved useful in the management of minimally invasive direct coronary artery bypass procedures.[139, 140] There have been a number of reports describing the usefulness of the pacing PAC when discontinuation of β blockade or mechanical stimulation of the heart by the surgeon failed to result in

an adequate heart rate during minimally invasive cardiac surgery.[140]

Suggested indications for the use of a PAC with pacing capability are as follows.[141]

1. Intermittent third-degree heart block
2. Second-degree heart block (Mobitz II)
3. Left bundle branch block (LBBB)
4. Digitalis toxicity
5. Severe bradycardia
6. Need for A-V sequential pacing
7. Need for intracardiac ECG

In addition, the following preoperative diagnoses have been shown to significantly predict the need for pacing catheters: sinus node dysfunction or bradydysrhythmias, history of transient complete A-V block, aortic stenosis, aortic insufficiency, and reoperation.[142]

Right Ventricular Ejection Fraction

Bing pioneered the technology responsible for our present ability to utilize indicator dilution techniques for the determination of ventricular volumes.[73] He developed a method that attempted to estimate the residual end-diastolic blood volume of the RV in normal and diseased human hearts. Following catheterization of the RV and the PA with a double-lumen catheter, Evan's blue was injected into the RV. The residual volumes were estimated from the slope of photographically recorded dye dilution curves.

Using Bing's original concepts, technologic advances in PAC technology have facilitated the measurement of RVEF and RV volumes by use of TD techniques.[120, 143, 144] This has occurred as a result of recent advances in the manufacture of thermistors for PACs that have a rapid response time of approximately 50 ms (normal, 300 to 1000 ms). The response time of these catheters is rapid enough to record beat-to-beat temperature variation and thus allow for calculation of RVEF. Kay and colleagues[57] validated this technique with radionuclear studies both in animal models and in patients after open heart surgery. Subsequently, Jardin et al.[27] and Rafferty[145] also validated this technique using echocardiography.

Using this "rapid response" catheter (7.5F, Baxter Healthcare) and an accompanying computer system (Monarch REF-1, Baxter Healthcare), computation of RVEF is easily accomplished from an experimental decay process of the thermal washout curve.[143] Normal RVEF (TD technique) is approximately 40%. RVEF, RV stroke volume, RV end-diastolic volume, and RV end-systolic volume may be calculated as follows:

$$\text{RV stroke volume} = \text{cardiac output/heart rate}$$
$$\text{RV end-diastolic volume} = \text{RV stroke volume/RVEF}$$
$$\text{RV end-systolic volume} = \text{RV end diastolic volume} - \text{RV stroke volume}$$

Thus, from the standard RVEF catheter the following hemodynamic measurements may be obtained: cardiac output, RVEF, and right atrial, right ventricular, as well as pulmonary artery and capillary wedge pressures. Hines and Barash[54] have demonstrated the ability to detect RV ischemia by monitoring RVEF and right ventricular end-diastolic pressure (RVEDP) in patients with right coronary artery disease. The *newest* modification of the RVEF system incorporates the measurement of both RVEF and continuous SvO₂ monitoring. Dormann et al.[146] evaluated the reproducibility and accuracy of this new system in patients undergoing CPB surgery. Catheter-derived mixed venous and arterial oximetry data were compared with simultaneous values using conventional laboratory co-oximetry methods. Their results demonstrated a significant correlation for SvO₂ between catheter-derived and laboratory co-oximetry data ($r^2 = -0.81$, $P < .01$). Their coefficient variation for each set of five repeated measurements for cardiac output was 8%, and for computed RVEF, was 15%.[146]

However, potential limitations do exist with the use of the thermal indicator technique. In patients with cardiac dysrhythmias such as atrial fibrillation (AF), variations in diastolic filling time may introduce error into the measurement of RVEF. However, since RVEF is computed with four to five beats, an average RVEF may be obtained. Conversely, a beat-to-beat RVEF can be calculated, so that minimal and maximal RVEFs are known. Second, in patients with regurgitant valvular lesions (tricuspid insufficiency), an erroneous RVEF may be seen because the technique measures forward ejection fraction.[53, 142]

The location of the injectate port further influences the accuracy of the cardiac output obtained via the TD technique. Comparison of RA and RV ejection sites, both in animals and humans, demonstrates that RV injection results in a highly variable and inaccurate measurement of output when compared with RA injection.[56, 147] Finally, by increasing the time necessary to equilibrate fully to temperature change, present techniques of thermistor mounting may artifactually lower the measurement of RVEF. Although the initial clinical data utilizing the "rapid response" PAC yielded promising results, cost and practical limitations have restricted its use in routine clinical practice. This catheter may be useful when acute changes in RVEF may occur such as following heart transplantation and management of pulmonary hypertension.

Continuous Cardiac Output Determinations Using Pulmonary Artery Catheter Modification

A method to measure continuous TD cardiac outputs has been developed. Rather than a cold bolus injectate to create a temperature signal, a filament is intermittently heated to provide a very small heat signal.[144, 148] To accomplish this, PACs have been modified such that a 10-cm thermal filament is located within the RV (Fig. 14–5). This filament is coiled over a portion of the PAC that lies in the RA and RV. The thermometer at the tip of the PAC detects changes in blood temperature, and the heat signal is then analyzed by stochastic techniques. Stochastic techniques differ from classic demonstrative techniques in that the statistical properties of the input and output signals are of more interest than the instantaneous values of the signals themselves.[148] Once in place, this thermal filament continually transfers a safe level of heat directly into the blood according to a pseudorandom binary sequence. Any resulting temperature change is then detected downstream in the PA and is cross-correlated with an input sequence to produce a TD washout curve. This TD curve is presented in millidegrees.[149] The cardiac output is then subsequently computed from the conservation of heat equation using the area under the curve.[148]

With this technique the average heat infused is usually

Continuous Cardiac Output: CCO Modified Swan-Ganz® Catheter

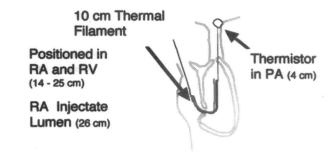

Figure 14–5. The continuous cardiac output technology uses thermodilution methods with a modified Swan-Ganz catheter. A 10-cm-long thermal filament on the catheter lies in the right atrium (RA) and the right ventricle (RV). A lumen exists in the RA, which can be used for fluid infusion or to obtain RA pressures. A standard thermistor lies 4 cm from the tip of the catheter and can be used for measuring PA pressures. (Courtesy of Baxter Healthcare, Edwards Division, Irvine, CA.)

less than 7.5 W. This temperature was selected so that the catheter surface temperature remains below 44°C regardless of blood flow conditions. Earlier studies suggest that long-term exposure at this temperature (44°C) has no detrimental effects on red blood cells, the myocardium,[150-152] or other blood component.[153] In practice, the actual filament surface temperature is continually measured and the delivered power is either reduced or terminated when the average temperature exceeds 44°C.[149]

Insertion of the PAC is performed by traditional methods allowing for placement of the thermistor in the PA outflow tract. Once the correct position of the PAC has been verified (using standard methods such as waveform or pressure form analysis), the catheter is connected to the monitor. Once this has been accomplished, the process of continuous cardiac output determination begins. The first cardiac output measurement is computed and displayed within several minutes. The heating sequence is repeated every 30 seconds; the displayed value is based on approximately six determinations and updated every 30 seconds.[154] Thus, the monitor actually provides a time-averaged, continuously updated rather than "instantaneous" cardiac output.

This method of measuring cardiac output (i.e., volumetric fluid flow using stochastic techniques) has been evaluated in a laboratory bench model[133] and in sheep.[155] Clinically, Yelderman et al.[149] have studied continuous cardiac output (CCO) as compared with BTD cardiac outputs in ICU patients. They found an acceptable correlation between TD (cardiac output) and CCO measurement ($r = .94$) in this patient population (range of cardiac output studied was 2.8 to 10.8 per minute).[149] One potential advantage of this system is that it is user-friendly, requiring no calculations and no injection of volume. In addition, it is possible to perform routine bolus cardiac output determinations through the same catheter. Another study demonstrated that the CCO catheter adequately measured cardiac output and SvO₂ in the clinical setting.[156] In a study comparing intermittent BTD with CCO during liver transplantation, CCO demonstrated logistical advantages and challenged the accuracy of BTD.[157]

Because BTD is not a true gold standard for cardiac output determination, new techniques compared with BTD may fail to achieve expected accuracy. However, good agreement has been found between CCO and BTD methods and between BTD and Fick methods with correlation coefficients on the order of $r = .94$ to $.97$ at steady state.[155, 156, 158] The absolute measurement bias in one study was 0.02 L, and the 95% confidence limits were 1.07 and -1.03 L. In conclusion, CCO, compared with BTD, is accurate and reliable, especially when the cardiac index is less than or equal to 4.5 L.min^{-1}·m^{-2}.[158, 159]

At present, increased cost is a major factor limiting the clinical application of this technology. In the setting of high cardiac output, the difference with BTD increases and the results must be cautiously interpreted.[160] In addition, studies have demonstrated clinically important time delays in the response of the CCO catheter. This delay must be considered when there are rapid alterations of the hemodynamic state.[161] The faster algorithm of stat CCO offers some advantage over trend CCO during an acute hemodynamic change. However, because of the averaging process for determining CCO, the response time of stat CCO is slower than that of mean arterial pressure and SvO$_2$.[156]

Miyasaka et al.[162] have advocated "thermodeprivation" as yet another potential approach to the determination of CCO. This technique employs the measurement of flow velocity in the pulmonary artery using a continuous arterial thermodeprivation system (KATS) catheter. This catheter is designed such that a continuously heated thermistor is incorporated into the tip of the PAC.[6] The heated thermistor is cooled by the surrounding blood; the decrease in temperature is proportional to the velocity of blood. This system is then calibrated with a simultaneous TD cardiac output and the velocity signal is subsequently converted into a quantitative flow value. The caveat here is that a constant blood vessel diameter (the vessel in which the PAC is placed) is assumed by the thermodeprivation method. As a result, variations in PA diameter or changes in the diameter of PA during monitoring (which may be seen with changes in volume status, positive end-expiratory pressure [PEEP], and so on) may prove to be a major limitation to the clinical usefulness of this technology. There has been one report of unsatisfactory continuous cardiac output measurement by thermodeprivation in cardiac surgical patients.[163] There was considerable error in the thermodeprivation measurements compared with BTD measurement (2 SD of the bias ranged from 1.2 to 4.5 L/minute in the operating room [OR] and 1.8 to 5.8 L/minute in the ICU). The main sources of error are the assumptions that the rheology of blood, the position of the thermistor, and PA diameter all remain constant through the perioperative period.[163]

A technique based on cyclic cooling of the blood in the RA and measurement of the temperature changes in the PA has been described.[164] This study demonstrated the feasibility of the new method to monitor cardiac output, and to detect changes greater than 0.25 L/minute.[164] Segal et al.[165, 166] recently evaluated a method for determining instantaneous and continuous cardiac output using a Doppler PAC. This method provides spaced average measurements of blood flow velocity in the PA, coupled with continuous measurement of the diameter of the PA. In this model quantitative flow is calculated by the use of the instantaneous, spaced average velocity (obtained from the velocity profile) and the instantaneous area (obtained from the vessel diameter). Siegel et al.[161] compared the results obtained with this Doppler PAC with measurements made by electromagnetic flow. Their results demonstrated that Doppler catheter-determined flow was highly predictive of electromagnetic flow in both continuous and pulsatile pump models ($r^2 = .89$, $r^2 = .97$ respectively).[161] This catheter system also provides instantaneous diameter measurements and mapping of instantaneous velocity profiles within the main PA. Although initial reports were encouraging, this technology failed for economic reasons and is not presently available.[167]

Indications

As originally reported in 1970, the primary indication for PAC was for hemodynamic assessment of patients following complicated MI.[168-170] Since these early reports, the potential benefits of the information gained from the PAC have extended its use to a variety of other clinical areas.[171-174] This expansion is attested to by the fact that an estimated 2 million PACs are sold annually in the United States. Among patients with complicated AMI, use of PAC increased from 1975 through 1988 with a decline in use in 1990.[175] However, the debate regarding the appropriate indications for PAC monitoring, which started over a decade ago, is still ongoing and is fueled by recent studies that have prompted a call for a moratorium in PAC use.[176]

The fact that a physician's database is improved by PA catheterization is evidenced by several reports documenting the difficulty of correlating physical signs with the severity of myocardial dysfunction.[64, 65, 68] Connors et al.[173] prospectively analyzed 62 consecutive PA catheterizations. They found that less than half of a group of clinicians correctly predicted PCWP or cardiac output, and 48% made at least one change in therapy based on data from the PAC.[173] Waller et al.[177] demonstrated that a group of experienced cardiac anesthesiologists and surgeons who were "blinded" to the results of PA catheterization during coronary artery bypass surgery were unaware of any problem during 65% of severe hemodynamic abnormalities. Similarly, Iberti and Fisher[68] showed that a group of physicians were unable to accurately predict hemodynamic data on clinical grounds, that 60% made at least one change in therapy, and 33% changed their diagnosis based on PA catheterization data.

The clinical utility and value of the PAC depend largely on interpretation of the information obtained. Clinical interpretation of data is influenced by the level of understanding of cardiopulmonary hemodynamics, technical skills, and professional integrity of the physician.[178] Clinician misinterpretation and misapplication of the data appear to be the greatest impediment to using PAC to alter pathophysiologic processes and improve outcome in critically ill patients.[179] Iberti et al.[180] have demonstrated an appalling lack of basic knowledge about information obtained from the PAC among ICU physicians. The development and maintenance of educational, credentialing, and continuous quality improvement policies involving the PAC is warranted and overdue.[181] In addition, widespread use of the PAC has significant economic ramifications. Data regarding cost-effectiveness of the PAC is extremely limited in terms of methodology and scope. However, economic impact and cost-effectiveness are moot prior to establishing clinical efficacy.[182]

Intuitively, an enhanced understanding of pathophysiologic processes in severe acute disease states will lead to an improved ability to guide therapeutic decision making, for example, in severe preeclampsia.[183] Whether enhanced understanding of patient hemodynamics translates into definable benefits for patients has recently come into question.[184] Although several studies have shown that PAC prompts changes in therapy in many patients, most data regarding outcomes are retrospective. Some reviewers suggest that the evidence demonstrates an absence of risk of injury from PA catheterization and provision of important clinical data and that PA catheterization meets Food and Drug Administration (FDA) requirements for safety and effectiveness.[185, 186] Recently, Leibowitz[187] reported that clinicians caring for over 500 patients with PACs in situ reported that the catheter was "felt to be helpful" in the management of 80% of these patients. A number of meta-analyses have been performed.[188] Sixteen randomized controlled trials were identified in this study. PAC-guided strategies revealed a modest risk reduction that did reach statistical significance. Risk reduction appears to be greatest in surgical series. Deficiencies of these trials regarding sample size calculations, unclear definition of concomitant therapies, blinding of physicians and patients, and outcome assessments have important implications for the proper design of future trials. Ethical difficulties have also hindered adequate trials. Competent physicians must be content to have their patients receive any of the various treatments in a randomized trial because, based on available data, none has proved preferable. If more than 70% of experts determine that PAC is indicated or contraindicated for a specific indication, a trial cannot ethically be performed for these indications.[189] However, we must do appropriate prospective studies to determine who benefits from PAC and who does not.[190]

In an attempt to address the issue of risk versus benefit of PACs, several organizations have published "guidelines" for the appropriate indications for PAC monitoring.[191-194] In an attempt to provide practice guidelines for PA catheterization, the American Society of Anesthesiologists (ASA) established a PA catheterization task force in 1991.[194] The mission of this group was to develop guidelines for the appropriate indications for PAC use. To fulfill its purpose, the task force reviewed a total of 860 clinical trials, controlled observational studies, uncontrolled case reports, and individual case reports. In addition, the task force focused its review on evidence of effectiveness based on clinical outcome. In its report, the task force reported that their survey of the literature demonstrated that PAC data appeared to change therapy in 30% to 60% of all cases reviewed. Although these studies demonstrated no effect on mortality in patients whose therapy was changed (25% of adults, 10% of children), the task force concluded that one of the major deficiencies in these studies was their small sample size, and this may account for the lack of change in outcome in these patient groups. In summary, based on the available evidence and the preponderance of expert opinion, management with PAC improves outcome in a number of patient populations: (1) in patients with AMI complicated by cardiogenic shock, progressive hypotension, or associated with mechanical complications; (2) in patients with congestive heart failure (CHF) refractory to empiric therapy; (3) in patients with pulmonary hypertension; and (4) in patients with shock or hemodynamic instability. Even if a benefit in terms of mortality is undemonstrable, more rapid diagnosis and achievement of therapeutic endpoints guided by PAC use can decrease morbidity and time needed for intensive care. If the patient is chosen carefully, the catheter inserted successfully and safely, the data obtained meticulously and interpreted correctly, and this interpretation leads to a change in therapy to which the patient responds appropriately, the patient will experience an improved outcome based on PAC use. However, this does not occur often enough to significantly improve outcome in the general patient population.[187]

To illustrate the potential clinical applications of PAC monitoring, its use in the following areas will be discussed:

(1) preoperative assessment, (2) perioperative monitoring (both cardiac and noncardiac surgery), (3) obstetric and gynecologic procedures, and (4) hemodynamic or nonsurgical indications.[195-210]

Preoperative Assessment

The preoperative use of the PAC provides physicians with data that may be used to guide patient therapy. Studies have suggested that this information gained from the PAC would often be undetected by clinical observation alone.[67] Orlando,[125] in a retrospective study of 148 consecutive patients over 65 years of age cleared for surgery by standard clinical assessment, found that preoperative invasive hemodynamic monitoring resulted in 23% of patients being classified as having severe cardiopulmonary compromise. As a result, these patients were identified as being at extremely high risk for the planned surgical procedure.[125] All eight of these patients who subsequently underwent surgery as originally planned died. Similarly, Babu et al.[208] examined a series of 75 elderly patients (average age, 68 years) who underwent preoperative PAC placement. In this patient population, 30 (40%) patients were found to have abnormal LV function (by PAC data) which was not detected by clinical evaluation alone.[208]

In a prospective study of elderly patients with hip fractures (N = 70; average age, 72 years), half of the patients (N = 35) were randomized for evaluation either by standard clinical examination combined with central venous pressure (CVP) placement, or PAC insertion.[211] The patients in the PAC group went to surgery only after correction of all hemodynamic abnormalities. Mortality in this group was 2.9% versus 29% in the CVP group.

In an attempt to answer the question of the potential positive effect of preoperative hemodynamic optimization using PAC data on outcome, Berlauk et al.[197] prospectively evaluated 89 patients scheduled for peripheral vascular surgery. In this study, patients were randomized into three groups: (1) preoperative optimization in the ICU 12 hours prior to surgery, (2) PAC insertion and hemodynamic manipulation 3 hours prior to surgery, or (3) control group (i.e., arterial line and CVP). Hemodynamic optimization was defined as a PCWP between 8 and 15 mmHg, a cardiac index (CI) greater than 2.8 L/minute/m², and a systemic vascular resistance (SVR) less than 1100 dynes-sec · cm⁻⁵. Patients in groups (1) and (2) were more hemodynamically stable intraoperatively and had a lower incidence of tachycardia, hypotension, and arrhythmias than group (3) patients. In addition, these groups had a lower incidence of postoperative cardiac morbidity and less early graft closure than did the control group ($P < .05$). However, PAC catheterization 12 hours before surgery did not result in any better outcome than catheterization 3 hours before surgery.

In a recent retrospective study, patients who had normal initial preoperative hemodynamic values or abnormal initial values that were normalized preoperatively experienced significantly fewer perioperative cardiovascular complications than those with abnormal initial values that were not normalized preoperatively.[212] These results suggest that there may be benefit to the practice of preoperative ICU admission, hemodynamic monitoring with a PAC, and "optimization" of cardiac function in selected patients undergoing major elective noncardiac surgery.

However, in a recent prospective study in which patients were randomized to receive preoperative monitoring and optimization with a PAC sited the night before surgery or standard care prior to aortic surgery, the incidence of post-operative cardiac, renal, and other complications was similar in both groups.[213] The authors suggested that routine use of PACs for perioperative monitoring during aortic surgery was not beneficial and may be associated with a higher rate of intraoperative complications. Variables such as cardiac risk factors and adenosine thallium scintigraphy may be more important predictors of cardiac events in such patients. Routine perioperative use of the PAC does not appear to be appropriate because of age alone.[214]

An observational study was unable to demonstrate any difference in outcome between elderly patients who did not undergo preoperative catheterization and unmatched patients who were admitted to the hospital during the same time period for other diagnoses.[215] The PAC task force of the ASA suggested that in this study, the similar outcomes may have been due to selection bias.[194]

Perioperative Monitoring

High-Risk General Surgical Patients

The presence of significant cardiac disease (defined as either a recent MI or clinical evidence of CHF) was one of the earliest indications for PAC insertion in noncardiac surgical patients. The presence of clinical CHF has been shown to place patients at increased risk for postoperative cardiac death following noncardiac surgery.[216-218]

In a 1972 report, Tarhan et al.[13] evaluated patients with a history of recurrent MIs who underwent noncardiac surgery. This study revealed a reinfarction rate of 37% within the first 3 months following infarction. In this study patients did not receive routine hemodynamic monitoring prior to their procedure.[13] In a later study of 733 patients, Rao et al.[219] studied the incidence of reinfarction in noncardiac surgical patients. In this study, PACs and arterial lines were inserted in all patients prior to surgery. Patients' hemodynamic status was optimized preoperatively using the information obtained from these monitors. Using this technique, Rao et al. reported a reinfarction rate (at 3 months) of only 5.8%. In spite of this study implying that PAC monitoring can decrease mortality in critically ill patients,[219] no scientific study has confirmed this impression.[220] Recent studies have evaluated the impact of PAC monitoring on mortality with emphasis on how the information is used.[220] Although a potential benefit from PAC monitoring has been noted, the limited sample size and selection criteria prevent definitive conclusions.[220] Many reported studies are retrospective, nonrandomized, unblinded, limited in scope or size, and founded on subjective endpoints. Large multicentered randomized controlled trials are required.

Major Vascular Surgery

Perhaps the major difficulty with trying to interpret the impact of PAC use in major vascular surgery is the absence of a control group for comparison (i.e., patients who do not receive a PAC). Routine use of PACs in elective abdominal aortic reconstruction remains controversial.[221, 222]

In an early report utilizing controls, Hesdorffer et al.[223] were able to demonstrate a reduction in mortality, perioperative hypertensive events, and renal failure in patients managed using an aggressive fluid loading protocol and a PAC who were undergoing aortic reconstruction. The main problem with this study is that the PAC was only a small part of the overall study design. Several other authors have suggested that utilizing PCWP measurements obtained from the

PAC to optimize preoperative volume status may prove beneficial in this patient population.[224, 225] In a prospective study, 41 patients (18 abdominal aortic aneurysm repairs, 23 other peripheral vascular procedures) who maintained their postoperative PCWP within 3 mmHg of their best preoperative level had a decrease in overall complication rate (14% vs 79%).[225] Berlauk et al. showed that optimization of hemodynamics in the ICU preoperatively reduced morbidity and mortality from 9.5% to 1.5%.[197] Others believe that the preoperative "tune-up" can be done more quickly and safely intraoperatively.[222] One recent prospective study demonstrated no change in postoperative cardiac, renal, and other complications following placement of the PAC the night before surgery and optimization of hemodynamic parameters.[213] A high incidence of unsuspected cardiorespiratory abnormalities severe enough to defer surgery have been detected in the over-65-years age group with the PAC.[67] This would suggest that the PAC is necessary to truly predict increased risk and poor outcome. However, more recent studies by Joyce et al.[201] and Isaacson et al.[202] reported different results. Using a randomized controlled protocol evaluation of patients without uncompensated renal disease or severe cardiac disease (left ventricular ejection fraction [LVEF] < 40%) undergoing abdominal aortic reconstruction, these authors were unable to show any difference in outcomes between patients monitored by PAC or CVP.[201, 202] In addition, it is likely that the general preparation of patients coming to the OR for aortic surgery has improved significantly over the last decade, particularly with regard to cardiac management and antihypertensive treatment.

In summary, the PAC may be useful in the management of some patients undergoing aortic surgery, although recent studies have identified patients who can be safely managed with arterial pressure and CVP monitoring alone.[201, 202, 214] Use of the PAC may lead to fewer complications in high-risk patients undergoing peripheral vascular surgery.

Neurosurgery

The main focus of all studies to date in the area of neurosurgery has been on the ability of PAC to detect air embolism.[226, 227] However, the use of the PAC to monitor and treat air embolism in neurosurgical patients does not appear to be appropriate.[214] Its use as a monitor is less sensitive than other techniques and its efficacy as a treatment modality is questionable. Of note, none of the studies has evaluated the impact of PAC use on clinical outcome.

Obstetrics and Gynecology

Once again, the major problems with studies performed using PAC in the obstetric and gynecologic patient population is the lack of historical controls.[195, 204-206, 228, 229] The major focus of PAC utilization has been in patients with severe preeclampsia.[204, 205] Available scientific data do not support use of the PAC in uncomplicated preeclampsia; however, most experts believe that PAC use may be helpful in the management of selected patients with severe preeclampsia.[214] Severe preeclampsia is characterized by elevated SVR, low or normal filling pressures, increased contractility (left ventricular stroke work index), and normal heart rate. The subsets of patients most likely to benefit from PAC monitoring were those with (1) refractory oliguria, (2) pulmonary edema, or (3) refractory hypertension.[214] The first two are considered indications by the American College of Obstetricians and Gynecologists.[230] Spapen et al.[228] reported on the potential of PAC monitoring to aid in the early recognition of an amniotic fluid embolus.

Hemodynamic Disorders

Historically, the use of PAC in ICUs has been widespread in both the medical and surgical settings. The data from the medical ICU has focused primarily on patients with MI. Once again, these uncontrolled studies have yielded inconsistent results.[14, 167] Opponents of PAC use in this setting argue that patients with an MI who were monitored by PAC had a higher in-hospital mortality, longer hospital stay, and shorter short-term survival than patients who did not have PAC inserted.[232, 233]

Data from the surgical intensive care literature support the ability of data from PAC to aid in diagnosis and to guide therapy.[171, 219, 223, 234, 235] However, the major question that remains is: does routine placement of a PAC in selected surgical ICU (SICU) patients reduce morbidity and mortality? In an attempt to answer this question, Scalea et al.[215] studied a group of geriatric blunt trauma patients. The authors showed that using routine placement of the PAC identified a group of patients in clinically unrecognized shock (46%). They demonstrated a reduction in mortality from 93% to 46%.[215] Shoemaker et al.[171] preoperatively randomized a high-risk general surgical population to receive either PAC or CVP placement. For the purpose of this study, patients were randomized into one of two treatment groups: (1) normal values of healthy subjects were used as therapeutic goals or (2) a protocol group in which median values of patients who had survived life-threatening postoperative shock were the therapeutic goals.[171] Controversy still exists about the result of this study (centering on whether the control and protocol groups were comparable), which revealed that the PAC protocol group had reduced mortality (4% versus 33%), fewer complications, fewer ICU hospital and ventilator days, and less total cost. Further research is required regarding goal-oriented use of the PAC to achieve supranormal oxygen delivery prior to high-risk surgery before a recommendation can be made.[236]

Other recent studies have demonstrated that in patients with sepsis and adult respiratory distress syndrome (ARDS) survival may be improved by therapy guided by the PAC. In a randomized prospective study, Tuchschmidt et al.[237] successfully employed the concept of achieving "supranormal" values in the treatment of 26 septic patients in the ICU. Similarly, Russell et al.[172] documented (retrospectively) improved outcome in patients with ARDS who had an elevated cardiac output. There are now several other publications from different institutions validating these higher goals for cardiac output.[171,238] Each of the groups of investigators focused on oxygen delivery and changed the long-established concept that a CI of 2.2 L/minute/m² is sufficient in all clinical situations. Carefully designed multicenter, randomized controlled trials are required to establish whether augmenting oxygen delivery improves organ-specific outcomes and survival in systemic inflammatory response syndrome (SIRS)–related organ dysfunction secondary to infection, trauma, or surgery.[236] However, hyperdynamic resuscitation has been shown to improve survival rates in life-threatening burns.[239] Unsustained or inadequate response to hyperdynamic resuscitation of burns has been associated with mortality.[240] However, only 8% of burn units in the United Kingdom, United States, Canada, Australia, and New Zealand use PACs in over half of their patients and few centers describe the use of predetermined goals to direct therapy following PAC insertion.[241] In conclusion, PAC use may be appropriate in septic shock unresponsive to early resuscitative measures.[242] Maintenance of normal hemodynamics in this group of patients appears to be the appropriate goal. Further research is needed to determine the proper role of the PAC in sepsis and septic shock.

RV dysfunction has been identified in septic shock by the use of an RVEF PAC, and RV contractility was improved by epinephrine.[243, 244] In a study of 27 septic shock patients, RV dysfunction was identified in 11 (41%).[245] In this specific patient population, fluid replacement alone did not succeed in stabilizing hemodynamic variables, necessitating inotropic therapy. The value of RVEDV derived from the RVEF PAC as an index of LV preload has been investigated.[246] RVEDV markedly overestimated LV preload with the conclusion that RVEDV should not be used as an absolute value for determining preload, as patients may be underresuscitated. The authors suggested use of transesophageal echocardiography (TEE) in conjunction with RVEF PAC to more accurately determine preload and cardiac performance in critically ill patients. In addition, Doppler ultrasound may be used as a screen to determine the need for PAC placement[247]: acceleration less than 200 cm/s² correlates well with CI less than 3.0 L/minute/m².

Invasive hemodynamic monitoring has become standard in the management of aneurysmal subarachnoid hemorrhage, facilitating the safe and effective use of hypervolemic, hypertensive therapy to treat or prevent cerebral vasospasm.[248] This study documented a 13% incidence of catheter-related sepsis, a 2% incidence of CHF, a 1.3% incidence of subclavian vein thrombosis, and a 1% incidence of pneumothorax in this patient population. A novel indication for the PAC has been described: pulmonary wedge aspiration cytology, allowing the tissue diagnosis of malignancy and enabling prompt institution of chemotherapy. The diagnosis in the case reported was made as part of the workup of pulmonary arterial hypertension.[249]

A prospective cohort study of 5735 patients with adjustment for treatment selection bias was designed to examine the association between the use of the PAC during the first 24 hours in the ICU and subsequent survival, length of stay, intensity of care, and cost of care.[176] The PAC was associated with increased mortality and increased utilization of resources. The cause of this apparent lack of benefit is unclear and the findings justify consideration of a randomized controlled trial of the PAC. Knowledge of the right heart PAC is not uniformly good among ICU physicians. Accreditation policies and teaching practices concerning this technique are undergoing urgent revision.[250] In addition, less invasive means of cardiovascular assessment are growing in popularity. For example, training intensive therapy unit (ITU) physicians in limited TEE, using a pediatric monoplane probe to evaluate LV function, has been shown to be rapidly and safely achievable, and to yield data pertinent to patient management, even in the early stages of skill acquisition.[251] Meta-analyses of clinical trials from 1979 to 1996 concluded that hemodynamic data obtained from the PAC appeared to be beneficial for the following indications[242, 252, 253]: (1) defining the status of underlying cardiovascular performance or the need for improvement; (2) direction of therapy when noninvasive monitoring may be inadequate, misleading, or the endpoints of resuscitation are difficult to define; (3) assessment of response to resuscitation; (4) potential reduction of secondary head or spinal cord injury in multisystem trauma; (5) direction of management of major trauma complicated by severe ARDS, oliguria or anuria, myocardial ischemia, CHF, or major thermal injury; and (6) establishing futility of care. There are few data to identify a grade A indication for the PAC in the care of critically ill patients.[253] Finding little evi-

Table 14–2. Guidelines for Safe Insertion of Pulmonary Artery (PA) Flow-Guided Catheters

1. Balance risk vs. benefit.
2. Slowly inflate the balloon while continuously monitoring the PA waveform.
3. Upon transition from the PA to the pulmonary capillary wedge pressure (PCWP) trace, immediately stop inflation.
4. If an overwedge pattern is observed, the balloon should be immediately deflated, and the catheter immediately withdrawn 1–2 cm (see Fig. 14–9). The balloon is slowly reinflated and a normal wedge pressure waveform is noted.
5. Minimize duration of PCWP measurements.
6. If the balloon inflates with <1.5 mL of gas, the catheter should be withdrawn at least 1–2 cm.
7. Spontaneous tip migration may occur; therefore continuously monitor the PA trace for "spontaneous wedging." If this occurs, withdraw the catheter 1–2 cm or until a normal PA tracing reappears.
8. Minimize the number of PCWP measurements in patients who are elderly, anticoagulated, or have pulmonary hypertension.
9. If PA diastolic pressure is <18 mmHg, use PA diastolic pressure rather than PCWP as an index of left ventricular filling pressure.

dence to support the use of PAC in the literature does not mean that it is neither efficacious nor effective. It may well be that information provided by PACs is important in the care process. However, there is little objective evidence to support this conclusion, and the challenge to clinicians is to design and conduct clinical trials capable of separating evidence from opinion.

Cardiac Surgery

Numerous uncontrolled observational studies have attempted to determine whether PACs change outcome in cardiac surgical patients.[177, 254, 255] Moore et al.[255] compared 20 consecutive patients with left main coronary artery stenosis undergoing coronary artery bypass grafting (CABG) without PAC monitoring with 28 patients undergoing surgery who had a preoperative PAC inserted. They demonstrated a decrease in mortality from 20% to 3.5% and concluded that this improvement was due to the use of vasodilators, inotropic agents, and propranolol. All of these modalities were facilitated by the information obtained using the PAC.

A more recent study by Tuman et al.[254] in 1094 patients undergoing cardiac surgery was unable to demonstrate any positive impact (i.e., a reduction in mortality, cardiac ischemia, or postoperative MI) in patients receiving elective or emergent PAC versus CVP placement. The lack of observed differences in outcome may have been due to patient demographics, as assignment to monitoring groups was made solely by the anesthesiologist assigned to the case. Similarly, a randomized controlled study by Pearson et al.[256] (N = 229) found no difference in death, length of ICU stay, or use of vasopressors between cardiac surgical patients monitored by PAC or CVP. Once again, the anesthesiologist in charge of the case could remove patients from the control (CVP) group and place them into the monitored PAC group at discretion. On balance, low-risk patients undergoing surgery do not appear to benefit from PAC use.[214] Studies examining high-risk patients undergoing cardiac surgery are lacking, making accurate determination of patient benefit difficult.

Insertion

Successful PAC insertion begins with preparation of the site for venipuncture (see Chapter 13 for details) and appropriate

balancing and calibration of pressure monitoring equipment. Following successful venipuncture (using the classic Seldinger technique),[257] a larger sheath and vessel dilator can be introduced into the vessel. After placement of the introducer, the dilator is removed and the larger intravascular sheath remains in place.[258] The PAC can then be inserted into the sheath and threaded into the central circulation. This method may be used whether the internal or external jugular, femoral, or antecubital veins are employed.

Selection of Insertion Site

A number of venous entry sites are employed for PA catheterization.[259–263] These include the internal and external jugular, subclavian, antecubital, and femoral veins. Ideally, the appropriate site should be easily accessible, a short distance from the RA, and be associated with minimal complications. Meticulous attention to detail is essential if complications are to be avoided (Table 14–2).

Based on these goals, most anesthesiologists inserting the PAC choose the internal jugular vein approach.[263] Advantages include simplicity, accessibility of the site during surgery, and a relatively short and direct pathway to the RA. Disadvantages include inadvertent carotid artery puncture with hematoma formation or dislodgment of atherosclerotic plaques, nerve injury, and, rarely, pneumothorax.[264–272] Insertion of the PAC through the femoral vein without the use of fluoroscopy has been shown to be safe and effective.[273]

Insertion Technique

With the introducer sheath in place, the Swan-Ganz catheter is inserted carefully and advanced until the tip lies in a central vein. Approximate distances from various insertion sites and the advantages and disadvantages of different insertion sites are listed in Tables 14–3 and 14–4. Intracardiac knotting is a consequence of inserting the PAC too far distally without the appropriate pressure trace being displayed on the monitor.

Location of the tip of the catheter in a central vein can be confirmed by pressure changes related to respiration or coughing. With the catheter in the RA, the balloon is inflated with 1.5 mL of air (never more or less), and the catheter slowly advanced. When the RA is entered, typical venous a, b, c, and v waves will be noted (RAP = 0–8 mmHg)[27] (Fig. 14–6). Further advancement of the catheter will produce a dramatic change in the pressure tracing as the tip of the catheter enters the RV. Within one cardiac cycle a pressure change from those characteristic of the atrium to a phasic pressure in the range of 25/0–5 mmHg, typical of the RV,

Table 14–3. Distances From Insertion Sites to Right Atrium, Pulmonary Artery, and Wedge Position

Insertion Site		Right Atrium	Right Ventricle	Pulmonary Artery
Internal jugular vein	Right	20 cm	30 cm	45 cm
	Left	25 cm	35 cm	50 cm
Antecubital vein	Right	50 cm	65 cm	80 cm
	Left	55 cm	70 cm	85 cm
Femoral vein		40 cm	50 cm	65 cm
Subclavian vein		10 cm	25 cm	40 cm

Table 14–4. A Comparison of Venous Access Routes

Route	Method of Cannulation	Advantages	Disadvantages
Peripheral external jugular vein	Percutaneous	Easy to learn Safe Does not interfere with cardiopulmonary resuscitation (CPR)	Valves may hinder catheter or guidewire insertion Stasis, thrombosis, and phlebitis are more common
Antecubital vein	Percutaneous/cutdown	Easy to learn Safe Preferred route with anticoagulant or thrombolytic therapy, because the site is easily compressible should bleeding occur	Stasis, thrombosis, infection, and venospasm are more common Catheter displacement is frequent
Central internal jugular vein	Percutaneous	Rapidly accessible Does not interfere with CPR Provides a straight route to the heart Less restrictive to patient movement	Air embolism, carotid artery puncture, tracheal injury may occur Pneumothorax (more common in the left than the right internal jugular vein) Thoracic duct injury (left internal jugular vein only)
Subclavian vein	Percutaneous	Rapidly accessible Allows free neck and arm movement Easier to keep sterile	Air embolism, more frequent pneumothorax and hemothorax; subclavian artery puncture; injury to nerve bundle may occur
Femoral vein	Percutaneous	Rapidly accessible Does not interfere with CPR	Sepsis, in situ thrombosis, pulmonary embolism may occur

should be observed. The catheter is then advanced through the RV (as quickly as possible to minimize the potential for dysrhythmias until it enters the main PA). Location can be verified by an increase in the diastolic pressure of 25/12 mmHg and a change in the morphology of the waveform. Usually there is no change in the systolic pressure. The catheter is advanced farther until it wedges in a branch of the PA. At this point, the trace will have the appearance of an atrial pressure pattern with a, b, c, and v wave components transmitted retrograde from the left atrium (PCWP = 8 to 12 mmHg).[274] In summary, pulmonary capillary wedge position is verified by (1) a characteristic waveform, (2) a mean pressure lower than the mean pulmonary artery pressure (PAP), and (3) the ability to withdraw arterialized blood.

Once the wedge position has been achieved, the balloon is deflated. This should produce a typical PAP tracing.[6] Reinflation of the balloon should reproduce the wedge tracing with 1.5 mL of air. If *less* than 1.5 mL of air results in a wedge tracing, the catheter should be withdrawn to the point where a 1.5-mL balloon inflation is associated with a PCWP. At *no time* should more air be injected into the balloon than is necessary to obtain PCWP. This will result in distal migration of the catheter. By emphasizing the aforementioned technique, PA catheterization can be accomplished in an expeditious and efficient manner (<2 minutes

in about 90% of patients). However, certain disease states such as low output, pulmonary hypertension, and congenital cardiac defects are commonly associated with difficult catheter insertions. In addition, unrecognized technical difficulties may also result in catheterization failure. These include air bubbles in the transducer or tubing that may dampen the pressure waves sufficiently to prevent recognition of the waveforms. Similarly, an improperly set calibration scale can also reduce the waveform deflection to such low levels that important pressure changes go unrecognized. Clotting within or at the tip of the catheter can prevent transmission of the characteristic waveform.

Interpretation of Hemodynamic Data

Pressure Measurements

The accurate interpretation of pressure measurements is central to defining the various subsets of patients with abnormal cardiovascular performance. Classically, intravascular pressures have been measured at end-exhalation because no airflow occurs and intrapleural pressure is considered static[275] (Fig. 14–7). In those patients in whom the point of end-exhalation is difficult to discern, direct measurement of res-

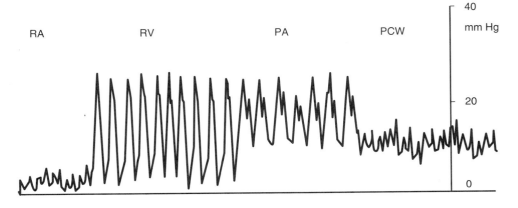

Figure 14–6. Pressure waveforms in relation to catheter position from right atrium to pulmonary capillary wedge position. RA, right atrial pressure; RV, right ventricular pressure; PA, pulmonary artery pressure; PCWP, pulmonary capillary wedge pressure.

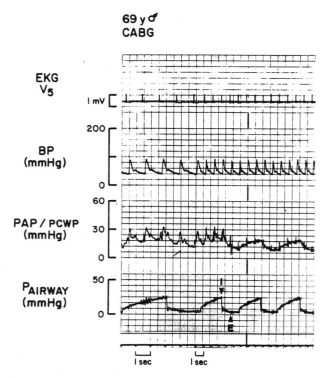

69 y ♂
CABG

EKG
V₅

BP
(mmHg)

PAP / PCWP
(mmHg)

P_AIRWAY
(mmHg)

Figure 14-7. Vascular measurements should be made at end-exhalation. This recording of an anesthetized patient receiving positive pressure ventilation shows a significant variation in pulmonary capillary wedge pressure during the respiratory cycle. EKG, electrocardiogram; BP, blood pressure; PA, pulmonary artery pressure; AP, airway pressure.

piratory variables (airway pressure, end-tidal CO_2, and so on) may be necessary.[7, 276] Numerous reports have documented the effects of airway pressure on the correlation between LAP and PCWP.[7, 275, 277-279] Spontaneous ventilation and noncompliant lungs *do not* alter the relationship.[7] In contrast, increased airway pressure, as seen with positive PEEP, continuous positive airway pressure (CPAP), airway obstruction, PAC tip placement above the LA, hypovolemia, and obesity all serve to increase the gradient between PCWP and LAP.[26, 28, 43, 279-283] As a result, controversy exists as to whether PEEP should be temporarily removed in order to accurately measure PCWP.[45, 283] Disadvantages of this technique include a temporary increase in the alveolar-arterial O_2 gradient and potential destabilization of the hemodynamic state.[45] Indeed, if a patient is receiving high levels of PEEP (>10 cm H_2O), spurious cardiovascular information may be obtained even with transient removal of PEEP.[34] Errors in interpretation may also occur as a result of transmural pressure gradients across a vessel. Downs[284] has suggested using direct measurement of intrapleural pressure as a means of more accurately assessing this transmural gradient. Finally, the relatively low resonant frequency of currently available clinical monitoring systems (catheter and tubing system) can be another significant cause of artifact.

Analysis of the pressure waveform may also yield information regarding cardiac pump function. Early reports by Kaplan and Wells[285] demonstrated in selected patients that abnormalities in the a, b, and c waves in the PCWP trace may be an early indicator of myocardial ischemia. In addition, acute papillary muscle dysfunction or rupture secondary to ischemia or infarction, respectively, may be detected by the onset of v waves in the PCWP trace. Large v waves may be seen in mitral regurgitation due to a dilated annulus, papillary muscle dysfunction, or ruptured chordae tendineae[286, 287] (Fig. 14-8). Unfortunately, the presence of v waves is not a clinically useful method for ischemia detection because it is not a specific marker. The pressure ratio of the v wave divided by the left ventricular systolic pressure has been found to correlate reasonably well with mitral regurgitant volume ($r = .75$).[288] The ratio is easily recorded during routine heart catheterization.[288]

Derived Cardiovascular Variables

At present, the anesthesiologist is confronted with a data dilemma. On the one hand, it is possible to obtain extensive physiologic measurements in the critically ill patient. On the other, the volume of data, the organization of the data, and the subsequent calculations necessary for clinical management can be overwhelming. Nowhere is this more obvious than in cardiovascular monitoring. The use of the pulmonary artery TD catheter has facilitated the clinician's ability to perform extensive hemodynamic assessments. Using these data, various circulatory disease states can now be defined in terms of pump failure, hypovolemia, and high or low resistance states. Assessment of cardiac performance using the derived indices of cardiac performance such as CI, stroke work index, SVR, PVR, and the O_2 transport provide the foundation for sound physiologic management of the critically ill patient[206, 284, 285, 289-293] (Table 14-5). To accommodate patients of varying body size, indexed systemic or pulmonary vascular resistance is often utilized. The sequential and repeated use of these measures provides the opportunity to use therapy aimed at treating specific hemodynamic abnormalities.

Cardiac Work

Although some estimation of ventricular function can be obtained by the shape of the ventricular pressure volume

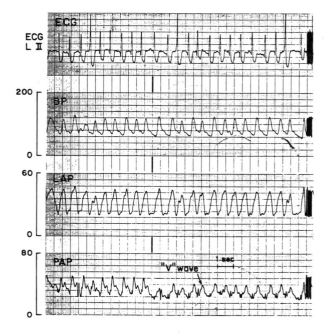

ECG
L II

BP

LAP

PAP

Figure 14-8. V waves are shown in the left atrial and pulmonary capillary wedge pressure tracing of a patient with mitral stenosis.

Table 14-5. Hemodynamic Calculations

Cardiac output (CO) L/min = heart rate × stroke volume

Cardiac index (CI) L/min/m² is calculated as follows:

$$CI = \frac{CO}{BSA}$$

Stroke volume (SV) or *stroke volume index* (SVI) overcomes some of the difficulties inherent in the use of CO or CI.

$$SV = mL/stroke\ \frac{CO}{Heart\ rate} \quad or \quad SVI = \frac{CI}{Heart\ rate}$$

$$SV = End\text{-}diastolic\ volume - end\text{-}systolic\ volume$$

Systemic vascular resistance (SVR) or *systemic vascular resistance index* (SVRI) is defined as:

$$SVR\ (RU) = \frac{MBP - RAP}{CO}$$

$$SVRI\ (RU/m^2) = \frac{MBP - RAP}{CI}$$

Pulmonary vascular resistance (PVR) or *pulmonary vascular resistance index* (PVRI) is defined as:

$$PVR\ (RU) = \frac{PAP - PCWP}{CO}$$

$$PVRI\ (RU/m^2) = \frac{PAP - PCWP}{CI}$$

Measurement of resistance is reported in one of two methods.

(1) Absolute resistance units (ARU) = dynes-sec · s · cm⁻⁵

(2) Hybrid resistance units (HRU) = RU

To convert HRU to ARU, multiply by 79.9

BSA, body surface area; RU, resistance units; MBP, mean blood pressure; RAP, right atrial pressure; PAP, pulmonary artery pressure; PCWP, pulmonary capillary wedge pressure.

loop and its relation to the pressure volume ordinates, the logistic difficulty in obtaining these data limits its clinical utility.[294-296] *Cardiac work* can serve as a more clinically useful index of cardiac performance. Work is a basic description of pump function and can be extrapolated from either a pressure volume loop or calculated by use of a formula. The amount of work performed is a function of the load carried and the distance moved (work = force × distance moved). In the OR or ICU, the most commonly employed formula for calculation of the LVSWI is:

$$LVSWI = \frac{(Mean\ BP - mean\ PCWP)}{body\ surface\ area} \times SVI \times 0.0136$$

where

LVSWI = left ventricular stroke work index (g-m/m² per beat)
SVI = stroke volume index (mL/m² per beat)
BP = mean aortic pressure (mmHg)
PCWP = mean pulmonary capillary wedge pressure (mmHg)
0.0136 = factor for converting mmHg · mL to g-m

Ventricular Function Curve

The ventricular function curve (VFC) defines the relationship between ventricular filling pressure and ventricular stroke work and is a unifying concept to explain the performance characteristics of a given ventricle. The LV function curves possess certain characteristics. Each has a steep ascending limb, which plateaus at higher filling pressures. Because the RV empties into a lower pressure system (PA), right VFCs have lower values for stroke work and may *not* possess a plateau. However, with either ventricle, the larger the input (end-diastolic volume), the greater the output (work)(within the limits of normal contractile performance).

Although more sophisticated indices of cardiac performance have been advocated, the VFC serves as one of the best clinical means of physiologically describing the performance of the intact heart. This is due, in part, to the fact that both ordinate (LVSWI) and abscissa (LVEDP, LAP, PCWP, and the like) are related qualitatively to the two major symptom complexes of patients with heart disease.

The graphic representation of the VFC is based on the work of Ross and Braunwald.[297] They constructed VFCs relating LV filling pressures and LVSWI. These curves were derived from data obtained under controlled conditions during cardiac catheterization. From these data the authors described three classes of ventricular function: normal function, mildly depressed ventricular function, and grossly depressed ventricular function.

The use of LVSWI rather than cardiac output or stroke volume has several advantages:

1. LVSWI defines the area within a pressure volume loop.
2. LVSWI includes measurements of both systolic and diastolic performance.
3. LVSWI contains the major variables that alter cardiac performance (e.g., heart rate, preload, afterload).

An upward shift to the left has been interpreted as an improvement in ventricular performance. A shift downward and to the right has been considered as a deteriorating ventricular performance. In addition to changes in *contractility*, many interventions, including alterations in preload, afterload, heart rate, and ventricular compliance, can produce shifts in the VFC. On this basis, some authorities have held that the use of LVSWI is too global to be informative. However, the directional changes of the VFC allow qualitative assessment of overall cardiac performance.

Derived Indices of Respiratory Performance

Derived indices, especially those concerning oxygen delivery, can play an important role in optimizing respiratory evaluation and support of critically ill patients.[198, 209, 292, 299] Nowhere is the interplay of respiratory and circulatory function more frequently assessed than in the selection of the optimal level of PEEP.[300] Just as there is no one perfect measure of cardiac function, no single parameter will define the optimal level of respiratory performance for all patients. The optimal level of PEEP has been variously defined as follows:

The best PaO_2 does not necessarily infer the optimal level of PEEP. As PaO_2 is increased by higher levels of PEEP, transport of oxygen to the tissues may actually decrease (secondary to decreased cardiac output). Similarly, the lowest alveolar-arterial oxygen gradient may be a function of an improvement in PaO_2 regardless of the effect on cardiac output. A reduction in intrapulmonary shunt to less than

Table 14-6. Complications (Case Reports) Associated With the Use of Pulmonary Artery (PA) Catheters

Venous Cannulation
Air embolization
Arterial puncture
Horner's syndrome
Hematoma
Nerve injury
Phrenic nerve blockade
Pneumothorax

Catheter Passage
Arrhythmias
Knotting
Knotting on papillary muscle
Pneumoperitoneum
Separation of introducer from hub
Bundle branch block

Catheter In Situ
Aberrant waveform due to balloon rupture
Bradycardia secondary to thermodilution cardiac output measurement
Cardiac valve injury
Catheter fracture
Deep venous thrombosis
Endobronchial hemorrhage
Endocarditis
False-positive lung imaging
False-positive echocardiography
Hemoptysis
Intraoperative transection of a catheter
Migration of pediatric PA catheter
PA perforation
Pulmonary infarction

15% has been thought to be a therapeutic goal that is consistent with adequate respiratory performance. Other reports emphasize that the best compliance coincides with optimal PEEP. Finally, an optimal level of PEEP has been defined as that which promotes the highest oxygen transport to the peripheral tissues.

Complications

Experience gained with more than a decade of use of the PAC in a wide variety of clinical situations has revealed a large variety of complications which can, and do, occur (Table 14-6). These range from minor sequelae of catheter use, without clinical significance, to those with a fatal outcome. As a matter of fact, Alschule[301] has termed "complications of vascular catheters" a new branch of medicine.

Swan, in his initial report describing 100 patients, noted only transient premature ventricular contractions, 2 cases of intravascular thrombosis, and 10 cases of balloon failure.[3] The last may have been related to the fact that catheters were reused. Despite numerous case reports that have detailed the occurrence of specific complications resulting from PAC insertion, few large series exist that quantify complication rates. More recent reports have focused on specific complications resulting from PAC insertion (Table 14-7).

For the purpose of this discussion, the complications arising from the use of a Swan-Ganz catheter can be usefully grouped in three categories:

1. Those associated with venous cannulation
2. Those associated with passing the catheter
3. Those occurring after the catheter is in place

Table 14-6 lists the variety of complications associated with the use of a Swan-Ganz catheter. Most complications are avoidable by meticulous attention to technique. Table 14-8 outlines associated factors and prevention and treatment.

Venous Cannulation

Arterial Puncture

The complications occurring during venous cannulation are, with a few exceptions, the same as those which may occur during insertion of any central venous catheter (CVC). The frequency of arterial puncture depends on several variables such as operator skill and experience, site of insertion, and the urgency of the situation. However, it should be noted that arterial puncture has been reported in conjunction with all insertion sites. The carotid artery can be punctured during attempts at cannulating the internal jugular vein.[271, 302, 303] Shah et al.[304] reported a 1.9% incidence of carotid artery punctures in more than 6000 patients receiving PACs. Another paper reported an incidence of 4 perforations in 1500 cannulations.[305] Methods to confirm that the insertion site is venous and not arterial include pressure waveform analysis, the usual comparison with blood in the arterial tubing, and blood gas laboratory measurements of P_{IO_2}.[306] Although most arterial punctures result in minimal morbidity, on occasion it has resulted in dissection of the right common carotid, subclavian, and innominate arteries[307] and, rarely, death has been reported.[269, 308] Early recognition followed by pressure over the puncture site will lead to immediate cessation of

Table 14-7. Reported Incidence of Adverse Effects Resulting From Pulmonary Artery (PA) Catheter Insertion

Complication	Reported Incidence (%)
Central Venous Access	
Arterial puncture	1.1-13
Bleeding at cutdown site (children)	5.3
Postoperative neuropathy	0.3-1.1
Pneumothorax	0.3-4.5
Air embolism	0.5
Catheterization	
Minor dysrhythmias*	4.7-68.9
Severe dysrhythmias (ventricular tachycardia or fibrillation)*	0.3-62.7
Right bundle branch block*	0.1-4.3
Complete heart block (in patients with prior left bundle branch block)*	8.0-8.5
Catheter Residence	
PA rupture*	0.1-1.5
Positive catheter tip cultures	1.4-34.8
Catheter-related sepsis	0.7-11.4
Thrombophlebitis	6.5
Venous thrombosis	0.5-66.7
Pulmonary infarction*	0.1-5.8
Mural thrombus*	28-61
Valvular/endocardial vegetations or endocarditis*	2.2-100
Deaths (attributed to PA catheter)*	0.02-1.5

*Complications thought to be more common (or exclusively associated) with PA catheterization than with central venous catheterization.

From Practice guidelines for pulmonary artery catheterization. A report by the American Society of Anesthesiologists Task Force on Pulmonary Artery Catheterization. Anesthesiology 1993; 78(2):380.

Table 14–8. Pulmonary Artery Catheter Complications, Associated Factors, and Prevention and Treatment

Complications	Associated or Causative Factors	Prevention/Treatment
Balloon rupture	Repeated inflations Excessive inflation volumes Prolonged catheterization Prolonged shelf life or absorption of lipoproteins resulting in weakened structural integrity of the balloon	Do not inflate the balloon if a rupture is suspected Use pulmonary artery diastolic pressure whenever possible, because diastolic pressure measurements do not require balloon inflation
Less Common Complications		
Pulmonary artery rupture	Distensive occlusion of the pulmonary artery Balloon inflation with fluid Excess catheter looping Pulmonary hypertension	Inflate the balloon slowly under continuous pulmonary arterial monitoring Discontinue inflation once pulmonary capillary wedge pressure is obtained Keep wedge time to a minimum (<8–15 s)
Complete heart block	Preexisting left bundle branch block Loop tightening (exerts direct pressure on the conduction system)	? Prophylactic pacemaker
Cardiac tissue injury	Forcible catheter withdrawal without deflated balloon Inadequate balloon inflation	Always deflate the balloon when withdrawing the catheter
Catheter knotting	Repeated catheter manipulation Catheter insertion with deflated balloon Large, dilated right ventricle	Avoid catheter redundancy Use estimates of average insertion lengths when catheterizing a patient without fluoroscopic guidance

bleeding without further consequence. However, large hematomas can occur leading to respiratory compromise, arterial compression, or exsanguination. The more serious sequelae are much more likely to occur if the large bore-introducer has been inserted into the artery. The incidence of this complication has been reported as 0.0995% in one series.[309] Arterial perforation in patients who are, or are subsequently to be, given heparin may result in cancellation of surgical procedures. Another possibility is that atherosclerotic plaques may be dislodged and embolize to the cerebral circulation. Puncture of the subclavian artery may be more insidious. Evidence of bleeding is not readily visible, nor can pressure be easily applied. The first evidence of subclavian artery puncture may be the appearance of a hemothorax on chest radiograph.

Presently, insertion techniques are aimed at increasing the ease of finding the vein and minimizing the risk of arterial injury. Techniques that result in engorgement of the internal jugular and subclavian veins such as use of Trendelenburg's position, coughing, Valsalva's maneuver, or the inspiratory phase of mechanical ventilation all contribute to a successful cannulation. Similarly, the use of a 20-gauge "finder" needle as a preliminary to locating the vein will produce a smaller hole in the event of an inadvertent arterial perforation. Once the vein has been located, this small needle can be left in place to serve as a visual guide for insertion of the larger needle. Unfortunately, arterial puncture can still occur with the second needle, although much less frequently.[310] The technique described by Civetta and Gobel[234] uses a 20-gauge spinal needle as the finder with a 16-gauge over-the-needle catheter threaded on the spinal needle prior to insertion. Schwartz and colleagues[269] have emphasized the importance of transducing the IV catheter or needle before the guidewire is passed. In their series, a number of patients sustained unrecognized carotid artery puncture with passage of an 8F sheath into the artery. In a subsequent group of patients in whom pressures were transduced, no sheaths were inserted in the carotid artery.

Previous arterial puncture often precludes subsequent use of the vein in the same location. Following the development of a hematoma, attempts at cannulation yield blood from the hematoma that cannot be distinguished from that of venipuncture. If arterial puncture occurs and a hematoma develops, we recommend use of another venous access site when feasible. If the carotid artery is entered prior to cardiac surgery, we recommend postponement due to heparinization and possible expansion of the hematoma. This may not be possible in urgent or emergent situations. In these cases, the neck is prepared and draped into the surgical field where the hematoma may be observed. Following heparinization, if the hematoma is enlarging, surgical exploration may be necessary before CPB.

Pneumothorax

Violation of the pleural space during attempts at venous cannulation is a well-recognized complication of both the subclavian and internal jugular vein approaches. The incidence of pneumothorax depends on both operator experience and cannulation site. In patients being mechanically ventilated, a simple pneumothorax may be converted into a tension pneumothorax, resulting in serious respiratory and circulatory compromise. In these patients, the insertion of a chest tube is indicated, with more urgency being demanded for a tension pneumothorax. If a chest tube is not immediately available, needle aspiration of the pleural space will relieve symptoms temporarily. If possible, a chest film should be obtained following PAC insertion, not only to confirm catheter position but to exclude the presence of pneumothorax. However, intraoperatively this is not routinely feasible. Because of differences in solubilities of gases, nitrous oxide will diffuse into any pneumothorax much faster than nitrogen can diffuse out. This can lead to a doubling or tripling of the size of the pneumothorax in a very few minutes, leading to the development of cardiovascular compromise. Clinically, unexplained rises in PCWP and pulmonary artery diastolic pressure (PADP) are the earliest signs of pneumothorax.[311] For this reason, attempts at subclavian cannulation are not advised intraoperatively or preoperatively when chest films cannot be obtained on a regular basis. In addition, hemothorax or hemopneumothorax can occur rarely when the subclavian or low internal jugular approach is used.[101]

Air Embolism

Despite the theoretical likelihood of air embolus occurring with some frequency during venous cannulation (especially through the large-bore introducer), very few reports have appeared in the literature documenting its occurrence.[312-314] Fatal air embolism has been reported to occur through smaller-bore CVCs connected to continuous flush systems.[306] Only three cases of clinically significant embolism have appeared in the literature that were associated with the insertion of a Swan-Ganz catheter.[313-315] Two of these were in conjunction with an introducer that had no provision for a self-sealing valve following removal of the catheter. The third was detected in a study in which Doppler monitors were placed over the right parasternal area specifically to study the occurrence of air embolism.[312] No clinical changes were noted at the time of embolization. Had it not been for the presence of the Doppler monitor, no suspicion of air embolus would have arisen. The utilization of Trendelenburg's position is probably responsible for preventing many air emboli. Nonetheless, air embolus probably occurs more frequently than we are aware of, but insufficient air enters the venous circulation to cause clinical symptoms. A recent report by Moorthy and colleagues[316] illustrates that venous air embolism can also occur during removal of the PAC.

Neurologic Deficit

Nerve injury during percutaneous venous catheterization is rare. Traumatic injury during attempts at venous cutdown has been reported.[317] As a result of trauma to the stellate ganglion, Horner's syndrome has been described during internal jugular catheterization.[318, 319] In a series examining neurologic deficits following open heart surgery, 4.1% of internal jugular vein catheterizations were associated with ipsilateral nerve deficit.[320] One report has emphasized the fact that complications of median sternotomy may also result in a similar neurologic presentation as that observed in venous cannulation.[321, 322] This makes identifying the precise cause of neurologic deficit difficult. However, when a peripheral neurologic deficit is observed, extensive workup is indicated. Both transient and permanent phrenic nerve injury has been reported with internal jugular and subclavian approaches.[322, 323] Brown[303] reported patients in whom an 8F introducer was inserted into the right common carotid artery. Cerebral embolization, rather than prolonged catheterization of the artery, led to a left hemiparesis.[303]

Passage of the Pulmonary Artery Catheter

Arrhythmias

The most common complication during catheter passage is the development of cardiac arrhythmias. Swan and Ganz[323] reported a 13% incidence of transient premature ventricular contractions in their original report. Since then, numerous studies have documented an incidence of isolated premature ventricular contractions ranging from 12% to 48%.[324-327] Those studies reporting the lower incidence relied on visual observation of an oscilloscopic ECG monitor during insertion, while investigators reporting the higher incidence of this complication (46% and 48%) relied on continuous ECG tracings for their data collection. As a result, the true incidence of premature ventricular contractions is probably closer to the latter. Ventricular tachycardia has been noted in as many as 33% of patients.[325] VF has been reported

as well. The incidence of arrhythmias may be related to the time required to float the catheter into the PA.[328] In a study by Lopez-Sendon[51] the presence of a recent right ventricular infarction (RVI) increased the incidence of VF during passage of the PAC (4.2% with RVI vs. 0.28%). In this same study, the incidence of VF was also higher during PAC insertion in patients suffering from AMI (1.07% versus a 0.85% overall rate of VF).

PAC-induced ventricular arrhythmias are most frequently characterized by right bundle branch block (RBBB) morphology and inferior frontal plane axis.[329] In a large series of insertions analyzed for new and complex arrhythmias, 5% of patients sustained a new RBBB.[330] Castellanos et al.[331] theorize that damage to the bundle of His may occur during passage of the PAC through the RV resulting in RBBB. In the majority of patients, this conduction abnormality has no significance. In one patient RBBB was seen only during balloon inflation.[332] However, in patients with preexisting LBBB, complete heart block may result with passage of the catheter through the RV chamber.[333] If catheterization is required for these patients, a pacing electrode should be available. Alternatively, transcutaneous pacing could be used in these situations. Using this approach, should complete heart block develop during insertion, the patient can be transcutaneously paced. A multipurpose (pacing) Swan-Ganz catheter may be placed in this situation. Parenthetically, the RV section of the pacing catheter shaft is stiffer and may actually predispose to RBBB. *Left* fascicular block or LBBB has also been reported with PAC insertion.

Clinically significant arrhythmias, including ventricular tachycardia and asystole, have also been reported on removal of PAC (63% incidence).[334, 335] The mechanism of production of these arrhythmias is the result of mechanical stimulation of the conduction pathways. Theoretically, the design of the catheter balloon prevents the tip of the catheter from contacting the ventricular surface. It was originally believed that this feature would eliminate arrhythmias during insertion. No doubt it has reduced the incidence of serious arrhythmias. Nonetheless, sufficient force is generated when the balloon or free portion of the catheter contacts the ventricular wall to stimulate the conduction system in a high percentage of patients. Production of arrhythmias can be minimized by passing the catheter rapidly once the RV is reached. Lidocaine 1.0 to 1.5 mg/kg IV, has been shown to be effective in reducing the occurrence of ventricular arrhythmias.[336, 337] We use lidocaine when previous catheter passage has resulted in hemodynamically significant arrhythmias. However, Salmenpera et al.[337] have shown that prophylactic use of lidocaine is ineffective.

In addition to the development of arrhythmias, a recent report demonstrates that the PAC may lodge in the coronary sinus during insertion.[318] Resistance to passage from RA to RV in conjunction with an observation of the systemic pressure trace should alert the clinician to this possibility. Similarly, Allyn et al.[338] reported the inadvertent passage of a PAC from the SVC through the LA and LV. Close observation of acute change in the waveform of the PAC should have alerted these authors to a potential change in PAC location.[338] Electrode separation from a multipurpose pacing PAC has been reported. As a result, the manufacturer has made specific recommendations for removal of this type of catheter.

Intracardiac Knotting

Several reports of intracardiac knotting of a PAC have appeared.[339-345] Most knots probably occur during insertion when coiling in the RA or RV can occur.[346] These knots may take the form of free, single, or double knots in the catheter, or more ominously, may incorporate intracardiac structures such as a papillary muscle and chordae tendineae, or the lead from a cardiac pacemaker.[347, 348] Knots may be diagnosed from postinsertion radiographs, or during attempts to remove the catheter, when resistance to withdrawal is felt.[342, 343]

The knot may be withdrawn through the original venotomy site.[349] More often, it becomes necessary to utilize one of a number of fluoroscopic techniques in the cardiac catheter laboratory in which the knot can be either tightened or untied or the catheter cut.[338, 350-352] Many successful nonsurgical techniques for removal of knotted and entrapped PACs have been described.[353, 354] Occasionally operative intervention becomes necessary.

The suspicion of coiling during insertion should be raised whenever an undue length of catheter has been inserted without achieving the expected intracardiac pressure tracing. Normal distances from insertion site to RA, RV, PA, and wedge position are shown in Table 14–3. When these reference points are exceeded by about 10 cm without the tip of the catheter reaching the appropriate location, the balloon should be deflated and the catheter withdrawn to the RA. If resistance is encountered, all attempts at withdrawal should cease and a chest film should be immediately obtained. Another sign suggestive of coiling is the occurrence of ventricular arrhythmias at a time when pressure tracings indicate the tip is still in the RA. Use of TEE to guide PAC placement in difficult cases has been described.[355]

Patients with a transvenous pacemaker in place who also require PA monitoring are at risk of having the catheter become entwined around the pacing leads. Insertion of a PAC in such a patient should be performed under fluoroscopy. Venous cannula obstruction by the PAC during CPB has been described.[356]

Isolated complications occurring during PAC insertion include torn chordae tendineae, probably caused by multiple attempts at insertion and withdrawal of the catheter while the balloon was still inflated.[357] Aberrant catheter locations have been reported, including the pleural space, the peritoneal cavity, the renal vein, the aorta, and the vertebral artery.[358] Most, if not all, of these complications probably could have been prevented by strict adherence to the previously described insertion techniques (see Table 14–2). Severe pulmonary hypertension secondary to embolization of a PAC fragment into the right PA has been described, which resolved with migration of the fragment to the lung periphery.[359]

The Catheter In Situ

Pulmonary Artery Perforation

Unquestionably, the most catastrophic complication resulting from PAC insertion is PA perforation and subsequent hemorrhage.[21, 360-380] Reports of this complication were rare for the first 10 years following introduction of the PAC (numbering only five). Since that time it has become much more commonly reported, and there are now more than 50 reported cases in the English-language literature.

The incidence of this complication varies between 0.03% and 0.2%.[381, 382] The latter study involved 32,442 patients and yielded an observed rate of 0.031% of PAC insertions. Risk factors include age greater than 60 years, PA hypertension, anticoagulant therapy, hypothermia, female sex, and manipulation of the heart by the surgeon.[380, 381] In one study 69% of patients were female and 50% had valvular heart disease.[383]

The right PA was injured in 93% of cases. Several significant risk factors for the development of PAC perforation have been identified. Advanced age, hypothermia, and pulmonary hypertension place the patient at greater risk for perforation.[380, 381] Furthermore, as noted, females have a higher incidence of perforation. Of 24 patients who had a PA perforation and in whom PA pressures were reported, 22 had pulmonary hypertension. In addition, deviations from standard insertion techniques have been noted in at least 10 of 56 reported cases as well.[380, 384-389]

The presenting sign of PA perforation in most cases is the sudden appearance of hemoptysis. Characteristically the blood is bright red and may vary in amount from less than 5 mL to massive bleeding.[368, 369] Usually this episode of bleeding is related to balloon inflation or catheter manipulation. However, hemoptysis may also be caused by flushing the catheter in the wedge position.[375] Acute pulmonary hypertension after wedging of a PAC may be a clue to PA perforation.[390] Use of an external balloon can limit balloon pressures within the PA and identify when excessive volumes are being forced into the PA balloon.[391]

Treatment of PAC perforation is largely supportive. If bleeding is massive, the patient must be intubated. If a double-lumen endotracheal tube is not available, an ordinary single-lumen endotracheal tube should be advanced into the mainstem bronchus of the noninvolved lung, usually the left. If the patient has received heparin, it should be reversed if possible. Massive blood and fluid replacement may be necessary, as well as operative intervention. The mortality rate is 70% in patients with hemothorax, and urgent thoracotomy is essential to survival in this setting.[382, 383] Conservative management strategies are associated with a high incidence of secondary, often fatal, hemorrhage. PEEP has been used, as well, in an attempt to compress the bleeding site.[392-394] PA perforation has been described as a complication following CPB. Rice et al.[395] reported a patient who sustained a PA perforation following CPB. In this situation, reversal of heparinization with protamine resulted in a resolution of the hemorrhage.

Controversy exists about what to do with the PAC once a PA perforation is suspected (i.e., do you have the balloon up, put more air in the balloon, or take the PAC out?). Barash et al.,[23] commenting on the early reports of PA perforation, suggested that pulling the PAC back with the balloon down about 5 to 10 cm was appropriate. The authors suggested that by doing this one could then inject some contrast media into the PAC to radiographically identify the precise location of the PA perforation. This could then be used to guide surgical interventions (i.e., wedge resection vs. pneumonectomy) if necessary.[21] Resnick et al.[396] recently reported on the ability of angiography to aid in the diagnosis and localization of PA perforation.

The common feature of PA perforation in most patients is distal location of the tip of the PAC (although it has been reported with a more central location as well)[397, 398] (Fig. 14–9). When the tip is located too far distal, balloon inflation can distend the vessel wall, subjecting it to large transmural pressures.[19] Distal catheter placement can occur as a result of failure to follow currently accepted insertion techniques or in the presence of pulmonary hypertension. The most frequently observed technical error is the use of less than 1.5 mL of air to inflate the balloon during PAC insertion. This allows the tip of the catheter to pass into smaller, more distal vessels. Subsequent balloon inflation with the full 1.5 mL will then overdistend the vessel, increasing the risk of PA perforation. The original descriptions of the PA insertion technique of PA perforation by Swan and Ganz and colleagues suggested advancing the tip of the catheter

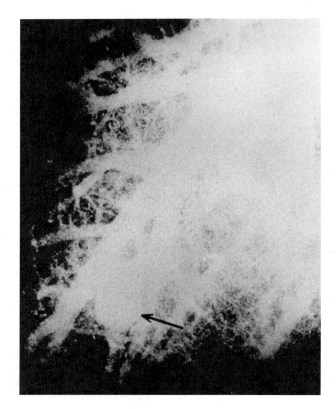

Figure 14-9. Postmortem barium gel studies showing extravasation of gel at the site of pulmonary artery perforation. The distal migration of the catheter presumably occurred with cardiac manipulation during cardiopulmonary bypass. (From Ikeda S, Yagi K, Schweiss JF, et al: In vitro reappraisal of the pulmonary artery catheter balloon volume-pressure relationship: Comparison of four different catheters. Can J Anaesth 1991; 38:648-653.)

1 to 3 cm with the balloon deflated after the initial wedge pressure was obtained.[1, 3, 4] However, this can also lead to distal placement.[399]

Pulmonary hypertension may lead to distal placement by distending smaller pulmonary arteries, thus allowing the catheter to wedge in a more distal location. PA hypertension can also lead to degenerative changes in the vessel wall such as sclerosis and aneurysmal dilation, which may further predispose the vessel to rupture. A case of PA perforation has

been reported secondary to pneumothorax, which caused mediastinal shift to the right, elevated PA pressures, and distal migration of the PAC.[400] RV perforation by a PAC during coronary artery bypass surgery has been described.[401]

The fact that the catheter tip is in a distal location may be identified by the phenomenon of *overwedging* (Fig. 14-10). Overwedging results from impingement of the tip of the catheter against the vessel wall or herniation of the balloon over the catheter tip.[23] The continuously rising pressure trace seen with this phenomenon results from the high-pressure flush system. Therefore, if overwedging is observed, the catheter should be withdrawn until a normal wedge tracing is obtained.

Several mechanisms that may be responsible for PA perforation have been described (Fig. 14-11). Inflation of the balloon with a distally located catheter tip can lead to direct tearing of the vessel. Eccentric balloon inflation, as demonstrated by several investigators, can expose the catheter tip and can actually propel it through the arterial wall.[399] This mechanism can be aggravated by the gradient existing with pulmonary hypertension.[23] The tip of the catheter may become lodged in a small vascular branch and may erode or perforate directly. Direct perforation may also occur during insertion. Migration of the catheter tip to more distal location during cardiac surgery has also been postulated as a potential mechanism.[402]

One safeguard that can clearly reduce the potential of PA perforation is to minimize the number of balloon inflations. In view of the fact that PADP agrees very well with PCWP (in the absence of pulmonary hypertension), we recommend that the PADP be used, whenever possible, as an indirect measurement of LAP.[23] If this is done the tip of the catheter can be left in a very proximal location, 4 to 5 cm beyond the pulmonic valve. If a true wedge pressure is required, the catheter can be floated into position through an external sheath which protects the catheter. Farber et al.[365] reported a patient who not only had PA perforation but also pneumothorax upon removal of the PAC. Culpepper and colleagues[361] also reported a patient who had massive hemoptysis and tension pneumothorax following insertion of a fiberoptic PAC. They hypothesized that perforation of a small artery and visceral pleura occurred following persistent wedging of the catheter. Since these early reports, several authors have demonstrated that the development of hemoptysis in patients with PAC in place should alert the clinician to the possibility of PA perforation.[360, 393] These authors also suggest that patients who survive the PA rupture (mortality rate of 40% to 70%) should undergo further studies

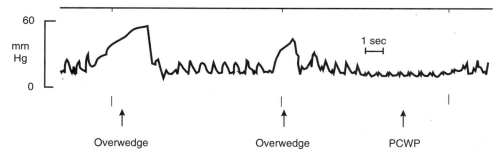

Figure 14-10. Intraoperative pulmonary artery pressure tracing demonstrating overwedging patterns observed with balloon inflation. This pattern results from the catheter tip impinging against the vessel wall, or balloon herniation over the catheter tip. The pulmonary artery catheter is withdrawn 3 cm and a normal transition from pulmonary artery to pulmonary capillary wedge pressure is obtained. (From Ikeda S, Yagi K, Schweiss JF, et al: In vitro reappraisal of the pulmonary artery catheter balloon volume-pressure relationship: Comparison of four different catheters. Can J Anaesth 1991; 38:648-653.)

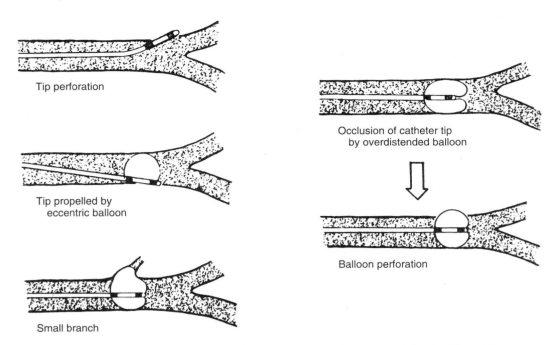

Figure 14–11. Possible mechanisms of pulmonary artery perforation. (From Ikeda S, Yagi K, Schweiss JF, et al: In vitro reappraisal of the pulmonary artery catheter balloon volume-pressure relationship: Comparison of four different catheters. Can J Anaesth 1991; 38:648–653.)

aimed at diagnosing a possible catheter-induced pseudoaneurysm.[310, 379] If such a pseudoaneurysm is found, it must be obliterated to prevent further bleeding.[403] Recently, immediate transcatheter steel coil embolization of a PAC-induced PA pseudoaneurysm has been described.[404–407] In a recent series, seven false aneurysms of the PA were diagnosed in five patients (four women, one man) age 67 to 81. All five patients underwent PAC placement to monitor cardiac surgery.[406]

Pulmonary Infarction

Early reports indicated that pulmonary infarction also resulted from distal placement of the catheter.[367, 408, 409] The mechanism responsible for distal placement has been described in the previous section. The sequelae of PA infarction may include deep venous thrombosis (DVT) with embolization, endothelial damage, or permanent wedging of the catheter tip in a distal PA. Clinical states characterized by low cardiac output may further predispose to this complication. Usually the diagnosis of pulmonary infarction is made by chest film.

As with PA perforation, prevention is directed at avoiding distal placement of the catheter, avoiding persistent balloon inflation, and use of a continuous high-pressure flush system with heparinized saline.

Thrombosis and Coagulopathies

Several studies have documented the fact that PACs are thrombogenic. Substantial thrombi (several hundred milligrams) will form on virtually 100% of catheters in vivo within 1 to 2 hours of insertion.[268, 317, 410–412] These thrombi are capable of causing both damped pressure tracings and yielding inaccurately low cardiac output measurements.

Connors et al.[270, 363] performed detailed postmortem examination on 32 consecutive patients brought to autopsy with a PAC in place. Thrombosis or hemorrhage related to

PAC was found in 29 (91%) patients.[270, 363] The incidence of thrombosis was higher after 36 hours of catheterization.

In addition, massive thromboses of the subclavian vein[317] and the SVC[413] have been reported. Devitt et al.[397] reported a case in which catheter thrombus was apparently stripped off the PAC during removal and embolized across a VSD to the cerebral and coronary circulations.

One hypothesis for the occurrence of pulmonary infarction or emboli is the development of thrombus on the catheter body. Although no report has directly shown embolization from such thrombi, much circumstantial evidence exists.[408, 412–414] In addition to the potential damage to the pulmonary parenchyma, Devitt et al. reported embolization across a VSD, the origin of which was thought to be from the PAC.[397] Early reports by Brunswick and Gionis[415] stated that starch crystals were seen on microscopic examination of the PAC clot. As a result, starch has been abolished in the subsequent manufacture of PACs. In an attempt to reduce thrombotic complications, heparin bonding of the catheters is now routine. Heparin bonding prevents thrombosis in a canine model and in humans.[411] A meta-analysis of randomized controlled trials has shown that heparin administration effectively reduces thrombus formation and may reduce PAC-related infection.[416] However, at present, no published study shows a lower morbidity when heparin-bonded catheters are inserted and one study suggested that the failure rate of PACs was not increased by the use of nonheparinized solutions, unlike arterial catheters.[417] Comparisons of cost-effectiveness of unfractionated heparin, low-molecular-weight heparin, and warfarin are also needed.[416] One study demonstrated an association between 8.5F femoral vein catheters and an increased incidence of DVT and the authors concluded that this technique should not be routine.[418] In addition, thrombosis has also been reported at insertion sites, such as the internal jugular vein.[419]

At the other end of the spectrum is the possibility of coagulopathies in patients with a PAC. Kim et al.[420] originally presented data to show thrombocytopenia related to PAC in a canine model. Richman et al.[421] confirmed these data in humans. Although platelet counts were decreased, no patient sustained a bleeding episode on this basis.

Infection

Septic complications of PACs have been documented by many investigators.[422-426] While evaluating these studies, it is important to remember that patients with PAC have other sources of infection present, for example, urinary catheters, IV catheters, and so on.[423, 424] While their occurrence is clearly demonstrated, the incidence and significance of these complications is less well known. It is difficult to separate colonization, contamination, and infection in published studies. Fortunately, reports of serious sequelae of positive catheter cultures are rare. The fortuitous surface antimicrobial activity of heparin-bonded catheters may account for the low incidence of catheter-related bacteremia (mean, 1.0%) compared with PACs of the same materials but not coated with benzalkonium-heparin (mean, 2.8%).[427] Elliott et al.[380] have provided a useful classification for the study of catheter sepsis. They defined *colonization* as a positive culture of the catheter tip without evidence of local or systemic infection. *Contamination* is defined as one of multiple blood cultures yielding a typical nonpathogen and culture of the catheter tip failing to grow any organisms. *Infection* can be (1) definite—positive blood and catheter cultures yielding the same organism; (2) probable—the same organism cultured from blood and catheter with no other probable source of infection; or (3) unrelated—if the same organism had been previously recovered from another source.

The reported incidence of catheter-related sepsis varies widely from 2% to 35%.[36, 383] Earlier reports disagreed on the impact of the duration of catheterization on rates of infection. The skin insertion wound is the major source of catheter contamination.[428] Sensitivity in diagnosis of PAC colonization can be improved by evaluating both the tip and intradermal segments.[429, 430] In the presence of an indwelling introducer the introducer tip should be used. Studies by Mermel et al.[101] and Raad et al.[431] have provided new evidence for the role of duration of placement as a predictor of PAC-related infections. Mermel et al. demonstrated an overall rate of local infection of 22% (65 of 297 catheters).[101] The authors further subdivided these PAC-related infections into those which occurred as a result of local infection of the introducer (58/297) or the intravascular portion of the PAC catheter (20/297); only two catheters (0.7%) caused bacteremia. Eighty percent of infected catheters (the introducer or the PAC itself) showed concordance with organisms cultured from skin of the insertion site. Of these, 17% were the result of a contaminated hub and 18% were organisms contaminating the extravascular portion of the catheter beneath the sleeve. The following were identified as increasing the relative risk (RR) of PA infection: (1) cutaneous colonization of the insertion site with more than 100 CFU (RR 5.5, $P < .001$), (2) insertion into an internal jugular vein (RR 4.3, $P < .001$), and (3) insertion in the OR using less stringent barrier precautions (RR 2.1, $P = .03$). Similarly, Raad et al.[431] found that 17% (12/71) of PACs in their study produced local infection and 5.6% (4/71) led to septicemia. These episodes of septicemia were directly related to the duration of PAC placement. Catheter-related septicemia occurred at rates of 2% and 16%, before and after 7 days of catheter placement, respectively. Further analysis of their data (life table analysis) showed that the cumulative risk of developing a catheter infection increased from 9% to 18% after *4 days* of placement of the PAC.[412] As a result of the data from these studies we recommend that the PAC be changed to a new site every 4 to 7 days. It is recommended that the use of a

guidewire technique for catheter replacement (PAC to CVC) is a safe alternative to de novo insertion of a CVC within 48 hours after initial insertion of the PAC.[432]

Recently, the use of sterile sleeves has been advocated for repositioning the PAC in a sterile fashion.[433-435] However, the precise benefit of these devices in substantially reducing PAC infections remains to be elucidated. A recent randomized study using a PAC that is completely shielded during balloon testing, preparation, and insertion (Arrow Hands-Off thermodilution catheter) has demonstrated a reduced incidence of systemic infections associated with prolonged PA catheterization.[436]

Not only are localized and systemic infections of concern but PACs may also be associated with an increased incidence of cardiac valve injury and endocarditis. Smith and coworkers reported ruptured chordae tendineae of the tricuspid valve as a result of withdrawing the PAC with the balloon inflated.[437, 438] Isolated case reports of erosion of the pulmonic[347, 439] and tricuspid valves[348] were followed by several series documenting an increased incidence of aseptic endocarditis. In a retrospective analysis Pace and Horton[440] noted three cases of aseptic endocarditis in 88 catheterized patients compared with 1 in 205 uncatheterized patients. Greene and Cummings[410] found four cases in 24 autopsies. An additional four cases occurred in the 270 noncatheterized patients. Subsequently, Greene et al.[441] reported that 1 in 493 patients dying prior to introduction of the PAC developed septic endocarditis, whereas 10 of 483 patients with PAC developed this condition. Routine PAC hemodynamic monitoring is not associated with an increased rate of prosthetic aortic graft infection.[442]

Ehrie et al.[443] noted that all six burn patients studied developed endocarditis and Sasaki et al.[444] documented a statistically significant increase in the incidence of this complication in 1105 burn patients following introduction of the PAC. In contrast, Katz et al.[199] were unable to find evidence of valvular damage.

Limitations

In addition to the complications associated with invasive monitoring, a major limitation of PACs is the assumption that intracardiac pressure measurements (PCWP) are a good approximation of the volume status of the ventricle. Preload can be clinically defined as being equal to end-diastolic volume. The use of PCWP to directly or indirectly assess preload assumes a linear relationship between ventricular end-diastolic volume and ventricular end-diastolic pressure. However, alterations in ventricular compliance can affect this pressure-volume relationship. Hansen et al.[445] demonstrated this poor correlation between PAP and LVEDV following CABG surgery. In this study, LVEDV was determined using concomitant determinations of ejection fraction, gated blood pool scintigraphy, and stroke volume (determined from TD cardiac output). The authors postulated that an altered ventricular pressure-volume relationship may reflect acute changes in ventricular complication in the first few hours following bypass surgery. Reductions in ventricular compliance (upward shift to the left) can be seen with myocardial ischemia, shock, RV overload, and pericardial effusion. Ventricular compliance is increased with vasodilators such as nitroglycerin and sodium nitroprusside.

Calvin et al.[446] made simultaneous pressure and volume measurements using radionuclear angiography in patients with sepsis and in another group with acute cardiac illnesses. They found no relationship between LVEDV and PCWP in either group ($r = .58$). The correlation decreased further when PEEP was employed ($r = .30$).[334] Beaupre et al.,[99] using 2-D echocardiography, reported similar findings in a group of anesthetized patients. They concluded that using PCWP as a guide to fluid therapy may be misleading.[99] This was further emphasized by Marmana and colleagues,[31] who examined the relationship of PCWP and LAP in patients undergoing coronary artery bypass surgery. In this study, PCWP was a poor predictor of LAP in the early postoperative period. They hypothesized that pulmonary venoconstriction resulting from increased pulmonary extravascular water (due to hemodilution of CPB) accounted for the difference between LAP and PCWP.[31]

Ellis and colleagues,[447] also using intraoperative radionuclear monitoring (gated pool), found alterations in ventricular diastolic and systolic performance that were not appreciated on routine hemodynamic monitoring. In patients with an LVEF less than 50% undergoing coronary artery bypass, a decreased ventricular compliance suggested that this group of patients required closer observation and increased cardiovascular support in the postbypass period. On the basis of additional radionuclear data showing a decline in LVEF from 70% to 49%, they also concluded that volume loading following CPB may be detrimental.

Significant diagnostic errors may result when PCWP is assumed to be directly related to LVEDV. For example, an elevated PCWP and a decreased cardiac output can be interpreted as LV failure. However, these hemodynamic findings may also reflect *ventricular interdependence*.[27] Ventricular interdependence occurs when the interventricular septum encroaches on the LV cavity. This can occur in acute respiratory failure, with high levels of PEEP, and so forth.[448, 449] The differential is made on the basis of knowledge of LVEDV. LVEDV is increased in LV failure, while it is decreased when ventricular interdependence is present (Table 14–9).

Future Directions

Noninvasive assessment of cardiovascular function by perioperative 2-D TEE offers the anesthesiologist monitoring techniques that overcome these limitations. These techniques will assume greater importance for the clinician in terms of patient care, research, and education. The potential appeal of these methods is a more precise physiologic definition of the patient's cardiac reserve without the risks associated with invasive tests. Just as invasive monitoring with the Swan-Ganz catheter has raised our awareness of cardiovascular physiology, these noninvasive procedures offer a unique method of supplementing our knowledge of the cardiovascular system. A satisfactory echocardiographic technique to monitor cardiac output has been difficult to develop.[424] PAC bolus TD remains the gold standard used for assessment of dual oximetry with carbon dioxide production (VCO_2) and oxygen consumption (VO_2) measured by a new metabolic monitor.[450]

Clinically, 2-D TEE is frequently being utilized in combination with the PAC. This combination provides the most sen-

sitive and specific methods for cardiac monitoring. In a 1990, Rafferty[145] highlighted the ability of the PAC and TEE to complement each other in the management of critically ill patients. In another study, there was complete agreement between PAC and TEE data in 36 (86%) of 42 patients in the diagnosis of illness of cardiac vs. noncardiac etiology.[451] The time taken from admission for PAC placement was 63 ± 45 minutes vs. 19 ± 7 minutes for TEE, which is clinically significant in the ITU setting.

PA catheterization has transformed the care of critically ill patients. It permits the direct measurement of vital hemodynamic and respiratory variables and permits rational application of therapeutic modalities. The existence of significant complications, however, mandates care in patient selection and in insertion and maintenance of the catheter. The age-old question of risk-benefit and the debate regarding the appropriate indications for PAC monitoring continue. The debate has been fueled by recent studies already alluded to. However, although precise data are lacking, all of us who rely on the information obtained from the PAC are convinced that it will continue to be an important tool in the management of the critically ill patient. It should not be forgotten that it is a tool only and that the ultimate monitoring system remains the clinician.

REFERENCES

1. Ganz W, Donoso R, Marcus HS, et al: A new technique for measurement of cardiac output by thermodilution in man. Am J Cardiol 1971; 27:392.
2. Lategola M, Rahn H: A self-guiding catheter for cardiac and pulmonary arterial catheterization and occlusion. Proc Soc Exp Biol Med 1953; 84:667.
3. Swan HJ: The role of hemodynamic monitoring in the management of the critically ill. Crit Care Med 1975; 75:83.
4. Swan HJC, Ganz W, Forrester J, et al: Catheterization of the heart in man with use of a flow-directed balloon-tipped catheter. N Engl J Med 1970; 283:447.
5. Applefeld JJ, Caruthers TE, Reno DJ, et al: Assessment of the sterility of long-term cardiac catheterization using thermodilution Swan-Ganz catheter. Chest 1978; 74:377.
6. Beique F, Ramsay J: The pulmonary artery catheter: A new look. Semin Anesth 1993; 2:315.
7. Berryhill RE, Benumof JL: PEEP-induced discrepancy between pulmonary arterial wedge pressure and left atrial pressure: The effects of controlled vs. spontaneous ventilation and compliant vs. noncompliant lungs in the dog. Anesthesiology 1979; 51:303–308.
8. Chun GM, Ellestad MH: Perforation of the pulmonary artery by a Swan-Ganz catheter. N Engl J Med 1971; 284:1041.
9. Keefer JR, Barash PG: Pulmonary artery catheterization: A decade of clinical progress? (editorial). Chest 1983; 84:241.
10. Lopez-Sendon J, Coma-Canella I, Gamallo C: Sensitivity and specificity of hemodynamic criteria in the diagnosis of acute right ventricular infarction. Circulation 1981; 64:515.
11. Nehme AE: Swan-Ganz catheter: Comparison of insertion techniques. Arch Surg 1980; 115:1194.
12. Page DW, Teres D, Hartshorn JW: Fatal hemorrhage from Swan-Ganz catheter (letter). N Engl J Med 1974; 291:260.
13. Tarhan S, Moffitt EA, Taylor WF, et al: Myocardial infarction after general anesthesia. JAMA 1972; 220:1451–1454.
14. Zion MM, Balkin J, Rosenmann D, et al: Use of pulmonary artery catheters in patients in the SPRINT Registry. Chest 1990; 98:1331–1335.
15. Swan-Ganz Flow Directed Thermodilution Catheters. American Edwards Laboratories. Product Information Bulletin 093-4/82.
16. Parlow JL, Milne B, Cervenko FW: Balloon flotation is more important than flow direction in determining the position of flow-directed pulmonary artery catheters. J Cardiothorac Vasc Anesth 1992; 6:20–33.
17. Eisenkraft JB, Eger EI: Nitrous oxide and Swan-Ganz catheters (letter). Anesth Analg 1982; 61:308.

Table 14–9. Hemodynamic Findings in Left Ventricular Failure and Ventricular Interdependence

	PCWP	Cardiac Output	LVEDV
Left ventricular failure	↑	↓	↑
Ventricular interdependence	↑	↓	↓

PCWP, pulmonary capillary wedge pressure; LVEDV; left ventricular end-diastolic volume.

18. Kaplan R, Abramowitz MD, Epstein BS: Nitrous oxide and air filled balloon-tipped catheters. Anesthesiology 1981; 55:71.

19. Hardy JF, Taillefer J: Inflating characteristics of Swan-Ganz catheter balloons: Clinical considerations. Anesth Analg 1983; 62: 363.

20. Hart U, Ward DR, Gillilian R, et al: Fatal pulmonary hemorrhage complicating Swan-Ganz catheterization. Surgery 1982; 91:24.

21. Basson MD: Hazards of pulmonary-artery catheterization (letter). N Engl J Med 1980; 302:807.

22. Ikeda S, Yagi K, Schweiss JF, et al: In vitro reappraisal of the pulmonary artery catheter balloon volume-pressure relationship: Comparison of four different catheters. Can J Anaesth 1991; 38: 648-653.

23. Barash PG, Nardi D, Hammond G, et al: Catheter-induced pulmonary artery perforation. Mechanisms, management, and modifications. J Thorac Cardiovasc Surg 1981; 82:5.

24. Goldhaber S: Pulmonary embolism thrombolysis. A clarion call for International Collaboration. J Am Cell Cardiol 1992; 2:246-247.

25. Woods M, Scott RN, Harken AH: Practical considerations for the use of a pulmonary artery thermistor catheter. Surgery 1976; 79:469.

26. Hobelmann CF Jr, Smith DE, Vergilio RW, et al: Left atrial and pulmonary artery wedge pressure difference with positive end-expiratory pressure. Surg Forum 1974; 25:232.

27. Jardin F, Farcot JC, Boisante L, et al: Influence of positive end-expiratory pressure on left ventricular performance. N Engl J Med 1981; 304:387.

28. Kane PB, Askanazi J, Neville JF Jr, et al: Artifacts in the measurement of pulmonary artery wedge pressure. Crit Care Med 1978; 6:36.

29. Manjuran RS, Agarwal JB, Roy SB: Relationship of pulmonary artery diastolic and pulmonary artery wedge pressures in mitral stenosis. Am Heart J 1975; 89:207.

30. Moser KM, Spragg RG: Use of the balloon-tipped pulmonary artery catheter in pulmonary disease. Ann Intern Med 1983; 98: 53.

31. Marmana RB, Hiro S, Levitsky S, et al: Inaccuracy of pulmonary capillary wedge pressure when compared to left atrial pressure in the early post surgical period. J Thorac Cardiovasc Surg 1982; 84:420.

32. Rotman M, Chen JTT, Senngen RP, et al: Pulmonary arterial diastolic pressure in acute myocardial infarction. Am J Cardiol 1974; 33:362.

33. Robotham JL, Rabson J, Permutt S, et al: Left ventricular hemodynamics during respiration. J Appl Physiol 1979; 47:1295.

34. Robotham JL, Lixfeld W, Holland L, et al: The effects of positive end-expiratory pressure on right and left ventricular performance. Am Rev Respir Dis 1980; 121:677.

35. Pichard AD, Diaz R, Marchant E, et al: Large v waves in the pulmonary capillary wedge pressure tracing without mitral regurgitation: The influence of the pressure/volume relationship on the v wave size. Clin Cardiol 1983; 6:534-541.

36. Boyd KD, Thomas SJ, Gold J, et al: A prospective study of complications of pulmonary artery catheterizations in 500 consecutive patients. Chest 1983; 84:245.

37. Bouchard RJ, Gault JH, Ross J Jr: Evaluation of pulmonary arterial end-diastolic pressure as an estimate of left ventricular end-diastolic pressure in patients with normal and abnormal left ventricular performance. Circulation 1971; 44:1072.

38. Braunwald E: On the difference between the heart's output and its contractile state. Circulation 1971; 43:171.

39. Shah DM, Browner BD, Dutton RE, et al: Cardiac output and pulmonary wedge pressure. Arch Surg 1977; 112:1161.

40. Sidulka A, Hakim TS: Wedge pressure in large vs. small pulmonary arteries to detect pulmonary venoconstriction. J Appl Physiol 1985; 59:1329-1332.

41. Shapiro HM, Smith G, Murray JA, et al: Errors in sampling pulmonary arterial blood with a Swan-Ganz catheter. Anesthesiology 1974; 40:291.

42. Morris AH, Chapman RH: Wedge pressure confirmation by aspiration of pulmonary capillary blood. Crit Care Med 1985; 13: 756-759.

43. Shasby DM, Dauber IM, Pfister S, et al: Swan-Ganz catheter location and left atrial pressure determine the accuracy of the wedge pressure when positive end-expiratory pressure is used. Chest 1981; 80:666.

44. Teboul JL, Besbes M, Andrivet P, et al: A bedside index assessing the reliability of pulmonary artery occlusion pressure measurements during ventilation with positive end expiratory pressure. J Crit Care 1992; 7:22-29.

45. Weisman IM, Rinaldo JE, Rogers RM: Positive end expiratory pressures in adult respiratory failure. N Engl J Med 1982; 307: 1381-1384.

46. Eisenberg PR, Jaffe AS, Schuster DP: Clinical evaluation compared to pulmonary artery catheterization in the hemodynamic assessment of critically ill patients. Crit Care Med 1984; 12: 549-553.

47. Dizon CT, Barash PG: The value of monitoring pulmonary artery pressure in clinical practice. Conn Med 1977; 41:622.

48. Forrester JS, Diamond G, McHugh TJ, et al: Filling pressures in the right and left sides of the heart in acute myocardial infarction. N Engl J Med 1971; 285:190.

49. Field J, Shiroff RA, Zelis RF, et al: Limitations in the use of the pulmonary capillary wedge pressure. Chest 1976; 70:451.

50. Levine HJ, Gaasch WH: Diastolic compliance of the left ventricle. I: Causes of a noncompliant ventricle. Mod Concepts Cardiovasc Dis 1978; 42:95.

51. Lopez-Sendon J, Lopez de Sa E, Gonzales Maqueda I, et al: Right ventricular infarction as a risk factor for ventricular fibrillation during pulmonary artery catheterization using Swan-Ganz catheters. Am Heart J 1990; 119:207-209.

52. Hines R, Rafferty T: Right ventricle: Toy or tool? Pro: A useful monitor. J Cardiothorac Vasc Anesth 1993; 7:236-240.

53. Spinale FG, Smith AC, Carabello BA, et al: Right ventricular function computed by thermodilution and ventriculography. J Thorac Cardiovasc Surg 1990; 99:141-152.

54. Hines R, Barash PG: Intraoperative right ventricular dysfunction detected with a right ventricular ejection fraction catheter. J Clin Monit Comput 1986; 2:206-208.

55. Armengol J, Man GC, Balsys AJ, et al: Effects of the respiratory cycle on cardiac output measurements: Reproducibility of data enhanced by timing the thermodilution injections in dogs. Crit Care Med 1981; 9:852.

56. Bromberger-Barnea B: Mechanical effects of inspiration on heart functions: A review. Fed Proc 1981; 40:2172.

57. Kay H, Afshari M, Barash P, et al: Measurement of ejection fraction by thermal dilution techniques. J Surg Rev 1983; 34: 337.

58. Cengiz M, Crapo RO, Gardner RM: The effect of ventilation on the accuracy of pulmonary artery and wedge pressure measurements. Crit Care Med 1983; 11:502.

59. Gamra H, Zhang HP, Clugston RA, et al: Thermodilution left-sided cardiac output for valve area determination after balloon mitral valvotomy. Am Heart J 1994; 128:934-400.

60. Andreen M: Computerized measurement of cardiac output by thermodilution: Methodological aspects. Acta Anaesthesiol Scand 1974; 18:297.

61. Kohanna FH, Cunningham JN Jr, Catinella, FP, et al: Cardiac output determination after cardiac operation. J Thorac Cardiovasc Surg 1981; 82:904.

62. Kressin N, Laravuso RB: Hemodynamic measurements in patients for coronary artery surgery: Cath lab vs. operating room (abstract). Anesthesiology 1983; 59:A6.

63. Shoemaker WC: The efficacy of central venous and pulmonary artery catheters and therapy based upon them in reducing mortality and morbidity. Arch Surg 1990; 125:1332-1338.

64. Shaver JA: Hemodynamic monitoring in the critically ill. N Engl J Med 1983; 308:277.

65. Shrader LL, McMillen MA, Watson CB, et al: Is routine preoperative hemodynamic evaluation of nonagenarians necessary? J Am Geriatr Soc 1991; 39:1-5.

66. Starr N, Estafanous FG, Goormastic M, et al: Operating room monitoring in adult open heart surgery: Results of a national survey (abstract). Anesthesiology 1982; 57:A157.

67. Del Guercio LRM, Cohn JD: Monitoring operative risk in the elderly. JAMA 1980; 243:1350.

68. Iberti TJ, Fisher CJ: A prospective study on the use of the pulmonary artery catheter in a medical intensive care unit — its effect on diagnosis and therapy. Crit Care Med 1983; 11:238.

69. Waller JL, Zaiden JR, Kaplan JA, et al: Hemodynamic responses to vascular cannulations before coronary bypass surgery. Anesth Analg 1980; 59:563.

70. Fegler G: Measurement of cardiac output in anaesthetized animals by a thermodilution method. Q J Exp Physiol 1954; 53: 153.

71. Forrester JS, Ganz W, Diamong G, et al: Thermodilution cardiac output determination with a single flow-directed catheter. Am Heart J 1972; 83:306.

72. Ganz W, Swan HJC: Measurement of blood flow by thermodilution. Am J Cardiol 1972; 29:241.

73. Bing R, Heimbecker R, Falholt W: An estimation of the residual volume of blood in the right ventricle and diseased hearts in vivo. Am Heart J 1951; 42:483–502.

74. Bilfinger TV, Lin CY, Anagnostopoulos CE: In vitro determination of accuracy of cardiac output measurements by thermal dilution. J Surg Res 1983; 33:409.

75. Branthwaite MA, Bradley RD: Measurement of cardiac output by thermal dilution in man. J Appl Physiol 1968; 24:434.

76. Fischer AP, Benis AM, Jurado RA, et al: Analysis of errors in measurement of cardiac output by simultaneous dye and thermal dilution in cardiothoracic surgical patients. Cardiovasc Res 1978; 12:190.

77. Hendriks FF, Schipperheyn JJ, Quanjer PH: Thermal dilution measurement of cardiac output in dogs using an analog computer. Basic Res Cardiol 1978; 73:459.

78. Hoel BL: Some aspects of the clinical use of thermodilution in measuring cardiac output. Scand J Clin Lab Invest 1978; 38: 383.

79. Jansen JR, Schreuder JJ, Bogaard, JM, et al: Thermodilution techniques for measurement of cardiac output during artificial ventilation. J Appl Physiol 1981; 51:584.

80. Merjavy JP, Hahn JW, Barner HB: Comparison of thermodilution cardiac output and electromagnetic flowmeter. Surg Forum 1974; 25:145.

81. Nelson LD, Houtchens BA: Automatic vs manual injections for thermodilution cardiac output determinations. Crit Care Med 1982; 10:190.

82. Olsson SB, Wassen R, Varnauskas E, et al: A simple analogue computer for cardiac output determination by thermodilution. Cardiovasc Res 1972; 6:303.

83. Olsson B, Pool J, Vandermoten P, et al: Validity and reproducibility of determination of cardiac output by thermodilution in man. Cardiology 1970; 55:136.

84. Sottile FD, Durbin CG, Hoyt JW, et al: Evaluation of pulmonary artery oximetry as a predictor of cardiac output (abstract). Anesthesiology 1982; 57:A127.

85. Espersen K, Jensen EW, Rosenborg D, et al: Comparison of cardiac output measurement techniques: Thermodilution, Doppler, CO$_2$-rebreathing and the direct Fick method. Acta Anaesthesiol Scand 1995; 39:245–511.

86. Maruschak GF, Potter AM, Schauble, JF, et al: Overestimation of pediatric cardiac output by thermal indicator loss. Circulation 1982; 65:380.

87. Mattea EJ, Paruta AN, Worthen LR: Sterility of prefilled syringes for thermal dilution cardiac output measurements (letter). Am J Hosp Pharm 1979; 36:1156.

88. Nelson LD, Anderson HB: Patient selection for iced versus room temperature injectate for thermodilution cardiac output determinations. Crit Care Med 1985; 13:182–184.

89. Nishikawa T, Dohi S: Slowing of heart rate during cardiac output measurement by thermodilution. Anesthesiology 1982; 57:538.

90. Griffin K, Benjamin E, DelGiudice R, et al: Thermodilution cardiac output measurement during simultaneous volume infusion through the venous infusion port of the pulmonary artery catheter. J Cardiothorac Vasc Anesth 1997; 11:437–499.

91. Runciman WB, Ilsley AH, Roberts JG: Thermodilution cardiac output—a systematic error. Anaesth Intensive Care 1981; 9: 135.

92. Levine BA, Strinek KR: Cardiac output determination by thermodilution technique: The method of choice in low flow states. Proc Soc Exp Biol Med 1981; 167:279.

93. Ross RM: Bedside calibration check of pulmonary artery catheters (letter). Chest 1981; 79:717.

94. Runciman WB, Ilsley AH, Roberts JG: An evaluation of thermodilution cardiac output measurement using the Swan-Ganz catheter. Anaesth Intensive Care 1981; 9:208.

95. Pesola GR, Ayala B, Plante L: Room-temperature thermodilution cardiac output: Proximal injectate lumen vs proximal infusion lumen. Am J Crit Care 1993; 2:132–133.

96. Medley RS, DeLapp TD, Fisher DG: Comparability of the thermodilution cardiac output method: Proximal injectate versus proximal infusion lumens [review]. Heart Lung 1992; 21:12–77.

97. Thrush DN, Varlotta D: Thermodilution cardiac output: Comparison between automated and manual injection of indicator. J Cardiothorac Vasc Anesth 1992; 6:17–99.

98. Dizon CT, Gezari WA, Barash PG, et al: Hand held thermodilution cardiac output injector. Crit Care Med 1977; 5:10.

99. Beaupre PN, Cahalan MK, Kremer PF, et al: Does pulmonary artery occlusion pressure adequately reflect left ventricular filling during anesthesia and surgery (abstract). Anesthesiology 1983; 59:A3.

100. Carlon GC, Howland WS, Kahn RC, et al: Usual complications during pulmonary artery catheterization. Crit Care Med 1978; 6: 364.

101. Mermel LA, McCormick RD, Springman SR, et al: The pathogenisis and epidemiology of catheter related infection with pulmonary artery Swan Ganz catheters: A prospective study utilizing molecular subtyping. Am J Med 1991; 91:197S–205S.

102. Michel L, McMichan JC, Bachy JL: Microbial colonization of indwelling central venous catheters: Statistical evaluation of potential contaminating factors. Am J Surg 1979; 137:745.

103. Michel L, Marsh HM, McMichan JC, et al: Infection of pulmonary artery catheters in critically ill patients. JAMA 1981; 245: 1032.

104. Todd MM: Atrial fibrillation induced by the right atrial injection of cold fluids during thermodilution cardiac output determination: A case report. Anesthesiology 1983; 59:253.

105. Esses G, Feinberg S, Panos T: Swan Ganz elbow (letter). Can Med Assoc J 1982; 126:1276.

106. Armstrong RF, St Andrew D, Cohen SL, et al: Continuous monitoring of mixed venous oxygen tension (P$_v$O$_2$) in cardiorespiratory disorders. Lancet 1978; 1:632.

107. Armstrong RF, Moxham J, Cohen SL, et al: Intravascular mixed venous oxygen tension monitoring. Br J Anaesth 1981; 53:89.

108. Kasnitz P, Druger GL, Yorra F, et al: Mixed venous oxygen tension and hyperlactatemia. JAMA 1976; 236:570.

109. Krauss XH, Verdouw PD, Hugenholtz PG, et al: On-line monitoring of mixed venous oxygen saturation after cardiothoracic surgery. Thorax 1975; 30:636.

110. Muir AL, Kirby BJ, King AJ, et al: Mixed venous oxygen saturation in relation to cardiac output in myocardial infarction. BMJ 1970; 4:276.

111. Prakash O, Meij SH, van der Borden SG, Clementi G, et al: Cardiovascular monitoring with special emphasis on mixed venous oxygen measurements. Acta Anaesthesiol Belg 1978; 29: 253–258.

112. Baele PL, McMichan JC, Marsh HM, et al: Continuous monitoring of mixed venous oxygen saturation in critically ill patients. Anesth Analg 1981; 61:513.

113. Jamieson WRE, Turnbull KW, Larrieu AJ, et al: Continuous monitoring of mixed venous oxygen saturation in cardiac surgery. Can J Surg 1982; 25:538.

114. Martin WE, Cheung PW, Johnson CC, et al: Continuous monitoring of mixed venous oxygen saturation in man. Anesth Analg 1973; 52:784.

115. Sperinde JM, Senelly KM: The oximetric Opticath system: Theory and development. *In* Fahey PJ (ed): Continuous Measurement of Oxygen Saturation in the High Risk Patient: Theory and Practice in Monitoring Mixed Venous Oxygen Saturation, vol 2. San Diego, Beach International, 1985, pp 59–80.

116. Waller JL, Kaplan JA, Bauman DI, et al: Clinical evaluation of a new fiberoptic catheter oximeter during cardiac surgery. Anesthesiology 1982; 61:676–679.

117. Hecker B, Brown D, Wilson D: A comparison of the pulmonary artery mixed venous oxygen saturation catheters during the changing conditions of cardiac surgery. J Cardiothorac Anesth 1989; 3:269–275.

118. Gettinger A, Glass D: In vivo comparison of two mixed venous oximetrics. Anesthesiology 1987; 66:373–375.

119. Armaganidis A, Dhainaut JF, Billard JL, et al: Accuracy assessment for three fiberoptic pulmonary artery catheters for SvO_2 monitoring. Intensive Care Med 1994; 20:484–488.

120. Dorman BH, Spinale FG, Kratz JM, et al: Use of a combined right ventricular ejection fraction-oximetry catheter system for coronary bypass surgery [see comments]. Crit Care Med 1992; 20:1650–1666.

121. Spinale FG, Smith AC, Carabello BA: Right ventricular function computed by thermodilution and ventriculography. J Thorac Cardiovasc Surg 1990; 99:141–52.

122. Nelson LD: Continuous venous oximetry in surgical patients. Ann Surg 1986; 302:329–333.

123. Norfleet ER, Watson CB: Continuous mixed venous oxygen saturation measurements: A significant advance in hemodynamic monitoring. Clin Monit 1985; 1:245–248.

124. Norwood SH, Nelson LD: Continuous monitoring of mixed venous oxygen saturation in pediatric cardiac surgery. Am Surg 1986; 52:114–115.

125. Orlando R: Continuous mixed venous oximetry in critically ill patients. Arch Surg 1986; 121:470–471.

126. Vedrinne C, Bastien O, De Varax R, et al: Predictive factors for usefulness of fiberoptic pulmonary artery catheter for continuous oxygen saturation in mixed venous blood monitoring in cardiac surgery. Anesth Analg 1997; 85:2–100.

127. Miller HC, Brown DJ, Miller GAH: Comparison of formulae used to estimate oxygen saturation of mixed venous blood from caval samples. Br Heart J 1974; 36:446.

128. Scheinman MM, Brown MA, Rapaport E: Critical assessment of use of central venous oxygen saturation as a mirror of mixed venous oxygen in severely ill cardiac patients. Circulation 1989; 40:165.

129. Meister SG, Helfant RH: Rapid bedside differentiation of ruptured interventricular septum from acute mitral insufficiency. N Engl J Med 1972; 287:1024.

130. Todres ID, Crone RK, Rogers MC, et al: Swan-Ganz catherization in the critically ill newborn. Crit Care Med 1979; 7:330–334.

131. Mihm F, Feeley TW, Rosenthal M, et al: The lack of effect of variable blood withdrawal rates on the measurement of mixed venous oxygen saturation. Chest 1980; 78:452.

132. Chatterjee K, Swan HJC, Ganz W, et al: Use of a balloon-tipped flotation electrode catheter for cardiac monitoring. Am J Cardiol 1975; 36:56.

133. Roth JV: Temporary transmyocardial pacing using epicardial pacing wires and pacing pulmonary artery catheters. J Cardiothorac Vasc Anesth 1382; 6:663–667.

134. Roth JV, Zaidman JR: Use of the pacing pulmonary arterial catheter to detect endocardial electrical activity during hypothermic cardioplegic arrest. J Clin Monit Comput 1988; 4:178–180.

135. Roth JV: Temporary transmyocardial pacing using epicardial pacing wires and pacing pulmonary artery catheters. J Cardiothorac Vasc Anesth 1992; 6:663–677.

136. Seltzer JL, Mora CT, McNulty SE: Evaluation of ventricular pacing with a new design in pulmonary artery catheter. Presented at Society of Cardiovascular Anesthesiologists Annual Meeting, Chicago, May 1986.

137. Lumb P: Atrioventricular sequential pacing with transluminal atrial and ventricular pacing probes inserted via a pulmonary artery catheter: A preliminary comparison with epicardial wires. J Clin Anesth 1989; 1:292–296.

138. Trankina MF, White R: Perioperative cardiac pacing using an atrioventricular pacing pulmonary artery catheter. J Cardiothorac Anesth 1989; 3:154–162.

139. Wasnick JD: Minimally invasive direct coronary artery bypass procedure and pacing pulmonary artery catheter (letter) [see comment]. J Cardiothorac Vasc Anesth 1996; 10:9755.

140. Wasnick JD, Hoffmann WJ, Acuff T: Anesthetic management of coronary artery bypass via mini-thoracotomy with video assistance. J Cardiothorac Vasc Anesth 1995; 9:731–733.

141. Zaidan JR: Experience with the pacing pulmonary artery catheter. Anesthesiology 1980; 3:S118.

142. Risk SC, Brandon D, D'Ambra MN, et al: Indications for the use of pacing pulmonary artery catheters in cardiac surgery. J Cardiothorac Vasc Anesth 1992; 6:275–299.

143. Mukherjee R, Spinale FG, VonRecum AF, et al: In vitro validation of right ventricular thermodilution ejection fraction system. Ann Biomed Eng 1991; 19:165–177.

144. Nelson LD: The new pulmonary arterial catheters. Right ventricular ejection fraction and continuous cardiac output. Crit Care Clin 1996; 12:795–818.

145. Rafferty TD: Transesophageal two dimensional echocardiography in the critically ill: Is the Swan-Ganz catheter redundant? Yale J Biol Med 1990; 64:375–385.

146. Dorman BH, Spinale FG, Kratz JM, et al: Use of combined right ventricular ejection fraction oximetry catheter system for coronary bypass surgery Chest 1992; 20:1650–1656.

147. Spinale FG, Zellner JL, Mukherjee R, et al: Placement consideration for measuring thermodilution right ventricular ejection fractions. Crit Care Med 1991; 19:417–421.

148. Yelderman ML: Continuous measurement of cardiac output with the use of stochastic system identification techniques. J Clin Monit Comput 1990; 6:322–332.

149. Yelderman ML, Ramsey MA, Quinn MD, et al: Continuous thermodilution cardiac output measurements in intensive care unit patients. J Cardiothorac Vasc Anesth 1992; 6:270–274.

150. Ham TH, Shen SC, Fleming EM, et al: Studies in destruction of red blood cells. IV. Thermal injury. Blood 1948; 3:373–403.

151. Henriques FC: Studies of thermal injury. V. The predictability and the significance of thermally induced rate processes leading to irreversible epidermal injury. Arch Pathol 1947; 43:489–502.

152. Henriques FC, Moritz AR: Studies of thermal injury. I. The conduction of heat to and through skin and the temperatures attained therein. A theoretical and an experimental investigation. Arch Pathol 1947; 43:531–549.

153. Gillis MF, Smith LG, Bingham DB: Final technical progress report on studies on the effects of additional endogenous heat relating to the artificial heart. US Dept of Health, Education, and Welfare publication No. (NIH) PH 43-66-1130-5. Government Printing Office, 1973.

154. Yelderman ML, Quinn MD, McKown RC: Thermal safety of a filamented pulmonary artery catheter. J Clin Monit 1992; 8:147.

155. Yelderman ML, Quinn, MD, McKown RC: Continuous thermodilution cardiac output measurements in sheep. J Thorac Cardiovasc Surg 1992; 104:315–320.

156. Lazor MA, Pierce ET, Stanley GD, et al: Evaluation of the accuracy and response time of STAT-mode continuous cardiac output. J Cardiothorac Vasc Anesth 1997; 11:432–466.

157. Greim CA, Roewer N, Thiel H, et al: Continuous cardiac output monitoring during adult liver transplantation: Thermal filament technique versus bolus thermodilution. Anesth Analg 1997; 85:483–488.

158. Thrush D, Downs JB, Smith RA: Continuous thermodilution cardiac output: Agreement with Fick and bolus thermodilution methods. J Cardiothorac Vasc Anesth 1995; 9:399–404.

159. Lefrant JY, Bruelle P, Ripart J, et al: Cardiac output measurement in critically ill patients: Comparison of continuous and conventional thermodilution techniques. Can J Anaesth 1995; 42:972–976.

160. Jacquet L, Hanique G, Glorieux D, et al: Analysis of the accuracy of continuous thermodilution cardiac output measurement. Comparison with intermittent thermodilution and Fick cardiac output measurement. Intensive Care Med 1996; 22:1125–1199.

161. Siegel LC, Hennessy MM, Pearl RG: Delayed time response of the continuous cardiac output pulmonary artery catheter. Anesth Analg 1996; 83:1173–1177.

162. Miyasaka K, Takata M, Miyasaka K: Flow velocity profile of the pulmonary artery measured by continuous cardiac output monitoring catheter. Can J Anaesth 1993; 40:183–187.

163. Uesugi F, Inada T, Inada K, et al: Continuous cardiac output measurement by thermodeprivation is unsatisfactory in cardiac surgical patients [letter]. J Cardiothorac Vasc Anesth 1996; 10:442–444.

164. Jansen JR, Johnson RW, Yan JY, et al: Near continuous cardiac output by thermodilution. J Clin Monit 1997; 13:233–299.

165. Segal J, Pearl RG, Ford AJ Jr, et al: Instantaneous and continuous cardiac output obtained with a Doppler pulmonary artery catheter. J Am Coll Cardiol 1989; 13:1382–1392.

166. Segal J, Gaudiani V, Nishimura T: Continuous determination of cardiac output using a flow directed Doppler pulmonary artery catheter. J Cardiothorac Vasc Anesth 1991; 5:309–315.

167. Iberti TJ, Silverstein JH: Continuous cardiac output measurements in critically ill patients. J Cardiothorac Vasc Anesth 1992; 6:267.

168. Forrester JS, Swan HJC: Acute myocardial infarction: A physiologic basis for therapy. Crit Care Med 1974; 2:283.

169. Forrester JS, Diamond G, Chatterjee K, et al: Medical therapy of acute myocardial infarction by application of hemodynamic subsets I. N Engl J Med 1976; 294(24): 1356.

170. Forrester JS, Diamond GA, Swan HJC: Bedside diagnosis of latent cardiac complications in acutely ill patients. JAMA 1972; 222:59.

171. Shoemaker WC, Appel PL, Kram HL: Prospective trial of supranormal values of survivors as therapeutic goals in high risk patients. Chest 1988; 94:1176–1186.

172. Russell JA, Ronco JJ, Lockat D, et al: Oxygen delivery and consumption and ventricular preload are greater in survivors of the adult respiratory distress syndrome. Am Rev Respir Dis 1990; 141:659–665.

173. Conners AF, Jr., McCaffree DR, Gray BA: Evaluation of right-heart catheterization in the critically ill patient without acute myocardial infarction. N Engl J Med 1983; 308:263.

174. Rice CL, Hobelman CF, John DA, et al: Central venous pressure or pulmonary capillary wedge pressure as the determinant of fluid replacement in aortic surgery. Surgery 1978; 84:437.

175. Yarzebski J, Goldberg RJ, Gore JM, et al: Temporal trends and factors associated with pulmonary artery catheterization in patients with acute myocardial infarction. Chest 1994; 105:1003–1088.

176. Connors AFJ, Speroff T, Dawson NV, et al: The effectiveness of right heart catheterization in the initial care of critically ill patients. JAMA 1996; 276:889–977.

177. Waller JL, Johnson SP, Kaplan JA: Usefulness of pulmonary artery catheters during aortocoronary bypass surgery. Anesth Analg 1982; 61:221.

178. Ermakov S, Hoyt JW: Pulmonary artery catheterization [review]. Crit Care Clin 1992; 8:773–806.

179. Nelson LD: The new pulmonary artery catheters: Continuous venous oximetry, right ventricular ejection fraction, and continuous cardiac output. New Horiz 1997; 5:251–258.

180. Iberti TJ, Fischer EP, Leibowitz AB: A multicenter study of physician's knowledge of the pulmonary artery catheter. Pulmonary Artery Catheter Study Group. JAMA 1990; 264:2928–2932.

181. Trottier SJ, Taylor RW: Physicians' attitudes toward and knowledge of the pulmonary artery catheter: Society of Critical Care Medicine membership survey. New Horiz 1997; 5:201–206.

182. Chalfin DB: The pulmonary artery catheter: Economic aspects. New Horiz 1997; 5:292–296.

183. Fox DB, Troiano NH, Graves CR: Use of the pulmonary artery catheter in severe preeclampsia: a review. Obstet Gynecol Surv 1996; 51:684–695.

184. Hollenberg SM, Hoyt J: Pulmonary artery catheters in cardiovascular disease. New Horiz 1997; 5:207–213.

185. Sprung CL, Eidelman LA: The issue of a U.S. Food and Drug Administration moratorium on the use of the pulmonary artery catheter. New Horiz 1997; 5:277–280.

186. Del Guercio LR: Does pulmonary artery catheter use change outcome? Yes. Crit Care Clin 1996; 12:553–557.

187. Leibowitz AB: Do pulmonary artery catheters improve patient outcome? No. Crit Care Clin 1996; 12:559–568.

188. Ivanov RI, Allen J, Sandham JD, et al. Pulmonary artery catheterization: A narrative and systematic critique of randomized controlled trials and recommendations for the future. New Horiz 1997; 5:268–276.

189. Sprung CL, Eidelman LA: Ethical issues of clinical trials for the pulmonary artery catheter [review]. New Horiz 1997; 5(3):264–277.

190. Connors AFJ: Right heart catheterization: Is it effective? [review]. New Horiz 1997; 5:195–200.

191. American College of Physicians/American College of Cardiology/American Heart Association Task Force on Clinical Privileges in Cardiology: Clinical competence in hemodynamic monitoring. J Am Coll Cardiol 1990; 15:1460–1464.

192. Technology Subcommittee of the Working Group on Critical Care, Ontario Ministry of Health: Hemodynamic monitoring: A technology assessment. Can Med Assoc J 1991; 145:114–121.

193. European Society of Intensive Care Medicine. Expert panel: The use of the pulmonary artery catheter. Intensive Care Med 1991; 17:i–viii.

194. Practice Guidelines for Pulmonary Artery Catheterization: A Report by the American Society of Anesthesiologists Task Force on Pulmonary Artery Catheterization. Anesthesiology 1993; 78: 380–394.

195. Berkowitz RL, Rafferty TD: Invasive hemodynamic monitoring in critically ill pregnant patients: Role of Swan-Ganz catheterization. Am J Obstet Gynecol 1980; 137:127.

196. Yang SC, P VK: Role of preoperative hemodynamic monitoring in intraoperative fluid management. Am Surg 1986; 52:536–540.

197. Berlauk JF, Abrams JH, Gilmour IJ, et al: Preoperative optimization of cardiovascular hemodynamics improves outcome in peripheral vascular surgery: A prospective, randomized clinical trial. Ann Surg 1991; 214:289–299.

198. Davies MJ, Cronin KD, Domaingue CM: Pulmonary artery catheterization. An assessment of risks and benefits in 220 surgical patients. Anaesth Intensive Care 1982; 10:9.

199. Katz RW, Pollack MM, Weibley RE: Pulmonary artery catheterization in pediatric intensive care. Adv Pediatr 1983; 30:169–190.

200. Kohanna FH, Cunningham JN Jr: Monitoring of cardiac output by thermodilution after open-heart surgery. J Thorac Cardiovasc Surg 1977; 73:451.

201. Isaacson IJ, Lowdon JD, Berry AJ, et al: The value of pulmonary artery and central venous monitoring in patients undergoing abdominal aortic reconstructive surgery: A comparative study of two selected, randomized groups. J Vasc Surg 1990; 12:754–760.

202. Joyce WP, Provan JL, Ameili FM, et al: The role of central hemodynamic monitoring in abdominal aortic surgery: A prospective randomized study. Eur J Vasc Surg 1990; 4:633–636.

203. Katz JD, Cronau LH, Barash PG, et al: Pulmonary artery flow-guided catheters in the perioperative period. JAMA 1977; 237: 2832.

204. Hjertberg R, Belfrage P, Hagnevick K: Hemodynamic measurements with Swan-Ganz catheter in women with severe proteinuric gestational hypertension (preeclampsia). Acta Obstet Gynecol Scand 1991; 70:193–199.

205. Clark ST, Cotton DB: Clinical indications for pullonary artery catheterization in the patient with severe preeclampsia. Am J Obstet Gynecol 1988; 158:453–458.

206. Cohn JD, Engler PE, Timpawat C, et al: Physiologic profiles in circulatory support and management of the critically ill. J Am Coll Emerg Physicians 1977; 6:479.

207. Benedetti TJ, Cotton DB, Read JC, et al: Hemodynamic observations in severe pre-eclampsia with a flow-directed pulmonary artery catheter. Am J Obstet Gynecol 1980; 136:465.

208. Babu SC, Sharma PVP, Raciti A, et al: Monitor-guided responses. Arch Surg 1980; 115:1384.

209. Aikawa N, Martyn JA, Burke JF: Pulmonary artery catheterization and thermodilution cardiac output determination in the management of critically burned patients. Am J Surg 1978; 136: 811.

210. Schrader LL, McMillen MA, Watson CB, et al: Is routine preoperative hemodynamic evaluation of nonagenarians necessary? J Am Geriatr Soc 1991; 39:1–5.

211. Schultz RJ, Whitfield GF, Lamura JJ, et al: Physiologic monitoring in patients with fractures of the hip. J Trauma 1985; 25: 309–316.

212. Flancbaum L, Ziegler DW, Choban PS: Preoperative intensive care unit admission and hemodynamic monitoring in patients scheduled for major elective noncardiac surgery: A retrospective review of 95 patients [see comments]. J Cardiothorac Vasc Anesth 1998; 12:3–9.

213. Valentine RJ, Duke ML, Inman MH, et al: Effectiveness of pulmonary artery catheters in aortic surgery: A randomized trial. J Vasc Surg 1998; 27:203–211.

214. Leibowitz AB, Beilin Y: Pulmonary artery catheters and outcome in the perioperative period. New Horiz 1997; 5:214–221.

215. Scalea TM, Simon H, Duncan AO, et al: Geriatric blunt multiple trauma: Improved survival with early invasive monitoring. J Trauma 1990; 30:129–136.

216. Goldman L, Caldera DL, Nussbaum SR, et al: Multifactorial index of cardiac risk in noncardiac surgical procedures. N Engl J Med 1997; 297:845–850.

217. Larsen SF, Ilesen KH, Jacobsen et al: Prediction of cardiac risk in noncardiac surgery. Eur Heart J 1987; 8:179–185.

218. Rao TLK, El-Etr AA: Myocardial reinfarction following anesthesia in patients with recent infarction. Anesth Analg 1981; 60: 271.

219. Rao TL, Jacobs KH, El-Er AA: Reinfarction following anesthesia in patients with myocardial infarction. Anesthesiology 1983; 59: 499–505.

220. Vender JS: Clinical utilization of pulmonary artery catheter monitoring [review]. Int Anesthesiol Clin 1993; 31:57–85.

221. Ellis JE: Con: Pulmonary artery catheters are not routinely indicated in patients undergoing elective abdominal aortic reconstruction [review]. J Cardiothorac Vasc Anesth 1993; 7:753–757.

222. Garnett RL: Pro: A pulmonary artery catheter should be used in all patients undergoing abdominal aortic surgery [review]. J Cardiothorac Vasc Anesth 1993; 7:750–752.

223. Hesdorffer CS, Milne JF, Meyers AM, et al: The value of Swan-Ganz catherization and volume loading in preventing renal failure in patients undergoing abdominal aneurysmectomy. Clin Nephrol 1987; 28:272–276.

224. Quinn K, Quebbeman EJ: Pulmonary artery pressure monitoring in the surgical intensive care unit. Arch Surg 1981; 116: 872–876.

225. Quintin L, Whalley DG, Wynands JE et al: The effects of vascular catheterizations upon heart rate and blood pressure before aorto-coronary bypass surgery. Can Anaesth Soc J 1981; 28:244.

226. Bedford RF, Marshall WK, Butler A, et al: Cardiac catheters for diagnosis and treatment of venous air embolism. J Neurosurg 1981; 55:610.

227. Noel TA: Air embolism removal from both pulmonary artery and right atrium during sitting craniotomy using a new catheter: Report of a case. Anesthesiology 1989; 70:709.

228. Spapen HD, Umbrain V, Brakemans, P, et al: Use of the Swan-Ganz catheter in amniotic fluid embolism (letter). Intensive Care Med 1988; 14:678.

229. Orr JW, Jr, Shinglefon HM, Soony ST, et al: Hemodynamic parameters following pelvic exenteration. Am J Obstet Gynecol 1983; 146:882–892.

230. American College of Obstetricians and Gynecologists Technical Bulletin No. 175. December 1992.

231. Neches WH, Park SC, Lenox CC, et al: Pulmonary artery wedge pressures in congenital heart disease. Cathet Cardiovasc Diagn 1977; 3:11–19.

232. Gore JM, Sloan K: Use of continuous monitoring of mixed venous saturation in the coronary care unit. Crit Care Med 1984; 86:757–761.

233. Gore J, Goldenberg R, Spodick D, et al: A community wide assessment of the use of pulmonary artery, catheters in patients with acute myocardial infarction. Chest 1987; 92:721–727.

234. Civetta JM, Gabel JC: Flow directed-pulmonary artery catheterization in surgical patients: Indications and modifications of technic. Ann Surg 1972; 176:753.

235. Whittemore AD, Clowes AD, Hechtman HB, et al: Aortic aneurysm repair: Reduced operative mortality associated with maintenance of optimal cardiac performance. Ann Surg 1980; 192: 414–421.

236. Matuschak GM: Supranormal oxygen delivery in critical illness. New Horiz 1997; 5:233–238.

237. Tuchschmidt J, Fried J, Astiz M, et al: Elevation of cardiac output and oxygen delivery improves outcome in septic shock. Chest 1992; 102:216–220.

238. Yu M, Levy MM, Smith P, et al: Effect of maximizing oxygen delivery on morbidity and mortality rates in critically ill patients: A prospective, randomized controlled study. Crit Care Med 1993; 21:830–838.

239. Schiller WR, Bay RC, Garren RL, et al: Hyperdynamic resuscitation improves survival in patients with life-threatening burns. J Burn Care Rehabil 1997; 18:10–16.

240. Schiller WR, Bay RC, Mclachlan JG, et al: Survival in major burn injuries is predicted by early response to Swan-Ganz-guided resuscitation. Am J Surg 1995; 170:696–699.

241. Mansfield MD, Kinsella J: Use of invasive cardiovascular monitoring in patients with burns greater than 30 per cent body surface area: A survey of 251 centres. Burns 1996; 22:549–551.

242. Parker MM, Peruzzi W: Pulmonary artery catheters in sepsis/septic shock. New Horiz 1997; 5:228–232.

243. Dhainaut JF, Pinsky MR, Nouria S, et al: Right ventricular function in human sepsis: A thermodilution study. Chest 1997; 112: 1043–1049.

244. Le Tulzo Y, Seguin P, Gacouin A, et al: Effects of epinephrine on right ventricular function in patients with severe septic shock and right ventricular failure: A preliminary descriptive study. Intensive Care Med 1997; 23:664–670.

245. Redl G, Germann P, Plattner H, et al: Right ventricular function in early septic shock states. Intensive Care Med 1993; 19:3–7.

246. Kraut EJ, Owings JT, Anderson JT, et al: Right ventricular volumes overestimate left ventricular preload in critically ill patients. J Trauma 1997; 42:839–845.

247. Nowzari F, Chendrasekhar A. Correlation of Doppler derived velocity change with cardiac index. J Trauma 1996; 40:580–582.

248. Rosenwasser RH, Jallo JI, Getch CC, et al: Complications of Swan-Ganz catheterization for hemodynamic monitoring in patients with subarachnoid hemorrhage [review]. Neurosurgery 1995; 37:872–875.

249. Bhuvaneswaran JS, Venkitachalam CG, Sandhyamani S: Pulmonary wedge aspiration cytology in the diagnosis of recurrent tumour embolism causing pulmonary arterial hypertension [review]. Int J Cardiol 1993; 39:209–212.

250. Gnaegi A, Feihl F, Perret C: Intensive care physicians' insufficient knowledge of right-heart catheterization at the bedside: time to act? [see comments]. Crit Care Med 1997; 25:213–220.

251. Benjamin E, Griffin K, Leibowitz AB, et al: Goal-directed transesophageal echocardiography performed by intensivists to assess left ventricular function: Comparison with pulmonary artery catheterization. J Cardiothorac Vasc Anesth 1998; 12:10–15.

252. Kirton OC, Civetta JM: Do pulmonary artery catheters alter outcome in trauma patients? New Horiz 1997; 5:222–227.

253. Cooper AB, Doig GS, Sibbald WJ: Pulmonary artery catheters in the critically ill. An overview using the methodology of evidence-based medicine [review]. Crit Care Clin 1996; 12:777–794.

254. Tuman KJ, McCarthy RJ, Spless BD, et al: Effect of pulmonary artery catherization on outcome in patients undergoing coronary artery surgery. Anesthesiology 1989; 70:199–206.

255. Moore CH, Lombardo TR, Allums JA, et al: Left main coronary artery stenosis: Hemodynamic monitoring to reduce mortality. Ann Thorac Surg 1978; 26:445.

256. Pearson KS, Gomez MN, Moyers JR, et al: A cost/benefit analysis of randomized invasive monitoring for patients undergoing cardiac surgery. Anesth Analg 1989; 69:336–341.

257. Seldinger SI: Catheter replacement of the needle in percutaneous arteriography. Acta Radiol 1953; 39:368–376.

258. Barash PG, Dizon CT: An introducer for intraoperative percutaneous insertion of a Swan-Ganz catheter. Anesth Analg 1977; 56:444.

259. Brahos GH: Central venous catheterization via the supraclavicular approach. J Trauma 1977; 17:872.

260. Dronen S, Thompson B, Nowak R, et al: Subclavian vein catheterization during cardiopulmonary resuscitation: A prospective comparison of the supraclavicular and infraclavicular percutaneous approaches. JAMA 1982; 247:3227.

261. Pego RF, Luria MH: Left subclavian vein puncture for insertion of Swan-Ganz catheters. Heart Lung 1979; 8:507.

262. DeLange SS, Boscoe MJ, Stanley TH: Percutaneous pulmonary artery catheterization via the arm before anaesthesia: Success rate, frequency of complications and arterial pressure and heart rate. Br J Anesth 1981; 53:1167.

263. Defalque RJ: Percutaneous catheterization of the internal jugular vein. Anesth Analg 1974; 53:116.

264. Ellison N, Jobes DR, Schwartz AJ, et al: Cannulation of the internal jugular vein: A cautionary note. Anesthesiology 1981; 55:337.

265. Ellison N, Schwartz AJ, Jobes DR, et al: Avoidance of carotid artery puncture sequelae during internal jugular cannulation. Anesth Analg 1982; 61:181.

266. Ellison N, Jobes DR, Schwartz AJ, et al: Cannulation of the internal jugular vein: Another cautionary note. Anesthesiology 1982; 57:345.

267. Ellison N, Jobes DR, Schwartz AJ: Internal jugular catheterization. Anaesthesia 1982; 37:605.

268. Elinger JH, Bedford RF, Buschi AJ: Do pulmonary artery catheters cause internal jugular vein thrombosis? (abstract). Anesthesiology 1982; 57:A118.

269. Schwartz AJ, Jobes DR, Greenhow DE, et al: Carotid artery puncture with internal jugular cannulation. Anesthesiology 1979; 51:S160.

270. Conners AF, Castele RJ, Farhat NZ, et al: Complications of right heart catheterization. Chest 1985; 88:567–572.

271. McNabb TG, Green LH, Parker FL: A potentially serious complication with Swan-Ganz catheter placement by the percutaneous internal jugular route. Br J Anaesth 1975; 47:895.

272. Birrer RB, Plotz CM: Bernard-Horner syndrome associated with Swan-Ganz catheter. N Y State J Med 1981; 81:362.

273. Wolrab C, Weber T, Tschernich H, et al: Assessment of left ventricular preload: Transesophageal echocardiography versus filling pressure. Acta Anaesthesiol Scand Suppl 1997; 111:283–286.

274. Kronberg GM, Quan SF, Schlobohm RM, et al: Anatomic locations of the tips of pulmonary-artery catheters in supine patients. Anesthesiology 1979; 51:467.

275. Maran AG: Variables in pulmonary capillary wedge pressure: Variation with intrathoracic pressure, graphic and digital recorders. Crit Care Med 1980; 8:102.

276. Berryhill RE, Benumof JL, Rauscher A: Pulmonary vascular pressure reading at the end of exhalation. Anesthesiology 1978; 49: 365–368.

277. Downs JB, Douglas ME: Assessment of cardiac filling pressure during continuous positive-pressure ventilation. Crit Care Med 1980; 8:285.

278. Geer RT: Interpretation of pulmonary-artery wedge pressure when PEEP is used. Anesthesiology 1977; 46:383.

279. Benumof JL, Saidman LJ, Arkin DB, et al: Where pulmonary arterial catheters go: Intrathoracic distribution. Anesthesiology 1977; 46:336.

280. Kane PB, Mon RL, Askanazi J, et al: Proceedings: The effects of PEEP and left atrial pressure on the correlation between pulmonary artery wedge pressure and left atrial pressure. Br J Anaesth 1976; 48:272.

281. Roy R: Pulmonary wedge catheterization during positive end-expiratory pressure ventilation in the dog. Anesthesiology 1977; 46:385.

282. Teeple E, Ghia JN: An elevated pulmonary wedge pressure resulting from an upper respiratory obstruction in an obese patient. Anesthesiology 1983; 59:66–68.

283. Vaitkus L: Discontinuing PEEP to measure pulmonary capillary wedge pressures. N Engl J Med 1983; 308:776.

284. Downs JB: A technique for direct measurement of intrapleural pressure. Crit Care Med 1976; 4:207.

285. Kaplan JA, Wells PH: Early diagnosis of myocardial ischemia using the pulmonary arterial catheter. Anesth Analg 1981; 60: 789–793.

286. Carlon GC, Kahn RC, Bertoni G, et al: Unexpected giant waves during pulmonary artery catheterization. Intensive Care Med 1979; 5:55.

287. Fuchs RN, Heuser RR, Yin FCP, et al: Limitations of pulmonary wedge v waves in diagnosing mitral regurgitation. Am J Cardiol 1982; 49:849.

288. Teien D, Jones M, Shiota T, et al: Relation of left atrial v-wave/left ventricular systolic pressure ratio to mitral regurgitant volume. Am Heart J 1995; 129:282–284.

289. Cohn JD, Engler PE, Del Guercio LRM: The automated physiologic profile. Crit Care Med 1975; 3:51–58.

290. Boutros AR, Lee C: Value of continuous monitoring of mixed venous blood oxygen saturation in the management of critically ill patient. Crit Care Med 1986; 14:130–134.

291. Sanchez R, Wee M: Perioperative myocardial ischemia: Early diagnosis using the pulmonary artery catheter. Cardiothorac Vasc Anesth 1991; 5:604–607.

292. VanRiper DF, Horrow JC, Kutalek SP, et al: Mixed venous oximetry during automatic implantable cardioverter defibrillator placement. J Cardiothorac Anesth 1990; 4:453–457.

293. Van Daele ME, Sutherland GR, Mitchell MM, et al: Do changes in pulmonary capillary wedge pressure adequately reflect myocardial ischemia during anesthesia? A correlative preoperative hemodynamic, electrocardiographic and transesophageal echocardiographic study. Circulation 1990; 81:865–871.

294. Braunwald E, Ross J Jr, Sonnenblick EH: Mechanisms of Contraction in the Normal and Failing Heart, ed 2. Boston, Little, Brown, 1976, p 130.

295. Scheinman M, Evans GT, Weiss A, et al: Relationship between pulmonary artery end-diastolic pressure and left ventricular filling pressure in patients in shock. Circulation 1973; 47:317.

296. Sonnenblick EH, Strobeck JE: Current concepts in cardiology: Derived indexes of ventricular and myocardial function. N Engl J Med 1977; 296:978.

297. Ross J Jr, Braunwald E: The study of left ventricular function in man by increasing resistance to ventricular ejection with angiotensin. Circulation 1964; 29:739–749.

298. Packman MI, Rackow EC: Optimal left heart filling pressure during fluid resuscitation of patients with hypovolemic and septic shock. Crit Care Med 1983; 11:165.

299. Barash PG: Circulatory strategies in acute respiratory failure. Curt Rev Respir Ther 1981; 21:163.

300. Covelli HD, Nessan VI, Tuttle WK III: Oxygen derived variables in acute respiratory failure. Crit Care Med 1983; 11:646.

301. Alschule M: A new branch of medicine: Complications of vascular catheter. Chest 1986; 89:242.

302. Matta B, Willatis S: A possible complication with a sheath introducer. Crit Care Med 1992; 47:534–535.

303. Brown CQ: Inadvertent prolonged cannulation of the carotid artery. Anesth Analg 1982; 61:150.

304. Shah KB, Rao TLK, Laughlin S, et al: A review of pulmonary artery catheterization in 6,245 patients. Anesthesiology 1984; 61:271–275.

305. Choh JH, Khazei AH, Ihm HJ, et al: Catheter induced pulmonary arterial perforation during open heart surgery. J Cardiovas Surg 1994; 35:61–64.

306. Landow L: Another problem in differentiating between carotid artery and jugular vein cannulation. Anesthesiology 1992; 76: 1061–1062.

307. Applebaum RM, Adelman MA, Kanschuger MS, et al: Transesophageal echocardiographic identification of a retrograde dissection of the ascending aorta caused by inadvertent cannulation of the common carotid artery. J Am Soc Echocardiogr 1997; 10:749–751.

308. Krespi YP, Komisar A, Lucente FE: Complications of internal jugular vein catheterization. Arch Otolaryngol 1981; 107:310.

309. Golden LR. Incidence and management of large-bore introducer sheath puncture of the carotid artery. J Cardiothorac Vasc Anesth 1995; 9:425–428.

310. Dodson T, Quindlen E, Crowell R, et al: Vertebral arteriovenous fistulas following insertion of central monitoring catheters. Surgery 1980; 87:343.

311. Kenny GN: Effect of haemothorax on pulmonary artery wedge pressure. A case report. Br J Anaesth 1979; 51:165.

312. Conahan TJ: Air embolization during percutaneous Swan-Ganz catheter placement. Anesthesiology 1979; 50:360.

313. Kopman EA: Preventing air embolism while inserting central catheters. Anesthesiology 1982; 57:349.

314. Peters JL, Armstrong, R: Air embolism occurring as a complication of central venous catheterization. Ann Surg 1978; 187:375.

315. Doblar DD, Hinkle JC, Fay ML, et al: Air embolism associated with pulmonary artery catheter introducer kit. Anesthesiology 1982; 56:307.

316. Moorthy SS, Tisinai KA, Speiser BS, et al: Cerebral air embolism during removal of a pulmonary artery catheter. Crit Care Med 1991; 19:981–983.

317. Dye LE, Segall PH, Russell RO Jr, et al: Deep venous thrombosis of the upper extremity associated with use of the Swan-Ganz catheter. Chest 1978; 73:673.

318. Cohen S, Whalen F: Another potential complication of a pulmonary artery catheter insertion. Anesthesiology 1991; 75:714.

319. Bradway WR, Gordon R, Ciudice J, et al: Thrombosis after pulmonary-artery catheterization via the internal jugular vein. N Engl J Med 1982; 306:1486.

320. Lederman R: Peripheral nerve injury after coronary artery bypass surgery. Neurosci Today 1981; 4:1.

321. Vander Salm TJ, Cereda JM, Cutler BS: Brachial plexus injury following median sternotomy. Part II. J Thorac Cardiovasc Surg 1982; 83:914.

322. Stock MC, Downs JB: Transient phrenic nerve blockade during internal jugular vein cannulation using the anterolateral approach. Anesthesiology 1982; 57:230.

323. Swan HJ, Ganz W: Complications with flow-directed balloon-tipped catheters. Ann Intern Med 1979; 91:494.

324. Sprung CL, Jacobs LJ, Caralis PV, et al: Ventricular arrhythmias during Swan-Ganz catheterization of the critically ill. Chest 1981; 79:413.

325. Sprung CL, Pozen RG, Rozanski JJ, et al: Advanced ventricular arrhythmias during bedside pulmonary artery catheterization. Am J Med 1982; 72:203.

326. Cairns JA, Holder D: Ventricular fibrillation due to passage of a Swan-Ganz catheter (letter). Am J Cardiol 1975; 35:589.

327. Damen J: Ventricular arrhythmias during insertion and removal of pulmonary artery catheters. Chest 1985; 88:190–193.

328. Iberti TJ, Benjamin E, Gruppi L, et al: Ventricular arrhythmias during pulmonary artery catheterization in the intensive care unit. Prospective study. Am J Med 1985; 78:451–454.

329. Wang TD, Chen WJ, Chen MF, et al: Rapid diagnosis of indwelling pulmonary artery catheter–induced ventricular arrhythmias by the characteristic left bundle branch block morphology and inferior frontal plane axis. Anaesth Intensive Care 1997; 25:77–79.

330. Luck JC, Engel TR: Transient right bundle branch block with Swan-Ganz catheterization. Am Heart J 1970; 92:263.

331. Castellanos A, Ramirez AV, Mayorga-Cortes A, et al: Left fascicular blocks during right-heart catheterization using the Swan-Ganz catheter. Circulation 1981; 64:1271.

332. Strasberg B, Berkowitz CE, Rosen KM: Right bundle branch block reflecting balloon inflation of Swan-Ganz catheter. Chest 1982; 81:368.

333. Abernathy WS: Complete heart block caused by the Swan-Ganz catheter. Chest 1974; 65:349.

334. Shimm DS, Rigsby L: Ventricular tachycardia associated with removal of a Swan-Ganz catheter. Postgrad Med 1980; 67:291.

335. Nakayama M, Aimono M, Kawana S, et al: Cardiac arrest during removal of a pulmonary artery catheter. Can J Anaesth 1996; 43:972–974.

336. Reitan J, Barash PG: Noninvasive monitoring: In Saidman L, Smith, NT (eds): Monitoring in Anesthesia, ed 2. London, Butterworths, 1981.

337. Salmenpera M, Peltola K, Rosenberg P: Does prophylactic lidocaine control cardiac arrhythmias associated with pulmonary artery catheterization? Anesthesiology 1982; 56:212.

338. Allyn J, Lichtenstein A, Koski EG, et al: Inadvertent passage of a pulmonary artery catheter from the superior vena cava through the left atrium and left ventricle into the aorta. Anesthesiology 1989; 70:1019–1021.

339. Thijs LG, Van-Heukelem HA, Bronsveld W, et al: Double intracardiac knotting of a Swan-Ganz catheter (letter). Br J Anaesth 1981; 53:672.

340. Tremblay N, Taillefer J, Hardy JF: Successful nonsurgical extraction of a knotted pulmonary artery catheter trapped in the right ventricle. Can J Anaesth 1992; 39:293–295.

341. Daum S, Schapira M: Intracardiac knot formation in a Swan-Ganz catheter. Anesth Analg 1973; 22:862.

342. Dach JL, Galbut DL, Lepage JR: The knotted Swan-Ganz catheter: New solution to a vexing problem. AJR 1981; 137:1274.

343. Fibuch EE, Tuohy GF: Intracardiac knotting of a flow-directed balloon-tipped catheter. Anesth Analg 1980; 59:217.

344. Graybar GB, Adler E, Smith W, et al: Knotting of a Swan-Ganz catheter (letter). Chest 1983; 84:240.

345. Iberti TJ, Jayagopal SG: Knotting of a Swan-Ganz catheter in pulmonary artery. Chest 1983; 83:711.

346. Andreasson S, Appelgren LK: Complication of Swan-Ganz catheter. Crit Care Med 1979; 7:256.

347. O'Toole JD, Wurtzbacher JJ, Wearner NE, et al: Pulmonary valve injury and insufficiency during pulmonary-artery catheterization. N Engl J Med 1979; 301:1167.

348. Boscoe MJ, Delange S: Damage of the tricuspid valve with a Swan-Ganz catheter. BMJ J 1981; 283:346.

349. Thomas HA.: The knotted Swan-Ganz catheter: A safer solution (letter). Am J Radiol 1982; 138:986.

350. McLoud TC, Putman CE: Radiology of the Swan-Ganz catheter and associated pulmonary complications. Radiology 1975; 116:19.

351. Block PC: Snaring of a Swan-Ganz catheter. J Thorac Cardiovasc Surg 1976; 71:917.

352. Greenfield DH, McMullan GK, Parisi AF, et al: Snare retrieval of a catheter fragment with inaccessible ends from the pulmonary artery. Cathet Cardiovasc Diagn 1978; 4:87.

353. Mehta N, Lochab SS, Tempe DK, et al: Successful nonsurgical removal of a knotted and entrapped pulmonary artery catheter. Cathet Cardiovasc Diagn 1998; 43:87–89.

354. Tan C, Bristow PJ, Segal P, et al: A technique to remove knotted pulmonary artery catheters. Anaesth Intensive Care 1997; 25:160–162.

355. Turnage WS, Fontanet H: Transesophageal echocardiography-guided pulmonary artery catheter placement [erratum appears in Anesth Analg 1994; 78:616]. Anesth Analg 1993; 77:858–859.

356. Oyarzun JR, Donahoo JS, McCormick JR, et al: Venous cannula obstruction by Swan-Ganz catheter during cardiopulmonary bypass. Ann Thorac Surg 1996; 62:266–267.

357. Kainuma M, Yamada M, Miyake T: Pulmonary artery catheter passing between the chordae tendineae of the tricuspid valve. Anesthesiology 1995; 83:1130–1131.

358. Kemmots UK: An inadvertent insertion of a Swan Ganz catheter into the intrathecal space. Anesthesiology 1985; 62:648–649.

359. Racionero MA, Prados C, Acitores I, et al: An infrequent complication of Swan-Ganz catheters (letter). Cardiovasc Surg 1995; 36:519–520.

360. Boncheck LI: Severe endobronchial hemorrhage. Ann Thorac Surg 1992; 53:738–742.

361. Culpepper JA, Setter M, Rinaldo RE: Massive hemoptysis and tension pneumothorax following pulmonary artery catheterization. Chest 1982; 3:380.

362. Deren MM, Barash PG, Hammond GL, et al: Perforation of the pulmonary artery requiring pneumonectomy after the use of a flow-directed Swan-Ganz catheter. Thorax 1979; 34:550.

363. Connors JP, Sandza JG, Shaw RC, et al: Lobar pulmonary hemorrhage. Arch Surg 1980; 115:883.

364. Colvin MP, Savege TM, Lewis CT: Pulmonary damage from a Swan-Ganz catheter. Br J Anaesth 1975; 47:1107.

365. Farber DL, Rose DM, Bassell GM, et al: Hemoptysis and pneumothorax after removal of a persistently wedged pulmonary artery catheter. Crit Care Med 1981; 9:494.

366. Feng WC, Singh AK, Drew T, et al: Swan Ganz catheter induced massive hemoptysis and pulmonary artery false aneurysm. Thorac Surg 1990; 50:644–646.

367. Foote GA, Schabel SI, Hodges M: Pulmonary complications of the flow-directed balloon-tipped catheter. N Engl J Med 1974; 209:927.

368. Forman MB, Obel IW: Pulmonary hemorrhage following Swan-Ganz catheterization in a patient without severe pulmonary hypertension. S Afr Med J 1980; 58:329.

369. Golden MS, Pinder T, Anderson WT, et al: Fatal pulmonary hemorrhage complicating use of flow-directed balloon-tipped catheter in a patient receiving anticoagulant therapy. Am J Cardiol 1973; 32:365.

370. Hardy JF, Morissett M, Taillefer J, et al: The pathophysiology of pulmonary artery ruptures by pulmonary artery balloon tipped catheters (abstract). Anesthesiology 1983; 59:A127.

371. Krantz EM, Viljoen JF: Haemoptysis following insertion of a Swan-Ganz catheter. Br J Anaesth 1979; 51:457.

372. Lapin ES, Murray JA: Hemoptysis with flow-directed cardiac catheterization. JAMA 1972; 220:1246.

373. Lee ME, Matloff JM and Hackner E: Catheter-induced pulmonary artery hemorrhage (letter). J Thorac Cardiovasc Surg 1982; 83:796.

374. McDanield DD, Stone JG, Faltas AN, et al: Catheter-induced pulmonary artery hemorrhage. Diagnosis and management in cardiac operations. J Thorac Cardiovasc Surg 1981; 82:1.

375. Melter R, Kint PP, Simoons M: Hemoptysis after flushing Swan-Ganz catheters in the wedge position. N Engl J Med 1981; 304:1171.

376. Ohn KC, Cottrell JE, Turndore H: Hemoptysis from a pulmonary-artery catheter. Anesthesiology 1979; 51:485.

377. Pape LA, Haffajee CI, Markis JE, et al: Fatal pulmonary hemorrhage after use of the flow-directed balloon-tipped catheter. Ann Intern Med 1979; 90:344.

378. Paulson DM, Scott SM, Sethi GK: Pulmonary hemorrhage associated with balloon flotation catheters: A report of a case and review of the literature. J Thorac Cardiovasc Surg 1980; 80:453.

379. Rubin SA, Puckett RP: Pulmonary artery-bronchial fistula: A new complication of Swan-Ganz catheterization. Chest 1979; 75:515.

380. Elliott CG, Zimmerman GA, Clemmer TP: Complications of pulmonary artery catheterization in the care of critically ill patients. Chest 1979; 76:647.

381. Sekkal S, Cornu E, Christides C, et al: Swan-Ganz catheter induced pulmonary artery perforation during cardiac surgery concerning two cases [review]. J Cardiovasc Surg 1996; 37:313–317.

382. Kearney TJ, Shabot MM: Pulmonary artery rupture associated with the Swan-Ganz catheter [see comments]. Chest 1995; 108:1349–1352.

383. Urschel JD, Myerowitz PD: Catheter-induced pulmonary artery rupture in the setting of cardiopulmonary bypass [see comments] [review]. Ann Thorac Surg 1993; 56:585–589.

384. Kron IL, Piepgrass W, Carabello B, et al: False aneurysm of the pulmonary artery: A complication of pulmonary artery catheterization. Ann Thorac Surg 1982; 33:629.

385. Lindgren KM, McShane K, Roberts WC: Acute rupture of the pulmonic valve by a balloon tipped catheter producing a musical diastolic murmur. Chest 1982; 81:251.

386. Lipp H, O'Donoghue K, Resnekov L: Intracardiac knotting of a flow-directed balloon catheter. N Engl J Med 1971; 284:220.

387. Mayerhofer KE, Billhart RA, Codini MA, et al: An aberrant wave form due to rupture of the balloon of the Swanz-Ganz catheter. N Engl J Med 1983; 308:594.

388. Moore RA, McNicholas K, Gallagher JD, et al: Migration of pediatric pulmonary artery catheters. Anesthesiology 1983; 58:102–104.

389. Kirton O, Varon AJ, Henry R, et al: Flow directed pulmonary artery catheter induced pseudoaneurysm: Urgent diagnosis and endovascular obliteration. Crit Care 1992; 20:1178–1373.

390. Duong TT, Aldea GS, Connelly GP, et al: Acute pulmonary hypertension after wedging of a pulmonary artery catheter as clues to pulmonary artery perforation. J Cardiothorac Vasc Anesth 1993; 7:508–509.

391. Westenskow DR, Silva FH: Device to limit inflation of a pulmonary artery catheter balloon. Crit Care Med 1993; 21:1365–1368.

392. Rao TLK, Gorski DW, Mathru M: Safety of pulmonary artery catheterization (abstract). Anesthesiology 1982; 57:A116.

393. Purut CM, Scott SM, Parham JV, et al: Intraoperative management of severe endobronchial hemorrhage. Ann Thorac Surg 1991; 51:304.

394. Puri VK, Carlson RW, Bander JJ, et al: Complications of vascular catheterization in the critically ill. Crit Care Med 1980; 8:495.

395. Rice PL, Piffarre R, El-Etr A, et al: Management of endobronchial hemorrhage during cardiopulmonary bypass. J Thorac Cardiovasc Surg 1981; 81:800.

396. Resnick JM, Engeler CE, Derauf BJ: Postmortem angiography of catheter induced pulmonary artery perforation. J Forensic Sci 1992; 37:1346–1351.

397. Devitt JH, Noble WH, Byrick RJ: A Swan-Ganz catheter related complication in a patient with Eisenmenger's syndrome. Anesthesiology 1982; 57:335.

398. Stein JM, Libson A: Pulmonary hemorrhage from pulmonary artery catheterization treated with endobronchial intubation. Anesthesiology 1981; 55:698.

399. Gomez-Arnau J, Juan-Montero G, Luengo C, et al: Retrograde dissection and rupture of pulmonary artery after catheter use in pulmonary hypertension. Crit Care Med 1982; 10:694.

400. Mangar D, Connell GR, Lessin JL, et al: Catheter-induced pulmonary artery haemorrhage resulting from a pneumothorax. Can J of Anaesth 1993; 40:1069–1072.

401. Lyew MA, Bacon DR, Nesarajah MS: Right ventricular perforation by a pulmonary artery catheter during coronary artery bypass surgery. Anesth Analg 1996; 82:1089–1090.

402. Johnson WE, Royster RL, Choplin RH, et al: Pulmonary artery catheter migration during cardiac surgery. Anesthesiology 1986; 64:258–262.

403. Yellin LB, Filler JJ, Barnette RE: Nominal hemoptysis heralds pseudoaneurysm induced by a pulmonary artery catheter. Anesthesiology 1991; 73:370–373.

404. Karak P, Dimick R, Hamrick KM, et al: Immediate transcatheter embolization of Swan-Ganz catheter–induced pulmonary artery pseudoaneurysm. Chest 1997; 111:1450–1452.

405. Tayoro J, Dequin PF, Delhommais A, et al: Rupture of pulmonary artery induced by Swan-Ganz catheter: Success of coil embolization. Intensive Care Med 1997; 23:198–200.

406. Ferretti GR, Thony F, Link KM, et al: False aneurysm of the pulmonary artery induced by a Swan-Ganz catheter: Clinical presentation and radiologic management [see comments]. AJR 1996; 167:941–945.

407. Ray CEJ, Kaufman JA, Geller SC, et al: Embolization of pulmonary catheter-induced pulmonary artery pseudoaneurysms. Chest 1996; 110:1370–1373.

408. Pokora TJ, Boros SJ, Brennom WS, et al: Fatal neonatal thrombosis associated with a pulmonary arterial catheter. Crit Care Med 1981; 9:618–619.

409. Reinke RT, Higgins CB, Atkin TW: Pulmonary infarction complicating the use of Swan-Ganz catheters. Br J Radiol 1975; 48:885.

410. Greene JF Jr, Cummings KC: Aseptic thrombotic endocardial vegetations. A complication of indwelling pulmonary artery catheters. JAMA 1973; 225:1525.

411. Hoar PF, Wilson RM, Mangano DT, et al: Heparin bonding reduces thrombogenicity of pulmonary-artery catheters. N Engl J Med 1981; 305:993.

412. Hoar PF, Stone JG, Wicks AE, et al: Thrombogenesis associated with Swan-Ganz catheters. Anesthesiology 1978; 48:445.

413. Snow P: Swan-Ganz catheter and superior vena cava syndrome (letter). JAMA 1980; 243:1525.

414. Bennegard I, Curelara B, Gustavsson LE, et al: Material thrombogenicity in central venous catheterization. Acta Anaesthesiol Scand 1982; 26:112.

415. Brunswick RA, Gionis TA: Starch as a cause of thrombus with Swan-Ganz catheters (letter). Chest 1982; 82:131.

416. Randolph AG, Cook DJ, Gonzales CA, et al: Benefit of heparin in central venous and pulmonary artery catheters: A meta-analysis of randomized controlled trials. Chest 1998; 113:165–171.

417. Zevola DR, Dioso J, Moggio R: Comparison of heparinized and nonheparinized solutions for maintaining patency of arterial and pulmonary artery catheters. Am J Crit Care 1997; 6:52–55.

418. Meredith JW, Young JS, O'Neil EA, et al: Femoral catheters and deep venous thrombosis: a prospective evaluation with venous duplex sonography. J Trauma 1993; 35:187–190.

419. Chastre J, Cornud F, Bouchama A, et al: Thrombosis as a complication of pulmonary-artery catheterization via the internal jugular vein: Prospective evaluation by phlebography. N Engl J Med 1982; 306:267.

420. Kim YL, Richman KA, Marshall BE: Thrombocytopenia associated with Swan-Ganz catheterization in patients. Anesthesiology 1980; 53:262.

421. Richman KA, Kim YL, Marshall BE: Thrombocytopenia and altered platelet kinetics associated with prolonged pulmonary-artery catheterization in the dog. Anesthesiology 1980; 53:101.

422. Bernardin G, Milhaud D, Roger PM, et al: Swan-Ganz catheter-related pulmonary valve infective endocarditis: A case report. Intensive Care Med 1994; 20:142–144.

423. Raphael P, Cogbill TH, Dunn EL, et al: Routine invasive hemodynamic monitoring does not increase risk of aortic graft infection. Heart Lung 1993; 22:121–124.

424. Perrino ACJ: Cardiac output monitoring by echocardiography: Should we pass on Swan-Ganz catheters? [review]. Yale J Biol Med 1993; 66:397–413.

425. Pinilla JC, Ross DF, Martin T, et al: Study of the incidence of intravascular catheter infection and associated septicemia in critically ill patients. Crit Care Med 1983; 11:21.

426. Singh S, Nelson N, Acosta I, et al: Catheter colonization and bacteremia with pulmonary and arterial catheters. Crit Care Med 1982; 10:736.

427. Mermel LA, Stolz SM, Maki DG: Surface antimicrobial activity of heparin-bonded and antiseptic-impregnated vascular catheters. J Infect Dis 1993; 167:920–924.

428. Egebo K, Toft P, Jakobsen CJ: Contamination of central venous catheters. The skin insertion wound is a major source of contamination. J Hosp Infect 1996; 32:99–104.

429. Rello J, Jubert P, Esandi ME, et al. Specific problems of arterial, Swan-Ganz, and hemodialysis catheters [review]. Nutrition 1997; 13:36S–41S.

430. Valles J, Rello J, Matas L, et al: Impact of using an indwelling introducer on diagnosis of Swan-Ganz pulmonary artery catheter colonization. Eur J Clin Microbiol Infect Dis 1996; 15:71–75.

431. Raad I, Umphrey J, Khan A, et al: The duration of placement as a predictor of peripheral and pulmonary arterial catheter infections. J Hosp Infect 1993; 23:17–26.

432. Bach A, Bohrer H, Geiss HK: Safety of a guidewire technique for replacement of pulmonary artery catheters. J Cardiothorac Vasc Anesth 1992; 6:711–714.

433. Bessette MC, Quintin L, Whalley, DG, et al: Swan-Ganz catheter contamination: A protective sleeve for repositioning. Can Anaesth Soc J 1981; 28:86.

434. Erceg GW: A sterile cover for repositioning a pulmonary-artery catheter. Anesthesiology 1980; 52:193.

435. Kopman EA, Sandza JG: Manipulation of the pulmonary-artery catheter after placement: Maintenance of sterility. Anesthesiology 1978; 48:373.

436. Cohen Y, Fosse JP, Karoubi P, et al: The "hands-off" catheter and the prevention of systemic infections associated with pulmonary artery catheter: A prospective study. Am J Respir Crit Care Med 1998; 157:284–287.

437. Smith WR, Glauser FL, Jemison P: Ruptured chordae of the tricuspid valve. The consequence of flow-directed Swan-Ganz catheterization. Chest 1976; 70:790.

438. Smith GB, Willatts SM: A hazard of Swan-Ganz catheterization. Anaesthesia 1981; 36:398.

439. Bernardin G, Milhaud D, Roger PM, et al: Swan-Ganz catheter-related pulmonary valve infective endocarditis: A case report. Intensive Care Med 1994; 20:142–144.

440. Pace NL, Horton W: Indwelling pulmonary artery catheters. Their relationships to aseptic thrombotic endocardial vegetations. JAMA 1975; 233:893.

441. Greene JF Jr, Fitzwater JE, Clemmer TP: Septic endocarditis and indwelling pulmonary artery catheters. JAMA 1975; 233:891.

442. Raphael P, Cogbill TH, Dunn EL, et al: Routine invasive hemodynamic monitoring does not increase risk of aortic graft infection. Heart Lung 1993; 22:121–124.

443. Ehrie M, Morgan AP, Moore FD, et al: Endocarditis with the indwelling balloon tipped pulmonary artery catheter in burn patients. J Trauma 1978; 18:664.

444. Sasaki TM, Panke TW, Dorethy JF, et al: The relationship of central venous and pulmonary artery catheter position to acute right-sided endocarditis in severe thermal injury. J Trauma 1979; 19:740.

445. Hansen R, Vrquerat C, Matthay M, et al: Poor correlation between pulmonary arterial pressure and left ventricular end diastolic volume after coronary artery bypass heart surgery. Anesthesiology 1986; 64:764–770.

446. Calvin JE, Driedger AA, Sibbald WJ: Does the pulmonary capillary wedge pressure predict left ventricular preload in critically ill patients? Crit Care Med 1981; 9:437.

447. Ellis RJ, Mangano DT, VanDyke DC: Relationship of wedge pressure to end-diastolic volume in patients undergoing myocardial revascularization. J Thorac Cardiovasc Surg 1979; 78:605.

448. King EG: Influence of mechanical ventilation and pulmonary disease on pulmonary artery pressure monitoring. Can Med Assoc J 1979; 121:901.

449. Raphael P, Cogbill TH, Dunn EL, et al: Routine invasive hemodynamic monitoring does not increase risk of aortic graft infection. Heart Lung 1993; 22:121–124.

450. Brandi LS, Bertolini R, Pieri M, et al: Comparison between cardiac output measured by thermodilution technique and calculated by O_2 and modified CO_2 Fick methods using a new metabolic monitor. Intensive Care Med 1997; 23:908–15.

451. Kaul S, Stratienko AA, Pollock SG, et al: Value of two-dimensional echocardiography for determining the basis of hemodynamic compromise in critically ill patients: A prospective study. J Am Soc Echocardiogr 1994; 7:598–606.

15 Perioperative Echocardiography

Kornel D. Balon, Jr., M.D.
Christopher J. Young, M.D.
Solomon Aronson, M.D., F.A.C.C., F.C.C.P.

During the past few years, transesophageal echocardiography (TEE) has rapidly become a valuable tool in the perioperative period. Its introduction has provided a new acoustic window to the heart and mediastinum, and it has evolved to become one of the most versatile modalities for diagnosis of cardiovascular diseases. Based on a combination of technological advancement and scientific investigation, countless applications of perioperative echocardiography have been developed. It has been shown TEE can be used safely in hemodynamically unstable patients and, in general, that it can circumvent the limitations of transthoracic echocardiography. In fact, prompt therapeutic interventions based on TEE findings can lead to improved survival and a satisfactory clinical outcome in these critically ill patients.[1, 2] Among the surgically treatable cardiac disorders that can be diagnosed accurately with the use of TEE are aortic dissection, cardiac tamponade, endocarditis, mechanical complications of myocardial infarction (including papillary muscle rupture and ventricular septal defect), and cardiac masses (including thrombus and tumor). Studies have demonstrated the ability of intraoperative echocardiography to alter surgical management and to predict outcome.[3-7] The main reason for the success of TEE is that it provides, with superb clarity and resolution, easily understandable images of cardiovascular abnormalities. Furthermore, TEE is relatively easy to perform and is without significant complications, even in the most critically ill patients.

The goals of this chapter are to familiarize the student of echocardiography with the basic principles of ultrasound and imaging techniques, to enhance understanding of the equipment used and the various considerations of the patient population as well as the echocardiographer, and to explain the diverse applications of pulsed wave and continuous-wave Doppler and two-dimensional (2-D) echocardiography.

Overview

Properties of Ultrasound

Ultrasound waves, by definition, are those sounds that are above the human audible range. For the purposes of echocardiography, these waves are directed into the thoracic cavity, where they are partially reflected by the structures contained inside. By interpretation of various characteristics of these reflections, various pieces of information can be derived about the tissues causing the reflections.

Wavelength, Frequency, and Velocity

A sound wave is a series of compressions and rarefactions. The combination of one compression and one rarefaction is designated as a single *cycle* (Fig. 15-1). The distance between the onset of one cycle and the onset of the next cycle is termed the *wavelength*. *Velocity* is the speed at which the waves propagate through a medium. As the waves travel by any fixed point in an ultrasound beam, the pressure cycles regularly and continuously between a high and a low value. The number of cycles per second (hertz) is called the *frequency* of the wave. Ultrasound is sound with frequency above 20,000 Hz, which is the upper limit of the human audible range. The relationship among the frequency (f), wavelength (l), and velocity (v) of a sound wave is defined by the formula:

$$v = f \times l \qquad (1)$$

Attenuation, Reflection, and Scatter

Waves interact with the medium in which they travel and with one another. Interaction among waves is called *interference*. Its density and homogeneity determine the manner in which waves interact with a medium. When a wave is propagating through an inhomogeneous medium (and all living tissue is essentially inhomogeneous), it is partly absorbed, partly reflected, and partly scattered. Reflected echoes, also referred to as specular echoes, are usually much stronger than scattered echoes. An inhomogeneous medium, such as a cardiac valve in a blood-filled heart chamber, produces strong specular reflections at the blood-valve interface. Conversely, media that are inhomogeneous at the microscopic level, such as muscle, produce more scatter than specular reflection. Any ultrasound beam traveling through tissues will be weakened or attenuated as it progresses.

Modern ultrasound transducers use piezoelectric crystals to transmit ultrasound and receive echoes. A high-frequency electric signal stimulates the crystal, which emits ultrasound. On the other hand, reflected ultrasound echoes striking the crystal's surface generate vibrations that are converted to electric impulses, amplified, processed, and then imaged on a television screen. Electronic circuits measure the time delay between the emitted and received echoes, and, using the known speed of ultrasound in tissue, convert this time delay into the precise distance between transducer and tissue.

The commonly used transducer emits a pulse of ultrasound waves for approximately one μs. It then "listens" for

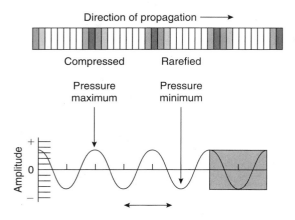

Direction of propagation ⟶

Compressed   Rarefied

Pressure maximum   Pressure minimum

Figure 15-1. Schematic depiction of sound wave.

the returning echoes for about 0.25 ms and pauses for 0.75 ms or less before repeating the cycle. Ultrasound takes about 0.1 ms to travel through 10 cm of human tissue and to be reflected or echoed back to the transducer. There is no time lost in the reflection process.

Imaging Techniques

M-Mode

The most basic form of ultrasound imaging is M-mode echocardiography. In this mode, the density and position of all tissues in the path of a narrow ultrasound beam (i.e., along a single line) are displayed as a scroll on a video screen. The scrolling produces an updated, continuously changing time plot of the studied tissue section, several seconds in duration. Since this is a timed *motion display* (normal cardiac tissue is always in motion), it is called M-mode. Because the image requires considerable interpretation and because only a very limited part of the heart is being observed at any one time, M-mode is not currently used as a primary imaging technique. This mode is, however, useful for the precise timing of events within the cardiac cycle and is often used in combination with color-flow Doppler imaging for the timing of abnormal flows. Quantitative measurements of size, distance, and velocity are also easily performed in the M-mode without the need for sophisticated analysis stations.

2-D Mode

By rapid, repetitive scanning along many different radii within an area in the shape of the fan (sector), echocardiography generates the 2-D image of a section of the heart. This image, which resembles an anatomic section, but which can be more easily interpreted, is called a 2-D scan. Information on structures and motion in the plane of a 2-D scan is updated 30 to 60 times per second, as opposed to the M-mode, which is updated 1000 times per second, making the latter mode more useful for detecting subtle changes in motion or dimension. This updating of the 2-D image produces a "live" (real-time) image of the heart. Scanning 2-D echo devices image the heart by using either a mechanically steered transducer or, as is common in many of the newer devices, an electronically steered ultrasound beam (phased-array transducer).

Doppler Echocardiography

Doppler echocardiography measures blood flow velocity in the heart and great vessels and is based on the effect described by the Austrian physicist Christian Doppler in 1842.[8] Most modern echo scanners combine Doppler capabilities with their 2-D imaging capabilities. After the desired view of the heart has been obtained by 2-D echocardiography, the Doppler beam, represented by a cursor, is superimposed on the 2-D image. As of this writing Doppler technology can be utilized in at least four different ways to measure blood velocities: pulsed wave, high repetition frequency, continuous wave, and color flow.

The Doppler Effect

The Doppler effect states that sound frequency increases as the sound source moves toward the observer and decreases as the source moves away (Fig. 15-2). In the circulatory system, the moving target is the red blood cell (Fig. 15-3). When an ultrasound beam with a known frequency (fo) is transmitted to the heart or great vessels, it is reflected by the red blood cells. The frequency of the reflected ultrasound waves (fr) increases when the red blood cells are moving toward the source of ultrasound. Conversely, the frequency of reflected ultrasound waves decreases when the red blood cells are moving away from the source. The change in frequency between the transmitted sound and the reflected sound is termed the *frequency shift* (Δf) or *Doppler shift* ($fr - fo$). The Doppler shift depends on the transmitted frequency (fo), the velocity of the moving target (v), and the angle (θ) between the ultrasound beam and the direction of the moving target as expressed in the *Doppler equation:*

$$\Delta f = \frac{2fo \times v \times \cos \theta}{c} \qquad (2)$$

where c is the speed of sound in blood (1560 m/s). The angle θ is 0 degree (i.e., the ultrasound beam is parallel with the direction of blood flow); the maximal frequency shift is measured because the cosine of 0 degree is 1. Note that as angle θ increases, the corresponding cosine becomes progressively less than 1, and this will result in underestimation of the Doppler shift (Δf) and, hence, peak velocity. The reason for this is peak flow velocity is derived from Δf by rearranging the Doppler equation:

$$v = \frac{c}{2} \times \frac{\Delta f}{fo} \qquad (3)$$

In clinical practice, the deviation from parallel of up to 20 degrees can be tolerated, since this only results in an error of 6% or less.

Pulsed-Wave Doppler

In the pulsed-wave mode, a single ultrasound crystal sends and receives sound beams. The crystal emits a short burst of ultrasound at a certain frequency (*pulse repetition frequency,* PRF). The ultrasound is reflected for moving red blood cells and is received by the same crystal. The time delay between the emission of the ultrasound signal burst and a sampling of the reflected signal determines the depth at which the velocities are sampled. The delay is proportional to the distance between the transducer and the loca-

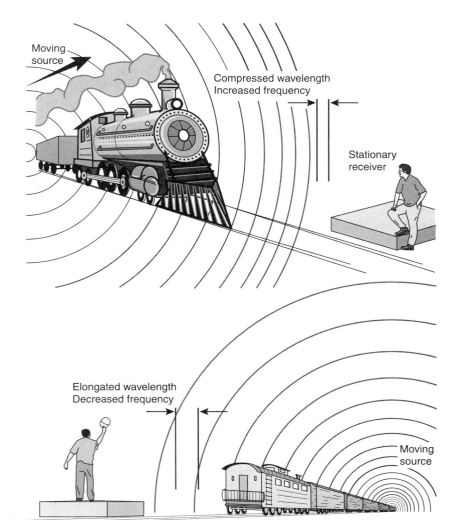

Figure 15-2. Representation of Doppler principle.

tion of the velocity measurements. To sample at a given depth (*D*), sufficient time must be allowed for the signal to travel a distance of 2 × *D* (from the transducer to the sample volume and back). The time delay, *Td*, between the emission of the signal and reception of the reflected signal, is related to *D*, and to the speed of sound in tissue (*c*) by the following formula:

$$D = \frac{c \times Td}{2} \qquad (4)$$

Therefore, the maximal frequency shift that can be determined by pulsed-wave Doppler is one half of the PRF, called the *Nyquist frequency.* If the frequency shift is higher than the Nyquist frequency, *aliasing* occurs; that is, the Doppler spectrum is cut off at the Nyquist frequency, and the remaining frequency shift is recorded on the opposite side of the baseline. Pulsed-wave Doppler measures flow velocities at a specific location within a "sample volume." The PRF varies inversely with the depth of the sample volume: the shallower the location of the sample volume, the higher the PRF and Nyquist frequency. In other words, higher velocities can be recorded without aliasing by the pulsed-wave Doppler if the sample volume is closer to the transducer.

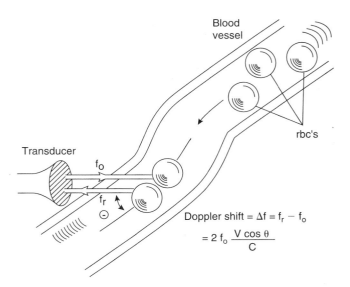

Figure 15-3. Drawing illustrating the Doppler effect. rbc's, red blood cells; f_o, transmitted frequency; f_r, reflected frequency; V, velocity of red blood cells; C, speed of ultrasound in blood.

High Pulse Repetition Frequency Doppler

On some instruments, pulsed-wave Doppler can be modified to a high PRF mode. While in conventional pulsed-wave Doppler only a single burst of ultrasound is considered to be in the body at any given time, in high PRF Doppler two to five sample volumes are simultaneously present in the tissues. Information coming back to the transducer may be coming back from depths of two, three, or four times the initial sample volume depth. The returning signals can be a mix of signals that have previously been emitted and have traveled to distant gates, and other signals that were just sent and returned from the first range gate.

The high PRF mode allows increasing the sampling frequency since the scanner does not wait for the return of the information from distant gates. It nonetheless receives that information back within the specified time-gate period. Higher velocities can be measured with this method than with pulsed-wave Doppler; however, the depth from which the velocity signals are reflected is unknown (range ambiguity).

Continuous-Wave Doppler

In the continuous-wave mode, the transducer has two crystals: one to send, the other to receive the reflected ultrasound waves continuously. Therefore, the PRF or the Nyquist phenomenon does not limit the maximal frequency shift that can be recorded by continuous-wave Doppler. Unlike pulsed-wave Doppler, continuous-wave Doppler measures all the frequency shifts (i.e., velocities) present along its beam path; hence, it is used to detect and to record the highest flow velocity available. Consequently, the region where flow dynamics are measured cannot be precisely localized.

Continuous-wave Doppler is particularly useful for the evaluation of patients with valvular lesions or congenital heart disease. It is also the preferred technique when attempting to derive hemodynamic information from Doppler signals.

Color-Flow Mapping

Color-flow imaging, based on pulsed-wave Doppler principles, displays intracavitary blood flow in three colors (red, blue, and green) or their combinations, depending on their velocity, direction, and extent of turbulence.[9] It uses multiple sampling sites along multiple ultrasound beams (*multigated*). At each sampling site (or *gate*), the frequency shift is measured, converted to a digital format, automatically correlated (*autocorrelation*) with a preset color scheme, and displayed as color flow superimposed on 2-D imaging. A location in the heart where the scanner has detected flow toward the transducer (the top of the image sector) is assigned the color red. Flow away from the direction of the top is assigned the color blue. This color assignment is completely arbitrary and determined by the equipment's manufacturer. In the most common color-flow coding scheme, the faster a velocity (up to a limit) becomes, the more intense that color becomes. Flow velocities that change by more than a preset value within a brief time interval (flow variance) have the color green added to either the red or the blue. Both rapidly accelerating laminar flow (change in flow speed) and turbulent flow (change in flow direction) satisfy the criteria for rapid changes in velocity. In summary, the brightness of the red or blue colors at any location and time is usually proportional to the corresponding flow velocity, while the hue is proportional to the temporal rate of change of the velocity.

Contrast Echocardiography

Contrast echocardiography is a recently developed clinical diagnostic tool that has been shown to be useful in the following areas: (1) identification of intracardiac shunt,[10] (2) identification of unknown cardiovascular structures,[11] (3) improved recording of Doppler-flow velocities,[12-14] (4) visualization of the endocardial border,[15, 16] and (5) assessment of myocardial perfusion.[17, 18] It uses injected contrast agents, typically nontoxic solutions containing gaseous microbubbles, which reflect the ultrasound beam emitted by the echo transducer. Thus, the imaged backscatter of the "tracer" microbubbles represents blood flow within the tissue on which the ultrasound beam is focused. Areas of impaired perfusion or no perfusion are, therefore, visualized.

Gramiak and Shah,[10] who described visualization of aortic valve incompetence at the time of left-sided heart catheterization, originally reported contrast echocardiography in 1968. Subsequently, contrast echocardiography has been used to image intracardiac shunts,[19-22] right- and left-sided heart incompetence,[10, 23-26] and pericardial effusions. In addition, left ventricular (LV) injections of hand-agitated microbubble solutions have been used to identify LV endocardial edges, cardiac output, and valvular regurgitation (semiquantitative).[10, 19-21, 23-26] More recently, echocardiographic contrast has gained popularity as a tool in helping determine myocardial perfusion, both by a patient's native blood flow[27] as well as by cardioplegia during extracorporeal circulation.[28]

Initially, contrast agents consisted of various solutions that had been agitated by hand to produce microbubbles that would serve as ultrasonic reflectors. Hand-agitated microbubbles, however, are relatively large and unstable (40 to 50 μm in diameter) and therefore preclude quantitative analysis of contrast-enhanced images.[29]

More recently, microbubbles produced by ultrasonic cavitation (sonication) have been shown to be superior to the hand-agitated microbubbles. Specifically, sonicated microbubbles have been shown to be smaller than hand-agitated microbubbles and, in fact, smaller than red blood cells. Indeed, sonicated microbubbles have been shown to be capable of passing, along with the red blood cells, through the microcapillary vascular bed and reflecting the echo beam. The smaller sonicated microbubbles, therefore, permit direct ultrasonic imaging of tissue perfusion and detection of valvular abnormalities.[30] In addition to their small size, the sonicated microbubbles have been shown to exhibit intracavitary velocities comparable to those of red blood cells as observed by Doppler.[31] Numerous investigations have postulated that, by controlling the size and stability of the microbubbles, quantitative measurements could be accomplished. Contrast ultrasonography has been shown to be capable of calculating absolute blood flow and volume in vitro and in vivo.[32-34] More recently, clinical contrast echo studies have safely used a commercially prepared air-filled albumin microsphere with known concentrations and size to visualize left-sided heart structures following intravenous (IV) injections.[35] The most recent studies have used IV injections of perfluorocarbon-exposed sonicated dextrose albumin (PESDA) microbubbles.[36] These studies suggest the possibility of noninvasive perfusion evaluation using contrast echocardiography. The ultimate quantitation of perfusion with contrast echo, however, will require further development of ultrasound contrast agents and ultrasound machines, along with application of mathematical models such as classic dye dilution theory.[37]

Imaging Artifacts and Pitfalls

An *artifact* is defined as any structure in an image that does not correspond to an anatomic tissue structure. These errors in interpretation of structures are due to inherent properties of ultrasound technology. Artifacts can be classified as missing structures, falsely perceived objects, general usage degradation, and structures with misregistered location.[38] Reverberations, a type of image degradation artifact, for example, occur when the ultrasonic beam travels through fluid, strikes the far wall of the image, and returns to the transducer. When the near side of the transducer functions as another reflecting surface, the ultrasonic beam will retrace itself, hit the far side of the image again, and return to the transducer. The added distance of travel produces another echo signal at twice the distance as the original signal. Reverberations may also occur from ultrasound beams reflecting from echo-producing structures within the heart. Reverberation artifacts occur commonly in the descending thoracic aorta and within a large ascending aorta. Acoustic shadowing, another type of image degradation artifact, may result from high-density structures such as calcium and prosthetic valves, which tend to lend themselves to bright echoes from the strong reflectors.

Side-lobe beams are generated from the edges of individual transducer elements and are projected in a different direction from the main ultrasonic beam. If a side-lobe beam is hitting an object, the echoes produced will be weaker. They nevertheless will be transmitted back to the transducer displayed as if they were generated from the main beam (i.e., in the center of the field). If the emitted echo beam is oscillating, then multiple side-lobe artifacts may be displayed as a curved line at the same level as the true object. A summary of these artifacts is listed in Table 15-1.

Pitfalls are errors in interpretation of an artifact or other normal structures mimicking pathologic entities and often can result in unnecessary clinical interventions. Pitfalls are generally categorized as false masses, fluid collections or cysts, misinterpretations of normal flow dynamics, and other easily misinterpreted structures, such as catheters and sutures.

The left atrial appendage (LAA) has pectinate muscles that are visualized during TEE as parallel muscle ridges that protrude into the LAA and may mimic thrombus. Because the LAA is a common site for thrombus formation, the echocardiographer must be able to distinguish the appearance of thrombus from pectinate muscle ridges. The tomographic slice of atrial tissue that separates the LAA from the left upper pulmonary vein appears as a globular mass that protrudes into the lumen of the left atrium (LA). This "mass," known as the warfarin ridge, undulates with the cardiac motion and can mimic tumor or thrombus. In addition, at the level of the LAA, a persistent left superior vena cava (SVC) may be seen as it courses posterior to the LA and drains into the coronary sinus (CS). This can often be confused with a pericardial cyst or abscess. Finally, an inverted LAA may mimic a thrombus and should be a consideration during open heart surgery when the LAA is mechanically blotted during de-airing.[39]

The anatomy of the right atrium (RA) frequently presents the echocardiographer with complex anatomic structures that can mimic pathologic conditions. For example, at the junction of the SVC and RA, the right valve of the sinus venosus forms the crista terminalis. This prominent muscular ridge commonly is seen extending into the RA at the superior lateral border and must be differentiated from thrombus. The RA also has trabeculations and pectinate muscles similar to those seen in the LA. At the junction of the inferior vena cava (IVC) and the RA, the eustachian valve is the embryologic remnant of the septum that directed IVC blood across the foramen ovale in utero.[40, 41] A lipomatous interatrial septum may also be confused with an infiltrative process within the heart.

A transverse five-chamber view at the level of the aortic valve does not achieve a cross section through the aortic valve in the plane parallel to its axis. Because of this, only the right and the noncoronary cusps of the aortic valve are fully visualized as they coapt at the level of the annulus. At this level, the left cusp of the aortic valve is imaged on end and may have an appearance similar to that of a valvular vegetation as it moves into and out of the imaging plane. Differentiation of this artifact from a true vegetation can best be achieved using multiplanar imaging to transect the valve in a plane directly parallel to its axis.

The orientation of the transverse aorta and the innominate vein as it courses anterior to the aorta gives the appearance of an aortic dissection. The utilization of color-flow and pulsed-wave Doppler spectral analysis can help differentiate flow patterns and rule out an aortic dissection. As the distal transverse aorta becomes the proximal descending aorta, the inferior vessel wall curves. A transverse image will yield an oblique slice through the aortic wall, which looks like a large atherosclerotic plaque extending into the lumen of the aorta. Multiple scanning can help to better visualize this portion of the aorta.

Various pericardial reflections, when fluid-filled, may mimic abscess or cystic cavities. One such space, the transverse sinus, exists between the anterior LA and the posterior wall of the ascending aorta. When a pericardial effusion is present, this space fills with fluid, and portions of the LAA and epicardium can be seen moving in and out of the imaging plane. If this space is not appreciated as extracardiac, an intracardiac tumor or thrombus may be incorrectly diagnosed. Table 15-2 summarizes the various pitfalls.

Examination

Instrumentation

Echo Scanners

The conversion of reflected ultrasound echoes into 2-D images is a process that involves numerous electronic and visual manipulations (Fig. 15-4). *Resolution* is the ability of the ultrasound to distinguish fine detail. The resolution of an echo system is the minimum distance that must separate two distinct reflectors so that they can be imaged as separate entities. Ultrasound echoes are received and converted to analog electronics signals by the transducer. Modern ultra-

Table 15-1. Artifacts

Missing structures
Problems with resolution
Entrapped air
Falsely perceived objects
Mirror images
Image degradation
Attenuation
Shadowing
Reverberation
Comet tail
Ring down
Bovie cautery
Structures with misregistered location
Side-lobe artifacts

Table 15-2. Pitfalls

False messages
    Atrial trabeculations
    Warfarin ridge
    Crista terminalis
    Right atrial superior vena cava (SVC)
    Lipomatous hypertrophy
    Eustachian valve
    Chiari's network
    Oblique cuts of aortic valve
    Inverted left atrial appendage
    Mitral valve annulus
    Innominate vein
Fluid collections, cysts
    Transverse sinus
    Effusions
    Oblique sinus
    Persistent left SVC
Physiologic valvular regurgitation
Other structures
    Catheters
    Pacer wires
    Sutures

sound transducers employ piezoelectric crystals to transmit ultrasound and perceived echoes. These signals undergo several modifications before being eventually displayed as an image. *Preprocessing* describes those modifications performed on analog or digital signals before input into the scanner's digital memory. These include dynamic range manipulation, gain attenuation, and time-gain compensation. The *dynamic range* of an ultrasound scanner is defined by the cutoff limits of echo signal intensity and can be adjusted by the operator. A wide dynamic range is needed for high resolution while a narrow dynamic range facilitates discrimination between true image signals and unwanted noise. The *gain* and *attenuation* controls increase or decrease the intensity of all signals in a proportional matter. The recent innovation, known as *lateral gain control*, allows the application of gain control to selected sectors of the ultrasound image. Any wave that travels to tissues is attenuated to a degree proportional to the travel distance. With this in mind, it is necessary to compensate for the fact that echoes that return from objects most distant are weaker than echoes that return from equally dense objects closer to the transducer. A mechanism called *time-gain compensation,* or depth compensation, is used to achieve this.

Leading-edge enhancement, or differentiation, is another type of preprocessing used to sharpen the video image. The reflected echo signal undergoes half-wave rectification. This is followed by a smoothing into a signal envelope. An amplifier then differentiates the leading edge of the smoothed signal envelope to its first mathematical derivative, and a narrower and brighter image spot is formed. Since a 2-D echo image is composed of multiple radially juxtaposed scan lines, excessive edge enhancement narrows bright spots and the direction of travel of the echo beam. For this reason, leading-edge enhancement is primarily performed on M-mode scans.

After the analog preprocessing is completed, ultrasound devices digitize the image data and a series of postprocessing manipulations. One early step in this process uses the scan converter to transform the information into a rectangular format for television screen display. The typical television display of an echo image consists of 128 columns by 512 rows for a total of 65,536 picture elements, or pixels.

Each unit of memory assigned to a pixel can store 1024 values of echo intensity, while the pixel itself can only display 64 shades of gray. Each gray level, therefore, represents multiple echo intensities. Thus gray-scale processing, greatly affects image quality.

Spatial processing is a very sophisticated type of averaging that involves modifications in the content of the pixel based on the content of its neighbors. This operation is done for all pixels, and the new pixels are stored in the new image memory area. This produces spatial smoothing of the image and is particularly useful for parts of the image in which no abrupt changes in the echo density occur. It also eliminates "noise." When detection of subtle changes in intensity is desired, as in endocardial border detection, an edge-enhancing convolution process is used.

Image Storage

All modern echo scanners allow the operator to store a single echo image on the display screen. This allows the

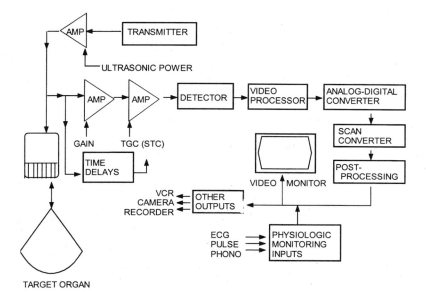

Figure 15-4. Schematic of a modern ultrasound scanner. The *arrows* indicate the directions for the flow of information or electronic power. AMP, electronic amplifier; TGC (STC), time gain compensation; VCR, videocassette recorder. (From Thys DM, Hillel Z: How it works; Basic concepts in echocardiography. *In* Bruijin NP, Clements F (eds): Intraoperative Use of Echocardiography. Philadelphia, JB Lippincott, 1991.)

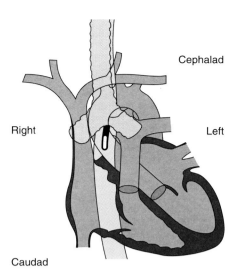

Color Figure 15–5. Position of transesophageal echocardiography probe relative to intrathoracic structures.

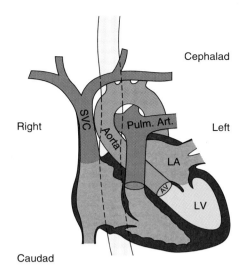

Color Figure 15–6. Schematic of cardiac anatomy.

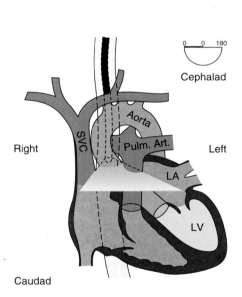

Color Figure 15–7. Anteroposterior view of imaging plane.

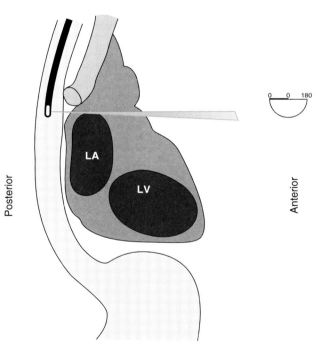

Color Figure 15–8. Lateral view of imaging plane.

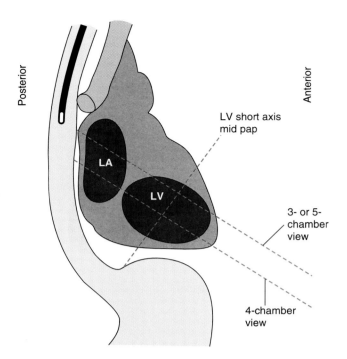

Color Figure 15-9. Schematic of planes of various imaging windows.

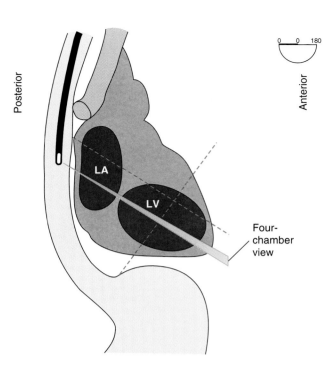

Color Figure 15-11. Lateral view of midesophageal four-chamber imaging plane.

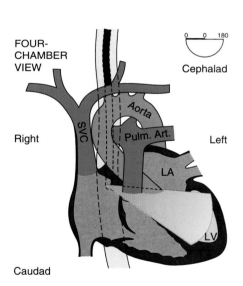

Color Figure 15-12. Anteroposterior view of midesophageal four-chamber imaging plane.

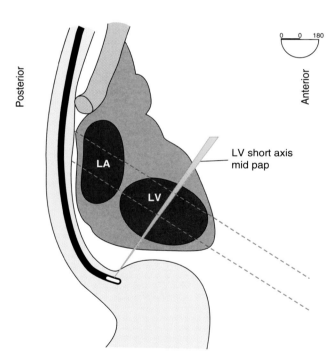

Color Figure 15-16. Lateral view of transgastric short axis mid-papillary imaging plane.

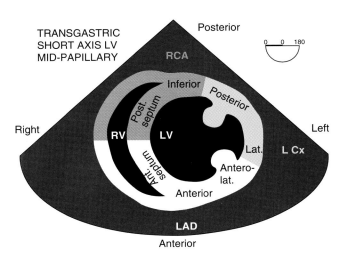

Color Figure 15-19. Schematic of transgastric short axis midpapillary view with segmental designations and coronary artery perfusion.

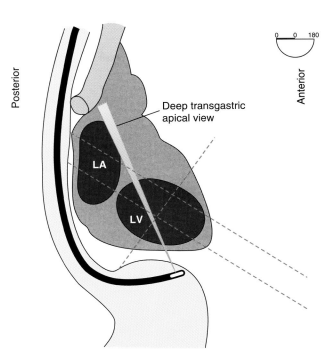

Color Figure 15-20. Lateral view of deep transgastric apical imaging plane.

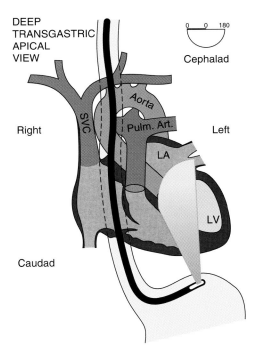

Color Figure 15-21. Anteroposterior view of deep transgastric apical imaging plane.

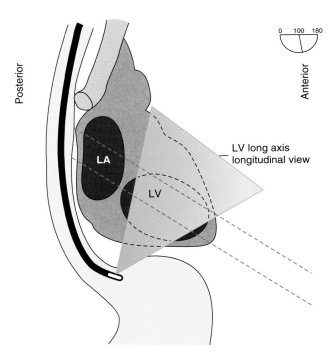

Color Figure 15-24. Longitudinal view of transgastric LV long axis imaging plane.

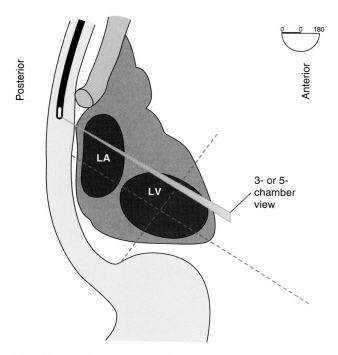

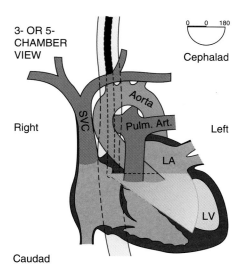

Color Figure 15-29. Anteroposterior view of midesophageal three- or five-chamber imaging plane.

Color Figure 15-28. Lateral view of midesophageal three- or five-chamber imaging plane.

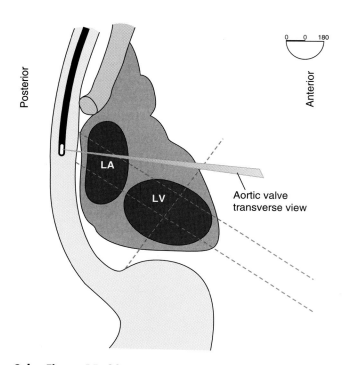

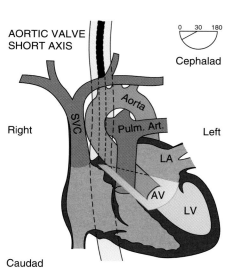

Color Figure 15-33. Lateral view of aortic valve transverse imaging plane.

Color Figure 15-34. Anteroposterior view of aortic valve short axis imaging plane.

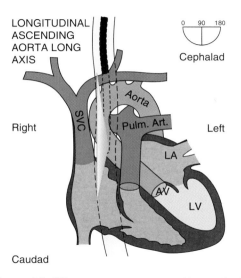

Color Figure 15–37. Anteroposterior view of longitudinal ascending aorta long axis imaging plane.

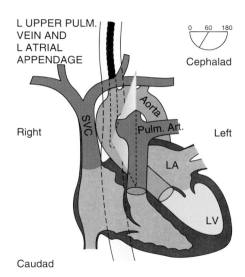

Color Figure 15–41. Anteroposterior view of left upper pulmonary vein and left atrial appendage imaging plane.

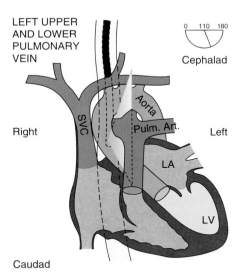

Color Figure 15–44. Anteroposterior view of left upper and lower pulmonary veins.

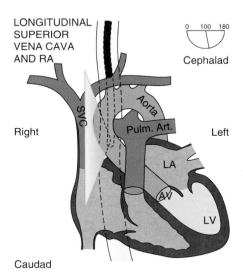

Color Figure 15–46. Anteroposterior view of bicaval imaging plane.

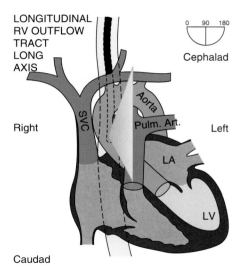

Color Figure 15-49. Anteroposterior view of longitudinal RV outflow tract long axis imaging plane.

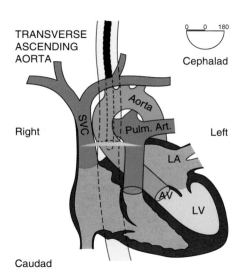

Color Figure 15-52. Anteroposterior view of transverse ascending aorta imaging plane.

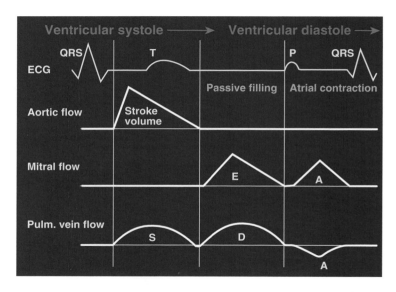

Color Figure 15-58. Flow patterns of the heart and their relation to the cardiac cycle.

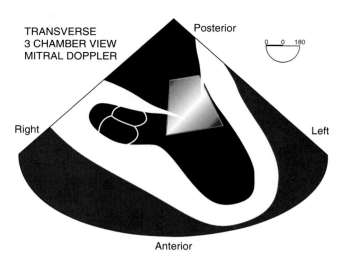

Color Figure 15-59. Schematic of the transverse three-chamber view and the area of interest for mitral pulsed wave Doppler interrogation.

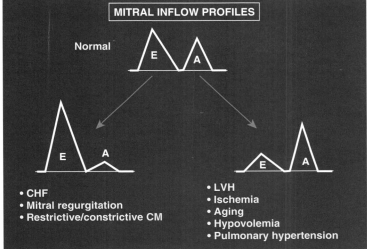

Color Figure 15–62. Mitral inflow profiles and physiologic basis for waveforms.

Color Figure 15–63. Mitral inflow profiles and respective differential diagnoses. CHF, congestive heart failure; CM, cardiomyopathy; LVH, left ventricular hypertrophy.

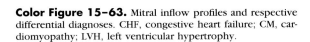

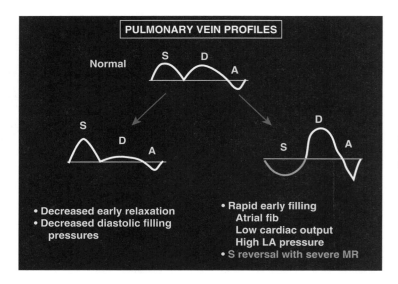

Color Figure 15-64. Pulmonary venous flow profiles with physiologic basis for waveforms and respective differential diagnoses.

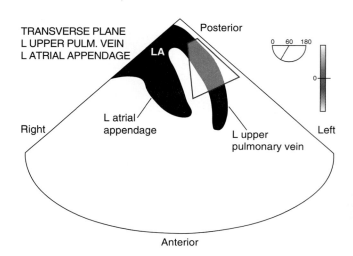

Color Figure 15-65. Schematic of left upper pulmonary vein and left atrial appendage and the area of interest for pulmonary venous flow pulsed wave Doppler interrogation.

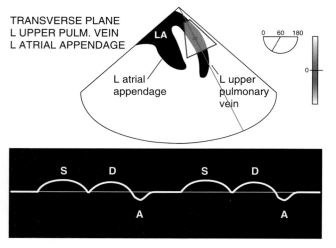

Color Figure 15-66. Schematic of the left upper pulmonary vein and left atrial appendage view and representative pulmonary venous pulsed wave Doppler flow profile.

scrutiny of any unusual transient anatomic or physiologic observations. Once frozen, an image can also be subjected to some simple quantitative measurements. With the continuous motion of the cardiac structures, it is often difficult, however, to capture the exact frame that is to be analyzed. For this reason, techniques to acquire several consecutive frames have been developed.

Cine Memory

One widely used technique for information storage is cine memory. This mode allows the capture of a sequence of several echo images into digital memory. Because of the digital storage technique, the quality of the stored images is high. They can then be displayed in several different ways. The frames can be displayed one by one as the operator manually controls the transition from one to the next, using the trackball found on all echo machines. In this mode, any amount of time can be spent on a single frame. The images may also be replayed continuously in a repeated endless-loop manner, at the same speed as the original recording speed or at a different speed.

Videotape

The video recorder is the most common long-term, mass storage medium used in echocardiography. Most echo scanners are equipped with ½-in. VHS, "super" VHS, or ¾-in. videocassette recorders (VCRs). Because VCRs store images in analog format, the quality of videotape images is currently inferior to the real-time display or the digital cine memory replay.

Other Storage Media

Most devices record the continuously scrolled information of M-mode and pulsed-wave Doppler using photographic or digital paper chart recorders. The scrolls can be subsequently used for quantitative analysis of these types of data. These devices can also provide prints of single-frame 2-D images.

Digital image storage is possible on magnetic disk. Standard floppy disks have a very limited storage capability, since the amount of information on any single video frame can be on the order of 1 MB. A new digital mass storage medium uses "write-once, read-many" digitally encoded laser disks. Using a large 810-MB memory, it can store 24,000 frames or 800 different cine loops, each 30 frames long.

Equipment

Basic requirement for TEE is a complete 2-D Doppler color flow echocardiographic instrument to which a transesophageal transducer has been attached. All endoscopic 2-D ultrasound transducers are constructed similarly. The conventional endoscope is fitted with a small 3.0- to 7.5-MHz side-viewing phased-array transducer at its tip. A lower frequency, such as 3.5 MHz, has greater penetration and is more suited for the transgastric view. It also increases the Doppler velocity limits. Conversely, the higher frequencies yield better resolution for detailed imaging. The tip can be directed by the adjustment of knobs placed at the proximal handle. In most adult probes there are two knobs; one allows anterior and posterior movement and the other permits side-to-side motion. The width of the adult transducer is 10 to 14 mm, miniaturized to 4 mm for pediatric use. The size of the adult probes requires the patient to weigh at least 20 kg.

While single-plane TEE instruments have been extremely useful, biplane devices that allow imaging of the heart and transverse and longitudinal planes provide incremental information. It has been shown that a multiplane TEE examination could in fact be performed using a biplane probe by improvised manipulation of the probe tip.[42] This, however, requires an extensive degree of probe rotation and lateral flexion coupled with bending of the probe tip forward and backward. Such practices prolong the examination time and could result in discomfort to the patient. The advent of multiplane TEE technology allows for easier and more effective imaging of the heart in multiple planes.[43-47] The multiplane transducer rotates 180 degrees. A finger pressure–sensitive switch at the proximal operator end accomplishes rotation of the transducer.

Patient and Echocardiographer Considerations

Preparation of the Anesthetized Patient

In the anesthetized patient, it is advisable to adhere to the following guidelines during TEE. The patient's airway must be protected to minimize the risks of aspiration of pharyngeal and gastric contents. The anesthesiologist must ensure maintenance of reasonable physiologic homeostasis during the stress of placing the TEE probe. This necessitates the use of appropriate physiologic monitoring and may require adjustments in the depth of general anesthesia and application of the techniques of administering local or regional anesthetics. Good communication and cooperation among personnel in the anesthesiology department, surgical personnel, and the echocardiographer are essential to ensure compatibility of TEE examinations with other necessary procedures. This includes not only placement of the probe but temporal organization of the echocardiographic studies and physical arrangement of the additional equipment and personnel (including the relatively bulky echocardiographic machine). A high level of diplomacy may be required, as the space near the head of an anesthetized patient is generally congested and in high demand. Although TEE has generally been accepted as a routine clinical procedure, oral if not written informed consent from the patient is sought at most centers.[48] Because the technique is semiinvasive, a benefit-risk calculation should precede the use of TEE in every individual patient. Operators not familiar with endoscopic techniques should be trained by colleagues experienced in TEE or endoscopy. Contraindications have to be carefully taken into consideration.

Technique of Probe Passage

The TEE probe is introduced in the same manner as a standard gastroscope. The probe is well lubricated and the function of the directional controls is tested prior to insertion. Because the presence of a TEE probe would complicate airway management during anesthetic induction, most anesthesiologists introduce TEE probes in anesthetized patients after tracheal intubation. To improve image quality, it is also useful to evacuate the stomach via suction prior to probe insertion. At scope introduction, the imaging surface of the transducer faces the tongue, which directs the ultrasound beam anteriorly toward the heart when the probe is in the esophagus. The head should be in the midline position with the neck slightly flexed. The endotracheal tube should be positioned to one side of the mouth, commonly the right, to provide sufficient room for the TEE probe. The usual technique is to place the well-lubricated probe in the posterior portion of the oropharynx. Looping the controls and proximal portion of the probe over the operator's neck and shoulder may stabilize the remainder of the probe. The operator's left hand then elevates the mandible by inserting the thumb behind the teeth, grasping the submandibular region with the fingers, and then gently lifting. The probe is then advanced against a slight but even resistance, until a loss of resistance is detected as the tip of the probe passes the inferior constrictor muscle of the pharynx. This usually occurs 10 cm past the lips in neonates to 20 cm past the lips in adults. Further manipulation of the probe is performed under echocardiographic guidance.

Difficult TEE probe insertion may be caused by the probe tip abutting the pyriform sinuses, vallecula, posterior tongue, or an esophageal diverticulum. Overinflation of the endotracheal tube cuff could also obstruct passage of the probe. Maneuvers that might aid the passage of the probe include changing the neck position, realigning the TEE probe, or applying additional jaw thrust to elevate the angles of the mandible. The probe may also be passed with the assistance of laryngoscopy. The probe should never be forced past an obstruction. This could result in airway trauma or esophageal perforation. If all of the aforementioned maneuvers fail, the presence of a pharyngeal or esophageal pathologic condition is suggested, and the procedure should be abandoned to avoid the risk of laceration or perforation of the esophagus.

After completion of the examination, the transducer is rinsed in running water to remove saliva and then immersed in glutaraldehyde solution (Cidex, Surgikos Inc., Arlington, TX) for at least 20 minutes to eradicate bacteria and viruses. The endoscope is then rinsed with tap water and allowed to air-dry. For long-term storage, the TEE scope should not be kept in its carrying case. A vertical wall rack with a clear protective cylinder is the best mechanism for interim storage. The wall rack should be mounted away from extremes of temperature or direct sunlight. While the TEE scope is stored, the transducer tip should be maintained in a straight rather than flexed position.[49]

Safety Guidelines and Contraindications

The patient's medical history, allergies, and medications are reviewed and any history of dysphagia or esophageal disease is investigated. To ensure the continued safety of TEE, the following recommendations are made. The probe should be inspected prior to each insertion for cleanliness and structural integrity. The TEE transducer must be inspected visually and manually for defects in the insulating covering (such as metallic protrusions, holes, dents, abrasions, or cracks). If possible, the electrical isolation should also be checked. Damage to the TEE scope may be prevented or markedly reduced by regular use of a bite-block. In addition to prolonging the life of the scope, the use of a bite-block protects a patient's teeth from damage during the procedure. The probe is inserted gently and, if resistance is met, the procedure is aborted. Minimal transducer energy is used and the image is frozen when not in use. Finally, when not imaging, the probe is left in the neutral, unlocked position to avoid prolonged pressure on the esophageal mucosa.

The need for endocarditis prophylaxis is controversial because no significant bacteremia or endocarditis is encountered with endoscopy unless a biopsy is performed.[50-53] Transient bacteremia, however, has been reported[54] to occur in 7% of TEE procedures and prophylaxis with IV antibiotic agents has been recommended at least for patients with high-risk (e.g., prosthetic valves) and intermediate-risk (e.g., dramatic mitral stenosis) conditions. Systemic antibiotic agents that the patient may be receiving for endocarditis may not adequately cover the oral pathogens introduced during TEE examination. The American Heart Association, however, has categorized endoscopy as a low-risk procedure not necessitating antibiotic agents.[55] Until an official policy is established, it is recommended that physicians follow the guidelines of the infectious disease review committee at their institution.

Absolute contraindications to TEE in intubated patients include esophageal stricture, diverticula, tumor, recent suture lines, and known esophageal interruption. Relative contraindications include symptomatic hiatal hernia, esophagitis, coagulopathy, esophageal varices, and unexplained upper gastrointestinal bleeding. It should be noted that, despite these relative contraindications, TEE has been used in patients undergoing hepatic transplantation without reported sequelae.[56]

Complications

Complications of TEE are rarely encountered. Death was reported in only 1 in 10,218 patients (0.0098%) with successful probe insertion in multicenter European studies,[57] comparable to the mortality rate with esophagogastroduodenoscopy (0.004%).[58, 59] Complications resulting from intraoperative TEE can be separated into two groups: injury from direct trauma to the airway and esophagus, and the indirect effect of TEE. In the first group, potential complications include esophageal bleeding, burning, tearing, and dysphagia. Immediate complications may also include chipped teeth and pharyngeal abrasions, while long-term complications may consist of unilateral vocal cord paralysis and ingestion of glutaraldehyde disinfectant solution.[60] Although in most patients even maximal flexion of the probe will not result in pressures above 17 mmHg, occasionally, even in the absence of esophageal disease, pressures greater than 60 mmHg will result.[61]

Further confirmation of the low incidence of esophageal injury from TEE is apparent in a few case reports of complications. In the world literature, there is only one report of a fatal esophageal perforation (this occurred in a patient with unsuspecting esophageal cancer),[57] and one report of a benign Mallory-Weiss tear following intraoperative TEE.[62] Hulyalkar and Ayd[63] confirmed that the incidence of postoperative occult or frank upper gastrointestinal bleeding was not increased in patients who underwent TEE. Additionally, the incidence of postoperative gastroscopy symptoms was comparable in the patients examined. Even the risk of a postoperative sore throat is more likely to be associated with endotracheal intubation than with TEE.[64]

In one of the earliest studies using TEE, transient vocal cord paralysis was reported in two patients undergoing neurosurgery in the sitting position with the head maximally flexed and with the presence of an armored endotracheal tube.[65] This complication was believed to be due to the pressure that the TEE probe exerted against the larynx. Since this initial report, no further problems of this kind have been reported with the use of the newer equipment. Other potential TEE complications in the adult population include tachy- and bradydysrhythmias,[66-68] possible splenic injury,[66] seizure, vomiting, hypotension,[69] and inability to place or remove the probe.[69-72]

Caution needs to be exercised when performing TEE in the pediatric population. One case report documented aortic compression by the TEE probe in two patients undergoing cardiac surgery.[73] Another case report brought attention to the possibility of bronchial obstruction by the TEE probe in a 5-year-old patient.[74] These cases point out the potential for airway obstruction and cardiovascular compromise when large TEE probes are used in small children. They also emphasize the need for development and availability of small TEE probes for use in this population.

The aforementioned hazards are certainly not the only

safety risks during TEE. Conversion of electrical to ultrasonic energy in the transducer also produces some heating, and the temperature of the transducer may rise above body temperature.[75, 76] To minimize the remote possibility of esophageal burns, the transmitter power supply to the transducer should always be kept to that minimum consistent with good image quality. During cooling on cardiopulmonary bypass, the temperature gradient between transducer and esophageal mucosa might become larger than is desirable, especially if circulatory insufficiency or shock compromises perfusion of the esophageal mucosa. It is recommended that the transmitting power be turned off during cardiopulmonary bypass when TEE monitoring is unnecessary.

The second group of complications that result from TEE includes hemodynamic and pulmonary effects of airway manipulation and, particularly for new TEE operators, distraction from patient care. Fortunately, in the anesthetized patient there are rarely hemodynamic consequences to esophageal placement of the probe, and there are no studies that specifically address this question. Most important for the anesthesiologist are the problems of distraction from patient care. Although these reports have not appeared in the literature, we have heard of several endotracheal tube disconnections during TEE that went unnoticed to the point of desaturation. Additionally, there have been instances in which severe hemodynamic abnormalities have been missed because of fascination with the images or the controls of the echocardiograph. It behooves new echo operators to enlist the assistance of an associate to watch the patient during the echo examination. After sufficient experience has been gained, the assistance of this associate will become unnecessary.

Training, Certification, and Quality Assurance

At present, no absolute minimum training criteria to perform intraoperative TEE have been established. A task force from the American College of Physicians, the American College of Cardiology, and the American Heart Association created the initial guidelines.[77] These guidelines are not specific for intraoperative echocardiography and were created by a group without representation by anesthesiologists. It was the position of this group that no distinction between intraoperative and nonintraoperative echocardiography should be made. Since its introduction to the operating room in the early 1980s, however, TEE has been increasingly utilized as an important technique for facilitating the hemodynamic management of patients during general anesthesia and accepted as an important diagnostic modality during cardiac surgery. In recognition of this fact, the American Society of Echocardiography (ASE) established the Council for Intraoperative Echocardiography in 1993 to serve as a forum to address issues related to the use of echocardiography in the operating room. In 1997, the council board decided to create a set of guidelines establishing what it considers a comprehensive intraoperative TEE examination.[78]

Despite the problems with defining competence, it is clear that intraoperative TEE is a new field in which anesthesiologists need specific training. Ideally, this training should begin with the dedicated training period. This is most easily accomplished during a cardiac fellowship but can be done by postgraduate physicians as well. Frequently, a symbiotic relationship with the cardiology division can be established in which the anesthesiologist can teach the fundamentals of airway management, operating room physiology, and the use of local anesthetics while learning the principles of echocardiography from the cardiologists.

The merger of the Society of Cardiovascular Anesthesiolo-

gists (SCA) examination and the ASE examination created the National Board of Echocardiography (NBE). NBE has worked in collaboration with the National Board of Medical Examiners (NBME) to develop an examination to allow physicians to test and demonstrate their knowledge of perioperative TEE based on an objective standard.

Quality assurance is another area for which no specific guidelines currently exist. It is clear that each intraoperative study should be recorded in a standardized manner and accompanied by a written report that becomes part of the patient's chart. Furthermore, TEE images should be copied and included in the chart, and careful records of any complications should be maintained. To ensure that the proper images are being obtained and that the interpretations are correct, the studies should be periodically reviewed. The relationship between cardiology and anesthesiology can be productive in this area as well.

Imaging and Echocardiographic Anatomic Considerations

Thorough knowledge of the heart as a complex, 3-D structure is necessary to make sense of the 2-D, planar images obtained with TEE (Figs. 15–5 through 15–8, see color Figures). The key to optimizing the benefit of intraoperative echocardiography is a thorough, systematic examination on every patient for whom TEE is used. A significant impact on patient management is occasionally made by unexpected findings, which turn up regularly. Merely focusing the examination on the supposed lesion of interest causes sonographic tunnel vision. This can lead to missed or improper diagnoses and can result in mismanagement. Routinely performing a complete examination also maximizes the echocardiographer's exposure and experience to normal and abnormal findings. This allows a more rapid attainment of ability to make judgments about the significance of what is seen.

Focusing one's attention on one particular structure at a time, such as one chamber or valve, enables performance of a coherent and competent echo examination. In order for one to fully appreciate the 3-D extent of the heart, utilizing 2-D echocardiography, the imaging plane must be moved, or swept, through the entire 3-D extent of the structure to examine it completely. This is done in the horizontal imaging planes by moving the probe up and down (proximally and distally) in the esophagus, and in the vertical planes by rotating it to the left or right.[79] Each structure should be examined in multiple imaging planes and from more than one transducer position.

The following terminology has been suggested by the ASE council to describe manipulation of the probe and transducer during the image acquisition.[78] *Advancing* the transducer means pushing the tip of the probe distally into the esophagus or stomach. *Withdrawing* the probe means pulling the tip in the opposite direction more approximately. Rotating the probe within the esophagus clockwise from interior to the patient's right will be called *turning to the right,* and rotating the probe clockwise in the opposite direction, *turning to the left.* Flexing the tip of the probe anteriorly with the large control wheel will be called *anteflexing,* and flexing it posteriorly in the opposite direction, *retroflexing.* Flexing the tip of the probe to the patient's right with the small control wheel will be called *flexing to the right,* and flexing in the opposite direction, *flexing to the left.* Finally, axially rotating the multiplane angle from 0 degree toward 180 degrees will be called *rotating forward,* and rotating in the opposite direction toward 0 degree will be called *rotating back.*

Although many recommendations exist as to the proper method of performing a complete TEE examination, it is important to keep in mind that the examination varies from examiner to examiner and institution to institution. In general, examination of a structure need not be performed continuously or completed before moving onto the next structure but may be broken up into different parts of the study for greater efficiency. For example, many will find it more practical to obtain all the midesophageal views before proceeding to the transgastric views. The examination, however, may be performed with an anatomic foundation (i.e., progressing from structure to structure within the heart) in order to provide a systematic approach. The cross-sectional views described are generally obtainable in most patients. Individual anatomic variation, however, can prevent ideal visualization in some patients. Because most of the structures to be examined are present in more than one cross section, a complete and comprehensive examination can still be performed in most patients.

Despite the lack of a standardized imaging protocol, the ASE council is in the process of releasing an outline of standardized images that should be acquired in a routine examination. As mentioned earlier, the order in which these images are obtained is left to individual practitioners, depending on their specific training and experience. It has been suggested that these views be divided into two general categories based upon where the transesophageal transducer lies within the alimentary tract, midesophageal or transgastric, with the preponderance of images being obtained in the midesophageal view. The great vessel windows are defined with relation to which specific portions of the aorta are being visualized. It is also helpful to divide the heart into coronal sections to further aid in the understanding of specific anatomic structures and their relationships with each

other. This is most applicable to studies of the LV. The segmental anatomy is divided into the basal, midpapillary, and apical levels. By combining these classifications with a description of the plane being obtained (i.e., transverse versus longitudinal), the echocardiographer has a mechanism to communicate findings with colleagues and to focus an examination as indicated by the initial findings. Table 15–3 lists the recommended views and the respective anatomic structures visualized.[78]

Comprehensive Transesophageal Echocardiographic Examination

What follows is a description of the examination suggested by the ASE council[78] of individual structures in the heart and great vessels, emphasizing the standard cross-sectional views that demonstrate each particular structure. In practice, however, performance of the examination will become a fusion of the structural and cross-sectional approaches tailored to individual preferences in training.

Left Ventricle

Ideally, multiple views from different transducer locations in long axis and short axis, global function, and regional wall motion will maximize the evaluation of the LV (Fig. 15–9, see color Figures) (Fig. 15–10). This can be accomplished quickly and easily in most patients using multiplane TEE by obtaining five standard views of the LV, three from the midesophageal window and two from the transgastric window.

Segmental models of the LV are needed to accurately describe a location and extent of regional wall motion abnor-

Table 15–3. Transesophageal Echocardiography Cross-Sectional Views

Window	Cross Section	Angle Range (degrees)	Structures Imaged
Midesophageal	Four-chamber	0–20	LV, LA, RV, MV, TV, IAS
	Mitral commissural	60–70	MV, LV, LA
	Two-chamber	80–100	LV, LA, LAA, MV, CS
	RV long axis	130–160	LV, LA, AV, LVOT, MV, ascending aorta
	AV short axis	70–90	RV, RA, TV, RVOT, PV
	Bicaval	30–60	AV, IAS
Transgastric	Basilar ventricular		
	Short axis	0–20	LV, MV
	Two-chamber	80–100	LV, MV, chordae tendineae, papillary muscles, CS
	Long axis	100–130	LVOT, AV, MV
	Midpapillary		
	Short axis	0–20	LV, RV, papillary muscles
	Two-chamber	80–100	LV, LA, papillary muscles
	RV long axis	100–120	RV, TV, RA, RVOT, PV
	Apical ventricular		
	Short axis	0–20	LV
	Long axis	0–20 (anteflexion)	LVOT, AV, MV
Great vessel	Ascending aorta		
	Short axis	0–30	Ascending aorta, SVC, PA, RPA
	Long axis	90–120	Ascending aorta, RPA
	Aortic arch		
	Short axis	90	Aortic arch, left brachiocephalic vein
	Long axis	0	Aortic arch, PA, PV, left brachiocephalic vein
	Descending aorta		
	Short axis	0	Descending thoracic aorta, left pleural space
	Long axis	90	Descending thoracic aorta, left pleural space

LV, left ventricle; LA, left atrium; RV, right ventricle; MV, mitral valve; TV, tricuspid valve; IAS, interatrial septum; LAA, left atrial appendage; CS, coronary sinus; AV, aortic valve; LVOT, left ventricular outflow tract; RVOT, right ventricular outflow tract; PV, pulmonary vein; SVC, superior vena cava; PA, pulmonary artery; RPA, right pulmonary artery.

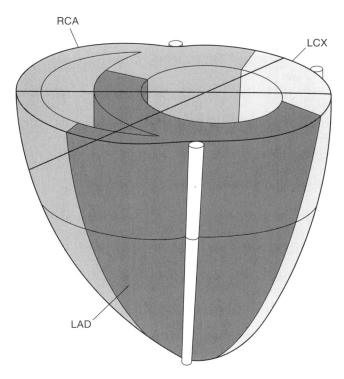

Figure 15–10. Schematic of ventricles with representation of coronary perfusion. RCA, right coronary artery; LAD, left anterior descending coronary artery; LCX, left circumflex coronary artery.

malities (RWMAs) detected by echocardiography, as well as correlating them with coronary artery anatomy. The development of biplane and then multiplane TEE has made imaging of the entire LV possible in most patients, justifying the use of more comprehensive segmental models. The ASE has recommended a 16-segment model for the LV dividing the basal and midlevels each into six segments and the apex into four. Another advantage of using this segmental model is that it promotes a common terminology among anesthesiologists, surgeons, and cardiologists in discussions about RWMAs of the LV.

As suggested by the council, the first step in obtaining the midesophageal views of the LV is to position the transducer posterior to the LA at the midlevel of the mitral valve (MV). The imaging plane is then oriented to simultaneously pass through the center of the mitral annulus and the apex of the LV. In many patients, the esophagus is lateral to this point and the tip of the probe must be flexed to the right to position the transducer directly posterior to the center of the mitral annulus. The LV is usually oriented with its apex somewhat more inferior than the base, and the tip of the probe must next be retroflexed to direct the imaging plane through the apex. Getting the proper amount of retroflexion is most easily accomplished by rotating to multiplane angle 90 degrees and then retroflexing until the apex of the LV is pointing straight down in the image display. The depth should be adjusted to include the entire LV, usually 16 cm. Care should be taken to avoid foreshortening of the ventricle. Rotating to multiplane angle 0 degree should keep the center of the mitral annulus and LV apex in view. The *midesophageal four-chamber view* can be obtained by rotating the multiplane angle forward from 0 degree until the aortic valve is no longer in view and the diameter of the tricuspid annulus is maximized (Figs. 15–11 and 15–12, see color Figures) (Figs. 15–13 and 15–14). This view usually presents between 10 to 30 degrees. The midesophageal four-chamber

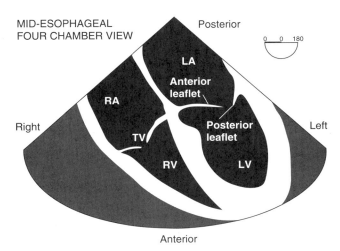

Figure 15–13. Schematic of midesophageal four chamber view.

view shows all three segments in each of the septal and lateral walls. The *midesophageal two-chamber view* can next be obtained by rotating the multiplane angle forward until the RA and the right ventricle (RV) disappear, usually between 90 and 110 degrees. The midesophageal two-chamber view of the LV shows the three segments in each of the anterior and inferior walls (Fig. 15–15). Finally, rotating the multiplane angle forward until the LV outflow tract, aortic valve, and the proximal ascending aorta come into view, usually between 130 and 160 degrees, develops the *midesophageal long axis view*. This view shows the basal and midanteroseptal segments, as well as the basal and midposterior segments. One can examine the entire LV without moving the probe, assuming the imaging plane is properly oriented through the center of the mitral annulus and the LV apex, simply by rotating the multiplane angle from 0 to 180 degrees.

The transgastric views of the LV suggested by the council are acquired by advancing the probe into the stomach and

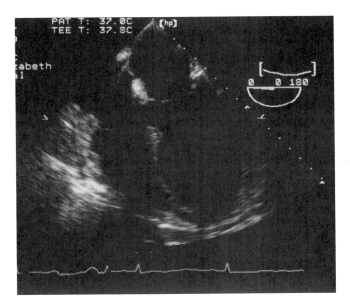

Figure 15–14. Midesophageal four-chamber view. (Courtesy of Kristine J. Hirsch, M.D., Halifax, NS, Canada.)

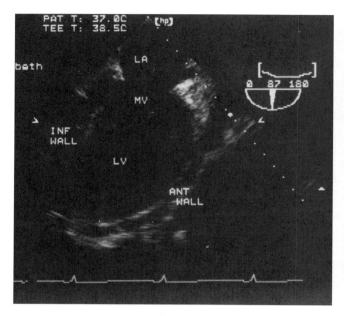

Figure 15–15. Midesophageal two-chamber view. (Courtesy of Kristine J. Hirsch, M.D., Halifax, NS, Canada.)

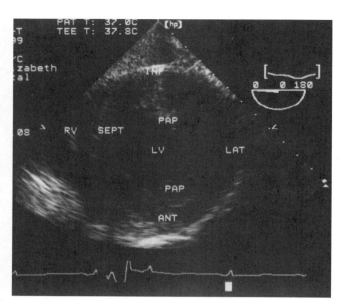

Figure 15–18. Transgastric short axis midpapillary view. (Courtesy of Kristine J. Hirsch, M.D., Halifax, NS, Canada.)

anteflexing the tip until the heart comes into view. At multiplane angle 0 degree, a short axis of the LV should appear and the probe is then turned to the right or left as needed to center the LV in the display. Again, the depth should be adjusted to include the entire LV, usually 12 cm. Next, the transducer is rotated forward to multiplane angle 90 degrees. This view should show the LV in the long axis with the apex to the left and the mitral annulus to the right of the display. The anteflexion of the probe should be adjusted until the long axis of the LV is horizontal on the display, taking care not to foreshorten the ventricle. Note the level on the LV over which the transducer (vertex of the image display) is located—basal, mid, or apical—and advance or withdraw the probe as needed to the midpapillary level. Now rotate back to multiplane angle 0 degree and the *transgastric short axis midpapillary view* will appear (Fig.

15–16, see color Figures) (Fig. 15–17 and 15–18). In some patients, advancing the probe develops *the apical transgastric short axis view* (Figs. 15–19, 15–20, 15–21, see color Figures) (Figs. 15–22 and 15–23).but in many the probe moves away from the heart and the image is lost. Withdrawing the probe until the mitral apparatus comes into view develops the *basal transgastric short axis view*. The transgastric short axis views have the disadvantage of showing only one level of the LV at a time. This view, however, has the advantage of simultaneously showing portions of the LV supplied by the right, circumflex, and the left anterior descending coronary arteries and is the most popular view for monitoring purposes (i.e., the midpapillary view). The size of the LV should be assessed for dilation and hypertrophy. At end-diastole, which is best determined by measuring at the onset of the R wave of the electrocardiogram (ECG), the normal LV diameter is less than 5.5 cm and the LV wall thickness is less than 1.2 cm. The *transgastric two-chamber*

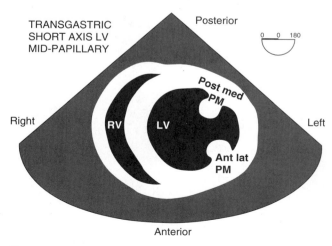

Figure 15–17. Schematic of transgastric short axis midpapillary view.

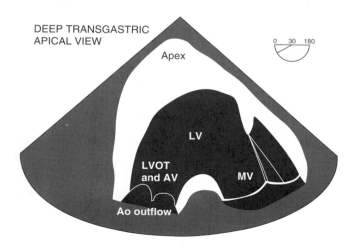

Figure 15–22. Schematic of deep transgastric apical view.

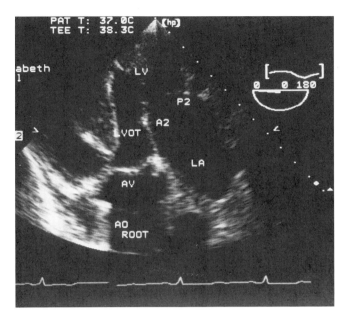

Figure 15-23. Deep transgastric apical view. (Courtesy of Kristine J. Hirsch, M.D.)

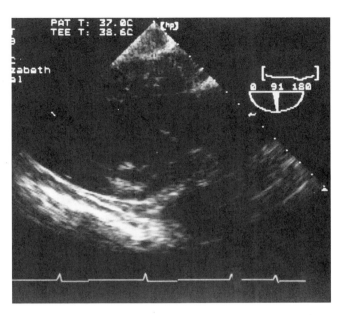

Figure 15-26. Transgastric LV long axis view. (Courtesy of Kristine J. Hirsch, M.D.)

view is developed by rotating the multiplane angle forward until the apex in the mitral annulus comes into view, usually close to 90 degrees (Fig. 15-24, see color Figures) (Figs. 15-25 and 15-26). The probe should be turned to the left or right as needed to open the LV chamber, that is, maximize its size in the image. This view usually shows the basal and midsegments of the inferior and anterior walls, but frequently not the apex.[78]

Mitral Valve

Under certain circumstances, such as during an MV repair procedure, a thorough echocardiographic anatomic examination of the mitral apparatus, delineating the nature and the location of the existent pathologic changes, becomes a necessity. A multiplane TEE examination is best suited to achieve this goal. Color-flow, pulsed-wave, and continuous-wave Doppler are necessary to find and quantitate the regurgitant or stenotic lesion. A thorough 2-D examination, however, of the entire MV is required (Fig. 15-27). As this examination is performed, the relationship of the chordal attachments between the papillary muscle and leaflets should be remembered and used to define the anatomic location of the leaflets visualized. The mitral leaflet section can be defined by visualizing a papillary or chordal attachment to a leaflet. Using multiple views, the leaflet surface anatomy is defined. In this section, the MV nomenclature proposed by Carpentier et al.[80] will be referred to as the MV anatomy is defined. This nomenclature is based on

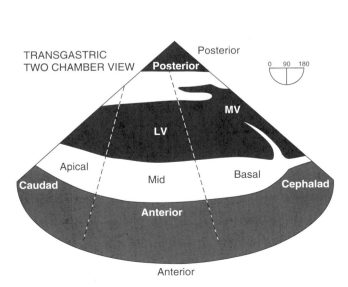

Figure 15-25. Schematic of transgastric LV long-axis view with segmental designations.

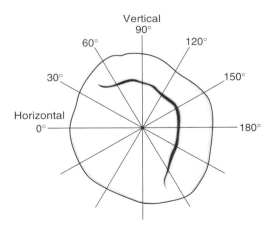

Figure 15-27. Schematic of the mitral valve with the intersect lines produced by multiplane TEE rotational scanning.

- Dividing the structures into what is perceived by the surgeon who observes the valve through a left atriotomy.

- The structures of the mitral apparatus in this orientation are defined as being anterior (A) or posterior (P) and being left or right as viewed by this surgical view; left-sided structures are noted by the numeral 1, and progressing to the right-sided structures, by the numeral 3.

Midesophageal Views

At the midesophageal level of the heart, five views are studied: (1) three-chamber view at 0 degree, (2) four-chamber view at 0 degree, (3) modified two-chamber view at 40 to 80 degrees, (4) two-chamber view, and (5) long axis view at 110 to 116 degrees.[81-83]

Three-Chamber View. The three-chamber view is obtained by advancing the TEE probe about 1 cm below the aortic valve basal view at 0 degree. This brings into view the left ventricular outflow tract (LVOT), LA, MV, LV, and a portion of the RV (Figs. 15–14 and 15–30; see color Figures 15–28 and 15–29.) In order for the plane of the TEE scan to pass through the LVOT, the scan must pass through an area in the region of basal A2 to the tip of A1 and the lateral portion of P2. The ventricular wall on the right of this screen is lateral to the anterolateral papillary muscle. This view often shows the chordae tendineae connecting the anterolateral papillary muscle to the anterior and posterior leaflet.

Four-Chamber View. From the three-chamber view, the probe is advanced slightly and anteflexed to obtain the classic four-chamber view at 0 degree as described above. The LVOT is no longer seen. The LA, LV, RA, and RV are seen. The papillary muscle, when seen, is again the anterolateral papillary muscle. To obtain this view, a plane must pass through the lateral base of A2 cutting through the tip of A1 and reaching more laterally to P2 and P3. The LV wall to the right of the screen is lateral and to the left is septal.

Modified Two-Chamber View. The modified two-chamber (commissural) view (Fig. 15–31) is best obtained by rotating the plane of the probe 40 to 80 degrees from the

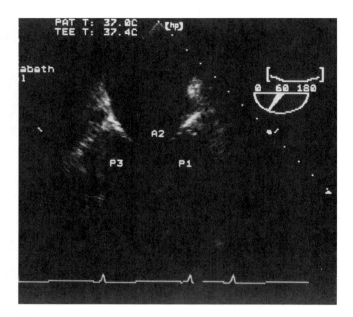

Figure 15–31. Midesophageal mitral valve commissural view with Carpentier designations of scallops. (Courtesy of Kristine J. Hirsch, M.D.)

three-chamber view. The goal is to obtain a view in which the three leaflet segments of the MV are seen: P3 on the left of the screen, P1 on the right, and the tip of A2 moving in and out between them during systole and diastole. With appropriate rotation of the probe, both the anterolateral and posteromedial papillary muscles with their chordal attachments are seen.

Two-Chamber View. The two-chamber view is obtained by further rotation of the plane of the probe between 80 and 100 degrees. The medial scallop of the posterior leaflet (P2) is seen on the left of the screen and the anterior leaflet on the right. The papillary muscle visualized on the left of the screen is the posteromedial papillary muscle.

Longitudinal View. The longitudinal axis view is obtained by rotating the plane of the probe between 110 and 140 degrees from the two-chamber view. This gives the best middle slice through A2 and P2. The middle scallop of the posterior leaflet is seen on the left of the screen and the middle portion of the anterior leaflet is seen on the right.

Transgastric Views

Basilar Ventricular Views. After examining the four-chamber view the probe is advanced until the transducer is to the level of the base of the LV. Further anteflexion, or rotation of the plane of the probe 0 to 15 degrees may be needed to obtain the classic "fish mouth" view of the MV orifice (Fig. 15–32). The anterior leaflet is seen on the left side of the screen, the posterior leaflet on the right, the medial commissure on the upper left of the screen, and lateral commissure on the lower right. With practice, color-flow Doppler can often be used to reveal the portion of the mitral leaflet coaptation where regurgitation occurs. An area of leaflet prolapse may be appreciated.

Rotation of the plane of the probe to 90 degrees often allows visualization of both papillary muscles and their chordal attachments to the MV leaflets. If both are not visual-

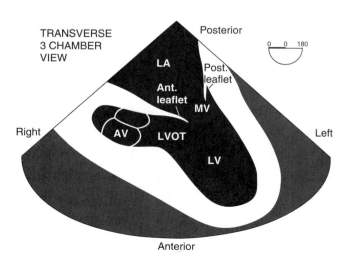

Figure 15–30. Schematic of midesophageal three-chamber view.

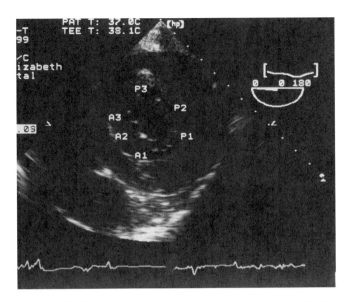

Figure 15–32. Transgastric basal view of mitral valve with Carpentier designations of scallops. (Courtesy of Kristine J. Hirsch, M.D., Halifax, NS, Canada.)

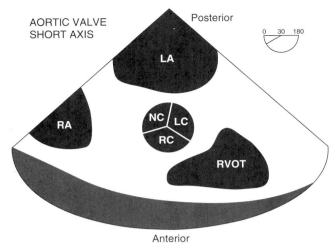

Figure 15–35. Schematic of aortic valve short axis view.

ized, they may be brought into view by rightward or leftward motion. Caution must be used in defining that MV leaflets are seen. In this view, posteromedial cords are seen overlapping anterior and posterior leaflet portions of A2, P2, and P3, as well as the medial commissure. Anterolateral cords are seen overlapping anterior and posterior leaflet portions of A1, P1, and P2, as well as the lateral commissure. This view is helpful in defining from which papillary muscle torn chordae originate (and hence what portion of the leaflet) and for assessing LV papillary muscle contractile function.

In this 90-degree view, the LVOT is often visualized in the lower right-hand corner. This provides access for measuring Doppler flow velocities across the LVOT and aortic valve for measuring gradient and continuity equation calculations.

Midventricular View. Advancing the probe further to 0 degree provides a *midpapillary muscle transgastric view of the LV and RV.* The location of the papillary muscle and determination of the number of heads is important here. This view is also very helpful in defining from which papillary muscle torn chordae originate (and hence what portion of the leaflet) and for assessing LV papillary muscle contractile function. This view is very similar to the basilar ventricular view and may be used to further delineate the anatomy of the MV and its associated structures.

Aortic Valve, Aortic Root, and Left Ventricular Outflow Tract

The aortic valve (AV) is a trileaflet, semilunar valve located close to the center of the heart. The aortic root includes the aortic valve annulus where it meets the LV, the AV itself, the sinuses of Valsalva, the coronary artery ostia, and the proximal ascending aorta. The LVOT is the outflow portion of the LV just proximal to the AV. The council recommends that all these structures be examined in detail with TEE using four standard cross-sectional views.

The *midesophageal AV short axis view* is obtained from the midesophageal window at 0-degree rotation (horizontal

plane), by advancing or withdrawing the probe until the AV comes into view (Figs. 15–33 and 15–34, see color Figures) (Figs. 15–35 and 15–36). The probe is then turned to the left or right as needed to bring the AV into the centerline of the display. Image depth is adjusted to bring the AV to the midrange of the image, usually 10 to 12 cm. The multiplane angle is then rotated forward until a symmetric image of the three leaflets of the AV comes into view. This view of the AV usually presents at about 30 to 60 degrees. This cross section is the only view that provides a simultaneous image of all three cusps of the AV. The leaflet adjacent to the atrial septum is the noncoronary cusp, the most anterior leaflet is the right coronary cusp, and the leaflet to the right side of the display from the other two is the left coronary cusp. In this window, it is important to evaluate the valve carefully in both systole and diastole. Each leaflet should be examined to

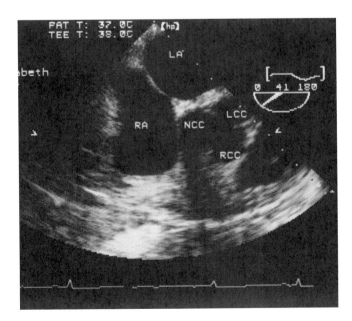

Figure 15–36. Aortic valve short axis view with anatomic designations of cusps. RCC, right coronary cusp; LCC, left coronary cusp; NCC, noncoronary cusp. (Courtesy of Kristine J. Hirsch, M.D., Halifax, NS, Canada.)

ensure independent movement throughout the cardiac cycle. Withdrawing the probe slightly will sweep the imaging plane superiorly just distal to the AV leaflets and bring the right and left coronary ostia into view, followed by the sinotubular junction in the short axis as the probe is further withdrawn. Advancing the probe through and then inferior to the AV will produce the short axis view of the LVOT. The midesophageal short axis view at the level of the AV leaflets can be used to measure the area of the AV by planimetry. Color-flow Doppler should be applied to this cross section to detect the presence, severity, and location of aortic regurgitation.

The *midesophageal long-axis view* of the AV is developed by keeping the AV in the centerline of the display wall and rotating forward until the LVOT, AV, and proximal ascending aorta line up in the image (Fig. 15–37, see color Figures) (Figs. 15–38 and 15–39). This usually exists at a multiplane angle of 120 to 160 degrees. The leaflet of the AV seen anteriorly or toward the bottom of the display is always the right coronary cusp. The leaflet seen posteriorly, however, in this cross section may be the left or the noncoronary cusp, depending on the exact location of the imaging plane as it passes through the valve. This is the best cross section for assessing the size of the aortic root by considering the diameters of the AV annulus, the sinuses of Valsalva, sinotubular junction, and proximal ascending aorta. Color-flow Doppler applied to this view allows detection of flow abnormalities in the LVOT, AV, and proximal ascending aorta.

The primary purpose of the two transgastric views of the AV is to direct the Doppler beam parallel to flow through the AV, which is not possible from the midesophageal window. They also provide good images of the ventricular aspect of the AV in some patients. The *basilar ventricular long axis view* is developed from the *basilar ventricular short axis view* by rotating the multiplane angle forward until the AV comes into view, usually 90 to 120 degrees. It may be necessary to turn the probe slightly to the right to help achieve the desired imaging plane orientation.

The transgastric ventricular views are obtained by advancing the probe deep into the stomach and positioning the probe adjacent to the LV apex. Flexing the probe anteriorly from this position develops the *transgastric ventricular long axis view* in many patients. The exact position of the probe and transducer is more difficult to determine and control

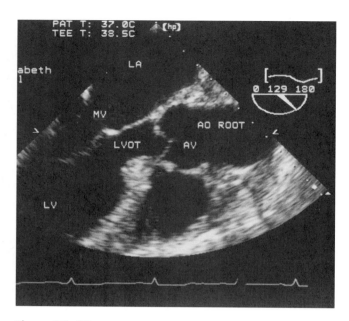

Figure 15–39. Longitudinal ascending aorta long axis view. (Courtesy of Kristine J. Hirsch, M.D., Halifax, NS, Canada.)

deep in the stomach, but some trial-and-error flexing, turning, advancing, withdrawing, and rotating of the probe result in development of this view in most patients. In the transgastric ventricular long axis view, the aortic valve is located in the far field at the bottom of the display, with LV outflow directed away from the transducer. Detailed assessment of valve anatomy is difficult in this view because the LVOT and AV are so far from the transducer, but, as has been alluded earlier, Doppler quantitation of flow velocities in the structures is usually possible.

LVOT flow is measured by placing the pulsed-wave Doppler sample volume just to the ventricular aspect of the aortic valve leaflets. Normal LVOT flow velocities are less than 1 m/s. Flow velocity through the AV is measured by directing the continuous-wave Doppler beam through the LVOT across the valve (Fig. 15–40). Color-flow Doppler imaging of the LVOT and AV may be helpful in directing the Doppler

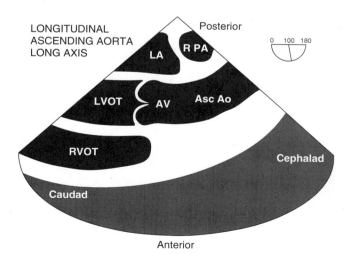

Figure 15–38. Schematic of longitudinal ascending aorta long axis view.

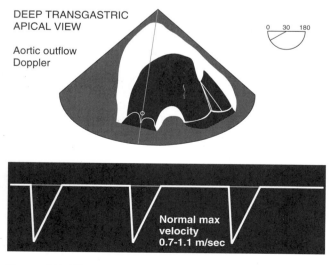

Figure 15–40. Schematic of deep transgastric apical view aortic outflow continuous-wave Doppler interrogation.

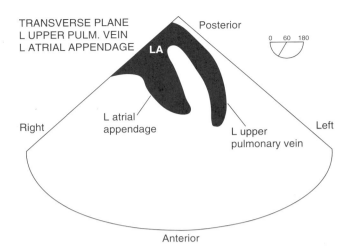

Figure 15-42. Schematic of left upper pulmonary vein and left atrial appendage.

beam through the area of maximum flow velocity in the AV.[78]

Left Atrium, Left Atrial Appendage, Pulmonary Veins, and Atrial Septum

Initial examination of the LA consists of a midesophageal four-chamber view with the multiplane angle at or near 0 degree and the image depth limited to approximately 10 cm. This allows optimal magnification of the LA near-field images. The LA is the chamber closest to the transducer and therefore appears at the top of the image display. After the LA is identified, the probe can be withdrawn several centimeters, then advanced several centimeters to image the entire LA from its most superior to most inferior extent. Near its superior and lateral aspect, the LA is seen to join the LAA (Fig. 15-41, see color Figures) (Figs. 15-42 and 15-43). The LAA may appear as a separate echolucent structure. This depends on the exact position and orientation of the trans-

ducer in the esophagus. Its continuity with the body of the LA, however, can be easily established with minor adjustments in probe position. The left upper pulmonary vein (LUPV) is identified by slightly withdrawing and turning the probe to the left. The LUPV is noted as an echolucent structure entering the LA from an anterior to posterior trajectory, just lateral to the LAA. Turning slightly further to the left and advancing 1 to 2 cm then identifies the left lower pulmonary vein (LLPV) (Fig. 15-44, see color Figures) (Fig. 15-45). Note that the LLPV enters the LA just below the LUPV and courses in a more lateral-to-medial direction. Consequently, flow within the LLPV tends to be at right angles to a Doppler beam originating from the TEE transducer, and thus is less suitable for quantitative spectral analysis. Imaging of the right upper pulmonary vein (RUPV) is then accomplished by turning the probe to the right at the level of the LAA. Like the LUPV, the RUPV can be seen to enter the LA in an anterior-to-posterior direction. The right lower pulmonary vein (RLPV) is then located by advancing the probe 1 to 2 cm farther as well as slightly turning the probe to the right. Like the LLPV, the RLPV enters the LA at right angles to the Doppler beam. Color-flow Doppler can be utilized to assist in identification of the pulmonary veins (PVs) as they enter the LA. The interatrial septum (IAS) is next examined at the midesophageal level by turning the probe slightly to the right of midline and withdrawing and advancing the probe to sweep through the entire superior-inferior extent of the structure. It consists of the thin fossa ovalis centrally and the thicker limbus regions anteriorly and posteriorly. The IAS should also be examined with color-flow Doppler to detect interatrial shunts. A definite identification of an interatrial shunt, however, may require the assistance of injected agitated saline (or other contrast agent), used in combination with a Valsalva maneuver.

The multiplane angle should next be rotated forward to about 90 degrees to the midesophageal two-chamber view to obtain orthogonal views of the LA, again limiting image depth to focus on the LA, LAA, and PVs. In this cross section, the LAA can be examined from its left-to-right limits by turning the probe from side to side. The LAA usually is seen clearly as an outpouching of the anterosuperior aspect of the LA. Turning the probe to the right and adjusting the multiplane angle until both the SVC and IVC come into view (~100-120 degrees) develops the *midesophageal bicaval view,* generally the most complete view of the IAS (Fig.

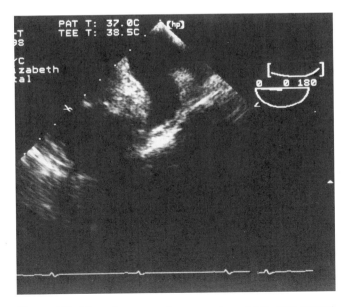

Figure 15-43. Left upper pulmonary vein and left atrial appendage. (Courtesy of Kristine J. Hirsch, M.D., Halifax, NS, Canada.)

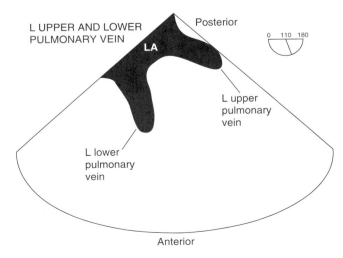

Figure 15-45. Schematic of left upper and lower pulmonary veins.

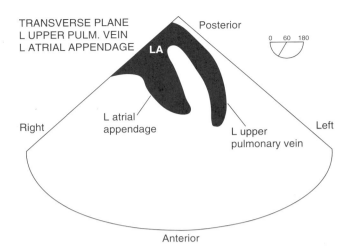

15–46, see color Figures) (Figs. 15–47 and 15–48). This view should be repeated with color-flow Doppler, and the other aforementioned methods to detect interatrial shunts. Finally, turning the probe slightly farther to the right will reveal the RUPV entering the LA.

The PV inflow should be examined by placing the pulsed-wave Doppler sample volume into any of the PVs 0.5 to 1.0 cm proximal to the LA. The LUPV is usually the easiest to identify and the most parallel to the Doppler beam. Once again, color-flow Doppler imaging may be useful in identifying PV flow and aligning the Doppler beam parallel to the flow.[78]

Right Ventricle

TEE examination of the RV should assess chamber size and function. Dilation of the RV with severe hypokinesia or akinesia of the RV free wall characterizes global RV dysfunction. Because of the asymmetry of the RV geometry and reduced muscular mass as compared to the LV, the contractile amplitude of the RV is less than that seen with the LV. Subtle regional dysfunction, therefore, is more difficult to diagnose, requiring either akinesia or dyskinesia to clearly establish the diagnosis of regional dysfunction.

The council recommends an examination of the RV utilizing four cross-sectional views: the *midesophageal RV four-chamber view*, the *midesophageal RV long-axis view*, the *transgastric short-axis view*, and the *transgastric RV long-axis view*. The midesophageal RV four-chamber view is obtained from the standard four-chamber view by turning the probe to the right until the tricuspid valve is in the center of the display. The image depth is adjusted to include the tricuspid annulus and the RV apex. This cross section shows the apical portion of the RV free wall to the right of the display and the basilar anterior free wall to the left. The midesophageal RV long axis view is developed by rotating forward, keeping the tricuspid valve visible until the right ventricular outflow tract (RVOT) opens up and the pulmonary valve and main pulmonary artery (PA) come into view. This usually becomes evident between 60 and 80 degrees. This cross section shows the conus region of the free wall of the RV to the right side of the display and the inferior portion of the anterior free wall to the left. RV end-diastolic and end-systolic areas of these views may be measured to calculate the fractional area of change as a gauge of RV function.

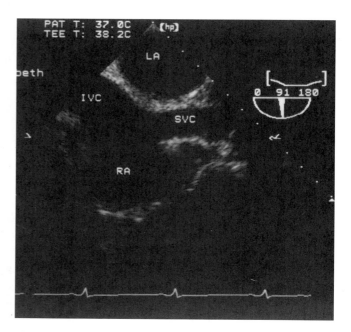

Figure 15–48. Bicaval view. (Courtesy of Kristine J. Hirsch, M.D., Halifax, NS, Canada.)

In the transgastric short axis view, the RV is seen to the left side of the display from the LV. The transgastric RV long-axis view is developed from this point by turning the probe to the right until the RV is located in the centerline of the display. This is followed by forward rotation until the apex of the RV appears in the left side of the display, usually about 100 to 120 degrees. This cross section provides good views of the posterior or diaphragmatic portion of the RV free wall, which is located in the near field.[78]

Tricuspid Valve

The tricuspid valve (TV) is composed of three leaflets (anterior, posterior, and septal), chordae tendineae, papillary muscles, annulus, and walls of the RV. In the esophageal four-chamber view, the TV is seen with the septal leaflet to the right of the display and the anterior leaflet to the left. The probe is advanced and withdrawn to sweep the imaging plane through the tricuspid annulus from its inferior to superior extent. Next, keeping the tricuspid annulus in the center of the display, the multiplane angle is rotated forward to develop the *midesophageal RV inflow-outflow view* (Fig. 15–49, see color Figures) (Figs. 15–50 and 15–51). This view presents the posterior leaflet to the left side of the display of the valve and the anterior leaflet to the right. These views are repeated with the color-flow Doppler to detect flow abnormalities of the TV.

The transgastric views of the TV are made by advancing the probe into the stomach and developing the *transgastric RV inflow view* as previously described. This cross section shows the TV with the RV to the left of the display and the RA to the right. This view also usually provides the best images of the tricuspid chordae tendineae, as they are perpendicular to the ultrasound beam. A short-axis view of the TV is developed by withdrawing the probe slightly toward the base of the heart until the tricuspid annulus is in the center of the display. This is followed by rotating the multiplane angle backward to about 30 degrees. In this cross section, the anterior leaflet is to the left in the far field, the posterior leaflet is to the left in the near field, and the septal

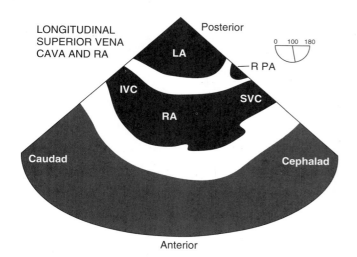

Figure 15–47. Schematic of bicaval window.

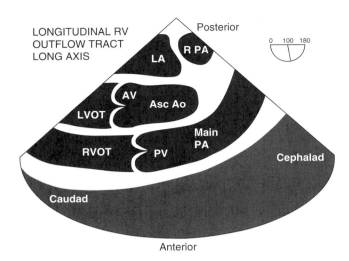

Figure 15-50. Schematic of longitudinal RV outflow tract long axis imaging plane.

leaflet is visible to the right side of the valve image. These views are repeated with color-flow Doppler of the valve.[84]

Right Atrium

The RA is well seen from the midesophageal window because of its close proximity to the esophagus. Typically, the midesophageal four-chamber view allows a direct comparison of the relative sizes of the RA and LA. Turning the probe to the right to the midesophageal RV four-chamber view brings the RA into the center of the display. Advancing and withdrawing the probe allow imaging of its entire inferior-to-superior extent. The midesophageal bicaval view (see Fig. 15-48), discussed earlier, provides good images of the RA appendage anteriorly. Turning the probe to the right and the left from the medial to the lateral borders of the RA completes its examination. The RA wall is typically thinner than the LA wall. The eustachian valve, a normal structure of variable size, is seen at the junction of the IVC and the RA. It is an embryologic remnant whose purpose was to direct flow across the then patent foramen ovale. It is formed by a fold of endocardium that arises from the lower end of the crista terminalis as it stretches across the posterior margin of the IVC to become continuous with the border of the fossa ovalis. Occasionally, the eustachian valve has mobile, serpiginous filaments attached to it, termed the *Chiari network,* which is considered a variation of normal. The venae cavae may be examined by sweeping from their junctions with the RA to their proximal portions by advancing or withdrawing the probe as appropriate. Frequently, venous catheters or pacemaker electrodes may be seen entering from the SVC and coursing through the tricuspid valve into the RV.[78]

Coronary Sinus

The CS is located in the atrioventricular groove along the posterior surface of the heart, partially incorporated into the atrial wall. It can be seen in long axis from the midesophageal four-chamber view by advancing or retroflexing the probe slightly through the inferior wall of the LA. A short axis image of the CS is seen in the midesophageal two-chamber view in or just superior to the inferior aspect of the atrioventricular groove. It may also be imaged by withdrawing the probe from the transgastric basilar short axis

view slightly until the CS is seen in long axis entering the RA. This view is particularly useful in facilitating the insertion of a cannula into the CS.[78]

Pulmonary Valve and Pulmonary Artery

Like the aortic valve, the pulmonary valve (PV) is a trileaflet, semilunar valve. Its leaflets, however, are thinner and in the far field, and therefore are more difficult to see with TEE. The orientation of the flow through the PV is roughly perpendicular to that of the aortic valve and is directed anteriorly to posteriorly and slightly right to left. TEE views of the PV suggested by the council are made from three cross sections. The midesophageal AV short-axis view provides a view of the PV and main PA to the right side of the display (Fig. 15-52, see color Figures) (Fig. 15-53). The multiplane angle is rotated back toward 0 degree and the probe anteflexed or slightly withdrawn to display the bifurcation of the main PA. The right PA should be visualized at the top of the display coursing off to the patient's right. The left PA arches over the left mainstem bronchus after bifurcation from the main PA and is often difficult to visualize with TEE. The midesophageal RV inflow-outflow view displays the PV in long axis and is useful for detecting a pulmonic regurgitation by color flow Doppler. The main PA and the PV are seen in the *upper esophageal aortic arch short axis view* in the left side of the display by turning the probe to the left and right until the structures come into view. Retroflexing the probe will often bring the PV into better view. This cross section usually allows the Doppler beam to be aligned parallel to the flow through the PV and main PA and is therefore useful in making spectral Doppler measurements of these structures.[84]

Aorta

Thoracic Aorta

The proximal and midascending aorta, mid- and distal aortic arch, and the entire descending thoracic aorta can be routinely imaged with multiplane TEE because these structures

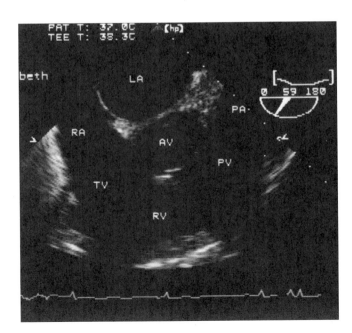

Figure 15-51. RV inflow-outflow view. (Courtesy of Kristine J. Hirsch, M.D., Halifax, NS, Canada.)

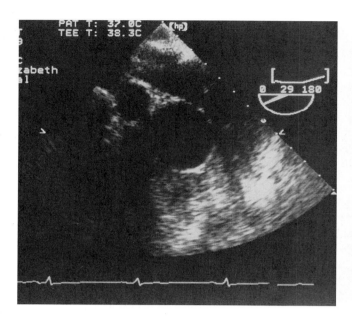

Figure 15-53. Transverse view of ascending aorta with bifurcation of PA to the right of the image. (Courtesy of Kristine J. Hirsch, M.D., Halifax, NS, Canada.)

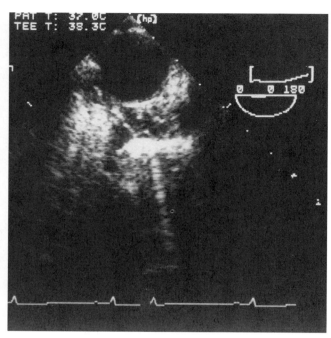

Figure 15-54. Short axis view of descending thoracic aorta. (Courtesy of Kristine J. Hirsch, M.D., Halifax, NS, Canada.)

are adjacent to the esophagus as it passes vertically through the mediastinum. The distal ascending aorta and proximal aortic arch, however, are usually not visualized with TEE because the air-filled trachea is interposed between these regions of the aorta and the esophagus. Epiaortic scanning can be used to examine these areas through a median sternotomy by covering a high-frequency transducer with a sterile sheath and placing it directly on the ascending aorta in the surgical field.[78]

Ascending Aorta

Assessment of the aorta is begun by examination of the proximal and midascending aorta. The transducer is advanced into the esophagus below the level of the carina (about 30 cm from the incisors) and turned to image anteriorly. The proximal and midascending aorta can be seen with TEE through the great vessel window at the level of the right PA, just superior to the midesophageal window. The *great vessel aortic short-axis view* of the ascending aorta is developed by rotating the multiplane angle forward until the vessel appears circular, about 20 to 40 degrees. Advancing and withdrawing the probe in the esophagus will image different levels of the aorta. Rotating the multiplane angle forward until the anterior and posterior walls of the aortic route appear parallel to one another will develop the *great vessel aortic long-axis view* of the ascending aorta. The diameter of the ascending aorta should be measured (usually <3.5 cm).[78]

Descending Aorta

After visualization of the ascending aorta, the multiplane angle is rotated back to 0 degree and the probe turned to the patient's left until the descending thoracic aorta appears in the near field of the display. This develops the *descending aorta short-axis view* (Fig. 15-54). With the multiplane angle at 0 degree (transverse plane), circular images of the descending thoracic aorta appear. Rotating forward from 0

to 90 degrees yields circular, oblique, and eventually the *descending aorta long-axis view* (Fig. 15-55) in which the walls of the descending aorta appear as two parallel lines.

The entire descending thoracic aorta and upper abdominal aorta can be examined by advancing and withdrawing the probe to different levels in the esophagus. The espha-

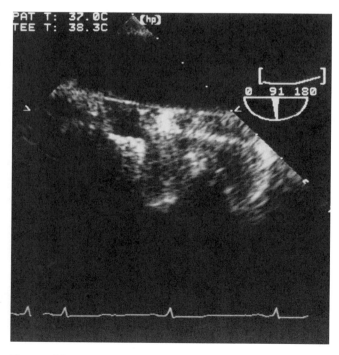

Figure 15-55. Long axis view of descending thoracic aorta. (Courtesy of Kristine J. Hirsch, M.D., Halifax, NS, Canada.)

gus is situated anterior to the aorta at the level of the diaphragm and then winds around within the thorax so that at the level of the transverse arch, the aorta is located anterior to the esophagus. As the probe is advanced distally in the esophagus, it must be turned to the left (posteriorly) to maintain the aorta in view. The mid- and distal abdominal aorta cannot be seen because it is difficult to maintain contact between the transducer and the aorta within the stomach.

Because of the changing relationships of the esophagus to the aorta and lack of internal landmarks, it is difficult to designate anterior and posterior or right-to-left orientations of the descending thoracic aorta with TEE imaging. Therefore, the depth of the transducer tip from the incisors is important to record. The level within the descending aorta may also be designated by the presence of an adjacent structure, such as the LA or the base of the LV.[78]

Aortic Arch

As the esophagus courses from the superior mediastinum into the posterior mediastinum, it encounters the distal arch and isthmic portion of the descending thoracic aorta. In this location it lies posterior and to the right of these segments of aorta. The aortic arch can be imaged by withdrawing the probe to the aortic arch window superior to the level of the descending thoracic aorta, about 18 to 20 cm from the incisors. Because the aortic arch lies slightly anterior to the esophagus, as the tip of the probe is withdrawn superiorly it should be turned slightly to the right (anterior) to keep the vessel in view. With the multiplane angle at 0 degree the *aortic arch long axis view* will be developed (Fig. 15–56). The proximal arch will be to the left of the display and the distal arch to the right. Rotating the multiplane angle forward to 90 degrees will develop the *aortic arch short axis view,* and turning the probe to the right and left will sweep the imaging plane proximally and distally through the arch.

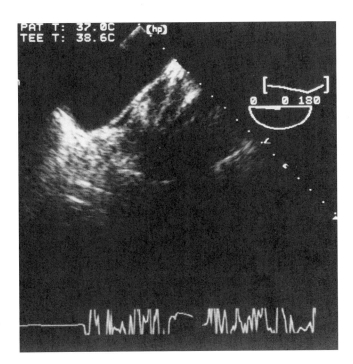

Figure 15–56. Long axis view of aortic arch. (Courtesy of Kristine J. Hirsch, M.D., Halifax, NS, Canada.)

In some individuals, the proximal left subclavian artery and left carotid artery can be imaged by withdrawing the transducer superiorly from the aortic arch long axis view. The right brachiocephalic artery is more difficult to image due to the interposition of the air-filled trachea. As the transducer is withdrawn, it can be turned to the left to follow the left subclavian artery distally. The left internal jugular vein lies anterior and to the left of the common carotid artery and sometimes can be seen. In the aortic arch short-axis view, the origin of the great vessels can often be identified at the superior aspect of the arch to the right of the display. The visualization rate of the arch vessels by TEE is lowest for the right brachiocephalic artery and highest for the left subclavian. The left brachiocephalic vein is also often seen anterior to the arch in both the aortic arch short-axis view and the aortic arch long-axis view.[78]

Global Ventricular Function

Evaluation of ventricular systolic and diastolic functions is an essential part of all echocardiographic examinations. Two-dimensional echocardiography allows visualization of the endocardial thickening of ventricular walls, by which global and regional ventricular functions are assessed. Determination of global systolic function is based on changes in ventricular size and volume. Regional (or segmental) wall motion analysis is fundamental in evaluating coronary artery disease and in performing stress echocardiography.

Estimation of Function

The development of quantitative analysis techniques for TEE applications has been fairly rapid because many of the mathematical models had already been used for transthoracic or epicardial echocardiography. The practical applications of quantitative TEE analysis have been limited by the necessity for time-consuming tracing and meticulous attention to detail that is essential to avoiding errors. The impending development of accurate, reliable on-line automated endocardial border detection is the factor that will probably bring quantitative analysis to the forefront of TEE analysis techniques.

In routine clinical work, however, the anesthesiologist-echocardiographer must make visual estimates of ventricular wall motion and overall function. These depend on the ability to interpret the images and correctly quantify subjective assessments of ventricular function. The variables most frequently used in the intraoperative setting to express LV global systolic function are ejection fraction (EF) and cardiac output.[85]

EF represents stroke volume (SV) as a percentage of end-diastolic LV volume; hence, its determination requires measurement of LV volume. Most of the current echocardiographic units have the capability of measuring volume by tracing the LV endocardial surface either manually or by automated edge detection. The ASE recommends the modified Simpson method to estimate ventricular volume from two orthogonal apical views.[76]

The fractional area of change of the LV and RV can be measured in virtually any true long- or short-axis cross sections of either ventricle and the estimates obtained are reasonable approximations of global EFs. EFs, however, are load-dependent and should be viewed cautiously as measures of overall ventricular performance. LV ejection fraction (LVEF) is an excellent predictor of survival in patients with coronary artery disease and is widely used in the perioperative assessment of high-risk patients.[86]

Cardiac output is the product of SV and heart rate. SV is determined either by 2-D volumetric measurement, as in calculation of EF, or by the Doppler method referred to below.

Segmental Left Ventricular Function

LV regional wall motion analysis is usually based on grading the contractility of individual segments.[76, 87] Ischemic segments of the heart do not contract normally. During acute ischemia, segmental wall motion abnormalities (SWMAs) precede and may occur in the absence of ST-segment changes.[88–90] It has been shown that when multiple TEE cross sections are monitored (not just the midpapillary cross section), the detection rate of SWMAs more than doubles.[91, 92]

Limitations of TEE in the detection of ischemia also should be recognized. When an area of myocardium is clearly in view, segmental contraction can be difficult to evaluate because the heart rotates markedly during systole. The same may be true during the discoordinated contraction that occurs due to bundle branch block or ventricular pacing. Consequently, a valid system for SWMA assessment first must compensate for global motion of the heart (typically by using a floating frame of reference), then evaluate both regional endocardial motion and myocardial thickening.[93] For these reasons, use of the floating reference system in the intraoperative period is recommended (Fig. 15–57). Consequently, the exact imaging plane for wall motion assessment is crucial. The short axis view of the LV at the level of the midpapillary muscles is used to ensure that the internal landmarks referenced in this circumstance are the anterolateral and posteromedial papillary muscles in monitoring of the muscular septal region. It must be recognized that although myocardial blood flow from the coronary arteries is best represented at the short axis midpapillary muscle level, there may be other myocardial regions that are underperfused and not adequately represented in one echocardiographic image plane.[94] A worsening of segmental wall motion and wall thickening (in the absence of similar global changes) of at least two classes is required to make the diagnosis of ische-

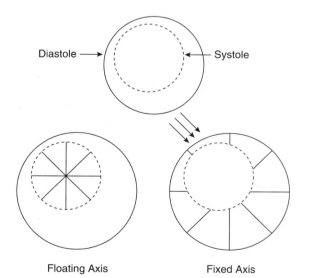

Figure 15–57. Comparison of fixed and floating axis systems. In the fixed axis system there is an apparent motion abnormality (delineated by the *arrows*). Conversely, in the floating axis system, the effects of translation are negated and no abnormality is observed.

Table 15–4. Classes of Segmental Ventricular Wall Motion

Class of Motion	Wall Thickening	Change in Radius*
Normal	Marked	>30% ⇓
Mild hypokinesis	Moderate	10%–30% ⇓
Severe hypokinesis	Minimal	<10%, >0% ⇓
Akinesis	None	None
Dyskinesis	Thinning	⇑

*Change in radius refers to the decrease in length during systole of imaginary radius from the endocardium to the center of the left ventricular cavity in the midpapillary cross section.

mia; less pronounced changes are not consistently interpreted, even by experts. The classes of wall motion are described in (Table 15–4).

Limitations

Interpretation of septal motion is the most problematic because it often is compounded by discoordinated contraction patterns. It is useful, in this instance, to apply a simple rule: when the septum is viable and nonischemic, it thickens appreciably during systole, although its inward motion may begin slightly before or after the inward motion of the other ventricular segments.[93, 95, 96] Thus, SWMAs can be detected during bundle branch block, ventricular pacing, and marked global movements of the heart but not by assessment of endocardial motion alone; wall thickening also must be assessed. Because not all hearts contract normally and not all parts of the normal heart contract to the same degree, not all SWMAs are indicative of myocardial ischemia.[97, 98] It is reasonable to assume, however, that most of the time an acute change in the regional contraction pattern of the heart during surgery is probably attributable to myocardial ischemia. An important exception to this rule may apply to models of acute coronary artery occlusion. In these models, it has been established that myocardial function becomes abnormal at the center of an ischemic zone. It is also true, however, that the myocardial regions adjacent to the ischemic zones become dysfunctional as well.[99, 100] The impairment of function in nonischemic tissue has been thought to be caused by a tethering effect. Tethering, or the attachment of noncontracting tissue that mechanically impairs contraction in adjacent tissue that is normally perfused, probably accounts for the consistent overestimation of infarct size by echocardiography when compared with postmortem studies.[101]

Another limitation of SWM analysis during surgery is that it does not differentiate stunned or hibernating myocardium from acute ischemia,[102] nor does it differentiate between increased oxygen demand and decreased oxygen supply as the cause of ischemia. Finally, it should be noted that areas of previous ischemia or scarring may become unmasked by changes in afterload and appear as new SWMAs.[103] This is particularly important in vascular surgery, during which major abrupt changes in afterload occur.

In addition to the drawbacks already mentioned, there remain other potential limitations to TEE monitoring intraoperatively. The most obvious of these is the fact that ischemia cannot be detected during critical periods such as induction, laryngoscopy, intubation, emergence, and extubation. In addition, the adequacy of SWM analysis may be influenced by artifact.[95] As mentioned earlier, artifacts can be produced by the ultrasound system itself or the particular tangential section being imaged.

Outcome Significance

Data regarding the significance of intraoperative detection of SWMAs suggest that transient abnormalities unaccompanied by hemodynamic or ECG evidence of ischemia may not represent significant myocardial ischemia and are usually not associated with postoperative morbidity.[104] Hypokinetic myocardial segments appear to be associated with minimal perfusion defects compared with the significant perfusion defects that accompany akinetic or dyskinetic segments. Hence, hypokinesia may be a less predictive marker for postoperative morbidity than akinesia or dyskinesia. Persistence of severe SWMAs, on the other hand, is clearly associated with myocardial ischemia and postoperative morbidity.[88, 105-107]

Intraoperative detection of new or worsened and persistent SWMAs during peripheral vascular surgery has been reported by several investigators to be associated with postoperative cardiac morbidity. The occurrence of new SWMAs during vascular surgery appears to be common[104-107]; however, in most cases they are transient and clinically insignificant. New SWMAs that are recognized to persist until the conclusion of surgery, in contrast, imply acute perioperative myocardial infarction.[88, 105-107] Intraoperative SWMAs, therefore, may be spurious, reversible with or without treatment, or irreversible. The reversible SWMAs may be associated with clinically insignificant, short periods of ischemia, whereas the irreversible SWMAs are associated with significant ischemia or infarction.

Intraoperative TEE has helped predict results of coronary artery bypass graft (CABG) surgery.[108] Following CABG to previously dysfunctional segments, immediate improvement of regional myocardial function (which is sustained) has been demonstrated.[109, 110] In addition, prebypass compensatory hypercontracting segments have been reported to revert toward normal immediately following successful CABG.[111] Persistent SWMAs following CABG appear to be related to adverse clinical outcomes, and lack of evidence of SWMAs following CABG has been shown to be associated with a postoperative course without cardiac morbidity.[102, 112]

Preload

In conventional hemodynamics, preload is often estimated by measuring filling pressures of the left side of the heart, such as pulmonary capillary wedge pressure (PCWP), LA pressure, or left ventricular end-diastolic pressure (LVEDP). In echocardiography, however, it can be determined by measuring LV end-diastolic dimensions. It has been shown that when compared with PCWP, end-diastolic volume (EDV) or end-diastolic area was superior as a predictor of cardiac index (CI) in patients undergoing CABG.[113] In fact, no significant correlation was found to exist between PCWP and CI. To gauge LA or LV filling pressures, echocardiography has primarily relied on Doppler measurement flow into LA from the PVs or LA, and out of the LA through the MV. Intraoperative TEE estimates of filling pressure appear to correlate well with PA catheter data.

Pulmonary Venous Flow

The normal Doppler velocity profile in the PV displays three flow peaks: a systolic peak indicating forward flow into the LA, a diastolic forward flow peak, and a reverse flow peak associated with atrial contraction. At normal LA pressure, the systolic increase in PV pressure is larger and more rapid than the LA pressure. At elevated filling pressures, however, the systolic pressure increase in the LA is equal to or more rapid than that in the PV, resulting in an early systolic peak. During diastole, forward flow velocity occurs after MV opening and in conjunction with the decrease in LA pressure. With atrial contraction, the increase in LA pressure may result in flow reversal into the PV, the extent and the duration of which are related to LV diastolic pressure, LA compliance, and heart rate. At elevated filling pressures, however, the systolic pressure increase in LA is equal to or more rapid than that in the PV, resulting in earlier peak of the systolic peak.[114, 115] LA pressures have been estimated from velocity measurements of PV flow. A correlation has been shown between TEE estimates of mean LA pressure and those obtained with LA and PA catheters.[116]

Transmitral Blood Flow

In patients with mitral regurgitation (MR), application of the Bernoulli equation to the maximum regurgitant Doppler velocity has been shown to provide a reliable and accurate method for the determination of LA pressure.[117, 118] When MR is absent, some have found excellent correlations between Doppler transmitral flow variables and PCWP, while others have found no relationship.[119-123] In a series of patients undergoing CABG, Nishimura et al.[123] observed that a reduction in early velocity and shortening of deceleration time of MV flow were significantly associated with reductions in preload. An increase in preload produced the opposite effect, while an increase in afterload produced variable effects. In most of the studies, PCWP has been estimated from transmitral flow velocity-time integrals.[123] Studies have been performed on patients with decreased LV systolic function undergoing coronary artery surgery. They have demonstrated high, statistically significant, correlations between PCWP and the deceleration time or deceleration slope of early diastolic filling as measured by transesophageal Doppler.[124] Specific methods of calculating LA pressure are discussed below.

End-Diastolic Ventricular Area

As already stated, it has been proposed that end-diastolic dimensions provide a better index of preload than the PCWP. TEE is often, however, for practical reasons, limited to a single short-axis view at the level of the papillary muscles. Some evidence suggests that short-axis end-diastolic areas measured at this level correlate reasonably well with measurements obtained by on-heart echocardiography,[125] and with end-diastolic volumes measured simultaneously using radionuclides.[126] This conclusion, however, was refuted by Urbanowicz et al.[127] At present, the debate as to the number of planes that are required to accurately represent ventricular volumes is ongoing and beyond the scope of this discussion.

Diastolic Function

Normal diastolic function allows adequate filling of the ventricles during rest and exercise without abnormal increase in diastolic pressures. Adequate diastolic filling ensures normal SV, according to the Frank-Starling mechanism. LV filling consists of a series of hemodynamic events that are affected by numerous intrinsic and extrinsic factors[128] (Table 15-5).

Definition of Diastole

During the interval between aortic valve closure and MV opening, LV relaxation occurs without change in LV volume, assuming that no intracardiac shunting is present. This active energy-dependent process causes pressure to decrease rap-

Table 15–5. Factors That Influence Left Ventricular (LV) Diastolic Chamber Distensibility

Factors extrinsic to the LV chamber
  Pericardial restraint
  Right ventricular loading
  Coronary vascular turgor (erectile effect)
  Extrinsic compression by tumor, pleural pressure, etc.
Factors intrinsic to the LV chamber
  Passive elasticity of LV wall (stiffness or compliance when myocytes are completely relaxed)
    Thickness of LV wall
    Composition of LV wall (muscle, fibrosis, amyloid, hemosiderin), including both endocardium and myocardium
    Temperature, osmolality
  Active elasticity of LV wall due to residual cross-bridge activation (cycling/latch state) through part or all of diastole
    Slope relaxation affecting early diastole only
    Incomplete relaxation affecting early, mid-, and end-diastolic distensibility
    Diastolic contracture, or rigor
  Elastic recoil (diastolic suction)
  Viscoelasticity (stress relaxation, creep)

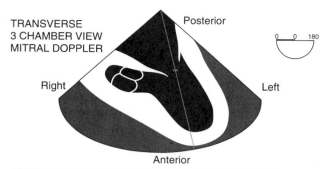

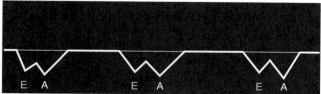

Figure 15–60. Schematic of the transverse three-chamber view and representative mitral inflow pulsed-wave Doppler profile.

idly in the LV after the end of contraction and during diastole. When LV pressure falls lower than LA pressure, the MV opens, and rapid early diastolic filling begins.[129, 130] Under normal circumstances, the predominant determinant of the driving force of early diastolic filling is the elastic recoil and the rate of relaxation of the LV. Normally, approximately 80% of LV filling occurs during this phase. This is followed by a period of slow filling known as diastasis. About 20% of filling occurs in the remaining late diastole as a result of active atrial contraction.

For each person, the proportion of LV filling during the early and late diastolic phases depends on elastic recoil, the rate of myocardial relaxation, chamber compliance, and LA pressure. The LV filling pattern is the result of the transmitral pressure gradient produced by the various factors. Transmitral Doppler recordings are the most frequently used method of evaluating diastolic LV filling and directly reflect the pressure difference between the LA and LV.[130–132] This measurement, in conjunction with PV flow velocity, representing LA filling, will assist in developing an analysis of diastolic function.[133, 134] (Figure 15–58, see color Figures).

Doppler Flow Velocities

When recording Doppler flow velocities, the echocardiographer must take into consideration several technical aspects of acquiring these velocities. First, the ultrasound beam needs to be parallel with the direction of blood flow to obtain the optimal flow signal. Because of the location of the papillary muscles, normal mitral inflow is directed toward the mid-to-distal portion of the posterolateral wall of the LV, which is approximately 20 degrees lateral to the apex. With dilatation of the LV, as in patients with dilated cardiomyopathy, mitral inflow is directed progressively more laterally and posteriorly.[135] The optimal transducer position, therefore, is approximately 20 degrees lateral to the apex in normal subjects and more lateral in those with LV enlargement.

The second consideration is sample volume size and location. To record peak mitral inflow velocities, the pulsed-wave Doppler technique is used, with a sample volume size of 1 to 2 mm between the tips of the mitral leaflets during diastole. The sample volume may be moved toward the mitral annulus to better record the duration of the atrial contraction velocity. For recording PV flow velocity, the sample

volume size is usually larger (2 to 4 mm) and is placed 1 to 2 cm into the LUPV.

Finally, the velocity scale and filter should be adjusted according to the peak velocities of the Doppler recording. Compared with mitral tricuspid flow velocities (range, 0.5 to 1.5 m/s), venous flow velocities are lower (range, 0.1 to 0.5 m/s), and because of this velocity scales should be expanded and the velocity filter should be low.

Transmitral Blood Flow

The initial classification of diastolic filling is usually attempted from peak mitral flow velocity at the early rapid filling wave (E), peak velocity of the late filling wave due to atrial contraction (A), and the E/A ratio (Fig. 15–59, see color Figures) (Figs. 15–60 and 15–61). Deviations from the

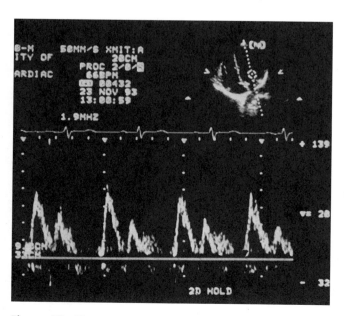

Figure 15–61. Pulsed-wave Doppler study of mitral inflow (transthoracic study).

normal diastolic velocity pattern have been described under various circumstances. Fusion of the E and A peaks occurs during tachycardia, whereas the A peak is absent during atrial fibrillation. Mitral regurgitation and stenosis each have their own flow signatures. The most commonly observed abnormality is a reversal of the E/A ratio, indicating impaired early LV filling (Figs. 15–62 and 15–63, see color Figures). This has been noted with advanced age, ischemic heart disease, hypertrophic cardiomyopathy, secondary LV hypertrophy, dilated cardiomyopathy, and RV pressure overload. Other factors affecting the E-peak velocity include the LA V-wave pressure, the LV relaxation rate, and the systemic arterial pressure. The E-peak varies directly with increasing LA pressure and inversely with increases in the time constant of relaxation or systemic arterial pressure.[136]

The contribution of atrial contraction to ventricular filling is ideally studied by measurement of mitral flow velocity. The area under the A-peak will be directly proportional to the fraction of the SV contributed by the atrial contraction. In cardiac surgical patients, it has been demonstrated that the decrease in CI occurring as a result of the loss of atrial contraction will be greater in patients with lower E/A ratios.[137] Others have used pulsed-wave Doppler echocardiography to document increased CI with atrioventricular versus ventricular pacing, or to optimize atrioventricular delay intervals during atrioventricular sequential pacing.[138-140]

Pulmonary Venous Blood Flow

Evaluation of PV flow is an integral part of assessing diastolic LV filling and is particularly useful in evaluating LV diastolic and LA systolic pressures. PV inflow into the LA is dependent on the pressure difference between the PV being sampled and the LA. There is, therefore, an inverse relationship between LA pressure and PV inflow. PV inflow is biphasic and occurs during the low points of the LA pressure curve.[141]

PA diastolic flow follows the pattern mitral inflow.[116, 142, 143] After rapid filling, LA pressure falls below PV pressure, allowing the LA to fill. During this time, the LA acts as a passive conduit between the PVs and the LV (Figs. 15–64 through 15–66, see color Figures) (Fig. 15–67). When impaired LV relaxation is present, LV pressure falls more slowly. This results in a decrease in the rate of decline in LA pressure, and, therefore, reduces the amount of diastolic LA filling.

PV systolic inflow is closely related to LA pressure, as well as to atrial compliance. Ventricular function, however, also plays a role because during systole the mitral annulus moves apically, which increases LA size and reduces LA pressure. When LA pressure is elevated, systolic filling of the LA from the PVs is reduced. A small amount of PV flow reversal usually occurs during atrial contraction when LA pressure exceeds PV pressure. The amount of atrial flow reversal depends on LA pressure prior to atrial contraction, as well as the additional pressure generated between this time and end-diastole. This is influenced by LV diastolic pressure (atrial afterload), as well as atrial volume (atrial preload) and atrial contractility.[144, 145]

Diastolic Filling Patterns

Normal Pattern

The rates of myocardial relaxation and compliance change with aging, so that different diastolic filling patterns are expected for different age groups. In normal young subjects, LV elastic recoil is vigorous and myocardial relaxation

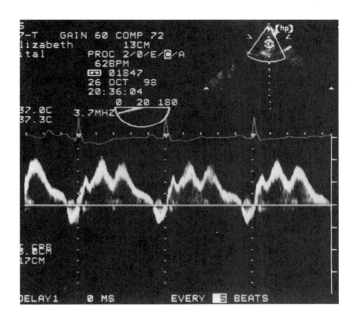

Figure 15–67. Pulsed-wave Doppler study of pulmonary venous inflow. (Courtesy of Kristine J. Hirsch, Halifax, NS, Canada.)

is swift; therefore, most filling is completed during early diastole, with only a small contribution at atrial contraction.[132, 146]

With aging, there is a gradual decrease in the rate of myocardial relaxation, as well as in elastic recoil, resulting in slow LV pressure declines and in slow filling. Because early LV filling is reduced, the contribution of atrial contraction to LV filling becomes more important. This results in a gradual increase in A-peak velocity with aging. PV flow velocities show similar changes with aging: diastolic forward flow velocity decreases as more filling of the LV occurs at atrial contraction and systolic forward flow velocity becomes more prominent.[147]

Abnormal Patterns

Impaired Myocardial Relaxation Pattern

In nearly all types of cardiac disease, the initial abnormality of diastolic filling is slowed or impaired myocardial relaxation that is more than that expected with aging.[146] LV hypertrophy and hypertrophic cardiomyopathy are examples in which this is true. Mitral E-peak velocity is decreased and A-peak velocity is increased, producing an E/A ratio of less than 1, with a prolonged deceleration time. PV forward flow velocity parallels mitral E-peak velocity and also decreases with compensatory increased flow in systole. The duration and velocity of the atrial flow reversal are usually normal, but they may be increased if LVEDP is high.

Restrictive Filling (or Decreased Compliance) Pattern

The term *restrictive diastolic filling,* or *restrictive physiology,* should be distinguished from restrictive cardiomyopathy. Restrictive physiology can be present in any cardiac abnormality or a combination of abnormalities that produce decreased LV compliance and markedly increased LA pressure. Patients with decompensated congestive heart failure (CHF), acute severe aortic regurgitation, and constrictive pericarditis all fall into this category. These patients present with an increase in LA pressure resulting in earlier opening of the MV and a greater initial transmitral gradient (high E-peak velocity). Atrial contraction increases LA pressure, but A-peak velocity and duration are shortened because LV pressure increases even more rapidly. Therefore, restrictive physiology is characterized by mitral flow velocities that show increased E-peak velocity, decreased A-peak velocity ($<<$E), and a shortened deceleration time. PV forward flow stops at mid- to late diastole, reflecting the rapid increase in LV pressure. At atrial contraction, the increase in LA pressure can produce the prolonged atrial flow reversal. Atrial flow reversal may not even be seen, however, if atrial contraction occurs when PV flow velocity is relatively high because of tachycardia.

Pseudonormalized Pattern

As diastolic function deteriorates, a transition from impaired relaxation to restrictive filling occurs. During this transition, the mitral inflow pattern goes through a phase that resembles a normal diastolic filling pattern, that is, a normal E/A ratio and normal deceleration time. This is the result of a moderately increased LA pressure superimposed on a relaxation abnormality.[148] This pseudonormal pattern can be distinguished from a new true normal pattern by the following[149]:

1. In patients with an LV of abnormal size or systolic dysfunction or with increased wall thickness, impaired relaxation is expected, and a normal E/A ratio suggests that increased LA pressure is masking the abnormal relaxation.

2. By demonstrating a shortening of mitral A-peak duration in the absence of a short P-R interval or by demonstrating prolonged atrial flow reversal exceeding mitral A-peak duration.

3. A reduction of preload by sitting or by Valsalva maneuver or sublingual nitroglycerin may be able to unmask the underlying impaired relaxation of the LV, decreasing the E/A ratio to less than 1.[150]

4. Color M-mode of mitral inflow can determine the rate of flow propagation in the LV.[151, 152] With worsening of diastolic function, myocardial relaxation is always impaired and flow propagation is slow, even when LA pressure and mitral E-peak velocity are increased.

Afterload

While afterload cannot be determined by echocardiography alone, the combination of ventricular dimensions with ventricular wall thickness and systolic arterial pressure yields end-systolic wall stress. Ventricular wall thickness is derived by calculating the difference between the epicardial and endocardial areas, whereas the ventricular dimension corresponds to the endocardial area.[153]

Elevations in wall stress have been observed in patients with LV enlargement caused by systemic hypertension, aortic stenosis, or aortic regurgitation.[154] Wall stress provides a better index of afterload than systemic vascular resistance (SVR) when forward stroke volume is not equal to the total ventricular ejection, as in MR or in the presence of a ventricular septal defect. Whether the same is true in patients without such lesions is unclear.

In cardiac surgical patients, poor correlations between SVR and end-systolic wall stress were observed.[155] In patients undergoing carotid artery surgery, wall stress was studied under various anesthetic measurements.[105] It was noted that,

during carotid artery cross-clamping, patients receiving high concentrations of volatile agents, with phenylephrine to maintain blood pressure, had significantly higher wall stress values than those receiving low concentrations of volatile agents without phenylephrine.

Contractility

Echocardiography has been utilized to estimate contractility in a variety of ways. It is best suited for the evaluation of contractility during the ejection phase of contraction, but the use of other approaches has also been explored.[112] The standard isovolumic phase index, dP/dt, cannot be obtained using TEE. Some information on the isovolumic phase can, however, be gathered by measuring the length of the pre-ejection period (PEP)[156, 157] and the maximal acceleration of blood flow into the aorta.[158-161] Currently available TEE imaging planes are not suitable for measurement of the latter.

Using echocardiography, contractility has most frequently been estimated with ejection-phase indices. Although a wide array of ejection-phase indices have been described, all require that end-diastolic and end-systolic dimensions be measured. In M-mode echocardiography, these dimensions will often be simple linear, internal dimensions of the LV cavity.

$$FS = \frac{LVIDD - LVISD}{LVIDD} \qquad (5)$$

The above expresses fractional shortening (*FS*), a basic ejection-phase index of contractility, where *LVIDD* represents the LV internal diastolic dimension and *LVISD* represents the LV internal systolic dimension.

With 2-D echocardiography, multiple tomographic cuts can be obtained and utilized to calculate ventricular volumes using a variety of formulas such as Simpson's rules.[162] Using the ventricular volumes, ejection fraction can then be calculated with the standard formula:

$$EF = (LVEDV - LVESV)/LVEDV \qquad (6)$$

where *EF* represents the ejection fraction, *LVEDV* represents the left ventricular end-diastolic volume, and *LVESV* represents the left ventricular systolic volume.

During intraoperative TEE, it is most convenient to monitor a single, short-axis view at the level of the midpapillary muscles. Once the end-diastolic and end-systolic endocardial areas have been delineated with the help of tracing software, contractility may be estimated by using the fractional area of contraction (FAC) or the ejection fraction area (EFA).

Hemodynamic Assessment

TEE has been used extensively for the evaluation of hemodynamics and global ventricular function. Some investigators have used TEE to measure standard hemodynamic variables (e.g., filling pressures, cardiac output) that were normally obtained by invasive cardiac catheterization, while others have used it to quantify cardiac dimensions, intracardiac flow rates, and overall cardiac performance. Now, echocardiography is the preferred method for determining various hemodynamic data noninvasively.[163]

M-mode and 2-D echocardiography alone can provide only indirect evidence of hemodynamic abnormalities, but this evidence may be the initial clue to such problems. However, this evidence remains qualitative at best. Intracardiac hemodynamic assessment requires Doppler echocardiography, and the accuracy of Doppler-derived hemodynamic measurements has been validated by comparison with simultaneously derived catheterization data.[164-167]

Pressure Gradients

The Bernoulli equation defines the complex relationship between the velocity of flow from one chamber to another and the pressure gradient between those chambers. For most clinical purposes, this relationship may be simplified to

$$P_1 - P_2 = 4V^2 \qquad (7)$$

where $P_1 - P_2$ is the pressure gradient in mmHg and V is the velocity of flow measured in meters per second by Doppler. Using the peak velocity yields the peak instantaneous gradient, while using the mean velocity of a stroke will give the mean pressure gradient. Most modern echo machines have automated the measurement of peak and mean velocities and the calculation of gradients. If the pressure of one chamber is known, calculation of the gradient between it and an adjacent chamber allows one to determine the pressure in the second chamber. This is simply the difference between the pressure in the first chamber and the gradient.[168]

Filling Pressures

To gauge LA or LV filling pressures, echocardiography has primarily relied on Doppler measurements of flow into the LA from the PVs or the LAA, and out of the LA through the MV. Intraoperative TEE estimates of filling pressure appear to correlate well with PA catheter data.[60]

Pulmonary Vein Flow

The normal Doppler velocity profile in the PV displays three flow peaks: a systolic peak indicating forward flow into the LA, a diastolic forward flow peak, and a reverse flow peak associated with atrial contraction. LA pressures have been estimated from velocity measurements of PV flow and have been shown to correlate with measurements obtained with LA and PA catheters.[116] Correlation also exists between TEE findings and filling pressures. This includes correlation between PCWP and evidence of PV flow reversal during atrial contraction,[143] as well as the relationship between pressure gradients and the shape of the IAS on TEE.[169]

Left Atrial Appendage Flow

In patients with sinus rhythm, LAA flow consists of two peaks: a forward contraction wave that coincides with atrial contraction and a retrograde filling wave that immediately follows atrial contraction and is associated with atrial relaxation.[170] It has also been shown that there exists a significant positive correlation between the maximum LAA area and the wedge pressure. This is in conjunction with a significant negative correlation between the LAA EF during atrial contraction and the wedge pressure.[171]

Mitral Flow

In patients with MR, application of the Bernoulli equation to the maximal regurgitant Doppler velocity has been shown to provide a reliable and accurate method for the determination of LA pressure.[117, 118] In the absence of MR, however, the correlation may be less clear.[119, 120, 122, 124] The data suggest that patients with decreased LV systolic function undergoing coronary artery surgery demonstrated high (statistically significant) correlations between PCWP and the deceleration time or deceleration slope of early diastolic filling as measured by transesophageal Doppler.

Calculation of Pressures

When trying to measure LV filling pressures by TEE, it is useful to begin by assessing whether significant MR is present. If it is, the Bernoulli equation is used to calculate LA pressure:

$$LA\ pressure = SBP - 4 \times MRV^2 \qquad (8)$$

where SBP is systolic blood pressure, and MRV is mitral regurgitant velocity. Additionally, if present, aortic regurgitation velocity reflects the diastolic pressure difference between the aorta and the LV. Therefore,

$$LVEDP = DBP - 4 \times (AR\ EDV)^2 \qquad (9)$$

where DBP is the diastolic blood pressure and $AR\ EDV$ represents the aortic regurgitant end-diastolic velocity.

If the EF has been calculated, it may not be necessary for MR to be present. With EFs less than 35%, the deceleration time of early diastolic filling provides an inaccurate estimate of PCWP. If DCT-E is less than 150 ms, PCWP is likely to be greater than 12 mmHg. If DCT-E is longer than 150 ms, PCWP is likely to be less than 10 mmHg. When the LVEF exceeds 35%, pulsed-wave Doppler analysis of mitral inflow alone is insufficient to derive PCWP.

In color M-mode Doppler, a spatiotemporal display of inflow velocity in the LV may assist in the derivation of PCWP.[151] The M-mode cursor is placed across the MV and color-flow velocity is recorded at high sweep speeds. On the display, flow propagation velocity (V_p) and time delay (TD) are measured. The LA pressure can then be calculated with the following equation[172]:

$$LA\ pressure = 5.27 \times (E/V_p) + 4.6\ mmHg \qquad (10)$$

where E is equal to peak early inflow velocity measured by pulsed-wave Doppler.

Another method of calculating PCWP is to use tissue Doppler imaging. The movement of tissue, such as myocardium, can be detected by Doppler analysis.[173] Compared to blood flow, tissue Doppler imaging is characterized by low velocity but high amplitude. Nagueh et al.[174] have described a technique to estimate LV filling pressure that combines pulsed-wave Doppler measurement of the mitral inflow with tissue Doppler imaging measurement of the mitral annulus. They observed that the best PCWP estimations were obtained with the following equation:

$$PCWP = 1.55 + 1.47 (E/E_a) \qquad (11)$$

where E is the peak early inflow velocity measured by pulsed-wave Doppler and E_a is the peak early diastolic mitral annulus velocity. The principal advantages of this new approach are that it is not dependent on EF and little influenced by tachycardia.

Cardiac Output and Stroke Volume

Flow across a fixed orifice is equal to the product of the cross-sectional area (CSA) of the orifice and flow velocity. Because flow velocity varies during ejection in a pulsatile system such as the cardiovascular system, individual velocities of the Doppler spectrum need to be summed (i.e., integrated) to measure the total volume of flow during a given ejection period. This sum of velocities is called the time velocity integral (TVI). This is equal to the area enclosed by the baseline and Doppler spectrum. It is also equal to the stroke distance (i.e., the distance blood travels with each beat of the heart). TVI can be measured readily with the built-in calculation package in the ultrasound unit by tracing the Doppler velocity signal. After TVI is determined, SV is calculated by multiplying TVI by CSA.

The location most frequently used to determine SV is the LVOT.[175] To accomplish this, the diameter (D) is measured at the level of the aortic annulus during systole. A line is drawn from where the anterior aortic cusp meets the ventricular septum to where the posterior aortic cusp meets the anterior mitral leaflet and perpendicular to the anterior aortic wall. Assuming a circular shape of the LVOT, the following formula is used to calculate the LVOT area:

$$LVOT \ area \ (cm^2) = (D/2)^2 \times \pi \quad (12)$$
$$= D^2 \times 0.785$$

Next, the LVOT velocity and the TVI are measured. A pulsed-wave sample volume is placed at the center of the aortic annulus, or 0.5 cm proximal to it in a patient with aortic stenosis. TVI (cm) is the area under the velocity curve and is equal to the sum of velocities (cm/s) during the ejection time (s). Calculation of SV across the LVOT follows:

$$SV = LVOT \ area \ (cm^2) \times TVI \quad (13)$$

Cardiac output is then obtained by multiplying SV by heart rate and CI by dividing cardiac output by body surface area.

Regurgitant Volume and Regurgitant Fraction

Regurgitant volume can be estimated by two different ways with echocardiography: by the volumetric method and by the proximal isovelocity surface area (PISA) method. The hydraulic orifice formula is used in both methods:

$$Flow = CSA \times velocity \ or \ volume = CSA \times TVI \quad (14)$$

Volumetric Method

Total forward volume across a regurgitant valve (Q total) is the sum of systemic SV (Qs) and regurgitant volume. Hence, regurgitant volume can be obtained by calculating the difference between the total forward SV and systemic SV.

$$Regurgitant \ volume = Q \ total - Qs \quad (15)$$

In MR, the Q total is the mitral inflow volume, calculated as a product of MV annulus area and mitral inflow TVI. Mitral inflow TVI is obtained by placing a sample volume at the center of the mitral annulus. Systemic SV (Qs) is obtained by multiplying the LVOT area by LVOT TVI. MV regurgitant volume is estimated as the mitral inflow volume minus the LVOT SV.[176] This calculation is not accurate (i.e., regurgitant volume is underestimated) if there is significant

aortic regurgitation. In aortic regurgitation, the aortic valve regurgitant volume is obtained by subtracting the mitral inflow SV (Qs) from the LVOT forward SV (Q total).

The regurgitant fraction is simply the percentage of regurgitant volume compared with the total flow across the regurgitant valve.

$$Regurgitant \ fraction = (regurgitant \ volume/Q \ total) \times 100\% \quad (16)$$

Proximal Isovelocity Surface Area Method

PISA involves the use of color-flow Doppler and is most commonly applied to MR or mitral stenosis (MS). As blood converges toward a narrow orifice, its velocity increases. When the velocity reaches the limit on the color-flow Doppler scale, it aliases and changes color from red to blue for flow toward the transducer (MR) in blue to red for flow away from the transducer (MS). This shift in color shows a hemispheric shell of blood converging toward the orifice called the PISA (Fig. 15-68). If the area of the hemisphere is determined (A_{PISA}) and multiplied by the aliasing velocity (V_{PISA}, known from the color-flow Doppler scale) the result is the instantaneous flow in milliliters per second. A_{PISA} is determined by measuring the radius of the PISA and using the formula for the area of a hemisphere:

$$A_{PISA} = 2\pi r^2 = 6.28r^2 \quad (17)$$

Next, peak instantaneous velocity of the orifice ($V_{orifice}$) is measured with continuous-wave Doppler. Now, the instantaneous flow (mL/s) is the same at the PISA as at the orifice, both of which are the products of area and velocity.

$$A_{PISA} \times V_{PISA} = A_{orifice} \times V_{orifice} \quad (18)$$

The area of the regurgitant orifice (cm²) for MR or the area of the MV and MS is determined by solving for $A_{orifice}$. This technique has limitations in that it makes two important assumptions that are not valid in many clinical situations. The first is that the orifice toward which the flow converges is circular and the second is that the blood converging on the orifice is not constrained by any adjacent structure such as the LV wall. Despite these limitations, in many situations

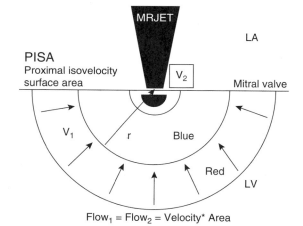

Figure 15-68. Schematic depicting the variables needed for the proximal isovelocity surface area (PISA) method of calculating mitral valvular areas.

PISA can provide important corroborative information about the severity of a valvular lesion.

Valvular Heart Disease

Assessment of the native cardiac valves and valvular heart disease remains one of the strongest indications for the use of TEE in the perioperative period. This includes evaluation of the anatomic and functional characteristics of the valves under varying physiologic conditions as a result of an abnormality and observation of the interaction of ventricular function with valvular function. Doppler hemodynamic measurements of the valves can give pressure gradients, estimated valve areas, estimates of filling and downstream pressures, cardiac output, and quantification of stenosis and regurgitation. In comparison with transthoracic echocardiography, TEE is particularly useful for assessing the MV with ease and accuracy and, to a lesser degree, the aortic valve.

Stenotic Lesions

All types of stenosis are characterized either by reduced orifice dimension in the case of valvular stenosis or reduced valvular inflow or outflow tract dimension for sub- or supravalvular stenosis. Furthermore, all parts of the valve apparatus and the inflow-outflow tracts can be a part of the pathologic condition and must be evaluated echocardiographically.

Mitral Stenosis

The most common cause of MS remains rheumatic heart disease, even in developed countries, while rarer causes include systemic lupus erythematosus, nonbacterial vegetations, tumors, thrombi, excessive mitral annular calcification, cor triatriatum, and supravalvular rings.[177, 178] The characteristic findings of rheumatic MS include thickened, rigid leaflets; commissure and chordal fusion and calcification; reduced leaflet mobility and diastolic doming; and leaflet tethering. Associated findings include enlargement of the LA; thrombus formation in the LA, especially the LAA; pulmonary hypertension; and tricuspid regurgitation, as well as right-sided heart enlargement and dysfunction.[179, 180] Hemodynamic evidence of increased upstream pressure, for example, spontaneous contrast or "smoke," can also manifest on TEE examination. Spontaneous contrast may be related to rouleaux formation resulting from a low flow state and strongly correlates with increased risk for thromboembolic phenomena.[181, 182] Therefore, full assessment includes observation of the mitral leaf-

lets and supporting structures (chordae, papillary muscles, commissures), the annulus, adjacent areas (LA and LAA, atrial septum, LVOT), the PVs, and the right-sided heart chambers. The first step in assessing the severity of MS should be to identify any coexisting valvular or ventricular abnormality since this can dramatically affect echocardiographic measurements.

In determining the grading or severity of the MS, direct planimetric measurement of the mitral orifice at the leaflet tips is often difficult because of difficulty obtaining an accurate short axis view using TEE.[183] As a result, most grading systems are related to morphologic grading of the stenosis as well as the hemodynamic effects. An example of a morphologic grading system (modified from Wilkins et al.[184] and Abascal et al.[185]) is given in Table 15-6.

Important pressure measures of stenosis severity include peak, mean, and end-diastolic pressure gradients across the valve. The pressure gradients are estimated using the modified Bernoulli equation, in which the diastolic pressure (DP) gradient is approximated by $4V^2$ with V being the measured inflow velocity at the appropriate time.[186] The velocity profile can be obtained from any transverse or longitudinal view where the direction of flow is along the axis of the ultrasound beam.

There are two commonly used methods for estimating mitral orifice area: the pressure half-time (PHT) method and the continuity equation. The PHT method correlates the rate of fall of the DP gradient with the orifice area. The more severe the MS, the slower the early diastolic (E wave) flow across the valve and the slower the falloff of the DP gradient. The rate of the DP gradient falloff is described by the PHT, that is, the time required for the initial gradient to fall to half its original value. The equation relating the mitral orifice area to the PHT is

$$MV\ area\ (cm^2) = 220/PHT\ (ms) \qquad (19)$$

The PHT is approximately 50 to 70 ms in normal patients and can range to over 300 ms in patients with severe MS.[187] This method correlates very well with cardiac catheterization estimates in patients without other left-sided heart valvular disease,[188, 189] LV hypertrophy, or significant LV systolic or diastolic function. Atrial dysrhythmias, prolonged P-R interval, and sinus tachycardia can all interfere with the reproducibility of measurements of PHT but do not directly affect the accuracy of the measurement. The PHT method is not valid in the presence of significant aortic regurgitation or LV dysfunction.[187]

An alternative method for estimating the mitral orifice area uses the continuity equation and works in the presence of LV dysfunction and hypertrophy; however, it is more

Table 15-6. Mitral Valve Morphology

Grade	Mobility	Leaflet Thickening	Subvalvular Thickening	Calcification
1	Highly mobile valve with restriction of leaflet tips only	Leaflets slightly increased in thickness (3-4 mm)	Minimal thickening	One area of increased echo brightness
2	Leaflet middle and base portions have normal mobility	Midleaflets normal; marked thickening of margins only (5-8 mm)	Thickening of chordal structures in up to one third of the chords	Scattered areas of brightness at the leaflet margins
3	Valve continues to move forward in diastole, mainly from the base	Thickening extending through the entire leaflet (5-8 mm)	Thickening extending to distal third of the chords	Brightness extending into the midportion of the leaflets
4	No or minimal forward movement of the leaflets in diastole	Marked thickening of all leaflet tissue (8-10 mm)	Extensive thickening/shortening of chords and papillary muscles	Extensive brightness throughout much of the leaflet tissue

time-consuming.[189] The continuity equation states that the SV across the MV equals the TVI of mitral inflow multiplied by the MV orifice area. Rearranging,

$$MV\ area\ =\ SV/TVI \qquad (20)$$

The SV can then be measured by using a similar calculation across either the aortic or pulmonary valve. Thus, the calculation requires measurement of two TVIs and a cross-sectional area on two separate valves under similar hemodynamic conditions, which may be difficult intraoperatively. If the aortic valve is used, the deep transgastric view of the LVOT and the aortic valve is the most appropriate view from which to obtain measurements. In the presence of significant coexisting MR, the MV area is underestimated.

The presence of pulmonary hypertension can be assessed by estimation of pulmonary systolic pressure from Doppler interrogation of tricuspid regurgitation. The peak tricuspid regurgitant jet velocity will give the peak pressure gradient across the TV during RV systole by application of the modified Bernoulli equation. Adding this pressure gradient to an estimate of actual measurement of RA pressure, the peak RV pressure can be estimated. This should correspond to the PA systolic pressure if there is no obstruction to RV outflow.[166]

In patients undergoing MV repair or replacement, the clinical implications of the echocardiographic examination are largely related to determination of the mechanical cause of the obstruction, the likelihood of successful repair of the valve, and the expected difficulty with mitral prosthesis introduction. One of the most important findings with regard to prosthesis introduction is the presence and severity of mitral annular calcification because this may significantly hinder the suturing of the prosthesis. The effects of coexisting cardiac disease (other valvular disease and ventricular dysfunction) may affect the patient's recovery, warranting complete documentation.

Aortic Stenosis

Many of the considerations for aortic valvular stenosis are similar to those for MS, but the windows for viewing the aortic valve are more limited and less optimally positioned for Doppler study. Only the deep transgastric view of the LVOT and the aortic valve is suitable for quantitative Doppler interrogation of the aortic valve and this view is not obtainable in every patient and under all conditions. The velocity of flow in aortic stenosis is much higher than for mitral disease because of the higher pressure gradients; consequently, continuous-wave Doppler is the modality of choice for quantitatively studying aortic stenosis.[190-192]

The primary disease states affecting the aortic valve include senescent aortic stenosis, congenital aortic stenosis (usually as a result of a bicuspid valve), and rheumatic aortic stenosis. Senescent (or degenerative) stenosis is characterized by the trileaflet aortic valve with rigid, calcified nodules in the sinuses that limit valve opening. Rheumatic stenosis (often coexistent with other valvular disease) has calcification and fusion of all three commissures of the trileaflet valve. Congenital aortic stenosis usually results from a bicuspid valve (occasionally unicuspid) with unequal leaflets, the larger of which may contain a raphe which can appear to be a fused commissure of a trileaflet valve. In congenital stenosis, the orifice is often ellipsoid in shape. The short-axis view of the aortic valve at the midesophageal level is often the best location for determining the number of leaflets as well as the annular ring. All types of aortic stenosis can also be associated with LV hypertrophy and poststenotic dilation

of the aorta. In addition to valvular disease, the subvalvular region can also be the site of stenotic narrowing of the outflow tract. Asymmetric septal hypertrophy (previously referred to as idiopathic hypertrophic subaortic stenosis), as well as isolated fibrous membranes and rings, can all be readily identified.[193-196]

The severity of the aortic stenosis may be directly assessed by planimetric measurement of the valve orifice, usually from the short axis view of the aortic valve. Accurate planimetry can be performed in more than 90% of patients.[197] Nomograms for aortic valve area as function of age and body surface area can then be used to determine the degree of severity.

The other important measure of stenosis severity is the transvalvular pressure gradient. Continuous-wave Doppler directed through the LVOT from the deep transgastric view can give accurate velocity, and, therefore, pressure gradient measurements. However, as previously noted, this view is not available in all circumstances. With accurate velocity profiles and the modified Bernoulli equation, the mean and peak gradients can be calculated from the mean and peak velocities, respectively.[166]

Complete assessment of the aortic valve must include observation of the viewable aorta, the LVOT, and the other cardiac valves because all may be involved with the aortic disease process, either primarily or secondarily.

Regurgitant Lesions

Mitral Regurgitation

Regurgitation of the MV can occur when one or more of the components of the MV do not function normally. Therefore, it is necessary to evaluate all parts of the valve leaflets, the annulus, the chordae tendineae, papillary muscles, and the adjacent myocardium (both the ventricle and the atrium). Common causes of MR include infective endocarditis, MV prolapse with or without chordal rupture, rheumatic disease, myxomatous disease, degenerative disease, myocardial infarction with or without papillary muscle dysfunction or chordal rupture, trauma, and mitral annular calcification or dilation. TEE is particularly effective at identifying chordal rupture and flail leaflets, compared with other modalities. MR may be classified as acute or chronic; and as valvular, supravalvular, or subvalvular.[198-204]

The hallmarks of rheumatic MR include thickened deformed leaflets relatively symmetrically, frequently with calcification of the subvalvular apparatus. The jet of regurgitation from rheumatic disease is usually centrally directed because of the symmetric pathologic changes. It is especially important to assess the other valves in rheumatic disease since multiple valves may be involved.[205]

Identifying the cause of the MR is vitally important because this has a significant effect on the feasibility of repair, the ease of replacement, and the prognosis and recovery of the patient. Because there are so many different causes of MR, morphologic assessment must be systematic and thorough; also, it is difficult to develop a simple grading system for describing MR.

After the cause of the MR has been identified, its severity can be determined by both quantitative and semiquantitative measures. TEE is extremely sensitive at detecting MR because of the proximity to the valve and the generally unobstructed view. As a result, trivial MR is commonly found even in normal patients and is often manifested by a small systolic flow reversal immediately posterior and superior to the mitral leaflets.[206] TEE often demonstrates larger jets of

MR than does transthoracic echocardiography and therefore the same severity markers may not be valid.[207]

Measures that have been proposed for semiquantitative measurement of MR severity include absolute jet cross-sectional area, relative jet area to the LA area, jet width, length of the jet, and PV systolic flow reversal (retrograde flow). The use of absolute jet area measured by TEE may offer a good measure of regurgitation severity. Maximal mosaic (that portion of the jet that aliases) jet area has been shown to correlate with angiographically derived data. Specifically, a maximal mosaic jet area less than 3 cm² correlates with mild regurgitation and greater than 6 cm² correlates with severe regurgitation.[208] Using the relative size of the jet area to the LA size has been shown to correlate well with catheterization assessments when transthoracic echocardiography is used, but the same has not been validated with TEE. The ratio values of less than 0.2 correlating with angiographically mild regurgitation and greater than 0.4 indicating severe regurgitation have not been confirmed for TEE measurements. In addition, this method is not valid with eccentric jets or those that sweep along the atrial walls.[209, 210]

Another approach has been to use the regurgitant jet diameter at its origin. A good correlation was found that when the regurgitant jet diameter exceeds 5.5 mm, severe MR is usually present. It was also shown that this method was not significantly affected by the driving pressure or the eccentricity of the jet. Potential limitations with this technique involve the assumption that the regurgitant orifice does not change during systole (which may not be valid), and the variations caused by technical factors such as gain settings.[211]

The presence of abnormal PV flow can also be used to assess the severity of the MR. Systolic flow reversal in the PV can be measured by pulsed-wave or color Doppler and correlates with severe MR. Moderate-to-severe MR has been shown when there is diminished anterograde flow during systole in the PVs as well. It must be remembered that discordant flow profiles have been noted between the right and left PVs when widely eccentric jets have been observed; therefore, a concerted effort must be made to interrogate all the PVs.[212-214]

Quantitative measures of MR include measures of regurgitant volume and fraction and in general are more involved than the semiquantitative measures. Both regurgitant fraction and volume can be directly calculated if the mitral and aortic SVs are known; that is, regurgitant volume is the difference between the aortic and mitral SVs and the regurgitant fraction is the regurgitant volume divided by the aortic SV. By using the continuity equation across each valve, the SVs can be measured at the annulus as the product of the TVI and the annulus cross-sectional area (estimated by πr^2 where r is the radius of the annulus). These measurements, while quantitative, cannot be done simultaneously, are time-consuming, and therefore may be of limited value with the variability of hemodynamics intraoperatively. In addition, this method is also susceptible to interference from other valvular and ventricular disease.[176, 215, 216]

Another quantitative method involves measurement of the volume flow rate proximal to the regurgitant orifice, or the PISA method. Since this method does not involve assessment of the distal jet of MR but measures the flow convergence proximal to the orifice, the PISA method is not as dependent on technical factors as the previously mentioned techniques. The flow of MR is calculated by multiplying the area of the PISA ($2pr^2$) by the aliasing velocity; then the effective regurgitant orifice area is calculated by dividing this flow by the peak velocity of the MR jet. This can then be used to calculate the regurgitant volume by multiplying the effective re-

gurgitant orifice area by the TVI of the MR. The regurgitant fraction is the regurgitant volume divided by the total SV for the MV. In severe MR, the effective regurgitant orifice area is usually greater than 0.4 cm² and the regurgitant volume is greater than 50 mL. As with many quantitative measures, the PISA calculation can be rather involved and can be subject to hemodynamic variability intraoperatively.[217-221]

It is worth restating that because of the wide number of possible causes and the presence of eccentric jets, as well as the plethora of quantitative and semiquantitative methods for assessing the severity of MR, full assessment of MR requires multiple views and methods. The echocardiographer should not rely on any one method exclusively but should generate a composite picture of the regurgitation based on all the available information.

The implications of the abnormality that is found can help determine the nature of any surgical intervention. Repair of the MV is possible for many lesions, including limited resection of mitral prolapse, excess tissue plication, limited excision of vegetation, chordal shortening, ring annuloplasty, resection of flail segments (usually the posterior leaflet is a better candidate), and more recent developments of artificial chordae and chordae transposition. Obviously, the type of repair indicated is highly dependent on the abnormality present, patient characteristics, and the skill of the surgeon.

Aortic Regurgitation

In addition to identifying the disease process itself, aortic regurgitation should be classified as congenital, acquired, or both, and may also be classified as acute or chronic. Common causes of aortic regurgitation include infectious endocarditis, leaflet perforation, prolapse and flail, myxomatous disease, perivalvular abscess, aortic root dilation, aortic dissection, rheumatic disease, Marfan's syndrome, and Ehlers-Danlos syndrome. Combinations of these disease states are also possible, so a complete examination is essential.[201, 222-224]

The severity of aortic regurgitation can be assessed by quantification of the diastolic flow reversal in the LVOT and aorta. As with aortic stenosis, aortic regurgitation is associated with higher pressure gradients and flow velocities than for mitral disease; therefore, continuous-wave Doppler is the most appropriate modality for quantifying aortic regurgitation.

One of the more important semiquantitative measures of regurgitation severity is the spatial extent (color Doppler) of the jet closest to the aortic valve. Specifically, the jet area and width have been shown to correlate well with angiographic measurements of severity. The jet width method has been shown to be both simple and descriptive. In one method, the ratio of the minimum subvalvular jet width to the maximum LVOT width is strongly sensitive; if the ratio is less than 0.25, the regurgitation is mild, and if the ratio is greater than 0.64, the regurgitation is severe. As with other such techniques, this method is valid only for centrally directed jets, which can be accurately measured; further, there is some variability from instrumentation factors. The use of jet area and length are more strongly load-dependent, that is, they are affected by changes in the DP gradient, LV compliance and filling pressure, and diastolic duration.[225, 226]

Quantitative methods for assessing aortic regurgitation severity are similar to those for MR and include measurement of regurgitant fraction and volume as well as continuous-wave Doppler profiles of the aortic regurgitation. Continuous-wave Doppler can measure the instantaneous pressure gradient and decay between the aorta and the LV. More severe aortic regurgitation leads to rapid decay of the pressure gradient and therefore more rapid falloff of the regurgitant velocity. This measurement, however, is only valid in the absence of significant LV dysfunction or rapid peripheral runoff, both of which may lead to decay of the pressure gradient by themselves. The rate of pressure decay can be quantified using the PHT previously described, performed using the deep transgastric view of the LVOT and aortic valve. An aortic PHT of less than 300 ms indicates severe regurgitation and a value greater than 600 ms is consistent with mild regurgitation.[227, 228]

The continuity equation is used as previously mentioned to calculate the regurgitant volume and fraction across the aortic valve, once again using the deep transgastric view, which may not be obtainable in all patients.[229] An additional limitation to this method lies in the fact that aortic velocities may exceed the limits of the pulsed-wave Doppler profile necessary for the calculation. In addition, coexistent left-sided valvular disease and shunting can invalidate the calculation. Because of these technical limitations, the continuity equation–based methods are infrequently used for quantitation of aortic regurgitation.

Tricuspid Regurgitation

The TV is larger than the MV and has three leaflets instead of two. Instead of two distinct papillary muscles, it has multiple separate papillary muscles and its annular ring is set inferior to the mitral annulus. Despite these differences, the TV has similar Doppler profiles to the MV but of slightly lower velocity. As with the MV, trivial tricuspid regurgitation may be noted in more than 90% of normal patients.[230] In general, most cases of tricuspid stenosis also involve tricuspid regurgitation. Causes of tricuspid regurgitation may involve annular dilation or intrinsic disease such as degenerative disease with prolapse, rheumatic disease, endocarditis, or rarely Ebstein's anomaly. The best view for visualization of the TV is from the distal esophagus in the transverse plane to include the anterior leaflets.[231, 232]

Semiquantitative measures of tricuspid regurgitation employing color Doppler have not been validated. Since the right side of the heart is of lower pressure and is more compliant than the left, it would be expected that significant regurgitation would lead to atrial dilation. Therefore, in the absence of atrial dilation, tricuspid regurgitation seen by TEE is probably not of clinical significance. Alternatively, with right-sided heart dilation, the tricuspid annulus may expand and thereby produce secondary regurgitation even with an otherwise normal TV. With wide-open tricuspid regurgitation, there may be mid-to-late systolic pressure equilibration between the RA and RV as evidenced by reduction of tricuspid regurgitation in later systole. The significance and implications of tricuspid regurgitation and the need for surgical intervention have not been as rigorously studied as has been the case for left-sided valvular disorders.

The presence of tricuspid regurgitation is useful for the noninvasive estimation of PA pressures. By measuring the peak velocity of the tricuspid regurgitation jet, the peak pressure gradient across the TV during systole can be calculated using the modified Bernoulli equation. This tricuspid pressure gradient can then be added to either a direct or an estimated RA (or central venous) pressure to calculate the RV peak systolic pressure. The peak RV systolic pressure is presumed to be the peak PA pressure in the absence of RVOT obstruction. This must be checked to validate that assumption because one possible cause of tricuspid regurgitation is annular dilation from RV pressure overload from obstruction to ventricular outflow.[165]

Prosthetic Valve and Surgical Repair Assessment

Complete discussion of the assessment of prosthetic valves and native valve repairs is well beyond the scope of this chapter; however, basic principles and pitfalls will be discussed. Obviously, the nature of the repair or the type of prosthesis used in combination with the baseline examination of the patient's condition will largely influence the goals of TEE evaluation in the perioperative period.

Valve Repair

The specific site of valve repair is of primary concern in the TEE examination, but it is also important to closely inspect the annulus even if it was not involved in the repair. The annulus should be examined structurally and with Doppler imaging to identify dehiscence and perivalvular leaks. The repaired structure should be closely examined as well as the other support structures. Leaflet mobility and morphology must be reassessed after the repair. Even if there was no concern before the repair regarding approximation with other structures, full TEE examination must be done again because the anatomic orientation may have changed with the repair. An example of this would be the new onset of systolic anterior motion of the MV after a prolapse repair. TEE is also very useful for identifying complications of repair such as perivalvular abscess, pseudoaneurysm, or thrombus formation.

Visualization of all structures and Doppler profiles seen prior to repair may not be possible because of reverberation off highly echogenic substances like sutures and any other prosthetic material used in the repair. Depending on the repair, complete assessment may not be possible because of this interference. Residual regurgitation is a frequent, almost expected outcome after valve repair, but characteristics of the regurgitation (direction, origin, and extent) may be significantly altered from baseline. In general, assessing MV repairs is easier and more successful than any other because of the optimal windows for evaluation of the valve.

Prosthetic Valves

All the considerations for examination of valvular repair apply to the TEE evaluation of prosthetic valves. In addition, extensive knowledge of the expected appearance and Doppler profiles of the specific type of prosthetic valve used is essential. In general, all prosthetic valves have a characteristic "normal," usually trivial amount of regurgitation that must be distinguished from perivalvular leaks, primary prosthetic malfunction, and traumatic leaks or shunts from the placement of the prosthetic valve. These "normal" regurgitant jets are usually centrally directed and low-velocity jets that may arise from several different origins. The normal jets of regurgitation must be distinguished from perivalvular leaks, not all of which are normal, whether or not they are more than trivial or mild in severity.

Similar measures of valve function can be derived from Doppler profiles; that is, measures of effective orifice area, pressure gradients, regurgitant fraction and volume, and PHTs are all feasible if the TEE views allow them. Several general trends have been noted with regard to these hemodynamic profiles. In the aortic position, homografts have larger effective orifice areas and smaller peak velocity and mean gradients than do heterografts and mechanical prostheses. Mechanical prostheses have the highest mean gradients and peak velocities, although there is considerable variation between prosthesis types. In addition, larger sizes of prostheses have smaller gradients, but again there is wide variability in the effect of increasing size on gradients depending on the type of prosthesis.[233]

Since pressure gradients are significantly load-dependent, the effective orifice may be the clearest way of assessing the adequacy of a prosthesis. Measurement of effective orifice area can be adversely affected by improper measurement of the sewing ring diameter and errors in velocity profile determination arising from nonparallel axes of flow and measurement (angle θ error). No one measurement should be used exclusively in the decision-making process.

When assessing aortic valve prostheses, it is imperative to also assess reversal of flow in the aorta to determine the severity of the aortic regurgitation. In the presence of flow reversal of the descending aorta, even aortic valve regurgitation that appears mild must be considered to be significant. In addition, it has been noted that prosthetic aortic regurgitation is usually underestimated by TEE as compared with TEE.

For mitral and tricuspid prostheses, the PHT method for determining effective orifice area can be used as for native disease, but the continuity equation approach may be more accurate.[187] The specific values to use for decision making will differ for different types of prostheses. TEE is very sensitive in identifying regurgitant jets for mitral and tricuspid prostheses. One means of distinguishing "normal" from pathologic regurgitant jets lies in the fact that "normal" is usually of lower velocity (nonaliasing, nonmosaic) as opposed to perivalvular jets. "Normal" jets do not normally cause any changes in pulmonary vein Doppler flow profiles. Periprosthetic regurgitant jets are often eccentric, high-velocity jets that may be difficult to fully visualize.[3, 234] TEE has been shown to have greater than 92% effectiveness for identifying mitral prosthetic abnormalities at the time of reoperation on the prosthesis.[235]

REFERENCES

1. Sohn DW, Shin GJ, Oh JK, et al: Role of transesophageal echocardiography and hemodynamically unstable patients. Mayo Clin Proc 1995; 70:925–931.
2. Brandt RR, Oh JK, Orszulak TA, et al: Role of emergency intraoperative transesophageal echocardiography. J Am Soc Echocardiogr 1998; 10:972–977.
3. Kyo SK, Takamoto S, Matsumura M, et al: Immediate and early postoperative evaluation of results of cardiac surgery by transesophageal two-dimensional Doppler echocardiography. Circulation 1987; 76(suppl):V-113.
4. Sheikh KH, Bengston JR, Rankin J, et al: Intraoperative transesophageal Doppler color-flow imaging used to guide patient selection and operative treatment of ischemic mitral regurgitation. Circulation 1991; 84:594.
5. Savage RM, Lytle BW, Aronson S, et al: Intraoperative echocardiography is indicated in high-risk coronary artery bypass grafting. Ann Thorac Surg 1997; 64:368–374.
6. Bergquist BD, Bellows WH, Leung JM: Transesophageal echocardiography in myocardial revascularization: II. Influence on intraoperative decision-making. Anesth Analg 1996; 82:1139–1145.
7. Deutsch HJ, Curtuis JM, Leischik R, et al: Diagnostic value of transesophageal echocardiography in cardiac surgery. Thorac Cardiovasc Surg 1991; 39:199–204.
8. Hatle L, Angelsen B: Doppler Ultrasound in Cardiology: Physical Principles and Clinical Applications, ed 2. Philadelphia: Lea & Febiger, 1985.
9. Omoto R, Kasai C: Physics and instrumentation of Doppler color flow mapping. Echocardiography 1987; 4:467–483.
10. Gramiak R, Shah PM: Echocardiography in the aortic root. Invest Radiol 1968; 3:356.
11. Seward JB, Tajik AJ, Spangler JG, et al: Echocardiographic contrast studies: Initial experience. Mayo Clin Proc 1975; 50:163–192.
12. Hagler DJ, Currie PJ, Seward JB, et al: Echocardiographic contrast enhancement of poor or weak continuous-wave Doppler signals. Echocardiography 1987; 4:63–67.
13. Nakatani S, Imanishi T, Terasawa A, et al: Clinical application of transpulmonary contrast enhanced Doppler technique in the assessment of severity of aortic stenosis. J Am Coll Cardiol 1992; 20:973–978.
14. von Bibra H, Sutherland G, Becher H, et al: Clinical evaluation of left heart Doppler contrast enhancement by a saccharide-based transpulmonary contrast agent. J Am Coll Cardiol 1995; 25:500–508.
15. Crouse LJ, Cheirif J, Hanly DE, et al: Opacification and border delineation improvement in patients with suboptimal endocardial border definition in routine echocardiography: Results of the Phase III Albunex Multi-Center Trial. J Am Coll Cardiol 1993; 22:1494–1500.
16. Schröder K, Agrawal R, Völler H, et al: Improvement of endocardial border delineation in suboptimal stressed echocardiograms using the new left heart contrast agent SH U 508 A. Int J Card Imaging 1994; 10:45–51.
17. Kaul S, Kelly P, Oliner JD, et al: Assessment of regional myocardial blood flow with myocardial contrast two-dimensional echocardiography. J Am Coll Cardiol 1989; 13:468–482.
18. Porter TR, D'Sa A, Turner C, et al: Myocardial contrast echocardiography for the assessment of coronary blood flow reserve: Validation in humans. J Am Coll Cardiol 1993; 21:349–355.
19. Sahn DJ, Allen HD, George W, et al: The utility of contrast echocardiographic techniques in the care of critically ill infants with cardiac and pulmonary disease. Circulation 1977; 56:959.
20. Allen HD, Sahn DJ, Goldberg SJ: New serial contrast technique for assessment of left-to-right shunting patent ductus arteriosus in the neonate. Am J Cardiol 1978; 41:288.
21. Ryssing E: Contrast echocardiography: The descending thoracic aorta and the left atrial posterior wall in neonates. Acta Paediatr Scand 1981; 70:735.
22. Zednikova M, Bayen MG, Yoshida Y, et al: Precordial contrast echocardiographic detection of patent ductus arteriosus in small preterm infants. Pediatr Cardiol 1982; 2:271.
23. Roelandt J, Meltzer RS, Serruys PW: Contrast echocardiography of the left ventricle. *In* Rijsterboroh H (ed): Echocardiography. Boston, Martinus Nijhoff, 1981, pp 219–232.
24. Roelandt J: Contrast echocardiography. J Ultrasound Med Bio 1982; 8:471.
25. Feigenbaum H, Stone JM, Lee DA, et al: Identification of ultrasound echoes from the left ventricle by use of intracardiac injections of indocyanine green. Circulation 1970; 41:615.
26. Reid CL, Kawanishi DT, McKay CR, et al: Accuracy of evaluation of the presence and severity of aortic and mitral regurgitation by contrast two-dimensional echocardiography. Am J Cardiol 1983; 52:375.
27. Sabia PJ, Powers ER, Ragosta M, et al: An association between collateral blood flow and myocardial viability in patients with recent myocardial infarction. N Engl J Med 1992; 327:1825–1831.
28. Aronson S, Lee BK, Zaroff JG, et al: Myocardial distribution of cardioplegic solution after retrograde delivery in patients undergoing cardiac surgical procedures. J Thorac Cardiovasc Surg 1993; 105:214–221.
29. Meltzer RS, Vered Z, Roelandt J, et al:. Systematic analysis of contrast echocardiograms. Am J Cardiol 1983; 52:375.
30. Feinstein SB, TenCate FJ, Zwehl W, et al: Two-dimensional contrast echocardiography: In vitro development and quantitative analysis of echo contrast agents. J Am Coll Cardiol 1984; 3:6.
31. Levine RA, Techolz LE, Goldman ME, et al: Microbubbles have intracardiac velocities similar to that of red blood cells. J Am Coll Cardiol 1984; 3:28.
32. Heidenreich PA, Weineck JG, Zaroff JG, et al: Contrast echo: In vitro flow calculations. Circulation 1989; 80(suppl 2):II-370.

33. Aronson S, Weincek JG, Zaroff JG, et al: Assessment of renal blood flow in the dog with contrast ultrasound. Anesth Analg 1990; 70:S10.

34. Heidenreich PA, Weineck JG, Zaroff JG, et al: Measurement of renal blood flow/volume with digital ultrasonography. Circulation 1989; 80(suppl 2):II-568.

35. Feinstein SB, Cheirif J, TenCate FJ, et al: Safety and efficacy of a new transpulmonary ultrasound contrast agent: Initial multicenter clinical results. J Am Coll Cardiol 1990; 16:316.

36. Porter TR, Xie F: Transient myocardial contrast after initial exposure to diagnostic ultrasound pressures with minute doses of intravenously injected microbubbles: Demonstration and potential mechanisms. Circulation 1995; 92:2391-2395.

37. Walker R, Weincek JG, Zaroff JG, et al: Pitfalls in quantitation of contrast echo: Threshold effects. J Am Soc Echocardiogr 1991; 4:301.

38. Seward JB, Khanderia BK, Oh JK, et al: Critical appraisal of transesophageal echocardiography: Limitations, pitfalls, and complications. J Am Soc Echocardiogr 1992; 5:288-305.

39. Aronson S, Ruo W, Sand M: Inverted left atrial appendage appearing as a left atrial mass with TEE during cardiac surgery. Anesthesiology 1992; 76:1054-1055.

40. Leon M, Pechacek LW, Solana LG, et al: Identification of a prominent eustachian valve by means of contrast two-dimensional echocardiography. Tex Heart Inst J 1983; 10:219-221.

41. Schrem SS, Freedberg RS, Gindea A, et al: I. The association between unusually large eustachian valves and atrioventricular valvular prolapse. Am Heart J 1990; 120:204-206.

42. Weintraub A, Richardson G, Hsu TL, et al: Multiplane transesophageal echocardiography. Clinical application of real-time, wide-angle, transesophageal two-dimensional echocardiography and color flow imaging. Echocardiography 1991; 8:677.

43. Flachskampf FA, Hoffman R, Hanrath P: Experience with the transesophageal echo transducer allowing full rotation of the viewing plain: The omniplane probe (abstract). J Am Coll Cardiol 1991; 17:34A.

44. Hoffman R, Flachskampf FA, Hanrath P: Planimetry of stenotic aortic valve area using multiplane transesophageal echocardiography. Circulation 1991; 84:II-129.

45. Daniel WG, Pearlman AS, Hausmann D, et al: Multiplane transesophageal echocardiography: Initial experience and potential applications (abstract). J Am Coll Cardiol 1992; 19:235A.

46. Pandian N, Hsu TL, Weintraub A, et al: Real-time multiplane transesophageal echocardiography using a prototype phased array TEE probe with 180 degree scan plane steering capability: Method, echo-anatomic correlations and early clinical experience (abstract). J Am Coll Cardiol 1992; 19:235A.

47. Schwartz S, Weintraub A, Simonetti J, et al: Multiplane transesophageal echocardiography: Clinical experience with prototype phased array and mechanical annular array probes. J Am Soc Echocardiogr 1992; 5:327.

48. Mitchell M, Sutherland G, Gussenhoven E, et al: Transesophageal echocardiography. J Am Soc Echocardiogr 1988; 1:5.

49. Phased Array Ultrasound Imaging Transducer for Transesophageal Echocardiography User's Guide. Andover, MA, Hewlett-Packard, 1987.

50. Botoman VA, Surawicz CM: Bacteremia with gastrointestinal endoscopic procedures. Gastrointest Endosc 1986; 32:342-346.

51. Norfleet RG, Mitchell PD, Mulholland DD, et al: Does bacteremia follow upper gastrointestinal endoscopy? Am J Gastroenterol 1981; 76:420-422.

52. Shorvon PJ, Eykyn SJ, Cotton PV: Gastrointestinal instrumentation, bacteremia, and endocarditis. Gut 1983; 24:1078-1093.

53. Perucca PJ, Meyer GW: Who should get endocarditis prophylaxis for upper gastrointestinal procedures? (editorial). Gastrointest Endosc 1985; 31:285-312.

54. Dennig K, Sedlmayr V, Seling B, et al: Bacteremia with transesophageal echocardiography (abstract). Circulation 1989; 80(suppl 2):II-473.

55. Dajani AS, Bisno AL, Chung KJ, et al: Prevention of bacterial endocarditis: Recommendations by the American Heart Association. JAMA 1990; 264:2919-2922.

56. Ellis JE, Lichtor JL, Feinstein SB, et al: Right heart dysfunction, pulmonary embolism, and paradoxical embolization during liver transplantation. Anesth Analg 1989; 68:777.

57. Daniel WG, Erbel R, Kasper W, et al: Safety of transesophageal echocardiography: A multi-center survey of 10,419 examinations. Circulation 1991; 83:817-821.

58. Silvis SE, Nebel O, Rogers G, et al: Endoscopic complications. JAMA 1976; 9:928-930.

59. Khandheria BK, Seward JB, Tajik AJ: Transesophageal echocardiography. In Braunwald E (ed): Heart Disease: A Textbook of Cardiovascular Medicine, ed 3. Philadelphia, WB Saunders, 1991.

60. Rafferty T, LaMantia K, Davis E, et al: Quality assurance for intraoperative transesophageal echocardiography monitoring: A report of 846 procedures. Anesth Analg 1993; 76:228-232.

61. Urbanowicz JH, Kernoff RS, Oppenheim G, et al: Transesophageal echocardiography and its potential for esophageal damage. Anesthesiology 1990; 72:40.

62. Dewhurst WE, Stragand JJ, Fleming BM: Mallory-Weiss tear complicating intraoperative transesophageal echocardiography in a patient undergoing aortic valve replacement. Anesthesiology 1990; 73:777.

63. Hulyalkar AR, Ayd JD: Low risk of gastroesophageal injury associated with transesophageal echocardiography during cardiac surgery. J Cardiothorac Vasc Anesth 1993; 2:175-177.

64. Owall A, Stahl L, Settergren G: Incidence of sore throat and patient complaints after intraoperative transesophageal echocardiography during cardiac surgery. J Cardiothorac Vasc Anesth 1992; 1:15-16.

65. Cucchiara RF, Nugent M, Seward JB, et al: Air embolism in upright neurosurgical patients: Detection and localization by two-dimensional transesophageal echocardiography. Anesthesiology 1984; 60:353.

66. Cahalan MK: Transesophageal echocardiography: Should I be using it? In Fortieth Annual Refresher Course Lectures and Clinical Update Program. New Orleans, American Society of Anesthesiologists, 1989, lecture 125.

67. Geibel A, Behroz A, Przewolka U, et al: Is transesophageal echocardiography a risk for patients with cardiac disease? (abstract). J Am Coll Cardiol 1988; 11:219A.

68. Seward JB, Khandheria BK, Oh JK, et al: Transesophageal echocardiography: Technique, anatomic correlations, implementation, and clinical applications. Mayo Clin Proc 1988; 63:649-680.

69. Pearson AC, Castello R, Labovitz AJ: Safety and utility of transesophageal echocardiography in the critically ill patient. Am Heart J 1990; 119:1083-1089.

70. Cyran SE, Kimball TR, Meyer RA, et al: Efficacy of intraoperative transesophageal echocardiography in children with congenital heart disease. Am J Cardiol 1989; 63:594-598.

71. Schluter M, Langenstein BA, Polster J, et al: Transesophageal cross-sectional echocardiography with a phased array transducer system: Technique and initial clinical results. Br Heart J 1982; 48:67-72.

72. Zenker G, Erbel R, Kramer G, et al: Transesophageal two-dimensional echocardiography in young patients with cerebral ischemic events. Stroke 1988; 19:345-348.

73. Lunn RJ, Oliver WC, Hagler DJ, et al: Aortic compression by transesophageal echocardiographic probe in infants and children undergoing cardiac surgery. Anesthesiology 1992; 77:587-590.

74. Gilbert TB, Panico FG, McGill WA, et al: Bronchial obstruction by transesophageal echocardiography probe in a pediatric cardiac patient. Anesth Analg 1992; 74:156-158.

75. O'Shea JP, D'Ambra MN, Magro C, et al: Transesophageal echocardiography: Is it safe to the esophagus? An in vivo study (abstract). Circulation 78(suppl 2):II-440, 1988.

76. Schiller NB, Shah PM, Crawford M, et al: Recommendations for quantitation of the left ventricle by two-dimensional echocardiography. American Society of Echocardiography Committee on Standards, Subcommittee on Quantitation of Two-Dimensional Echocardiograms. J Am Soc Echocardiogr 1989; 2:358-367.

77. Popp RL, Winters WL: Clinical competence in adult echocardiography. J Am Coll Cardiol 1990; 15:1465.

78. Shanewise JS, Cheung AT, Aronson S, et al: ASE/SCA Guidelines for performing a comprehensive intraoperative multiplane transesophageal echocardiographic examination: Recommendations of the American Society of Echocardiography Council For Intraoperative Echocardiography and the Society of Cardiovas-

cular Anesthesiologists Task Force for certification in perioperative Transesophageal echocardiography. J Am Soc Echocardiogr 1999; 12:884–900.

79. Shanewise JS: Normal 2D echo and color flow Doppler. *In* Introduction for Anesthesiologists—Basic Transesophageal Echo. San Diego, Society of Cardiovascular Anesthesiologists/American Society of Echocardiography, 1999.

80. Carpentier AF, Lessana A, Relland J, et al: The "Physio-Ring": an advanced concept in mitral valve annuloplasty. Ann Thorac Surg 1995; 60:1177–1186.

81. Foster GP, Isselbacher EM, Rose AR, et al: Accurate localization of mitral regurgitant defects using multiplane transesophageal echocardiography. Ann Thorac Surg 1998; 65:1025–1031.

82. Grewal SG, Malkowski MJ, Kramer CM, et al: Multiplane transesophageal echocardiographic identification of the involved scallop in patients with a flail mitral valve leaflet: Intraoperative correlation. J Am Soc Echocardiogr 1998; 11:966–971.

83. Bollen BA: Basic evaluation of mitral valve regurgitation. *In* Introduction for Anesthesiologists—Basic Transesophageal Echo. San Diego, Society of Cardiovascular Anesthesiologists/American Society of Echocardiography, 1999.

84. Shanewise JS: Basic evaluation of tricuspid and pulmonic valve dysfunction. *In* Introduction for Anesthesiologists—Basic Transesophageal Echo. San Diego, Society of Cardiovascular Anesthesiologists/American Society of Echocardiography, 1999.

85. Bergquist BD, Leung JM, Bellows WH: Transesophageal echocardiography in myocardial revascularization: I. Accuracy of intraoperative real-time interpretation. Anesth Analg 1996; 82:1132–1138.

86. Abel MD, Nishimura RA, Callahan MJ, et al: Evaluation of intraoperative transesophageal two-dimensional echocardiography. Anesthesiology 1987; 66:64–68.

87. Shiina A, Tajik AJ, Smith HC, et al: Prognostic significance of regional wall motion abnormality in patients with prior myocardial infarction: A prospective correlated study of two-dimensional echocardiography and angiography. Mayo Clin Proc 1986; 61:254–262.

88. Smith JS, Cahalan MK, Benefiel DJ, et al: Intraoperative detection of myocardial ischemia in high-risk patients: Electrocardiography vs. two-dimensional transesophageal echocardiography. Circulation 1985; 72:1015–1021.

89. Leung JM, et al: Prognostic importance of post bypass regional wall motion abnormalities in patients undergoing coronary artery bypass graft surgery. Anesthesiology 1989; 71:16–25.

90. van Daele ME, Sutherland MB, Mitchell MM, et al: Do changes in pulmonary capillary wedge pressure adequately reflect myocardial ischemia during anesthesia? A correlative preoperative hemodynamic, electrocardiographic, and transesophageal echocardiographic study. Circulation 1990; 81:865–871.

91. Shah PM, Kyo S, Matsumura M, Omoto R: Utility of biplane transesophageal echocardiography in left ventricular wall motion analysis. J Cardiothorac Vasc Anesth 1991; 5:316–319.

92. Rouine-Rapp K, Ionescu P, Balea M: Detection of intraoperative segmental wall motion abnormalities by transesophageal echocardiography: The incremental value of additional cross sections and transverse and longitudinal planes. Anesth Analg 1996; 83:1141–1148.

93. Lehman KG, Korrester AL, MacKenzie WB, et al: Onset of altered intraventricular septal motion during cardiac surgery. Circulation 1990; 82:1325.

94. Chung F, Seyone C, Rakowski H: Transesophageal echocardiography may fail to diagnose perioperative myocardial infarction. Can J Anaesth 1991; 38:98.

95. Clements FM, de Bruijn NP: Perioperative evaluation of regional wall motion by transesophageal two-dimensional echocardiography. Anesth Analg 1987; 66:249.

96. Rosenthal A, Kawasuji M, Takemura H, et al: Transesophageal echocardiography monitoring during coronary artery bypass surgery. Jpn Circ J 1991; 55:109.

97. Sheehan FH, Feneley MP, Debruijn NP, et al: Quantitative analysis of regional wall thickening by transesophageal echocardiography. J Thorac Cardiovasc Surg 1992; 103:347.

98. Cahalan MK: Intraoperative assessment of systolic ventricular function. *In* 2nd Annual Comprehensive Review of Intraoperative Echo. San Diego, Society of Cardiovascular Anesthesiologists/American Society of Echocardiography, 1999.

99. Lieberman AN, Weiss JL, Juqdutt BD, et al: Two-dimensional echocardiography and infarct size: Relationship of regional wall motion and thickening to the extent of myocardial infarction in the dog. Circulation 1981; 63:739–746.

100. Luma JAC, Becker LA, Melin JA, et al: Impaired thickening of non-ischemic myocardial during acute regional ischemia in the dog. Circulation 1985; 71:1048.

101. Force T, Kemper A, Perkins L, et al: Overestimation of infarct size by quantitative two-dimensional echocardiography: The role of tethering and of analytic procedures. Circulation 1986; 73:1360.

102. Braunwald E, Kloner RA: The stunned myocardium: Prolonged, post ischemic ventricular dysfunction. Circulation 1982; 66:1146.

103. Buffington CW, Coyle RJ: Altered load dependence of post ischemic myocardium. Anesthesiology 1991; 75:464.

104. London MJ, Tubau JF, Wong MG, et al: The "natural history" of segmental wall motion abnormalities in patients undergoing non-cardiac surgery. Anesthesiology 1990; 73:64.

105. Smith JS, Roizen MF, Cahalan MK, et al: Does anesthetic technique making difference? Augmentation of systolic blood pressure during carotid endarterectomy: Effects of phenylephrine versus light anesthesia and of isoflurane versus halothane on the incidence of myocardial ischemia. Anesthesiology 1988; 69:846.

106. Roizen MF, Beaupre PN, Alpert RA, et al: Monitoring with two-dimensional transesophageal echocardiography. Comparison of myocardial function in patients undergoing supraceliac, suprarenal-infraceliac, or infrarenal aortic occlusion. J Vasc Surg 1984; 2:300.

107. Gewertz BL, Kremser PC, Zarins CK, et al: Transesophageal echocardiographic monitoring of myocardial ischemia during vascular surgery. J Vasc Surg 1987; 5:607.

108. Wickey GS, Larach DR, Keifer JC, et al: Combined interpretation of transesophageal echocardiography, electrocardiography, and pulmonary artery wedge waveform to detect myocardial ischemia. J Cardiothorac Vasc Anesth 1990; 4:102–104.

109. Simon P, Mohl W, Neumann F, et al: Effects of coronary artery bypass grafting on global and regional myocardial function: Intraoperative echo assessment. J Thorac Cardiovasc Surg 1992; 104:40.

110. Koolen JJ, Visser CA, Van Wezel HB, et al: Influence of coronary artery bypass surgery on regional left ventricular wall motion: An intraoperative two-dimensional transesophageal echocardiography study. J Cardiothorac Vasc Anesth 1987; 1:276.

111. Voci P, Billotta F, Aronson S, et al: Changes in myocardial segmental wall motion, systolic wall thickening, and ejection fraction immediately following CABG: An echocardiographic analysis comparing dysfunctional and normal myocardium. J Am Soc Echocardiogr 1991; 4:289.

112. Konstadt S, Reich DL, Thys DM, et al: Transesophageal echocardiography. *In* Kaplan JA (ed): Cardiac Anesthesia. Philadelphia, WB Saunders, 1993, pp 342–385.

113. Thys DM, Hillel Z, Goldman ME, et al: A comparison of hemodynamic indices derived by invasive monitoring and two-dimensional echocardiography. Anesthesiology 1987; 67:630.

114. Jensen JL, Williams FE, Beilby BJ, et al: Feasibility of obtaining pulmonary venous flow velocity in cardiac patients using trans-thoracic pulsed-wave Doppler technique. J Am Soc Echocardiogr 1997; 10:60–66.

115. Appleton, CP: Hemodynamic determinants of Doppler pulmonary venous flow velocity components: New insights from studies in lightly sedated normal dogs. J Am Coll Cardiol 1997; 30:1562–1574.

116. Kuecherer HF, Muhuideen IA, Kususmoto FM, et al: Estimation of mean left atrial pressure from transesophageal pulsed Doppler echocardiography of pulmonary venous flow. Circulation 1990; 82:1127–1139.

117. Gorcsan J, Snow FR, Paulsen W, et al: Noninvasive estimation of left atrial pressure in patients with congestive heart failure and mitral regurgitation by Doppler echocardiography. Am Heart J 1991; 121:858–863.

118. Ge Z, Zhang Y, Fan D, et al: Simultaneous measurement of left a show pressure by Doppler echocardiography and catheterization. Int J Cardiol 1992; 37:243–251.

119. Channer KS, Culling WI, Wilde P, et al: Estimation of left ventricular end diastolic pressure by pulsed Doppler ultrasound. Lancet 1986; 1:1500–1507.

120. Stork TV, Muller RM, Piske GJ, et al: Noninvasive determination of pulmonary artery wedge pressure: Compared analysis of pulsed Doppler echocardiography and right heart catheterization. Crit Care Med 1990; 18:1158–1163.

121. Ettles DF, Davies J, Williams GJ, et al: Can left ventricular and diastolic pressure be estimated by pulsed Doppler ultrasound? Int J Cardiol 1988; 20:239–245.

122. Kuecherer H, Ruffmann K, Kuebler W: Determination of left ventricular filling parameters by pulsed Doppler echocardiography: A noninvasive method to predict-pressures in patients with coronary artery disease. Am Heart J 1988; 116:1017–1021.

123. Nishimura RA, Abel MD, Housmans PR, et al: Mitral flow velocity curves as a function of different loading conditions: Evaluation by intraoperative transesophageal Doppler echocardiography. J Am Soc Echocardiogr 1989; 2:79.

124. Giannuzzi P, Imparato A, Temporelli PL, et al: Doppler derived mitral deceleration time of early filling as a strong predictor of pulmonary capillary wedge pressure in post infarction patients with left ventricular systolic dysfunction. J Am Coll Cardiol 1994; 23:1630–1637.

125. Konstadt SN, Thys D, Mindich BP, et al: Validation of quantitative intraoperative transesophageal echocardiography. Anesthesiology 1986; 65:418.

126. Clements FM, Harpole D, Quill T, et al: Simultaneous measurements of cardiac volumes, areas and ejection fractions by transesophageal echocardiography and first-pass radionuclide angiography (abstract). Anesthesiology 1988; 69:A4.

127. Urbanowicz JH, Shaaban MJ, Cohen NH, et al: Comparison of transesophageal echocardiographic and scintigraphic estimates of left ventricular end diastolic volume index and ejection fraction in patients following coronary artery bypass grafting. Anesthesiology 1990; 72:607.

128. Grossman W: Evaluation of systolic and diastolic function of the myocardium. In Grossman W (ed): Cardiac Catheterization and Angiography, ed 3. Philadelphia, Lea & Febiger, 1986, pp 301–319.

129. Ishida Y, Meisner JS, Tsujioka K, et al: Left ventricular filling dynamics: Influence of left ventricular relaxation and left atrial pressure. Circulation 1986; 74:187–196.

130. Curtois M, Kovacs SJ, Ludbrook PA: Transmitral pressure-flow velocity relation: Importance of regional pressure gradient in the left ventricle during diastole. Circulation 1988; 78:661–771.

131. Appleton CP, Hatle LK, Popp RL: Relation of transmitral flow velocity patterns to left ventricular diastolic function: New insights from a combined hemodynamic and Doppler echocardiographic study. J Am Coll Cardiol 1988; 12:426–440.

132. Oh JK, Appleton CP, Hatle LK, et al: The noninvasive assessment of left ventricular diastolic function with two-dimensional and Doppler echocardiography. J Am Soc Echocardiogr 1997; 10:246–270.

133. Jensen JL, Williams FE, Beilby BJ, et al: Feasibility of obtaining pulmonary venous flow velocity in cardiac patients using transthoracic pulsed-wave Doppler technique. J Am Soc Echocardiogr 1997; 10:60–66.

134. Rossvoll O, Hatle LK: Pulmonary venous flow velocities recorded by transthoracic Doppler ultrasound: Relation to left ventricular diastolic pressures. J Am Coll Cardiol 1993; 21:1687–1696.

135. Appleton CP, Jensen JL, Hatle LK, et al: Doppler evaluation of left and right ventricular diastolic function: A technical guide for obtaining optimal flow velocity recordings. J Am Soc Echocardiogr 1997; 10:271–292.

136. Choong CY, Abascal V, Thomas JD, et al: Combined influence of ventricular loading and relaxation on the transmitral flow velocity profile in dogs measured by Doppler echocardiography. Circulation 1988; 78:672.

137. Konstadt SN, Reich DL, Thys DM, et al: Importance of atrial systole to ventricular filling predicted by transesophageal echocardiography. Anesthesiology 1990; 72:971–976.

138. Stewart WJ, Dicola VC, Harthorne W, et al: Doppler ultrasound measurement of cardiac output in patients with physiologic pacemakers. Am J Cardiol 1984; 54:308.

139. Haskell RJ, French WJ: Optimum AV interval in dual chamber pacemakers. Pacing Clin Electrophysiol 1986; 9:670.

140. Pearson AC, Janosik DL, Redd RM, et al: Prediction of hemodynamic benefit of physiologic pacing from baseline Doppler echocardiographic parameters (abstract). Pacing Clin Electrophysiol 1987; 10:127A.

141. Rakowski H, Appleton CP, Chan KL, et al: Canadian consensus recommendations for the measurement and reporting of diastolic dysfunction by echocardiography. J Am Soc Echocardiogr 1996; 9:736–760.

142. Keren G, Sherez J, Megedish R, et al: Pulmonary venous flow pattern: Its relationship to cardiac dynamics: A pulsed Doppler echocardiographic study. Circulation 1985; 71:1105–1112.

143. Nishimura RA, Abel MD, Hatle LK, et al: Relation of pulmonary vein to mitral flow velocities by transesophageal Doppler echocardiography: Effect of different loading conditions. Circulation 1990; 81:1488–1497.

144. Basnight MA, Gonzalez MS, Kershenovich SC, et al: Pulmonary venous flow velocity: Relation to hemodynamics, mitral flow velocity and left atrial volume and ejection fraction. J Am Soc Echocardiogr 1991; 4:547–558.

145. Hoit BD, Shao Y, Gabel M, et al: Influence of loading conditions and contractile state on pulmonary venous flow: Validation by Doppler velocimetry. Circulation 1992; 86:651–659.

146. Appleton CP, Hatle LK: The natural history of left ventricular filling abnormalities: Assessment by two-dimensional and Doppler echocardiography. Echocardiography 1992; 9:437–457.

147. Klein AL, Burstow, DJ, Tajik AJ, et al: Effects of age on left ventricular dimensions and filling dynamics in 117 normal persons. Mayo Clin Proc 1994; 69:212–224.

148. Nishimura RA, Schwartz RS, Holmes DR, et al: Failure of calcium channel blockers to improve ventricular relaxation in humans. J Am Coll Cardiol 1993; 21:182–188.

149. Assessment of diastolic function. In Oh JK, Seward JB, Tajik AJ (eds): The Echo Manual. Philadelphia, Lippincott-Raven, 1999; 45–57.

150. Dumesnil JG, Gaudreault G, Honos GN, et al: Use of Valsalva maneuver to unmask left ventricular diastolic function abnormalities by Doppler echocardiography in patients with coronary artery disease or systemic hypertension. Am J Cardiol 1991; 68:515–519.

151. Takatsuji H, Mikami T, Urasawa K, et al: A new approach for evaluation of left ventricular diastolic function: Spatial and temporal analysis of left ventricular filling flow propagation by color M-mode Doppler echocardiography. J Am Coll Cardiol 1996; 27:365–371.

152. Stugaard M, Steen T, Lundervold A, et al: Visual assessment of intraventricular flow from color M-mode Doppler images. Int J Card Imaging 1994; 10:279–287.

153. Reichek N, Wilson J, St John Sutton M, et al: Noninvasive determination of left ventricular end-systolic stress: Validation of the method and initial application. Circulation 1982; 65:99.

154. Hartford M, Wilstand JCM, Wallentin I, et al: Left ventricular wall stress and systolic function in untreated primary hypertension. Hypertension 1985; 7:97.

155. Lang RL, Borow KM, Newman A, et al: Systemic vascular resistance: An unreliable index of afterload. Circulation 1986; 74: 1114.

156. Weissler AM: To systolic time intervals. N Engl J Med 1977; 96: 321.

157. Lewis RP, Rittgers SE, Forester WF, et al: A critical review of the systolic time intervals. Circulation 1977; 56:146.

158. Noble MIM, Trenchard D, Guz A: Left ventricular ejection in conscious dogs: 1. Measurement and significance of the maximum acceleration of blood from the left ventricle. Circ Res 1966; 19:139.

159. Bennett ED, Else W, Miller GAH, et al: Maximum acceleration of blood from the left ventricle in patients with ischemic heart disease. Clin Sci Mol Med 1974; 46:49.

160. Mehta N, Bennett ED: Impaired left ventricular function in acute myocardial infarction assessed by Doppler measurement of ascending aorta blood velocity and maximum acceleration. Am J Cardiol 1986; 57:1052.

161. Sabbah HN, Khaja F, Brymer JF, et al: Noninvasive evaluation of left ventricular performance based on peak aortic blood accel-

eration measured with a continuous-wave Doppler velocity meter. Circulation 1986; 74:323.

162. Folland ED, Parisi AF, Moynihan PF, et al: Assessment of left ventricular ejection fraction and volumes by real-time, two-dimensional echocardiography. Circulation 1979; 60:760.

163. Thys DM: Cardiac hemodynamics and quantitative echo. *In* 2nd Annual Comprehensive Review of Intraoperative Echo. San Diego, Society of Cardiovascular Anesthesiologists/American Society of Echocardiography, 1999.

164. Callahan MJ, Tajik AJ, Su-Fan Q, et al: Validation of instantaneous pressure gradients measured by continuous-wave Doppler in experimentally induced aortic stenosis. Am J Cardiol 1985; 56:989–993.

165. Currie PJ, Seward JB, Chan KL: Continuous wave Doppler determination of right ventricular pressure: A simultaneous Doppler catheterization study in 127 patients. J Am Coll Cardiol 1985; 6:750–756.

166. Currie PJ, Hagler DJ, Seward JB, et al: Instantaneous pressure gradient: A simultaneous Doppler and dual catheter correlative study. J Am Coll Cardiol 1986; 7:800–806.

167. Burstow DJ, Nishimura RA, Bailey KR, et al: Continuous-wave Doppler echocardiographic measurement of prosthetic valve gradients: A simultaneous Doppler catheter correlative study. Circulation 1989; 80:504–514.

168. Shanewise J: Hemodynamic workshop. *In* 2nd Annual Comprehensive Review of Intraoperative Echo. San Diego, Society of Cardiovascular Anesthesiologists/American Society of Echocardiography, 1999.

169. Kusumoto FM, Muhiudeen IA, Kuecherer HF, et al: Response of the interatrial septum to transatrial pressure gradients and its potential for predicting pulmonary capillary wedge pressure: An intraoperative study using transesophageal echocardiography in patients during mechanical ventilation. J Am Coll Cardiol 1993; 21:721–728.

170. Jue J, Winslow T, Fazio G, et al: Pulsed Doppler characterization of left atrial appendage flow. J Am Soc Echocardiogr 1993; 6:237–244.

171. Tabata T, Oki T, Fukuda N, et al: Influence of left atrial pressure on left atrial appendage flow velocity patterns in patients in sinus rhythm. J Am Soc Echocardiogr 1996; 9:857–864.

172. Garcia MJ, Ares MA, Asher C, et al: Color M-mode flow velocity propagation: An index of early left ventricular filling that combined with pulsed Doppler peak E velocity may predict capillary wedge pressure. J Am Coll Cardiol 1997; 29:448–454.

173. Uematsu M, Miyatake K, Tanaka N, et al: Myocardial velocity gradient as a new indicator of regional left ventricular contraction: Detection by a two-dimensional tissue Doppler imaging technique. J Am Coll Cardiol 1995; 26:217–223.

174. Nagueh SF, Mikati I, Kopelen HA, et al: Doppler estimation of left ventricular filling pressure in sinus tachycardia: A new application of tissue Doppler imaging. Circulation 1998; 98:1644–1650.

175. Zoghbi WA, Quinones MA: Determination of cardiac output by Doppler echocardiography: A critical appraisal. Herz 1986; 11:258–268.

176. Rokey R, Sterling LL, Zoghbi WA, et al: Determination of regurgitant fraction in isolated mitral or aortic regurgitation by pulsed Doppler two-dimensional echocardiography. J Am Coll Cardiol 1986; 7:1273–1278.

177. Annegers JF, Pillman NL, Weidman WH, et al: Rheumatic fever in Rochester, Minnesota, 1935–78. Mayo Clin Proc 1982; 57:753.

178. Nihoyannopoulos P, Gomez PM, Joshi J, et al: Cardiac abnormalities in systemic lupus erythematosus: Association with raised anticardiolipin antibodies. Circulation 1990; 82:369–375.

179. Pomerance A: Chronic rheumatic and other inflammatory disease. *In* Pomerance A, Davies MJ (eds): The Pathology of the Heart. Oxford, Blackwell, 1975, pp 307–326.

180. Roberts WC: Morphologic features of the normal and abnormal mitral valve. Am J Cardiol 1983; 51:1005–1028.

181. Chen Y-T, Kan M-N, Chen J-S, et al: Contributing factors to formation of left atrial spontaneous echo contrast in mitral valvular disease. J Ultrasound Med 1990; 9:151–155.

182. Daniel WG, Nellessen U, Schröder E, et al: Left atrial spontane-ous contrast in mitral valve disease: An indicator for increased thromboembolic risk. J Am Coll Cardiol 1988; 11:1204–1211.

183. Olson LJ, Freeman WK, Enriquez-Sarano M et al: Transesophageal echocardiographic evaluation of native valvular heart disease. *In* Freeman WK, Seward JB, Khandheria BK, et al (eds): Transesophageal Echocardiography. Boston, Little, Brown, 1994, p 192.

184. Wilkins GT, Weyman AE, Abascal VM, et al: Percutaneous balloon dilatation of the mitral valve: An analysis of echocardiographic variables related to outcome and the mechanism of dilatation. Br Heart J 1988; 60:299–308.

185. Abascal VM, Wilkins GT, Choong CY, et al: Mitral regurgitation after percutaneous balloon mitral valvuloplasty in adults: Evaluation by pulsed Doppler echocardiography. J Am Coll Cardiol 1988; 11:257–263.

186. Olson LJ, Tajik AJ: Echocardiographic evaluation of valvular heart disease. *In* Marcus ML, Schelbert HR, Skorton DJ, et al (eds): Cardiac Imaging: A Companion to Braunwald's Heart Disease. Philadelphia, WB Saunders, 1991, pp 430–433.

187. Hatle L, Angelson B, Tromsdal A: Noninvasive assessment of atrioventricular pressure half-time by Doppler ultrasound. Circulation 1979; 60:1096–1104.

188. Moro E, Nicolosi GL, Zanuttini D, et al: Influence of aortic regurgitation on the assessment of pressure half time and derived mitral-valve area in patients with mitral stenosis. Eur Heart J 1988; 9:1010–1017.

189. Nakatani S, Masuyama T, Kodama K, et al: Value and limitations of Doppler echocardiography in the quantification of stenotic mitral valve area: Comparison of pressure half time and the continuity equation methods. Circulation 1988; 77:78–85.

190. Dittrich HC, McCann HA, Walsh TP, et al: Transesophageal echocardiography in the evaluation of prosthetic and native aortic valves. Am J Cardiol 1990; 66:758–761.

191. Schwinger ME, Kronzon I: Improved evaluation of left ventricular outflow tract obstruction by transesophageal echocardiography. J Am Soc Echocardiogr 1989; 2:191–194.

192. Mügge A, Daniel WG, Wolpers HG, et al: Improved visualization of discrete subvalvular aortic stenosis by transesophageal color-coded Doppler echocardiography. Am Heart J 1989; 117:474–475.

193. Davies MJ: Pathology of Cardiac Valves. London, Butterworths, 1980, pp 18–35.

194. Pomerance A: Pathogenesis of aortic stenosis and its relation to age. Br Heart J 1972; 34:569–574.

195. Passik CS, Ackermann DM, Pluth JR, Edwards WD: Temporal changes in the causes of aortic stenosis: A surgical pathologic study of 646 cases. Mayo Clin Proc 1987; 62:119–123.

196. Subramanian R, Olson LJ, Edwards WD: Surgical pathology of pure aortic stenosis: A study of 374 cases. Mayo Clin Proc 1987; 62:119–123.

197. Chandrasekaran K, Foley R, Weintraub A, et al: Evidence that transesophageal echocardiography can reliably and directly measure the aortic valve area in patients with aortic stenosis—a new application that is independent of LV function and does not require Doppler data (abstract). J Am Coll Cardiol 1991; 17:20A.

198. Daniel WG, Mügge A, Martin RP, et al: Improvement in the diagnosis of abscesses associated with endocarditis by transesophageal echocardiography. N Engl J Med 1991; 324:795–800.

199. Shively BK, Gurule FT, Roldan CA, et al: Diagnostic value of transesophageal compared with transthoracic echocardiography in infective endocarditis. J Am Coll Cardiol 1991; 18:391–397.

200. Klodas E, Edwards WD, Khandheria BK: Use of transesophageal echocardiography for improving detection of valvular vegetations in subacute bacterial endocarditis. J Am Soc Echocardiogr 1989; 2:386–389.

201. Ballal RS, Mahan EF III, Nanda NC, Sanyal R: Aortic and mitral valve perforation: Diagnosis by transesophageal echocardiography and Doppler color flow imaging. Am Heart J 1991; 121:214–217.

202. Turabian M, Chan K-L: Rupture of mitral chordae tendineae resulting from blunt chest trauma: Diagnosis by transesophageal echocardiography. Can J Cardiol 1990; 6:180–182.

203. Hozumi T, Yoshikawa J, Yoshida K, et al: Direct visualization of ruptured chordae tendineae by transesophageal two-dimen-

sional echocardiography. J Am Coll Cardiol 1990; 16:1315-1319.

204. Schlüter M, Kremer P, Hanrath P: Transesophageal 2-D echocardiographic feature of flail mitral leaflet due to ruptured chordae tendineae. Am Heart J 1984; 108:609-610.

205. Bryam MT, Roberts WC: Frequency and extent of calcific deposits in purely regurgitant mitral valves: Analysis of 108 operatively excised valves. Am J Cardiol 1983; 52:1059-1061.

206. Akamatsu S, Uematsu H, Yamamoto M, et al: Evaluation of physiological mitral regurgitant flow with transesophageal Doppler echocardiography. Japan Circ J 1989; 53:663.

207. Smith MD, Harrison MR, Pinton R, et al: Regurgitant jet size by transesophageal compared with transthoracic Doppler color flow imaging. Circulation 1998; 83:79-86.

208. Castello R, Lenzen P, Aguirre F, Labovitz AJ: Quantitation of mitral regurgitation by transesophageal echocardiography with Doppler color-flow mapping: Correlation with cardiac catheterization. J Am Coll Cardiol 1992; 123:1245-1251.

209. Helmcke F, Nanda NC, Hsuing MC, et al: Color Doppler assessment of mitral regurgitation with orthogonal planes. Circulation 1987; 75:175-183.

210. Sahn DJ: Instrumentation and physical factors related to visualization of stenotic and regurgitant jets by Doppler color flow mapping. J Am Coll Cardiol 1988; 12:1354-1365.

211. Tribouilloy C, Shen WF, Quere J-P, et al: Assessment of severity of mitral regurgitation by measuring regurgitant width at its origin with transesophageal Doppler color flow imaging. Circulation 1992; 85:1248-1253.

212. Klein AL, Tajik AJ: Doppler assessment of pulmonary venous flow in healthy subjects and in patients with heart disease. J Am Soc Echocardiogr 1991; 4:379-392.

213. Castello R, Pearson AC, Lenzen P, Labovitz AJ: Effect of mitral regurgitation on pulmonary venous velocities derived from transesophageal echocardiography color-guided pulsed Doppler imaging. J Am Coll Cardiol 1991; 17:1499-1506.

214. Klein AL, Obarski TP, Stewart WJ, et al: Transesophageal Doppler echocardiography of pulmonary venous flow: A new marker of mitral regurgitation severity. J Am Coll Cardiol 1991; 18:518-526.

215. Enriquez-Sarano M, Bailey KR, Seward JB, et al: Quantitative Doppler assessment of valvular regurgitation. Circulation 1993; 87:841-848.

216. Enriquez-Sarano M, Tajik AJ, Bailey KR, Seward JB: Color flow imaging compared with quantitative Doppler assessment of severity of mitral regurgitation: Influence of eccentricity of jet and mechanism of regurgitation. J Am Coll Cardiol 1993; 21:1211-1219.

217. Lopez JF, Hanson S, Orchard RC, Tan L: Quantification of mitral valvular incompetence. Cathet Cardiovasc Diagn 1985; 11:139-152.

218. Giesler M, Grossmann G, Schmidt A, et al: Color Doppler echocardiographic determination of mitral regurgitation from the proximal velocity profile of the flow convergence region. Am J Cardiol 1993; 71:217-224.

219. Chen C, Koschyk D, Brockhoff C, et al: Noninvasive estimation of regurgitant flow rate and volume in patients with mitral regurgitation by Doppler color mapping of accelerating flow field. J Am Coll Cardiol 1993; 21:374-383.

220. Utsonomiya T, Ogawa T, Tang HA, et al: Doppler color flow mapping of proximal isovelocity surface area: A new method for measuring volume flow rate across a narrowed orifice. J Am Soc Echocardiogr 1991; 4:338-348.

221. Recusani F, Bargiggia GS, Yogananthan AP, et al: A new method for quantification of regurgitant flow rate using color Doppler flow imaging of the flow convergence region proximal to a discrete orifice: An in vitro study. Circulation 1991; 83:594-604.

222. Olson LJ, Subramanian R, Edwards WD: Surgical pathology of pure aortic insufficiency: A study of 225 cases. Mayo Clin Proc 1984; 59:835-841.

223. Pyeritz RE, McKusick VA: The Marfan syndrome: Diagnosis and management. N Engl J Med 1979; 300:772-777.

224. Leier CV, Call TD, Fulkerson PK, Wooley CF: The spectrum of cardiac defects in the Ehlers-Danlos syndrome, types I and III. Ann Intern Med 1980; 92:171-178.

225. Perry GJ, Helmcke F, Nanda NC, et al: Evaluation of aortic insufficiency by Doppler color flow mapping. J Am Coll Cardiol 1987; 9:952-959.

226. Welch GH Jr, Braunwald E, Sarnott SJ: Hemodynamic effects of quantitatively varied experimental aortic regurgitation. Circ Res 1957; 5:546-551.

227. Grayburn PA, Handshoe R, Smith MD, et al: Quantitative assessment of the hemodynamic consequences of aortic regurgitation by means of continuous wave Doppler recordings. J Am Coll Cardiol 1987; 10:135-141.

228. Labovitz AJ, Ferrara RP, Kern MJ, et al: Quantitative evaluation of aortic insufficiency by continuous wave Doppler echocardiography. J Am Coll Cardiol 1986; 8:1341-1347.

229. Yeung AC, Plappert T, St John Sutton MG: Calculation of aortic regurgitation orifice area by Doppler echocardiography: A new application of the continuity equation. Circulation 1988; 78 (suppl 2):II-39.

230. Silver MD, Lam JHC, Ranganathan N, et al: Morphology of the human tricuspid valve. Circulation 1971; 43:333-348.

231. Banks T, Fletcher R, Ali N: Infective endocarditis in heroin addicts. Am J Cardiol 1977; 40:438-444.

232. McKinsey DS, Ratts TE, Bisno AL: Underlying cardiac lesions in adults with infective endocarditis: The changing spectrum. Am J Med 1987; 82:681-688.

233. Miller FA Jr, Callahan JA, Taylor CL, et al: Normal aortic valve prosthesis hemodynamics: 609 prospective Doppler examinations. Circulation 1989; 80(suppl 2):II-169.

234. Abbruzzese PA, Meloni L, Cardu G, et al: Intraoperative transesophageal echocardiography and periprosthetic leaks. J Thorac Cardiovasc Surg 1991; 101:556-557.

235. Khandheria BK, Seward JB, Oh JK, et al: Value and limitations of transesophageal echocardiography in assessment of mitral valve prostheses. Circulation 1991; 83:1956-1986.

PART FOUR

Respiratory System

16 Monitoring the Function of the Respiratory System

Thomas J. Gal, M.D.

Monitoring the function of the respiratory system is of great importance to the anesthesiologist because the problems associated with inadequate ventilation, if unrecognized, can contribute significantly to anesthetic morbidity. Some monitoring techniques are sophisticated and invasive while others rely on more simple clinical observation. In this chapter the wide range of techniques available to monitor respiratory function and ventilation is considered, with an emphasis on the physiologic principles that form the basis of the measurements. The goal is to enhance the clinician's understanding of the indications, interpretations, and limitations of such respiratory measurements.

Respiratory Mechanics

Respiratory mechanics concerns the study of the function of the respiratory system as an air pump. It involves the analysis of the means whereby forces are generated to move air and thus physically transport air to and from the alveoli. Contraction of the respiratory muscles produces the force necessary to move air in and out of the lungs. This force must in turn overcome three basic opposing forces: inertia, elastance, and resistance.

Respiratory Muscles

Contraction of the inspiratory muscles produces expansion of the chest and fills the lungs with air. The principal muscle of inspiration, the diaphragm, contracts and descends to expand the chest longitudinally and to elevate the lower ribs. This action is responsible for more than two thirds of the air movement during quiet inspiration. The remaining volume is due to contraction of the external intercostals to further elevate the ribs and enlarge both the transverse and anteroposterior chest dimensions. Expiration during quiet breathing results essentially from the passive recoil of the lungs and chest wall. Only during higher levels of ventilation or when air movement is impeded do the internal intercostals and abdominal muscles contract to depress the ribs and compress the abdominal contents to provide active expiratory effort. The expiratory muscles, however, play important roles in other breathing-related activities, such as talking, singing, and coughing.

All measurements of pulmonary function that require patient effort are influenced by respiratory muscle strength. This can be evaluated specifically by measurements of maximal static respiratory pressures. These pressures are generated against an occluded airway during a maximal forced effort and can be measured with simple aneroid gauges.[1]

The inspiratory muscles are at their optimal length near residual volume. Thus, maximum inspiratory pressure (PImax) is usually measured after a forced exhalation. Similarly, maximum expiratory pressure (PEmax) is measured at total lung capacity where expiratory muscles are stretched to their optimal length by a full inspiration. Typical values for PImax in healthy young males are about -125 cm H_2O, while PEmax can be as high as $+200$ cm H_2O.

Values for PEmax less than $+40$ cm H_2O suggest impaired coughing ability,[2] whereas PImax values of -25 cm H_2O or less indicate severely impaired ability to take a deep breath. The latter value is often utilized as a criterion for extubation; however, observations in healthy volunteers during partial curarization suggest that this level of adequate ventilatory ability is too low to ensure adequate airway integrity.[3]

Forces Opposing Airflow

The movement of air in and out of the lungs is opposed by basic forces that must be overcome. These opposing forces are inertia, elastance, and resistance. During most breathing activities, inertia, which comprises the impedance to acceleration of gas and tissue, is negligible. Elastance and its reciprocal compliance are reflections of the relationships of pressure to volume when there is no airflow. Hence such measurements are referred to as *static*. Resistance, on the other hand, is highly dependent on the rate of change of lung volume, that is, flow. Such measurements during active breathing are referred to as *dynamic*.

Static

The respiratory system and its component lung and chest wall are elastic. That is, they tend to regain their original size and configuration following deformation when deforming forces are removed. Both lung and chest wall have positions of equilibrium. These are the volumes that they tend to assume in the absence of external forces acting upon them, and the volumes to which they continuously attempt to return when displaced. The equilibrium position of the lung is at residual volume (RV). To sustain any volume in the lung above RV, force must be applied to the lung and the lung will recoil with an equal and opposite force. At all volumes above RV, the lung recoils inward. The equilibrium position of the chest wall is at a relatively large volume, about 60% of total lung capacity (TLC). To sustain any volume in the chest wall below this point, the wall must be contracted and it will tend to recoil outward, opposite in direction from the lung. To sustain any volume in the chest wall above its equilibrium point, the wall must be actively enlarged and its recoils inward, in the same direction as the lung.

In the intact respiratory system, the lung and chest wall are coupled and work together. Behavior of the respiratory system is determined by the individual properties of the lung and chest wall. The equilibrium position of the respiratory system will be at that volume in which the tendency of the lung to recoil inward is balanced by the tendency of the wall to recoil outward (Fig. 16–1). To sustain any volume in the respiratory system other than this resting volume, which is the functional residual capacity (FRC), a force must be applied to displace both lung and chest wall. The recoil pressure of the respiratory system (Prs) that develops is the algebraic sum of the individual recoil pressures of the lung (PL) and the chest wall (Pw). Thus:

$$Prs = PL + Pw; \text{ at FRC } Prs = 0$$

The lung is a distensible elastic body enclosed in an elastic container, the thoracic cavity. Just as a spring is described by the force required to stretch it to a certain length, so can the respiratory system be described by the static pressure required to change its volume. This relation between changes in volume and changes in pressure is termed compliance ($\Delta V/\Delta P$). For the various components of the respiratory system, compliance is determined by relating the change in volume to a given distending pressure. These various pressures are:

1. Transpulmonary pressure (PL) or pressure across lung
$$PL = PA - Ppl$$

where
  PA = alveolar pressure; it is the same as mouth pressure under condition of zero flow
  Ppl = intrapleural pressure, usually estimated by esophageal pressure

2. Pressure across chest wall (Pw)
$$Pw = Ppl - Pbs$$

where
  Pbs = pressure at body surface (atmospheric)

3. Transthoracic or pressure across respiratory system (Prs)
$$Prs = PA - Pbs$$

Because the pressure-volume (P-V) curves for the respiratory system are curvilinear (see Fig. 16–1), compliance will vary from one portion of the curve to another, depending on the range of lung volume. Therefore, values are usually obtained in the range of 1 L above FRC where the P-V relationships are most linear.

The measurement of Ppl has long since been estimated by a special thin-walled balloon in the midesophagus. The balloon was 10 cm long and was usually filled with 0.5 mL of air.[4] More recently a 127-cm-long nasogastric tube incorporating a similar balloon has become available commercially,[5] and made the measurement more accessible to the clinician (Fig. 16–2). The pressure across the lung (PL) is thus measured by connecting the balloon to one port of a differential pressure transducer while the other port of the transducer senses mouth pressure.

It is important to make the distinction between static and dynamic compliance. When no gas flow occurs and pressure and volume are kept constant, the measurement is termed *static compliance.* Such would be the case if the patient's lung were inflated by a device, such as a supersyringe, and then held. *Dynamic compliance,* on the other hand, relates pressure and tidal volume at the moment inspiration changes to expiration and flow ceases only momentarily. Ideally these two compliance measurements are similar. However, if flow is impeded for some reason—for instance, by bronchoconstriction or a kink in the endotracheal tube—dynamic compliance is influenced by resistance to flow and does not reflect the true static compliance. Dynamic and static compliance differ by an amount related to flow resistance at endinspiration. The difference in pressures (peak versus plateau) can be readily appreciated in circuits utilizing a ventilator equipped with an inspiratory hold or pause with no flow or by merely clamping the expiratory tubing. The relationship between delivered volume and plateau pressure during this pause is often referred to as the "quasi-static" or "effective" compliance (Fig. 16–3).

Dynamics

Dynamics deals with conditions of airflow and describes the relationships between pressure and flow in the respiratory system. Therefore, resistance (R) is computed from pressure differences responsible for flow and the simultaneous measurement of airflow (R = $\Delta P/\dot{V}$).

Various components of the respiratory system contribute to the total resistance to airflow. These include an elastic component, the chest wall, and a nonelastic component termed pulmonary resistance, which for practical purposes is synonymous with airway resistance (Raw). Approximately 60% of total respiratory resistance is Raw; the remaining 40%

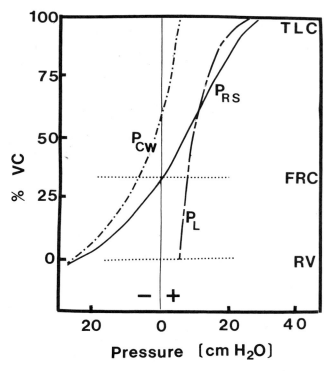

Figure 16–1. Recoil pressure curves for lung (P$_1$), chest wall (P$_{cw}$), and total respiratory system (P$_{rs}$) are plotted as a function of lung volume, in this case vital capacity (VC). FRC, functional residual capacity; RV, residual volume; TLC, total lung capacity.

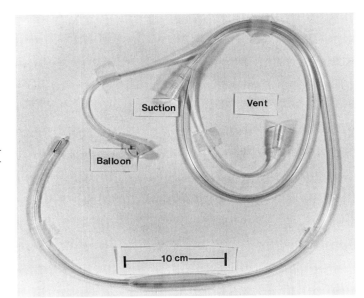

Figure 16-2. Commercially available nasogastric tube incorporating the 10-cm esophageal balloon used to measure pleural pressures. (Courtesy of NCC Division, Mallinkrodt Inc., Argyle, NY.)

is accounted for by the chest wall. It is important to note that the "chest wall" in physiologic terms includes not only the bony thorax but also the diaphragm and abdominal contents. Therefore, changes in muscle tone may affect measurements of total respiratory system resistance without actually altering airway resistance.

One other important factor to consider about Raw is the fact that resistance to airflow is determined by the size of the airways. Airways are largest at high lung volumes and smallest at low volumes, such as residual volume. Passive changes in Raw can thus occur with changes in lung volume

in the absence of bronchodilation or constriction. Because the relationship of Raw to lung volume is not linear, the reciprocal of Raw, conductance (Gaw), is related to lung volume in a linear manner and is utilized to identify the presence of bronchostriction or bronchodilation. Such determinants of Raw are, by convention, made at FRC.

Methods of Measuring Resistance

Flow-Pressure-Volume Method

Simultaneous recordings of the three variables, flow, pressure, and tidal volume (Fig. 16-4), provide the basis for this analysis. The change in pressure (ΔP) and change in flow ($\Delta\dot{V}$) between two points where volume is identical are used to calculate resistance. This method of analysis is termed the isovolume technique. Another more complex technique relating pressure flow and volume is termed the Comroe-Nissel-Nims technique.[6] With this method, static compliance is first calculated by dividing the total inspired volume by the pressure measured immediately prior to exhalation. Next, the point on the flow trace at which the expiratory flow is 0.5 L/second is noted and the volume of gas remaining in the lungs at this point also is measured. Dividing this volume by the compliance value gives a pressure associated with a flow of 0.5 L/second and thus provides the calculation of resistance. In either of these cases, the use of airway or mouth pressure yields total respiratory system resistance, whereas the use of PL yields pulmonary resistance.

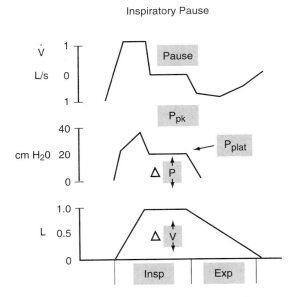

Inspiratory Pause

Figure 16-3. Diagrammatic representation of flow ($\dot{V}$) in liters per second pressure (P) in centimeters H_2O and tidal volume in liters typical of a cycle of mechanical ventilation incorporating an inspiratory pause. During the pause, peak pressure (P_{pk}) decreases to the plateau pressure (P_{plat}). The ratio of delivered volume (ΔV) to this pressure (ΔP) is the quasi-static compliance.

Passive Exhalation Method

The time it takes for the volume of the respiratory system to decrease to 37% of its initial preexpiratory value is termed the time constant (tk). This tk is essentially equal to the product of resistance and compliance. In this method, compliance is determined in similar manner as in the Comroe-Nissel-Nims technique, by relating V to P prior to exhalation. If the time interval to exhale to 370 mL (Fig. 16-5) is then

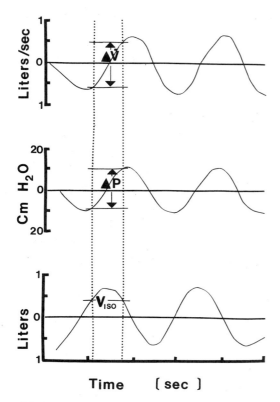

Figure 16-4. Simultaneous record of flow ($\dot{V}$), pressure (P), and volume (V) for determination of resistance by the isovolume technique. Change in pressure (P) and change in flow ($\dot{V}$) between two points where volume is identical (V_{iso}) provide an estimate of resistance.

measured and divided by this compliance value, another calculation of total respiratory system resistance is provided.

Forced Oscillation

Total respiratory resistance can be measured during quiet breathing by imposing rapid small-line wave oscillations at the mouth and recording the resultant sine wave flows and pressure. Such oscillations are produced by a loudspeaker or valveless pump. To measure the pressure change due to resistance, the components due to compliance and inertia must be eliminated. This is done by choosing the resonant frequency of the respiratory system (3 to 8 Hz) where compliance and inertia are 180 degrees out of phase (i.e., equal magnitude and opposite sign) and cancel out. The oscillating pressure wave is then due to resistance alone.[7] One of the major advantages of this technique is that it requires very little patient cooperation. However, to be a true reflection of changes in airway tone, lung volume changes must be taken into account.

Body Plethysmography

This technique, first described by Dubois et al.,[8] has the advantage of specifically determining Raw and simultaneously providing a measurement of thoracic gas volume. The patient must sit in a closed box and breathe via a mouthpiece. During panting-like breaths (two to three

breaths per second), flow at the mouth measured by a pneumotachograph is displayed on the y-axis of an oscilloscope, while box pressure is displayed on the x-axis. The slope of this loop is usually measured between 0 and 5 L/second to compute resistance (Fig. 16-6A). When the airway is occluded during such panting, pressure at the mouth is displayed on the y-axis and related to box pressure to estimate thoracic gas volume, which in most cases is the FRC (Fig. 16-6B).

Flow Interrupter Technique

A rapid noninvasive and convenient means of estimating respiratory system resistance utilizes rapid airway occlusion. The technique requires that pressure and flow at the mouth or airway opening be monitored while flow is suddenly interrupted at the end of an inspiration (Fig. 16-7). Such a condition occurs with the inspiratory pause phase on most anesthesia ventilators. A measure of total respiratory resistance (Rrs) is obtained by dividing the peak or maximal pressure (Pmax) by the flow (V) immediately prior to the occlusion or pause. The Pmax at end-inspiration is the total dynamic pressure required for delivery of the set tidal volume (VT) at the set flow rate. As the end-inspiratory occlusion or pause takes place, Pmax immediately decreases to P1 followed by a slower decay to a plateau value (P2). The latter represents static elastic recoil pressure at the end-inspiratory lung volume and serves as the basis for calculating compliance. The immediate decrease in pressure from Pmax to P1, with interruption of flow, reflects the intrinsic flow resistance of the airways, including the tracheal tube.

A calculation of this airway resistance or interrupter resistance (Rint) is obtained by subtracting P1 from Pmax and dividing by flow (see Fig. 16-7). If one subtracts P2 from P1 and divides by flow, the other component of Rrs, the effective additional resistance (ΔRrs), is estimated. The

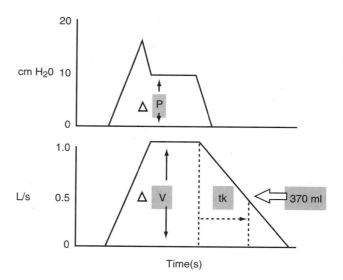

Figure 16-5. Illustration of the passive exhalation method for estimating resistance. Compliance (C) is calculated as volume per change in pressure (V/P) prior to exhalation. tk, Time required to exhale to 37% of preexpiratory volume (i.e., 370 mL). Resistance (R) is calculated from equation: R × C = tk.

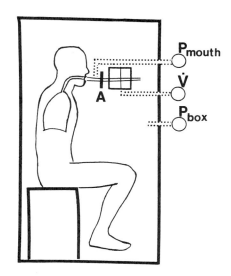

A: Shutter open   **B: Shutter closed**

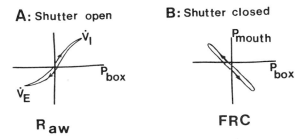

R_{aw} FRC

Figure 16-6. *A* and *B*, Constant volume body plethysmograph used to determine airway resistance and thoracic gas volume by utilizing relationships of flow, box pressure, and mouth pressure during panting with shutter open and closed.

ΔRrs is also referred to as tissue resistance (Rti) and reflects the viscoelastic properties of lung tissue and inequalities in regional time constants.[9] The accuracy of estimating these components of flow resistance—and in particular ΔRrs—is highly dependent on a sufficiently long pause to allow pressure differences due to regional lung inhomogeneities to equilibrate at a stable P2.

The intrinsic flow resistance (Rint) decreases with increasing inflation volumes because airway caliber is passively increased. On the other hand, tissue resistance or ΔRrs increases to a greater extent with inflation such that total Rrs is greater also.

Conventional wisdom suggests that as inspiratory flow increases Rrs should increase as well, especially in patients with obstructive airway disease. Actually with inflation volumes of 0.5 L or more, Rrs was noted to decrease as flow was increased, and reached a value at a flow of 1.0 L/second, which was about half that at 0.25 L/second.[10] A comparable relationship between flow and Rrs was shown in 16 normal anesthetized paralyzed subjects[11] and in 8 patients with adult respiratory distress syndrome.[12]

This decrease in Rrs with increasing flow is clinically relevant because it occurs in the flow range commonly used in the care of patients (0.75 to 1.0 L/second) and with commonly used tidal volumes (10 mL/kg). It appears that the increased airway resistance (Rint) with increased flow is offset by a greater decrease in ΔRrs or tissue resistance that occurs as either flow rates or breathing frequencies increase.

Since total Rrs in chronic obstructive pulmonary disease (COPD) is nearly three times that of normal, it follows that both Rint, the airway resistance component, and ΔRrs, the tissue component, are increased. Time constant inequalities that affect ΔRrs play a greater role in COPD patients than in healthy individuals and contribute considerably to the increased dynamic work of breathing. The magnitude of this tissue resistance is greatest with low inspiratory flows and large tidal volumes. Thus, the rapid shallow breathing pattern characteristic of COPD patients, especially with ventilatory failure, may represent an attempt to reduce the work of breathing.

Measurement of Lung Volumes

In a clinical setting there are only a few volumes that are worthwhile monitoring (Table 16-1). The simplest of these is resting V_T. In patients connected to a ventilator or anesthetic circuit, it is important to place the measuring device (to be discussed later) on the expiratory side of the circuit and as close to the patient as possible. The latter is important to minimize the effects of added gas flow from continuous positive pressure circuits or fresh gas flow from the anesthesia machine.

$$Rrs = (Pmax - P_2)/\dot{V}$$

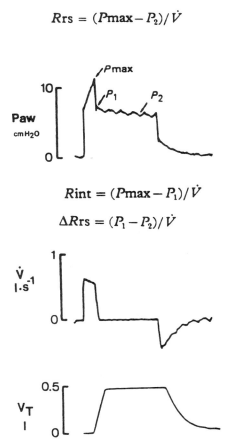

$$Rint = (Pmax - P_1)/\dot{V}$$

$$\Delta Rrs = (P_1 - P_2)/\dot{V}$$

Figure 16-7. Tracing of flow ($\dot{V}$), airway opening (P), and changes in lung volume (V) to illustrate rapid occlusion at end-inspiration during constant flow inflation. Pressure immediately decreases from its maximal value (P_{max}) to an intermediate pressure (P_1) and then slowly decays to a plateau value (P_2). The various components of total respiratory resistance (R_{rs}) are calculated from these pressures and $\dot{V}$ (see text for further explanation).

Table 16–1. Pulmonary Function Tests

	Values*
Forced vital capacity (FVC)	5000 mL
Forced expiratory volume in 1 second (FEV$_1$)	4000 mL
FEV$_1$/FVC	>75%
Functional residual capacity (FRC)	3000 mL
Slow vital capacity (VC)	5000 mL
Inspiratory capacity (IC)	3000 mL
Total lung capacity (TLC)	6000 mL
Expiratory reserve volume (ERV)	1500 mL
Residual volume (RV)	1500 mL
Dead space (VD)	150 mL
Dead space to tidal volume ratio (VD/VT)	≦ 0.33
Maximum voluntary ventilation (MVV)	170 L/min
Lung compliance (CL)	0.2 L/cm H$_2$O
Airway resistance (Raw)	1.5 cm H$_2$O/L/s
Diffusing capacity (DL) (single breath, CO monoxide)	31 mL CO/min/mmHg
Inspiratory pressure (PImax)	−125 cm H$_2$O
Expiratory pressure (PEmax)	+200 cm H$_2$O
Peak expiratory flow rate (PEFR)	500 L/min

* Typical values for a young, healthy, 70-kg male.

Vital Capacity

The vital capacity (VC) in the normal adult is basically a measure of stature; that is, it correlates strongly with height. The volume represents the difference between the limits of maximum voluntary inspiration (TLC and voluntary expiration [residual volume]). Devices for measuring this volume are discussed later.

Normally, VC is more than 10 times the resting VT. The relationship between the two is often used to estimate ventilatory reserve. In disease, VC is reduced by abnormalities of the bony thorax, increased lung stiffness, abdominal distention, muscle weakness, and a loss of functional alveoli. Other factors, such as pain, fatigue, and poor effort, may prevent the maximum full inspiration and expiratory effort required for normal measured volumes.

Functional Residual Capacity

FRC refers to the gas remaining in the lungs at the end of a normal expiration, or, more precisely, the volume at which the recoil of the lung and thorax oppose each other equally (see Fig. 16–1). In most clinical situations a reduction in FRC is associated with increased lung recoil, that is, decreased compliance.[13] Thus, there appears to be little advantage to measuring FRC in the usual clinical setting of the operating room or intensive care unit.

The techniques available for determining FRC are also somewhat difficult to apply in these areas. The most accurate technique utilizes the body plethysmograph, as during Raw determinations. This technique is virtually impossible in the unconscious artificially ventilated patient because of the requirements for confinement in an airtight box. Lung volume in this case is estimated by using Boyle's law to relate changes in box pressure to changes in mouth pressure during panting against a closed airway (see Fig. 16–6B).

Multiple Breath Nitrogen Washout

This open circuit technique measures the washout of nitrogen (N$_2$) from the lungs after a switch from air breathing to 100% O$_2$. Although the volume of the lungs (FRC) is unknown, the gas content is 80% N$_2$. Thus, if the total volume of N$_2$ in the lungs could be measured, the volume of the alveolar gas (FRC) could be calculated. The expired gas can be collected into a large spirometer and its final N$_2$ content determined or, as is now more common, N$_2$ concentration and volume are continuously measured until the expired N$_2$ concentration is 1.5% or less. Although this can be achieved in 2 to 3 minutes in some healthy subjects, in patients with obstructive lung disease it may take 7 to 10 minutes or even longer. As a consequence of the slower N$_2$ washout, FRC is usually underestimated in such patients, in contrast to values obtained for the true thoracic gas volume with the body plethysmograph.

Helium Dilution

This closed circuit technique has been used most frequently during anesthesia and in other clinical settings. Essentially the patient's alveolar gas is allowed to equilibrate with a closed circuit (e.g., a bag) containing a known amount of helium (He$_I$). At the beginning of rebreathing there is no helium in the lung (He$_I$ = 0). All helium is in the circuit or bag. At the end of a period of rebreathing helium, the concentration is equal in both. Since initial (He$_I$) and final (He$_F$) helium concentrations are measured and volume of the bag or circuit is known, the volume of the lungs (FRC) can be calculated:

$$\text{FRC (He}_I) = \text{bag volume (HE}_I) = \text{He}_F \text{ (FRC + bag volume)}$$

Much like N$_2$ washout, the completeness of helium dilution requires communication of all lung areas with the circuit. In disease states, particularly when there is airway obstruction, the technique again understimates the true FRC.

Effects of General Anesthesia on Respiratory Mechanics

This section discusses the effects of general anesthesia on lung volumes (FRC), pressure-volume, and pressure-flow behavior of the respiratory system. In normal recumbent humans FRC is reduced by about 500 mL after the induction of general anesthesia. The changes occur within a minute and are not further affected by muscle paralysis. Although the exact mechanism is uncertain, simultaneous determination by N$_2$ washout and body plethysmography agree and suggest that the changes are probably not due simply to gas trapped in closed distal airways.[14] The degree of changes appears related to body habitus and shape of the chest wall, which allows for differing degrees of diaphragmatic displacement.

The pressure-volume curve of the respiratory system tends to shift to the right 20 to 30 minutes after induction of anesthesia. Thus compliance is decreased. The decrease in lung compliance is due to the decreased FRC. In a sense the changes can be likened to tightly strapping the chest. The altered function of the chest wall, therefore, secondarily affects the mechanical properties of the lungs.

The changes in pressure-flow relationships of the respiratory system with anesthesia are much less understood. Pulmonary resistance increases and may be due largely to placement of the endotracheal tube, to reflex changes in airway smooth muscle tone, to airway secretions, and to increased lung recoil.

Measurements of Ventilation

Flow and Volume

Peak Flowmeter

A measurement widely used in the management of variable airflow limitation is the peak expiratory flow rate, the maximal flow generated during a forced expiration begun at the position of full inspiration. This flow can be measured conveniently with hand-held flowmeters (Fig. 16–8) and is markedly affected by changes in the caliber of large airways. Because repeat measurements are relatively easy to obtain, peak flow rates are often used to monitor responses to bronchodilator therapy in asthma attacks.[15]

The original instrument, the Wright Peak Flowmeter, and all subsequent devices essentially measure a pressure drop that is directly related to flow in the presence of a fixed resistance. Normal peak flow values in young healthy males are greater than 500 L/minute.[16] Values less than 200 L/minute in the surgical candidate suggest impaired cough efficiency and the increased likelihood of postoperative complications.[17] The test is much less unpleasant and exhausting than the full forced vital capacity (FVC) maneuver; therefore, it provides the clinician with a valuable tool to identify gross pulmonary disability at the bedside. It is important, however, to understand that the measurement depends on effort and thus can be influenced by patient cooperation and other factors, such as muscle weakness.

Pneumotachography

Of the devices available to measure flow, the pneumotachograph is perhaps the best known. A low mechanical resistance, usually in the form of a screen, is placed directly in the stream of gas flow. The pressure gradient across this resistance is sensed by a differential pressure transducer. This pressure drop is linearly related to flows as long as flow is laminar. To ensure such linearity, it is important to select the pneumotach that is linear in the flow rates likely to be experienced (e.g., for forced expiration, 6 to 10 L/second; for quiet adult tidal volumes, 0 to 1 L/second).

The pressure gradient is not only dependent on flow rate but also on the density and viscosity of the gas mixture, as well as its temperature. Furthermore, condensation of moisture increases screen resistance and may cause turbulence.

The latter is usually eliminated by electrically heating the screen. Despite these limitations, the rapid response, small dead space, and low resistance of the pneumotachograph make it useful for many applications for flow measurement. Also, by integrating this flow electronically with respect to time, one can derive a measurement of volume.

Hot Wire Spirometers

A heated wire or thermistor will be cooled by a gas stream to an extent dependent on the flow rate and thermal conductivity of the gas. Such devices tend to be robust, are easily sterilized, and are suitable for applications not requiring a high degree of accuracy. They do, however, rapidly diminish in sensitivity if coated with foreign debris, such as airway secretions.

Ultrasonic Flowmeters

The velocity of gas flow can be measured utilizing ultrasound. The basis for such ultrasonic flowmeters is the measurement of the change in the speed of sound. Two piezoelectric crystals aligned at angles to the gas flow alternately transmit and receive bursts of oscillations at a frequency of 100 kHZ. Such flowmeters have advantages over pneumotachographs in certain situations because of their low resistance. They also lack problems with moisture, positive pressure, or motion artifact, and tend to be more stable, that is, exhibit less drift over long periods of use.

Thoracoabdominal Movement

Konno and Mead[18] have measured movements of the chest wall and abdomen and demonstrated their relationship to V_T during obstructed respiration. Various transducers and devices have measured the changes in physical shape and, hence, electric properties of the chest and abdomen during respiration. These devices have consisted of mercury in rubber strain gauges, magnetometers, impedance electrodes, and most recently, the inductance plethysmograph (Respitrace, Ambulatory Monitoring Inc., Ardsley, NY).[19] The device consists of two insulated coils, one of which encircles the abdomen and the other the rib cage. The coils are contained within a netlike garment and are excited by a high-frequency oscillation. The inductance of the coils changes with respiration as a function of changes in cross-sectional

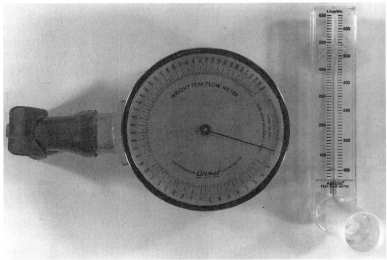

Figure 16–8. Hand-held peak flowmeters for bedside measurement. The original Wright meter is on the left while an inexpensive model is pictured on the right. (Health Scan Products, Inc., Cedar Grove, NJ.)

area of the compartment enclosed within. The instrument is useful to detect apnea and eliminates the need for a mouthpiece or mask. For measurement of volumes, however, devices such as the Respitrace must be regarded as semiquantitative unless rigorous calibrations with a spirometer are repeatedly carried out.

Collection Devices

Gas Meters

Dry gas meters (Parkinson-Cowan) have been utilized to measure minute ventilation for extended periods. The meters have large internal volumes and have an intolerable amount of dead space to allow rebreathing. Rather, gas must be collected via a one-way valve on the expiratory limb or in a Douglas bag which is then emptied into the meters. The gas volumes are collected at ambient temperature and pressure-saturated with H_2O vapor (ATPS); but for precision, respiratory volumes are expressed at body temperature and pressure saturated with H_2O vapor (BTPS). Many tables are available for such conversion factors, which are calculated as follows:

$$\text{BTPS vol} = \text{ATPS vol} \times \frac{(273 \times T_b °C)}{(273 \times T_{atm} °C)} \times \frac{(P_{atm} - P_{H_2O} T_b)}{(P_{atm} - P_{H_2O} T_{atm})}$$

where
T_b = body temperature
T_{atm} = atmospheric temperature
P_{H_2O} = vapor pressure of H_2O at T_b or T_{atm}
P_{atm} = atmospheric or barometric pressure

Spirometers

The classic Collins water seal spirometers are reliable, accurate, and serve as the reference standard for volume measurements. However, they are cumbersome and poorly suited for use in the operating room or intensive care unit. Dry spirometers, such as the rolling seal or wedge types, have similar problems of bulk but have better frequency responses, a characteristic that render them more useful for forced respiratory maneuvers. In addition, they often have electrical circuitry capable of differentiating the volume signal to obtain flow. The principal shortcoming of dry spirometers lies in the difficulty in applying them to systems in which rebreathing takes place or additional fresh gas is added to the volume inspired.

Mechanical Respirometers

In contrast to the limitations of conventional spirometers, mechanical respirometers provide less expensive, more convenient access to the breathing circuit. Such devices estimate volume from rotation of a low-friction inertia vane. The widely used Wright respirometer contains a geared system that converts rotation of the vane into movements of hands over a dial. Tangential slots around the vane ensure that flow is recorded in only one direction. Thus it may be inserted between the endotracheal tube and breathing circuit. The small dead space (20 to 25 mL) and relatively low resistance render it suitable for spontaneously breathing patients. The instrument is more accurate at flows of about 20 L/minute. These flows are typical of quiet expiration in adults. Because of inertia, resistance, and momentum of the vane, the Wright respirometer tends to overread at higher flows (>1 L/sec-

ond) and underread at lower flows. These effects may be magnified if the density of the gas mixture differs from usual because inertial and momentum forces are highly influenced by gas density. For the most part clinical changes in gas composition have relatively little effect, but water condensation may be a problem with extended use, as is also the case with accumulation of foreign material.

These problems of the Wright respirometer are shared by a number of similar devices. Such is the case with the larger, widely used Dräger respirometer. The latter senses flow in either direction and must, of necessity, be placed in an area of unidirectional flow—hence, its conventional location on the expiratory limb of an anesthesia circuit system. Such placement of the respirometer renders it prone to overreading because of increases in fresh gas delivery to the system, particularly when such delivered flows are large (e.g., 10/L/minute).[20]

Pressure Monitoring

Airway pressure (Paw) may be simply measured with the aneroid gauges present in anesthesia or ventilator circuits. These simple measurements are usually sufficiently accurate to make some assessment of patient or system mechanics. However, for most accurate assessment of patient mechanics, pressures should be sensed as close to the patient as possible and ideally at the inlet to an endotracheal tube. Automated measurement of Paw from the same sites can be obtained with simple strain gauge transducers, such as those used to measure blood pressure. If an esophageal balloon is used to measure Ppl, a differential pressure transducer, that is, one with two ports, will be needed. The negative or subambient Ppl must be referenced to mouth pressure (Pm) to derive the transpulmonary (PL) pressure. Thus PL = Pm − Ppl.

Mean Airway Pressure

The instantaneous positive pressure applied to the airway varies during each respiratory cycle. The physiologic effects of such pressure depend not only on the instantaneous magnitude of the pressure but also on the length of time it is applied to the airway. A clinically useful composite of all the pressures transmitted to the airway during mechanical ventilation is the mean airway pressure ($\overline{Paw}$), or the average pressure present in the airways. The $\overline{Paw}$ can be thought of simply as the area under the pressure curve. This can be estimated graphically or by electronic integration of the signal from a pressure transducer. In either case $\overline{Paw}$ is computed by dividing the area under the pressure curve by the total time for each entire respiratory cycle (i.e., inspiration plus expiration).

Many factors influence the values of $\overline{Paw}$. Perhaps the most obvious is the deliberate use of high driving pressures or excessive ventilatory volumes. Prolongation of the inspiratory time also increases $\overline{Paw}$, since the inspiratory portion of the pressure curve has the largest area per unit time.

Essentially, the area under the pressure curve varies directly with the duration of inspiration and inversely with the length of expiration. Thus, any increase in the ratio of inspiratory time to expiratory time (I/E ratio) will increase $\overline{Paw}$ if the total respiratory cycle is unchanged. One such prolongation of inspiration occurs with an end-inspiratory pause in which the lungs are held inflated at a fixed level of pressure or volume for a time. The longer this time, the greater the area under the pressure curve and the higher the $\overline{Paw}$.

Expiratory resistance, or "retard," has been employed in mechanical ventilation to mimic pursed-lips breathing with the hopes of allowing more uniform lung emptying. The technique involves placement of a variable resistance in the exhalation circuit to slow expiratory flow. Thus, expiratory pressures decrease more slowly and contribute to increasing Paw.

Positive end-expiratory pressure (PEEP), is a maneuver in which airway pressure is not allowed to decrease to atmospheric pressure at the end of exhalation. The elevated baseline pressure that results with PEEP also contributes to an increased Paw. Conversely, if negative pressure were applied during exhalation to produce negative end-expiratory pressure, Paw would decrease.

For the most part Paw is considered to be synonymous with mean alveolar pressure (PA). This PA is closely related to the efficiency of ventilation, oxygenation, and the cardiovascular effects of mechanical ventilation, as well as lung distention and barotrauma. For the most part, Paw can be assumed to equal PA unless differences arise because of inspiratory or expiratory flow resistance losses.[21] The same PA may be achieved with the application of PEEP or by extending the inspiratory time with an end-inspiratory pause. However, these two methods of achieving the same PA have different effects on gas exchange. PEEP predictably increases dead space while the inspiratory pause appears to improve the efficiency of alveolar ventilation by producing a lower maximal PA for a greater portion of the total respiratory cycle. This appears to promote recruitment of refractory but potentially functional lung areas.

Peak Airway Pressure

Much importance has been ascribed to peak airway pressure (PAP) as the major factor in producing alveolar disruption, commonly referred to as barotrauma. The relationship of PAP to barotrauma is rather circumstantial because PA and lung volume are usually increased at the same time.[22] The measurement of PAP is to a great extent an artifact of the site at which it is sampled. As such it reflects more of the mechanical characteristics of the breathing circuits and endotracheal tube than the actual PA associated with lung expansion.

Although increases in PAP are often viewed as a sign of airway smooth muscle constriction, that is, bronchospasm, many other factors may be responsible (Fig. 16-9). Endobronchial intubation, for example, may result in dramatic increases in Paw during mechanical ventilation because gas delivery is confined to only one lung. The presence of the tube at the carina may also stimulate the very abundant and sensitive irritant receptors in this area, and may actually produce reflex bronchospasm. More commonly, such irritation is manifested by persistent coughing and straining and the need for high inflation pressures. The use of neuromuscular blockers can differentiate reflex from actual bronchoconstriction. Excessive inflation pressures may also result from inspissated secretions or overinflation of the cuff. Usually, such obstruction is associated with audible noises throughout both inspiratory and expiratory phases of respiration. Diagnosis may be inferred by failed attempts to pass a suction catheter; it may be verified only with fiberoptic bronchoscopy. Clinicians may be alerted to the possibility of such obstruction if peak pressures are extremely high, but plateau pressures during inspiratory pauses are much lower, because the latter more directly reflect Paw or PA distal to the endotracheal tube.

It is also important to note that simply increasing the rate

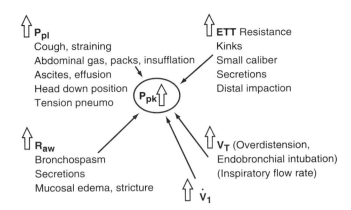

Increased Peak Airway Pressure

Figure 16-9. Increases in peak pressure (P_{pk}) may be due to increases in pleural pressure (P_{pl}), airway resistance (R_{aw}), endotracheal tube (ETT) resistance, tidal volume (V_T), and inspiratory flow ($\dot{V}_l$).

of delivery of the same V_T, that is, by increasing inspiratory flow, may produce an increase in PAP. In contrast, with distal airway obstruction, both PAP and plateau pressure will usually increase. The only situation that can produce this same concomitant increase in PAP and plateau pressure is the delivery of excessively large tidal volumes (>15 mL/kg). The latter explains the clinical picture with endobronchial intubation. The normal V_T is excessive for the single lung and therefore is associated with a high Paw. The pressure increases not only as the simple result of added volume, but the end-inspiratory hyperinflation also may place many lung regions on the flatter portion of their normal pressure-volume curve.

Pressure-Volume Relationships

The effects of circuit distensibility or compliance in reducing the actual amount of delivered volume is well recognized. This distention of tubing can be minimized by the use of stiffer circuit material. However, another factor, compression of gases with the tubing, is not prevented. The latter is a function of circuit size (including humidifier) and the pressure at end-inspiration. The discrepancies due to gas compression become important when small tidal volumes are used, particularly in the face of high inflation pressures. This gas, which is compressed during inspiration, is added to the measured expired volume to produce an overestimate of volume. The gas composition is also diluted by the same added gas, resulting in decreased tension from expired gases such as CO_2.

Figure 16-3 illustrates typical flow, volume, and pressure relationships that might exist in the patient circuit during cycling of a mechanical ventilator. Maximum (peak) Paw and plateau or static pressures can readily be measured, and, in conjunction with V_T measurements, can be used to estimate dynamic compliance (Cdyn) and static compliance (Cst):

$$Cdyn = V_T/peak\ pressure$$

$$Cst = V_T/plateau\ pressure$$

Plateau pressure can be estimated during the period of no

Pulse Method

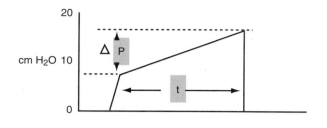

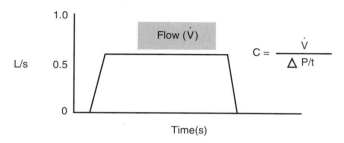

$$C = \frac{\dot{V}}{\Delta\,P/t}$$

Time(s)

Figure 16–10. Illustration of the pulse method for estimating compliance (C) by dividing the constant flow (V) by the rate of rise of pressure (P/t).

flow, that is, inspiratory pause available on most ventilators. If this is not available, the expiratory limb of the circuit may be clamped. The value is often referred to as quasi-static because it is not truly a static measurement as might be obtained by inflation with a supersyringe or passive deflation against an occlusion.

Another useful form of quasi-static compliance measurement applicable to ventilator patients receiving constant inspiratory flow is based on the pressure rise per unit time during such flow.[23] This pulse method is based on the principle that when a constant flow is introduced to the respiratory system, the rate of increase in pressure is inversely related to the compliance of the system:[24]

$$\text{Compliance} = \frac{\text{Flow}}{\Delta\,\text{Pressure/time}}$$

since

$$\text{Flow} = \Delta\,\text{Volume/time}$$

$$\text{Compliance} = \frac{\Delta\,\text{Volume}}{\Delta\,\text{Pressure}}$$

Values for compliance estimated by this method in all patients were nearly identical to those obtained by relating delivered V_T to the plateau pressure and are considered quasi-static. The estimation of compliance by this pulse method is illustrated in Figure 16–10.

Compliance can also be estimated from pressure-volume loops provided by a new pressure-based flow sensor and respiratory gas monitor (Capnomac Ultima, Datex Inc., Helsinki, Finland). The pressure on the x-axis at the delivery of a V_T on the y-axis (Fig. 16–11A) can be used to calculate compliance, where ΔV_T approximates dynamic compliance. Changes in flow resistance can be estimated by the character of the flow-volume curves (Fig. 16–11B). Both of these mea-

surements can be helpful in subjectively assessing the adequacy of ventilation in the anesthetized patient.

Monitoring Gas Exchange

Capnometry and Capnography

Analysis of CO_2 in the respired gases has become commonplace in the operating room setting. The actual measurement of CO_2 concentration is termed capnometry. Capnography, on the other hand, refers to the display of this concentration on a screen or recording chart, usually as a function of time. This latter ability to actually see the CO_2 waveforms enhances their interpretations in contrast to the simple digital readout of CO_2 concentrations that constitutes capnometry. Nevertheless, the simple readout of CO_2 concentration with capnometry can alert the anesthesiologist to an increase or decrease in or absence of CO_2 (Table 16–2).

The most common systems available for breath-by-breath CO_2 analysis utilize the infrared absorption of gases. Infrared light of a certain wavelength (2600 or 4300 nm) passes through a reference gas sample containing no CO_2 or a known amount. The light also passes through the gas sample to be analyzed. The CO_2 absorbs the infrared energy in proportion to its concentration. Photocells sense a difference in intensity between light transmitted through the reference chamber and that through the sample gas, which is related to the CO_2 concentration in the sample chamber.

Instruments monitor CO_2 either by direct in-line measurement at the sample site by a flowthrough device or by aspiration of the gas sample into a separate monitor. The in-line sensors, such as those available from Siemens Corporation and Hewlett-Packard, are placed directly in the breathing system with a special adapter and ideally as close to the patient as possible. Such sensors are fragile, expensive, somewhat cumbersome, and have a relatively large dead space. On the other hand, moisture is not a problem and there is no limitation on where the actual monitor console needs to be placed. Such monitors also do not require standard gases for calibration.

Analyzers that continually withdraw gas samples are more common. It is important to realize that this sample gas (up to 250 mL/minute) must be returned to the anesthesia system or scavenger to avoid pollution due to anesthetic gases. Such analyzers are plagued by excess moisture and require that the small-diameter sampling tube be as short as possible to improve response time. The response time is inherently shorter with in-line sensors that analyze gas directly in the airway and thus lack the delay and mixing of gases associated with suction and transport to a remote infrared analyzer.

Normally, CO_2 concentrations are displayed with respect to time (Fig. 16–12). However, the expired volume may also substitute for time on the abscissa. Such curves requires more effort and equipment but may yield more information regarding respiratory dead space.[25]

There are two components to this dead space, which is sometimes referred to as "physiologic dead space": the airway dead space (V_{Dan}) and the alveolar dead space (V_{DAV}). The V_{Dan} (sometimes called anatomic dead space) consists of the airway compartment from the lips to the alveolar-gas interface. It relates to body size, surface, and respiratory system compliance and is about 85 mL in the average-sized adult. Increased lung volume (FRC) is associated with a passive increase in V_{Daw} in bronchodilation.

V_{DAV} is the result of all causes distal to the alveolar-gas

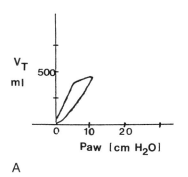

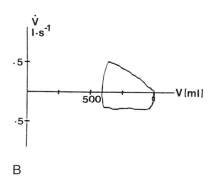

Figure 16–11. Typical normal pressure-volume (*A*) and flow-volume (*B*) curves recorded in a paralyzed mechanically ventilated patient with the pressure-based flow sensor of the Capnomac Ultima. (Datex Inc., Helsinki, Finland.)

interface. It results from the increased spread of ventilation-perfusion quotient ratios ($\dot{V}/\dot{Q}$) and a temporal mismatch of airway time constants and pulmonary blood flow.

During each breath, gases emerge sequentially from the conducting airways which make up the VDan and then finally from the alveoli. The characteristic CO_2 waveform displayed in Figure 16–12 exhibits three basic concentrations during inspiration. During the initial phase (A) the CO_2 level remains near the previous inspiratory level and reflects gas cleared from the VDan. In phase B, which follows, there is an admixture of residual dead space gas and alveolar gas that is beginning to emerge from lung areas having relatively short conducting airways. The CO_2 level rises rapidly in phase B to approach alveolar levels. The final phase C is often referred to as the alveolar plateau because it represents gas washed out of the alveoli. The slope of this phase is increased when there is nonhomogeneous mixing of gas, such as with airway obstruction. It also increases with exercise and hypermetabolic states. For the most part, a steep alveolar CO_2 slope indicates that ventilatory efficiency depends on the magnitude of VT. Thus, unless VT is adequate (>10 mL/kg) the CO_2 concentration at end-expiration will not approach the arterial CO_2. During exhalation, gas flow is fast initially and later leaves at slower flows. Blood flow, on the other hand, tends to increase as expiration proceeds such that more CO_2 is delivered to air spaces. This effect is more pronounced during positive pressure ventilation. Because of this upward slope of the alveolar plateau, end-tidal CO_2 tension (PETCO$_2$) exceeds the mean alveolar CO_2 pressure (PACO$_2$). Normally, however, there is sufficient mixing with dead space gas such that PETCO$_2$ is somewhat less than arterial CO_2 tension (PaCO$_2$).

Clinically, PETCO$_2$ is used to provide a noninvasive estimate of PaCO$_2$. Under ideal conditions, even in the presence of general anesthesia, the difference between them is negligible.[26] The most significant determinant of a gradient between PaCO$_2$ and PETCO$_2$ is the presence of lung disease characterized by the extremes of high $\dot{V}/\dot{Q}$ relationships that behave functionally as dead space areas. These poorly or nonperfused lung units have a PaCO$_2$ of nearly zero. Thus the weighted average of all lung units will yield a low PETCO$_2$.

The other major sources of abnormally low PETCO$_2$ values involve sampling errors. The most obvious is a system leak such that some of the exhaled volume is lost and not subject to sampling. Most leaks are obvious but some, such as a poorly sealed endotracheal tube cuff, may require more intense scrutiny. The other sampling problem relates solely to aspirating devices and the relationship of sampling volume to patient VT. In adults, the expired tidal volumes are usually sufficient to supply the aspirated sample. Dilution of this sample with CO_2-free fresh gas can occur if the sample site is far from the patient's airway, or if exhaled volumes decrease as with shallow breathing. The implications of this problem in pediatric systems with high fresh gas flows are obvious.

Table 16–2. Etiologies of Changes in Carbon Dioxide Detected by Capnometry

End-Expired CO₂ Absent
Endotracheal (ET) tube misplacement
    Extubation
    Esophageal intubation
Complete tube obstruction
Circuit disconnection
Apnea
Circulatory arrest
Low End-Expired CO₂
Hyperventilation
Pulmonary hypoperfusion
    Decreased cardiac output
    Pulmonary embolism (air, thrombus)
    Congenital right-to-left shunt
Leaking shallow breathing
Rapid shallow breathing (panting)
High End-Expired CO₂
Hypoventilation
Increased CO₂ production
CO₂ rebreathing (increased inspired CO₂)
    Exhausted CO₂ absorber
    Faulty unidirectional valves

Dead Space

Respiratory dead space is most often considered in physiologic terms, that is, the volume of inspired and expired gas that does not partake of gas exchange in the alveoli. Physiologic dead space (VD) has two components: VDan and VDA. The capnograph allows estimation of VDan (see Fig. 16–12) by what is often referred to as the equal area method, first described by Aitken and Clark Kennedy.[27] Essentially, VDan is identified by the vertical line which subdivides phase B into two equal portions by assuming this volume represents the abrupt transition between the conducting dead space and the alveolar gas component. Unfortunately, this technique tends to overestimate VDan in situations in which the slope of the alveolar phase is increased (i.e., hypermetabolic states and asynchronous alveolar emptying with lung diseases).

The alveolar component of VD is not measured directly but rather determined from simultaneous measurements of

Exhaled CO₂ Waveform

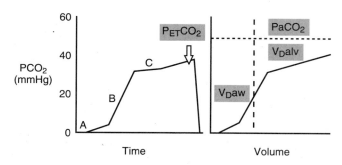

Figure 16–12. Characteristic waveform of exhaled CO₂ plotted as a function of time and of volume. PaCO₂, arterial CO₂ tension; PETCO₂, end-tidal CO₂ tension; VDaw, airway (anatomic) dead space; V_Dalv, alveolar dead space.

VDan and VD. The latter, which exceeds VDan by inclusion of VDA, is now usually defined by the mixing equation originally devised by Christian Bohr but later modified by Enghoff, who substituted PaCO₂ in the equation

$$V_D = V_T \times \frac{(Pa_{CO_2} - P\bar{E}_{CO_2})}{(Pa_{CO_2} - PI_{CO_2})}$$

where

$P\bar{E}_{CO_2}$ = mixed expired CO₂ tension
PI_{CO_2} = inspired CO₂ tension

Clinical measurement of VD requires a sample of arterial blood flow (PaCO₂). Mixed expired gases are collected over several minutes in a large bag or spirometer to measure P̄E_{CO_2}. VT can be conveniently measured with a Wright respirometer. Since there is usually no rebreathing involved, PI_{CO_2} is usually assumed to be zero. It is also important to subtract apparatus dead space (face mask, valves, tubing) to obtain accurate measurements of VD.

In normals this VD constitutes less than one third of VT (i.e., VD/VT ≤ 0.33). The calculation of VD/VT helps to estimate the relationship between alveolar ventilation and minute ventilation, or more specifically the efficiency of ventilation. Such information can be very useful in determining whether to institute or discontinue mechanical ventilation.

Clinical Applications and Limitations

The useful information presented by capnography provides particular insight into the mechanical and gas exchange functions of the lung. However, changes in metabolic and cardiovascular function are also detectable. For example, malignant hyperthermia with its increased CO₂ production may present early with a rise in end-tidal CO₂ and particularly with a more prominent slope of the alveolar plateau. Capnography can also indicate the quality of the circulation. If PETCO₂ suddenly begins to decrease, it could be the result of decreased blood flow to the lungs secondary to hypovolemia, embolism, or myocardial dysfunction. Perhaps the greatest emphasis on capnography concerns its potential use in identifying malfunction of breathing systems such as the anesthesia circuit (see Chapter 17).

Assessing Adequacy of Oxygenation

Techniques for measuring and sampling delivered oxygen concentrations are discussed elsewhere (see Chapter 17). The end result, the arterial O₂ tension (PaO₂) requires, of course, analysis of arterial blood. To fully understand the implications of a given value of PaO₂, one must examine its relationship to the alveolar O₂ tension (PAO₂) by utilizing the alveolar air equation, which describes the gas content in lung alveoli and, in particular, the PAO₂. PAO₂ can be calculated beginning with the partial pressure of oxygen in the trachea (PIO₂). The partial pressure of water vapor at body temperature (47 mmHg) must be included in the calculation because as dry gas enters the airway, it is warmed to body temperature and humidified prior to reaching the alveoli:

$$PI_{O_2} = FI_{O_2}(P_b - 47)$$

where

FIO₂ = fractional O₂ concentration in inspired air
Pb = atmospheric (barometric) pressure (760 mmHg at sea level)

Since CO₂ is added to the alveolar gas from the blood, the PaCO₂ must be subtracted. The PaCO₂ is usually substituted because the PACO₂ cannot easily be measured. The PACO₂ must also be corrected for by the respiratory exchange ratio (R) since less CO₂ is produced than oxygen consumed (normally R = 0.8). Thus, in a normal subject breathing ambient air at sea level, the PAO₂ can be estimated if we assume a normal PaCO₂ of 40 mmHg:

$$PA_{O_2} = PI_{O_2} - Pa_{CO_2}/R$$

$$PA_{O_2} = 0.21 (760 - 47) - 40/0.8 = 100 \text{ mmHg}$$

This shortened form of the equation produces a small (5%) underestimation of PAO₂ when R = 0.8. If R = 1.0, there is no error.

If ventilation and pulmonary blood flow were matched perfectly, the PaO₂ would be the same as the PAO₂. However, regional variation in both prevents this ideal situation from developing. Thus, even in healthy subjects, the PaO₂ is 10 to 15 mmHg less than PAO₂. This difference is referred to as the alveolar-arterial gradient for oxygen (PAO₂ − PaO₂). Its magnitude reflects the degree of inefficient gas exchange on the part of the lung. Since this gradient is exaggerated by disease, the interpretation of a value of PaO₂ is only valid when the PAO₂ is considered as well.

Data from two patients illustrate this point. Both patients have identical PaO₂ values (65 mmHg) while breathing room air. In patient A, however, the PaCO₂ value is 56 mmHg, whereas in patient B the PaCO₂ is 28 mmHg. The PAO₂ value in patient A is calculated as (760 − 47) − 56/0.8 = 80 mmHg. The alveolar-arterial gradient is thus 15 mmHg. This is still within the normal range and does not indicate lung disease. The specimen was drawn from a healthy young patient following a large dose of a narcotic. In patient B, the PaO₂ value is 0.21 (760 − 47) − 28/0.8 = 115. The alveolar-arterial in this case is 50 mmHg, nearly four times the normal value, and clearly indicates abnormal oxygen transfer. The patient in this example was breathing very rapidly with signs of marked dyspnea and had pneumonia.

The normal PAO₂ − PaO₂ tends to increase in normals and in the presence of pulmonary disease as FIO₂ is increased. This tends to limit its usefulness in assessing gas exchange in patients whose FIO₂ is changed. One attempt to standardize PaO_2 values was suggested by dividing PaO_2 by FIO_2.[28] This produces rather confusing units and fails to account for differences in $PaCO_2$. Another index of gas exchange less affected by the FIO_2 is the ratio of arterial to alveolar O_2 (PaO_2/PAO_2).[29] Although not as stable as originally suggested, this ratio is still far more constant than the alveolar-arterial gradient. It is most stable above PaO_2 values of 200 mmHg, that is, when FIO_2 exceeds 0.3.[30] In normals the values are about 0.7 to 0.8.[30]

Estimation of Shunt

The most common causes of arterial hypoxemia are low or decreased ventilation-perfusion relationships ($\dot{V}/\dot{Q}$) in numerous regional lung units. As these regional units are underventilated and normally perfused, there is a low PAO_2 and also a decreased PaO_2 in the blood leaving to enter the systemic circulation. If increasing the FIO_2 has little or no effect in increasing PaO_2, right-to-left shunting is assumed to be the cause of the low PaO_2. A regional lung unit is the site of shunting when it has essentially zero ventilation and relatively persistent perfusion, such that $\dot{V}/\dot{Q}$ approaches zero. Blood flows past such a alveolus whose PaO_2 is zero and retains its low mixed venous O_2 tension ($P\bar{v}O_2$) prior to entering the systemic circulation.

The calculation of this shunt (Qs/Qt) has been utilized as an indicator of the lungs' ability to oxygenate blood. To calculate shunt, one must know barometric pressure, PaO_2, $PaCO_2$, hemoglobin concentration, and ($P\bar{v}O_2$). Thus, equipment consists of a barometer, blood gas analyzer, blood sampling devices, and either a pulmonary artery or central venous catheter to obtain $P\bar{v}O_2$. It is also necessary to ensure that the patient is breathing 100% O_2 for at least 20 minutes. The formula used to calculate shunt is:

$$Qs/Qt = \frac{Cc'O_2 - CaO_2}{Cc'O_2 - C\bar{v}O_2}$$

where

$Cc'O_2$ = oxygen content of pulmonary end-capillary blood
$Ca'O_2$ = arterial oxygen concentration
$C\bar{v}O_2$ = mixed venous oxygen concentration

Since perfused capillaries ventilated with O_2 are exposed to the PAO_2, the latter must be calculated from the alveolar air equation. The PAO_2 is multiplied by the solubility coefficient (0.003) to calculate dissolved O_2. Because each gram of hemoglobin (Hb) also holds 1.39 mL of O_2 when fully saturated, $Cc'O_2 = (Hb \times 1.39) + (PAO_2 \times 0.003)$. The $Cc'O_2$ represents an ideal O_2 content in the pulmonary end capillaries, which assumes that the Hb concentration in that vascular bed is equal to that of arterial blood and that the O_2 tension of the capillary blood is equal to the ideal PAO_2 calculated from the alveolar air equation. This ideal PAO_2 is not always achieved in all lung areas and the variable inaccuracies that arise from this assumption may result in larger than expected calculations of Qs/Qt.[31]

Arterial Hb is not fully saturated (S); therefore, CaO_2 = (Hb $\times$ 1.39 $\times$ %S) + ($PaO_2 \times 0.003$).

$C\bar{v}O_2$ is calculated similarly except that it is multiplied by 0.003 to estimated dissolved O_2. Thus, $C\bar{v}O_2$ = (Hb $\times$ 1.39 $\times$ %S) + ($P\bar{v}O_2 \times 0.003$).

The accuracy of the Qs/Qt calculation also depends on many other variables such as cardiac output, respiratory quotient, the quality of the mixed venous sample, or an assumed arteriovenous O_2 content difference. Thus, many clinicians prefer the simpler use of alveolar-arterial oxygen ($A-aO_2$) difference rather than shunt to assess adequacy of oxygenation. Others have proposed shortcut methods for calculating percent shunt, assuming unchanged cardiac output and FIO_2 of 1.0[32]:

$$\% \text{ Shunt} = \frac{A-aO_2 \text{ difference}}{10}$$

The importance of cardiac output must be emphasized in patients with acute respiratory failure, who often experience reduction in cardiac output secondary to continuous positive pressure breathing. Cardiac output profoundly affects PaO_2 for a given level of shunting. Wide swings in a patient's PaO_2 can occur without an actual change in pulmonary status but rather as a result of changes in cardiac output. The same increases and decreases in cardiac output can raise or lower the calculated Qs/Qt values. Thus, neither Qs/Qt nor alveolar-arterial O_2 differences can be meaningfully interpreted unless cardiac output changes are considered.

Diffusion

The role of diffusion in producing abnormalities in gas exchange is of little importance and for practical purposes can be ignored under resting conditions. Limitation of diffusion would consist of an oxygen gradient between alveolar and end-capillary O_2 tensions. This is normally zero. Only if cardiac output is increased and FIO_2 decreased does such a gradient develop. Examples of such situations would be high levels of exercise and breathing at altitudes above 10,000 ft.

Diffusing capacity of the lungs (DL) is defined as the rate at which a gas enters the blood divided by its driving pressure. The latter again is the gradient between alveolar and end-capillary tensions. The units in which DL is expressed are milliliters per minute per millimeters Hg. Measurement of DL does provide information about the amount of functioning capillaries in contact with ventilated air spaces as may occur in certain pulmonary vascular and parenchymal disease states. The brief inhalation of nontoxic low concentrations of carbon monoxide (CO) has become standard in most pulmonary function laboratories for this purpose. The equipment requirements and the large variations in normal values for each of the techniques (single-breath, steady-state, rebreathing) render the measurement well outside the usual clinical realm and well beyond the scope of this discussion. For a comprehensive discussion of the interpretation and significance of such testing the reader is referred to an excellent review.[33]

CO has several features that make the gas useful to measure DL. It has 200 times the affinity for hemoglobin compared to oxygen. Thus, CO will not build up rapidly in plasma. Most important, however, is the low CO concentration in the blood under normal conditions, such that pulmonary capillary tension can be assumed to be zero. Of the techniques utilizing CO, the rebreathing method is least influenced by changes in $\dot{V}/\dot{Q}$ distributions.

To measure CO diffusing capacity of the lungs (DLCO), three values must be obtained. These are the milliliters CO transferred from alveoli to blood per minute, the mean alveolar CO tension (PACO), and the pulmonary capillary CO tension (PcCO):

$$DLCO = \frac{CO \text{ mL/min/mmHg}}{PACO - PcCO}$$

In the *single-breath method,* the patient inspires a dilute mixture of CO and holds the breath for 10 seconds. During this period, CO leaves alveolar gas to enter the blood in proportion to the diffusing capacity. The milliliter of CO transferred is calculated from percent CO in alveolar gas at the beginning and end of the breath-hold by infrared analysis. To do this, FRC must be calculated from the helium dilution and then added to the inspiratory volume. The $Pcco$ is essentially zero and can be ignored. $Pcco$ is not the simple average of Pco at the beginning and end of the breath-hold but must be calculated by a special equation that considers alveolar volume as reflected by the ratio of inspired to expired helium concentrations.[34]

The single-breath method requires very little patient cooperation and is relatively simple to perform because it requires no blood samples. It is relatively insensitive to backpressure of CO in the blood and only mildly affected by $\dot{V}/\dot{Q}$ inequalities. Disadvantages include the extensive mathematical computations and the requirement for a 1.3 L or greater inspired volume with a breath-hold. The latter may not be feasible in the dyspneic patient or in the exercising subject.

The steady-state method is regarded as more physiologic than the single-breath test because it can be measured in such patients. The patient breathes a low (0.1%) concentration of CO for about 30 seconds or until a steady state is established. The rate of CO disappearance from alveoli to blood is measured along with $Paco$. Unfortunately, with steady-state methods, $Paco$ is again difficult to measure and must be estimated using an assumed value for arterial blood samples and the sensitivity of the measurement to maldistribution of $\dot{V}/\dot{Q}$, which may lead to small errors in estimates of $Paco$ and the ratio of dead space gas volume to tidal gas volume (VD/VT), but large variations in $Dlco$. On the other hand, the steady-state technique requires less equipment and fewer calculations. Little patient cooperation is needed because measurements are made during normal tidal breathing. Therefore, steady-state $Dlco$ can be measured during many activities, including general anesthesia.

Another technique for measuring $Dlco$ is the rebreathing method. Here the patient exhales either to residual volume or to FRC. Then a known volume of test gas is breathed at a rate of about one breath per second for 30 seconds, while gas concentrations (He, O_2, CO) are monitored continuously. The rate of CO uptake is calculated from the known system volume and the rate of CO disappearance. The pressure gradient for CO is calculated from the exponential disappearance, assuming $Pcco$ is zero. This measurement can be performed in patients with small vital capacities (1.3 L) and in most clinical settings. It appears to be the least sensitive to inequalities of $\dot{V}/\dot{Q}$. Although some patients have difficulty breathing at the fixed rate required, rebreathing appears to be the technique of choice when the single-breath method cannot be used.[35]

In general, however, rebreathing steady-state and single-breath techniques give rather similar results. Normal values, depending on individual laboratories, range from 20 to 30 mL/minute/mmHg. Increases in $Dlco$ occur with body, size, age, lung volume, exercise, body position, and $Paco_2$ and Pao_2. Therefore, changes in these variables must be considered when interpreting $Dlco$ values.

Oxygen Cost of Breathing

During normal breathing the oxygen cost of breathing (Vo_2R) makes up only a small amount (<5%) of total O_2 consumption. As levels of ventilation increase, the power output of the respiratory muscles increases and Vo_2R as-

sumes a greater magnitude.[36] Such increases in Vo_2R are common in patients who require mechanical ventilation and have been attributed to the increased ventilation required by the catabolic states, as well as the increased work of breathing and inefficiency of respiratory muscles. A reasonable estimate of this increased Vo_2R can be made by measuring the difference in O_2 consumption (Vo_2) during spontaneous ventilation and that in the relaxed patient receiving mechanical ventilation.

The measurement of Vo_2 in ventilated patients has proved rather difficult. As a result, in many critical care unit patients, studies have calculated Vo_2 from the Fick equation:

$$Vo_2 = CO \times C(a-v)o_2$$

where
    CO = cardiac output
    $C(a-v)o_2$ = arteriovenous oxygen content difference

This has significant limitations because of the coupling which may occur between O_2 delivery and consumption.[37]

Prior clinical determinations of Vo_2 have utilized measurements of inspired and expired gas concentrations (O_2, CO_2, N_2). Collection of expired gas required a spirometer[38] or meterologic balloon.[39] More recently, metabolic carts with rapid analyses of inspired and expired gases have made such clinical measurements of Vo_2 more feasible. Similarly rapid anesthetic gas analyzers presently available enable similar, albeit approximate, calculations in anesthetized patients.

The O_2 consumed by aerobic metabolism is entirely dependent upon O_2 uptake from inspired gas. For a normal person at rest, this O_2 uptake (Vo_2) is usually about 250 mL/minute. This volume inspired per unit time is equal to the volume of inspired gas times the fractional concentration of O_2 (i.e., $VI \times FIO_2$). Likewise, the exhaled oxygen volume equals the product of exhaled volume and fractional expired O_2 concentration ($VE \times FEO_2$). The O_2 uptake equals the difference between the inspired and expired O_2:

$$Vo_2 = (VI \times FIO_2) - (VE \times FEO_2)$$

The measurement of both VI and VE at the same time is somewhat impractical. Therefore, VE, which is more easily measured, is utilized in the equation to calculate Vo_2:

$$Vo_2 = VE_{(STPD)} \left[\frac{FIO_2 (1 - FEO_2 - FECO_2)}{1 - FIO_2 - FICO_2} - FEO_2 \right]$$

Because variations in VE relationships to VI may be produced by changes in the respiratory quotient (i.e., the ratio of CO_2 production to O_2 consumption), another calculation, which utilizes the rate of nitrogen exchange in the lungs, is utilized. Because no uptake or elimination of N_2 occurs in a steady state, the inhaled N_2 volume ($VI \times FIN_2$) is equal to the exhaled N_2 volume ($VE \times FEN_2$). The equation utilizing FEN_2 and inspired nitrogen FIN_2 concentrations can serve as a check on the validity of the above calculation with O_2 and CO_2:

$$Vo_2 = VE_{(STPD)} \left[\frac{FEN_2 \times FIO_2}{FIN_2} - FEO_2 \right]$$

It is important to note that both calculations report Vo_2 in terms of VE defined as standard temperature, pressure dry (STPD). This normalization for temperature and pressure allows comparisons to be made for Vo_2 at different altitudes and hence barometric pressures, since the volume occupied by any gas depends on temperature and pressure:

$$V_{STPD} = V_{ATPS} \times \frac{Pb - P_{H_2O}}{760} \times \frac{273}{273 + T}$$

where

V_{STPD} = volume of gas at standard temperature and pressure, dry

V_{ATPS} = volume of gas at ambient temperature and pressure, saturated with water vapor

Pb = barometric pressure

P_{H_2O} = vapor pressure of water at T

273 = absolute O°C

T = ambient or room temperature

A similar formula can be utilized to correct to V_{STPD} from the volume of gas measured at ambient temperature and pressure, dry (V_{ATPD}). The latter is merely substituted in the equation for V_{ATPS}.

Simple Monitoring of Ventilation Without Instrumentation

In the early days of anesthesia with diethyl ether, most patients breathed spontaneously and ventilation was monitored by simple inspection of neck, chest, and abdomen. These were correlated with gas movement by observation of the rebreathing bag. Normal quiet breathing in the supine position is primarily abdominal; that is, it consists of diaphragmatic descent. Rib cage movement is nonexistent until higher levels of breathing occur or when mechanical ventilation is utilized. In the presence of respiratory obstruction, diaphragmatic power overcomes the action of the rib cage and the rib cage may be drawn in paradoxically. This phenomenon is particularly evident in an infant or child, whose thorax is far more flexible than that of an adult. The same paradoxical chest movement occurs with respiratory muscle weakness and is most evident with high levels of spinal cord injury.

In addition to simple patient observation, the adequacy of ventilation can be estimated by listening to breath sounds through esophageal or precordial stethoscopes. When placed on the precordium, the stethoscope can provide adequate transmission of heart sounds; but breath sounds may be inaudible, especially during spontaneous breathing. In this case, the relatively low flow rates (<0.2 L/second) are difficult to hear. When placed over the jugular notch, however, the turbulent flows around the larynx are easily heard and can provide clear evidence of laryngeal spasm, even when mild. Without question, the simplest and most reliable of the respiratory monitors is the esophageal stethoscope, which conveys both heart and breath sounds clearly. Wheezing, leaks, and accumulation of secretions can be readily identified. In addition, the absence of breath sounds is a simple reliable monitor of disconnection in the presence of mechanical ventilation. This event should trigger a response to check out other components of the breathing circuit, such as ventilator bellows and pressure gauges.

Monitoring movement of the breathing bag has been a mainstay of simple monitoring practice during spontaneous or manually controlled ventilation. One must be careful not to be deceived by errors produced by excessively high fresh gas flows or aspiration of gas from the circuit either for analysis or by the scavenging system. Thus, regardless of

how simple such respiratory monitoring methods are, each has the potential for misinterpretation. A sound understanding of physiologic and mechanical concepts is of equal importance to the understanding of the more sophisticated techniques.

REFERENCES

1. Black LF, Hyatt RE: Maximal respiratory pressures: Normal values and relationship to age and sex. Am Rev Respir Dis 1971; 103: 641–650.
2. O'Donoghue WJ, Baker JP, Bell F, et al: Respiratory failure in neuromuscular disease management in a respiratory intensive care unit. JAMA 1971; 235:733–735.
3. Pavlin EG, Holle RH, Schoene R: Recovery of airway protection compared to ventilation in humans after paralysis with curare. Anesthesiology 1989; 70:379–380.
4. Milic-Emili J, Mead J, Turner JM, et al: Improved technique for estimating pleural pressure from esophageal balloons. J Appl Physiol 1964; 19:207–211.
5. Leatherman NE: An improved balloon system for monitoring intraesophageal pressure in acutely ill patients. Crit Care Med 1978; 6:189–192.
6. Comroe JH, Nissell OL, Nims RG: A simple method for concurrent measurement of compliance and resistance to breathing in anesthetized animals and man. J Appl Physiol 1954; 7:225–228.
7. Fisher AB, Dubois AB, Hyde RW: Evaluation of the oscillation technique for the determination of resistance to breathing. J Clin Invest 1968; 47:2045–2057.
8. Dubois AB, Botelho SY, Comroe JH: A new method for measuring airway resistance in man using a body plethysmograph: Values in normal subjects and in patients with respiratory disease. J Clin Invest 1956; 35:326–335.
9. Bates JHT, Milic-Emili J: The flow interruption technique for measuring respiratory resistance. J Crit Care 1991; 6:227–238.
10. Tantucci C, Corbeil C, Chasse M, et al: Flow resistance in patients with chronic obstructive pulmonary disease in acute respiratory failure. Am Rev Respir Dis 1991; 144:384–389.
11. D'Angelo E, Robatto FM, Calerinin E, et al: Pulmonary and chest wall mechanics in anesthetized paralyzed humans. J Appl Physiol 1991; 70:2602–2610.
12. Eissa NT, Ranieri VM, Corbeic C, et al: Analysis of behavior of the respiratory system in ARDS: Effects of flow, volume, and time. J Appl Physiol 1991; 70:2719–2729.
13. Katz JA, Zinn SE, Ozanne GM, et al: Pulmonary chest wall and lung-thorax elastance in acute respiratory failure. Chest 1981; 80:304–311.
14. Westbrook PR, Stubbs SE, Sessler AD, et al: Effects of anesthesia and multiple paralysis on respiratory mechanics in normal man. J Appl Physiol 1973; 34:81–86.
15. Banner AS, Shah RS, Addington WW: Rapid prediction of need for hospitalization in acute asthma. JAMA 1976; 235:1337–1338.
16. Leiner GC, Abramowitz S, Small MJ et al: Expiratory peak flow rate, standard values for normal subjects, use as a clinical test of ventilatory function. Am Rev Respir Dis 1963; 88:644–651.
17. Stein M, Koota GM, Simon M, et al: Pulmonary evaluation of surgical patients. JAMA 1962; 181:6765–6770.
18. Konno K, Mead J: Measurement of the separate volume changes of the rib cage and abdomen during breathing. J Appl Physiol 1967; 22:407–422.
19. Cohn MA, Rao ASV, Broudy M, et al: The respiratory inductive plethysmograph; a new noninvasive monitor of respiration. Bull Eur Physiopathol Respir 1982; 18:643–658.
20. Mapleson WW: Physical aspects of automatic ventilators some application of basic principles. In Mushin MA, Rendell-Baker L, Thompson PW, et al (eds): Automatic Ventilation of the Lungs, ed 3. Oxford, Blackwell Scientific, 1980, pp 132–151.
21. Marini JJ: Positive end expiratory pressure and adult respiratory distress syndrome. J Crit Care 1992; 7:137–141.
22. Manning HL: Peak airway pressure. Why the fuss? Chest 1994; 105:242–247.

23. Surratt PM, Owens O: A pulse method of measuring respiratory system compliance in ventilated patients. Chest 1981; 80:34–38.

24. Rattenborg CC, Holaday DA: Constant flow inflation of the lungs, theoretical analysis. Acta Anaesthesiol Scand 1967; 23:211–223.

25. Fletcher R: Deadspace, during anesthesia. Acta Anaesthesiol Scand Suppl 1990; 94:46–50.

26. Whitesall R, Assidao C, Gollman D, et al: Relationship between arterial and peak expired carbon dioxide pressure during anesthesia and factors influencing the difference. Anesth Analg 1981; 60:508–512.

27. Aitken RS, Clark Kennedy AE: On the fluctuation in the composition of the alveolar air during the respiratory cycle in muscle exercise. J Physiol (Lond) 1928; 65:389–411.

28. Model JH, Graves SA, Ketover A: Clinical course of 91 consecutive near drowning victims. Chest 1976; 70:231.

29. Gilbert R, Keighley JF: The arterial-alveolar oxygen tension ratio. An index of gas exchange applicable to varying inspired oxygen concentrations. Am Rev Respir Dis 1974; 109:142–145.

30. Gilbert R, Auchinsloss JH, Kuppinger M, et al: Stability of the arterial-alveolar oxygen partial pressure ratio. Effects of low ventilation-perfusion ratios. Crit Care Med 1979; 7:267–272.

31. Marshall BE: Anesthesia for one lung ventilation. Anesthesiology 1988; 69:630–631.

32. Chiang ST: A nonogram for venous shunt (Q_s/Q_T) calculation. Thorax 1968; 23:563.

33. Staub NC: Alveolar-arterial oxygen tension gradient due to diffusion. J Appl Physiol 1963; 18:673–680.

34. Forster RE, Dubois AB, Briscoe WE, et al: The Lung: Physiologic Basis of Pulmonary Function Tests, ed 3. St. Louis, Mosby–Year Book, 1986.

35. Davies NJH: Does the lung work? 4. What does the transfer of carbon-monoxide mean? Br J Dis Chest 1982; 76:105–124.

36. Bradley ME, Leith DE: Ventilatory muscle training and oxygen cost of sustained hyperventilation. J Appl Physiol 1978; 45:855–892.

37. Stock MC: The oxygen cost of breathing. Chest 1992; 101:1486–1487.

38. Wilson RS, Sullivan SF, Malm JR, et al: Oxygen cost of breathing following anesthesia and cardiac surgery. Anesthesiology 1973; 39:38–93.

39. Field S, Kelly SM, Macklem PT: The oxygen cost of breathing in patients with cardiorespiratory disease. Am Rev Respir Dis 1982; 129:9–13.

17 Monitoring the Anesthesia Machine and Respiratory Gases

William T. Ross, Jr., M.D., M.B.A.

General Description of a Modern Continuous Flow Anesthesia Machine

Continuous flow anesthesia machines available for use in today's practice of anesthesia have evolved from experience and the thoughtful application of sound principles from several disciplines. This evolution can be traced through published reports of innovative technology spanning more than a hundred years. More important, reports describing failures of anesthesia machines and unexpected results from their operation have resulted in modifications leading to development of the anesthesia machines presently available for clinical use. To understand the implications of a departure of anesthesia equipment from its expected function (whether from malfunction or misuse), one needs to think in terms of the manner in which the equipment can fail. The operation of equipment after failure of a portion of the assembled apparatus is referred to as a failure mode. Understanding likely failure modes significantly enhances appreciation of the equipment with which one works. More complete and specific information about the construction of modern anesthesia machines may be found in the several excellent texts[1-3] and manufacturers' publications,[4-7] as well as in the extensive literature concerning anesthesia equipment.

The continuous flow anesthesia machine (Fig. 17-1) is a device that allows the anesthesiologist to accurately combine several gases (or vapors) to provide the gas mixtures used in the conduct of clinical anesthesia. The two major suppliers of anesthesia machines in the United States are Datex-Ohmeda (Madison, WI) and North American Dräger (Telford, PA). These machines, designed originally to be freestanding, mobile devices, are equipped with high-pressure vessels, typically E cylinders, each containing a few hundred liters of gas at high pressure.

Gas Supply

The gases most often available on anesthesia machines are oxygen and nitrous oxide. Provision for other compressed gases such as air, helium, or carbon dioxide may be found on some machines. Most hospitals in the United States now supply some or all of the gases used in anesthesia through built-in piping systems. The compressed gas cylinders present on machines in current practice are best regarded as

a reserve supply, available for use in the event of a failure of the hospital medical gas piping system. As such they permit the anesthesia in progress to be brought to a controlled conclusion. The widespread dependence on plumbing systems as the primary gas supply is so established that it is unwise to begin subsequent anesthetics with only E cylinders available. Reserve stocks of E cylinders are often maintained by hospital departments such as respiratory therapy or central supply not under the control of the anesthesia department. Stock levels may easily be too low to sustain continuation of a surgical schedule. Additionally, anesthesia ventilators utilize oxygen as the driving gas to produce tidal ventilation. Their use markedly increases the consumption of compressed oxygen[8] and places further demand on the supply and exchange of cylinders.

When full, high-pressure cylinders containing only gaseous oxygen or air are filled to pressures of approximately 2000 psig. Therefore, the amount of oxygen or air contained in a cylinder is proportional to the pressure in the cylinder. As a result, the amount of oxygen or air in a compressed gas cylinder may be accurately estimated when the pressure within the cylinder is known and the temperature of the cylinder and its contents remains constant. By contrast, a "full" cylinder of N_2O contains liquid N_2O with gaseous N_2O occupying the headspace above the liquid. N_2O has a vapor pressure of approximately 750 psig at room temperature. The amount of liquid N_2O (or any fluid, for that matter) contained in a cylinder may be accurately estimated by knowing the weight of N_2O (weight of cylinder plus N_2O less the tare weight of the cylinder) contained within the cylinder. In practice, the weighing of cylinders is awkward and is rarely performed except as a demonstration in a teaching environment. In addition, the tare weight of cylinders is typically unknown. Furthermore, during periods of using N_2O the vaporization of liquid N_2O to gas results in sufficient cooling of the cylinder and its contents to significantly reduce the vapor pressure of the liquid remaining within the cylinder. The pressure measured in cylinders of N_2O that have been subjected to significant cooling will be found to be as much as several hundred pounds below the expected 750 psig even though they still contain liquid N_2O.[9] Consequently the amount of N_2O remaining in cylinders in clinical practice is not accurately known.

Pressure and Flow Controls

A pressure of 50 psig is used as the intermediate or "working" pressure within the plumbing of the intermediate pressure section of anesthesia machines; that is, proximal to flowmeter control valves or on/off controls such as the oxy-

This chapter draws extensively from Phillip JM, Feinstein DM, Raemer DB: Monitoring anesthetic and respiratory gases. *In* Blitt CD, Hines RL (eds): Monitoring in Anesthesia and Critical Care Medicine. New York, Churchill Livingstone, 1995, pp 363–383.

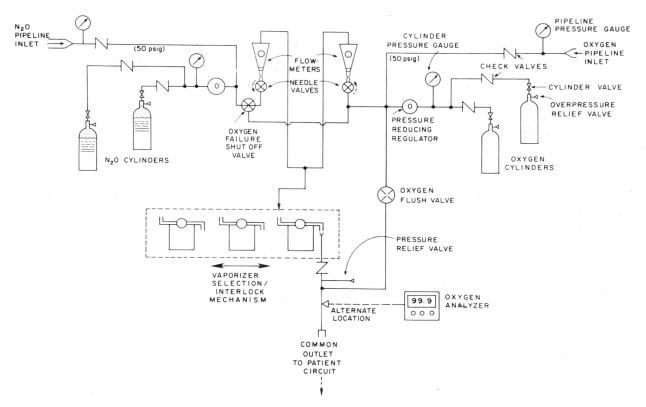

Figure 17–1. Schematic diagram of a "generic" continuous flow anesthesia machine. This diagram illustrates common design features rather than a specific machine.

gen flush valve. The flows set by flow control valves are monitored by observing their associated flowmeters. The flow control valves used in anesthesia machines regulate gas flow function as variable resistors and can provide, at any given setting, constant gas flow at their outlets only if presented with constant inlet pressure. Expressed mathematically, this relationship is fundamentally the same as Ohm's law for electrical circuits:

$$\text{Flow} = \frac{\text{Pressure}}{\text{Resistance}}$$

This relation dictates a requirement to accurately reduce the high pressure available in high-pressure cylinders to a constant working pressure. Such a requirement can be met by pressure-reducing regulators adjusted to maintain a constant outlet pressure of 50 psig (or slightly less) while a variable (up to ~2000 psig) but greater pressure is presented to the inlet. Likewise, variations in the pressure of gases in the gas piping system will result in proportional variations in the flow of that gas through a flow control valve. For example, a 10% variation in supply pressure will produce a similar variation in the gas flow exiting the flow control valve in the absence of compensating adjustments of the flow control valve. Ohmeda anesthesia machines in production today are constructed with the intermediate pressure section of the machine incorporating an additional stage of regulated pressure reduction to a pressure lower than the pipeline supply pressure of 50 psig. This design achieves superior regulation of the pressure being presented to the needle valves controlling gas flow through the flowmeters.[5]

Vaporizers

Agent-specific vaporizers are used to accurately add measured concentrations of volatile anesthetics to the gas stream. These devices must be used only with the anesthetic agent for which they were designed. Anesthetic machines having more than a single vaporizer should have an interlock-exclusion mechanism to prevent more than one vaporizer from being used at a time. The interlock mechanism also serves to isolate vaporizers not selected for use from the gas stream by disconnecting both the inlet and outlet of unselected vaporizers from the gas stream. This feature prevents vapor originating from an upstream vaporizer from being carried downstream and mixing with liquid anesthetic in the downstream vaporizer. Isolation of unselected vaporizers from the gas stream also prevents the addition of small amounts of volatile anesthetics to the gas stream as a result of continuing evaporation of volatile anesthetics. A patent channel connecting the anesthetic reservoir to the gas stream is present even though the vaporizer is turned off.[10]

Oxygen Flush Circuit

The oxygen flush circuit permits the flushing of the patient breathing circuit with a high flow of oxygen. It should be noted that the operation of the flush valve simply admits a high flow of oxygen to the outlet of the machine and neither turns off vaporizers nor provides a high flow of the anesthetic-containing gas mixture. Certain older machines had flush valves that were linked to include other functions such as deselecting vaporizers.

Most Ohmeda anesthesia machines of recent manufacture have a check valve installed between the outlet of vaporizers and the junction of the oxygen flush line with the fresh gas stream (i.e., near the fresh gas outlet of the machine). This feature prevents retrograde flow of appreciable volumes of gas back into the machine with the application of positive pressure at the machine outlet as occurs with positive pressure ventilation. It also isolates vaporizers from the "pumping effect" of pressure fluctuations on the constancy of vaporizer output.[11]

Fresh Gas Outlet

Access to the gas stream exiting the anesthesia machine is provided at the fresh gas port. This outlet is equipped with a standard, tapered 15-mm connector through which gas can be delivered to the patient breathing circuit.

Rationale for Monitoring the Anesthesia Machine

Fundamentally, anesthesia machines fail to perform the functions for which they were designed when they provide incorrect concentrations (or proportions) of the various gases they are supposed to combine or when they deliver an incorrect absolute amount of gas. These situations can lead to disastrous consequences if oxygen is greatly reduced or absent from the gas mixture. Other serious failures can occur with less dire consequences; for example, the omission of the anesthetic agent from the gas mixture can result in failure to achieve or maintain the anesthetic state. Because gas flowing from the anesthesia machine is relied upon to fill reservoir bags in anesthetic circuits and ventilators, leaks permitting the loss of gas from the breathing circuit can result in a failure to ventilate.

Monitoring of the anesthesia machine, as well as the anesthetized patient, can provide early, timely recognition of problems; this recognition is essential to their prompt correction. Early detection of changes in the status of the anesthesia machine will help minimize the likelihood of an adverse outcome.

Oxygen Delivery

There is little debate that assurance of adequate delivery of oxygen to the patient breathing circuit is a crucial function of anesthesia machine monitoring. The assumption that operator vigilance would prevent the occasional accidental delivery of hypoxic or anoxic breathing mixtures has proved inaccurate.[12, 13] This observation has resulted in extensive efforts to design machines that do not permit the delivery of hypoxic gas mixtures. Several different approaches have been taken to implement this feature.

One early approach was to construct machines so that the flow of oxygen could not be reduced to less than some minimum value. In this way anoxic mixtures are prevented, although hypoxic mixtures may be accepted at some N_2O flowmeter settings.

Beginning in the 1960s anesthesia machines were equipped with fail-safe mechanisms[4, 5, 7] designed to automatically halt the delivery of gases other than oxygen in the event of failure of the oxygen supply pressure within the intermediate-pressure section of the machine. It must be noted, however, that this system responds to *oxygen supply*

pressure rather than to the flow of oxygen. Anesthetists must understand that with older machines, not equipped with oxygen proportion controllers, it is possible to administer hypoxic gas mixtures continuously by adjusting oxygen to low (or even to zero) flow even though the machine is equipped with a fail-safe mechanism. To check the operation of the fail-safe device, oxygen and N_2O are turned on and the source (i.e., cylinder or piped in) of oxygen pressure is removed. The flow of N_2O should decline in proportion to the fall in oxygen pressure and be interrupted entirely as oxygen pressure falls below approximately 25 psig. The abruptness of cessation of N_2O flow varies with the particular implementation of the fail-safe function and may even vary among individual machines of the same model. Ohmeda refers to its fail-safe mechanism as a "pressure sensing shut-off valve," whereas Dräger designates theirs as an "oxygen failure protection device" (OFPD). Testing the operation of these devices is not checked during the checkout procedures described below.

Another design strategy has been to design machines that are not capable of delivering mixtures of gases containing less than 25% to 30% oxygen. Ohmeda and North American Dräger have implemented this function by pursuing different schemes to monitor or control the concentration of oxygen being supplied to the patient breathing circuit. Initially, North American Dräger offered pneumatic devices called oxygen ratio monitors (ORMs) which triggered an alarm when oxygen mixtures containing less than 30% oxygen were selected. More recently Dräger has offered oxygen ratio monitor controllers (ORMcs) which will control the concentration of oxygen actually delivered by the anesthesia machine when the operator attempts to select combinations of flows of oxygen and N_2O that would result in the delivery of less than 25% to 30% oxygen. This device automatically adjusts the flow of N_2O downward when the operator decreases the oxygen flow to a point that would result in a gas mixture containing less than 25% to 30% oxygen without the action of the ORMc. Conversely, if the operator attempts to deliver a gas mixture containing less than 25% to 30% oxygen by increasing the flow of N_2O, the ORMc operates to limit the flow of N_2O.

Ohmeda machines incorporate a mechanical linkage (Link 25) between the oxygen and N_2O flow control valves to produce a similar result. The Link 25 causes a proportional increase in the flow of oxygen when a flow adjustment is made to increase the flow of N_2O so that the resulting gas mixture would otherwise contain more than 70% N_2O. The device also operates in an inverse manner so that an adjustment in the flow of oxygen downward results in a proportional reduction in the flow of N_2O so that the concentration of oxygen in the resulting gas mixture remains at or above 30%. The combination of fail-safe devices and oxygen proportion controllers on machines of recent manufacture works in tandem to make the administration of hypoxic gas mixtures very unlikely.

Oxygen Analyzers

All gas machines should have the capability to analyze the gas supplied to the patient for oxygen. Oxygen analyzers are durable, inexpensive, and reliable devices that specifically identify as well as quantitate the fraction of oxygen in the gas stream (see also Chapter 18). This may be accomplished by placing the oxygen analyzer sensor in the inspiratory limb of the patient breathing circuit or, alternatively, in the fresh gas line proximal to the breathing circuit.[14] The location of the oxygen analyzer sensor in the inspiratory limb of the patient breathing circuit is particularly advantageous when low-flow anesthetic techniques are employed with circle absorber breathing circuits because it indicates the actual concentration of oxygen being presented to the patient. This concentration varies with time and will be affected by the patient's oxygen consumption, uptake of gases other than oxygen from the breathing circuit (e.g., N_2O), and the total fresh gas flow.

On modern anesthesia machines oxygen analysis is accomplished by a separate device for analysis of oxygen in the gas mixture being supplied to the patient *in addition to* analysis of respiratory gases in the breathing circuit, which may include determinations of inspiratory and expiratory oxygen concentrations. The redundancy afforded by such a scheme greatly enhances safety for patients and *must not be used as an argument for eliminating basic oxygen analysis from anesthesia machines.* Furthermore, such an arrangement permits an analytic check of the oxygen supplied by a machine during machine checkout separate from any information that may be obtained from associated respiratory gas analysis devices. During anesthetic administration a basic oxygen analyzer provides a running crosscheck for fraction of inspired oxygen (F_{IO_2}) data being supplied by a respiratory gas analyzer.

Approaches to the Monitoring of Anesthesia Machines

Monitoring the anesthesia machine for the conduct of anesthesia includes tasks that must be done before the device is used for patient care, during the conduct of the anesthetic, and following completion of the anesthetic.

Preanesthetic Check

A preanesthetic checkout of the anesthesia apparatus is a prerequisite of the reliable conduct of safe anesthesia. When planning to conduct an anesthetic one must understand the general capabilities of the anesthesia machine to be used. At a minimum the anesthesiologist needs to know, with a high degree of certainty, whether the machine has monitors that can be turned off independently from the gas flows available on the machine and whether the machine can produce hypoxic mixtures under any circumstances, despite monitoring devices.

While a number of anesthesia machine checkout procedures have been recommended, the Food and Drug Administration (FDA) published and widely disseminated an anesthesia machine checkout procedure in 1986 that was endorsed and promoted by the American Society of Anesthesiologists.[15] Several limitations of this procedure became apparent, and the FDA Center for Devices and Radiologic Health issued a revised Anesthesia Apparatus Checkout procedure in 1993. This document[16] appears as Figure 17–2. This checkout procedure has been widely applied and accepted.

When combined with effective preventive or progressive maintenance programs, the application of systematically applied checkout practices should help maintain a low incidence of critical machine failures. Its repeated use will improve the practitioner's familiarity with and understanding of the workings of anesthesia machines.

The introductory statement in the FDA checkout recommendations notes that the recommendations are valid only for anesthesia systems that conform to current standards. Presently, the applicable American Society for Testing and Materials (ASTM) standard is designated F 1161-88 and entitled *Standard Specification for Minimum Performance and Safety Requirements for Components and Systems of Anesthesia Gas Machines.*[17] Standards are further discussed in a later section.

The introductory statement further acknowledges that standards for the design and construction of anesthesia machines may change and that machines that antedate the current standard may be in service. It goes on to encourage modification of the checkout procedure in order to ensure its utility in the face of variations in equipment design, as well as local variations in clinical practice, with the caution that such procedural modifications be instituted with appropriate review. This statement is clearly intended to provide flexibility of application in real-world situations, provided that any modifications are applied with responsible attention to technical detail by anesthesiologists and institutions.

The testing and checkout procedures described here and in the FDA checkout procedure are abbreviated or operational test procedures. The results of such testing will suggest when further servicing of an anesthesia machine is needed. These checkout procedures cannot replace service and periodic preventive maintenance by trained service personnel. In some instances the checkout procedures may be at variance with checkout procedures recommended by the equipment manufacturer. It is best to discuss such differences with the supplier or manufacturer and use the result of those discussions to establish an institution's checkout procedures.

Preliminary Visual Inspection

An initial visual survey of the machine should be conducted. During a walk-around inspection the operator should verify that the apparatus has had a thorough preventive maintenance inspection within the interval established by the institution for such periodic inspections. This information should be available on an inspection sticker affixed to the machine in an obvious location. Other items to be checked during the visual inspection are the settings of controls and the presence of obvious damage to machine components or the absence of components. Flowmeters should be observed for damage and for the presence of bobbins, floats, or balls resting on the *bottom* of each flowmeter. Any sign of obvious damage to the machine should alert the anesthesiologist to the possibility of a breach of integrity of the device. For example, a damaged flowmeter shield should cause the operator to carefully seek evidence of damage to the flowmeter itself. In addition to inspection to detect obvious gross damage, the checkout includes functional testing (as for leaks; see below) and a search for the cause(s) of damage in order to prevent recurrences. Even if damage is determined to be superficial, it should be reported in an effective manner so the general condition of the machine may be maintained by assigned repair personnel. Signal wires, power cords, and gas and vacuum tubing should be inspected for cracks or other damage. If there is any question concerning damage to these items they should be replaced promptly.

Initially the machine can be expected to be found with the pipeline-supplied gases connected and with all flowmeters and vaporizers turned off; however, the operator must determine that adjustable controls on the machine are set to appropriate positions to proceed with the initial checkout. A consistent confirmation of the setting of all adjustable controls will assure that controls have not been left in some unexpected configuration and will permit the development of work habits which will become personal routines promot-

Anesthesia Apparatus Checkout Recommendations, 1993

This checkout, or a reasonable equivalent, should be conducted before administration of anesthesia. These recommendations are only valid for an anesthesia system that conforms to current and relevant standards and includes an ascending bellows ventilator and at least the following monitors: capnograph, pulse oximeter, oxygen analyzer, respiratory volume monitor (spirometer) and breathing system pressure monitor with high and low pressure alarms. This is a guideline which users are encouraged to modify to accommodate differences in equipment design and variations in local clinical practice. Such local modifications should have appropriate peer review. Refer to the operators manual for specific procedures and precautions.

Emergency Ventilation Equipment
*1. **Verify Backup Ventilation Equipment is Available & Functioning**

High Pressure System
*2. **Check Oxygen Cylinder Supply**
   a. Open O_2 cylinder and verify at least half full (about 1000 psi).
   b. Close cylinder.
*3. **Check Central Pipeline Supplies**
   a. Check that hoses are connected and pipeline gauges read about 50 psi.

Low Pressure System
*4. **Check Initial Status of Low Pressure System**
   a. Close flow control valves and turn vaporizers off.
   b. Check fill level and tighten vaporizers' filler caps.
*5. **Perform Leak Check of Machine Low Pressure System**
   a. Verify that the machine master switch and flow control valves are OFF.
   b. Attach "Suction Bulb" to common (fresh) gas outlet.
   c. Squeeze bulb repeatedly until fully collapsed.
   d. Verify bulb stays *fully* collapsed for at least 10 seconds.
   e. Open one vaporizer at a time and repeat 'c' and 'd' as above.
   f. Remove suction bulb, and reconnect fresh gas hose.
*6. **Turn On Machine Master Switch**
   and all other necessary electrical equipment.
*7. **Test Flowmeters**
   a. Adjust flow of all gases through their full range, checking for smooth operation of floats and undamaged flowtubes.
   b. Attempt to create a hypoxic O_2/N_2O mixture and verify correct changes in flow and/or alarm.

Scavenging System
*8. **Adjust and Check Scavenging System**
   a. Ensure proper connections between the scavenging system and both APL (pop-off) valve and ventilator relief valve.
   b. Adjust waste gas vacuum (if possible).
   c. Fully open APL valve and occlude Y-piece.
   d. With minimum O_2 flow, allow scavenger reservoir bag to collapse completely and verify that absorber pressure gauge reads about zero.
   e. With the O_2 flush activated, allow the scavenger reservoir bag to distend fully, and then verify that absorber pressure gauge reads < 10 cm H_2O.

Breathing System
*9. **Calibrate O_2 Monitor**
   a. Ensure monitor reads 21% in room air.
   b. Verify low O_2 alarm is enabled and functioning.
   c. Reinstall sensor in circuit and flush breathing system with O_2.
   d. Verify that monitor now reads greater than 90%.
10. **Check Initial Status of Breathing System**
   a. Set selector switch to "Bag" mode.
   b. Check that breathing circuit is complete, undamaged and unobstructed.

   c. Verify that CO_2 absorbent is adequate.
   d. Install breathing circuit accessory equipment (e.g., humidifier, PEEP valve) to be used during the case.
11. **Perform Leak Check of the Breathing System**
   a. Set all gas flows to zero (or minimum).
   b. Close APL (pop-off) valve and occlude Y-piece.
   c. Pressurize breathing system to about 30 cm H_2O with O_2 flush.
   d. Ensure that pressure remains fixed for at least 10 seconds.
   e. Open APL (pop-off) valve and ensure that pressure decreases.

Manual and Automatic Ventilation Systems
12. **Test Ventilation Systems and Unidirectional Valves**
   a. Place a second breathing bag on Y-piece.
   b. Set appropriate ventilator parameters for next patient.
   c. Switch to automatic ventilation (Ventilator) mode.
   d. Turn ventilator ON and fill bellows and breathing bag with O_2 flush.
   e. Set O_2 flow to minimum, other gas flows to zero.
   f. Verify that during inspiration bellows delivers appropriate tidal volume and that during expiration bellows fills completely.
   g. Set fresh gas flow to about 5 L/min.
   h. Verify that the ventilator bellows and simulated lungs fill and empty appropriately without sustained pressure at end expiration.
   i. *Check for proper action of unidirectional valves.*
   j. Exercise breathing circuit accessories to ensure proper function.
   k. Turn ventilator OFF and switch to manual ventilation (Bag/APL) mode.
   l. Ventilate manually and assure inflation and deflation of artificial lungs and appropriate feel of system resistance and compliance.
   m. Remove second breathing bag from Y-piece.

Monitors
13. **Check, Calibrate and/or Set Alarm Limits of all Monitors**
   Capnometer   Pulse Oximeter
   Oxygen Analyzer   Respiratory Volume Monitor (Spirometer)
   Pressure Monitor with High and Low Airway Pressure Alarms

Final Position
14. **Check Final Status of Machine**
   a. Vaporizers off.
   b. APL valve open.
   c. Selector switch to "Bag"
   d. All flowmeters to zero (or minimum).
   e. Patient suction level adequate.
   f. Breathing system ready to use.

If an anesthesia provider uses the same machine in successive cases, these steps need not be repeated or may be abbreviated after the initial checkout.

Figure 17-2. *Anesthesia Apparatus Checkout Recommendations, 1993,* published by the Food and Drug Administration.

ing efficient, thorough machine review prior to beginning each anesthetic procedure.

Check of Backup Emergency Ventilation Equipment (Item 1 of the Checklist)

While it may be argued that backup ventilation equipment is not, strictly speaking, a part of the anesthesia machine, its presence is essential to providing safe anesthetic care. It seems wise to include it in the checkout of devices necessary for the conduct of anesthetics. The preliminary inspection should include a check that backup ventilation equipment is available and functional. The equipment should include a bag-and-valve apparatus to permit positive pressure ventilation that, especially for perioperative patient care, should be supplied with oxygen. Many facilities will provide oxygen from a source separate from the anesthesia machine but readily available in the operating room (OR).

Specific functional checks of portions of anesthesia machines found in the body of the FDA-recommended checkout procedure include the following:

- Manual ventilation capability
- The high-pressure section
- The low-pressure section
- The scavenging apparatus
- The patient breathing circuit
- Mechanical ventilation capability
- Operation and initial settings of monitors
- Initial settings of anesthesia machine controls

See Figure 17–2.

Check of High-Pressure (Cylinder) Oxygen Supply (Item 2)

Cylinders mounted on the machine should be examined in their yokes for proper mounting and the presence of only one seat washer. The pressure of gas available in the cylinders mounted on the machine should be determined. If the high-pressure (cylinder) gauges indicate no pressure in the high-pressure section of the machine, the high-pressure part of the machine is depressurized; turning on a cylinder will indicate the pressure available in that cylinder.

On machines with multiple gas cylinders attached to high-pressure manifolds, an important condition routinely occurs that prevents the ready determination of gas pressure available in individual cylinders (see Fig. 17–1).

With the machine connected to the pipeline gas supply, 50 to 55 psig will be applied to the plumbing within the machine proximal to the valves controlling the flow of gas to the flowmeters (intermediate-pressure section). In a typical machine, the pressure-reducing regulator valves have been set to deliver gas to the machine from the high-pressure cylinders at a slightly lower pressure. This feature keeps the outlet valve of the reducing regulator closed so long as the design pressure (i.e., 50 to 55 psig) is maintained within the internal plumbing of the intermediate-pressure section of the machine by the piped-in gases. Thus, use of gas from cylinders is minimized, even if the cylinder valves remain open, as long as there is adequate pipeline pressure. In practice, however, reductions of intermediate-section pressure may occur during periods of demand for high flow from the pipeline system such as with ventilator operation or during use of flush valves.

Because the high-pressure yokes are equipped with check valves to permit cylinders to be changed without losing gas while the remaining cylinder valve(s) remain open to provide an uninterrupted supply of gas, and to prevent transfilling of high-pressure cylinders containing gas at unequal pressures, high-pressure gas will be trapped between the yoke check valve and the reducing regulator. The high pressure indicated by the cylinder gauges can be released by removing the machine from the pipeline gas supply *and* permitting flow from the regulator (with cylinder valves off) to depressurize the high- and intermediate-pressure sections of the anesthesia machine. This latter step is not required by the FDA checkout procedure but is described here to provide a more complete description of anesthesia machine operation. The valve on each oxygen cylinder should be

opened in turn while the cylinder pressure gauge is observed. If more than one cylinder is present, the second cylinder's valve may also be opened to see if the pressure in it is greater than that in the first cylinder. If an increase in pressure is seen after the cylinder valve of the second cylinder is opened, the pressure indicated is the pressure present in that cylinder. If no increase in pressure is observed, one cannot tell what the pressure is in the second cylinder unless the high- and intermediate-pressure sections of the anesthesia machine are depressurized as described above. It is acceptable to begin an anesthetic if at least one oxygen cylinder contains 600 to 1000 psig.

Following the pressure check of oxygen cylinders the respective cylinder valves should be closed. This step prevents unrecognized use of oxygen from the cylinders if the pipeline pressure transiently drops below approximately 50 psig. Optionally, the pressure in high-pressure cylinders of other gases may be checked in a similar way.

Check of Pipeline Supplies of Medical Gases (Item 3)

The pipeline gas supply connections to the machine and respective pipeline pressures of 50 to 55 psig should be verified. Medical gas systems commonly have the pressure of oxygen 3 to 5 psig greater than the pressures for N_2O and compressed air. This practice ensures that inadvertent cross-connection of oxygen pipelines with either of these gases favors the flow of oxygen into N_2O or air piping rather than favoring the flow of N_2O or air into the oxygen piping. Such cross-connections have resulted from plumbing errors within pipeline systems, as well as from malfunction of devices connected to more than one gas in the piping system.[18]

Recommendations have been made to minimize gas leaks, particularly to prevent N_2O contamination of the OR atmosphere.[19] In response to this concern, connections between the anesthesia machine and the medical gas piping system are made with diameter index safety system (DISS) connectors tightened lightly, but more than fingertight, with a wrench. Quick connectors are not standardized for use in medical gas piping systems and are prone to leakage and damage while disconnected.

Check of the Low-Pressure Section (Items 4 to 7)

The low-pressure section of the anesthesia machine is that portion of the machine from the flow control valves (including the oxygen flush valve) to the fresh gas outlet. It includes flowmeters, vaporizers, and all associated plumbing. Testing of this portion of the machine is complicated by the use of unidirectional (check) valves at various locations in the low-pressure section of the machine. Check valves have been used by manufacturers in the assembly of various models of their machines. Check valves are used extensively in anesthesia machines to prevent reverse flow of gas in various portions of the machine. They are usually placed as follows:

1. In the common gas line near the fresh gas outlet to the patient breathing circuit just proximal to the point at which the oxygen flush line joins the gas stream[20]
2. At the outlet of vaporizers to minimize the pumping[11] effect of mechanical ventilation on vaporizer output

Outlet check valves are most often present in machines

manufactured by Ohmeda. The operation of check valves is typically not tested in the daily checkout of anesthesia machines but should be tested by maintenance personnel during periodic preventive maintenance.

Understanding Pneumatic Systems Containing Check Valves

Although the testing of pneumatic assemblies for leaks is quite straightforward, some configurations of components can isolate one segment of an assembly from other segments. With respect to anesthesia machines, this can be particularly perplexing when a portion of the apparatus under test contains unidirectional or check valves. Figure 17–3A illustrates a segment of tubing connected in series with a flow control valve and a flow measuring device. The tubing may be tested for leakage most simply by placing a plug equipped with a pressure gauge in the downstream end. Flow is admitted to the tube by the flow control valve until a predetermined pressure is reached and then the flow is reduced to zero. (For testing the low-pressure section of anesthesia machines the test pressure should be 30 cm H_2O.) If the segment of tubing is free from leaks the pressure

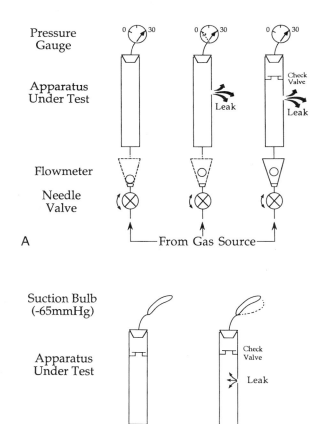

indicated will remain at 30 cm H_2O. On the other hand, if there is a leak the pressure will fall promptly. In this case the magnitude of the leak can be measured by increasing gas flow to the point that the testing pressure of 30 cm H_2O is achieved and, by fine flow adjustments, exactly maintained. The flow indicated is the leak rate at the test pressure (e.g., 300 mL/minute at 30 cm H_2O).

When the segment of tubing under test includes a check valve downstream from the leak, simple pressure testing may not detect the leak. If the segment under test is pressurized, pressure will increase on both sides of the check valve. When inlet flow ceases, the leak permits the loss of pressure in the portion of the apparatus upstream from the check valve. The fall in pressure in the upstream part of the apparatus causes the check valve to close and prevents loss of pressure in the portion of the apparatus downstream from the check valve, leading to the erroneous interpretation that the entire segment of tubing under test is free from leaks. If, as described in the preceding paragraph, the pressure in the tubing segment under test is brought up to the test pressure using the needle valve, the leak rate is equal to the flow at which the test pressure remains constant.

Figure 17–3B depicts another way to test a segment of tubing with an intrinsic check valve. This method permits the identification of leaks and allows go/no-go decisions to be made. Initially all gas flow into the segment of tubing under test is turned off and a suction bulb is attached to the downstream outlet of the tubing being tested. The bulb is squeezed repeatedly until it remains collapsed. At this point the interior of the tubing has a negative pressure of about −65 mmHg. If the plumbing being tested has no leak, the bulb will remain collapsed. If a leak is present, regardless of whether it is upstream or downstream from the check valve, ambient air will be sucked into the segment of tubing being tested and the bulb will expand. The machine will have passed the test if the bulb remains collapsed for 10 seconds or more. With typical sphygmomanometer bulbs this represents a leak rate of less than approximately 120 mL/minute.

The test device for negative pressure testing for leaks can be assembled using a squeeze bulb similar to those used with sphygmomanometers but having its check valve arranged so that releasing the bulb results in negative pressure at the inlet to the bulb. The inlet to the bulb should be connected to a short piece of tubing, to the other end of which is attached a 15-mm standard tapered connector (endotracheal tube connector) suitable for attachment to the fresh gas outlet of the machine being checked. This test device should be tested periodically to ensure that it continues to be able to provide a negative pressure of approximately −65 mmHg. Bulbs assembled with the associated connectors for negative pressure testing are commercially available.

Flowmeters (Item 7)

With the machine master switch turned on, the function of the flowmeters is tested. The floats should be observed to move smoothly within the bore of each flowmeter over the full length of the flowmeter tube and should return smoothly to the base of the tube when the flow control valve is closed. Floats are designed to rotate during use. Failure to rotate results in sticking or interference between the float and the tube wall, causing erroneous readings.

The oxygen-proportioning system is tested by setting typical flows of oxygen and N_2O, attempting to reduce the flow of oxygen to the point at which a hypoxic mixture would result, and observing that there is a proportional reduction

Figure 17–3. *A* and *B*, The effect of a check valve on procedures used to test a segment of tubing for leaks. See text for discussion.

in the flow of N_2O. This check should confirm that delivered oxygen concentrations are always greater than 25%.

Adjustment and Check of Scavenging System (Item 8)

It is usually convenient to check and adjust the waste gas scavenging system during the early part of machine check-out. The interface between the patient breathing circuit and the conduit to the removal route should be inspected for integrity and lack of occlusion. A common cause of partial obstruction in the scavenging system is collection of water in dependent loops of the scavenger connecting tubing. If a closed scavenging system with a reservoir bag is in use, the scavenger must be adjusted to provide proper flow so the reservoir bag on the scavenging system is emptied only at the highest flows that the operator expects to use. Usually this will be in the neighborhood of 10 L/minute. With the Y connection to which the patient will be connected occluded and the adjustable pressure-limiting (APL) valve open, a 10-L/minute flow is admitted to the breathing circuit while the scavenging suction is turned off. This procedure slightly increases the pressure within the breathing circuit. Operation of the oxygen flush valve should produce a pressure increase of less than 10 cm H_2O within the breathing circuit. These steps provide a functional test of the positive pressure relief valve in a closed scavenging system and prove that the outlet of any other type of scavenging system is patent.

Similarly, with zero fresh gas flow into the patient breathing circuit, the scavenger suction on, the patient connection occluded, and the APL valve open, there should be less than 2 cm H_2O negative pressure measured in the patient breathing circuit with proper functioning of the negative pressure relief valve in the scavenging system. Other scavenging systems, such as passive systems that carry waste gases to the return vent of a nonrecirculating air-conditioning system, may[7] or may not be equipped with pressure relief valves. These systems rely on patent, large-bore (typically 19-mm) tubing as a conduit. Occlusion of this tubing or the direct application of suction to it must be avoided to prevent excessive positive or negative pressure from being applied to the patient breathing circuit.[21]

Open scavenging systems are in common use today. They rely on the presence of high flow (~25 L/minute) suction applied to a large canister. The presence of multiple vent holes, or relief ports, in the canister permits room air to be drawn inside without creating negative pressure in the interior of the canister. Waste anesthetic gases from the patient breathing circuit or ventilator are conducted to the interior of the canister, where they are forced by the high flow of room air into the suction system. These systems are mechanically simple and minimize the likelihood that either positive or negative pressure will be inadvertently applied to the patient breathing circuit.

Oxygen Analyzer (Item 9)

The initial check of the oxygen analyzer should follow the manufacturer's instructions and, after a suitable warm-up interval, confirm that it reads, or can be adjusted to read, close to 21% when the sensor is positioned in ambient air, well away from sources of gases that might change the ambient oxygen concentration. The sensor should be repositioned to its place on the anesthesia machine, the circuit flushed with a high flow of 100% oxygen and the monitor observed to

read 100% ±10%. If the analyzer calibration control is adjusted while the sensor is exposed to 100% oxygen, the analyzer should be further checked to confirm a reading of 21% ±2% in room air.

To confirm that oxygen is the only gas present in the fresh gas being supplied to the patient breathing circuit, the breathing circuit should be flushed with 100% oxygen, following which a flow of 3 to 5 L/minute of oxygen is continued. A reading of 100% ±10% should be noted on the oxygen analyzer. No odor (suggesting that a vaporizer is leaking or has been left on) should be detectable by a sniff of the gas exiting the downstream end of the inspiratory limb of the breathing circuit.

Concerns have been expressed regarding recommendations that anesthetists breathe from the anesthetic circuit. If one prefers, the composition of the gas being delivered from the anesthesia machine to the patient breathing circuit may be determined by using the oxygen analyzer or a respiratory gas analyzer if at hand. Devices for analyzing respiratory gases are discussed in detail in a later section.

Breathing System Setup and Check of Carbon Dioxide Absorbent (Item 10)

The circle absorption breathing system should be inspected to ensure that it is intact, undamaged, and that all accessories for the conduct of the proposed anesthetic are attached. The breathing circuit should be tested with accessories connected and the ventilator bag selector valve set to the BAG position.

If the CO_2 absorbent contains an indicator, inspection of the canister can suggest whether the absorbent has been expended. Because different indicators may be used in different formulations of absorbing compounds, the anesthesiologist must be aware of the expected color changes with the product in use.[22] The color change reflects a change in pH on the surface of the granules of absorbent. This change is most marked at the end of a period of use and the color change may not persist overnight.

Changes of absorbent should be scheduled at regular intervals, which should be shortened as suggested by color changes at the *end* of periods of use. Most CO_2-absorbing circle systems are equipped with two canisters in series with the gas flow in the circle. Net flow through the canisters is from top to bottom in current machines. When the color change indicating consumption of the absorbent extends into the downstream canister of the absorber assembly, the absorbent should be changed in the upstream canister and that canister placed in the downstream (lower) position in the gas stream.

Leak Testing of the Circle Absorption Breathing System (Item 11)

When machines having a minimum flow of oxygen (typically in the range of 200 to 500 mL/minute) are tested for leaks, it will not be possible to measure leaks that are less than the minimum flow without disconnecting the machine from the pipeline gas supply. As a practical matter, leaks of 500 mL/minute or less may be accepted so long as low-flow or closed-circuit techniques are not used and sufficient total flow is available to ensure adequate ventilation of the patient. Any machine with leaks greater than 2 L/minute, including leaks in the breathing circuit, should be removed from service for repair. It is recommended that test pressures within anesthetic machines and breathing circuits be limited to less than 100 cm H_2O.

The procedures described below will measure the total of all leaks in gas machines (downstream from the flowmeters) having no check valves between the flowmeters and the fresh gas outlet *and* in the breathing circuit. With gas flows turned off, the Y connector occluded, and the APL valve closed, the breathing circuit can be pressurized to 30 cm H_2O using the oxygen flush valve. Once a pressure of 30 cm H_2O has been achieved, it should remain near 30 cm H_2O for 10 seconds. If it does not, a significant leak is present. Alternatively, machines having a continuing minimum flow of oxygen should demonstrate a continuing increase in pressure in the breathing circuit. If it appears that the pressure developed will continue to rise beyond 30 cm H_2O, it may be inferred that the anesthesia machine *and* the patient breathing circuit have no major leaks and that any leak present is less than the continuing minimum oxygen flow rate. A continuing minimum flow of oxygen of 500 mL/minute into an adult CO_2-absorbing breathing circuit will require about 10 seconds to cause a rise in pressure from 30 cm H_2O to 32 cm H_2O in the circle system. After this test the occlusion at the Y connector should be removed.

Check of Manual and Mechanical Ventilating Capability (Item 12)

A second breathing bag attached to the Y connector will serve to simulate a patient's "lungs." With the ventilator bag selector valve set to the BAG position and a flow of approximately 5 L/minute established, the APL valve is adjusted to a pressure of 5 to 10 cm H_2O within the breathing circuit. By alternately squeezing the "lung" bag and the breathing bag attached to the circuit, one should demonstrate

1. Sequential inflation and deflation of the test "lung" without sustained positive pressure
2. Appropriate feel of breathing system resistance
3. Proper movement of the unidirectional valves in the breathing circuit

The mechanical ventilation function, is checked by switching the ventilator bag selector valve to the VENTILATOR position; a low (1 L/minute or less) flow of oxygen is set, the ventilator remains turned OFF, and the breathing circuit (now including the ventilator bellows) and test "lung" are filled using the oxygen flush valve, if necessary. The ventilator bellows (standing bellows ventilator assumed) should remain filled with less than 4 cm H_2O, continuing positive pressure in the breathing circuit. The ventilator is turned ON, and it is verified that the test "lung" inflates during the inspiratory phase of the ventilator cycle and that deflation of the "lung" is not restricted during the expiratory phase. It is convenient to use ventilator settings of 500 mL tidal volume with a rate of 10 breaths/minute and a fresh gas flow of 5 L/minute of oxygen for this ventilator checkout. The use of consistent, specific settings makes variations in results easier to identify. The breathing circuit pressure gauge and spirometer verify that pressure and flow are developed in the breathing circuit as the ventilator cycles. This portion of the checkout is completed by removing the test "lung," selecting the BAG position of the ventilator bag selector valve, opening the APL valve, reducing the oxygen flow, and setting the ventilator and the ventilation monitor to a tidal volume and rate suitable for the next patient to be anesthetized.

Monitoring Equipment (Item 13)

Electrical monitoring equipment for both physiologic and machine variables is turned on and checked for proper operation as part of the checklist. Certain apparatuses such as older physiologic monitors, certain oxygen analyzers, and gas analyzers require a warm-up interval to assure stable operation. The warm-up is related either to some components reaching thermal equilibrium or to "conditioning" of electrodes. The appropriate procedures for activation and calibration of equipment are detailed in the operator's manual for each piece of equipment. If the correct procedure is followed, a need for considerable calibration suggests the possibility of significant drift or erratic behavior of the monitor or its associated sensor.

Intraoperative Monitoring of Anesthesia Machines

Monitoring during anesthesia administration requires careful attention to the status of the patient on a continuing basis. The following discussion addresses only those tasks that directly involve monitoring of the anesthesia machine. Patient monitoring per se is addressed in other chapters.

Intraoperative monitoring can be thought of as systematic verification of pressures within various portions of the machine, of proper gas flows, and of proper gas proportions, including vaporized volatile anesthetics. The operator should establish a pattern for scanning the different sources of data and should expect to check those more frequently that vary substantially over short intervals or that are judged to be particularly crucial. As conditions change during the conduct of the anesthetic, the order of the scan and the priority assigned to various monitoring tasks may require adjustment. For example, the initial portion of anesthetic administration demands frequent appraisal of the concentration of anesthetic agents while uptake of the anesthetic proceeds toward equilibrium as influenced by physiologic parameters (e.g., cardiovascular responses, pattern of ventilation, absence of patient movement in response to surgical stimulation) and by measurement of the changing concentration of volatile agents in exhaled gas (e.g., mass or Raman spectroscopy, or infrared [IR] absorption).

During a later phase of anesthetic maintenance, with the patient more nearly in equilibrium with the anesthetic agent, the anesthetic concentration might be monitored less frequently and attention (i.e., priority) might be directed toward lower-priority tasks such as ensuring that an adequate amount of liquid anesthetic is present in its vaporizer. Such examples illustrate the issues encountered in understanding and describing the details of monitoring tasks occurring during anesthesia administration (see Chapter 3). Various circumstances may dramatically affect the identification and description of criteria one might use to set priorities to establish variables to be tracked most closely, as well as to set tolerances. Tolerances are the limits of individual variables that would be accepted before triggering action to adjust the variable being monitored (e.g., volatile anesthetic concentration) or adjustments of related variables (e.g., the administration of fluids).

Monitoring a number of variables requires ongoing assessment of the stream of continually presented data. Experienced clinicians can perform such tasks fairly well, but the presentation of increasingly large volumes of information threatens to overload them. This is demonstrated when alarms sound on OR equipment not related to the administration of the anesthetic, and the anesthesiologist responds by searching the anesthetic machine for the source of the alarm. Manufacturers of anesthesia machines have responded to this problem by developing schemes for prioritizing the alarms presented and having them appear in central or common locations with instructions to direct the operator's attention to the appropriate portion(s) of the anesthetic apparatus.

Although reports indicate that critical incidents have different origins, causes are attributed most often to human error rather than to machine failure per se.[2, 12, 13, 23] Understanding this, anesthetists should confirm their prior actions and continuously scan the entire clinical setting, including the anesthesia machine, for information. The anesthesiologist who is idle for very long during the conduct of anesthesia is, at the least, falling behind in the gathering of information and runs the risk of missing important changes in the status of the anesthetic being conducted.

Table 17–1 provides a broad outline of anesthesia machine parameters to be evaluated periodically during the conduct of clinical anesthesia.

Pipeline pressure should be monitored periodically and confirmed to remain at 50 psig ± 5 psi. Major fluctuations may result from high resistance in the supply lines (e.g., multiple check valves in the pipeline system) producing a large pressure drop when higher flows are called for, as when an oxygen-powered ventilator cycles or when the oxygen flush is activated. When such pressure drops are particularly extensive, fail-safe systems may be activated, resulting in intermittent changes in the flow of N_2O or other gases. This situation indicates inadequate capacity of the oxygen pipeline system and should be corrected. It may interfere with the proper operation of oxygen-powered equipment, particularly anesthesia ventilators, and does not permit the high flow of oxygen necessary to provide rapid oxygen flushing of the patient breathing circuit. Low pipeline pressures can indicate a faulty pipeline regulator, exhaustion of the pipeline source of gas, or, rarely, substantial leaks within the pipeline system.

Close monitoring of pressure within the high-pressure portion of the anesthesia machine during the use of the cylinder gas supplies allows the operator to estimate the amount of gas remaining in the machine. This information, together with knowledge of the flow rate being employed, can be used to calculate the expected duration of the remaining gas supply. When carried out carefully and early, this calculation can enable either additional cylinders to be delivered in a timely manner or the anesthetic technique to be modified to conserve the available supply. Such estimates can be limited in several ways. The operator must recognize that the quantity of N_2O remaining within the cylinders cannot be accurately estimated (see previous discussion). If oxygen-powered equipment is used (e.g., ventilators) or the

oxygen flush valve is operated, increased and unmeasured oxygen expenditure occurs.

The flow of each of the gases constituting the gas mixture being supplied to the anesthetized patient is usually monitored by the anesthesiologist observing flowmeters for each gas. Although the anesthesiologist continues to be the primary monitor of gas flow, automated flow monitoring and controlling devices are becoming widespread. As described earlier, anesthesia machines presently in production and meeting the ASTM F 1161-88 standard are equipped with oxygen ratio control devices. These devices often provide the first indication that an attempt to select an incorrect proportion of oxygen has occurred. It is important for the user of an anesthesia machine to recognize that these devices rely on the critical assumption that correctly identified gases are being supplied to the apparatus. If the incorrect gas is supplied,[5, 14, 24] these mechanical, pneumatic devices cannot properly report or control the proportion of oxygen actually being delivered by the anesthesia machine. For this reason, it is particularly crucial that *analytic* instruments be included on anesthesia machines to measure oxygen concentration. Knowledge of the concentration of oxygen is so fundamental to the safe conduct of anesthesia that the use of monitors dedicated specifically to the analysis of oxygen should be incorporated in anesthesia machines even though respiratory gas analysis is also available. Information about oxygen concentration is available indirectly by calculation using the flows of individual gases being employed, directly from an oxygen analyzer (or other analytic instrument), and from on-line analysis of respiratory gas within the patient breathing circuit.

Adjustment of flowmeter settings can be made in a manner that minimizes the likelihood of accidental creation of hypoxic gas mixtures. It is suggested that anesthesiologists develop the habit of increasing the flow of oxygen first, when they increase total flow, and of decreasing the flow of oxygen last when they decrease total flow.

Breathing Circuit Pressure Monitoring

Monitoring pressures within the patient breathing circuit may confirm proper pressures, identify improper machine function, or indicate certain physiologic or physical problems with the patient or tracheal tube used to provide access to the patient's airway. Within the last 5 years it has become increasingly common to have graphic display of airway pressures depicting airway pressure waveforms with respect to time during positive pressure ventilation. Sufficiently detailed information about pressures within the patient breathing circuit can be obtained from graphic displays or from careful observation of the pressure gauge in the circuit. These data allow the anesthesiologist to recognize leaks, ventilator malfunctions, disconnection of either the patient or of components of the anesthetic apparatus, changes in the physiologic condition of the patient (e.g., bronchospasm), occlusion of tubing within the anesthetic system (including the tracheal tube and scavenging system), and a closed APL valve during spontaneous ventilation.

Positive Pressure

The fact that positive pressure has been developed within the patient's airway does not ensure that adequate ventilation has been achieved. Although adequacy of ventilation can be accurately assessed by measuring arterial CO_2 pressure (Pa_{CO_2}), measurement of end-tidal CO_2 and exhaled

Table 17–1. Variables Requiring Monitoring During Anesthesia

Pipeline pressure of all gases connected to the anesthesia machine
Pressure within the high-pressure section of the anesthesia machine
Flowmeter indication for each gas
Concentration of oxygen within the patient breathing circuit
Pressure and flow of gas within the patient breathing circuit (i.e., ventilation)
Concentration of anesthetic agents and other gases within the patient breathing circuit
Operation of the waste gas scavenging system

tidal or minute ventilation is practical and virtually continuous in clinical settings.

Electromechanical spirometers are readily available and have found widespread acceptance. The location of pressure- and flow-measuring apparatus within the patient breathing circuit is an important determinant of the information these devices can provide. Spirometers are usually placed in the expiratory limb of the circle absorbing system. In this position they measure the sum of the volume of gas exhaled by the patient plus the volume of fresh gas flowing through the spirometer during the interval of measurement. Pressure-measuring devices are typically located downstream from the exhalation unidirectional valve (between it and the inspiratory unidirectional valve). Conditions that cause a sustained elevation of pressure within the patient's airway and in the adjacent segment of the breathing circuit, such as a positive end-expiratory pressure (PEEP) valve, will not be indicated on the pressure gauge positioned in the usual location in the patient breathing circuit. The PEEP valve, positioned upstream from the expiratory unidirectional valve, in combination with a competent inspiratory unidirectional valve, serves to isolate the segment of the breathing circuit contiguous with the patient's airway from the pressure gauge.

Negative Pressure

Negative pressures within the patient breathing circuit are abnormal and should be investigated and corrected promptly. Some causes are low total gas flow in combination with too rapid descent of hanging bellows in older anesthesia ventilators, application of too great a suction to the gas scavenging system, or failure of the negative pressure relief valve of a closed scavenging system. This last effect may result in the removal of such large volumes of gas from the patient breathing circuit that the patient cannot be ventilated properly. Ventilators utilizing hanging (ascending during inspiration) bellows may create sufficient negative airway pressure during exhalation that patients having airways with poor elastic support suffer airway closure and interference with gas exchange. This situation is managed by admitting a fresh gas flow to the breathing circuit that exceeds the maximum rate of filling of the bellows during its descent or adjusting the ventilator to slow the rate of descent of the bellows. A major hazard of the hanging bellows arrangement is that, in the event of a disconnection of the patient or failure of the ventilator, the bellows continues to move normally and is more likely to escape notice than is a standing bellows ventilator.

Monitoring Respiratory Gases

The routine monitoring of respiratory gases (O_2, CO_2, N_2O, N_2, and volatile anesthetics) during the conduct of general anesthesia is widely employed in the United States. The American Society of Anesthesiologists' *Standard for Basic Anesthetic Monitoring* (effective July 1, 1999) (Fig. 17–4) calls for measurement of oxygen concentration in the patient breathing system (when an anesthesia machine is employed) and quantitative assessment of oxygenation such as by pulse oximetry during the conduct of all anesthetics. Assessment of ventilation by measurement of the volume of exhaled gas and monitoring for the presence of exhaled CO_2 is "strongly encouraged." The standard requires quantitative measurement of end-tidal CO_2 whenever the patient has a tracheal tube or laryngeal mask airway in place. It also specifies that ventilators shall be equipped with disconnect alarms.

When practicing modern anesthesia, the practitioner functions at the interface between the delivery system (the anesthesia machine) and the requirements and responses (physiology) of the patient. This is perhaps most evident when the composition of the gases in the breathing circuit is measured and the rate of change of their concentrations is tracked. The gases commonly measured in the patient breathing circuit are oxygen (O_2), N_2O, CO_2, and volatile anesthetic agents. For example, a patient with compromised myocardial contractility will manifest a more rapid rise of alveolar anesthetic agent concentration toward the inspired concentration than will a "normal" patient. A secondary consequence of myocardial compromise is further reduction of cardiac output due to the myocardial depressant effect of the anesthetic agent. The breath-to-breath measurement of anesthetic concentration in respiratory gases permits the anesthetist to adjust concentrations, so that higher-than-necessary concentrations are not administered, and to control the concentration of agents to that necessary to achieve an anesthetic state satisfactory for the procedure being performed.

Similarly, anesthetics alter the patient's respiratory status. A balance between CO_2 production and CO_2 removal through respiration determines end-tidal P_{CO_2}. If respiration remains constant, end-tidal P_{CO_2} will increase under conditions of increased CO_2 production such as fever or the addition of CO_2 as the insufflating gas during laparoscopy.

Measurement of end-tidal nitrogen can assist in understanding the extent to which a patient has been denitrogenated. Intraoperative increases in exhaled nitrogen provide evidence of air embolism or of a leak in the bellows of the Dräger AV-E anesthesia ventilator that is powered by a mixture of air and oxygen. Measurement of CO_2 in exhaled gas provides clear evidence of the state of ventilation of the patient so long as the delivery of CO_2 to the alveoli remains constant.[25, 26] Circulatory failure will result in reduced end-tidal CO_2 due to greatly diminished delivery of CO_2 to the lungs.

Because of substantial effects of sampling site on the concentration of different gases in different portions of the anesthetic circuit, it is important to understand expected concentrations in the patient breathing circuit and particularly the influences of uptake, ventilation, and fresh gas flow. End-tidal sampling of respiratory gases of small infants may require special attention because of their small tidal volume compared with the flow rate of sidestream gas analysis equipment and fresh gas flow.

Several practical devices to analyze the composition of respiratory gas in conjunction with anesthetic administration have been developed and used in clinical practice. These devices are based on

- IR spectroscopy
- Raman spectroscopy
- Mass spectroscopy
- Photoacoustic spectroscopy

Experience over the past 10 years has shown that practical devices to monitor respiratory gases should have the characteristics listed in Table 17–2.

Mass spectroscopy instruments were introduced into clinical practice in the early 1980s to measure respiratory gases during anesthesia. Instruments were available for single (one patient) OR use, as well as for utilizing time-shared, multiplexed sampling systems to conduct gas samples from several patients (ORs) to a single mass spectroscopy instrument. Mass spectroscopy instruments required a high vacuum for operation. They required constant upkeep to ensure multi-

STANDARDS FOR BASIC ANESTHETIC MONITORING

(Approved by House of Delegates on October 21, 1986 and last amended on October 21, 1998)

These standards apply to all anesthesia care although, in emergency circumstances, appropriate life support measures take precedence. These standards may be exceeded at any time based on the judgment of the responsible anesthesiologist. They are intended to encourage quality patient care, but observing them cannot guarantee any specific patient outcome. They are subject to revision from time to time, as warranted by the evolution of technology and practice. They apply to all general anesthetics, regional anesthetics and monitored anesthesia care. This set of standards addresses only the issue of basic anesthetic monitoring, which is one component of anesthesia care. In certain rare or unusual circumstances, 1) some of these methods of monitoring may be clinically impractical, and 2) appropriate use of the described monitoring methods may fail to detect untoward clinical developments. Brief interruptions of continual† monitoring may be unavoidable. *Under extenuating circumstances, the responsible anesthesiologist may waive the requirements marked with an asterisk (*); it is recommended that when this is done, it should be so stated (including the reasons) in a note in the patient's medical record.* These standards are not intended for application to the care of the obstetrical patient in labor or in the conduct of pain management.

STANDARD I

Qualified anesthesia personnel shall be present in the room throughout the conduct of all general anesthetics, regional anesthetics and monitored anesthesia care.

OBJECTIVE

Because of the rapid changes in patient status during anesthesia, qualified anesthesia personnel shall be continuously present to monitor the patient and provide anesthesia care. In the event there is a direct known hazard, e.g., radiation, to the anesthesia personnel which might require intermittent remote observation of the patient, some provision for monitoring the patient must be made. In the event that an emergency requires the temporary absence of the person primarily responsible for the anesthetic, the best judgment of the anesthesiologist will be exercised in comparing the emergency with the anesthetized patient's condition and in the selection of the person left responsible for the anesthetic during the temporary absence.

STANDARD II

During all anesthetics, the patient's oxygenation, ventilation, circulation and temperature shall be continually evaluated.

OXYGENATION

OBJECTIVE

To ensure adequate oxygen concentration in the inspired gas and the blood during all anesthetics.

METHODS

1) Inspired gas: During every administration of general anesthesia using an anesthesia machine, the concentration of oxygen in the patient breathing system shall be measured by an oxygen analyzer with a low oxygen concentration limit alarm in use.*

2) Blood oxygenation: During all anesthetics, a quantitative method of assessing oxygenation such as pulse oximetry shall be employed.* Adequate illumination and exposure of the patient are necessary to assess color.*

VENTILATION

OBJECTIVE

To ensure adequate ventilation of the patient during all anesthetics.

METHODS

1) Every patient receiving general anesthesia shall have the adequacy of ventilation continually evaluated. Qualitative clinical signs such as chest excursion, observation of the reservoir breathing bag and auscultation of breath sounds are useful. Continual monitoring for the presence of expired carbon dioxide shall be performed unless invalidated by the nature of the patient, procedure or equipment. Quantiative monitoring of the volume of expired gas is strongly encouraged.*

2) When an endotracheal tube or laryngeal mask is inserted, its correct positioning must be verified by clinical assessment and by identification of carbon dioxide in the expired gas. Continual end-tidal carbon dioxide analysis, in use from the time of endotracheal tube/laryngeal mask placement, until extubation/removal or initiating transfer to a postoperative care location, shall be performed using a quantiative method such as capnography, capnometry or mass spectroscopy.*

3) When ventilation is controlled by a mechanical ventilator, there shall be in continuous use a device that is capable of detecting disconnection of components of the breathing system. The device must give an audible signal when its alarm threshold is exceeded.

4) During regional anesthesia and monitored anesthesia care, the adequacy of ventilation shall be evaluated, at least, by continual observation of qualitative clinical signs.

CIRCULATION

OBJECTIVE

To ensure the adequacy of the patient's circulatory function during all anesthetics.

METHODS

1) Every patient receiving anesthesia shall have the electrocardiogram continuously displayed from the beginning of anesthesia until preparing to leave the anesthetizing location.*

2) Every patient receiving anesthesia shall have arterial blood pressure and heart rate determined and evaluated at least every five minutes.*

3) Every patient receiving general anesthesia shall have, in addition to the above, circulatory function continually evaluated by at least one of the following: palpation of a pulse, auscultation of heart sounds, monitoring of a tracing of intraarterial pressure, ultrasound peripheral pulse monitoring, or pulse plethysmography or oximetry.

BODY TEMPERATURE

OBJECTIVE

To aid in the maintenance of appropriate body temperature during all anesthetics.

METHODS

Every patient receiving anesthesia shall have temperature monitored when clinically significant changes in body temperature are intended, anticipated or suspected.

---

† Note that "continual" is defined as "repeated regularly and frequently in steady rapid succession" where "continuous" means "prolonged without any interruption at any time."

To become effective July 1, 1999

Figure 17-4. *Standard for Basic Anesthetic Monitoring.* Approved by ASA House of Delegates on October 21, 1986, and last amended on October 21, 1998.

Table 17–2. Characteristics of Anesthetic Respiratory Gas Monitors

Ease of use, setup
Simultaneous, accurate, real-time measurement of physiologically important gases in the anesthetic system:
O_2
CO_2
N_2O
N_2
Volatile (halogenated) anesthetic agents
Breath-to-breath measurement of gas concentrations
Display of waveforms of gas concentration vs. time
Readout of inspired and end-tidal gas concentrations

plex sampling system reliability, to maintain the very high vacuum in the detector, and to prevent or correct detector contamination. These instruments are no longer being produced commercially for applications in anesthesia, although some remain in service. Ehrenwerth and Eisenkraft[3] provide a detailed description of clinical mass spectroscopy. Of the techniques employed to analyze respiratory gases during anesthesia, mass and Raman spectroscopic analyses are widely used in the United States.

The instruments currently commercially available for clinical application to respiratory gas analysis are principally IR and Raman spectroscopic instruments. Raman spectroscopic instruments are able to detect and measure oxygen using Raman spectroscopy, while IR spectrometers incorporate any of several techniques of oxygen analysis. Raman spectroscopy measures nitrogen directly.

Oxygen cannot be detected using IR spectroscopy but can be detected by oxygen-specific analyzers such as fuel cell or polarographic electrode devices. Ohmeda respiratory gas monitors use slow-responding oxygen-sensing electrodes through which the gas stream is gated by a valve slaved to respond to the presence or absence of CO_2. The flow of gas is permitted to continue only while CO_2 is present (exhaled gas) over a period of several breaths. The measured value for oxygen thus obtained is the concentration of oxygen in exhaled gas. The scheme is then reversed by sampling only while CO_2 in the gas stream is low or zero. Oxygen measured in this way corresponds to the inspired concentration of oxygen.

The breath-to-breath analysis of respiratory gases for oxygen is technically demanding due to the long response time of polarographic and fuel cell oxygen detectors. A paramagnetic oxygen sensor with rapid response has been developed. It exploits the paramagnetic property of O_2 molecules. In this device the sample gas stream and a reference stream of air (thus maintaining a constant oxygen concentration in the reference gas stream) are admitted to opposite sides of the diaphragm of a sensitive differential transducer. Downstream from the pressure transducer, both gas streams pass through an electromagnetic field that has a rapidly reversing polarity. The pressure in the gas streams increases in proportion to the oxygen concentration because of increased resistance to flow resulting from the interaction of paramagnetic O_2 with the magnetic field. The resulting pressure difference is proportional to the oxygen concentration in the sample stream and is converted electronically to display oxygen concentration or partial pressure.

Infrared Spectroscopy

IR spectroscopy analyzes concentration of CO_2, N_2O, and the volatile anesthetic agents. These instruments take advantage of the fact that these gases absorb IR energy in proportion to the concentration of the gas present in the measurement cell. The optical bench consists of an IR source producing a beam of IR illumination of specific wavelengths directed through a cuvette or measurement cell. The intensity of the IR light exiting the cell is compared with a reference beam from the same source but not passing through the gas sample cell. The phenomenon of IR absorption by CO_2, N_2O, and the volatile anesthetic agents follows the Beer-Lambert law, which states that the concentration (C) of the gas being analyzed is proportional to the negative logarithm of 1 minus the fraction of the incident light absorbed (A_a):

$$C = \frac{-\ln(1 - A_a)}{aD}$$

and inversely proportional to the product of D is the length of the light path within the measurement cell and a is the absorption coefficient for the particular gas being measured.

To better understand the basic construction of modern IR gas analyzers, some characteristics of IR spectra need to be considered. Light of a specific wavelength is obtained by passing light from a source (resistive lamp) through filters on a rotating wheel arranged to sequentially pass only specific wavelengths to illuminate the gas sample cuvette. The wavelengths chosen are those which are strongly absorbed by the gas(es) being assayed. For CO_2 the chosen wavelength is 4.3 μm. For N_2O, there are two absorption peaks, at 3.9 μm and 4.5 μm. The absorption peaks for these two gases are sharp enough and sufficiently different in wavelength that they may be identified by the characteristic wavelength at which IR absorption occurs. On the other hand, the volatile anesthetic agents all have absorption peaks at approximately 3.3 μm that cannot be distinguished from each other. In addition, they demonstrate absorption peaks in the range between 9 and 12 μm, which are sufficiently distinct to permit identification of the agent in use. By using the longer wavelength to identify the agent and the shorter wavelength to quantitate the volatile agent, IR instruments such as the Ohmeda 5250-RGM are able to identify and measure the concentration of the volatile agents. Such instruments represent a considerable improvement over instruments that require the operator to tell the machine which agent to measure. Currently available (2000) IR gas monitors do not simultaneously identify multiple volatile anesthetic agents.

A source of error for which compensation must be provided is "collision broadening." This phenomenon results from interaction between gas molecules in mixtures of gases. For example, the measured concentration of CO_2 or N_2O will be systematically increased or decreased by as much as 10% of the actual concentration when both are present or in the presence of high concentrations of oxygen. A number of IR gas analyzers of recent design measure the interfering gas and apply required corrections automatically.

Raman Spectroscopy

Raman spectroscopy is another analytic technique that has been adapted for use in clinical anesthesia. These devices draw a gas sample continuously into a measurement cell arranged so that a beam of monochromatic light traverses the cell. The light source is a helium-neon (He-Ne) laser. The characteristic of the sample gas exploited by this technique is that molecules which interact with the incident beam absorb photons and subsequently re-emit a small fraction ($\sim 10^{-6}$) of the absorbed photons at angles to the incident beam with the wavelength shifted to a lower (less energetic) wavelength. The wavelength shift is characteristic of the gas being illuminated (analyzed), and the intensity of the emitted light is proportional to the concentration of the gas being analyzed. In practice, the detectors are located at right angles to the axis of the incident beam.

The current example of a Raman instrument is the Rascal II, a product of Ohmeda. The original Rascal instrument developed by Albion, Inc. required considerable maintenance. It had high power requirements. Its laser measurement cell unit (or "resonator") was prone to contamination and required frequent service or replacement. The Rascal II has much lower power requirements owing to an improved laser. Its gas sampling system and sample cell have been redesigned to be much less subject to contamination. Individual instruments can be fitted to analyze up to four volatile agents, and these can be selected from all of the currently available agents. In addition, the Rascal II uses the Raman technique to analyze O_2, N_2, N_2O, and CO_2.

Rascal II instruments are designed to measure mixtures of the volatile anesthetic agents simultaneously. Because of the very low level of scattered light being detected, this instrument requires that the gas-measuring cell remain free from contamination and have a system of drying and filtering through which the sampled gas passes en route to the measurement cell. Temperature compensation of the laser, measurement cells, and detectors is provided to control the effects of temperature on the optical geometry of the detector. The pressure within the measurement cell is tightly compensated to improve the accuracy of measurement and to minimize the effect of variations in ambient pressure, pumping pressure fluctuations, and sampling tube resistance. In order to control the total resistance in the gas sampling system, the manufacturer specifies the internal diameter and length of the sampling tubing. Changes—especially unrecognized changes—in the characteristics of the sampling tubing will affect the resistance of the sampling system and the overall operation of the instrument, leading to a need for frequent, open-case recalibrations. To minimize this problem, sample-tubing supplies should be standardized.

Clinical Capnography

A graph of the partial pressure (or concentration) of CO_2 in exhaled gas plotted over time is referred to as a capnogram. Instruments providing such graphic displays of CO_2 in exhaled gas in real time are called capnographs and the technique used to measure CO_2 in this way is called capnography. Instruments displaying only numerical end-tidal P_{CO_2} (PETCO$_2$) values are called capnometers and the technique is referred to as capnometry. The shape of the capnogram reveals much about the integrity of the breathing circuit and physiology of the patient's cardiorespiratory system.[27] For monitoring during clinical anesthesia, capnography is preferred over capnometry. (See also Chapter 16.)

The Normal Capnogram

The characteristic features of a normal capnogram are shown in Figure 17-5. At the end of normal inhalation, the CO_2 tension in perfused alveoli is in equilibrium with and equal to that in end-capillary blood, while a small volume of gas in unperfused alveoli is in equilibrium with inspired gas, assumed to be zero. The gas filling the airways down to a point proximal to the alveoli contains no CO_2 (inspired gas). At the start of exhalation (point A) the airway gas sampled is the CO_2-free anatomic dead space, so the measured CO_2

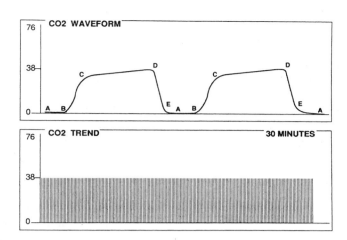

Figure 17-5. A normal capnogram is shown in the top panel. Exhalation begins at point A. Segment A-B represents tracheal dead space. Segment C is the early rise in CO_2 concentration as alveolar gas makes its way to the airway. Segment C is the alveolar plateau. Point D, the maximum CO_2 value in the capnogram, is the end-tidal value of CO_2. Inhalation of CO_2 free gas begins immediately after point D and continues to point E. Shown on the bottom panel is the trend display.

remains zero. As exhalation continues (segment A-B), CO_2-containing gas from the respiratory tree enters the trachea and displaces dead-space gas. CO_2 arrives at the airway and first appears on the capnogram at point B, from where it increases. In a normal capnogram, the increase in CO_2 is a sharp, smooth upstroke (segment B-C). Then, the minimally changing CO_2 concentration produces a nearly horizontal alveolar plateau (segment C-D), the terminal portion of which reveals the concentration of CO_2 in end-tidal exhaled gas (point D). Near the end of the exhalation when the expiratory flow rate approaches zero, the end-tidal CO_2 measured approaches the ventilation-weighted average of ventilated lung units. The highest value is end-tidal CO_2 (point D). End-tidal CO_2 approximates alveolar CO_2, which in turn approximates Pa_{CO_2} (neglecting gas exhaled from nonperfused alveoli which reduces the CO_2 concentration measured in exhaled gas relative to the Pa_{CO_2}).[28] At the next inhalation, airway CO_2 again decreases toward zero (point E). Unless there is CO_2 in inspired gas, the capnogram trace passes point A, indicating an inspired CO_2 concentration of zero.

Capnogram Display

The capnogram may be displayed as a "normal" trace (with a time base in the range of 2 to 3 cm/second), as a low-speed trace (time base ~1 to 2 cm/second), or as a trend display (time base < 0.1 cm/second). Some monitors show two or more traces simultaneously. Low-speed wave and trend displays obscure details of individual breaths but highlight evolving events. Normally, each breath should rise to the same end-tidal value and fall to the zero baseline. Alterations of trend and changes in fine detail of the capnogram wave indicate abnormal patient physiology or a malfunctioning gas delivery system.

Differential Diagnosis of Abnormal Capnograms

Because the essence of pulmonary ventilation and gas exchange is elimination of CO_2 from the lung, the capnogram is the most reliable and effective monitor to determine the

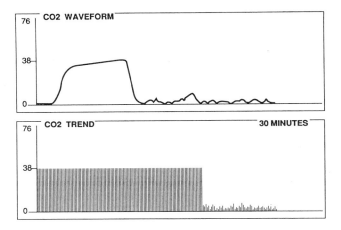

Figure 17–6. Sudden decrease of PETCO₂ to near-zero values. The trend display demonstrates the sudden occurrence of low PETCO₂ values after a period of normal PETCO₂. The real-time capnogram is disrupted, showing the lack of proper sampling of CO_2 in the airway. Critical events that may present with this pattern include esophageal intubation, complete airway disconnection, ventilator malfunction, or a totally obstructed airway.

presence of pulmonary ventilation and gas exchange. The integrity and function of both the patient's cardiorespiratory system and the breathing circuit are all reflected in the capnogram,[28, 29] and malfunctions often can be detected by changes in it.[28] The following brief discussions focus on major categories of capnographic abnormalities.

Decrease in Partial Pressure of End-Tidal Carbon Dioxide

Sudden Decrease to Near-Zero Concentration

A sudden drop of end-tidal CO_2 (Fig. 17–6) to zero or near zero usually heralds imminent disaster. The possibility of capnograph malfunction must be considered but never assumed. Critical events that may present this way include esophageal intubation,[30] complete airway disconnection, ventilator failure, and a totally obstructed endotracheal tube.[31] Each of these events results in the sudden disappearance of CO_2 at the patient's airway, and nothing in the capnogram distinguishes one event from another. Only after auscultation of the chest and verification of pulmonary ventilation should the possibility of monitor malfunction be entertained. Even patient color and oxygen saturation may remain acceptable for quite some time after the cessation of adequate ventilation. Once a failure of ventilation has been ruled out as the source of the flat capnogram, monitor malfunction and sampling system blockage can be considered. Because potentially fatal airway disasters may occur at any time without warning, continuous capnography during general anesthesia is recommended to greatly improve early detection of problems and help one avoid catastrophic events.

Sudden Decrease to Low but Non-Zero Concentration

Figure 17–7 demonstrates a fall in PETCO₂ (point D in Fig. 17–5) to values approaching but not reaching zero, indicating that a full exhalation is no longer being detected at the airway. Exhaled gas may be escaping through a poorly fitting mask. If an endotracheal tube is in place, a loose-fitting tra-

cheal tube (i.e., a leaking or defective endotracheal tube cuff) should be considered. Mainstream capnography systems may produce a similar capnogram if the transducer is partially displaced.

Examination of airway pressure may be helpful in diagnosing the cause of such sudden drops in PETCO₂. If the airway pressure is low during mechanical ventilation, there is probably a leak somewhere in the delivery system. If the airway pressure is high during mechanical ventilation, there is probably a partial obstruction of the endotracheal tube resulting in lower tidal volume being delivered to the patient, high airway pressure in the circuit, and obstruction to full exhalation of alveolar gas. In this instance, the drop in PETCO₂ occurs because the exhalation is not completed before the next mechanical breath begins.

Exponential Decrease

An exponential drop in PETCO₂ that occurs within a short time (e.g., a dozen breaths) almost always signals a sudden catastrophic event in the patient's cardiorespiratory system (Fig. 17–8). The physiologic basis for this capnogram is an increase in physiologic dead-space ventilation or a decrease in CO_2 returning from tissues to the lungs. Possible causative events include hypotension from blood loss, vena caval compression, circulatory arrest, and pulmonary arterial occlusion by thrombus or air embolism. Immediate diagnosis and treatment are required for all of these conditions. Air embolism is likely whenever the surgical site or an open intravenous site is at a negative pressure relative to venous pressure.

The most common noncatastrophic cause of rapid exponential decrease in PETCO₂ is an increase in ventilation caused by ventilator or fresh gas flow adjustment. However, this benign diagnosis should be entertained only after catastrophic events have been ruled out.

Sustained Low Concentrations

Without Good Plateaus. Occasionally, with no apparent abnormality in the breathing circuit or the patient's cardiorespiratory status, the capnogram shows sustained low PETCO₂ values without a good alveolar plateau (Fig. 17–9).

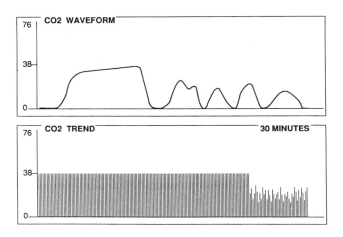

Figure 17–7. Sudden decrease of PETCO₂ to low, non-zero values. Full exhalation is no longer being detected by the capnograph. A leak in the airway system or poorly fitting anesthesia mask may be the culprit. Note the disappearance of the alveolar plateau on the real-time capnogram and the irregular, non-zero value of PETCO₂ on the trend display.

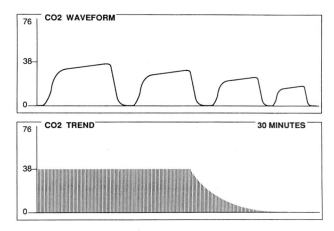

Figure 17–8. Exponential decrease of $PETCO_2$. This pattern almost always signals a sudden and potentially catastrophic loss of pulmonary perfusion in the patient, such as that caused by cardiorespiratory arrest, severe pulmonary hypoperfusion, or pulmonary embolism. Note the normal shape of the capnogram in real time but the exponential decay of the $PETCO_2$ on the trend display.

The absence of a good alveolar plateau suggests incomplete lung emptying before the next inspiration, or that exhaled gas is diluted with fresh gas during exhalation. The latter can occur with small tidal volumes and a high gas sample rate. Several maneuvers are available to differentiate these possibilities.

Incomplete lung emptying may be suggested by adventitial sounds (e.g., wheezing or rhonchi showing small airway obstruction from bronchospasm or secretions). If rhonchi are present, tracheal suctioning often corrects the partial obstruction and restores full exhalation and the CO_2 waveform. Bronchospasm may be treated with bronchodilators, anticholinergics, or halogenated anesthetic vapors. Expiratory obstruction may be caused by a tube kink or obstruction from many other causes, including a tracheal tube cuff herniating into the tube lumen. Passing a suction catheter down the tracheal tube usually confirms or eliminates this possibility.

After partial airway obstruction is eliminated as a cause, excess airway sampling must be considered. Most clinical devices that measure end-tidal CO_2 operate at sample flow rates of 150 to 200 mL/minute. When small tidal volumes and large sampling flow rates are employed, sampling during the low- or no-flow condition at the end of exhalation entrains gas from the inspiratory limb of the breathing circuit, resulting in artifactual dilution of CO_2 concentration available to the sampling line near the end of the expiratory plateau. In small newborns, sample rates of 50 mL/minute or less may not eliminate this artifact. Sampling near the carina using a small catheter within the lumen of the endotracheal tube or using specially constructed endotracheal tubes having a dedicated sampling channel have been used to improve sampling fidelity.

With Good Plateaus. In some circumstances of apparently normal ventilation, the capnogram will demonstrate a low $PETCO_2$ with brisk rise and fall of the capnographic wave and a fairly flat alveolar plateau (Fig. 17–10). There may be a large discrepancy between end-tidal CO_2 and $PaCO_2$, which may indicate capnograph malfunction or miscalibration. It is most often associated with a large physiologic dead space in the patient. The anesthetist may check capnograph accuracy by breathing into the gas sampler and

ensuring that the reading is between 34 and 46 mmHg. Many conditions are associated with a large arterial-to-end-tidal CO_2 gradient. Indeed, anesthesia itself tends to increase this gradient to an average of 4 mmHg.[32] Pulmonary disease, pneumonia, and bronchopulmonary dysplasia in children can increase the arterial-to-alveolar CO_2 gradient. Pulmonary artery hypoperfusion from hypovolemia and high airway pressures (e.g., sitting neurosurgical procedures with dehydration, vasodilators, and hyperventilation) commonly result in wide $PaCO_2$ to $PETCO_2$ gradients.

Gradually Decreasing Concentration

When the capnogram retains its normal morphology but $PETCO_2$ (Fig. 17–11) falls slowly over minutes or hours, possible causes include falling body temperature, relative hyperventilation, or decreasing systemic or pulmonary perfusion.

As body temperature falls, so does metabolism and CO_2 production. If ventilation is not decreased, alveolar and arterial PCO_2 will fall. A gradual fall in $PETCO_2$ can result from growing physiologic dead space and from decreased CO_2 return from tissues arising from insufficient cardiac output secondary to myocardial depression or hypovolemia.

If ventilation is increased by ventilator or fresh gas flow adjustment, $PETCO_2$ will gradually fall toward a new equilibrium value. This common clinical occurrence is especially obvious when increased minute ventilation is temporally correlated with the end-tidal CO_2 trend.

Increase in Partial Pressure of End-Tidal Carbon Dioxide

Gradual Increase in Concentration

A rise in $PETCO_2$, with unchanged capnogram morphology (Fig. 17–12), may be associated with decreased minute ventilation, increased CO_2 production, or absorption of insufflating CO_2 during laparoscopy.[33]

Minute ventilation decreases from partial airway obstruction, small leaks in the ventilator,[34] or a change in ventilator or fresh gas flow settings. CO_2 production increases with hyperthermia of any cause, including excessive heating, sepsis, or malignant hyperthermia. When end-tidal CO_2 rises

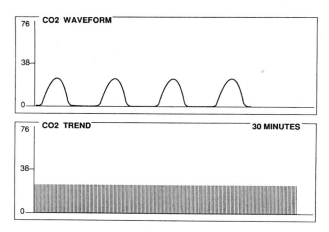

Figure 17–9. Sustained low $PETCO_2$ without good plateaus. When this pattern exists on the capnogram, the $PETCO_2$ does not represent a good estimate of alveolar CO_2 concentration. Often, a gentle squeeze on the breathing bag will produce a full exhalation and the resulting "ventilated $PETCO_2$" may be used as an estimate of $PaCO_2$.

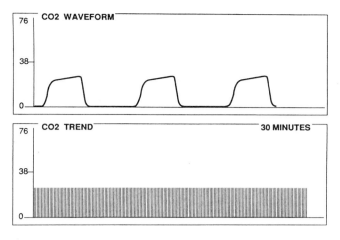

Figure 17–10. Sustained low PETCO$_2$ with good alveolar plateaus. This pattern suggests hyperventilation. Other possibilities include a wide arterial-alveolar CO$_2$ gradient in the patient due to excessive physiologic dead-space ventilation. The only way to differentiate these two possibilities is to measure the PaCO$_2$.

rapidly despite steady-state ventilation, malignant hyperthermia must be considered immediately.[35, 36]

CO$_2$ absorption from exogenous sources, such as insufflating CO$_2$ during laparoscopy,[33] may mimic increased endogenous CO$_2$ production, causing end-tidal CO$_2$ to rise slowly.

Sudden Increase in Concentration

Sudden, transient increases in PETCO$_2$ may be caused by any factor that acutely increases the amount of CO$_2$ reaching the pulmonary circulation. Common causes include intravenous bicarbonate injection, release of a surgical limb tourniquet, or release of an aortic cross-clamp.

Sudden Increase in Both the Capnogram Baseline and End-Tidal Carbon Dioxide Tension

A sudden rise in the baseline of the capnogram with an approximately equal rise in PETCO$_2$ value usually indicates some contamination in the sample cell (in the instrument or in the airway, depending on the system employed), usually with water, mucus, or dirt. Cleaning the sample cell or replacing the sample inlet filter may restore proper performance.

Gradual Increase in Both the Capnogram Baseline and End-Tidal Carbon Dioxide Tension

A gradual rise in both baseline and PETCO$_2$ values indicates that previously exhaled CO$_2$ is being rebreathed from the circuit (Fig. 17–13). In this situation, the inspiratory portion of the capnogram fails to reach the zero baseline, and there may actually be a premature rise in CO$_2$ concentration during the inspiratory phase of ventilation. This rise precedes the characteristic sharp upstroke associated with exhalation. The PETCO$_2$ value usually increases until a new equilibrium alveolar CO$_2$ tension (PaCO$_2$) is reached, at which time elimination once again equals production.

Some anesthesia circuits, such as the Mapleson D and the Jackson-Rees circuits commonly used in pediatric anesthesia, are partial rebreathing circuits by design.[37, 38] The user of these circuits should be aware of the characteristic capnogram resulting from their use. The exact amount of rebreath-

ing depends on complex interactions between exhaled tidal volume, volume of sidestream sampling for gas analysis, fresh gas flow, expiratory reservoir volume, APL valve setting, APL valve location, and the expiratory pause time.[37] When using partial rebreathing circuits, these complex interactions make exact prediction of PETCO$_2$ and PaCO$_2$ difficult or impossible. If there is a good alveolar plateau on the capnogram, the PETCO$_2$ value provides a good estimate of PaCO$_2$. Arterial CO$_2$ is then related to alveolar CO$_2$ in the usual manner, being higher by an amount that depends upon physiologic dead space. Undesired rebreathing in a partial rebreathing circuit can be reduced by increasing fresh gas flow, using larger tidal volumes, and allowing more time for exhalation.

Non-zero inspiratory CO$_2$ in a circle system invariably indicates a circuit malfunction. The most common causes are faulty valves (allowing bidirectional gas flow), a CO$_2$ absorber bypass circuit enabled, or exhausted CO$_2$ absorbent. Visual inspection of the CO$_2$ canister, valves, and bypass switch (if present) usually identifies these conditions. Occasionally the chemical indicator in soda lime fails to reindicate depletion after the soda lime stands overnight.[39] Therefore it is good practice to observe the CO$_2$ absorbent for color change after a period of use (such as in the afternoon) rather than after a period of non-use (such as in the early morning).

Corporate Events Affecting Gas Monitoring Equipment

The development of respiratory gas monitoring equipment has been the result of the development of different technologies by different companies. There is presently (i.e., late 1999) considerable consolidation occurring in the industry. The following is provided to help the reader appreciate the role commerce has in influencing the supply of highly technical equipment. Undoubtedly there will be further changes in both the suppliers of our equipment and in the development of even more robust monitors. The original Rascal instrument was developed by Albion. The trademarks and rights to the technology were bought by Ohmeda, a division of BOC Group, Inc. in the late 1980s. Extensive improvement in the instrument resulted in the Rascal II as marketed by Ohmeda. Ohmeda has refined the development of IR gas analysis for capnography and anesthetic agent analysis (in-

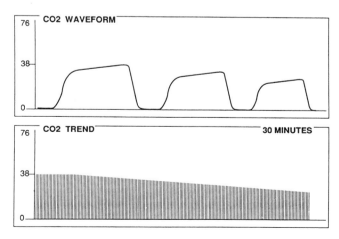

Figure 17–11. Gradually decreasing PETCO$_2$. Possible causes include hyperventilation, a falling body temperature, or slowly decreasing cardiac output.

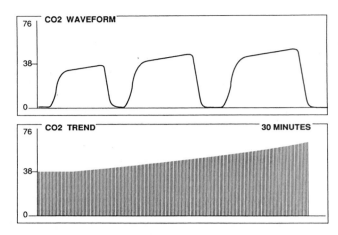

Figure 17–12. Gradually increasing PETCO$_2$. This may be associated with a partial airway obstruction, a rising body temperature, or hypoventilation due to a partial leak in the breathing circuit. If the rise is rapid, malignant hyperthermia should be considered.

cluding N$_2$O). In the 1980s, in Europe, the Finnish company Datex-Engstrom, a division of Instrumentarium Corporation, was developing and marketing instruments for respiratory gas and physiologic monitoring. Datex had developed the rapidly responding paramagnetic oxygen analyzer. In April 1998, Instrumentarium completed acquisition of Ohmeda Medical Systems from BOC Group to form Datex-Ohmeda. The new company will be well positioned to further refine and market IR gas analysis equipment. Since the formation of Datex-Ohmeda, the Rascal II has been out of production, although its maintenance is still supported. Hewlett-Packard is another U.S. manufacturer of respiratory gas analysis equipment.

Hazards of Respiratory Gas Monitoring

Respiratory gas monitoring has become increasingly common in anesthesia practice. Although this monitoring modality is noninvasive, it is not without hazards. Additional fittings and devices in the breathing circuit can be sources of disconnection, leak, or obstruction.[40] Sampled gas must be disposed of safely. If sampled gas is returned to the breathing circuit, the danger of infectious contamination must be considered. If sampled gas is not returned to the breathing circuit, its loss has further ramifications. In low-flow anesthesia, circuit gas composition becomes difficult to predict (but, of course, it is measured).[41] Also, circuit volume may decrease, eventually resulting in negative airway pressure[42] leading to the potential for reduction or failure of ventilation. This reduction in ventilation is a particular concern in the anesthetic care of infants and small children who may have minute ventilation which is less than the minute volume of gas removed from the breathing circuit by sidestream respiratory gas analyzers. Negative airway pressure has occurred during cardiopulmonary bypass[42] when fresh gas flow to the anesthetic circuit has been reduced.

Some respiratory gas monitoring systems discontinue sampling when in standby mode, while others merely discontinue analysis while continuing to remove gas from the breathing circuit. As with any monitored variable, incorrect data or misinterpretation[40] can lead to incorrect treatment and potential patient harm.

Gaba et al.[13] presented a useful framework for developing a conceptual understanding of the manner in which anesthetic accidents evolve (see Chapter 3). They described the important elements leading to anesthetic mishaps in terms of the complexity of the interactions between "equipment, the anesthesiologist and the patient" and the tightness of the coupling between the various elements of a complex system. They further described a view in which simple incidents might interact and propagate within a complex system to develop into critical events or, when combined with a "substantive negative outcome," produce events that are generally recognized as accidents. Suggested strategies for recovery from such situations are the following steps:

1. Recognition and verification of a developing incident
2. Determining the extent of the threat
3. Supporting life-sustaining functions
4. Application of initial diagnostic and corrective action(s)
5. Follow-up with specific diagnoses and treatments
6. Adequate follow-up to ensure continued correction throughout recovery

Innovative Approaches to Anesthetic Machine Design

With respect to the degree of sophistication of the monitoring of functions of anesthesia machines, development of anesthesia machines is proceeding rapidly. Today, anesthesia machines are being produced by only two domestic manufacturers: Ohmeda and Dräger. The ongoing evolution of integration of the monitoring of machine functions and patient physiologic variables is clearly apparent. Integrated monitoring is designed so that turning on the machine master switch initiates monitoring of machine functions, and one cannot use the machine without the monitoring apparatus functioning, human "ingenuity" notwithstanding! For example, modern anesthesia machines have a backup battery powering the machine monitoring functions. In the event the machine is not connected to the 120 V alternating current electrical service, and battery power is used to power the monitoring functions, an advisory warning is provided to

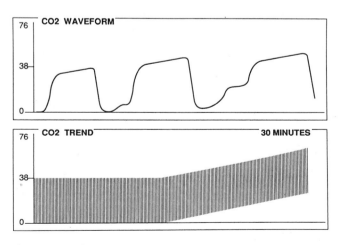

Figure 17–13. Gradual increase in both the baseline and end-tidal CO$_2$ concentration. This pattern demonstrates that previously exhaled CO$_2$ is being rebreathed from the breathing circuit. The inspired minimum fails to reach the zero baseline and the PETCO$_2$ steadily rises.

inform the operator of the limited power available from the battery.

Another direction apparent in the development of anesthesia machines is the implementation of hardware designed so that it is not possible to administer gas mixtures containing less than 25% to 30% oxygen. Both manufacturers now provide machines that prevent the administration of less than 25% to 30% oxygen.

Considerable attention is now being devoted to the manner in which the monitored information is displayed. As noted earlier, the anesthesiologist who is faced with nearly simultaneous multiple alarms can become overloaded with data—some data appearing to conflict to the point that effective responses to the alarms are seriously degraded. Alarms may be assigned priorities so the anesthesiologist has an opportunity to rapidly assess and plan a response to monitor-generated messages. Schreiber and Schreiber[6] described a scheme in which all possible alarm conditions are prioritized into a three-level classification:

1. Warning: requires immediate operator response

2. Caution: requires prompt operator response

3. Advisory: requires operator awareness that a condition exists

The Schreibers provided a detailed description of the display of such prioritized alarms in the form of audible, visual, and printed, or cathode ray tube–T–displayed messages, including the suppression of lower-priority audible alarms until the higher-priority alarm conditions are corrected. This type of prioritized alarm indication is available on Dräger and Ohmeda anesthesia machines. Alarms with prioritized indications are called for in the ASTM standard F 1161-88 where they are designated as:

Category I—high priority
Category II—medium priority
Category III—low priority

It may soon be the norm to have monitored variables that fall outside of predetermined limits displayed in a central location on the anesthesia machine. Suggested courses of action might also be presented. The integration of the information resulting from the monitoring of anesthesia machine functions with information resulting from physiologic monitoring of the patient will undoubtedly receive much attention.

In 1978, Cooper et al.[43] reported the development of a demonstration anesthesia system, which incorporated new applications of electronic control of mechanical and pneumatic functions. They used electronically controlled digital valves to adjust the flow of gases and an electronically controlled injector for control of the amount of volatile anesthetic added to the gas mixture in this innovatively designed anesthesia machine. For a variety of reasons, some of which were identified in their report, as well as high costs related to product liability, development, and proof of concept costs by potential manufacturers, the concepts used in the design of this apparatus have not been incorporated into the design of even the newest anesthesia machines. Additional sophisticated prototypes[44, 45] have demonstrated further refinement of computer control and display of "standard" anesthesia machine functions and monitoring variables.

Loeb et al.[44] developed and described the Utah Anesthesia Workstation. This device is a standard anesthesia machine enhanced with computer-driven display, control, and monitoring of gas flows and pressures, as well as display, control,

and monitoring of ventilation. The workstation control function can be operated in any of three modes. It can function as a conventional "manual" anesthesia machine, in an "electronic control" mode, or in an "autopilot" mode. In the electronic control mode the anesthesiologist selects the *flows* for oxygen, N_2O, and anesthetic vapor. In the autopilot mode the anesthesiologist selects the *concentration* desired and the computer calculates and sets the flows necessary to achieve them. The workstation provides elaborate monitoring of the progress of the anesthetic, displays pressures, flows, and CO_2 concentration on a breath-by-breath basis and has been demonstrated to detect common and uncommon problems with the anesthetics being conducted.

Standards and Guidelines

The ASTM, the International Standards Organization (ISO), and the European Committee for Standardization (CEN) are each working toward standards for anesthesia workstations. This process is, conceptually, a much more complex undertaking than are the existing standards for anesthesia machines and other individual anesthesia devices and items of equipment. It will involve standardized specification of most mechanical and pneumatic components presently included on anesthesia machines as well as ventilators, vaporizers, and scavenging devices. In addition to specifying the manner in which these components will be monitored, the developing standards must describe schemes for integrating the information obtained into sophisticated alarm and warning systems. The need to specify detailed data protocols for routing anesthesia data, along with physiologic data, for display, analysis, and record-keeping, are all issues to be resolved by these ambitious efforts.

The continuing evolution of anesthesia machines is confirmed by the ongoing development of new standards to describe their construction (see above). The role of standards and guidelines in shaping the way anesthesia machines and related devices are used should be understood by those who use and who are involved in the acquisition of these devices.

Organizations

A number of organizations have written standards concerning various aspects related to the construction and use of anesthesia machines and of apparatuses that support the conduct of anesthetic practice. Standards characteristically represent the combined efforts of several groups (e.g., manufacturers, users, distributors, and regulators) concerned with a particular issue. As such, published standards represent consensus documents agreed to and developed by the conferees that admittedly have differing, even competing, interests. While standards may seem flawed from some perspectives, they are pragmatic instruments developed by knowledgeable people and are useful in the everyday world of commerce and practice.

Standards do not, by themselves, have the force of law. They may be adopted voluntarily or, in other instances, be given the force of law by state or local codes or laws. For example, the National Fire Protection Association (NFPA) documents are often cited by building codes and therefore compliance with NFPA standards becomes mandatory before a building can be certified to meet the requirements of the state or local building code.

In general, whether mandated by law or not, compliance with published standards by practitioners and institutions ensures adherence to good practice as agreed upon by those intimately familiar with the field. In most instances standards undergo periodic review and revision. Most institutions will need to plan for compliance with revisions of standards from time to time. This can be accomplished most easily if they stay abreast of trends in the field and develop practical plans for compliance with evolving standards. The responsibility for decision making in institutional policy, risk management, and purchasing will reside with informed anesthesia clinicians, administrators, risk managers, and biomedical engineers.

Compressed Gas Association

The Compressed Gas Association (CGA) is a voluntary organization of the manufacturers of compressed gases and products related to the use of compressed gases. This group has published standards describing the color-coding of compressed gas cylinders, safety connecting systems (DISS, thread index safety system) to prevent the accidental cross-connection of gas cylinders and piping systems, the construction of cylinders for service as high-pressure gas storage vessels, and the pin index safety system to prevent the connection of improper gas cylinders to yokes intended for specific gases. Some of the CGA standards provide examples of very specific methodologies to be used; for example, the descriptions of safety systems for interconnection of gas vessels and piping systems describe the fittings in such detail that different manufacturers are able to produce connectors that are compatible and interchangeable.

National Fire Protection Association

The NFPA has prepared standards that are widely applicable to building design and construction, including, but not limited to, healthcare facilities. In the course of its work, the NFPA has written standards dealing with electrical safety, the handling of medical gases, and medical gas piping systems that are the most widely recognized standards applied to healthcare facilities. While these standards do not relate directly to anesthesia machines, understanding the underlying principles is of vital importance to those who provide anesthesia care.

American Society for Testing and Materials

The ASTM assembles knowledgeable committees to define and publish standards to permit the interchange of information and ideas between groups having interests in a wide variety of technical disciplines. Since 1983 the work of the ASTM relating to anesthesia equipment and machines has been assigned to the ASTM F29 committee. This committee has published a standard for performance and safety for components and systems of anesthesia gas machines.[17]

Other Organizations

The U.S. Department of Transportation has developed detailed regulations governing the manufacture, marking, testing, and transportation of containers for gases and other fluids. These regulations include the compressed gas cylinders utilized in the practice of anesthesia. The Underwriter's Laboratories (UL) has published standards that pertain to devices and components used in conjunction with anesthesia machines.

A number of mechanisms and organizations have appeared that promote the safety of medical devices and the dissemination of information concerning problems with or failure of various medical devices, including anesthesia machines. The Anesthesia Patient Safety Foundation is prominent as an organization assuming responsibility for overseeing safety issues related to anesthesia, including those issues which pertain directly to anesthesia machines.

The Safe Medical Devices Act of 1990 requires user facilities to report to the FDA instances in which medical devices have contributed to serious injury, illness, or death of a patient. Lees[47] has summarized the important elements of this act.

Appendix 1 lists addresses, phone numbers, and websites of organizations that write standards or guidelines applicable to the use of anesthesia machines. Appendix 2 lists organizations reporting equipment problems and promoting safe anesthesia practices. Most publish a directory of available publications and will provide information concerning their areas of expertise.

REFERENCES

1. Dorsch JA, Dorsch SE: Understanding Anesthesia Equipment, ed 4. Baltimore, Williams & Wilkins, 1999.
2. Petty C: The Anesthesia Machine. New York, Churchill Livingstone, 1987.
3. Eisenkraft JB, Raemer DB: Monitoring Gases in the Anesthesia Delivery System. In Ehrenwerth J, Eisenkraft JB (eds): Anesthesia Equipment: Principles and Applications. St Louis, Mosby–Year Book, 1993.
4. Schreiber P: Safety Guidelines for Anesthesia Systems. Telford, PA, North American Dräger, 1984.
5. Bowie E, Huffman LM: The Anesthesia Machine: Essentials for Understanding. Madison, WI, Ohmeda/BOC Healthcare Group, 1985.
6. Schreiber P, Schreiber J: Anesthesia System Risk Analysis and Risk Reduction. Telford, PA, North American Dräger, 1987.
7. Cicman J, Himmelwright C, Skibo V, et al: Operating Principles of Narkomed Anesthesia Systems. Telford, PA, North American Dräger, 1993.
8. Grogono AW, Travis JT: Anesthesia ventilators. In Ehrenwerth J. Eisenkraft JB (eds): Anesthesia Equipment: Principles and Applications. St Louis, Mosby–Year Book, 1993, pp 140–171.
9. Jones PL: Some observations on nitrous oxide cylinders during emptying. Br J Anaesth 1974; 46:534–538.
10. Cook TL, Eger EI, Behl RS: Is your vaporizer off? Anesth Analg 1977; 56:793–800.
11. Keet JE, Valentine GW, Riccio JS: An arrangement to prevent pressure effect on the Vernitrol vaporizer. Anesthesiology 1963; 24:734–737.
12. Cooper J, Newbower R, Long C, et al: Preventable anesthesia mishaps: A study of human factors. Anesthesiology 1978; 49:399–406.
13. Gaba DM, Maxwell M, DeAnda A: Anesthetic mishaps: Breaking the chain of accident evolution. Anesthesiology 1987; 66:670–676.
14. Mazze RI: Therapeutic misadventures with oxygen delivery systems: The need for continuous in-line oxygen monitors. Anesth Analg 1972; 51:787–792.
15. Anesthesia Apparatus Checkout Recommendations. American Society of Anesthesiologists Newsletter, October 1986; 50:5–6.
16. Anesthesia Apparatus Checkout Recommendations, 1993. US Dept of Health and Human Services. Rockville, MD, Division of Technical Development, Center for Devices and Radiological Health, Food and Drug Administration. http://www.fda.gov/cdrh/humfac/anesckot.html

17. Standard Specification for Minimum Performance and Safety Requirements for Components and Systems of Anesthesia Gas Machines. Designation: F 1161-88. Philadelphia, PA, American Society for Testing and Materials, 1989.
18. Bageant RA, Hoyt JW, Epstein RM: Error in a pipeline gas concentration: An unanticipated consequence of a defective check valve. Anesthesiology 1981; 54:166-169.
19. Whitcher C, Piziali RL: Monitoring occupational exposure to inhalational anesthetics. Anesth Analg 1977; 56:778-785.
20. Comm G, Rendell-Baker L: Back pressure check valves a hazard. Anesthesiology 1982; 56:327-328.
21. Hamilton RC, Byrne J: Another cause of gas scavenging line obstruction. Anesthesiology 1979; 51:365-366.
22. How to monitor Sodasorb exhaustion. Lexington, MA, Sodalines. Dewey and Almy Division of WR Grace, June 1987.
23. Epstein RM, Rackow H, Lee ASJ, et al: Prevention of accidental breathing of anoxic gas mixtures during anesthesia. Anesthesiology 1962; 23:1-4.
24. Cooper JB, Newbower RS, Kitz RJ: An analysis of major errors and equipment failures in anesthesia management: Considerations for prevention and detection. Anesthesiology 1984; 60:34-42.
25. Well ME, Bisera J, Trevino RP, et al: Cardiac output and end-tidal carbon dioxide. Crit Care Med 1985; 13:907-909.
26. Spargo PM: The use of end-tidal PCO_2 monitoring to detect pulmonary embolism during Swan-Ganz catheter removal (abstract). Anesthesiology 1985; 63:A293.
27. Swedlow DB: Capnometry and capnography: An anesthesia disaster warning system. Semin Anesth 1986; 5:194.
28. Gravenstein JS, Paulus DA, Hayes TJ: Capnography in Clinical Practice. Boston, Butterworths, 1988.
29. Smalhout B, Kalenda Z: An Atlas of Capnography, vol 1. Zeist, Netherlands, Kerckebosch-Zeist, 1975.
30. Linko K, Paloheimo M, Tammisto T: Capnography for detection of accidental oesophageal intubation. Acta Anaesthesiol Scand 1983; 27:199.
31. Murray IP, Modell JH: Early detection of endotracheal tube accidents by monitoring carbon dioxide concentration in respiratory gas. Anesthesiology 1983; 59:344.
32. Raemer DB: Monitoring respiratory function. In Rogers MC, Tinker JH, Covino BG, et al (eds): Principles and Practice of Anesthesiology. St Louis, Mosby-Year Book, 1992.
33. Shulman D, Aronson HB: Capnography in the early diagnosis of carbon dioxide embolism during laparoscopy. Can Anaesth Soc J 1984; 31:455.
34. Osborn IJ, Raison JC, Beaumont JO, et al: Respiratory causes of "sudden unexplained arrhythmia" in post-thoracotomy patients. Surgery 1971; 69:24.
35. Baudendistel L, Goudsouzian N, Coté C, et al: End-tidal CO_2 monitoring: Its use in the diagnosis and management of malignant hyperthermia. Anaesthesia 1984; 39:1000.
36. Triner L, Sherman J: Potential value of expiratory carbon dioxide measurement in patients considered to be susceptible to malignant hyperthermia. Anesthesiology 1981; 55:482.
37. Gravenstein N, Lampotang MS, Beneken JEW: Factors influencing capnography in the Bain circuit. J Clin Monit Comput 1985; 1:6.
38. Nightingale DA, Richards CC, Glass A: An evaluation of rebreathing in a modified T-piece system during controlled ventilation in anesthetized children. Br J Anaesth 1975; 37:762.
39. Sato T: New aspects of carbon dioxide absorption in anesthetic circuit. Med J Osaka Univ 1971; 22:173.
40. Cooper JB, Newbower RS, Long CD, et al: Preventable anesthesia mishaps: A study of human factors. Anesthesiology 1978; 49:399.
41. Huffman LM, Riddle RT: Mass spectrometer and/or capnograph use during low-flow, closed circuit anesthesia administration. Anesthesiology 1987; 66:439.
42. Mushlin PS, Mark JB, Elliott WR, et al: Inadvertent development of subatmospheric airway pressure during cardiopulmonary bypass. Anesthesiology 1989; 71:459.
43. Cooper JB, Newbower RS, Moore JW, et al: A new anesthesia delivery system. Anesthesiology 1978; 49:310-318.
44. Loeb RG, Brunner JX, Westenskow OR, et al: The Utah Anesthesia Workstation. Anesthesiology 1989; 70:999-1007.
45. Sykes MK, Sugg BR, Hahn CEW, et al: A new microprocessor-controlled anaesthetic machine. Br J Anaesth 1989; 62:445-455.

Appendix 1

Organizations Which Have Developed Standards Applicable to Anesthesia Machines and Equipment

Compressed Gas Association (CGA)
1735 Jefferson Davis Highway Suite 1004
Arlington, VA 22202-4102
(703) 412-0900
http://www.cganet.com/

American Society for Testing and Materials (ASTM)
100 Barr Harbor Drive
West Conshohocken, PA 19428-2959
(610) 823-9585
http://www.astm.org/

International Organization for Standardization (ISO)
http://www.iso.ch/
ISO is represented in the United States by the member body:
American National Standards Institute (ANSI)
11 West 42nd Street
New York, NY 10036
(212) 642-4900
http://www.ansi.org/

National Fire Protection Association (NFPA)
1 Batterymarch Park
Quincy, MA 02269-9101
(617) 770-3000
http://www.nfpa.org/

Underwriter's Laboratories, Inc. (UL)
333 Pfingsten Road
Northbrook, IL 60062-2096
(847) 272-8800
http://www.ul.com/

Appendix 2

Organizations Reporting Equipment Problems and Promoting Safe Anesthesia Practices

Anesthesia Patient Safety Foundation (APSF)
520 N. Northwest Highway
Park Ridge, IL 60068
(708) 825-5586
http://www.apsf.org/

Emergency Care Research Institute (ECRI)
  (publisher of *Health Devices*)
5200 Butler Pike
Plymouth Meeting, PA 19462
(610) 825-6000
http://www.ecri.org/

18 Monitoring of Oxygen

Kevin K. Tremper, M.D., Ph.D.
Steven J. Barker, M.D., Ph.D.

While reading this sentence you are consuming approximately 10^{18} molecules of oxygen per second. This phenomenal oxygen transport to the tissues is required to maintain aerobic metabolism in the average 70-kg adult at rest. As single-celled animals evolved to multicelled organisms and eventually to large mammals, an immense problem of oxygen distribution had to be solved.

There are two limitations on oxygen delivery in cellular life in an aqueous environment. First, molecular diffusion of gases in liquids is an extremely slow process. Second, the solubility of oxygen in water is very low. The diffusion constant (diffusivity) of oxygen in water is approximately 10^{-5} cm²/second. For single-celled creatures, oxygen can diffuse rapidly from the cell wall to the mitochondria because the diffusion distance is short. As the number of cells grows and the diffusion distance increases, the rate of oxygen transport limits aerobic metabolism. It would take nearly a day for an oxygen molecule to diffuse 1 cm in water by pure molecular diffusion. Consequently, as multicellular organisms evolved, they developed a more efficient transport system to distribute oxygen by bulk flow to each cell. Because the solubility of oxygen in water is low, the transport system also needed a mechanism to increase the oxygen-carrying capacity of an aqueous medium. The result in vertebrate life is the cardiovascular system and blood, using hemoglobin as a carrier to increase the oxygen capacity of the transport medium.

Over the past several decades, a number of oxygen transport variables have been developed to quantitate the effectiveness of the oxygen delivery system. Since the 1970s, both invasive and noninvasive continuous monitoring systems have been developed to assess the adequacy of oxygen transport. These devices monitor oxygenation by different means and at different points in the oxygen transport system. In this chapter, the commonly measured and calculated oxygen transport variables are described, and available oxygen monitoring techniques are reviewed in depth. For each technique, the physics and engineering behind the measurement, as well as the physiologic interpretation of the measured variable, are discussed. Each technique has its limitations in the detection of hypoxia.

Analysis of Inspired Oxygen

Inspired oxygen in an anesthetic circuit can be measured by a mass spectrometer, a Raman spectrometer, or an analyzer that measures oxygen only. Mass and Raman spectrometers are discussed elsewhere in this text. Several types of oxygen-only analyzers have been used in clinical practice, including polarographic, paramagnetic, and galvanic (fuel cell) devices. The polarographic Clark electrode is the most commonly used device for P_{O_2} measurement and is described below (Fig. 18–1). The reader is referred to other texts for a description of the paramagnetic and galvanic analyzers.[1, 2] All present-generation machines have integrated inspired oxygen analyzers that are activated whenever the machine is turned on.

Monitoring the oxygen concentration in the anesthetic or ventilator circuit is mandatory. Although this does not ensure an adequate arterial oxygen tension (Pa_{O_2}), it confirms that hypoxic oxygen concentrations are not delivered to the patient's airway.

Polarographic Analyzers

Polarographic analyzers are based on the principle of the Clark electrode. The breakdown (reduction) of oxygen occurs at a charged metal cathode (a "rest" voltage of 0.5 to 0.8 V) in the polarographic electrode, and the current produced by the reaction alters the conductivity of an electrolyte solution of potassium chlorine. Essential components are a silver anode, a platinum or gold cathode, and a gas-permeable membrane. The specific rest voltage causes only oxygen to react. When a gas sample contains oxygen, the current flow is proportional to the P_{O_2} in the electrolyte solution. Response times for these analyzers are about 10 to 60 seconds.

If accuracy at concentrations of oxygen of less than 50% is desired, these analyzers are calibrated using room air. Accuracy in the 90% to 100% range requires calibration on 100% oxygen. Regular preventive maintenance is required because the electrode membrane and electrolyte have a limited life span. This is the same electrode used in conventional blood gas machines.

Clinical Use

Ideally, an inspired oxygen analyzer should be accurate to ±2% and capable of response within 2 to 10 seconds. It should be unaffected by the relative humidity within the 30% to 90% range. Analyzers should be compensated for both temperature and pressure. Exposure to anesthetic gases should not affect their accuracy. Halothane is known to cause P_{O_2} electrodes to drift upward. The degree of this drift depends on the concentration of halothane and the composition of the electrode membrane. Calibration is best per-

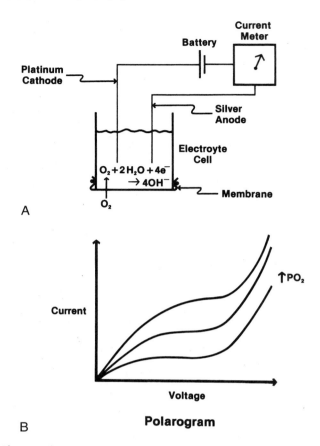

A

B

Polarogram

Figure 18-1. *A,* Schematic of a Clark polarographic oxygen electrode. The circuit consists of a voltage source (battery) and a current meter connecting platinum and silver electrodes. The electrodes are immersed in an electrolyte cell. A membrane permeable to oxygen, but not to the electrolyte, covers one surface of the cell. Oxygen diffuses through the membrane and reacts at the platinum cathode with water to produce hydroxyl ions. The ammeter measures the current produced by the electrons consumed in this reaction at the cathode. *B,* A plot of current produced as a function of the voltage between the two electrodes (polarizing voltage). This plot is called a polarogram. In the range near 660 mV there is a plateau in the polarogram. The plateau occurs at higher currents as the P_{O_2} in the cell is increased. Most polarographic oxygen electrodes use 600- to 800-mV polarizing voltage to obtain a stable current at each P_{O_2}.

formed using dry 100% oxygen. After calibration, accuracy should be maintained for at least 8 hours.

High- and low-concentration alarms are essential features of most oxygen analyzers. Both visual and auditory alarms must be present and functional during use of an anesthesia machine or ventilator. Although oxygen analyzers can detect disconnections in fresh gas lines, they are unable to detect disconnection of the patient's endotracheal tube from the anesthetic breathing circuit unless the sensor is placed in the expiratory limb of the circle system.[3]

Quantitative Oxygen Transport Variables

Oxygen Content

Oxygen content is defined as the volume of oxygen (milliliters) carried in 100 mL of blood. It is a basic variable that is found in all oxygen transport calculations. Although oxygen content can be measured directly by the volumetric method

of Van Slyke and Neill,[4] it is usually calculated from this equation:

$$CaO_2 = Hb \times 1.37 \times HbO_2 + 0.0034 \times PaO_2 \quad (18.1)$$

where

CaO_2 = arterial oxygen content (a denotes an arterial sample) in mL/dL (also called vol%)
Hb = hemoglobin concentration in g/dL
1.37 = volume of oxygen (mL) carried by 1 g of fully saturated hemoglobin
HbO_2 = fractional hemoglobin saturation (discussed later)
0.0034 = solubility coefficient of oxygen in plasma (mL of oxygen per dL plasma per mmHg)
PaO_2 = arterial oxygen tension in mmHg

With a normal hemoglobin of 15 g/dL and normal PaO_2 and HbO_2 values of 95 mmHg and 95%, respectively, the CaO_2 is 20 mL/dL. Coincidentally, this is very similar to the oxygen content of room air at sea level. Thus, the cardiovascular system produces the same oxygen content near each cell that would exist if the cells were surrounded by room air. Methods of measuring both HbO_2 and P_{O_2} are discussed below.

In Equation 18.1, the oxygen content is very sensitive to the hemoglobin concentration and HbO_2 whereas it is relatively insensitive to the P_{O_2} because of the small solubility coefficient for oxygen in plasma. However, the oxygen saturation itself depends nonlinearly on P_{O_2}. Because oxygen content is proportional to hemoglobin concentration, if the arterial hemoglobin is fully saturated, the content can be roughly estimated as equaling slightly less than half the hematocrit. The hematocrit equals approximately three times the hemoglobin concentration.

Oxygen Delivery

The overall flow rate of oxygen to the tissues is called the oxygen delivery (O_2del), determined as the CaO_2 times the cardiac output. At a cardiac output of 5 L/minute for a 70-kg adult, normal O_2del is 1000 mL of oxygen per minute (20 mL of oxygen 100 mL or 200 mL of oxygen per L × 5 L/minute = 1000 mL of oxygen per minute). Because normal cardiac output depends on the size of the patient, cardiac output is indexed to body surface area: cardiac index (CI) = cardiac output/body surface area (m^2). The range for CI is 2.5 to 3.4 L/minute/m^2. The O_2del index (Equation 18.2) is defined as the arterial oxygen content times the CI:

$$O_2del\ index = CaO_2 \times CI\ (mL\ oxygen/min/m^2)$$

$$Normal\ O_2del\ index = 20\ mL/dL \times 10\ dL/L \times 3\ L/min/m^2$$

$$= 600\ mL/min/m^2 \quad (18.2)$$

The O_2del index is an overall assessment of oxygen transport to the tissues, but it does not ensure adequate oxygen supply to any specific organ. The O_2del to each organ can be defined as the CaO_2 times the blood flow to the specific organ.

Oxygen Consumption

Human tissues consume an average of 5 mL of oxygen from every 100 mL of blood flow. Because the normal CaO_2 is 20 mL/dL of blood, 75% of the oxygen remains in the venous blood. The oxygen consumption (V_{O_2}) of the body (Equation 18.3) can be calculated by subtracting the mixed venous blood oxygen content (Cv_{O_2}) from the Ca_{O_2} and multiplying this difference by the cardiac output:

$$V_{O_2} = (Ca_{O_2} - Cv_{O_2}) \times \text{cardiac output} \qquad (18.3)$$

As with oxygen delivery, oxygen consumption is indexed so that the normal value is independent of patient size:

$$V_{O_2} \text{ index} = V_{O_2} (Ca_{O_2} - Cv_{O_2}) \times Cl$$

$$\begin{aligned} V_{O_2} \text{ index} = (20 \text{ mL/dL} - 15 \text{ mL/dL}) \\ \times 3 \text{ L/min/m}^2 \times 10 \text{ dL/L} \end{aligned}$$

$$V_{O_2} \text{ index} = 150 \text{ mL/min/m}^2$$

The normal range of the oxygen consumption index is 115 to 165 mL/min/m². These values are for healthy resting humans and increase up to 10 times with exercise, shivering, hyperthermia, or sepsis. V_{O_2} index decreases during anesthesia and hypothermia.

Mixed Venous Oxygen

Mixed venous blood is sampled from the pulmonary artery to ensure proper mixing. A mixed venous sample does not reflect the oxygen returned to the heart from any specific organ. The normal Cv_{O_2} is 15 mL/dL, which corresponds to a mixed venous saturation of 75% and a P_{O_2} of 40 mmHg. Mixed venous blood oxygen tension ($\overline{Pv}_{O_2}$) should reflect tissue P_{O_2}. Although tissue P_{O_2} values vary greatly, the mean P_{O_2} of interstitial fluid is the same as the $\overline{Pv}_{O_2}$, that is, 40 mmHg.[5]

Oxygen Extraction

The oxygen extraction ratio (O_2 ext) is a supply-demand balance for oxygenation:

$$O_2\text{ext} = Ca_{O_2} - Cv_{O_2}/Ca_{O_2} \times 100\% \qquad (18.4)$$

The O_2ext is actually the ratio of V_{O_2} to O_2del:

$$O_2\text{ext} = (Ca_{O_2} - Cv_{O_2}) \times Cl/Ca_{O_2} \times Cl \times 100\%$$

Because Cl appears in both the numerator and the denominator of the above equation, it need not be measured to calculate O_2ext. For this reason, O_2ext was an especially useful variable prior to the availability of thermodilution pulmonary artery catheters. The normal O_2ext is only 25%, so there appears to be a wide margin of safety for oxygen transport. In fact, the body can easily extract up to 50% of the delivered oxygen without obligatory tissue hypoxia. When the O_2ext exceeds 50%, there is an increasing incidence of tissue hypoxia because of the low P_{O_2} (the 50% hemoglobin saturation, or P-50, of adult hemoglobin is normally 26.7 mmHg).

Hypoxia: Definitions

Hypoxia is defined as inadequate tissue oxygenation due to either inadequate blood flow or low Ca_{O_2}. Hypoxia due to inadequate blood flow is ischemic hypoxia. Hypoxia due to low oxygen content is hypoxemic hypoxia. Ca_{O_2} can be reduced as a result of decreased hemoglobin (anemic hypox-

emia), Pa_{O_2} (hypoxemic hypoxemia), or Hb_{O_2} (toxic hypoxemia). Toxic hypoxemia (decreased fractional hemoglobin saturation) results from increased methemoglobin (MetHb) or carboxyhemoglobin (CoHb) and is discussed later.

Measurement of Oxygen Tension

Clark PO_2 Electrode

Oxygen partial pressure (or *tension*) in a liquid is defined as the P_{O_2} in the equilibrium gas phase. When several phases are in contact at equilibrium (e.g., lipid, water, and gas), the P_{O_2} will be equal in all phases, but the oxygen concentration in each phase will be proportional to its solubility in that phase. In 1956, Leland Clark developed the polarographic oxygen electrode for measuring P_{O_2} (described earlier in this chapter).[6] With the addition of the Severinghaus carbon dioxide electrode in 1958, the blood gas machine was developed, and care of the critical patient was revolutionized.[7]

PO_2 Optode

The phenomenon of photoluminescence quenching has been used to develop sensors for measuring P_{O_2}, called the "optode."[8, 9] When light shines on a luminescent material, specific light frequencies are absorbed, exciting electrons to a higher energy state (Fig. 18-2). These electrons then fall spontaneously into a lower energy state by emitting a photon of a frequency different from that of the original light. In some luminescent dyes, this light emission is "quenched" by the presence of oxygen. When the excited electron falls into a lower energy state, its energy can be either emitted as a photon (luminescence) or absorbed by an oxygen molecule, thereby increasing the energy of the latter (see Fig. 18-2). For these photoluminescence-quenching dyes, the amount of oxygen present can be related to the luminescent intensity. The empirical relationship governing this phenomenon is known at the Stern-Volmer equation.[8]

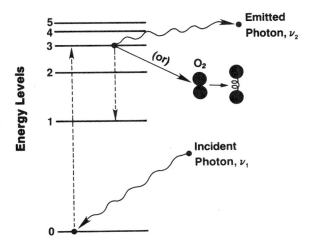

Figure 18-2. The photoluminescence-quenching phenomenon. An electron of the fluorescent dye is excited to a higher energy level by an incident photon (ν_1). This excited electron can return to a lower energy level either by emitting a photon (ν_2) or by interacting with and raising an oxygen molecule to a higher vibrational energy level. (From Barker SJ, Tremper KK, Hyatt J, et al: Continuous fiberoptic arterial oxygen tension measurements in dogs. J Clin Monit Comput 1987; 3:48–52.)

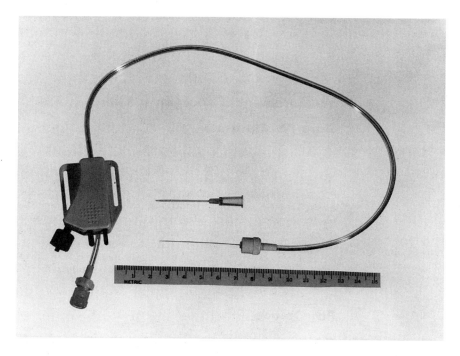

Figure 18-3. An optode probe and the 20-gauge cannula through which it is inserted. (From Barker SJ, Tremper KK, Hyatt J, et al: Continuous fiberoptic arterial oxygen tension measurements in dogs. J Clin Monit Comput 1987; 3:48-52.)

$$I\,(PO_2) = I_0/(1 + K \times PO_2) \qquad (18.5)$$

where

I = intensity of the luminescent signal at the PO_2 being measured

I_0 = intensity of the luminescent signal in the absence of oxygen

PO_2 = oxygen partial pressure

K = quenching constant

The advantages of the optode as a PO_2 measuring device are its simplicity and size. The sensor consists of a small fiberoptic strand with a dye encapsulated at the tip, and it can be easily miniaturized. Figure 18-3 shows an optode that easily fits through a 22-gauge intravenous cannula.[9] Another advantage of optode technology is that pH-sensitive dyes are also available; therefore, a three-fiber optode sensor can measure PO_2, partial pressure of carbon dioxide (PCO_2), and pH simultaneously.[10]

Continuous Oxygen Tension Monitoring

Invasive PO$_2$ Monitoring

Clark Electrode

The primary problem in continuous invasive PaO_2 monitoring is miniaturization of the Clark electrode to fit through an arterial cannula. There are two approaches to this problem. One is to insert only the platinum cathode in the arterial cannula and place the reference anode on the skin surface. The platinum cathode is surrounded by a thin layer of electrolyte and covered with an oxygen-permeable membrane.[11-13] The second approach involves miniaturization of the entire anode-cathode electrode for intra-arterial insertion.[13-16]

Studies of intra-arterial PO_2 monitoring using Clark electrodes have yielded conflicting results. It is often difficult to compare such studies because the data are usually analyzed by linear regression and correlation coefficients. The correlation coefficient is extremely sensitive to the x and y range over which the data are collected. Furthermore, a high correlation coefficient (r close to 1.0) implies a high degree of association between the methods (i.e., when one goes up, the other will go up), but it does not imply that one method can replace the other.

As an alternative, Altman and Bland recommended using the mean and standard deviation of the difference between the two methods of measurement as an assessment of agreement.[17-19] The mean difference is called the "bias," and the standard deviation is the "precision." The bias indicates a consistent overestimate or underestimate of one method relative to the other, or the systematic error, while the precision represents the scatter, or random, error. Note that a larger precision implies a less precise measurement. For example, Figure 18-4 is a scattergram plot of data from an intra-arterial Clark electrode used in neonatal patients.[15] The abscissa of this plot is PaO_2 determined on arterial samples by a blood gas analyzer, and the ordinate is the intra-arterial electrode PaO_2. Although these data yield a correlation coefficient of 0.88, y varies greatly on x over the entire range of PaO_2. For example, at a PaO_2 of 40 mmHg, the intra-arterial probe PO_2 values vary from the mid-20s to 70 mmHg, with one data point as high as 100 mmHg.

Umbilical artery Clark electrodes in neonates have been associated with a number of complications, including thrombus formation, embolism, vascular perforation, infarction, lower extremity ischemia, and infection. Probe size has also caused problems in the use of Clark electrodes for both umbilical and radial arterial monitoring. Damping of the arterial pressure waveform and inaccurate blood pressure measurements are commonly reported.[15, 16] Other reported problems include calibration drift and systematic underestimation of PaO_2. The causes of these errors are not understood, but they may involve decreased blood flow around the electrode tip or clot formation on the electrode surface.

Optode PO$_2$ Sensors

The above discussion of optode principles suggests that these sensors lend themselves to miniaturization more readily

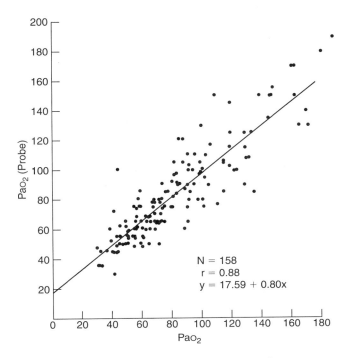

Figure 18–4. Relation between Pao₂ and intravascular oxygen tension (probe) measurements. (From Malalis L, Bhat R, Vidyasagar D: Comparison of intravascular Po₂ with transcutaneous and Pao₂ values. Crit Care Med 1983; 11:110–113.)

Table 18–1. Statistical Comparison of Arterial Oxygen Tensions Obtained by Optode and by Blood Gas Analysis in 12 Surgical Patients

Variable	0–700 mmHg	0–150 mmHg
n	96	38
r	.970	.923
Linear regression		
Slope	1.07	1.05
Intercept	−10.6	−8.5
Bias	−1.10	3.74
Precision	19.0	11.7

From Barker SJ, Tremper KK: Intra-arterial PO₂ monitoring. Int Anesthesiol Clin 1987; 25:199–208.

than the Clark electrode. In fact, three-component optodes (pH, Pco₂, Po₂) have been incorporated into a probe with a diameter of 0.5 to 0.6 mm. Such a sensor will pass easily through a 20-gauge cannula without preventing the aspiration of blood samples or monitoring of pressure waveforms.[20] There have been multiple studies conducted to evaluate the accuracy and reliability of these continuous blood gas monitors, primarily in the intensive care unit (ICU) setting (Table 18–1).[21-23] Although the devices are inherently accurate when used as continuous intravascular monitors, there are occurrences in which the device shows an unexpected drop in Po₂ coincident with a rise in Pco₂ and a fallen pH.[21] This has been attributed to thrombosis formation at the tip of the sensor. There are also brief periods when the Po₂ drops

precipitously to a value that is more consistent with tissue or venous values. This may be associated with the sensor tip being placed against the wall of the vessel or possibly decreasing flow in that artery.[21]

These problems have led to the development of an on-line extravascular system to measure blood gases using optode technology (Fig. 18–5). Although this device is not a continuous monitor, it allows intermittent on-demand blood gas measurement with a high level of accuracy. To date there are no large-scale studies that would determine whether these devices are cost-effective in the management of the critically ill. Because there will always be the necessity to have a traditional blood gas machine available to confirm the accuracy of these devices, those costs cannot necessarily be removed. Two recent articles have reviewed the state of the art of intravascular blood gas monitoring.[22, 23]

Noninvasive PO₂ Monitoring

Transcutaneous PO₂

In 1972, two researchers reported that Po₂ values similar to Pao₂ could be obtained by heating a Clark electrode and placing it on the skin surface of a newborn infant.[24, 25] Over the next decade, this technique, transcutaneous oxygen monitoring, became routine in the care of premature infants at risk of both hypoxia and hyperoxia.[26, 27] In the late 1970s, transcutaneous Po₂ (Ptco₂) values were found to be significantly lower than Pao₂ values during episodes of hemody-

Figure 18–5. A schematic representation of an extravascular monitoring system. The sensor cassette is inserted close to the wrist into the patient's arterial line tubing. When a blood gas is desired blood is withdrawn into the sensor cassette via the sampling syringe. (From Mahutte CK: On-line arterial blood gas analysis with optodes: Current status. J Clin Biochem 1998; 31: 119–130.)

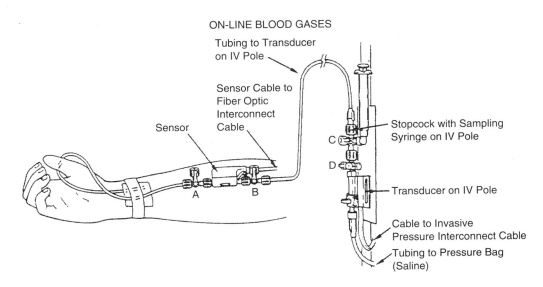

namic instability.[28, 29] Although this discovery lessened the usefulness of $PtcO_2$ as a PaO_2 monitor, it did give the user a valuable indicator of peripheral perfusion.

$PtcO_2$ is the oxygen tension of heated skin. To obtain a measurable PO_2 at the skin surface with a fast response time, the skin must be heated to at least 43°C. The stratum corneum, composed of lipid in a protein matrix, is normally a very efficient barrier to gas transport. When heated above 41°C, the structural characteristics of this layer change, allowing oxygen to diffuse through it readily.[30, 31] In the epidermis, heating causes vasodilation of the dermal capillaries, which is said to "arterialize" this capillary blood.

The perfusion of this hyperemic epidermal capillary bed depends on adequate blood flow to the dermal vasculature. Consequently, if the cardiac output decreases, skin blood flow and oxygen delivery to the transcutaneous sensor decrease. Figure 18–6 illustrates the relation between PaO_2 and $PtcO_2$ during induced hypoxemia (hypoxemic hypoxia) followed by hemorrhagic shock (ischemic hypoxia) in an animal study.[32] During the shock state, $PtcO_2$ decreased with

Table 18–2. Changes in $PtcO_2$ Index With Age and Cardiac Output

$PtcO_2$ Index* ($PtcO_2/PaO_2$)	Age Group
1.14	Premature infants
1.0	Newborn
0.84	Pediatric
0.8	Adult
0.7	Older adult (>65 yr)

$PtcO_2$ Index†	Cardiac Index (L/min/m²)
0.8	>2.2
0.5	1.5–2.2
0.1	<1.5

* All of these $PtcO_2$ index values have a standard deviation of approximately 0.1.

† These data are from adult patients.

decreasing cardiac output even though PaO_2 was relatively unchanged.

This effect of cardiac output on the $PtcO_2$-PaO_2 relationship can be quantitated in terms of a transcutaneous oxygen index:

$$PtcO_2 \text{ index} = PtcO_2/PaO_2 \qquad (18.6)$$

$PtcO_2$ index has been used as an indicator of peripheral perfusion analogous to the alveolar-arterial PO_2 gradient for the assessment of pulmonary function.[33] Table 18–2 shows the $PtcO_2$ index as a function of CI found in adult patients in critical care units. Under stable hemodynamic conditions, the normal $PtcO_2$ index for adult patients was 0.79, whereas this index fell to 0.49 when the CI decreased below 2.2 L/minute/m².[33] A review of the published $PtcO_2$ values on hemodynamically stable patients in various age groups revealed that the $PtcO_2$ index decreases progressively with age from premature infants to elderly patients (see Table 18–2). Glenski and Cucchiara[34] also found that the $PtcO_2$ index is relatively independent of probe location as long as the probe is on the central body rather than on an extremity.

A study showed that $PtcO_2$ also depends on $PaCO_2$, and that during hyperventilation both skin blood flow and $PtcO_2$ index are significantly decreased.[35] Voluntary hyperventilation in healthy subjects decreased $PtcO_2$ index to values as low as 0.1. $PtcO_2$ is thus a noninvasive monitor of peripheral tissue PO_2, and as such it depends on all parameters that affect oxygen delivery.

In summary, $PtcO_2$ values follow the trend of PaO_2 under conditions of adequate cardiac output and decrease relative to PaO_2 under conditions of low cardiac output states or hyperventilation. Thus, $PtcO_2$ may aid in the diagnosis and treatment of low-flow shock conditions. The limitations of $PtcO_2$ monitoring include calibration and electrode maintenance, warm-up time, and the possibility of skin burns. Because of the availability of simpler techniques (pulse oximetry), $PtcO_2$ currently is not widely used clinically.

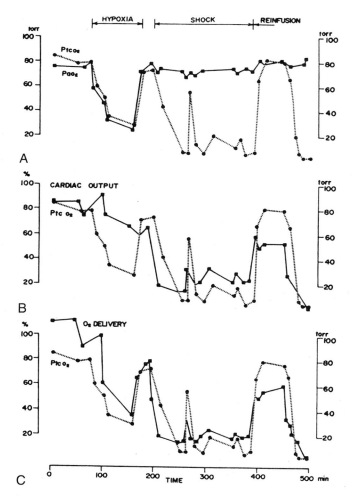

Figure 18–6. Hypoxia and hypovolemic shock study in dogs. *A*, Serial transcutaneous oxygen tension ($PtcO_2$) and arterial oxygen tension (PaO_2). *B*, $PtcO_2$ and cardiac output. *C*, $PtcO_2$ and oxygen delivery throughout a representative experiment. Note $PtcO_2$ values follow the PaO_2 values during hypoxia, but not during shock; $PtcO_2$ values follow cardiac output during shock, but not during hypoxia; however, $PtcO_2$ values most closely follow oxygen delivery throughout the entire experiment. (From Tremper KK, Waxman K, Shoemaker WC: Effects of hypoxia and shock on transcutaneous PO_2 values in dogs. Crit Care Med 1979; 7:529–531.)

Measurement of Hemoglobin Saturation

Hemoglobin Saturation vs. Oxygen Saturation

Oxygen saturation is defined as the blood oxygen content divided by the oxygen capacity times 100%. Oxygen content was originally measured volumetrically by the method of

Van Slyke and Neill.[4] *Oxygen capacity* is defined as the oxygen content of the blood after it has been equilibrated with room air ($PO_2 = 159$ mmHg). When this definition was formed, the maximum blood oxygen content clinically achieved occurred at room air PO_2 because increased inspired oxygen concentrations were not available. From the oxygen content formula (see Equation 18.1), we see that this definition of oxygen saturation includes contributions from both hemoglobin-bound and dissolved oxygen. Adult blood usually contains four species of hemoglobin: oxyhemoglobin (O_2Hb), reduced hemoglobin (RHb), methemoglobin (MetHb), and carboxyhemoglobin (COHb). COHb and MetHb are found in low concentrations except in pathologic states. Because these dyshemoglobins do not transport oxygen, they do not contribute to the oxygen content or to the definition of oxygen saturation given previously. When spectrophotometric methods for measuring hemoglobin species concentration became available, hemoglobin saturation could be more easily determined. The term *functional hemoglobin saturation* (SaO_2) is defined as

$$SaO_2 = [O_2Hb]/[O_2Hb] + [RHb] \times 100\% \quad (18.7)$$

where brackets denote concentration. This definition of hemoglobin saturation does not include MetHb or COHb because they do not contribute to oxygen transport. *Fractional hemoglobin saturation* (HbO_2), which is also called oxyhemoglobin fraction, is defined as

$$HbO_2 = [O_2Hb]/[O_2Hb] + [RHb] \\ + [COHb] + [MetHb] \times 100\% \quad (18.8)$$

This definition of hemoglobin saturation—that is, the ratio of oxyhemoglobin to total hemoglobin—is the saturation used in the calculation of oxygen content and delivery (see Equation 18.2). It is important to remember these definitions when evaluating the clinical utility and limitations of hemoglobin saturation monitors.

Hemoglobin Saturation Measurement: Beer's Law

Spectrophotometry was first used to determine the hemoglobin concentration of blood in the 1930s.[36] This method is based on the Lambert-Beer law (Equation 18.9), which relates the concentration of a solute to the intensity of light transmitted through the solution (Fig. 18–7).

$$I_{trans} = I_{in} \, e^{-DC\alpha\lambda} \quad (18.9)$$

where

I_{trans} = intensity of transmitted light
I_{in} = intensity of incident light
e = base of natural logarithm (2.718)
D = distance light is transmitted through the liquid
C = concentration of the solute (hemoglobin)
$\alpha\lambda$ = extinction coefficient of the solute (a constant for a given solute at a specific light wavelength λ)*

Thus, if a known solute is dissolved in a clear solvent in a cuvette of known dimensions, the solute concentration can be calculated if the incident and transmitted light intensity are measured (see Fig. 18–7). The extinction coefficient $\alpha\lambda$

---

*This law further states that the absorbance from multiple solutes in solution is the sum of the absorbances of the various solutes times their respective concentrations, for example, $C_1\alpha_{\lambda 1} + C_2\alpha_{\lambda 2} + C_3\alpha_{\lambda 3}$, and so forth.

BEER'S LAW

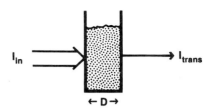

$$I_{trans} = I_{in}e^{-(D \times C \times \alpha_\lambda)}$$

I_{trans} = **intensity of light transmitted**
I_{in} = **intensity of incident light**
D = **distance light is transmitted through the liquid**
C = **concentration of solute (oxyhemoglobin)**
α_λ = **extinction coefficient of the solute (a constant)**

Figure 18–7. Beer's law: The concentration of a solute dissolved in a solvent can be calculated from the logarithmic relationship between the incident (I_{in}) and transmitted (I_{trans}) light intensity and the solute concentration. *D*, distance light is transmitted through the liquid. (Modified from Tremper KK, Barker SJ: Pulse oximetry and oxygen transport. *In* Payne JP, Severinghaus JW [eds]: Pulse Oximetry. Berlin, Springer-Verlag, 1986, pp 19–27.)

is independent of the concentration, but is a function of the light wavelength used (Fig. 18–8).

Laboratory oximeters use this principle to determine hemoglobin concentration by measuring the intensity of light transmitted through a hemoglobin dispersion produced from lysed red blood cells.[37] For each wavelength of light used, an independent Lambert-Beer equation can be written. If the number of equations is equal to the number of solutes (i.e., hemoglobin species), we can solve for the concentration of each type. Therefore, at least four wavelengths of light are required to determine the concentrations of four species of hemoglobin (see Fig. 18–8). For the Lambert-Beer law to be valid, both the solvent and the cuvette must be transparent at the light wavelengths used, the light path length must be known exactly, and no other absorbers can be present in the solution. It is difficult to fulfill all of these requirements in clinical devices. Consequently, although these devices are theoretically based on the Lambert-Beer law, empirical corrections are required to improve their accuracy.

Invasive Hemoglobin Saturation Monitoring

Mixed Venous Hemoglobin Saturation

Mixed venous oxygen tension ($P\bar{v}O_2$) and mixed venous hemoglobin saturation ($S\bar{v}O_2$) reflect global tissue oxygenation and the ability of the cardiopulmonary system to transport sufficient oxygen to meet body oxygen needs. Thus, continuous mixed venous oxygen monitoring should be useful clinically. In 1973, a fiberoptic system was reported to accurately measure $S\bar{v}O_2$ in humans.[38] This device used optical fibers incorporated into a pulmonary artery catheter to estimate the hemoglobin saturation from a reflected light signal. Light at red and infrared wavelengths was transmitted down one set of fiberoptic channels while the reflected signal from intact circulating red blood cells was transmitted back via other fibers to an external photodetector.[38] Although this

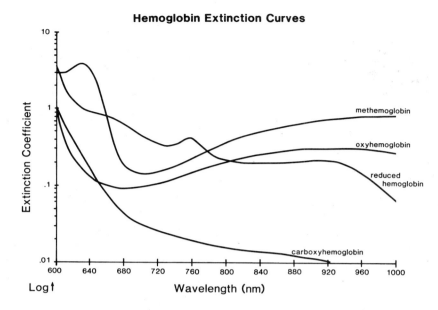

Hemoglobin Extinction Curves

Figure 18-8. Transmitted light absorbance spectra of four hemoglobin species: oxyhemoglobin, reduced hemoglobin, carboxyhemoglobin, and methemoglobin. (From Barker SJ, Tremper KK: Pulse oximetry: Applications and limitations. Int Anesthesiol Clin 1987; 25:155–175.)

first system appeared to work, it was not commercially produced because of the technical problems of inserting a pulmonary artery catheter that was made relatively stiff by the fiberoptic bundles.

In the late 1970s, Oximetrix, Inc. (Division of Abbott Laboratories, Mountain View, CA) developed two fiberoptic reflectance systems for measuring hemoglobin saturation. The first system, introduced in 1977, employed a 7F double-lumen umbilical artery catheter to be used in monitoring critically ill newborn infants.[39] The second system, introduced in 1981, used a 7.5F pulmonary artery catheter with thermodilution capability for cardiac output measurement in addition to continuous mixed venous monitoring.[40] These new systems used three wavelengths of light to calculate saturation. However, a minimum of four wavelengths are required to calculate hemoglobin saturation from Beer's law in the presence of MetHb and COHb. The Oximetrix mixed venous saturation monitor can accurately measure functional hemoglobin saturation in the absence of significant dyshemoglobin concentrations.[40] However, an experimental study has shown that methemoglobinemia produces significant errors in the saturation measurement.[41] See Pulse Oximetry, below.

American Edwards Corporation, (Irvine, CA) has also produced a mixed venous saturation pulmonary artery catheter that uses two wavelengths of light. This device requires manual entry of the total hemoglobin to improve accuracy, whereas the Oximetrix system can accurately measure mixed venous saturation over a wide range of hematocrits.[42, 43]

Continuous $S\bar{v}O_2$ monitoring detects acute changes in the relationship of O_2del to V_O_2 (decreased supply, increased demand, or both). Three causes of reduced O_2del decrease $S\bar{v}O_2$: decreased cardiac output, decreased hemoglobin, and decreased SaO_2. Abnormal hemoglobins also fail to deliver oxygen to tissue. Clinical situations in which increasing V_O_2 causes decreasing $S\bar{v}O_2$ are shivering, malignant hyperthermia, exercise, agitation, fever, and thyroid storm. Monitoring $S\bar{v}O_2$ has been recommended in cardiac surgery patients and other critically ill patients at risk of acute cardiopulmonary decompensation.[44-46] It has also been recommended as a valuable adjunct in the management of ventilator-dependent patients on positive end-expiratory pressure (PEEP). As PEEP increases, arterial saturation improves. Eventually, PEEP de-

creases venous return and cardiac output, causing a decrease in $S\bar{v}O_2$.

$S\bar{v}O_2$ monitoring will not determine the source of an imbalance between O_2del and V_O_2, nor does it detect regional ischemia. Monitoring of $S\bar{v}O_2$ requires the insertion of a pulmonary artery catheter and hence is inappropriate in many patients.

Noninvasive Hemoglobin Saturation Monitoring

Pulse Oximetry

No monitor of oxygen transport has had a greater impact on the practice of anesthesiology than the pulse oximeter. Unknown in the operating room before the 1980s, the pulse oximeter is now a standard of care for all anesthetics.[47, 48] Its operation requires no special training or new skills on the part of the user. It is noninvasive and almost free of risk. The pulse oximeter gives continuous, real-time estimates of SaO_2, which can warn of hypoxemia from many causes, including loss of airway patency, loss of oxygen supply, and increases in venous admixture.

Figure 18-9 illustrates the stages of the oxygen transport system, showing that the pulse oximeter, like the optode already discussed, monitors oxygen at the level of the arterial blood. Respired gas monitors can confirm only that oxygen is being delivered to the lungs, but the pulse oximeter also monitors the function of the lungs in transporting this oxygen to the arterial blood. Pulse oximetry does not guarantee that oxygen is being delivered to or utilized by the tissues. This can be determined only by monitors functioning further down the oxygen transport chain, such as $PtcO_2$ (see above). This section reviews the physical and engineering principles of pulse oximetry, as well as recent refinements such as adaptive signal filtering to reduce motion-induced errors. The pulse oximeter's accuracy, clinical applications, and limitations are also discussed.

Historical Development of Pulse Oximetry. Although the pulse oximeter became a standard for basic anesthetic

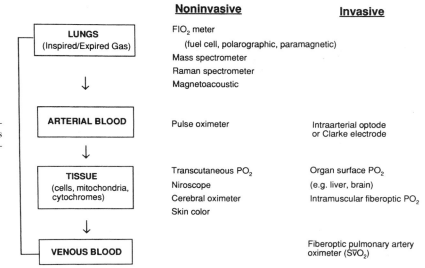

Figure 18–9. Block diagram of the oxygen transport system. Both invasive and noninvasive monitors of oxygenation are listed for each level in the transport process.

monitoring in the operating room in the 1980s, in vivo oximeters actually date back to the 1930s.[49, 50] In 1935, Carl Matthes developed the first instrument that measured SaO_2 by transilluminating tissue. Matthes' device used two wavelengths of light, one visible and one infrared, much like the modern-day pulse oximeter. This instrument could follow saturation trends but was difficult to calibrate. J.R. Squires developed a similar instrument that calibrated itself by compressing the ear to eliminate blood, a technique that was used later in the first commercially marketed in vivo oximeters.

Glen Millikan created the first lightweight ear oximeter in the early 1940s for aviation research. Millikan coined the term *oximeter* to describe his device, which was used to measure hemoglobin saturation in pilots flying at high altitudes. The first report in the anesthesiology literature of the operating room application of an in vivo oximeter was published in 1951.[51] Figure 18–10 shows a detailed record of the hemoglobin saturation obtained from an ear oximeter plotted versus time during a tonsillectomy. Even though this record shows a dramatic fall in saturation during the induction of anesthesia (described, curiously, as "breath holding") the device drew little attention from anesthesiologists until much later. None of these early in vivo oximeters made use of the pulsatile quality of arterial blood, hence none of them were "pulse oximeters."

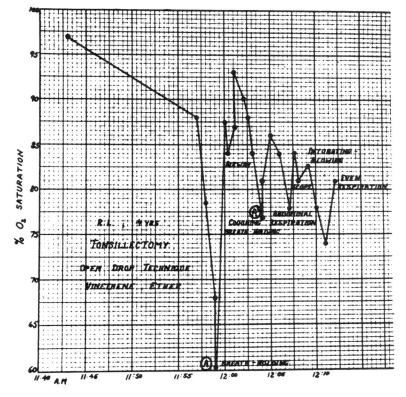

Figure 18–10. Ear oximeter hemoglobin saturation plotted as a function of time for a 4-year-old child undergoing general anesthesia for tonsillectomy. The anesthesia technique was open-drop ether with no supplemental oxygen. Note the significant desaturation associated with "breath holding" during induction of anesthesia. Saturation does not return to its preinduction baseline value at any time during the record. (From Steven RC, Slater HM, Johnson AL, et al: The oximeter: A technical aid for the anesthesiologist. Anesthesiology 1951; 12:548.)

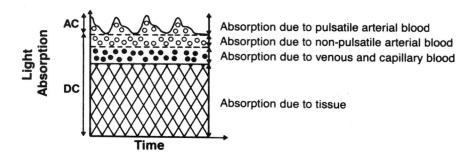

Figure 18–11. A schematic of the light absorbances of living tissue plotted vs. time. The fixed (DC) absorbance results from solid tissues, venous and capillary blood, and the nonpulsatile arterial blood. The AC component is caused by pulsations in the arterial blood volume. (Modified from Ohmeda Pulse Oximeter Model 3700 Service Manual. Boulder, CO, Ohmeda, 1986, p 22.)

The first pulse oximeter was invented by Takuo Aoyagi in the mid-1970s. While developing a method to measure intravenous dye washout curves using light transmission through the ear, Aoyagi discovered that his light-absorbance curves contained fluctuations caused by the arterial pulse. In dealing with this "artifact," he discovered that the relative amplitudes of the fluctuations at the two light wavelengths varied with arterial hemoglobin saturation. This fortuitous discovery soon led him to the creation of the first two-wavelength pulse oximeter, which was marketed by Nihon Kohden Corporation (Osata, Japan). Aoyagi's oximeter used filtered light sources and fiberoptic transmission cables between the instrument and the ear sensor, rendering it somewhat awkward for use in the operating room.

The next breakthrough in pulse oximetry came in the late 1970s, when Scott Wilbur of the Biox Corporation (now Datex-Ohmeda) developed the first ear sensor that used light-emitting diodes (LEDs) and solid-state photodetectors built into the sensor itself. The fiberoptic cables of previous ear oximeters were replaced by a thin electrical cable.[52] The accuracy of the pulse oximeter was also improved by the incorporation of digital microprocessors in the instrument. Further electronic improvements were made by both Biox and Nellcor in the early 1980s, and the pulse oximeter was ready to take its place as a standard operating room monitor. The instrument had now become reliable and easy to use, as well as relatively inexpensive. It gained rapid acceptance and quickly became a standard of care in the operating room by 1987. Today no anesthesiologist would feel comfortable inducing general anesthesia without a functioning pulse oximeter. An excellent review of the history of pulse oximetry and the development of blood gas analysis has been written by Severinghaus and Astrup.[53]

Physical Principles of Pulse Oximetry. Pulse oximeters estimate SaO_2 by measuring the transmission of light at two wavelengths through a pulsatile vascular tissue bed. In principle, the pulse oximeter uses the finger, ear, or other tissue as a "cuvette" containing hemoglobin (see Beer's law, above). However, living tissue contains many light absorbers other than arterial hemoglobin, including skin, soft tissue, bone, and venous and capillary blood. Early in vivo oximeters, such as Millikan's, compensated for this additional tissue absorbance by compressing the soft tissues during a calibration cycle to eliminate all blood. The absorbance of the bloodless tissue was then used as a baseline. Some of these oximeters heated the tissue during measurement to render it hyperemic and thus obtain an absorbance more dependent on arterial blood.

The pulse oximeter distinguishes the light absorbance of arterial blood from that of other absorbers in the tissue in a novel way. As shown in Figure 18–11, light absorbance in tissue can be divided into a constant, or direct current (DC), component and a pulsating, or alternating current (AC), component. Conventional pulse oximetry relies on the assumption that the AC component represents arterial blood, which is the only pulsatile absorber. Any other fluctuating light absorbers will therefore constitute sources of error. The consequences of and recent modifications to this assumption are discussed below under Motion Artifact and Adaptive Digital Signal Filtering.

Current pulse oximeters use two wavelengths of light, usually 660 nm (red) and 940 nm (near infrared). The pulse oximeter measures the AC component of the light absorbance at each wavelength and then divides it by the corresponding DC component (Fig. 18–12), yielding the *pulse added absorbances:* $S_{660} = AC_{660}/DC_{660}$ and $S_{940} = AC_{940}/DC_{940}$. The pulse added absorbances at the two wavelengths are independent of the intensity of incident light. The oximeter then calculates the ratio R of the two pulse added absorbances:

$$R = (AC_{660}/DC_{660})/(AC_{940}/DC_{940}) \qquad (18.10)$$

It can be shown from the Lambert-Beer law that in the absence of dyshemoglobins (COHb, MetHb) the ratio R is uniquely related to the SaO_2. Although the pulse oximeter saturation (SpO_2) can be mathematically derived from the value of R via the theory described above, the oximeter actually uses an empirical calibration curve relating SpO_2 to

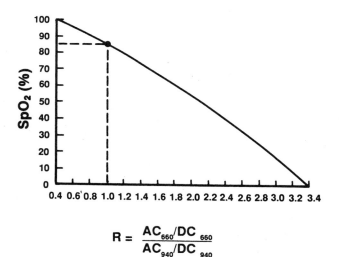

Figure 18–12. A typical pulse oximeter calibration algorithm, in which SpO_2 is plotted vs. the ratio R. The value of R varies from roughly 0.4 at 100% saturation to 3.4 at 0% saturation. An R value of 1.0 corresponds to an SpO_2 reading of 85%. Although a similar curve can be derived from the Lambert-Beer law, the curve used is actually a composite of experimental data obtained on healthy adult volunteers. (Adapted from Pologe JA: Pulse oximetry: Technical aspects of machine design. Int Anesthesiol Clin 1987; 25:142.)

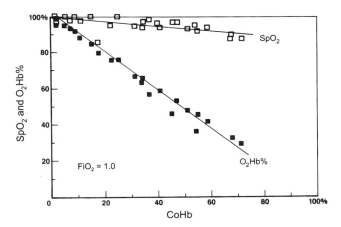

Figure 18–13. SpO₂ and fractional saturation (O₂Hb%) plotted vs. carboxyhemoglobin level (COHb%) for dogs inhaling carbon monoxide 200 ppm. SpO₂ seriously overestimates arterial fractional hemoglobin oxygen saturation in the presence of COHb and remains greater than 90% even for COHb% = 70. The pulse oximeter "sees" COHb as though it were mostly O₂Hb. (From Barker SJ, Tremper KK: The effect of carbon monoxide inhalation on pulse oximeter signal detection. Anesthesiology 1987; 66:677–679.)

R, such as the one shown in Figure 18-12. The calibration curves used in all pulse oximeters today are based on experimental data obtained from human volunteers. This empirical calibration is stored in the microprocessor memory of the pulse oximeter. Although the pulse oximeter does not require user calibration, this does not imply that the instrument calibrates itself for each patient. In fact, the oximeter assumes the same calibration curve for every patient.

Sources of Error. Given the physics and design principles already outlined, the major sources of error in SpO₂ readings are easily predictable. This section examines the most common sources of error, as well as some of the design approaches used to minimize these errors. The user must be well aware of these problems in order to know when to expect erroneous data.

Dyshemoglobins and Intravenous Dyes. Because the pulse oximeter measures light absorbance at two wavelengths, it can deal with unknown concentrations of only two solutes, that is, the two hemoglobin species O₂Hb and RHb (Equations 18.7 and 18.8). If any light-absorbing species other than O₂Hb and RHb is present, the pulse oximeter cannot accurately estimate saturation. As shown by the light absorbance spectra in Figure 18-8, both COHb and MetHb absorb light at one or both of the wavelengths used by the pulse oximeter. Significant concentrations of either of these dyshemoglobins can be expected to produce erroneous SpO₂ values. The fact that "functional saturation" (SaO₂) does not depend explicitly on dyshemoglobin concentrations does not imply that SaO₂ can be determined by a two-wavelength oximeter. In the presence of these additional hemoglobins, no oximeter can measure the concentrations of any hemoglobin species using only two wavelengths of light (Equation 18.8).

The effects of COHb on SpO₂ values have been determined experimentally in dogs.[54] Figure 18-13 shows SpO₂ from pulse oximetry as well as fractional saturation (O₂Hb%) determined by in vitro oximetry, both plotted as functions of COHb (expressed as a percentage of total hemoglobin, COHb%). Even when COHb% reaches levels greater than 70, displayed SpO₂ values remain greater than 90%. The pulse

oximeter thus interprets COHb as though it were composed mostly of O₂Hb, a fact that can be predicted from the absorbance spectra of Figure 18-8. At the wavelength of 660 nm, COHb has roughly the same absorbance as O₂Hb; at 940 nm, COHb is relatively transparent. This is consistent with the clinical observation that patients with carboxyhemoglobinemia have a bright-red or "plethoric" skin color.

The effects of MetHb on SpO₂ values have been similarly evaluated in animal experiments.[41] Figure 18-14 shows SpO₂ and O₂Hb%, again measured by in vitro oximetry, plotted as functions of MetHb%. As in the case of COHb (see Fig. 18-13), the presence of MetHb causes the pulse oximeter to overestimate fractional hemoglobin saturation. However, the behavior of SpO₂ with MetHb is different, in that the SpO₂ values tend to decrease with increasing MetHb until reaching a plateau at about 85%. For MetHb% values greater than roughly 30, there is no further decrease in SpO₂. When the O₂Hb concentration is further decreased by decreasing the fraction of inspired oxygen (FiO₂) at fixed MetHb levels (i.e., increasing the RHb concentration), SpO₂ represents neither functional nor fractional saturation. This fact is again consistent with the light absorbance spectra of Figure 18-8, which show that MetHb has high absorbance values at both wavelengths of light used by the pulse oximeter. This high absorbance, which tends to give MetHb its characteristic brown color, adds to both the numerator and denominator of the ratio R given by Equation 18.10. Increasing both the numerator and denominator of this ratio by a fixed amount tends to drive the value of R toward 1.0. The calibration curve of Fig. 18-12 shows that an R value of 1.0 corresponds to an SpO₂ value of 85%. This may explain why the pulse oximeter tends to read near 85% saturation in the presence of high MetHb levels.[41]

Fetal hemoglobin (HbF) appears to have little effect upon the accuracy of pulse oximetry. This is because the extinction coefficients of HbF at the two wavelengths used by the

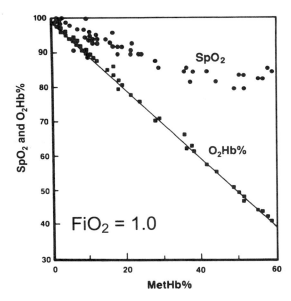

Figure 18–14. SpO₂ and fractional saturation (O₂Hb%) vs. methemoglobin level (MetHb%) for dogs with drug-induced (by benzocaine spray) methemoglobinemia. Although SpO₂ shows a downward trend with increasing MetHb%, O₂Hb% is consistently overestimated and it appears that a plateau is reached at SpO₂ = 85%. When FiO₂ is decreased during this experiment, SpO₂ measures neither functional nor fractional saturation. (From Barker SJ, Tremper KK, Hyatt J, et al: Effects of methemoglobinemia on pulse oximetry and mixed venous oximetry.)

pulse oximeter (660 and 940 nm) are not very different from the corresponding values for adult hemoglobin (HbA). This is fortunate because the percentage of HbF present in neonatal blood varies with gestational age and is not accurately predictable. On the other hand, HbF does produce small errors in multiwavelength in vitro oximeters. The oxygenated state of HbF is interpreted by these laboratory oximeters as consisting partially of COHb.[55]

Theoretical considerations suggest that sickle cell hemoglobin (Hb S) should also have little effect on pulse oximeter accuracy, but this is difficult to confirm experimentally. It would be unethical to subject homozygous (SS) patients intentionally to hypoxemia in order to determine pulse oximeter accuracy. There are a few clinical studies involving SS patients, either in their normal health or during a sickle cell crisis. However, these studies have produced conflicting results. Among other problems, it is not clear what should be the gold standard with which to compare SpO_2 values in SS patients. One study, which concluded that SpO_2 overestimated SaO_2 with a bias of 6.9%, used an in vitro multiwavelength CO oximeter as the comparison standard.[56] However, the standard laboratory CO oximeter is designed to function in the presence of only four types of hemoglobin: RHb, O_2Hb, COHb, and MetHb. Its accuracy in the presence of Hb S must be confirmed before it is used as a standard for pulse oximetry. Some studies have used as a standard the SaO_2 calculated from the PaO_2, which is measured by standard blood gas electrodes. This method is highly suspect if standard oxygen-hemoglobin dissociation curves are employed, because it is well known that SS patients have abnormal dissociation curves. At least two studies have actually measured the O_2 dissociation curves of individual SS subjects and then used these to calculate SaO_2 from PaO_2.[57, 58] These studies concluded that pulse oximeter accuracy is maintained in the presence of SS disease, as long as differences in O_2 dissociation curves are accounted for. All clinical studies of these high-risk patients have the disadvantage of a limited range of available SaO_2 values.

The ratio R, and hence the SpO_2 value, can be affected by any substance present in the blood that absorbs light at 660 or 940 nm. Dyes injected intravenously for diagnostic purposes can therefore have significant effects on SpO_2. Intravenous methylene blue can produce sudden large decreases in SpO_2 values in normal subjects.[59] Indigo carmine yields small decreases in SpO_2, and indocyanine green has an intermediate effect. Bilirubin appears to have no significant effect on SpO_2 at concentrations seen clinically.[60] Nail polish has variable effects upon SpO_2 values, usually producing falsely low readings.[61] Relatively opaque, acrylic nail polish can prevent the pulse oximeter from detecting any pulsatile absorbance at all. This problem can be averted by simply rotating the sensor 90 degrees, so that the coated fingernail does not fall within the light path. Alternatively, an earlobe may be used as the site for sensor placement.

Wavelength Uncertainty. The LEDs used as light sources by the pulse oximeter are not ideal monochromatic (i.e., single-wavelength) radiators; they emit light energy over a narrow but finite range of wavelengths. The center wavelength, or wavelength of peak energy radiation, varies measurably for diodes of the same specification. This variation can easily be ±15 nm. Figure 18–8 shows that a change in wavelength by this amount yields a significantly different extinction coefficient, particularly at the 660-nm wavelength. Pulse oximeter manufacturers have developed two approaches to this problem. The simplest method is to determine the center wavelength of all LEDs and to reject those that are outside of a specified wavelength range, for example, 660 ± 5 nm. This method is effective but expensive

because of the large number of LEDs that must be discarded. The second method is to store multiple calibration algorithms in the pulse oximeter software, corresponding to several different LED center wavelengths. The electrical connector on the sensor cable is then pin-coded so that the appropriate algorithm is selected for a given sensor. Neither of these methods entirely eliminates the effects of wavelength variation. Center wavelength variability does not affect the pulse oximeter's ability to follow changes in saturation, but it will produce between-sensor differences in the absolute value of SpO_2.[62]

Signal-to-Noise Ratio. The amplitude of the fluctuating, or AC, component of the light absorbance may be less than 1% of the amplitude of the DC component. Any influence that decreases the AC absorbance component, increases the DC component, or adds an artifactual AC component not related to arterial pulsations will worsen the signal-to-noise ratio. The AC signal is decreased in low-perfusion states; the DC signal is increased by ambient light reaching the detector; and artifactual AC signals are caused by motion of the patient (e.g., shivering), fluctuating external light sources, or venous pulsations (e.g., tricuspid regurgitation).

The photodiode light detector used in the pulse oximeter sensor cannot discriminate one wavelength of light from another; it is effectively "color blind." The detector therefore responds to ambient room light, as well as to light from either of the LEDs. In most pulse oximeters, this problem is alleviated by activating the red and infrared LEDs in an alternating sequence. During a part of this sequence, both LEDs are turned off and the photodetector determines the ambient background light. This sequence is repeated many times per second (e.g., 480 Hz) in an attempt to eliminate light interference from rapidly changing ambient sources. Despite this design, ambient light artifact can create problems with the pulse oximeter signal-to-noise ratio. This difficulty can be minimized by covering the sensor with an opaque shield of some sort, such as a surgical drape or towel.

If the peripheral pulse is weak, as during shock, the AC absorbance signal becomes extremely small compared with the DC signal. The pulse oximeter has an automatic gain control that adjusts either the LED light intensity or the photodetector amplifier gain to compensate for changes in AC signal amplitude. When the pulsatile absorbance is small, the pulse oximeter maximizes its amplifier gain or LED brightness. Unfortunately, this process also amplifies background noise from all sources, including ambient light. At the highest amplifier gain, the pulse oximeter may interpret components of the background noise as a pulsatile absorbance and generate an SpO_2 value from this artifact.[52] This phenomenon could be easily demonstrated in early pulse oximeters by placing a piece of paper between the photodetector and the LEDs in the sensor. Many first-generation pulse oximeters would amplify the background noise and display a pulse and SpO_2 value from the paper.

The low signal-to-noise ratio problem is also demonstrated by the so-called penumbra effect.[63] If a pulse oximeter finger sensor is partially dislodged or malpositioned in such a manner that the light passes through the fingertip at a grazing incidence, the oximeter may display a correct heart rate but an erroneous SpO_2 value. The SpO_2 value from a malpositioned sensor is usually falsely low during normoxemia, but it may be falsely high during hypoxemia.[64] For example, one very common pulse oximeter with a malpositioned finger sensor yielded an SpO_2 value of 91% in a subject whose actual saturation was 70%.[64] This behavior may be another example of the $R = 1.0$ phenomenon (Equation 18.10), discussed above.

All pulse oximeters display some sort of visual indicator

or pulsatile absorbance signal. This may be a simple one-dimensional laddergram display or a two-dimensional absorbance-vs-time plethysmogram. In most pulse oximeters, the displayed waveform represents the signal output after amplification and therefore does not correspond to the actual amplitude of the absorbance pulsations. However, a few manufacturers have chosen to display a waveform whose height represents the pulsatile absorbance before amplification. The user must therefore determine what the waveform measures, but in general it cannot be assumed that waveform amplitude has any relation to pulse amplitude. The pulse oximeter is not a quantitative monitor of peripheral perfusion, and it cannot be relied upon to warn of impending ischemia.

The behavior of pulse oximeters during shock or low-perfusion states has been examined in both humans and animals.[65-71] During hemorrhagic shock, the pulse oximeter may display no SpO$_2$ value at all, or give a falsely low estimate. One ICU study showed that loss of signal was associated with low cardiac output, extremes in systemic vascular resistance, hypothermia, and extreme anemia.[65] A study of failure rates in the operating room found that pulse oximeters (Nellcor N-100, Ohmeda 3700) failed in 1.12% of all patients.[66] Failure in this case was defined as the lack of an SpO$_2$ value for a cumulative period of 30 minutes or greater. If the original finger sensor failed to function in a particular patient, other probe sites (ear, nose) were tried before the test was declared a failure. Higher failure rates were associated with poor preoperative physical status, long operations, and advanced age. A more recent study employed computerized anesthesia records, and found that 9% of all cases (n = 9203) had gaps in SpO$_2$ data of 10 minutes or more.[72] Higher failure rates were associated with higher American Society of Anesthesiologists (ASA) physical status number, hypotension, and hypothermia.

Several studies have aimed at determining the thresholds for loss of signal during low-perfusion states. Lawson et al.[67] produced gradual occlusion of blood flow with a pressure cuff while monitoring flow at the fingertip with a laser-Doppler flow probe. They found in healthy volunteers that the pulse oximeter lost signal when blood flow had decreased to an average of 8.6% of its baseline value, which occurred at an average cuff pressure of 96% of systolic pressure. Upon cuff deflation the signal returned at a blood flow of 4% of baseline. Severinghaus and Spellman[72] studied pulse oximeter behavior during several types of reduction in finger blood flow, including blood pressure cuff, brachial artery pressure clamp, and arm elevation. Failure occurred at higher mean arterial pressures with the arterial clamp than with gravitational hypotension, showing the importance of pulsatility of the blood volume. These studies demonstrate that the pulse oximeter functions well over a wide range of blood flows and blood pressures in the extremity. Because it is designed to function independently of changes in flow or pressure, the pulse oximeter cannot be used to measure the adequacy of peripheral perfusion, even though there have been attempts to do so.[68-70, 74]

The electrosurgical unit (ESU), or "Bovie," is another potent source of artifact. Although the ESU does not generate light, the electromagnetic radiation from its electrode is very intense and fills the operating room whenever the device is activated. The electrical cable leading from the pulse oximeter sensor to the instrument acts as an antenna that responds to the electromagnetic radiation from the ESU. This interference can be clearly seen on the electrocardiogram (ECG) waveform, where it usually drowns the ECG in a sea of noise. Early-generation pulse oximeters were similarly affected: the SpO$_2$ value would disappear upon ESU activation, and a new value would not appear until 10 to 20 seconds

after deactivation. Newer pulse oximeters have greatly improved in this respect. In most clinical situations, they continue to display and update SpO$_2$ and heart rate values during ESU use. However, most pulse oximeters continue to display their last "valid" SpO$_2$ value for some time during loss-of-signal periods. Therefore, the user can assume that the pulse oximeter is actually measuring SpO$_2$ during ESU activation only if a reasonable plethysmograph waveform is displayed during these periods.

Motion Artifact and Adaptive Digital Signal Filtering. Artifacts caused by patient motion have plagued pulse oximetry, particularly in the recovery room and ICU. While loss of signal and erroneous readings due to motion occur infrequently in the operating room (1% to 2%), they can cause a false alarm incidence exceeding 50% in recovery room and ICU settings.[75] Patient motion, such as shivering, causes a large fluctuating absorbance signal that is incorrectly interpreted by the pulse oximeter algorithm. Instrument manufacturers have approached this problem in the past by two methods: (1) increasing signal averaging time, and (2) ECG synchronization. In the first approach, the value of the ratio R is stored on a beat-to-beat basis and averaged for several seconds. This running average is less sensitive to patient motion but is also slower to respond to sudden changes in saturation. The reduction in false alarm rate is thus accompanied by a slower response to true alarms. In the second approach, developed by Nellcor, the pulse oximeter compares the pulsatile absorbance signal with a simultaneous ECG waveform to ensure that arterial pulsations are synchronized with the ECG.[76] When this "C-lock" feature of the Nellcor N-200 is used, absorbance pulsations that are not correlated with an ECG R wave are rejected and do not influence the SpO$_2$ value. Although this feature has been available for years, C-lock has not significantly improved the reliability of the pulse oximeter during patient motion.

A more elegant solution to the motion problem is to determine the "noise signal," then subtract the noise from the total signal, leaving a noise-free signal from which to calculate the SpO$_2$. This "adaptive filtering" technique requires that the noise signal be identified and distinguished from the "true" signal, a step that has not been accomplished until recently. Masimo Inc. (Newport Beach, CA) has employed this approach to develop an algorithm called Signal Extraction Technology (SET), which improves pulse oximeter performance in the presence of motion artifact.[77, 78] The method is based on two assumptions. (1) Most of the noise associated with motion artifact is produced by pulsations in venous blood volume resulting from movement. The conventional pulse oximeter assumes that only arterial blood pulsates. Pulsating venous blood will produce an additional fluctuating absorbance which will cause errors in the calculation of R and hence SpO$_2$. (2) Since motion artifact is produced by venous pulsations, the second assumption is that the saturation values from these pulsations will be less than arterial values. (That is, venous blood has a lower saturation than arterial blood.) The Masimo SET electronically scans all possible values of the ratio R, corresponding to 0% through 100% saturation, and calculates the signal intensity at each possible R value, as shown in Figure 18–15. In this example of a "discrete saturation transform," there is an intensity peak at 80% saturation and another peak at 97% saturation. The higher peak corresponds to the arterial pulsations and is used to calculate SpO$_2$. The lower peak at 80% presumably represents the venous pulsations. This entire sequence is repeated once per second on the most recent 6 seconds of raw data. The Masimo SET SpO$_2$ value thus represents a 6-second running average of SaO$_2$, updated every second.

This new technology has been evaluated in a volunteer

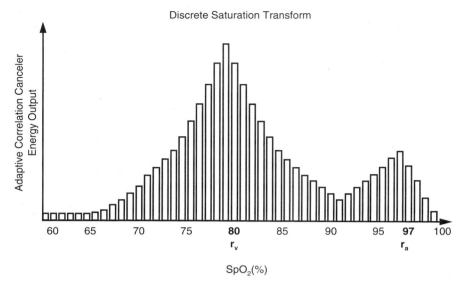

Discrete Saturation Transform

Figure 18–15. Discrete saturation transform: a plot of adaptive correlation canceler energy output vs. possible SpO$_2$ values. Two peaks occur in the energy output. The right-hand peak (r$_a$ = 97%) corresponds to the arterial saturation and yields the displayed SpO$_2$ value. The left-hand peak (r$_v$ = 80%) may correspond to the saturation of the venous blood, although this has not been confirmed experimentally. (Data courtesy of Masimo, Inc., Newport Beach, CA.) (From Barker SJ, Shah NK: Effects of motion on the performance of pulse oximeters in volunteers. Anesthesiology 1996; 85:780.)

experiment in which motion was induced in one hand while the other hand served as a stationary control.[77] The Masimo SET instrument was compared with the Nellcor N-200 and N-3000 pulse oximeters. In this experiment the Masimo instrument demonstrated greater accuracy during motion, remaining within 7% of the control SpO$_2$ value 99% of the time, as compared with 76% and 87% for the N-200 and N-3000 devices. The difference was even more dramatic if the oximeter sensors were connected to their instruments after the motion was initiated: 97%, 68%, and 47%, respectively.[77]

These findings are supported by a clinical study in the postanesthesia care unit (PACU), comparing the Masimo SET with a Nellicor N-200 in patients who experienced motion artifact upon initial application of the pulse oximeter. In 100 patients, there were 27 false alarms for the Masimo vs. 94 for the N-200. While both oximeters exhibited losses of signal and falsely low SpO$_2$ values, the incidence and duration of these events were significantly less in the Masimo instrument.[78] These two studies show promising results for the next generation of pulse oximeters. If the improved performance is confirmed in clinical use, this will promote wider application of pulse oximetry in settings previously limited by patient motion. Additional studies will determine whether this new approach yields better performance in settings of low perfusion, such as shock or post cardiopulmonary bypass.

Clinical Applications: Accuracy and Response

Methods-Comparison Studies. This section reviews clinical applications of pulse oximetry, particularly in the operating room and recovery room. We also discuss the physiologic limitations of pulse oximetry; that is, what clinical changes can and cannot be determined from saturation monitoring. In reviewing studies of pulse oximeter accuracy, some simple statistical tools are needed. Clinical studies of pulse oximeter accuracy are examples of methods-comparison studies, in which two independent methods are used to measure the same variable simultaneously. One of the two methods is generally a new or unproven technique (in this case, pulse oximetry) and the other method is considered a gold standard. The gold standard for pulse oximeter studies is usually a multi-wavelength in vitro CO oximeter, such as the Instrumentation Laboratory model IL 482 (Lexington, MA) or Radiometer OSM-3 (Copenhagen, Denmark). Such devices claim an uncertainty on the order of ±1% (1 SD) for

measurements of fractional saturation [Equation (18.8)]. Because the accuracy of today's pulse oximeters may be comparable to this figure (generally ±2%), we must remember that both methods in such comparison studies have uncertainty. Thus there is rarely a true gold standard of absolute accuracy for any monitor.

The most commonly recommended statistics for evaluating methods-comparison studies are the "bias and precision" as defined by Bland and Altman.[18] The *bias* is defined to be the mean difference between a number of simultaneous measurements by the two methods, and the *precision* is the standard deviation of this difference. (We have suggested calling the latter quantity the "imprecision," because a larger value implies a less precise measurement.) In this text, we define the difference between measurements as the pulse oximeter SpO$_2$ value minus the CO oximeter O$_2$Hb% value. In some of the literature, particularly in Europe, the opposite sign is used. The bias will measure systematic error, that is, the tendency of one of the two methods to consistently overestimate or underestimate relative to the other. The precision represents the variability or random error between the two methods. If both the systematic and random errors are within acceptable limits, then the methods-comparison study can conclude that one method can replace the other.

Unfortunately, many published methods-comparison studies do not include bias and precision values. Some do not even include a scattergram, or graphical representation of the method A versus method B data. The reported statistics often include Pearson's correlation coefficient r and a linear regression slope and intercept of the data. Although sometimes useful, these statistics are not the most informative for evaluating methods-comparison data. The correlation coefficient is not a measure of the agreement between two variables; it is a measure of their association. It is affected by the range of values covered by the data as well as by the agreement between the two methods. Similarly, linear regression slope and intercept are meaningless if the data points fall within a narrow range of values.

Most pulse oximeter manufacturers claim an accuracy of ±2% (1 SD) for SpO$_2$ values between 70% and 100%. The uncertainty increases to ±3% for SpO$_2$ values between 50% and 70%, and no accuracy is specified for SpO$_2$ values below 50%. This implies that for saturations above 70%, the SpO$_2$ value should be within 2% of the actual saturation 68% of the time, and within 4% (2 SD) 95% of the time. Table 18–3 summarizes the results from 12 studies of pulse oximeter

Table 18-3. Pulse Oximeter Experimental and Clinical Accuracy Data

Reference	Manufacturer*	r	s	I	N	SEE% (S_{yx})	Range (% High–Low)	Bias ± Prec.
Experimental Studies in Adult Volunteers								
Yelderman	N-100	0.98	1.03	−2.33	79	1.83	98–65	
Chapman	Biox II	0.96	0.79	17.9	117	2.72	100–54	
Kagle	Ohmeda 3700 (XJI)	0.99	0.96	4.59	48	2.7†	99–60	
	N-100	0.99	0.96	5.34	48	2.7†	99–60	
Severinghaus	N-100				60		70–40	6.6 ± 10.8
	N-200				60		70–40	−4.5 ± 8.2
	Ohmeda 3700				60		70–40	2.7 ± 5.8
	CR (.28)				60		70–40	1.4 ± 5.9
	PC (1600)				60		70–40	0.0 ± 3.5
	NO (3.3)				120		70–40	1.1 ± 5.4
	MQ (7)				36		70–40	−2.9 ± 5.2
	Datex				59		70–40	−1.6 ± 5.4
Nickerson	Ohmeda 3700				165		100–65	−2.6 ± 2.1
	CR				165		100–65	−1.0 ± 2.8
	N-100				165		100–65	−0.4 ± 1.7
	NO				165		100–65	−1.0 ± 1.6
Clinical Studies in Adult Patients								
Tremper‡	Biox III	0.57	0.93	5.22	383	3.09	100–81	1.4 ± 3.1
Mihm	N-100	0.96	0.97	1.51	131		100–56	
Cecil	Ohmeda 3700	0.83	0.95	0.42	333		100–62	−0.31 ± 2.44
	N-100	0.80	0.78	21.2	330		100–62	0.59 ± 3.02
Clinical Studies in Pediatric Patients								
Fait	N-100	0.89	1.05	−6.56	192		100–70	
Boxer	N-100	0.95	1.01	0.15	108		95–35	−0.87 ± 3.7
Clinical Studies in Neonatal Patients								
Mok	N-100	0.84	0.65	27.8	27		100–43	1.4
Durand		0.86	0.68	29.6	108	2	100–78	−0.2 ± 2.5

The values r, s, and I are linear regression correlation coefficients, slopes, and intercepts, respectively; N, number of data pairs; SEE (S_{yx}), the standard error of the estimate; Bias, the mean difference between SpO_2 and SaO_2; Prec, the standard deviation of the differences.

* All manufacturers' specified accuracies are similar; 1 SD = ±2%, 100% to 70–80%, 1 SD = ±3%, 70–80% to 50%, and unspecified <50%. Manufacturers: N-100 and N-200 (Nellcor); Biox II, Biox III, and Ohmeda 3700 (Ohmeda); CR (Critikon); PC 1600 (Physio-Control); NO (Novametrix); MQ (Marquest); and Datex. The software revision is in parentheses following the manufacturer abbreviation when this information was provided in the referenced study. (Nellcor N100 Technical Manual. Hayward, CA, Nellcor Corporation; Ohmeda 3700 Pulse Oximeter Technical Manual. Boulder, CO, Ohmeda Division of BOC; Novametrix 500 Pulse Oximeter Technical Manual. Wallingford, CT, Novametrix Medical Equipment.)

† These values of S_{yx} are determined from the authors' 99% confidence intervals.

‡ The SpO_2 data were collected in patients with pulmonary artery catheters for simultaneous cardiac output determinations. Therefore, these patients were probably more critically ill than those in the other studies.

Modified from Tremper KK, Barker SJ: Pulse oximetry. Anesthesiology 1989; 70:98–108 [see table references].

accuracy: 5 in healthy volunteers, 3 in adult patients, and 2 each in pediatric and neonatal patients.[49] As shown in the table, the various authors have presented their data in different ways. In addition to correlation and linear regression, some authors also provide standard error of the estimate $S_{y,x}$ which is the standard deviation of the y-values about the linear regression line.

Response to Rapid SpO_2 Changes. Two of the volunteer studies shown in Table 18-3 are of special interest in that they evaluated both accuracy and response times to relatively sudden changes in hemoglobin saturation.[79, 80] Both studies discovered errors in pulse oximeter calibration algorithms, which were subsequently revised by some of the manufacturers. As a result of these "after-market" software revisions, seemingly identical pulse oximeters may actually function differently. Reports of experimental studies should therefore specify not only the pulse oximeter manufacturer and model number but also the software version installed.

The pulse oximeter response times to sudden changes in saturation are much shorter for ear than finger probes, as shown in Figure 18-16.[79] The time for a 50% response to rapid desaturation or resaturation ranged from 10 to 20 seconds for the ear probe, whereas for the finger probes it varied between 24 and 50 seconds. Similar results were obtained in another study comparing response times of finger probes to those of both ear probes and reflectance sensors on the forehead.[81] Both studies showed wide variations among subjects in response times for finger sensors. These time delays and their variability should be considered in the selection of sensor sites in clinical situations wherein SpO_2 can change rapidly, for example, in the operating room. On the other hand, clinical studies also find that finger sensors are currently the most reliable in obtaining SpO_2 values during periods of hemodynamic instability.[82]

The pulse oximeter's response to sudden SaO_2 changes is also affected by the signal-averaging time of the instrument, which is often user-selectable. The SpO_2 value will respond more quickly to a rapidly changing SaO_2 if a short averaging time is selected. On the other hand, if the signal-to-noise ratio is marginal or frequent artifacts (e.g., electrocautery) are present, a longer averaging time will yield more accurate SpO_2 values. The user must determine the appropriate averaging time on the basis of the clinical setting. The default averaging time, the value applied when the instrument is first turned on, also varies among manufacturers. The user should know this default value for his or her particular instrument.

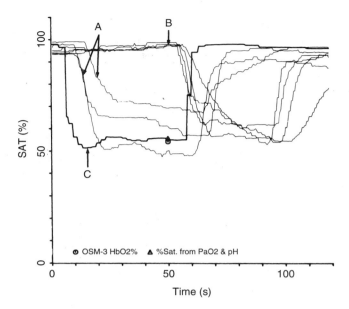

Figure 18-16. Tracings of SpO_2 vs. time for seven pulse oximeters during a rapid and brief desaturation in a healthy volunteer. Tracings labeled *A* represent three ear sensors; tracings *B* are four finger sensors; tracing *C* is the actual saturation calculated from expired oxygen tension measured by mass spectrometry. The ear sensors register the desaturation with a 10- to 15-second time lag, whereas the finger sensors show a nearly 50-second time lag in this volunteer. (Adapted from Severinghaus JW, Naifeh KH: Accuracy of response of six pulse oximeters to profound hypoxia. Anesthesiology 1987; 67:553.)

Pulse Oximeter Accuracy. The accuracy of pulse oximetry found in most clinical studies is comparable to the manufacturers' specifications, as shown in Table 18-3. However, the user must be aware that the specified uncertainty of $\pm 2\%$ to $\pm 3\%$ refers to 1 SD, or a confidence interval of 68%. That is, 68% of a large number of measurements made simultaneously by a gold standard would fall within 1 SD of the SpO_2 value. If the desired confidence interval is 95%, the uncertainty becomes 2 SD, or $\pm 4\%$ to $\pm 6\%$.

Clinical studies of accuracy generally pool data from multiple patients to determine the uncertainty in SpO_2 values. This procedure yields a more pessimistic view of accuracy than would be obtained by studying results for individual patients. If a pulse oximeter sensor is placed on a patient and the SpO_2 value is 95%, there is a 68% probability that the patient's true saturation lies between 93% and 97% (± 1 SD). On the other hand, if the displayed SpO_2 value on that same patient decreases from 95% to 93%, the fact that the patient's saturation is actually falling is more certain than is the original absolute SpO_2 value. This variability among patients is a price we pay for the convenience of having the pulse oximeter precalibrated with a universal algorithm. This calibration algorithm represents an average of data from a large number of healthy adult volunteers. Alternatively, manufacturers could have required user calibration on each individual patient. This would have yielded a more accurate pulse oximeter, but it would have removed one of the most attractive features of pulse oximetry, namely, the absence of user calibration and the immediate availability of SpO_2 data when the sensor is placed on the patient.

To use any monitor intelligently, the clinician must know when to suspect a problem with the accuracy of the data and what actions to take next. In the case of pulse oximetry, these actions depend on the reason the SpO_2 value is considered suspicious. As already noted, the current gold standard for validation of SpO_2 is in vitro multiwavelength CO oximetry. Laboratory CO oximeters can determine either functional or fractional hemoglobin saturation even in the presence of MetHb or COHb. If the user suspects significant dyshemoglobinemia, as in a patient with a smoke inhalation injury, then CO oximeter analysis of an arterial blood specimen is mandatory. But if the SpO_2 value is suspicious with little possibility of a dyshemoglobinemia, an arterial blood gas analysis with calculation of SaO_2 will suffice. An example of this is the healthy patient with dark skin pigmentation whose SpO_2 values fall in the low 90s despite adequate ventilation with an adequate FIO_2. The clinician must remember that the SaO_2 value given by a blood gas analyzer is calculated from the measured PaO_2 and an assumed oxygen-hemoglobin dissociation curve, as shown in Figure 18-17.

Clinical Effectiveness of Pulse Oximetry. Since the pulse oximeter became a minimum standard of anesthesia care in the operating room in 1986,[83] it has been unethical to perform randomized controlled studies of its clinical effectiveness in that setting in the United States.[47] Before pulse oximetry was a minimum standard, several such studies were performed. Coté et al.[84] studied 152 pediatric patients during anesthesia and surgery. In one half of these patients, the SpO_2 data were unavailable to the anesthesiologist. The study found that major events, defined as SpO_2 less than 85% for more than 30 seconds, occurred significantly more often in those patients for whom the SpO_2 values were unavailable. Most of these major events occurred in patients under 2 years of age. A study of adult patients undergoing gynecologic surgery demonstrated SpO_2 values of less than 90% in 10% of all procedures and values of less than 85% in 5% of procedures.

After the pulse oximeter became a standard of care in the operating room, it had a major impact in other clinical settings as well. Two studies monitored SpO_2 during transport from the operating room to the recovery room and found a

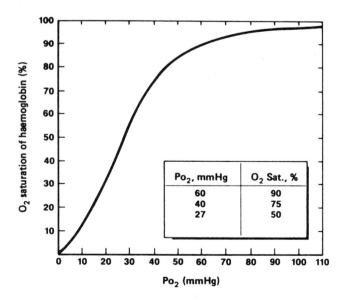

Figure 18-17. The oxyhemoglobin dissociation curve. Hemoglobin saturation is plotted as a function of arterial oxygen tension (PaO_2, mmHg). Under normal conditions for adults, a PaO_2 of 27 mmHg yields a saturation (O_2 Sat. %) of 50% (P = 50). The curve is shifted to the right by acidosis, hypercarbia, increases in 2,3,-diphosphoglycerate (2,3-DPG), and hyperthermia.

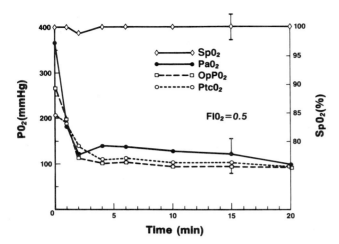

Figure 18-18. Four oxygenation variables plotted vs. time from the onset of endobronchial intubation (Time 0) in a dog at $FIO_2 = 0.5$. Arterial oxygen tension (PaO_2), optode intra-arterial oxygen tension ($OpPO_2$), and transcutaneous oxygen tension ($PtcO_2$) all decreased rapidly during the firts 2 minutes of endobronchial intubation, whereas the SpO_2 value did not change significantly at any time. (From Barker SJ, Tremper KK, Hyatt J, et al: Comparison of three oxygen monitors in detecting endobronchial intubation. J Clin Monit Comput 1988; 4:241.)

high incidence of desaturation, to values less than 90% in patients who did not receive supplemental oxygen.[85, 86] These studies lend strong support to a uniform policy of transporting all patients from the operating room with supplemental oxygen. Clinical studies also suggest that SpO_2 should be continuously monitored in most patients in the recovery room. A study of postoperative pediatric patients showed no correlation between SpO_2 and a traditional postanesthesia score based on motor activity, respirations, blood pressure, mental status, and color.[87] The authors concluded that pediatric patients in the recovery room should be monitored continuously by pulse oximetry or given supplemental oxygen regardless of their apparent state of wakefulness. In another study, 14% of adult patients in the recovery room experienced SpO_2 values less than 90%.[87] A higher incidence of desaturation was associated with obesity, extensive surgery, advanced age, and poor preoperative physical status. Most patients are more likely to experience hypoxemia in the recovery room than in the operating room. In general, patients in the recovery room do not have a protected airway and are not receiving mechanically assisted ventilation, yet they have not recovered completely from the depressant effects of anesthesia and surgery.

Limitations of Saturation Monitoring. A properly functioning pulse oximeter warns of developing hypoxemia. However, at the increased FIO_2 normally used in the operating room, SpO_2 does not provide early warning of decreasing PaO_2. It is clear from the oxyhemoglobin dissociation curve (see Fig. 18-17) that PaO_2 must decrease to less than 80 mmHg before saturation falls significantly. An excellent example of this limitation is the detection of accidental endobronchial intubation. Figure 18-18 shows data from four different oxygenation monitors plotted as functions of time for a dog undergoing general anesthesia at an FIO_2 of 0.5.[88] In addition to SpO_2, the plot shows PaO_2 values from sequential arterial blood samples, $PtcO_2$, and the oxygen tension from an intra-arterial fiberoptic optode blood gas sensor ($OpPO_2$. At 0 minutes on the time axis, the endotracheal

tube was guided from the trachea into the left mainstem bronchus via fiberoptic bronchoscopy. Within 3 minutes, the PaO_2, $PtcO_2$ and $OpPO_2$ values all fell significantly. However, the SpO_2 value never decreased below 98% during the entire experiment. In this situation, the pulse oximeter provided no indication that an endobronchial intubation had taken place, whereas the other monitoring techniques all showed significant changes. Only when the experiment was repeated for FIO_2 values of 0.3 or less did the pulse oximeter display consistent saturation decreases of 6% or more. This illustrates an important physiologic limitation of saturation monitoring: when an increased FIO_2 is used, the PaO_2 value can decrease far below its baseline before the pulse oximeter will alert the clinician. Metaphorically, the pulse oximeter is a sentry standing on the edge of the cliff of desaturation. It gives no warning as we approach the edge of the cliff; it only tells us when we have fallen off.

Finally, no discussion of a clinical monitor is complete without a description of the risks and complications of the monitoring process. Because the pulse oximeter is a noninvasive device that does not (normally) produce heat or radiation, these risks might be expected to be nonexistent. Unfortunately, owing to the possibility of human error, this is not true. In a case report, a Physio-Control pulse oximeter sensor was mistakenly connected to an Ohmeda instrument.[89] The two oximeters use the same electrical connector, but the internal pin connections are entirely different. This resulted in severe thermal burns to both the finger and the earlobe of a newborn infant. The lesson from this case is that compatibility between sensor and instrument must be ensured before a sensor is placed on a patient.

Another risk of pulse oximetry is potential tissue ischemia caused by disposable tape-on sensors. These sensors must be applied with caution, considering that soft tissue often swells during lengthy operations. Any inelastic adhesive device wrapped around the circumference of a digit can act as a tourniquet, particularly if the extremity is dependent or if peripheral edema may occur.

Pulse Oximetry: Conclusions. The pulse oximeter is the most significant advance in oxygen monitoring since the development of the blood gas analyzer. It is the only oxygen monitor that provides continuous, real-time, noninvasive data on arterial oxygenation. Because it is noninvasive and nearly risk-free when used properly, the pulse oximeter should be used in all clinical settings in which there is any risk of arterial hypoxemia. It is already a minimum standard of care in the operating room, and it is rapidly becoming a standard in other critical care settings. Hypoxia remains the most common cause of anesthesia-related preventable mortality.[89, 90] The avoidance of hypoxia is a fundamental goal of the anesthesiologist, and an understanding of both the physics and physiology of continuous saturation monitoring by pulse oximetry can help the anesthesiologist to accomplish this task.

Tissue Oximetry (Near-Infrared Spectroscopy)

We have described how infrared light may be used to determine hemoglobin saturation in arterial blood by analyzing the pulse added absorbance and in venous blood by analyzing the reflected absorbance in the pulmonary artery all based on the similar physics of absorbance spectroscopy. A mean value of the hemoglobin saturation of the blood within a volume of tissue may also be obtained by either measuring light transmitted through the tissue or reflected from the tissue. Because the hemoglobin is within the arterial, capillary, and venous vascular beds, the resulting signal will be a weighted average of all three compartments. The largest volume of blood is within the venous compartment that drains from the tissue; therefore, the signal principally follows the mean venous hemoglobin saturation and has been called tissue oximetry. Hemoglobin is not the only constituent in tissue that changes its light absorbance properties with its state of oxygenation. Within the mitochondria, cytochrome aa_3 (cytaa_3) at the end of the oxygen transport chain also has a light absorbant spectrum in the near-infrared range. Therefore, in theory a near-infrared device could actually measure the oxidative state of the mitochondria within the cells. In 1977 Franz Jobsis[92] described a spectrophotometric technique to measure the saturation of cytaa_3 in the cerebral tissue of living cats. This experimental technique has several technical limitations, including a requirement for high-intensity light, an unknown light path length, and substantial interference of the light absorption by hemoglobin. More recently experimental techniques have been used in infants to measure the oxidative state of both hemoglobin and cytaa_3 in cerebral tissue.[83] Again, it is difficult to set an absolute value of "tissue" saturation because of the problems in determining light path length, which is an essential element of the Lambert-Beer law. There are also simultaneous variations in blood volume and blood saturation that can alter the reading, and finally the inability to empirically calibrate the device because there is no gold standard.[94]

Two approaches have been taken in developing devices to measure brain oxygenation with near-infrared light. The first approach attempts to monitor concentrations of hemoglobin, oxyhemoglobin, and cytaa_3 directly from reflected light. A variety of sophisticated methods have been incorporated into these concentration monitoring devices in an attempt to overcome the aforementioned problems. The specifics of these have been reviewed in an article by Wahr et al.[94] The current production device using these technologies is expensive and has been applied to date primarily in research studies.[94] The second type of device attempts to measure the mean hemoglobin saturation within the tissue between the light source and the detector. In theory, because the device uses the ratio of oxyhemoglobin to reduced hemoglobin, the path length should cancel. In addition, this device does not attempt to measure cytaa_3 saturation specifically and just the global saturation of the hemoglobins within the tissue sample. To form a ratio, this technique uses two frequencies of light analogous to pulse oximetry.[95-97] One of the criticisms of this technique is that the probes that are placed on the skull may be measuring the hemoglobin saturation of the blood in the subcutaneous tissue and not penetrating to the cerebral tissue. In an attempt to minimize this effect, the device measures absorbance ratios with two different light sources at different spacings, subtracting one from the other to eliminate the potential surface absorbance effect[94, 98] (Fig. 18-19). This dual light source technique has been used in the INVOS Monitor (INVOS-3100, Somanetics Inc., Troy, MI) which is the only commercially available saturation measuring device. Although there is no gold standard, the INVOS Monitor has been shown to match predicted (theoretical) decreases in cerebral saturation in volunteers breathing hypoxic gas mixtures.[98]

Several other clinical studies have examined this monitor in situations in which cerebral oxygenation is at substantial risk, that is, during carotid endarterectomy and during cardiopulmonary bypass with or without circulatory arrest.[99-102] Ausman et al.[99] found that five patients in whom the saturation remained above 35% during circulatory arrest had no demonstrable neurologic insult, while the one patient whose saturation fell below 35% had evidence of global hypoxic injury at the postmortem examination. In a subsequent case

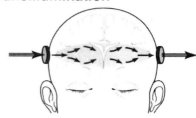

A. Transillumination

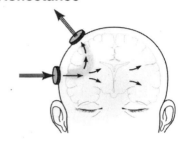

B. Reflectance

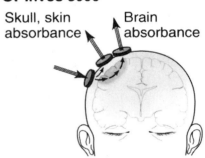

C. Invos 3000

Skull, skin absorbance   Brain absorbance

Figure 18-19. Light absorption may be measured in a transillumination mode *(A)* or in a reflectance mode *(B, C)*. The mode of monitoring determines the proportion of cerebral tissue that will contribute to the light absorbance signal. The Invos 3000 *(C)* uses two light receivers in an attempt to differentiate between light absorbance due to skull and overlying tissues and light absorbance due to cerebral tissue. (From Wahr JA, Tremper KK, Samra SS, et al: Near-infrared spectroscopy: Theory and applications. J Cardiothorac Vasc Anesth April 1996; 10:406-418.)

reported in 1996 no neurologic dysfunction was seen in a patient monitored during circulatory arrest whose cerebral saturation value was below 34% for 15 minutes.[101] On the other hand, Brown et al.[102] reported a poor correlation between the INVOS saturation values compared with jugular bulb venous saturation and patients undergoing elective cardiac surgery. None of these patients had severe desaturations or postoperative neurologic deficits. Samra et al.[100] studied 38 patients undergoing carotid endarterectomies comparing contralateral and ipsilateral saturation values before, during, and after cross-clamping of the carotid. They noted a statistically significant decrease in cerebral saturation on the ipsilateral side of slightly more than 6% in the 38 patients studied, although there was substantial patient-to-patient variability in saturation values. None of these patients had postoperative neurologic dysfunction.[100]

Although cerebral oxygen monitoring is currently not a standard of care in any setting, these data suggest that the device may be useful during procedures in which the cerebral circulation and oxygenation are at extreme risk. Unfortunately, there are insufficient data to date to determine the saturation level at which cerebral ischemia will occur. Therefore, it is not possible to determine sensitivity and specificity in detecting cerebral tissue at risk of damage.

REFERENCES

1. Tremper KK, Barker SJ: Monitoring of oxygen. *In* Lake CL (ed): Clinical Monitoring for Anesthesia and Critical Care, ed 2. Philadelphia, WB Saunders, 1994, pp 196–212.
2. Westenskow DR, Jordan WS, Jordan R, et al: Evaluation of oxygen monitors for use during anesthesia. Anesth Analg 1981; 60:53–56.
3. McGarrigle R, White S: Oxygen analyzers can detect disconnections. Anesth Analg 1985; 63:464–465.
4. Van Slyke DD, Neill JM: The determination of gases in blood and other solutions by vacuum extraction and manometric measurement. Int J Biol Chem 1924; 61:523–557.
5. Guyton AC: Transport of oxygen and carbon dioxide in the blood and body fluids. *In* Guyton A (ed): Textbook of Medical Physiology. Philadelphia, WB Saunders, 1981, pp 504–514.
6. Clark LC: Monitor and control of tissue O_2 tensions. Trans Am Soc Artif Intern Organs 1956; 2:41–48.
7. Severinghaus JW, Bradley AF: Electrodes for blood PO_2 and PCO_2 determination. J Appl Physiol 1958; 13:515–520.
8. Gehrich JL, Lubbers DW, Opitz N, et al: Optical fluorescence and its application to an intravascular blood gas monitoring system. IEEE Trans Biomed Eng 1986; 33:117–132.
9. Barker SJ, Tremper KK, Hyatt J, et al: Continuous fiberoptic arterial oxygen tension measurements in dogs. J Clin Monit Comput 1987; 3:48–52.
10. Shapiro BA, Cane RD, Chomka CM, et al: Preliminary evaluation of an intra-arterial blood gas system in dogs and humans. Crit Care Med 1989; 17:455–460.
11. Kollmeyer KR, Tsang RC: Complications of umbilical oxygen electrodes. J Pediatr 1974; 84:894–897.
12. Harris TR, Nugent M: Continuous arterial oxygen tension monitoring in the newborn infant. J Pediatr 1973; 82:929–939.
13. Katayama M, Murray GC, Uchida T, et al: Intra-arterial continuous monitoring by an ultra fine microelectrode (abstract). Crit Care Med 1987; 15(4):357.
14. Bratanow N, Polk K, Bland R, et al: Continuous polarographic monitoring of intra-arterial oxygen in the perioperative period. Crit Care Med 1985; 13:859–860.
15. Malalis L, Bhat R, Vidyasagar D: Comparison of intravascular PO_2 with transcutaneous and PaO_2 values. Crit Care Med 1983; 11:110–113.
16. Rithalia SVS, Bennett PJ, Tinker J: The performance characteristics of an intra-arterial oxygen electrode. Intens Care Med 1981; 7:305–307.
17. Altman DG, Bland JM: Measurement in medicine: The analysis of method comparison studies. Statistician 1983; 32:307–317.
18. Bland JM, Altman DG: Statistical methods for assessing agreement between two methods of clinical measurement. Lancet 1986; 1:307–310.
19. Altman DG: Statistics and ethics in medical research. Vol 6. Presentation of results. BMJ 1980; 2:1542–1544.
20. Barker SJ, Hyatt J: Continuous measurement of intraarterial pHa, $PaCO_2$, and PaO_2 in the operating room. Anesth Analg 1991; 73:43–48.
21. Mahutte CK, Sassoon CS, Muro JR: Progress in the development of a fluorescent intravascular blood gas system. J Clin Monit Comput 1990; 6(2):147–157.
22. Wahr JA, Tremper KK: Continuous intravascular blood gas monitoring state of the art. J Cardiothorac Vasc Anesth 1994; 8:342–353.
23. Mahutte CK: On-line arterial blood gas analysis with optodes: Current status. J Clin Biochem 1998; 31:119–130.
24. Eberhard P, Hammacher K, Mindt W: Perkutane Messung des Sauerstoffpartialdruckes: Methodik und Anwendungen (abstract). Stuttgart Proc Med Tech 1972; 26.
25. Huch A, Huch R, Meinzer K, et al: Eine schwüle, behitze Ptoberflächenelektrode zur kontinuierlichen Überwachung des PO_2 beim Menschen: Elektrodenaufbau und Eigenschaften (Abstract). Stuttgart Proc Med Tech 1972; 26.
26. Huch R, Huch A, Albani M, et al: Transcutaneous PO_2 monitoring in routine management of infants and children with cardiorespiratory problems. Pediatrics 1976; 57:681–688.
27. Peabody JL, Willis MM, Gregory GA, et al: Clinical limitations and advantages of transcutaneous oxygen electrodes. Acta Anaesthesiol Scand Suppl 1978; 68:76–81.
28. Marshall TA, Kattwinkel J, Berry FA, et al: Transcutaneous oxygen monitoring of neonates during surgery. J Pediatr Surg 1980; 15:797–803.
29. Versmold HT, Linderkamp O, Holzman M, et al: Transcutaneous monitoring of PO_2 in newborn infants. Where are the limits? Influences of blood pressure, blood volume, blood flow, viscosity, and acid base state. Birth Defects 1979; 4:286–294.
30. Baumgardner JE, Graves DJ, Newfeld GR, et al: Gas flux through human skin: Effects of temperature, stripping and inspired tension. J Appl Physiol 1985; 5:1536–1545.
31. Van Duzee BF: Thermal analysis of human stratum corneum. J Invest Dermatol 1975; 65:404–408.
32. Tremper KK, Waxman K, Shoemaker WC: Effects of hypoxia and shock on transcutaneous PO_2 values in dogs. Crit Care Med 1979; 7:526–531.
33. Tremper KK, Shoemaker WC: Transcutaneous oxygen monitoring of critically ill adults, with and without low flow shock. Crit Care Med 1981; 9:706–709.
34. Glenski JA, Cucchiara RF: Transcutaneous O_2 and CO_2 monitoring of neurosurgical patient: Detection of air embolism. Anesthesiology 1986; 64:546–550.
35. Barker SJ, Hyatt J, Clark C, et al: Hyperventilation reduces transcutaneous oxygen tension and skin blood flow. Anesthesiology 1991; 75:619–624.
36. Severinghaus JW: Historical development of oxygenation monitoring. *In* Payne JP, Severinghaus JW (eds): Pulse Oximetry. Berlin, Springer-Verlag, 1986.
37. Brown LJ: A new instrument for the simultaneous measurement of total hemoglobin, % oxyhemoglobin, % carboxyhemoglobin, % methemoglobin, and oxygen content in whole blood. IEEE Trans Biomed Eng 1980; 27:132–138.
38. Martin WE, Cheung PW, Johnson CC, et al: Continuous monitoring of mixed venous oxygen saturation in man. Anesth Analg 1973; 52:784–793.
39. Wilkinson AR, Phibbs RH, Gregory GA: Continuous measurement of oxygen saturation in sick newborn infants. J Pediatr 1978; 93:1016–1019.
40. Beale PL, McMichan JC, Marsh HM, et al: Continuous monitoring of mixed venous oxygen saturation in critically ill patients. Anesth Analg 1982; 61:513–517.
41. Barker SJ, Tremper KK, Hyatt J, et al: Effects of methemoglobinemia on pulse oximetry and mixed venous oximetry. Anesthesiology 1989; 70:112–117.
42. Gettinger A, Detraglia MC, Glass DD: In vivo comparison of two mixed venous saturation catheters. Anesthesiology 1987; 66:373–375.
43. Lee SE, Tremper KK, Barker SJ: Effects of anemia on pulse oximetry and continuous mixed venous oxygen saturation monitoring in dogs. Anesth Analg 1988; 67:S130.
44. Jamieson WRE, Turnbull KW, Larrieu AJ, et al: Continuous monitoring of mixed venous oxygen saturation in cardiac surgery. Can J Surg 1982: 25:538–543.
45. Schmidt CR, Frank LP, Forsythe MJ, et al: Continuous SvO_2 measurement and oxygen transport patterns in cardiac surgery patients. Crit Care Med 1984; 12:523–557.
46. Waller JL, Kaplan JA, Bauman DI, et al: Clinical evaluation of a new fiberoptic catheter oximeter during cardiac surgery. Anesth Analg 1982; 61:676–679.
47. Eichorn JH, Cooper JB, Cullen BF, et al: Standards for patient monitoring during anesthesia at Harvard Medical School. JAMA 1986; 256:1017–1020.
48. American Society of Anesthesiologist: Standards for Basic Intra-Operative Monitoring. Anesthesia Patient Safety Foundation. 1987; March 3.
49. Tremper, KK, Barker SJ: Pulse oximetry. Anesthesiology 1989; 70:98–108.
50. Severinghaus JW, Astrup PB: History of blood gas analysis. Anesth Clin 1987; 25:1–215.

51. Stephen CR, Slater HM, Johnson AL, et al: The oximeter-A technical aid for the anesthesiologist. Anesthesiology 1951; 12: 541–555.

52. Wukitsch MW, Tobler D, Pologe J, et al: Pulse oximetry: An analysis of theory, technology and practice. J Clin Monit Comput 1988; 4:290–301.

53. Severinghaus JW, Astrup PB: History of blood gas analysis. VI. Oximetry. J Clin Monit Comput 1986; 2:270–288.

54. Barker SJ, Tremper KK: The effect of carbon monoxide inhalation on pulse oximeter signal detection. Anesthesiology 1987; 66:677–679.

55. Cornelissen PJH, van Del WC, de Jong PA: Correction factors for hemoglobin derivatives in fetal blood as measured with the IL282 CO-Oximeter. Clin Chem 1983; 29:1555–1556.

56. Craft JA, Alessandrini E, Kenney LB, et al: Comparison of oxygenation measurements in pediatric patients during sickle cell crises. J Pediatr 1994; 124:93–95.

57. Rackoff WR, Kunkel N, Silber JH, et al: Pulse oximetry and factors associated with hemoglobin oxygen desaturation in children with sickle cell disease. Blood 1993; 81:3422–3427.

58. Weston-Smith SG, Glass UH, Acharya J, Pearson TC: Pulse oximetry in sickle cell disease. Clin Lab Haematol 1989; 11:185–188.

59. Scheller MS, Unger RJ, Kelner MJ: Effects of intravenously administered dyes on pulse oximetry readings. Anesthesiology 1986; 65:550–552.

60. Veyckemans F, Baele P, Guillaume JE, et al: Hyperbilirubinemia does not interfere with hemoglobin saturation measured by pulse oximetry. Anesthesiology 1989; 70:118–122.

61. Coté CJ, Goldstein A, Fuschsman WH, et al: The effect of nail polish on pulse oximetry. Anesth Analg 1988; 67:683–686.

62. Pologe JA: Pulse oximetry: Technical aspects of machine design. Int Anesthesiol Clin 1987; 25:137–153.

63. Kelleher JF, Ruff RH: The penumbra effect: Vasomotion-dependent pulse oximeter artifact due to probe malposition. Anesthesiology 1989; 71:787–791.

64. Barker SJ, Hyatt J, Shah NK, et al: The effect of sensor malpositioning on pulse oximeter accuracy during hypoxemia. Anesthesiology 1993; 79:248–254.

65. Tremper KK, Hufstedler S, Barker SJ, et al: Accuracy of a pulse oximeter in the critically ill adult: Effect of temperature and hemodynamics (abstract). Anesthesiology 1985; 63:A175.

66. Freund PR, Overand PT, Cooper J, et al: A prospective study of intraoperative pulse oximetry failure. J Clin Monit Comput 1991; 7:253–258.

67. Lawson D, Norley I, Korbon G: Blood flow limits and pulse oximeter signal detection. Anesthesiology 1987; 67:599–603.

68. Narang VPS: Utility of the pulse oximeter during cardiopulmonary resuscitation. Anesthesiology 1986; 65:239–240.

69. Nowak GS, Moorthy SS, McNiece WL: Use of pulse oximetry for assessment of collateral arterial flow. Anesthesiology 1986; 64:527.

70. Skeehan TM, Hensley FA Jr: Axillary artery compression and the prone position. Anesth Analg 1986; 65:518–519.

71. Barrington KJ, Ryan CA, Finer NN: Pulse oximetry during hemorrhagic hypotension and cardiopulmonary resuscitation in the rabbit. J Crit Care 1986; 1:242–246.

72. Reich DL, Timcenko A, Bodian CA, et al: Predictors of pulse oximetry data failure. Anesthesiology 1996; 84:859–864.

73. Severinghaus JW, Spellman MJ Jr: Pulse oximeter failure thresholds in hypotension and vasoconstriction. Anesthesiology 1990; 73:532–537.

74. Graham B, Paulus DA, Caffee HH: Pulse oximetry for vascular monitoring in upper extremity replantation surgery. J Hand Surg [Am] 1986; 11:687–692.

75. Lawless ST: Crying wolf: False alarms in a pediatric intensive care unit. Crit Care Med 1994; 981–985.

76. Nellcor N-200 Pulse Oximetry Note Number 6. C-LOCK ECG Synchronization Principles of Operation. Hayward, CA, Nellcor, 1988.

77. Barker SJ, Shah NK: Effects of motion on the performance of pulse oximeters in volunteers. Anesthesiology 1997; 86:101–108.

78. Dumas C, Wahr JA, Tremper KK: Clinical evaluation of a proto-

79. Severinghaus JW, Naifeh KH: Accuracy of response of six pulse oximeters to profound hypoxia. Anesthesiology 1987; 67:551–558.

80. Kagle DM, Alexander CM, Berko RS, et al: Evaluation of the Ohmeda 3700 pulse oximeter: Steady-state and transient response characteristics. Anesthesiology 1987; 66:376–380.

81. Barker SJ, Hyatt J: Forehead reflectance pulse oximetry: Time response to rapid saturation change (abstract). Anesthesiology 1990; 73(3A):A544.

82. Barker SJ, Le N, Hyatt J: Failure rates of transmission and reflectance pulse oximetry for various sensor sites. J Clin Monit Comput 1991; 7:102–103.

83. American Society of Anesthesiologists: Standards for basic intraoperative monitoring. Anesthesia Patient Safety Newsletter, March 1987; p 3.

84. Coté CJ, Goldstein EA, Coté MA, et al: A single blind study of pulse oximetry in children. Anesthesiology 1988; 68:184–188.

85. Pullerits J, Burrows FA, Roy WL: Arterial desaturation in healthy children during transfer to the recovery room. Can J Anaesth 1987; 34:470–473.

86. Tyler IL, Tantisira B, Winter PM, et al: Continuous monitoring of arterial oxygen saturation with pulse oximetry during transfer to the recovery room. Anesth Analg 1985; 64:1108–1112.

87. Soliman IE, Patel RI, Ehrenpreis MB, et al: Recovery scores do not correlate with post-operative hypoxemia in children. Anesth Analg 1988; 67:53–56.

88. Barker SJ, Tremper KK, Hyatt J, et al: Comparison of three oxygen monitors in detecting endobronchial intubation. J Clin Monit Comput 1988; 4:240–243.

89. Murphy KG, Segunda JA, Rockoff MA: Severe burns from a pulse oximeter. Anesthesiology 1990; 73:350–352.

90. Keenan RL, Boyan CP: Cardiac arrest due to anesthesia: A study of incidence and causes. JAMA 1985; 253:2373–2377.

91. Taylor G, Larson CP Jr, Prestwich R: Unexpected cardiac arrest during anesthesia and surgery: An environmental study. JAMA 1976; 236:2758–2760.

92. Jobsis FF: Noninvasive infrared monitoring of cerebral and myocardial oxygen sufficiency and circulatory parameters. Science 1977; 198:1264–1267.

93. Cope M, Delpy DT: System for long-term measurement of cerebral blood and tissue oxygenation on newborn infants by infrared transillumination. Med Biol Eng Comput 1988; 26:289–294.

94. Wahr JA, Tremper KK, Samra S, et al: Near-infrared spectroscopy: Theory and applications. J Cardiothorac Vasc Anesth 1996; 10:406–418.

95. Sevick E, Chance B, Leigh J, et al: Quantitation of time and frequency resolved optical spectra for the determination of tissue oxygenation. Anal Biochem 1991; 195:330–351.

96. Haida M, Chance B: A method to estimate the ratio of absorption coefficients of two wavelengths using phase moduclated near infrared light spectroscopy. Adv Exp Med Biol 1994; 345: 829–835.

97. Kiu H, Boas DA, Beauvoit B, et al: Absorption and scattering properties in a highly absorbing turbid medium. Proc Opt Soc Am 1994; 21:272–277.

98. McCormick PW, Stewart M, Goetting MG, et al: Noninvasive cerebral optical spectroscopy for monitoring cerebral oxygen delivery and hemodynamics. Crit Care Med 1991; 19:89–97.

99. Ausman JI, McCormick PW, Stewart M, et al: Cerebral oxygen metabolism during hypothermic circulatory arrest in humans. J Neurosurg 1993; 79:810–815.

100. Samra SK, Dorje P, Zelenock GB, et al: Cerebral oximetry in patients undergoing carotid endarterectomy under regional anesthesia. Stroke 1996; 27:49–55.

101. Samra SK, Chandler WF: Cerebral oximetry during circulatory arrest for aneurysm surgery. J Neurosurg Anesthesiol 1997; 9:154–158.

102. Brown R, Wright G, Royston D: A comparison of two systems for assessing cerebral venous oxyhemoglobin saturation during cardiopulmonary bypass in humans. Anaesthesia 1993; 48:697–700.

19 Arterial Blood Gas Analysis and Monitoring

Charles G. Durbin, Jr., M.D., F.C.C.M.

Interest in arterial blood gases covers a span of several hundred years. Since the discovery of oxygen in air by Joseph Priestley in 1774, humans have been fascinated by the function of this gas in biologic systems. In 1799 Sir Humphrey Davy succeeded in proving that both oxygen and carbon dioxide were present in blood. The full significance of these discoveries, however, was not apparent until the middle of the 20th century.

The value and physiologic interpretation of chemical measurements throughout history have depended on the specific devices used to make the measurements. Improved technology has always driven and expanded the understanding of physiologic processes. The clinical utility of blood gases and acid-base information today depends on the methods of measurement. New understanding of blood gases and acid-base data continue to be shaped by new equipment used to obtain the values of these variables.

For the past 30 years, serial determination of arterial and venous blood gases and hemoglobin saturation have been used to avoid critical events, titrate therapy, and manage a wide variety of clinical conditions. It is essential that the capabilities and limitations of the technology used to determine these variables be kept foremost in mind when using the measured data in clinical applications and patient care decisions.

Blood Oxygen Measurement

Oxygen is essential to all life forms. Oxidation of carbon-containing compounds is fundamental to production of energy for survival, growth, and reproduction. Oxygen deprivation leads to dysfunction and death of higher organisms within a short time. Humans have essentially no reserves of this essential gas, and interruption of ventilation for as little as 10 minutes results in severe organ damage. Much of modern critical care therapy involves maintenance and manipulation of oxygen uptake and delivery. Several methods of oxygen measurement have been developed and are in widespread use.

Techniques

The most common device used today for measurement of arterial oxygen partial pressure (PaO_2) is the Clark electrode. Prior to 1952 when Leland Clark covered a platinum wire with cellophane to exclude proteins, the polarographic technique of measuring oxygen concentration in fluids was discovered by Jaroslav Heyrovsky[1] in 1922. Heyrovsky won the Nobel prize for chemistry in 1959. In 1954 Clark[2] combined the reference electrode in the same package, eliminating drift and improving response time and accuracy; this innovation remains the standard for PaO_2 analysis today. Oxygen ionizes in water and the unpaired electron interacts with the electrode to produce an electrical charge alteration directly related to the oxygen concentration. Prior to development of this technique, there were no clinically useful ways available to measure PaO_2. Although chemical release of gases and vacuum extration techniques (Van Slyke method) accurately measure blood oxygen (and carbon dioxide) content, they are cumbersome and time-consuming to use.[3] With miniaturization of the Clark electrode, smaller samples are necessary to produce accurate results. Indwelling devices have been produced that are able to determine PaO_2 continuously.

Oxygen concentration can be determined by a number of additional techniques. Mass spectroscopy involves analysis of gas mixtures by ionization and dispersion by a magnetic field that separates and identifies the components by their charge-to-mass ratios. Another method uses Raman light scattering, a technique based on exciting the outer shell electrons of the gas and detecting the characteristic light emitted when the electrons return to their unexcited state. These techniques are mainly used for determining concentrations in gas mixtures, not gases dissolved in liquids. Gas separated by a semipermeable membrane in contact with blood will equilibrate with the gases present in the blood. Mass spectroscopic techniques have been used to indirectly determine blood gases by analyzing the gas that equilibrates with arterial blood.

While measurement of PaO_2 is important, the discovery that hemoglobin was capable of loosely binding great quantities of oxygen was monumental to understanding the physiology of the whole organism. Recognition of the nonlinear relationship of PaO_2 to blood content of oxygen required identification of the role of hemoglobin in this process. In 1903, Christian Bohr demonstrated the sigmoid shape of the oxyhemoglobin dissociation curve of whole blood. He also described the effect of CO_2 tension on the position of this curve. A leftward shift of the curve, facilitating uptake of O_2, occurs when CO_2 is released in the lungs. This is known today as the Bohr effect. While PaO_2 is important in determining the activity of oxygen as it relates to the dissolved portion of the gas, the majority of the body's supply of oxygen is determined by the quantity of oxygen bound to hemoglobin.

Measurement of the percentage of oxygen saturation of hemoglobin is simple. Since the various species of hemoglobin have different absorption curves in the visible and infrared spectrum (Fig. 19-1), measurement of absorption at several different wavelengths makes calculation of the relative amount of each species possible. The advent of microcom-

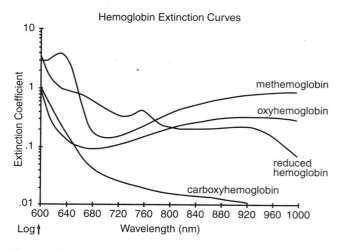

Hemoglobin Extinction Curves

Figure 19–1. Absorption spectra of various species of hemoglobin. By comparing the total absorbance at several different wavelengths, the percentage of each can be estimated. (From Barker SJ, Tremper KK: Pulse oximetry: Applications and limitations. Int Anesthesiol Clin 1987; 25:155–175.)

puters and light-emitting diodes has allowed real-time, noninvasive determination of arterial oxyhemoglobin saturation by pulse oximetry, which is described in detail in Chapter 18. Reflective oximetry through optical fibers embedded in pulmonary artery catheters has been used to continuously determine mixed venous oxygen saturation (see Chapter 14).

Measuring and Monitoring Blood Gases

Usually, blood gases (BGs) are analyzed intermittently, reflecting a single physiologic moment in time. Analysis is often performed at a distant site with a time delay of minutes to hours, thus increasing the disparity between the measurement and the patient's physiologic condition. Repeated measurements are used to determine trends and response to therapy and to understand the patient's physiology. The term "to monitor" means to watch closely and a device or measurement used to watch the patient is called a monitor. The frequency of repeated measurements needed to detect a specific event is determined by the duration of the event. For instance, cardiac arrest caused by anoxia requires less than 1 minute to occur. Intermittent BG measurements performed every several hours would be unlikely to detect the anoxia preceding the arrest, and this form of BG "monitoring" is not appropriate to prevent cardiac arrest from anoxia. Because a decline in arterial oxygen content will precede anoxic cardiac arrest, continuous (rather than intermittent) monitoring of PaO_2 (or saturation) could be used to detect this event and allow intervention prior to occurrence of the poor outcome.[4]

Intermittent measurements are useful to confirm diagnoses and follow longer clinical changes. For instance, the progression of gas exchange abnormalities following aspiration of gastric contents is easily followed with infrequent measurements of arterial BGs. The improvement in oxygenation may be apparent within minutes of increasing the positive end-expiratory pressure (PEEP) or inspired oxygen concentration (FIO_2). BG monitoring may be performed intermittently or continuously with indwelling devices. One noninvasive alternative to indwelling continuous monitoring mentioned previously is pulse oximetry.

Continuous indwelling arterial BG sensors have been developed for use clinically.[5-8] One type is a fiberoptic device that can be placed through a 20-gauge arterial catheter and provide continuous measurement of arterial PO_2, PCO_2, and pH.[9, 10] Optical sensors rely on a color change of an analyte within the fiberoptic system which interacts with the blood component measured. These optode devices have been placed into clinical use.[11, 12] They appear to be stable, accurate, and tolerant of the abuses of the clinical environment for at least several days.[13] The monitors attached to these devices are bulky and expensive, and the value and reliability of this form of monitoring is yet to be determined. Being continuous monitors, however, they provide ongoing information unavailable by any other method. When used selectively, these devices may be cost-effective, reducing the need for other forms of BG sampling and shortening hospital length of stay.[14]

On-demand, in-line testing, and point-of-care determination of BGs are techniques designed to reduce the time for obtaining results during intermittent BG determinations.[15, 16] These techniques are clinically acceptable but less accurate than laboratory-maintained BG analyzers.[17] The contribution they make to patient care and costs is not yet clear. It is apparent that BGs are sampled more frequently with these devices, and this may lead to worsening of the problems of iatrogenic anemia and additional blood transfusions. Point-of-care testing is discussed in more detail in Chapter 24.

Hazards and Pitfalls of Oxygen Partial Pressure Monitoring

Sampling Errors

Samples for intermittent BG measurement are collected by direct arterial puncture with a small-gauge, sterile needle, or from an indwelling arterial catheter. Indications for insertion, techniques for placement, and complications from arterial catheters are discussed in Chapter 13. Direct arterial puncture is performed after raising a skin wheal with a small amount of local anesthetic not containing epinephrine. A small metal needle with a syringe rinsed with a solution containing 0.1 to 1.0 mg/L of heparin is inserted into a palpable artery after sterilizing the skin. Alternatively, a dry pellet of heparin in the syringe can be used to prevent the blood sample from clotting. This is more expensive but avoids the heparin solution contamination problems discussed below. A butterfly needle may be used as an alternative to a hypodermic needle attached to a small (1 to 3 mL) syringe. Pulsatile flow is noted confirming arterial entry. After an adequate sample is withdrawn (0.2 to 1.5 mL, depending on the specific analyzer), the needle is removed and manual pressure applied over the puncture site.

The arterial puncture site should be examined for the development of a hematoma. Infection from a single arterial puncture is rare; pain from hematoma formation is common. Spasm, arterial clot, and ischemia may occur and must be treated to prevent permanent disability. This direct sampling technique is more hazardous in patients who are receiving therapeutic anticoagulation. An indwelling arterial catheter may be of less risk under this circumstance. Raynaud's disease and other arterial occlusive conditions are relative contraindications to repeated direct arterial punctures.

When a blood sample is obtained from an arterial catheter, care must be taken to avoid contamination of the sample with the catheter flush solution. Three times the dead-space amount of fluid must be withdrawn and discarded to produce an uncontaminated sample. A simple way to do this is to note the volume that is withdrawn until blood just appears in the aspirating syringe; this is approximately 80% of the dead-space volume. Removing three to four times this volume guarantees an adequate sample.[18]

Sample Handling

The syringe containing the blood sample should be capped, sealed without any visible air bubbles, and immediately processed in a BG analyzer. If there is to be a delay before performing the analysis (>30 minutes), the sample should be cooled in ice to reduce the metabolic activity of the white blood cells and diffusion of gases through the syringe. While the metabolic activity of white blood cells is normally of little consequence, in patients with leukemia or other causes of an elevated white blood cell count, the changes caused by metabolism may be quite significant.[19, 20] The effects of dilution of the sample with heparin flush solution are indicated in Table 19–1. The most significant abnormality induced by this type of contamination is in the $PaCO_2$ measurement. Because the CO_2 content is directly proportional to the PCO_2 of the blood and very little CO_2 is present in the flush solution, the measured PCO_2 is markedly reduced in the contaminated sample. The bicarbonate concentration is similarly affected because it is merely calculated from the Henderson-Hasselbalch equation. There are commercially prepared heparin-coated syringes in both glass and plastic that obviate the problem of contamination by the heparin solution.

Because plastic is permeable to O_2 and CO_2, some recommend glass syringes for BG sampling. The rate of change BG values in blood contained in plastic syringes is slow and not important if samples are analyzed in a short time.

Variability of Oxygen Measurements

When deciding to make an intervention based on a measurement of PaO_2, it is important to keep in mind the variability of this value as determined from the analyzer. If laboratory or commercially prepared standards are used for quality control, the variability of PO_2 on repeated measurements on the same machine is very small, a standard deviation of 1 to 4 mmHg at clinical levels of PaO_2. This variability depends on the composition of the standard and its temperature. Warm fluorocarbon solutions demonstrate the least variation, and cool aqueous solutions, the most.[21] Failure to meet these

accuracy levels should initiate machine repair as part of a required quality control procedure. Variation between different analyzers is much greater, however. As much as a 10- to 15-mmHg difference in PaO_2 around a "true" PaO_2 of 60 mmHg may occur between different analyzers.[21]

Another source of variability in PaO_2 results from patient factors. With continuous intra-arterial monitoring, the PaO_2 varies quite widely in response to minor interventions and minimal clinical changes. Occasionally, large changes are seen without discernible causes. Some of the variations in the continuous monitors are attributed to the sensor impinging intermittently on the wall of the artery, but others are undoubtedly related to patient factors and reflect true changes.[22] Accuracy and precision of the continuous monitors cannot be determined during use as there is no "gold standard" continuous measurement method with which to compare. Similar variations have been identified in many healthy, normal people using pulse oximetry. Repeated, intermittent arterial BGs in clinically stable patients often show marked variation.[23] The amount of variability which is normal is not known. When an intermittent determined PaO_2 value is interpreted, the potential for this large variability must be borne in mind. Interpretation of the significance of a change must be based on developing trends correlated with other observations rather than on the absolute value obtained.

Temperature Correction of Arterial Oxygen Tension

As blood is cooled, solubility of oxygen is increased. Since BG analyzers are conventionally maintained at 37°C, some suggest that the oxygen value obtained be back-corrected to the patient's actual body temperature. Temperature correction of PaO_2 is usually performed in hypothermic patients. Because O_2 solubility is increased with hypothermia, the partial pressure determined by the analyzer will be higher than that obtained with an analyzer maintained at the same temperature as the patient. Temperature correction, therefore, will lower this value. Physiologically, because metabolic activity is reduced by lower body temperature, the need for oxygen delivery should parallel its availability. Hypothermia also increases hemoglobin's affinity for oxygen, making release more difficult. Temperature correcting the PaO_2 of a hypothermic patient may artifactually indicate the need for increased oxygen in the inspired mixture. However, the risks of administration of extra oxygen (increasing the FIO_2) are minimal, and the extra margin of safety is justified when correcting hypothermic samples. Patients with fevers would appear to have a slightly higher PaO_2 when the sample is temperature-corrected. The impact is much less because of the minimal change (2° to 4°C) that is clinically possible with hyperthermia compared to hypothermia where 10° to 12°C decrease in body temperature is frequent.

Clinical Use of Oxygen Monitoring

Oxygen-Hemoglobin Saturation Relationship

As discussed above, blood contains a large amount of oxygen due to the presence of hemoglobin. Hemoglobin consists of four heme subunit proteins clustered around a ferrous ion. There are four binding sites in each molecule of hemoglobin, one on each subunit. As the first O_2 molecule is bound, the

Table 19–1. Effect of Heparin Solution on Blood Gas Values

Blood Heparin Flush	100% 0%	50% 50%	0% 100%
With Normal Blood Gases*			
PCO_2 (mmHg)	44.9	18.8	3.2
PO_2 (mmHg)	143.5	152.5	171.4
pH	7.41	7.44	6.11
HCO_3^- (mEq/L)	28.2	12.7	0.1
With Low Oxygen and Bicarbonate*			
PCO_2 (mmHg)	16.2	7.2	0.1
PO_2 (mmHg)	45.1	48.1	171.4
pH	7.25	7.25	6.11
HCO_3^- (mEq/L)	16.2	7.2	0.1

*The top section illustrates the effect on a relatively normal sample; the bottom section shows the effect on a hypoxic sample with metabolic acidosis. The major effects of dilution are on the PCO_2 measurement and HCO_3^- calculation.

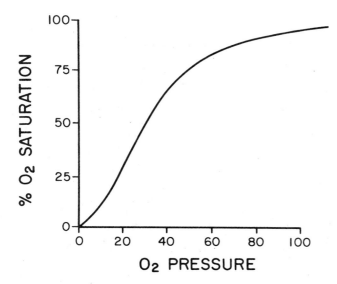

Figure 19-2. The relationship between the P_{O_2} and the percentage saturation of hemoglobin is demonstrated. The sigmoid shape of the curve is due to increased ease of binding of successive O_2 molecules.

other chains rotate and the binding of the next O_2 molecule is facilitated. This change in subunit configuration occurs with the addition of each successive O_2 molecule until all four binding sites are occupied.[24, 25] This allosteric cooperation accounts for the shape of the oxyhemoglobin dissociation curve (Fig. 19-2).

The relationship between oxygen saturation and P_{O_2} is important to remember in clinical practice. A simple rule of thumb is that at a P_{O_2} of 40 mmHg, hemoglobin is about 70% saturated; at 60 mmHg, it is about 90% saturated. The "40, 50, 60/70, 80, 90 rule" is illustrated in the following easy-to-recall form:

P_{O_2} (mmHg)	40	50	60
% Saturation	70	80	90

Measurement of Hemoglobin Saturation

Measurement of hemoglobin saturation is easily carried out by determining the light absorbance in the visual and infrared spectral range by photodetection in a co-oximeter. Oxygenated hemoglobin absorbs light in a different pattern than deoxygenated hemoglobin. The absorbance spectra for these species are illustrated in Figure 19-3. By comparing the absorbance at several wavelengths, the percentage of saturated hemoglobin can be calculated. Current co-oximeters use at least four different wavelengths and calculate carboxyhemoglobin and methemoglobin percentages as well as the percentage of oxygen saturation of normal hemoglobin.

Alterations in Oxygen-Hemoglobin Association Relationship

Various conditions, such as those listed in Table 19-2, affect the position of the oxyhemoglobin dissociation curve. Major factors shifting the curve to the right (reducing hemoglobin affinity for oxygen) are acidosis (respiratory or metabolic),

fever, and increased 2,3-diphosphoglycerate (2,3-DPG). Minor factors include increased hemoglobin concentration, exogenous cortisol, hyperaldosteronism, and hyperthyroidism. Factors that shift the curve to the left (producing more avid binding of oxygen) are cold, alkalosis, reduced 2,3-DPG, anemia, hypothyroidism, carboxyhemoglobin, and methemoglobin.[26] Genetic hemoglobin variants have various effects on the curve. The clinical significance of these changes in hemoglobin-oxygen affinity have not been established.[27] Conjugated hemoglobins used as blood substitutes have very high oxygen affinity P_{50} (50% saturation point) <10 mmHg but cause no apparent problems with oxygen delivery in animals.[28, 29]

The P-50 Value

A useful way to describe the shift in the oxyhemoglobin dissociation curve quantitatively is to calculate or experimentally determine the P_{O_2} at which the blood sample is 50% saturated. This is called the P-50 value. A normal value is about 27 mmHg. If the P-50 is greater than this, the curve is shifted to the right. If it is less, the curve is shifted to the left. The magnitude of the shift is indicated by the distance from this normal value.

Oxygen Content

The oxyhemoglobin dissociation curve allows determination of the amount of oxygen carried by hemoglobin, the reservoir of oxygen. The actual amount of molecular O_2 dissolved in blood or plasma is directly related to the P_{O_2} and is quite small in relation to the amount bound to hemoglobin. This is illustrated in the following equation which describes the amount of oxygen in arterial blood:

$$CaO_2 = (Hb \times 1.37 \times SaO_2) + 0.0031 \times PaO_2$$
$$\text{Total content} = \text{bound} + \text{dissolved}$$

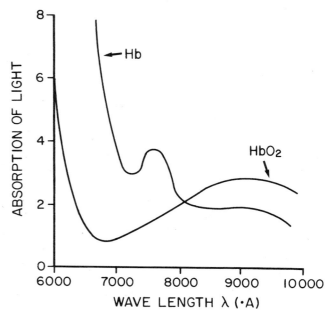

Figure 19-3. Absorption of light of oxygenated and deoxygenated hemoglobin. Comparing the absorption at several wavelengths allows calculation of the percentage oxygen saturation.

Table 19-2. Factors Affecting Hemoglobin-Oxygen Affinity

Causes of Increased Oxygen Affinity
Hypothermia
Respiratory alkalosis
Metabolic alkalosis
Decreased 2,3-diphosphoglycerate (2,3-DPG)
Decreased serum phosphate
Anemia
Hypothyroidism
Factors That Decrease Oxygen Affinity
Fever
Respiratory acidosis
Metabolic acidosis
Increased 2,3-DPG
Steroid administration
Hyperaldosteronism
Hyperthyroidism
Polycythemia

where

C_aO_2 = the oxygen content in liters of oxygen per 100 mL of whole blood
Hb = the hemoglobin content in g/dL of blood
1.37 = the milliliters of oxygen in a fully saturated gram of hemoglobin
S_aO_2 = arterial saturation
0.0031 = the amount of oxygen dissolved in plasma for each millimeter of mercury of P_O_2.

Oxygen Transport

When describing the amount of oxygen that is available to the body, the concept of oxygen transport is often used:

$$\text{Oxygen transport} = C_aO_2 \times CO \times 10$$

where CO is cardiac output. More appropriately called oxygen availability, this product estimates the total available arterial oxygen (in milliliters) per minute. In states in which oxygen transport is inadequate, this variable allows a rational therapeutic approach to be taken by addressing each of the components of the delivery system independently.

Although this oxygen transport variable is useful in a conceptual sense, there are several problems with using it clinically. Because hemoglobin is almost fully saturated if P_aO_2 is greater than 60 mmHg, tissues can only use more oxygen if they can increase flow (cardiac output) or increase extraction (resulting in a lower venous saturation). When flow or cardiac output is limited, extraction is increased. The tissues are able to extract only part of the available oxygen; this fraction varies among different tissues. The heart is efficient at removing the available oxygen and removes as much as 90% of the oxygen delivered (coronary sinus hemoglobin saturation may fall as low as 5%).[30] Other organs may suffer at a much higher venous oxygen content. The brain begins to fail at a venous blood oxygen tension ($P\bar{v}O_2$) around 20 mmHg at which point venous blood is still about 40% saturated.

Arteriovenous Oxygen Content Difference

Comparing the oxygen content of the venous blood with the amount available in the arterial blood gives a measure of the utilization of oxygen. $C(a-v)O_2$, or the arteriovenous oxygen content difference, is easily calculated if a mixed venous blood sample can be obtained (usually from a pulmonary artery or central venous catheter). $C(a-v)O_2$ is usually 5 to 6 vol% but it may increase to 8 to 10 vol% in stress states (increased total body oxygen extraction). A problem with this parameter, as well as the oxygen availability parameter described previously, is that the physiology of the entire body is averaged in the calculations. Critical regional differences in supply and demand matching are not reflected in these overall indices. $P\bar{v}O_2$ gives some indication of total body oxygen supply and demand balance.

Oxygen Utilization Coefficient

A measure of the efficiency of extraction of oxygen is the ratio of oxygen consumption divided by oxygen transport. This is termed the utilization coefficient (UC). This estimate of the ratio of supply to demand can be approximated by subtracting mixed venous oxygen saturation, $S\bar{v}O_2$, from 1:

$$UC = 1 - S\bar{v}O_2$$

This assumes an arterial saturation of greater than 92%. Usually UC falls between 0.2 and 0.3; when it reaches 0.5 (meaning that half of the delivered oxygen is used), tissue hypoxia is likely.

Arterial Oxygenation

Alveolar-Arterial Oxygen Partial Pressure Difference

The expected P_aO_2 varies with the inspired fraction of oxygen. The relationship between the ideal alveolar concentration of oxygen and the inspired oxygen fraction is shown by the alveolar air equation:

$$P_AO_2 = F_IO_2(Pb - 47) - P_aCO_2/R$$

where

P_AO_2 = the ideal alveolar partial pressure of oxygen
F_IO_2 = the inspired oxygen fraction
Pb = the barometric pressure in mmHg
47 = the vapor pressure of H_2O in mmHg at 37°C
P_aCO_2 = the partial pressure of carbon dioxide in the blood
R = the respiratory quotient (the volume of CO_2 produced for each volume of oxygen consumed).

The term P_aCO_2/R is a measure of the oxygen that is being removed by the blood flowing through the lungs in relation to the amount of oxygen being brought into the lungs by ventilation. The difference between this ideal value for oxygen, P_AO_2, and the actual measured value, P_aO_2, is called the alveolar-arterial oxygen difference or the alveolar-arterial gradient for oxygen or $P_AO_2 - P_aO_2$.

Calculating and following the alveolar-arterial gradient is a clinical tool to monitor deficits in oxygenation. Changes in this parameter are produced by several mechanisms. $P_AO_2 - P_aO_2$ is dependent on F_IO_2 (as indicated in the previous equation). A "normal" gradient is about 5 to 10 mmHg on room air, but it increases to 50 to 70 mmHg on an F_IO_2 of 1.0. Other causes of an increased gradient include abnormal cardiac function with a decreased cardiac output, lung disease with increased resistance to diffusion of oxygen, ventilation-perfusion mismatching, or intrapulmonary or intracardiac shunting. Decreased PAO_2-PaO_2 is seen with increased cardiac output, systemic sepsis, left-to-right intracardiac shunts, and failure to utilize oxygen in the tissues, as occurs in cyanide or carbon monoxide poisoning.

Calculation of PAO_2-PaO_2 is useful when changing the FIO_2 of a patient on mechanical ventilation. For example, a PaO_2 of 246 mmHg is obtained from an intubated, ventilated patient. The FIO_2 is 1.0. The PAO_2-PaO_2 is calculated:

$$PAO_2 = 1.0(760 - 47) - 40/0.8$$

assuming the Pb is 760 mmHg, the $PaCO_2$ is normal (40 torr), and R is 0.8.

$$PAO_2 = 663$$

$$PAO_2 - PaO_2 = 663 - 246 = 417$$

To change the FIO_2 to produce a PaO_2 of 100 mmHg, the same equation is solved for FIO_2:

$$PAO_2 - PaO_2 = 417$$

$$\text{Setting } PaO_2 = 100$$

$$PAO_2 = 517$$

$$517 = FIO_2(760 - 47) - 40/0.8$$

$$FIO_2 = (517 + 40/0.8)/(760 - 47) = 0.80$$

The assumptions made in this calculation are that equilibration had taken place before the first blood sample was obtained and that no change occurred in PAO_2-PaO_2. As implied previously, the PAO_2-PaO_2 changes with changes in FIO_2. Since, in this example, the new FIO_2 was lower than the previous setting, the gradient would also be lower, thus providing a margin of safety.

Oxygenation Ratio

A method to eliminate the effects of changes in PAO_2-PaO_2 caused by changes in FIO_2 is to divide the PaO_2 by the FIO_2. This number is referred to as the oxygenation ratio. To use this parameter in the example shown previously:

$$PaO_2/FIO_2 = 246/1.0 = 246$$

to obtain a $PaO_2 = 100$, then

$$100/FIO_2 = 246$$

$$FIO_2 = 100/246 = 0.41$$

This result differs significantly from the previous method (a lower new FIO_2 was obtained) and reflects the fact that the PAO_2-PaO_2 falls as FIO_2 is reduced.

Arterial-Alveolar Oxygen Ratio

Another index of gas exchange is the ratio of arterial to alveolar O_2 (PaO_2/PAO_2).[31] This index, like the oxygenation ratio above, is less affected by FIO_2, more constant than PAO_2-PaO_2, and most constant above alveolar oxygen values

of 200 mmHg ($FIO_2 > 0.3$).[32] Normal PaO_2/PAO_2 values range from 0.7 to 0.8. It offers no advantage in comparison to the oxygenation ratio. Factors such as cardiac output and oxygen consumption affect this and the other monitors already discussed. Lung abnormalities are not specifically quantitated.

Venous Admixture (Shunt Fraction)

The best estimate of oxygenation defect is provided by venous admixture or interpulmonary shunt calculation. The formula for this is

$$\dot{Q}s/\dot{Q}t = (CaO_2 - CcO_2)/(C\bar{v}O_2 - CcO_2)$$

where
CaO_2 = arterial content of oxygen
$C\bar{v}O_2$ = mixed venous content of oxygen
CcO_2 = estimated pulmonary capillary content of oxygen.

This takes into account the effects of changes in cardiac output (as reflected in $C\bar{v}O_2$) and oxygen consumption. Unlike the parameters above, this index provides a useful reflection of the degree of pulmonary abnormality independent of changes in other oxygen delivery variables. The factors influencing the values of the calculated parameters of oxygenation are listed in Table 19-3.

Hypoxia

Physiologic Effects

Oxygen is essential to all tissues for energy generation through oxidative phosphorylation in the Krebs cycle. Anaerobic metabolism is much less efficient and not satisfactory for most organs for long periods. Oxygen is transported by the blood (bound to hemoglobin and freely dissolved) and must diffuse from the red blood cell to the mitochondria. There are almost no tissue stores of oxygen in the body. Oxygen must be continuously delivered in order to maintain organ function and prevent cellular death. The driving force for oxygen delivery from blood to tissues is diffusion down a partial pressure gradient from the end capillary to the mitochondrion. The PO_2 in the mitochondrion is probably less than 2 mmHg.[33] An absolute low level of PaO_2 that is likely to produce injury is not possible to determine. Venous blood leaving a tissue is thought to reflect the driving pressure of the most oxygen-limited mitochondria in that tissue. Oxygen extraction from blood by the (normal) brain seems to fail when jugular venous blood reaches about 20 mmHg. This may occur at PaO_2 of 25 to 35 mmHg depending on the hemoglobin type, concentration, and blood flow. Other or-

Table 19-3. Factors Affecting Clinical Indices of Oxygenation

Index	Factors Influencing Value		
	FIO_2	CARDIAC OUTPUT	OXYGEN CONSUMPTION
Alveolar-arterial gradient	Yes	Yes	Yes
Oxygenation ratio	No	Yes	Yes
Alveolar-arterial ratio	No	Yes	Yes
Venous admixture	No	No	No

Table 19-4. Effect of Hypercarbia on Arterial Oxygen Tension*

	PaO_2 (mmHg)	
$PaCO_2$ (mmHg)	ROOM AIR	30% FIO_2
40	92	156
50	80	144
60	68	132
70	56	120
80	44	108
90	32	96
100	20	84

*The predicted PaO_2 due to a rise in $PaCO_2$ on room air (21% FIO_2) and on 30% FIO_2. A normal, unchanging alevolar-to-arterial gradient is assumed in performing the calculations.

gans may tolerate lower venous (and arterial) oxygen partial pressures.

Theoretically, there are three distinct potential contributors to tissue hypoxia. Hypoxemia (low PaO_2), anemia hypoxia (low hemoglobin leading to inadequate oxygen content), and ischemic hypoxia (low blood flow leading to tissue hypoxia). These three factors are included in the calculated parameter, *oxygen transport*, described in a previous section of this chapter.

Anemic hypoxia is important when the amount of hemoglobin is reduced. The absolute tolerable lower limits of anemia vary among patients and are very dependent on the ability to compensate by increasing flow, that is, vasodilation of critical tissue beds and increasing cardiac output. While healthy people may survive short periods with hemoglobin levels of 2 to 3 g/dL without organ failure, patients with reduced cardiac reserve or increased tissue demand may sustain injury at 8 g/dL.

Ischemic hypoxia is the most important source of clinical concern. While blood flow is necessary for delivery of oxygen and other nutrients, it is also essential for removal of the toxic products of metabolism. Complete interruption of blood flow to an organ, ischemic anoxia, results in rapid disruption of organ function and, if it persists for more than a short period, organ death. The tolerance to ischemic anoxia varies from organ to organ. Irreversible brain injury occurs after only 3 to 5 minutes of total ischemic anoxia. The heart may resume normal function after several hours without blood flow.

While much of the discussion in this chapter is related to determination and treatment of hypoxemia (diminished PO_2), probably more significant is the lack of oxygen at the tissue level. As noted in the above discussion, there are several independent contributors to inadequate tissue oxygen flow. Arterial BGs are just one of them. A more inclusive method of monitoring would be to measure the tissue oxygen state directly. Indwelling arterial devices used for BG monitoring can be inserted directly into tissues to estimate tissue partial pressure of oxygen.[34] Changes with anemia and shock can be identified with these devices. The significance of the data obtained is not entirely clear at the present time, but clinical experience with these monitors is accumulating and they appear to be useful.[35]

There are two distinct concerns related to PaO_2 that need to be addressed: hypoxemia and high FIO_2. Although the definition of hypoxemia varies from organ to organ, a PaO_2 of 55 mmHg or less or a saturation of 88% is usually considered to be a useful definition of hypoxemia.[36] At this point on the oxyhemoglobin dissociation curve, there is still a large quantity of bound oxygen (90% of total capacity). In

healthy individuals, PaO_2 declines with increasing age, reaching a nadir of around 80 ± 5 mmHg at age 70. The use of high FIO_2 to achieve this desired level of PaO_2 may be associated with development of pulmonary oxygen toxicity.[37] Abnormalities of gas exchange and pathologic changes in lung structure occur with high FIO_2. In extreme cases, the adult respiratory distress syndrome (ARDS) follows prolonged use of elevated FIO_2.[38-40]

Causes of Hypoxemia

Hypercarbia

The cause of low PaO_2 easiest to understand is hypercarbia in a patient breathing room air. It can be seen from the alveolar gas equation described earlier in this chapter that a high $PaCO_2$ results in a low PaO_2 when the FIO_2 is low, even with normal pulmonary function. The effect of increasing $PaCO_2$ is shown in Table 19-4. By simply increasing the FIO_2, this cause of hypoxia can be overcome. For example, the PaO_2 of a patient with a $PaCO_2$ of 80 mmHg would only be 44 mmHg on room air; this would improve dramatically to 108 mmHg by increasing the FIO_2 slightly to 0.30. Hypoventilation leading to hypercarbia is often seen as a consequence of general anesthesia, especially when narcotics are employed. The practice of administering an increased FIO_2 to patients recovering from anesthesia is based on this consideration.[41]

Decreased Inspired Oxygen

A second cause of low PaO_2 that can be entirely explained by the alveolar gas equation is the effect of decreased FIO_2, such as occurs at high altitude. Table 19-5 illustrates the effect on PaO_2 of increased height above sea level. As with hypercarbia, this cause of hypoxemia can be overcome by increasing the FIO_2. This is the reason that mountain climbers and pilots wear oxygen masks at high altitudes.

Diffusion Defects

The idea that thickened gas exchange membranes caused a mechanical diffusion defect for oxygen was a popular belief in the past. Since oxygen is more limited by diffusion than CO_2, an increase in the thickness of the alveolar-capillary

Table 19-5. Effect of Increased Altitude and Decreased Barometric Pressure on Oxygen Tension*

Altitude (ft)	Barometric Pressure	Alveolar PO_2	Arterial PO_2
0	760	149	99
2000	707	138	88
4000	656	127	77
6000	609	118	68
8000	564	108	58
10,000	523	100	50
12,000	483	91	41
14,000	446	83	41
16,000	412	76	34
18,000	379	69	27
20,000	349	63	21
30,000	226	37	0

*The fall in barometric pressure is shown as altitude increases. The PAO_2 and estimated PaO_2 are shown. The PAO_2–PaO_2 is assumed to be 0, the $PaCO_2$ is assumed to be 40 (0–12,000 ft) or 25 mmHg (12,000–30,000 ft), and the respiratory quotient is assumed to be 0.8.

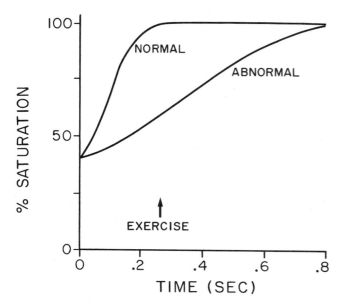

Figure 19-4. The time spent by a red blood cell in transit through the pulmonary bed. Full saturation with oxygen is obtained in about one third of this time. Even in extremely abnormal alveoli with thickened walls, saturation is complete during the normal passage. Exercise shortens transit time and may cause desaturation in the extremely diseased lung by this mechanism. See text for details.

membrane could theoretically decrease PaO_2 by preventing adequate O_2 passage through the lung into the blood. A pulmonary function test, carbon monoxide diffusion capacity, was purported to correlate with an increase in the thickness of this membrane (see Chapter 16). This led to the concept of alveolar-capillary block, which was used to explain the hypoxemia seen in a wide variety of pulmonary diseases.

The clinical significance of this pathophysiologic mechanism has been questioned. In Figure 19-4, it can be seen that during transit through the pulmonary circulation the average red blood cell is fully saturated in less than 0.25 second, one-third the time spent in contact with the gas exchange membrane. Even in those patients having diseases with massive thickening of this membrane (interstitial fibrosis, alveolar proteinosis), oxygen transport is complete during the normal red blood cell transit time. It is only during periods when transit time is reduced (such as with increased cardiac output from exercise or fever) that desaturation occurs. This cause of arterial hypoxia can be easily overcome by slight increases in the FIO_2. The use of portable, low-flow oxygen delivery devices has markedly improved the lifestyle of patients suffering from diseases causing this form of oxygenation failure.

Ventilation-Perfusion Mismatching

The most important cause of oxygenation failure is ventilation-to-perfusion mismatching ($\dot{V}/\dot{Q}$ mismatching). One extreme example of this problem is "shunt" in which there is perfusion of areas that have no ventilation. Unlike the causes of hypoxia discussed in the preceding paragraphs, this cause of hypoxia is not overcome by simply increasing the FIO_2. To separate the effects of $\dot{V}/\dot{Q}$ mismatching from true shunt, 100% O_2 may be administered; any residual oxygenation deficit is due to true shunt rather than $\dot{V}/\dot{Q}$ mismatching. The series of curves in Figure 19-5 illustrate the relationship of

FIO_2 to PaO_2 with various degrees of intrapulmonary shunt (extrapulmonary venous-to-systemic shunts behave in an analogous manner). Thirty percent inspired oxygen fails to correct the hypoxia caused by a shunt greater than 15%.

Therapeutic Approaches to Hypoxemia

Diseases that lead to $\dot{V}/\dot{Q}$ mismatching and shunt include cardiogenic pulmonary edema, ARDS, pneumonia, pulmonary embolism, volume overload, inhalation burn injury, respiratory distress syndrome of the newborn, use of antineoplastic agents, and other diverse conditions. The therapeutic goal is treatment of the primary problem; however, maintenance of an acceptable PaO_2 is essential to recovery. The main therapies used to increase PaO_2 are increased FIO_2 and raised airway pressure. The goal in treatment of this class of disease is to maintain oxygenation on a nontoxic FIO_2. Pulmonary oxygen toxicity occurs in less than 24 hours at an FIO_2 of 100%.[42] FIO_2 levels of 40% to 60% are probably acceptable at sea level indefinitely.

PEEP is a useful and popular method of raising airway pressure. PEEP decreases shunt and increases lung volume by recruiting collapsed alveoli.[43] The effectiveness of this form of therapy is increased if the lung abnormality is uniformly distributed throughout both lungs. Because cardiac output may decrease with the application of PEEP, the actual PaO_2 may decrease owing to a lower PvO_2, despite improvement in lung function and reduction of intrapulmonary shunt.

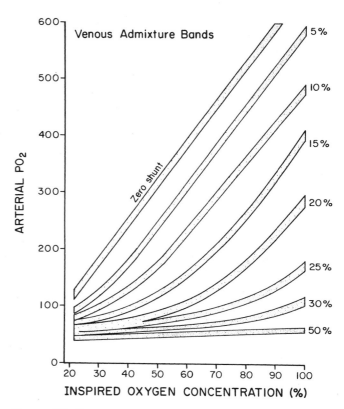

Figure 19-5. Bands showing the range of PaO_2 expected with various amounts of venous admixture or shunt. Knowing the PaO_2 and the inspired oxygen allows a guess at the percentage of shunt present. (Modified from Nunn JF: Applied Respiratory Physiology. Cambridge, Butterworths, 1987, p 371.)

Table 19–6 lists several methods that have been suggested when deciding on the "best" PEEP level. At one extreme is the experience of Kirby and coworkers[44] and extended by DiRusso and others,[45] who believe that PEEP is therapeutic and should be used to maximum effect regardless of the cardiovascular or barotraumatic effects. The other side of the debate is illustrated by Petty and Fowler,[46] who suggest that PEEP is toxic and should be employed only if high levels of FIO_2 are ineffective in preventing severe hypoxemia. (Petty and Fowler's work is done at an altitude over 5000 ft, where an FIO_2 of 100% is equivalent to an FIO_2 of only 78% at sea level.) Possibly owing to early use of some low level of end-expiratory pressure (10 to 12 cm of H_2O) in patients at risk for developing hypoxic lung disease, it appears that the incidence and severity of ARDS is declining.

Volutrauma is replacing barotrauma as a concern during mechanical ventilation in patients with ARDS.[47, 48] The concept that ARDS is a patchy disease is borne out in sequential computed tomographic (CT) studies of the chest. The use of large tidal volumes applied to the few remaining normal alveoli may lead to alveolar rupture and a worsening of the disease. A pressure-volume curve can be used to determine an upper and lower inflection point. The PEEP level should be at or above the lower inflection point to maximize alveolar recruitment.[49] Peak pressure, which determines tidal volume, should be below the upper inflection point to minimize volutrauma risk.[50] Using tidal volumes of 3 to 5 mL/kg instead of the more common 10 to 12 mL/kg has been suggested as a way of preventing this problem. Allowing the $PaCO_2$ to rise (permissive hypercapnia),[51, 52] use of inhaled nitric oxide,[53] partial liquid ventilation,[54] surfactant administration,[55] and extracorporeal membrane oxygenation and CO_2 removal are experimental treatment modalities being evaluated in patients with ARDS.[56, 57]

Because the side effects of positive pressure ventilation and PEEP are significant and always affect the cardiovascular system,[58] monitoring of cardiac function is usually indicated when these modalities are employed. This is often assisted by use of a flow-directed pulmonary artery catheter, which may be used to optimize cardiac filling, cardiac output, and shunt fraction ($\dot{Q}s/\dot{Q}t$). The insertion techniques, use, and complications of this device are described in Chapter 14.

Table 19–6. Methods Proposed to Determine the Ideal Level of Positive End-Expiratory Pressure (PEEP)

PaO_2 is acceptable
Static lung compliance is maximum[a]
Intrapulmonary shunt is $\leq 15\%$[b]
Intrapulmonary shunt is $\leq 20\%$[c]
PEEP is lowest, and FIO_2 is up to 80%[d]
FIO_2 is $\leq 40\%$
Smallest end-tidal-to-arterial CO_2 gradient[e]
PEEP is above lower inflection point of static pressure/volume curve[f]

[a]Suter PM, Fairley HB, Isenberg MC: Optimum end expiratory pressure in patients with acute pulmonary failure. N Engl J Med 1975; 292:284–289.
[b]Gallagher J, Civetta JM: Goal-directed therapy of acute respiratory failure. Anesth Analg 1980; 59:831–834.
[c]DiRusso SM, Nelson LD, Safcsak K, et al: Survival in patients with severe adult respiratory distress syndrome treated with high-level positive end-expiratory pressure. Crit Care Med 1995; 23:1485–1496.
[d]Petty TL, Fowler AA: Another look at ARDS. Chest 1982; 82:98–104.
[e]Murray IP, Modell JH, Gallagher TJ, et al: Titration of PEEP by the arterial minus end-tidal carbon dioxide gradient. Chest 1984; 85:100–104.
[f]Dambrosio M, Roupie E, Mollett JJ, et al: Effects of positive end expiratory pressure and tidal volumes on alveolar recruitment and hyperinflation. Anesthesiology 1997; 87:495–503.

Calculation of $\dot{Q}s/\dot{Q}t$ is performed with the following equation:

$$\dot{Q}s/\dot{Q}t = (CaO_2 - CcO_2)/(C\bar{v}O_2 - CcO_2)$$

where CaO_2 is calculated from arterial saturation and measured hemoglobin, and $C\bar{v}O_2$ is calculated from a mixed venous sample obtained from the distal port of the pulmonary artery catheter. Care must be taken to aspirate this sample slowly (usually over 20 to 30 seconds) to avoid arterializing the blood. CcO_2, is estimated from the following equation:

$$CcO_2 = 1.37 \times Hb \times 100\% + 0.0031 \times PaO_2$$

This calculation is performed assuming that pulmonary capillary blood is fully oxygen-saturated and that there is no alveolar-pulmonary capillary gradient for oxygen. These assumptions are not perfectly correct, but the errors introduced are small and inconsequential for clinical management decisions.

The usefulness of the shunt calculation is that it removes the effect of changes in cardiac output from the intrapulmonary effects of airway pressure therapy. Although there is no a priori reason to believe that shunt is the pathologic problem in ARDS, those clinicians who monitor and treat changes in shunt fraction report the lowest mortality in this condition.[59, 60] The use of PEEP to improve pulmonary compliance makes physiologic sense. However, mechanical difficulties in measuring pulmonary compliance and conflicting results by various investigators have made it a less useful parameter to optimize PEEP. Most authors agree that PEEP should be used to avoid high concentrations of inspired oxygen.

The cardiac effects of PEEP (or more correctly, increased mean airway pressure) include reduced venous return, increased right ventricular afterload,[61] decreased left ventricular afterload, and leftward shift of the intraventricular septum.[62] Possible effects of PEEP are reduced cardiac compliance[63] and reduced contractility.[64] Some authors have actually shown an increase in contractility with elevated airway pressure.[65] Since airway pressure may be reflected in vascular pressures, the absolute values of filling pressure are altered when increased airway pressures are employed. As much as half of the PEEP may be reflected in the ventricular filling pressure and should be subtracted from the measured value.[66] Cardiac status should be assessed by observing the changes in filling pressures and cardiac output occurring after volume challenges and not on the actual values determined from pulmonary artery monitoring.

The effects of changes in the level of PEEP on the cardiovascular system are rapid, occurring in less than a minute. The effects on arterial BGs are more gradual, requiring at least 10 to 15 minutes to reach a new steady state. The same is true for FIO_2, although evidence suggests that a shorter equilibration time period may be acceptable to assess the results of a change in FIO_2.[67]

Hyperoxia

Hyperoxia ($PaO_2 > 75$ mmHg) in the premature infant is associated with the development of blindness due to retrolental fibroplasia. The exact cause of this problem is not known and oxygen may be one of several factors responsible.[68] Hyperoxia (at >1.5 atm as seen in divers or in patients in hyperbaric chambers) stimulates the central nervous system and causes seizures.

Table 19-7. Therapeutic Uses of Increased Fraction of Inspired Oxygen

Carbon monoxide poisoning
Venous air embolism
Arterial air (or other gas) embolism
Fetal distress (maternal hyperoxia)
Acute myocardial ischemia
Cerebral ischemia
Pneumothorax
Pneumocephalus
Fluorocarbon blood substitute
Anaerobic infections

There are several short-term therapeutic uses of hyperoxia (Table 19-7). Administration of 100% oxygen is therapeutic in carbon monoxide poisoning. Hyperbaric oxygen may also be employed in this circumstance (if a hyperbaric chamber is readily available). Systemic or venous air embolism is an indication for high FIO_2 to reduce the size of the bubble. Denitrogenation of the blood creates a pressure gradient for nitrogen to leave the bubble. Tension pneumocephalus[69] or pneumothorax may be improved by a high PaO_2, but direct removal of the trapped air is the normal therapeutic approach. In prolonged or difficult obstetric delivery, fetal metabolic status may be improved when maternal PaO_2 is elevated above 200 mmHg. When a fluorocarbon blood substitute (Fluosol) is used to replace red blood cells, 100% oxygen must be used to raise the amount of dissolved oxygen to acceptable levels (at least 5 vol%).[70] Administration of high FIO_2 is practiced in patients with chest pain presumed due to myocardial infarction or ischemia to prevent hypoxia from early pulmonary edema and to improve cardiac oxygenation. Hyperoxia has been shown to improve cerebral function in patients after cerebral artery occlusion, but the risks from oxygen toxicity have not made this a standard practice for long-term (>24 hours) treatment.[71]

Acid-Base Monitoring

Investigations into pH and CO_2 measurements originated with concerns over fermentation in the 1800s. Louis Pasteur demonstrated that control of acidity was essential to proper brewing and creation of wine from grapes. Wilhelm Ostwald developed the hydrogen electrode capable of measuring H^+ ions, and his student, Walther Nernst, developed the mathematics of the theory of electrochemical activity. The Nernst equation forms the basis for all ion-specific electrodes, including pH and PCO_2. Early equipment was improved, used on blood, and the theoretical bases of acid-base equilibrium refined by Phyllis T. Kerridge, Karl Albert Hasselbalch, Poul Astrup, and others. The volumetric techniques developed by Van Slyke enabled researchers and clinicians to determine the blood content of CO_2 accurately. Analysis of as little as 50 to 100 μL of blood for PCO_2, pH, and PO_2 is possible today. Indwelling microelectrodes are capable of continuous monitoring of these values.

pH is measured by determining the potential difference between a silver–silver chloride reference cell and a mercury–mercury chloride test cell separated by a pH-sensitive glass membrane. The value by convention is determined at 37°C. A modification of the pH electrode is used to measure PCO_2. The entire electrode is covered with polytef (Teflon), which is freely permeable to CO_2; the change in potential difference between the CO_2-impermeable glass electrode and the Teflon-covered pH electrode is used to determine PCO_2.

Miniature electrodes and optodes similar to those used for measurement of oxygen have been used for continuous monitoring of arterial and venous PCO_2 and pH.

The discussion about acid-base monitoring and clinical implications is based on the assumption that total body metabolic activity is reflected by plasma. This compartment only approximates what is happening in each separate tissue. Monitors of tissue pH, PCO_2, K^+, and PO_2 can be used in human tissues to assess local homeostasis and abnormalities. Tissue probes are closer to the intracellular environment where the abnormalities originate and have their most significant effects. Other technologies, such as magnetic resonance imaging (MRI), accurately identify intracellular metabolic derangements by identifying abnormalities of intercellular energy stores. This technology, currently a research tool, will soon be available at the bedside to direct clinical interventions.

Buffers and Carbon Dioxide Transport

The end products of cellular respiration are carbon dioxide and water. The human body produces about 12,000 mEq of acid in the form of CO_2 every 24 hours. This tremendous load is excreted by the lungs in the form of volatile acid (CO_2), and body pH is tightly maintained. A smaller amount of fixed acid is excreted by the kidneys. This amounts to about 1 mEq/kg of body mass each day. These two systems are responsible for the control of body acid-base balance and maintenance of optimal pH for metabolic health of individual organs and the whole body.

In order for ventilation to be efficient in acid removal, metabolic CO_2 must be transported to the lungs. CO_2 is relatively insoluble in blood and is predominantly carried as bicarbonate, which is produced by reaction with water, as shown in the following chemical equation:

$$CO_2 + H_2O \rightarrow H_2CO_3 \rightarrow H^+ + HCO_3^-$$

In order for this system of CO_2 transport to work, the normally slow conversion of CO_2 to bicarbonate is facilitated by the enzyme carbonic anhydrase located primarily in red blood cells. Hemoglobin and other proteins serve as carriers for some of the CO_2 produced. The relative amounts of CO_2 carried in each of these forms is indicated in Table 19-8.

Hemoglobin acts as a buffer when oxygen is released at the tissue level. This allows some of the H^+ produced from carbonic acid to be neutralized by hemoglobin. This is referred to as the Haldane effect. As illustrated in Figure 19-6, when a solution of oxygenated free hemoglobin at pH 7.3 is deoxygenated, the solution pH increases to 7.5. As oxygen is released at the tissues, the buffering effect of hemoglobin allows less pH change than would otherwise occur with the production of carbonic acid. This makes hemoglobin a most important buffer.

Table 19-8. Forms and Amount of Carbon Dioxide Carried in Whole Venous Blood*

CO₂ Species	mmol/L
Dissolved CO_2	1.27
Carbonic acid (undissociated)	0.0012
HCO_3^-	20.3
Carbamino compounds (hemoglobin)	1.7
Total	23.3

*O_2 saturation is 70%; hemoglobin is 12–14 g/dL.

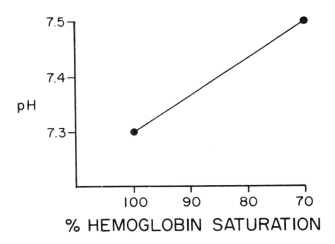

Figure 19-6. The effect of desaturating a solution of hemoglobin. The pH increases as the oxygen saturation decreases. This is referred to as the Haldane effect.

Most of the important actions of the CO_2 transport system occur inside red blood cells. Major ion and chemical shifts are indicated in Figure 19-7. In order to maintain electrical neutrality inside the red blood cell, Cl^- is exchanged for HCO_3^-. This is termed the chloride shift (or Hamberger effect). K^+ is excreted from the cell as well. The total number of particles in the red blood cell increases as a result of these events, and water passively enters the cell along an osmotic gradient. The red blood cell swells, resulting in a venous hematocrit level that is slightly greater than the arterial (6% to 10%) change. Venous potassium levels are similarly elevated. These differences should be kept in mind when analyzing blood drawn from arterial catheters and comparing the results with normal venous values.

Buffer Systems

Buffer systems consist of a weak acid or base and its salt. These systems change in pH by increasing or decreasing the amount of their dissociated form when a stronger acid or base is added to the system. The general behavior of such buffers is illustrated for a theoretic buffer system in Figure 19-8. As acid or base is added to the system, the pH tends to remain unchanged. A buffer system is most resistant to changes in pH and is most efficient at buffering around its pK. The pK is the pH at which the weak acid or base is half dissociated.

The general chemical dissociation formula for a weak base is shown in the following equation:

$$BOH \rightarrow OH^- + B^+$$

where

BOH = a weak base
OH^- = the hydrogen ion acceptor
B^+ = a cation available to form a salt.

When a strong acid is combined with a weak base, the following equation describes the buffer system formed:

$$\text{Strong base} + \text{weak base} \rightarrow \text{weak acid} + \text{neutral salt}$$

pH is defined as the negative logarithm of the H^+ concentration of an aqueous solution. K is the ionization constant

for an acid or a base. K can be defined in the following way for a weak acid:

$$K[HA] \rightarrow [H^+] \times [A^-]$$

where

$[HA]$ = the concentration of the unionized acid
$[H^+]$ = the concentration of the H^+
$[A^-]$ = the concentration of the salt-forming radical (or base).

Rearranging this equation yields

$$[H^+] = K[HA]/[A^-]$$

Taking the negative logarithm of both sides yields

$$-\text{Log } [H^+] = pH = -\log K + \log \{[A^-]/[HA]\}$$

By convention, pK is the negative logarithm of K. pH can be defined in terms of any of its buffer pairs, as suggested by the following general formula:

$$pH = pK + \log \{[\text{base}]/[\text{acid}]\}$$

Since bicarbonate is present in the blood in large quantities, the use of carbonic acid in this equation yields the following description of blood pH:

$$pH = pK + \log \{[HCO_3^-]/[H_2CO_3]\}$$

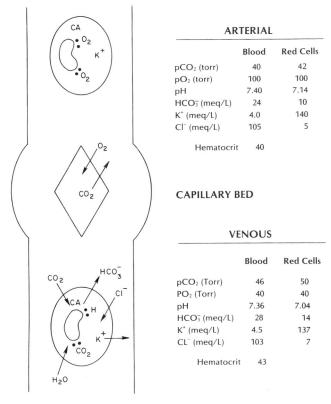

ARTERIAL		
	Blood	Red Cells
pCO_2 (torr)	40	42
pO_2 (torr)	100	100
pH	7.40	7.14
HCO_3^- (meq/L)	24	10
K^+ (meq/L)	4.0	140
Cl^- (meq/L)	105	5
Hematocrit	40	

CAPILLARY BED

VENOUS		
	Blood	Red Cells
pCO_2 (Torr)	46	50
PO_2 (Torr)	40	40
pH	7.36	7.04
HCO_3^- (meq/L)	28	14
K^+ (meq/L)	4.5	137
CL^- (meq/L)	103	7
Hematocrit	43	

Figure 19-7. The transition of blood from arterial to venous. The chemical composition and blood gas changes are illustrated. An important change is the increase in levels of hematocrit and potassium. Other details are explained in the text. CA, carbonic anhydrase.

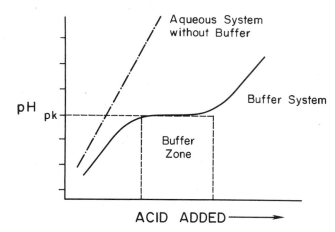

Figure 19-8. The performance of a "typical" buffer system. A buffer system is most resistant to change near its pK. The effect on pH of an aqueous system without buffer is contrasted in the dotted line.

The pK for this reaction is 3.5, far from the usual blood pH.[72] By expressing this equation in terms of CO_2 (since there is approximately 600 times more CO_2 than H_2CO_3 present in blood), the apparent pK becomes 6.1, and the classic Henderson-Hasselbalch form of the equation is

$$pH = 6.1 + \log \{[HCO_3^-]/(s \cdot P_{CO_2})\}$$

where s = the solubility constant for CO_2. Even at this pK, this buffer system would not be a very satisfactory one to maintain a physiologic pH of 7.40. However, since the CO_2 can be continually removed from the system, the pH can be easily regulated. This is called an open system.

The importance of ventilation in the maintenance of acid-base balance is demonstrated during apnea when the blood pH rapidly falls to very low levels in several minutes. This is illustrated in Figure 19-9. To change the pH by an equivalent amount using renal compensatory mechanisms takes days to weeks to achieve.

Hazards and Pitfalls

Temperature Correction of pH and Carbon Dioxide Tension

Solubility of carbon dioxide as well as oxygen in blood depends on blood temperature. The ionization state and configuration of proteins, including albumin, are also affected by temperature, generally becoming more basic as temperature falls. BG analyzers are maintained at 37°C. Whether to correct the values obtained from patients with abnormal body temperatures to 37°C has been debated for many years. Temperature-correction formulas have been derived by cooling or heating a normal sample of plasma or whole blood and measuring BGs in analyzers maintained at the same temperature as the sample. Mathematical formulas were developed to produce normal values in an analyzer at the same temperature as the anerobically cooled or heated normal blood sample.[73] Deviations in calculated values are assumed to indicate an abnormality.

Several clinical and experimental arguments suggest that temperature correction of BGs is inappropriate. Study of poikilothermic animals demonstrates that when their blood is obtained at different temperatures and processed in an arterial BG analyzer at 37°C, the values obtained are identical and equal to "normal" values obtained and analyzed at 37°C. In humans in cold environments, blood obtained from cold distal arteries has the same values as blood obtained from warm central arteries when both are analyzed at 37°C. If the values were temperature-corrected, the cold sample would be alkalotic (lower P_{aCO_2}) and have a lower P_{aO_2}.

The effects of temperature on enzyme system activities parallel changes in measured H^+ activity. To maintain neutrality, that is, the same relative activity of $[H^+]$ and $[OH^-]$, the solution must become slightly alkalotic as temperature decreases. A major contributor to this change with hypothermia is the ionization of histidine's alpha-imidazole locus on hemoglobin. Another is the increased solubility of CO_2. A "normal" value should be obtained when the sample is warmed; deviations from normal should be considered pathologic. This is termed the "alpha-stat" approach (from the alpha-imidazole locus of hemoglobin). According to this approach no mathematical correction of in vitro values is necessary or appropriate.[74, 75]

Clinical evidence also refutes routine temperature correction of BGs. Profoundly hypothermic animals given sodium bicarbonate to normalize temperature-corrected BGs invariably develop profound alkalemia and suffer myocardial damage on rewarming.[76] Hypothermic patients given little or no bicarbonate during cardiopulmonary bypass have normal acid-base balance when returned to normothermia.[77]

Accuracy of Measurements of Carbon Dioxide Tension and pH

The pH and P_{CO_2} electrodes are rugged, reliable, and accurate. Laboratory standards of accuracy require that the range of values for known standards when repeatedly tested be less than 5 mmHg for P_{CO_2} and less than 0.04 for pH. The clinical use of pH is somewhat confusing because it represents logarithmic changes in H^+ concentrations. As seen in

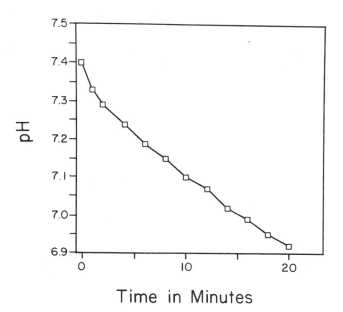

Figure 19-9. pH changes over time during apnea. The importance of the respiratory system to acid-base balance is discussed in the text.

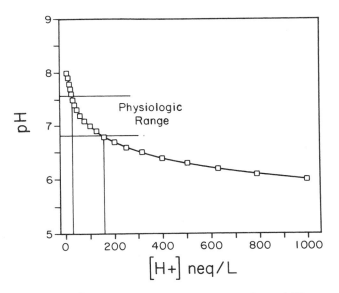

Figure 19-10. The relationship between pH and actual H^+ concentration. The normal range is quite wide.

Figure 19-10, the H^+ concentration changes by a factor of 10 between pH of 7.00 and 8.00. At a normal pH of 7.40, the H^+ concentration is about 40 nEq/L. When we consider how tightly controlled most body chemicals are (such as potassium or sodium), it is surprising to see that H^+ is allowed to vary normally between 32 and 45 nEq/L (pH 7.35 to 7.45).

Arterial versus Venous Acid-Base Balance

Because there is very little difference between arterial and venous PCO_2, usually only 4 to 5 mmHg, a venous sample can be used to evaluate acid-base status.[78] Bicarbonate is calculated from the pH and is also only slightly lower in venous samples. Malignant hyperthermia may be confirmed in the operating room by a venous blood sample since this hypermetabolic state is characterized by early development of a mixed metabolic and respiratory acidosis.[79] Although a rise in end-tidal PCO_2 may trigger an investigation, venous acid-base balance is an excellent monitor for this syndrome.[80] In the case of a patient with cardiorespiratory arrest when external chest compressions are being performed, a large discrepancy between arterial and venous BGs may exist.[81] The venous PCO_2 may reflect the adequacy (or inadequacy) of the artificial circulation and tissue acid-base status and predict outcome.[82] The end-tidal PCO_2 may be a useful monitor of tissue acidosis, as it reflects venous and tissue PCO_2 in this circumstance.[83, 84]

Acid-Base Monitoring

Respiratory disorders are defined from the value of the $PaCO_2$. If the $PaCO_2$ is greater than 45 mmHg, then a respiratory acidosis is present. This is often called hypoventilation; however, this word carries the connotation of a patient who is breathing slowly and shallowly. Patients may, in fact, be hyperventilating in a clinical sense (breathing rapidly or deeply with an elevated minute ventilation) with hyper-

carbia. In order to avoid confusion, increased $PaCO_2$ is called "respiratory acidosis," "hypercarbia," or "hypercapnia" throughout the remainder of this chapter. Respiratory alkalosis is defined as a $PaCO_2$ less than 35 mmHg. This should not be referred to as "hyperventilation" but as "hypocapnia," "hypocarbia," or "respiratory alkalosis." In referring to the various components of acid-base balance derangement, processes are identified with the suffix "-osis" regardless of the blood pH. The pH of the blood is suffixed with "-emia." For example, a patient with a low pH due to metabolic acidosis may have partial respiratory compensation (pH <7.35 and $PaCO_2$ <35); this would be described as acidemia (low blood pH) from metabolic acidosis (the metabolic process) with respiratory alkalosis or hypocapnia (the respiratory process).

The major problem in dealing with the interpretation of acid-base information is separation of the metabolic and respiratory components. For every primary disorder, there is a partial or complete compensatory response in the other system. When a disorder is treated, it is essential to identify the initiating (primary) disturbance, as this may require therapy. Treatment must not be directed at the compensatory response.

Many systems of analysis have been developed to deal with the problem of identifying the primary disorder and secondary response. Several of these approaches are described later in this chapter. None of the systems is completely effective in identifying the primary disorder. Whenever there is more than a single primary disorder, no system is capable of sorting out the components and directing therapy. The clinical status of the patient and the response to attempted correction of a disturbance provide the information needed to correctly diagnose the condition and direct treatment.

When BG results are reported from an automated analyzer, the PCO_2 and the pH are measured accurately. The values for bicarbonate, standard bicarbonate, total CO_2, buffer base, or base excess are calculated from nomograms based on the Henderson-Hasselbalch equation or other nomograms derived from the behavior of blood or plasma in vitro. These derived parameters were devised in attempts to separate the metabolic or fixed component (renal) from the respiratory component ($PaCO_2$) of the acid-base status. Table 19-9 lists the normal values for some of these proposed parameters. Most of these indices attempt to mathematically remove the respiratory component of the disorder by assuming a PCO_2 of 40 mmHg as normal. This is done by analyzing the sample after equilibrating with a gas mixture having a $PaCO_2$ of 40 mmHg and a PO_2 of 100 mmHg (for base excess) at normal body temperature (37°C). The actual value of $PaCO_2$ and pH are plotted graphically or used to calculate the corrected value of the HCO_3^-, buffer-base, and base excess.

Total CO_2 includes bicarbonate and dissolved CO_2. It is based on extraction techniques and is not very different from plasma bicarbonate (dissolved CO_2 is only 1/20th the

Table 19-9. Metabolic Indices of Acid-Base Balance

Index	Reference Values (mEq/L)
Plasma bicarbonate	22-26
Total CO_2	23-27
CO_2 combining power	21-27
Standard bicarbonate	21-25
Whole buffer base	45-50
Base excess	−3-+3

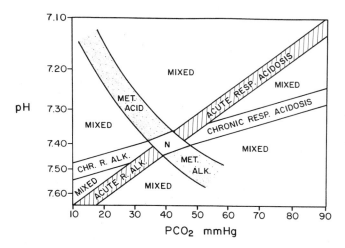

Figure 19-11. Significance bands describing the expected range of compensation for the primary disorders. See text for details. (Modified from Levesque RP: Acid-base disorders: Application of total body carbon dioxide titration in anesthesia. Anesth Analg 1975; 54:307.)

amount of bicarbonate).[85] No correction is made for the respiratory system contribution in either of these indices.

CO_2 combining power was suggested as a way to account for the respiratory contribution to the disorder. Plasma is equilibrated with gas having a P_{CO_2} of 40 mmHg. The total CO_2 (and bicarbonate) is determined and should approximate the "corrected" metabolic contribution to acid-base balance. Theoretic problems with this calculated variable are that it is based only on the plasma component of blood (as indicated previously, hemoglobin plays a significant buffering role clinically), and it is an in vitro correction factor.

Standard bicarbonate, proposed by Astrup, is the bicarbonate of whole blood equilibrated under standard conditions of P_{CO_2} and temperature and includes the in vitro buffering contribution of hemoglobin.[86]

Whole buffer base is the "unmeasured" buffers (amino acids in proteins) added to plasma bicarbonate. It does not take into account the contribution from changes in hemoglobin oxygenation, which may buffer pH at the tissue level. Whole buffer base is normally 45 to 50 mEq/L. It is not calculated under standard conditions.

Base excess is the amount of acid (or base) needed to return a sample of whole blood to normal pH under standard conditions of P_{CO_2}, P_{O_2}, and temperature.[87] It is also an

in vitro method for estimating the body's metabolic attempt to correct for abnormalities in acid-base status. The normal value for base excess is 0.

All these methods describe in vitro techniques to define the metabolic components of an acid-base disorder. Deviations from normal values are proposed to indicate a metabolic derangement. A problem of interpretation of all of these values is caused by the fact that compensation does occur and "normal" values are not necessarily appropriate.[88]

The use of graphic "significance bands" as described by Arbus and associates[89] helps identify the primary disorder and the expected compensatory response range. As seen in Figure 19-11, the six primary disorders can be identified in graphic form.[90] These disorders are acute respiratory alkalosis, chronic respiratory alkalosis, metabolic alkalosis, acute respiratory acidosis, chronic respiratory acidosis, and metabolic acidosis.

To use the graphic method to identify the types of derangements present, plot the pH against the Pa_{CO_2}. The intersection identifies the type of problem. For example, a pH of 7.54 with a Pa_{CO_2} of 25 mmHg indicates "acute respiratory alkalosis" with appropriate metabolic compensation. The areas marked "mixed" identify situations in which more than one primary disorder is present or the degree of compensation is inappropriate or incomplete. There is no system to separate the components when more than a single primary disorder is present. The clinical situation must be known to appropriately diagnose the problem. Further information can be obtained by making interventions and repeating the measurements. Only primary derangements should be treated, and then only if certain limits are exceeded and symptoms are present.

The data used to design the significance bands in Figure 19-11 were obtained by observing groups of patients with only one primary disorder and recording their range of compensation. These data have been collected and summarized.[91] Table 19-10 summarizes the in vivo compensation that occurs in response to a primary disorder. To use this information, simply use the correction factor to predict the compensated value. Any deviation from this expected value indicates a second (or third) primary disorder which may require independent assessment and treatment.

Respiratory Disorders

Acute Respiratory Acidosis

Disorders that decrease the efficiency of pulmonary carbon dioxide excretion may increase Pa_{CO_2}. Acute changes in the

Table 19-10. Compensatory Responses to the Six Primary Disorders*

Disorder	Compensatory Response (Expected)	Magnitude of Response (Predicted)
Respiratory alkalosis, acute	Decreased HCO_3^-	$[HCO_3^-]$ decreases 2 mEq/L for each 10-mmHg decrease in Pa_{CO_2}
Respiratory alkalosis, chronic	Decreased HCO_3^-	$[HCO_3^-]$ decreases 5 mEq/L for each 10-mmHg decrease in Pa_{CO_2}
Metabolic alkalosis	Increased Pa_{CO_2}	$Pa_{CO_2} = 0.9 \times [HCO_3^-] + 9$
		$Pa_{CO_2} = 0.9 \times [HCO_3^-] + 15.6$
		$Pa_{CO_2} = $ base excess $+ 40.6$
Respiratory acidosis, acute	Increased HCO_3^-	$[HCO_3^-]$ increases 1 mEq/L for each 10-mmHg increase in Pa_{CO_2}
Respiratory acidosis, chronic	Increased HCO_3^-	$[HCO_3^-]$ increases 3.5 mEq/L for each 10-mmHg increase in Pa_{CO_2}
Metabolic acidosis	Decreased Pa_{CO_2}	$Pa_{CO_2} = 1.5 \times [HCO_3^-] + 8$
		$Pa_{CO_2} = 1.8 \times ($base excess $-24) + 8$
		$Pa_{CO_2} = $ last 2 decimal fractions of the pH

*The direction of the expected response is indicated as well as several rules of thumb for determining the magnitude of the compensatory response.

metabolic component result in pH being returned toward normal. Normal people with acute elevation in $PaCO_2$ show about 1 mEq/L increase in bicarbonate for each 10-mmHg increase in $PaCO_2$ (about 0.8 base excess units) owing to tissue and hemoglobin buffers.[92] Renal regulation takes much longer but is far more complete.

The causes of acute respiratory acidosis include drug effects on the respiratory center or neuromuscular transmission and upper or lower airway obstruction. Narcotics and sedatives, general anesthetics, bronchospasm, upper airway occlusion, and rebreathing of exhaled CO_2 are causes of acute CO_2 retention (Table 19–11).

The physiologic effects of acute hypercapnia are usually fairly benign. If hypoxia is avoided, hypercapnia increases heart rate and blood pressure through sympathetic stimulation. It shifts the hemoglobin saturation curve to the right. Dysrhythmias and enhanced cardiac contractility may result. Serum potassium increases slightly. During severe bronochospasm, a normal $PaCO_2$ may be impossible to achieve without causing barotrauma. Despite a prolonged, markedly elevated $PaCO_2$ and correspondingly low pH in these patients, no serious long-term problems have been seen following resolution of bronchospasm.[93] Patients with reduced lung compliance associated with severe ARDS have been hypoventilated using "permissive hypercarbia" in an effort to avoid volutrauma and the cardiovascular effects of the high airway pressures that would be necessary to achieve normal $PaCO_2$.[94-96] If $PaCO_2$ increases above 80 to 90 mmHg, coma from CO_2 narcosis may occur. In patients with head injury or brain tumors, increased cerebral blood flow from elevated $PaCO_2$ may cause increased intracranial pressure and herniation of brain across rigid intracranial structures.

Treatment of acute hypercapnia is directed at relief of the underlying cause rather than the pH change. Occasionally, it is necessary to correct the pH with exogenous base. The use of sodium bicarbonate is controversial in that additional CO_2 is liberated and unless ventilation can be increased, the pH will remain unchanged or actually fall further. Also, since the CO_2 can freely diffuse into cells, the intercellular pH will fall even if there is no change in blood pH. Nonbicarbonate buffers such as tromethamine (Tham) have been suggested for use with hypercarbia.[97, 98] Carbicarb (a mixture of sodium carbonate and sodium bicarbonate) has been tested and found not to increase $PaCO_2$ as much as sodium bicarbonate.[99]

Chronic Respiratory Acidosis

When an elevated $PaCO_2$ persists for longer than 6 to 10 hours, the metabolic compensation is more complete. Hypercapnia causing acidemia stimulates retention of bicarbonate. Compensation does not return blood pH to normal if $PaCO_2$ is greater than 55 mmHg. An increase of 3.5 mEq/L bicarbonate (3 base excess units) for every 10-mmHg rise in $PaCO_2$ is seen in response to this primary disorder.[100] CO_2 retention is a result of $\dot{V}/\dot{Q}$ mismatch in chronic lung disease. End-stage restrictive lung disease (such as kyphoscoliosis) may also result in hypercapnia.[101] Ondine's curse and the pickwickian syndrome are conditions in which the central nervous system center controlling respiratory drive becomes less sensitive to changes in pH, with a resultant elevation in $PaCO_2$. As a consequence of this abnormality, pulmonary hypertension and right heart failure frequently follow prolonged elevations of $PaCO_2$. Hypoxemia on room air (described previously) also occurs as a consequence of markedly elevated $PaCO_2$.

The treatment of the elevated CO_2 should be directed at the underlying cause. If severe and progressive, mechanical ventilation will be required. Occasionally, noninvasive ventilation or bilevel continuous positive airway pressure (CPAP) may stabilize patients with chronic respiratory failure.[102] Ventilatory muscle weakness, fatigue, and malnourishment contribute to elevated CO_2 in chronic pulmonary disease.[103, 104] Diaphragm rest and nutritional improvement can favorably affect gas exchange. Conditioning exercises may also improve muscle strength and endurance.[105] High glucose loads during parenteral feeding can increase CO_2 production by stimulating fat synthesis and may worsen respiratory failure.[106] Drugs that have been used to reduce $PaCO_2$ include estrogens, caffeine, aminophylline, and doxapram hydrochloride.[107] Surgical procedures to correct airway obstruction and obesity have been successful in treating the pickwickian syndrome. Positive pressure ventilation reverses the CO_2 retention, but this may mean indefinite commitment to artificial ventilation. The use of noninvasive ventilation or bilevel CPAP, especially at night during sleep, may improve function and prolong life in those terminal patients with very high $PaCO_2$ levels.[108-110]

Acute Respiratory Alkalosis

$PaCO_2$ decreases when alveolar ventilation exceeds carbon dioxide production (Table 19–12). This results in a rise in pH. An immediate change in total CO_2 and base excess follows the change in $PaCO_2$. This amounts to a decrease of 2 mEq/L of bicarbonate (1.8 base excess units) for each 10-mmHg change in $PaCO_2$. This immediate compensation is not due to renal mechanisms; it is most likely due to local tissue factors. After several hours, renal retention of acid begins. This results in a fall in calculated bicarbonate (or a negative base excess) and if hypocarbia continues, the disorder becomes chronic with more complete compensation.

As seen in Table 19–12, many of the causes of hypocapnia have no specific therapy. Induced respiratory alkalosis reduces cerebral blood flow and may improve intracranial compliance in patients with brain tumors. The routine use of mechanical hyperventilation in head injury has been questioned.[111, 112] Patients with neurologic injury may spontaneously hyperventilate to a lower than normal $PaCO_2$; no treat-

Table 19–11. Causes of Respiratory Acidosis

Chronic obstructive pulmonary disease
Acute bronchospasm
Primary alevolar hypoventilation
 Ondine's curse
 Pickwickian syndrome
High-level spinal cord injury
Myasthenia gravis
Multiple sclerosis
Muscular dystrophies
Bulbar polio
Guillain-Barré syndrome
Narcotic drug effects
Neuromuscular blocking drugs
Airway obstruction
General anesthetics
Mechanical ventilation
Rebreathing
 Intentional
 Equipment failure

Table 19–12. Causes of Respiratory Alkalosis*

> Hypoxemia
> Decreased pulmonary compliance
> > Pulmonary edema
> > Adult respiratory distress syndrome
> > Pulmonary fibrosis
> Infection
> > Septic syndrome
> > Pneumonia
> > Fever
> Bronchospasm (early)
> Pulmonary embolism
> Drugs
> > Doxapram HCl
> > Theophylline
> > Progesterone
> > Salicylates
> Pregnancy
> Central nervous system disorders
> Cirrhosis
> Excessive mechanical ventilation
> Anxiety
> Psychogenic

*Some of these may require primary treatment; however, low $PaCO_2$ is usually never itself treated.

ment would be appropriate because this is a normal protective response. Anxiety can often be treated with anxiolytic agents or reassuring discussions with the patient. Hypoxia (PaO_2 <55 torr) stimulates the peripheral chemoreceptors located in the aorta and carotid arteries, resulting in an increase in minute ventilation. Other disorders may be treated, but therapy is not directed at the hypocapnia per se.

Chronic Respiratory Alkalosis

When hypocapnia persists for several hours or longer, renal mechanisms are activated and further compensation occurs. Renal compensation occurs naturally in inhabitants of high altitudes. Some patients can completely compensate for respiratory alkalosis and obtain a normal pH. This is unusual with other disorders. For every 10-mmHg fall in $PaCO_2$, there is up to a 5-mEq/L decrease in bicarbonate (4 base excess units), as seen in Table 19–10.[113] It may take several weeks to normalize pH in this circumstance.

Metabolic Acidosis

When acid products decrease the serum bicarbonate, the respiratory center and peripheral chemoreceptors are stimulated and ventilation increases. This response is proportional to the degree of change in bicarbonate and may be delayed 12 to 24 hours. This delay is due to the slow transfer of bicarbonate across the blood-train barrier. Central nervous system pH changes due to changing blood bicarbonate concentrations occur after blood pH changes. When the brain is involved in the process causing metabolic acidosis, this delay is absent. The expected $PaCO_2$ in compensation for a decreased bicarbonate is about $1.5 \times [HCO_3^-] + 8$.[114] Another rule of thumb is that the $PaCO_2$ should be equal to the first two decimal fractions of the pH (i.e., a pH of 7.25 should result in producing a $PaCO_2$ of about 25) (see Table 19–10).

Anion Gap

The causes of metabolic acidosis are listed in Table 19–13. The anion gap is a tool useful in explaining the root cause of an acid-base disorder.[115] It is calculated as the serum sodium minus the sum of the chloride and bicarbonate.

$$\text{Anion gap} = [Na^+] - ([Cl^-] + [HCO_3^-])$$

This gap accounts for unmeasured anions, including negatively charged proteins, phosphate, sulfate, and others. These are divided into two groups: those with lactic or other acid accumulation, called "high anion gap"; and those with bicarbonate loss balanced by chloride, "normal anion gap." A normal anion gap is between 8 and 12 mEq/L. Calculation of the anion gap may allow differentiation of the causes of the metabolic disorder.

The underlying cause of the acidosis should be treated if possible. The following formula is useful to calculate the required amount of base to administer if correction of a deficit is deemed desirable; usually a blood pH less than 7.15 requires treatment:

Bicarbonate dose (mEq) = base excess $\times$ 0.2 $\times$ weight (kg)

or

Bicarbonate dose (mEq) = $(24 - [HCO_3^-]) \times 0.2$ weight (kg)

These approximations allow about half the deficit in plasma to be corrected. The effect of treatment on acid-base parameters should be closely monitored. Recent data suggest that aggressive correction of the deficit in metabolic acidosis may be associated with paradoxical central nervous system depression and respiratory arrest.[116] Concern for the levels and balance of potassium, phosphate, chloride, and magnesium should also be considered in these disorders and during therapy.

Metabolic Alkalosis

Because metabolic disorders develop slowly and respiratory compensation occurs immediately, there is no distinction between chronic and acute metabolic derangements. Despite this fact, the respiratory response elicited by metabolic alkalosis is quite variable. No definite reasons for this variability have been identified. A normal or low $PaCO_2$ suggests a

Table 19–13. Causes of Metabolic Acidosis

Normal Anion Gap	Elevated Anion Gap
Renal tubular acidosis	Renal failure
Diarrhea	Ketoacidosis
Carbonic anhydrase inhibitors	Starvation
Ureteral diversions	Ethanol ingestion
Hyperalimentation	Methanol ingestion
Renal failure (early)	Ethylene glycol ingestion
Acid ingestion	Salicylates
Hyperchloremia	Lactic acidosis
	Nephrotic syndrome
	Seizures
	Circulatory failure
	Cyanide poisoning
	Carbon monoxide poisoning

Table 19–14. Causes of Metabolic Alkalosis

Diuretic use
Nasogastric suction
Vomiting
Diarrhea (containing chloride)
Antacid administration
Transfusions (citrate)
Drugs
  Carbenicillin
  Penicillin
Hypokalemia
Hypercalcemia
Primary hyperaldosteronism

coexisting respiratory alkalosis. Several formulas have been proposed to predict the respiratory compensation seen in metabolic alkalosis. The $Paco_2$ was equal to $0.9 \times [HCO_3^-] + 12$ (range, 9 to 16) in a group of patients in whom alkalosis was induced by a variety of methods.[117] Other authors have found less of a compensatory respiratory acidosis, as indicated in Table 19–10.[118]

There are many causes of this common abnormality of acid-base balance. Some are listed in Table 19–14. Diuretic use with hypokalemia and hypochloremia is a frequent cause. Acid and chloride loss from the gastrointestinal tract, antacid administration, certain antibiotics, and some endocrine abnormalities are also implicated. Some causes are treatable by replacement of chloride and potassium. There are several significant, undesired side effects of metabolic alkalosis. These include increased total body oxygen consumption, myocardial depression, and increased frequency of cardiac arrhythmias.

Combined Acid-Base Disorders

The disorders described in the preceding sections were single primary disorders with the appropriate, expected compensatory responses. More than one primary disorder may be present. This is suggested when the expected compensation to the first disorder is not seen. No system of analysis is effective in identifying multiple disorders; trends and the response to interventions can give clues.

Physicochemical Approach to Blood Gases (Stewart's Approach)

The preceding discussion of acid-base balance was based on the Henderson-Hasselbalch equation for defining the relationship between Pco_2, pH, and the weak anion, $[HCO_3^-]$. The clinical interpretation of this equation is that these three variables are each able to vary independently of each other, which is not true. Both pH and $[HCO_3^-]$ are determined by Pco_2 and other factors not included in the Henderson-Hasselbalch equation, namely, proteins and organic acids. The use of buffer-base and of base excess mentioned above were attempts to account for some of the discrepancies from reality by using this simplified approach. They have not been totally successful and the use of the anion gap was proposed as a method to enhance the understanding of other factors not included in the Henderson-Hasselbalch approach. Peter Stewart[119] suggested a more comprehensive, quantitative physicochemical approach to describing acid-base balance. His theory begins with the following general conditions:

1. Electroneutrality is maintained: the sum of positive charges must equal the sum of negative charges.
2. Dissociation equilibria of all incompletely dissociated substances must always be satisfied, that is, $[H^+] \times [A^-] = K_a \times [HA]$.
3. Mass is conserved: specifically, the total concentration of an incompletely dissociated substance can always be accounted for as the sum of the concentrations of its dissociated and undissociated forms, for example, $[A_{tot}]_n = [HA]_n + [A^-]_n$.

This leads to three sets of variables that can be changed primarily and independently:

1. Pco_2, regulated by alveolar gas, which is controlled by the relationship of ventilation to CO_2 production. CO_2 is able to freely cross all body compartments and thus all compartments are open systems (through the lung) for CO_2.
2. Strong ion difference (SID), which is the difference between the sum of all strong anions and the sum of all strong cations; $SID = [Na^+] + [K^+] + 2[Ca^{2+}] + 2[Mg^{2+}] - [Cl^-] - [\text{other strong anions}]$. These are regulated through the kidney and are open systems for water and electrolytes.
3. The total of all nonvolatile weak acids present, $[A_{tot}]_{1...n}$. In plasma this is primarily inorganic phosphate and serum proteins, including the most important, which is albumin.

None of the other variables commonly thought of, that is, $[H^+]$, $[HCO_3^-]$, total CO_2 content, or any weak base, can be changed primarily or individually. They are all dependent variables which will change if and when one or more of the independent variables change. This implies that pH is a dependent variable and not a primary determinant of acid-base balance. Therapies directed at improving acid-base abnormalities can only be applied to the independent variables.

To arrive at meaningful solutions to the above equations

Table 19–15. Primary Disorders of Acid-Base Equilibrium Using Stewart's Approach

Respiratory Disorders		Nonrespiratory Disorders		
		ABNORMAL STRONG ION DIFFERENCE	WEAK ACIDS ABNORMALITIES	
	Abnormal Pco_2		Serum albumin	Inorganic phosphate
Alkalosis	Hypocapnia	Increased	Hypoalbuminemia	—
Acidosis	Hypercapnia	Decreased	Hyperalbuminemia	Hyperphosphatemia
			Other proteins	

Based on Stewart PA: Independent and dependent variables of acid-base control. Respir Physiol 1978; 33:9–26.

Table 19–16. Factors Influencing Strong Ion Difference

	Change in Concentration of All Anions	Imbalance of Strong Ions
Alkalosis	Concentration (water deficit)	Chloride deficit
Acidosis	Dilution (water excess)	Chloride excess
		Unmeasured anions*

*Unmeasured anions include lactate, keto acids, exogenous acids (salicylates, etc.).

requires solving a series of simultaneous equations with many coefficients and factors. Several guesses and approximations are necessary to solve these equations, as well as the power of a computer.[120, 121] The final equation for acid-base balance can be written

$$SID + [H^+] - [OH^-] - [HCO_3^-] - [CO_3^=] - [Alb^{-X}] - [Pi^{-X}] = 0$$

where $[Alb^{-X}]$ is the concentration of negative charge from albumin and $[Pi^{-X}]$ is the negative charge concentration from the inorganic phosphates. Substituting known estimates for the contributions from albumin and inorganic phosphates allows calculation of the dependent variables in terms of the other factors.[122]

In a given system, the values of all the dependent variables are determined by the independent variables. The Henderson-Hasselbalch relationship is an example of this dependent variable interrelationship for PCO_2, pH and $[HCO_3^-]$. If any two are known the third can be calculated. The equation cannot explain why, at the given PCO_2, any particular set of values of pH and $[HCO_3^-]$ exists; the higher-order equations explain these in terms of SID, PCO_2, [Alb], and [Pi]. The failure of the Henderson-Hasselbalch relationship to produce insight into many acid-base disturbances has led to other measures of metabolic balance and to the development of the concept of anion gap to help explain the perceived anomalies.

Stewart's approach brings insight to several areas of physiology.[123] Body fluid compartments separated by membranes in which gradients of acid are maintained is one such area. The production of acid in tissues such as the gastric mucosa is not dependent on a hydrogen pump; rather, the acidosis is created by decreasing the SID, primarily by Cl^- manipulation. Hydrogen is at most a passive participant in the process. Acid-base disturbances are classified differently using Stewart's approach into the seven primary disorders listed in Table 19–15. There are several causes of SID disorders; these are detailed in Table 19–16. Included is the category of acidosis caused by unmeasured anions, equivalent to the contributors to an increased anion gap acidosis.

Stewart's approach is exciting in that it allows a comprehensive view of diagnosis and, perhaps, better treatment of acid-base disorders in complicated patients. It explains satisfactorily some previously observed clinical phenomena. The hypoalbuminemia of cirrhosis and malnutrition explains the alkalosis observed. The influence of changes in sodium on acid-base status is clarified. There remain several unanswered questions about this theory. Some of these are: What are the expected (compensatory) responses to abnormalities in each independent variable? What are the limits of compensation? Are there differences in compensation in each system depending on the duration of primary abnormality? How can multiple disorders be separated? Why is there failure of a

low pH to elicit compensatory hyperventilation with hyperchloremia following normal saline resuscitation? What abnormalities need to be corrected? What is the best way to correct identified abnormalities in each component?

As our understanding of the physiology and pathophysiology of acid-base control is better elucidated, these and other questions should become clear. The basic approach offered by Peter Stewart is a giant step forward in our understanding.

REFERENCES

1. Heyrovsky J: Electrolysis with the dropping mercury electrode. Chem Listy 1922; 16:256–304.
2. Clark LC Jr: Measurement of oxygen tension: A historical perspective. Crit Care Med 1981; 9:960–962.
3. Van Slyke DD, O'Neil JM: The determination of gases in blood and other solutions by vacuum extraction and manometric measurement. J Biol Chem 1924; 61:523.
4. Oropello JM, Manasia A, Hannon E, et al: Continuous fiberoptic arterial and venous blood gas monitoring in hemorrhagic shock. Chest 1996; 109:1049–1055.
5. Shapiro BA, Cane RD: Preliminary evaluation of an inter-arterial blood gas system in dogs and humans. Crit Care Med 1989; 17: 455–460.
6. Peterson JI, Fitzgerald RV, Buckhold DK: Fiberoptic probe for measurement of oxygen partial pressure. Anal Chem 1984; 56: 62–67.
7. Abraham E, Gallagher TJ, Fink S: Clinical evaluation of a multi-parameter intra-arterial blood-gas sensor. Intensive Care Med 1996; 22:507–513.
8. Roupie EE, Brochard L, Lemaire FJ: Clinical evaluation of a continuous intra-arterial blood gas system in critically ill patients. Intensive Care Med 1996; 22:1162–1168.
9. Zimmerman JL, Dellinger RP: Initial evaluation of a new intra-arterial blood gas system in humans. Crit Care Med 1993; 21: 495–500.
10. Eberhart RC: Indwelling blood compatible chemical sensors. Surg Clin North Am 1985; 65:1025–1040.
11. Ishikawa S, Makita K, Nakazawa K, et al: Continuous intra-arterial blood gas monitoring during oesophagectomy. Can J Anaesth 1998; 45:273–276.
12. Zollinger A, Spahn DR, Singer T, et al: Accuracy and clinical performance of a continuous intra-arterial blood-gas monitoring system during thoracoscopic surgery. Br J Anaesth 1997; 79: 47–52.
13. Shapiro BA, Mahutte CK, Crane RD, et al: Clinical performance of a blood gas monitor: A prospective, multicenter trial. Crit Care Med 1993; 21:487–494.
14. Shapiro BA: In vivo monitoring of arterial blood gases and pH. Respir Care 1992; 37:1087–1095.
15. Shapiro BA: Clinical and economic performance criteria for intraarterial and extraarterial blood gas monitors, with comparison with in vitro testing. Am J Clin Pathol 1995; 104(suppl 1): S100–106.
16. Shapiro BA: Intra-arterial and extra-arterial pH, PCO_2 and PO_2 monitors. Acta Anaesth Scand Suppl 1995; 104:69–74.
17. Franklin ML, Peruzzi WT, Moen SG, et al: Evaluation of an on-demand, ex vivo bedside blood gas monitor on pulmonary artery blood gas determinations. Anesth Analg 1996; 83:500–504.
18. Bourke DL: Errors in intraoperative hematocrit determination. Anesthesiology 1976; 45:357–359.
19. Fox MJ, Brody JS, Weintraub LR, et al: Leukocyte larceny: A cause of spurious hypoxemia. Am J Med 1979; 67:742–746.
20. Mizock BA, Franklin C, Lindesmith P, et al: Confirmation of spurious hypoxemia using continuous blood gas analysis in a patient with chronic myelogenous leukemia. Leuk Res 1995; 19:1001–1004.
21. Ong ST, David D, Snow M, et al: Effect of variations in room temperature on measured values of blood gas quality-control materials. Clin Chem 1983; 29:502–505.

22. Mahutte CK: On-line arterial blood gas analysis with optodes: Current status. Clin Biochem 1998; 31:119–130.

23. Thorson SH, Marini JJ, Pierson DJ, et al: Variability of arterial blood gas values in stable patients in the ICU. Chest 1983; 84:14–18.

24. Perutz NF: Stereochemistry of cooperative effects in hemoglobin. Nature 1970; 228:726–739.

25. Perutz NF: Hemoglobin structure and respiratory transport. Sci Am December 1978; 239:92–125.

26. Shappell SD, Lenfant CJM: Adaptive, genetic, and iatrogenic alterations of the oxyhemoglobin-dissociation curve. Anesthesiology 1972; 37:127–139.

27. Schumacker PT, Long GR, Wood LDH: Tissue oxygen extraction during hypovolemia: Role of hemoglobin P_{50}. J Appl Physiol 1987; 62:1801–1807.

28. Standl TG, Reeker W, Redmann G, et al: Haemodynamic changes and skeletal muscle oxygen tension during complete blood exchange with ultrapurified polymerized bovine haemoglobin. Intensive Care Med 1997; 23:865–872.

29. Nolte D, Botzlar A, Pickelmann S, et al: Effects of diaspirin-cross-linked hemoglobin (DCLHb) on the microcirculation of striated skin muscle in the hamster: A study on safety and toxicity. J Lab Clin Med 1997; 130:314–327.

30. Rubio R, Berne RM: Regulation of coronary blood flow. Prog Cardiovasc Dis 1975; 43:105–122.

31. Gilbert R, Keighley JF: The arterial-alveolar oxygen tension ratio. An index of gas exchange applicable to varying inspired oxygen concentrations. Am Rev Respir Dis 1974; 109:142–145.

32. Gilbert R, Auchincloss JH, Kuppinger M, et al: Stability of the arterial/alveolar oxygen partial pressure ratio. Crit Care Med 1979; 7:267–272.

33. Nunn JF: Applied Respiratory Physiology, ed 3. London, Butterworths, 1987, pp 241, 473.

34. Hoffman WE, Charbel FT, Edelman G: Brain tissue oxygen, carbon dioxide, and pH in neurosurgical patients at risk for ischemia. Anesth Analg 1996; 82:582–586.

35. Drucker W, Pearce F, Glass-Heidenreich L, et al: Subcutaneous tissue oxygen pressure: A reliable index of peripheral perfusion in humans after injury. J Trauma 1996; 40(suppl 3):S116–122.

36. Block AJ, Cherniac RM, Christopher KL, et al: Problems in prescribing and supplying oxygen for medicare patients. Am Rev Respir Dis 1986; 134:340–341.

37. Durbin, CG Jr: Pulmonary oxygen toxicity. Respir Care 1993; 39:1–12.

38. Deneke SM, Fanburg BL: Normobaric oxygen toxicity of the lung. N Engl J Med 1980; 303:76–86.

39. Golde AR, Mahoney JL: The oxygen optode: An improved method of assessing flap blood flow and viability. J Otolaryngol 1994; 23:138–144.

40. Powell CC, Schultz SC, Burris DG, et al: Subcutaneous oxygen tension: A useful adjunct in assessment of perfusion status. Crit Care Med 1995; 23:867–873.

41. Marshall BE, Wyche MQ: Hypoxemia during and after anesthesia. Anesthesiology 1972; 37:178–209.

42. Davis WB, Rennard SI, Bitterman PB, et al: Pulmonary oxygen toxicity: Early reversible changes in human alveolar structures induced by hyperoxia. N Engl J Med 1983; 309:878–883.

43. Roes DM, Downes JB, Heenan TJ: Temporal responses of functional residual capacity and oxygen tension to changes in positive end-expiratory pressure. Crit Care Med 1981; 9:79–82.

44. Kirby RR, Downs JB, Civetta JM, et al: High level and expiratory pressure (PEEP) in acute respiratory failure. Chest 1975; 67:156–163.

45. DiRusso SM, Nelson LD, Safcsak K, et al: Survival in patients with severe adult respiratory distress syndrome treated with high-level positive end-expiratory pressure. Crit Care Med 1995; 23:1485–1496.

46. Petty TL, Fowler AA: Another look at ARDS. Chest 1982; 82:98–104.

47. Finfer S, Rocker G: Alveolar overdistension is an important mechanism of persistent lung damage following severe protracted ARDS. Anaesth Intensive Care 1996; 24:569–573.

48. Dreyfuss D, Saumon G: Barotrauma is volutrauma, but which volume is the one responsible? Intensive Care Med 1992; 18:139–141.

49. Dambrosio M, Roupie E, Mollet JJ, et al: Effects of positive end-expiratory pressure and different tidal volumes on alveolar recruitment and hyperinflation. Anesthesiology 1997; 87:495–503.

50. Servillo G, Svantesson C, Beydon L, et al: Pressure-volume curves in acute respiratory failure: Automated low flow inflation versus occlusion. Am J Respir Crit Care Med 1997; 155:1629–1636.

51. Kalfon P, Rao GS, Gallart L, et al: Permissive hypercapnia with and without expiratory washout in patients with severe acute respiratory distress syndrome. Anesthesiology 1997; 87:6–17.

52. Thorens JB, Jolliet P, Ritz M, et al: Effects of rapid permissive hypercapnia on hemodynamics, gas exchange, and oxygen transport and consumption during mechanical ventilation for the acute respiratory distress syndrome. Intensive Care Med 1996; 22:182–196.

53. Rossaint R, Kelly K, Kaisers U: Present role of nitric oxide inhalation in severe lung failure. Acta Anaesth Scand Suppl 1996; 109:88–92.

54. Weis CM, Wolfson MR, Shaffer TH: Liquid-assisted ventilation: Physiology and clinical application. Ann Med 1997; 29:509–517.

55. Jobe AH, Ikegami M: Surfactant for acute respiratory distress syndrome. Adv Intern Med 1997; 42:203–230.

56. Pappert D, Falke KJ: Indications, modifications and technique of ECMO with or without NO-therapy. Acta Anaesth Scand Suppl 1996; 109:117–120.

57. Tao W, Brunston RL Jr, Bidani A, et al: Significant reduction in minute ventilation and peak inspiratory pressures with arterio-venous CO_2 removal during severe respiratory failure. Crit Care Med 1997; 25:689–695.

58. Dofinsky PM, Whitcomb ME: The effect of PEEP on cardiac output. Chest 1983; 84:210–216.

59. Gallagher J, Civetta JM: Goal-directed therapy of acute respiratory failure. Anesth Analg 1980; 59:831–834.

60. Miller RS, Nelson LD, DiRusso SM, et al: High-level positive end-expiratory pressure management in trauma-associated adult respiratory distress syndrome. J Trauma 1992; 33:284–290.

61. Luce JM: The cardiovascular effects of mechanical ventilation and positive end-expiratory pressure. JAMA 1984; 252:807–811.

62. Jardin F, Farcot JC, Boisante L, et al: Influence of positive end-expiratory pressure on left ventricular performance. N Engl J Med 1981; 304:387–392.

63. Haynes JB, Carson SD, Whitney WP, et al: Positive end-expiratory pressure shifts left ventricular pressure-area curves. J Appl Physiol 1980; 48:670–676.

64. Prewitt RM, Wood LDH: The effect of positive end-expiratory pressure on ventricular function in dogs. Am J Physiol 1979; 236:H534–544.

65. Buda AJ, Pinsky MR, Ingels NB, et al: Effects of intrathoracic pressure on left ventricular performance. N Engl J Med 1979; 301:453–459.

66. Chapin JC, Downs JB, Douglas ME, et al: Lung expansion, airway pressure transmission, and positive end-expiratory pressure. Arch Surg 1979; 114:1193–1197.

67. Mathews PJ: The validity of Pao_2 values 3, 6, and 9 minutes after an Fio_2 change in mechanically ventilated heart-surgery patients. Respir Care 1987; 32:1029–1034.

68. Lucey JF, Dangman B: A reexamination of the role of oxygen in retrolental fibroplasia. Pediatrics 1984; 73:82–96.

69. Kitahata LM, Katz JD: Tension pneumocephalus after posterior fossa craniotomy: A complication of the sitting position. Anesthesiology 1976; 44:448–450.

70. Faithfull NS: Fluorocarbons: Current status and future applications. Anaesthesia 1987; 42:234–242.

71. Kapp JR: Neurological response to hyperbaric oxygen—a criterion for cerebral revascularization. Surg Neurol 1981; 15:43–46.

72. Roughton JWF: Transport of oxygen and carbon dioxide. *In* Fenn WO, Rahn H (eds): Handbook of Physiology, Section 3: Respiration, vol 1. Washington, DC, American Physiological Society, 1964, p 800.

73. Andritsch RF, Muravchick S, Gold MI: Temperature correction of arterial blood gas parameters: A comparative review of methodology. Anesthesiology 1981; 55:311–316.

74. Ream AK, Reitz BA, Silverberg G: Temperature correction of $Paco_2$ and pH in estimating acid-base: An example of the emperor's new clothes? Anesthesiology 1982; 56:41–44.
75. Rahn H, Reeves RB, Howell BJ: Hydrogen ion regulation, temperature, and evolution. Am Rev Respir Dis 1975; 112:162–165.
76. Becker H, Vinten-Johansen J, Buckberg GD, et al: Myocardial damage caused by keeping pH 7.40 during deep systemic hypothermia. J Thorac Cardiovasc Surg 1981; 82:810–820.
77. Blayo MC, LeCompte Y, Pocidalo JJ: Control of acid-base status during hypothermia in man. Respir Physiol 1980; 42:287–298.
78. Brandenburg MA, Dire DJ: Comparison of arterial and venous blood gas values in the initial emergency department evaluation of patients with ketoacidosis. Ann Emerg Med 1998; 31:458–465.
79. Durbin CG: Malignant hyperthermia syndrome: Identification and management. In Berry FA (ed): Anesthetic Management of Difficult and Routine Pediatric Patients. New York, Churchill Livingstone, 1986, pp 414–415.
80. Michalek-Sauberer A, Fricker R, Gradwohl I, et al: A case of suspected malignant hyperthermia during desflurane administration. Anesth Analg 1997; 85:461–462.
81. Blumenthal SR, Voorhees WD: The relationship of carbon dioxide excretion during cardiopulmonary resuscitation to regional blood flow and survival. Resuscitation 1997; 35:135–143.
82. Levine RL, Wayne MA, Miller CC: End-tidal carbon dioxide and outcome of out-of-hospital cardiac arrest. N Engl J Med 1997; 337:301–306.
83. Garnett AR, Ornato JP, Gonzalez ER, et al: End-tidal carbon dioxide monitoring during cardiopulmonary resuscitation. JAMA 1987; 257:512–515.
84. Androgue HJ, Rashad MN, Gorin AB, et al: Assessing acid-base status in circulatory failure. Differences between arterial and central venous blood. N Engl J Med 1989; 320:1312–1316.
85. Van Styke DD, Cullen GE: Studies of acidosis. 1. Bicarbonate concentration of blood plasma: Its significance and its determination as measure of acidosis. J Biol Chem 1917; 30:289–346.
86. Astrup P: New approach to acid-base metabolism. Clin Chem 1961; 7:1–15.
87. Astrup P, Jorgensen K, Siggaard Andersen O, et al: Acid-base metabolism: A new approach. Lancet 1960; 1:1035–1039.
88. Schwartz WB, Relman AS: A critique of the parameters used in the evaluation of acid-base disorders. N Engl J Med 1963; 268:1382–1388.
89. Arbus CS, Hebert LA, Levesque PR, et al: Characterization and clinical application of the "significance band" for acute respiratory alkalosis. N Engl J Med 1969; 280:117–123.
90. Levesque PR: Acid-base disorders: Application of total body carbon dioxide titration in anesthesia. Anesth Analg 1975; 54:299–307.
91. Narins RG, Emmett M: Simple and mixed acid-base disorders: A practical approach. Medicine (Baltimore) 1980; 59:161–187.
92. Brackett NC, Cohn JJ, Schwartz WB: Carbon dioxide titration curve of normal man: Effect of increasing degrees of acute hypercapnia on acid-base equilibrium. N Engl J Med 1965; 272:6–12.
93. Travaline JM, Krachman S, D'Alonzo GE: Mechanical ventilation in severe asthma: When and how. J Respir Dis 1995; 16:609–611, 616.
94. Williams TJ, Tuxen DV, Scheinkestel CD, et al: Risk factors for morbidity in mechanically ventilated patients with acute severe asthma. Am Rev Respir Dis 1992; 146:607–615.
95. Kacmarek RM, Hickling KG: Permissive hypercapnia. Respir Care 1993; 38:373–387.
96. Simon RJ, Ivatury RR: The expanding role of permissive hypercapnia in patients with ARDS. Trauma Q 1996; 12:257–271.
97. Minuck M, Sharma GP: Comparison of Tham and sodium bicarbonate in resuscitation of the heart after ventricular fibrillation in dogs. Anesth Analg 1977; 56:38–45.
98. Manfredi F, Sieker HO, Spoto AP, et al: Severe carbon dioxide intoxication: Treatment with organic buffer (trishydroxymethyl aminomethane). JAMA 1960; 173:999–1003.
99. Gazmuri RJ, von Planta M, Weil MH, et al: Cardiac effects of carbon dioxide–consuming and carbon dioxide–generating buffers during cardiopulmonary resuscitation. J Am Coll Cardiol 1990; 15:482–490.
100. Brackett NC, Wingo CF, Muren O, et al: Acid-base response to chronic hypercapnia in man. N Engl J Med 1969; 280:124–130.
101. West JB: Causes of carbon dioxide retention in lung disease. N Engl J Med 1971; 284:1232–1236.
102. Poponick JM, Renston JP, Emerman CL: Successful use of nasal BiPAP in three patients previously requiring intubation and mechanical ventilation. J Emerg Med 1997; 15:785–788.
103. Arora NS, Rochester DF: Respiratory muscle strength and maximal voluntary ventilation in undernourished patients. Am Rev Respir Dis 1982; 126:5–8.
104. Hunter MAB, Cary MA, Larsh HW: The nutritional status of patients with chronic obstructive pulmonary disease. Am Rev Respir Dis 1981; 124:376–391.
105. Sonnes LJ, Davis JA: Increased exercise performance in patients with severe COPD following inspiratory resistive training. Chest 1982; 82:436–439.
106. Covelli HD, Black JW, Olsen MS, et al: Respiratory failure precipitated by high carbohydrate loads. Ann Intern Med 1981; 95:579–581.
107. Aubier M, De Troyer A, Sampson M, et al: Aminophylline improves diaphragm contractility. N Engl J Med 1981; 305:249–277.
108. Hill NS: Noninvasive ventilation. Does it work, for whom, and how? Am Rev Respir Dis 1993; 147:1050–1055.
109. Strumpf DA, Millman RP, Carlisle CC, et al: Nocturnal positive-pressure ventilation via nasal mask in patients with severe chronic obstructive pulmonary disease. Am Rev Respir Dis 1991; 144:234–239.
110. Meecham-Jons DJ, Paul EA, Jones PW: Nasal pressure support ventilation plus oxygen compared with oxygen therapy alone in hypercapnic COPD. Am J Respir Crit Care Med 1995; 152:538–544.
111. Allen CH, Ward JD: An evidence-based approach to management of increased intracranial pressure. Crit Care Clin 1998; 14:485–495.
112. Dexter F: Research synthesis of controlled studies evaluating the effect of hypocapnia and airway protection on cerebral outcome. J Neurosurg Anesth 1997; 9:217–222.
113. Lahiri S, Milledge JS: Acid-base in Sherpa altitude residents and lowlanders at 4880 M. Respir Physiol 1967; 2:323–334.
114. Albert MS, Dell RB, Winters RW: Quantitative displacement acid-base equilibrium in metabolic acidosis. Ann Intern Med 1967; 66:312–322.
115. Emmet M, Narins RG: Clinical use of the anion gap. Medicine (Baltimore) 1977; 56:38–54.
116. Morris LR, Murphy MB, Kitabchi AE: Bicarbonate therapy in severe diabetic ketoacidosis. Ann Intern Med 1986; 105:836–840.
117. Fulop M: Hypercapnia in metabolic alkalosis. N Y State J Med 1976; 76:19–22.
118. Goldring RM, Cannon PJ, Heinemann HO, et al: Respiratory adjustment to chronic metabolic alkalosis in man. J Clin Invest 1968; 47:188–202.
119. Stewart PA: Independent and dependent variables of acid-base control. Respir Physiol 1978; 33:9–26.
120. Fencl V, Leith DE: Stewart's quantitative acid-base chemistry: Applications to biology and medicine. Resp Physiol 1992; 91:1–16.
121. Figge J, Mydosh T, Fencl V: The role of serum proteins in acid-base equilibria. J Lab Clin Med 1991; 117:453–467.
122. Figge J, Mydosh T, Fencl V: Serum proteins and acid-base equilibria: A follow-up. J Lab Clin Med 1992; 120:713–719.
123. Jennings DB: The physiocochemistry of [H^+] and respiratory control: Roles of PCO_2, strong ions, and their hormonal regulators. Can J Physiol Pharmacol 1994; 72:1499–1512.

PART FIVE

Other Monitoring Applications

20 Monitoring of Temperature and Heart and Lung Sounds

Carol L. Lake, M.D., M.B.A.

Stethoscopes

Strange noises emanating from the body had been noted in the 17th and 18th centuries. Initial efforts to hear these noises were by direct application of the physician's ear to the patient's chest or abdomen. Laennec, faced with the inability to directly auscultate the heart of an obese patient, recalled that a cylinder amplified sounds. Rolling a piece of paper into a cylinder, Laennec applied one end of it to the patient's chest and the other to his ear—the first stethoscope.[1]

Indications

Although multiple modalities to monitor circulation and ventilation have supplanted the routine use of precordial and esophageal stethoscopes, the stethoscope still provides an uncomplicated, nonelectric method to qualitatively assess heart and lung function.[2, 3] Acoustic and electronic stethoscopes, including some with earphones rather than earplugs, may ultimately replace the traditional stethoscope for all auscultatory activities.

Types

Precordial. Precordial weighted stethoscopes are available in small, medium, and large sizes for application with double-sided tape disks to the precordium or sternal notch. Various types of rubber or plastic tubing connect the stethoscope to monaural or standard binaural earpieces. The presence and quality of heart and lung sounds are commonly assessed using precordial stethoscopes.

Esophageal. An esophageal stethoscope, an inexpensive, simple monitoring device of heart and lung sounds, was introduced into anesthesia practice more than three decades ago[4] (Fig. 20–1A). It consists of a catheter fitted with openings in the distal 2 to 3 cm that are covered by a rubber cuff. Esophageal stethoscopes do not require electricity or complicated technological interpretation. Examples of clinical situations detected with esophageal stethoscopes, but not as readily with other circulatory or respiratory monitors, are wheezing, dysrhythmias, ventilator disconnection or malfunction, and abnormal heart tones, including murmurs.[3] More sophisticated versions of the esophageal stethoscope incorporate thermistors (Fig. 20–1C), electrocardiograph (ECG) electrodes (Fig. 20–1B), and Doppler transducers for determination of cardiac output.[5] The advantages of monitoring the ECG from the esophagus[6] are discussed in Chapter 12. In addition to the risks of esophageal damage from passage of the probe, the possibility of esophageal burns from leakage currents is present when they are connected to electrically powered ECG and temperature modules.[7]

Doppler. Doppler probes of 2.4 MHz transmit and reflect ultrasound from the heart of both infants and adults. The optimal location for cardiac monitoring is the third or fourth intercostal space to the right of the sternum. However, placement should be at a point where sound transmission is best, particularly in response to rapid injection of fluid through a central venous catheter. Precordial Dopplers are usually used for detection of venous air embolism rather than routine cardiac monitoring. Unlike the normal cardiac sounds, air embolism causes a characteristic high-pitched scratching noise.[8] An unfortunate disadvantage of Doppler technology is interference by electrocautery.

Complications from Use of Stethoscopes

Loss of an esophageal stethoscope into the stomach coincident to placement of a nasogastric tube and a second esophageal stethoscope has been reported.[9] Stethoscopes may fracture with retention of fragments in the gastrointestinal tract. Misidentification of the esophagus containing a stethoscope for the trachea or the internal jugular vein containing a ventriculojugular shunt catheter has been reported in children.[10] Misplacement of stethoscopes into the trachea instead of the esophagus causes significant gas leakage around the endotracheal tube cuff that may preclude adequate ventilation.[11] Loss of the cuff of the esophageal stethoscope can occur, especially with repeated use. Inadvertent fixation of the stethoscope during surgical repairs around the nasopharynx or esophagus can be avoided by using a precordial device or verifying mobility of the stethoscope during surgical procedures in the area. Esophageal stethoscopes are flammable at clinically used oxygen and nitrous oxide concentrations if a source of ignition is nearby.[12]

Monitoring of Temperature

Physiology of Thermoregulation

Heat Gain

Body heat is primarily produced by metabolism in the liver and skeletal muscles. Basal heat production ranges from 65 to 85 kcal/hour. Heat is produced by voluntary muscle activity (exercise), involuntary muscle activity (shivering), and nonshivering thermogenesis (NST). During moderate work or

357

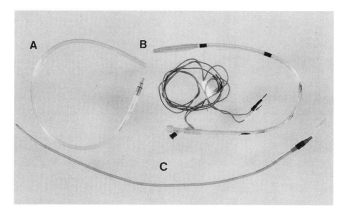

Figure 20–1. Esophageal stethoscopes of various types. *A* is an adult stethoscope. Stethoscope *B* is modified with two electrodes for monitoring the electrocardiogram. Stethoscope *C* has an integral thermistor for monitoring esophageal temperature.

exercise, heat production increases to 300 kcal/hour. With maximal work, heat production increases to 600 kcal/hour or more. Heat generated from muscular contraction is transferred to blood flowing through the muscle bed. The temperature of the body core, as well as of blood exiting from the liver or lower extremities, increases during exercise.

NST, an oxygen-consuming, heat-producing mechanism stimulated by the sympathetic nervous system, is the major mechanism for heat production in infants. It results from byproducts of glucose metabolism, fatty acid metabolism, and gluconeogenesis. In infants fatty acids are liberated from triglycerides due to lipase release (stimulated by norepinephrine) in brown fat and oxidized in muscle, white fat, brain and liver or reesterified or oxidized in brown fat. Brown fat, constituting 2% to 6% of body weight, is located between the scapulae, around kidneys, adrenals, vertebrae, neck blood vessels, mediastinum, and in the axillae. It causes the infant's neck and interscapular skin to be warmer than other body parts during cold exposure. Microscopically, brown fat contains numerous mitochondria, densely packed with cristae and respiratory chain components.[13] NST is more energy-efficient than shivering thermogenesis, which is, nevertheless, fully developed in infants. It is unaffected by neuromuscular blockade[14] but is blocked by sympathectomy, ganglionic blockade, and β-adrenergic blockade.

Heat Loss

Physiologic Mechanisms. Convection, conduction, and radiation from the skin surface and lungs normally dissipate the heat produced and protect the body from thermal damage. The thermoregulatory center is located in the anterior and posterior hypothalamus, the anterior temperature-sensitive area known as the Aronsohn-Sachs center, and the posterior, temperature-insensitive area, known as the Krehl-Isenschmidt center.[15] The hypothalamic temperature changes as heated blood from muscle flows into the area. The posterior hypothalamus receives sensory input of temperature changes, while the anterior hypothalamus adjusts the mechanisms controlling heat loss and production. An increase in hypothalamic temperature induces systemic dilatation of skin vessels and secretion of sweat to offset the increase, a process known as the Benzinger reflex.[14] Cold impulses arriving in the posterior hypothalamus induce shivering to initiate heat production. However, in the presence of normal or increased body temperature, the anterior hypothalamus overrides the posterior center, preventing heat production. Because hypothalamic temperature is integral to thermal equilibrium, its temperature should probably be regarded as the "core temperature."

In addition to the central thermoreceptors, peripheral thermoreceptors are found in the skin. From these receptors, cold impulses (activated at skin temperatures of <40°C and maximal at 30° to 35°C) travel through the A delta nerve fibers while warm impulses are carried by the C fibers (activated at 30° to 35°C and maximal at 40° to 45°C).[16]

Alterations in the core temperature away from its set point initiate changes in heat production or heat loss. In order to maintain a balance between heat production and heat loss, the autonomic nervous system varies the blood supply to the body surface, causing shivering or sweating. If the environmental temperature is cool, a thermal gradient between the body surface and the environment allows rapid dissipation. If environmental temperature is increased to body surface temperature or greater, heat is lost only by vaporization of sweat. Maximal rates of sweat vaporization are limited by atmospheric humidity, air movement, and rate of sweating. At conditions of increased humidity, heat loss through sweat vaporization is limited and body temperature increases. Practically, the amount of heat loss through sweating is about 650 kcal/hour.

In addition to sweating, cardiovascular changes occur in humans exposed to hot environments (Table 20-1). These changes include increased cardiac output, tachycardia, decreased hepatic and splanchnic blood flow, decreased sys-

Table 20–1. Physiologic Consequences of Temperature Alterations

Increased Environmental Temperature
Increased respiratory work
Increased cardiac work
Increased oxygen demand
Hypovolemia
Acidosis (respiratory and metabolic)

Decreased Environmental Temperature
Patient discomfort
Increased oxygen demand (shivering)
Decreased drug disposition
Decreased myocardial contractility and compliance
Impaired coronary autoregulation (coronary perfusion dependent on diastolic pressure)
Decreased total myocardial oxygen consumption (oxygen consumption per beat same or increased)
Cardiac dysrhythmias (atrial and ventricular, ventricular fibrillation around 28°C, asystole with profound hypothermia), J point elevation on ECG, conduction disturbances (increased P–R interval, A-V block, widening of the QRS complex, bradycardia, and Osborne wave (secondary wave following S wave)
Peripheral vasoconstriction (increased systemic vascular resistance, decreased microcirculatory flow, increased hematocrit)
Decreased cerebral blood flow and CMRO$_2$
Central nervous system depression, delirium, and coma (EEG slowing between 30°–35°C, decreased EEG amplitude <30°C, isoelectricity of increasing duration <22°C)
Decreased oxygen availability (oxyhemoglobin dissociation curve shifted to left)
Sympathetic stimulation
Hyperglycemia
Thrombocytopenia and impaired platelet thromboxane synthesis
Decreased anesthetic requirements and delayed anesthetic emergence

ECG, electrocardiogram; A-V, atrioventricular; EEG, electroencephalogram.

temic vascular resistance, and reduced effective volume. In adequately conditioned and heat-acclimatized humans, maximal cardiac output increases, peak heart rate decreases, stroke volume increases, and sweat composition and volume change to limit volume and sodium loss. However, these compensatory mechanisms are overwhelmed by prolonged exposure to high environmental temperatures. Sweating ceases, cardiac output and stroke volume decrease, and cutaneous blood flow is reduced while core temperature increases. The end result is heat stroke, which is characterized by a rectal temperature greater than 41.1°C, delirium, and coma.[17] Even physically conditioned and heat-acclimatized individuals may suffer heat stroke during extreme exertion.

Nonphysiologic Mechanisms. *Heat Loss in Infants.* Infants have considerable difficulty maintaining their core temperature in the face of changing ambient temperatures. They have a small body mass acting as a heat generator, but a large surface area for heat loss (ratio of surface to mass = 3:1). Heat loss is also increased in infants because of their lack of subcutaneous tissue and decreased motor tone.

Thermoregulation increases oxygen consumption in infants in proportion to the ambient-to-skin surface temperature gradient.[17] Thus, the thermoregulatory range of infants is significantly limited compared with that of the adult. Minimum ambient temperature for thermoregulation is 22°C in an infant compared with 0°C in an adult. Minimal oxygen consumption in infants occurs at environmental temperatures of 32° to 34°C, the neutral thermal state, in which there is less than a 2°C gradient between environmental and abdominal skin temperature.[18] Thus, the usual recommendations are to maintain operating room temperature at 27°C for premature infants, 26°C for infants up to 6 months of age, and at 25°C for infants from 6 months to 24 months of age. However, most operating room personnel are most comfortable with relative humidities of less than 50%, temperatures of 18°C, and an air exchange rate of 25/hour or greater.[19]

Heat Loss in Adults. Heat transfer occurs only when there is a temperature difference between two surfaces. In humans heat loss occurs in two phases: (1) transfer of heat from body core to skin surface (internal temperature gradient) and (2) heat dissipation (the external temperature gradient). Heat loss is determined by the skin and environmental temperatures, the thermal transfer coefficient, and the surface area. Tissue thickness, body size, and blood flow determine thermal transfer coefficients. Heat transfer from the core to the surface of the body creates an internal temperature gradient. Vasoconstriction decreases cutaneous blood flow and increases tissue insulation, attempting to increase the internal temperature gradient and reduce conductive and convective heat loss.

Heat loss across the external temperature gradient is affected by evaporation, convection, conduction, and radiation. Evaporative heat losses through the skin and respiratory systems depend on minute ventilation, airflow velocity, and relative humidity (specifically the difference between vapor pressures in the environment and on the skin surface). The transfer of heat to the air currents (convection) is influenced by air velocity, specific heat of the flowing gas, surface area, and ambient temperature. Because of high air turnover rates in operating rooms, convection causes about 25% of body heat loss.[20] Trapping a layer of air between the skin and the environment reduces heat loss by convection.

Heat loss by conduction depends on a temperature gradient between contacting surfaces and is affected by surface area and the thermal conductivity of the surface. Wetting

increases conduction by 25- to 30-fold. Radiant heat loss is the transfer of heat between two objects in the form of electromagnetic energy. It is independent of environmental temperature but is dependent on the radiating surface area and proportional to the temperature difference between skin and surrounding environment.[20] Radiation is the largest source of heat loss (65%) for the human body, particularly in infants (50% versus 20% in adults).

Indications for Temperature Measurement

The measurement of body temperature by some route is a standard of care during all anesthetic procedures. Both the risk of malignant hyperthermia (MH) and accidental hypothermia necessitate continuous observation of temperature. However, a recent study noted that fewer than 15% of anesthesiologists routinely monitor the temperature of patients receiving regional anesthesia.[21] A specific indication for temperature monitoring is induced hypothermia, either by surface or perfusion (extracorporeal circulation) cooling.

Measurements of skin, core, and mean body temperature are typically made in the perioperative period. Accurate assessments of skin temperature require measurements at four or more sites.[22] Body temperature in neutral or warm environments is calculated as:

$$T_{body} = (0.66 \times T_{core}) + (0.34 \times T_{skin})$$

where T_{core} is core temperature, T_{body} is mean body temperature, and T_{skin} is mean skin temperature.[23] Total body heat (TBH) is determined as:

$$TBH = \text{Mean temperature} \times \text{weight (kg)} \times \text{specific heat}$$

where the specific heat of the human body is 3.475 kJ°C^{-1}.[24]

Methods

John Hunter in 1776 was the first to measure body temperature by using a mercury-in-glass thermometer placed under the tongue. Today glass thermometers are rarely used clinically, having been replaced by thermistors inserted at various body sites.

Thermistors and Thermocouples

A thermistor or thermally sensitive resistor includes semiconductive elements (heavy metal oxides such as manganese, iron, zinc, cobalt, nickel) in which electrical resistance varies with temperature. Electrodes are attached to a bead of the metal oxide which is sealed into a small measuring tip. Large changes in resistance correspond to changes in temperature, allowing a rapid response time. Thermistors are usually accurate to ±5°C over a range from −80° to +150°C, but narrower ranges improve linearity.[25]

In a thermocouple, voltage is produced by the electromotive force (Seebeck effect) between two dissimilar metals (usually copper and constantan, a mixture of copper and nickel) that depends on the temperature difference between two junctions maintained at different temperatures, a standard thermoneutral or "cold" junction and the probe end of the thermocouple. One of the junctions is maintained as the "reference" junction while the other becomes the "measuring" junction, located within the probe. The electromotive force generated is proportional to the temperature difference between the two junctions.[25] Thermocouples have several advantages, including small size and reproducibility. A problem with thermocouples involving the reference junction is the Peltier effect, occurring when a current passed around the thermocouple circuit creates cold at one junction and heat at the other, so that the reference junction does not remain thermoneutral.

Liquid Crystal Devices

Adhesive liquid crystal temperature detectors measure skin temperature over ranges of 34° to 40°C (92° to 104°F) (Fig. 20-2). Skin temperature on the forehead is usually close to oral temperature but demonstrates considerable individual variation. Although temperatures measured with liquid crystal thermometry correlate well with forehead skin temperature, their correlation with temperatures monitored at other sites is poor ($r = .54$ to esophageal or tympanic probes).[26] Vaughan and colleagues[27] reported that compared with tympanic membrane thermometry, liquid crystal strips failed to accurately track temperature trends in postanesthetic patients. Their data suggest that temperature in the body shell is an unreliable indicator of core temperature.[27] Skin thermistors are also unreliable indicators of MH because peripheral vasoconstriction is an initial feature of the syndrome.

Despite their inaccuracy, the convenience of liquid crystal thermometers makes them useful for continuous temperature monitoring in operating rooms, postanesthesia care units, and during regional anesthesia or sympathetic blockade of peripheral nerve blocks. For perioperative use the sensors are applied to the forehead, while during sympathetic blocks they are applied to the involved extremity. Advantages include safety (completely noninvasive) and low cost. Disadvantages include difficulties with adhesion secondary to skin secretions, susceptibility to external thermal influences such as radiant heat lamps or air currents, allergic reactions to adhesive backing, and inaccuracy and imprecision.[26-28]

Infrared Thermometry

Another method of clinical thermometry is an infrared tympanic probe, which determines temperature by measuring the infrared radiation given off by an object. It consists of an otoscope-like probe covered by a disposable speculum that is introduced into the external auditory canal like an otoscope. The sensor in the probe gathers emitted infrared radiation for about 1 second and then transfers that information to an analog-to-digital converter and microprocessor. A liquid crystal displays the resultant temperature on a base module. Accuracy of this technology has been documented with in vitro water baths as well as in vivo. Clinical trials demonstrate a correlation coefficient of the infrared tympanic probe with pulmonary artery thermistor or esophageal temperature of .9833.[16, 29] Aural canal and tympanic thermometry accurately assess hypothalamic temperature. Advantages of this technology include the speed of determination, reduced potential for cross-contamination, and the absence of need for direct contact and temperature equilibrium of the device with the measuring surface.

Sites

Sites used for measurement of body temperature include the skin, nasopharynx, esophagus, bladder, rectum, axilla, and tympanic membrane. Central sites for temperature monitoring include the esophagus, nasopharynx, tympanic membrane, and pulmonary artery. Intermediate sites are the bladder and rectum. The skin is the most common peripheral site.

The choice of site depends on the purpose of the measurement. Usually it is either specific organ temperature or core (total body) temperature that is needed. Temperatures measured in the tympanic membrane or nasopharynx estimate brain temperature. Esophageal temperature approximates myocardial temperature. Cork and coworkers[30] reported the greatest precision (correlation between tympanic membrane and other sites) and accuracy (accuracy defined by difference from the tympanic membrane temperature) for temperature measurements in the urinary bladder, nasopharynx, and esophagus. Axilla, great toe, and forehead temperatures are less accurate than the other sites.[30]

Tympanic Membrane

The efficacy and convenience of tympanic thermometry was documented more than two decades ago. Measurement of tympanic membrane temperature as an index of brain temperature is particularly relevant because thermal homeostasis depends on anterior hypothalamic temperature.[31] At the tympanic membrane, the thermoelectric sensor is in the vicinity of the internal carotid artery, the major cerebral blood supply.[32] The tympanic membrane and surrounding structures

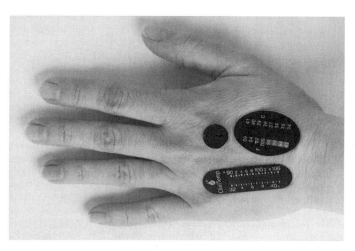

Figure 20-2. Three types of liquid crystal thermometers measuring skin temperature on the hand. For perioperative monitoring, these devices are usually placed on the patient's forehead.

are supplied by branches of the external carotid artery, including the internal maxillary and posterior auricular arteries. Tympanic temperatures parallel temperatures measured from an ideally placed esophageal thermistor except that tympanic temperatures are lower by about 0.2°C.[32] The tympanic membrane may be the optimal site during profound hypothermic circulatory arrest.[33]

An otoscopic examination to document patency of the auditory canal should precede tympanic or external auditory canal thermometry. The presence of cerumen may render measurements inaccurate.

Nasopharyngeal

Nasopharyngeal temperatures estimate brain temperature, particularly when the thermistor is carefully positioned behind the soft palate. However, air leakage around tracheal tube cuffs affects nasopharyngeal probe accuracy. Another disadvantage is the possibility of epistaxis or adenoidal bleeding in children.

Esophageal

Esophageal temperatures are affected by ventilation (particularly when the thermistor is placed at the mid- or upper esophagus,[34] thoracotomy, or rapid infusion of cold fluids or blood that cools the heart and great vessels. Variations of 1° to 6°C have been reported, depending on the location of the tip of the probe within the esophagus,[32, 34, 35] tracheal intubation or extubation, and intrathoracic manipulation. Kaufman[35] noted that the coolest portion of the esophagus is the point where both heart and breath sounds were best heard and the warmest point is 12 to 16 cm past the position of best cardiorespiratory sounds. Compared with the lower esophagus, temperature at the tracheal bifurcation is about 1°C lower and at the atrium about 0.5°C lower.[36] The ideal location for the thermistor is about 45 cm from the nostril so that its tip is between the heart and descending thoracic aorta and below the pulmonary veins.[37] However, this suggestion assumes that the distance between the teeth and the heart is similar in all individuals. Accurate positioning of the probe in relation to the heart is achieved by auscultation through an integral esophageal stethoscope (see Fig. 20–10). Whitby and Dunkin[34] noted that in the lower esophagus temperatures approximated cerebral temperatures in the absence of rapid infusions of cold fluids or an open thorax.

Contraindications to esophageal temperature measurements are bronchoscopy, esophagoscopy, laryngoscopy, certain facial or oral surgical procedures, and patients with esophageal disorders (varices, Zenker's diverticulum).[38] However, Ritter and coworkers inserted esophageal stethoscopes in patients with varices undergoing hepatic transplantation without any incidents of bleeding. Normal esophageal temperature ranges from 36.9° to 37.7°C.[25]

Bladder

Urinary catheters with thermistor tips have been available for more than a decade, providing a safe, continuous, and convenient method for temperature measurement.[39] Both urine volume and bladder temperature are simultaneously measured. Bladder temperature is usually 0.2°C higher than rectal temperature, 0.7° greater than esophageal temperature, and 3.5° higher than skin temperature (thumb).[40] During extracorporeal cooling and rewarming, temperature in the urinary bladder changes more rapidly than rectal temperature.[41] Lilly et al.[39] noted an excellent correlation between urinary bladder and esophageal, rectal, and pulmonary artery temperatures, the strongest correlation being with pulmonary artery temperatures during extracorporeal rewarming. Nevertheless, the advantages of bladder temperature monitoring may be outweighed by the risks of bladder catheterization if a urinary catheter is not otherwise indicated.

Rectum

The rectum is distant from either the central nervous system or the heart; therefore, it has little thermal significance. Several sources of inaccuracy of rectal temperatures are the presence of heat-producing bacteria in the rectum, insulation by feces, or cold blood returning from the legs.[42] Temperatures measured in the rectum often differ substantially from those measured in other areas. For this reason, rectal temperatures should be considered erroneous if they differ from other points. However, rectal temperatures may be useful indicators of the temperature of poorly perfused tissues[25] (Fig. 20–3). Rectal thermometry is relatively contraindicated during surgical procedures in the lower pelvis or during organ transplantation because of the risk of infection in an immunocompromised patient. The risk of rectal perforation should always be considered during placement of probes, particularly in infants and children. Normal rectal temperatures are 36.9° to 37.7°C.[25]

Skin

Skin temperature is lower than core temperature and the skin-to-core gradient decreases during general anesthesia[43] (Fig. 20–4). Factors altering thermal conduction, convection, and radiation affect skin temperature so that the measured temperature is a balance between metabolic heat production and cutaneous loss. The forehead and axilla are common skin sites for monitoring temperature. Axillary temperature normally ranges from 35.3° to 36.7°C.[25] However, measurement is affected by pressure on the probe and sweat production.

Other Sites

During cardiopulmonary bypass, temperatures of the venous blood returning to the extracorporeal circuit and arterial blood leaving the circuit are routinely measured. Muscle temperatures can be measured with a 25-gauge needle thermistor. Because a special probe is required, muscle temperatures are infrequently measured. However, muscle temperatures are quite responsive to blood flow. During extracorporeal cooling and rewarming, muscle remains warmer during hypothermia and cooler after rewarming.

Temperature can be measured in the pulmonary artery through the thermistor used for thermodilution cardiac output determinations. However, temperatures from this site are affected by ventilation, use of topical pericardial hypothermia, and cold cardioplegia solutions. In the absence of topical hypothermia and cardioplegia, pulmonary artery temperatures are indicative of core temperature. After discontinuation of cardiopulmonary bypass, pulmonary artery temperatures tend to be lower than temperatures from nasopharyngeal, rectal, and other sites.[44]

In the perioperative period, the temperature of the great toe of cardiac surgical patients has been advocated as an indicator of peripheral perfusion because of the dependence of its temperature on cutaneous blood flow. It also correlates well with cardiac output.[45] However, this temperature is not indicative of skin temperature.[46]

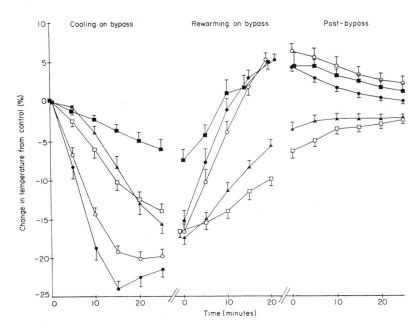

Figure 20-3. Changes in temperature as percentage of control temperature during extracorporeal cooling and rewarming. Cooling and rewarming occurred most rapidly in the esophagus. Rewarming also occurred more rapidly in the nasopharynx (*open circles*) than in bladder (*solid triangles*), rectum (*open squares*), or skin (*solid squares*). Bladder temperature decreased more slowly during cooling and increased more slowly during rewarming than esophageal temperature (*solid circles*). Bladder temperature remained below nasopharyngeal, esophageal, and skin temperatures after bypass. (From Bone ME, Feneck RO: Bladder temperature as an estimate of body temperature during cardiopulmonary bypass. Anaesthesia 1988; 43:181–185.)

Complications of Temperature Measurement

Tympanic membrane temperature probes have a reported complication rate of less than 3% with the primary complication being bleeding from the external auditory canal.[47] Other complications from the tympanic site include tympanic membrane perforation.[48] As described earlier, burns are possible when temperature probes are electrically operated and leakage currents are present.[8]

Alterations in Temperature in the Perioperative Period

Induced Hypothermia

Hypothermia has been used in both neurosurgery and cardiac surgery to decrease the metabolic rate and allow complex intracranial and intracardiac repairs. However, it is infrequently used in neurosurgery because of the prolonged time required for surface cooling and rewarming or the requisite anticoagulation if extracorporeal techniques are used. Some degree of hypothermia is used in most centers during cardiopulmonary bypass in both adult and pediatric patients. Profound hypothermia to esophageal temperatures of 10° to 12°C is used in children with congenital cardiac lesions and occasionally in adults with lesions of the aortic arch. Hypothermia with circulatory arrest provides ideal surgical conditions, decreases the duration of cardiopulmonary bypass, and prevents myocardial rewarming from washout of cardioplegia solutions by noncoronary collateral circulation.

Cold induces intense stimulation of thermoregulatory mechanisms, including sympathetic stimulation, vasoconstriction, shivering, and specific responses in cardiorespiratory, central nervous, renal, hepatic, and endocrine systems. Anesthesia blunts both the sympathetic and shivering responses to hypothermia.

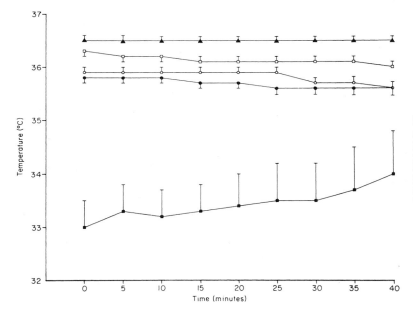

Figure 20-4. During the prebypass period, skin temperature (*solid squares*) is lower than internal body temperatures measured in the esophagus (*solid circles*), nasopharynx (*open circles*), rectum (*open squares*), and bladder (*solid triangles*). (From Bone ME, Feneck RO: Bladder temperature as an estimate of body temperature during cardiopulmonary bypass. Anaesthesia 1988; 43: 181–185.)

During surgery hypothermia is induced by either surface or core cooling. Core cooling with an extracorporeal circuit causes significant differences in the temperature measured at various sites (see Fig. 20-3). The rate of decrease in temperature is greatest in the esophagus and least in the rectum.[40] During perfusion cooling, bladder temperature is similar to rectal temperature but differs significantly from nasopharyngeal, esophageal, and skin temperatures.[40] During hypothermia, renal oxygen consumption decreases more rapidly than oxygen consumption in other organs, decreasing renal blood flow.

During perfusion rewarming, esophageal and nasopharyngeal temperatures demonstrated the greatest rate of rise, with increases in bladder and rectal temperatures occurring more slowly[40] (see Fig. 20-3). Lilly and colleagues noted that urinary bladder temperature consistently increased faster than rectal temperature and correlated well with pulmonary artery temperature during extracorporeal rewarming.[39] Changes in esophageal and nasopharyngeal temperatures reflect blood flow from the extracorporeal circuit to the vital organs. Temperatures measured from these sites tend to overshoot the control values during rewarming.[40]

After perfusion hypothermia and rewarming, core temperature often decreases (afterdrop) after cessation of extracorporeal circulation. *Afterdrop* is defined as the difference between the nasopharyngeal temperature at the termination of bypass and the lowest nasopharyngeal temperature reached after bypass).[44] Ramsay and coworkers[44] noted that the urinary bladder temperature at termination of bypass most closely indicated the amount of afterdrop and was minimized by a bladder temperature greater than 36.2°C. Rajek and colleagues[49] demonstrated that the core-to-peripheral temperature gradient at the end of rewarming and the afterdrop were greater with perfusion hypothermia to a nasopharyngeal temperature of 27°C than to 31°C. The use of warm forced air over the face, head, and shoulders, coupled with a water mattress, reduced the afterdrop as compared with no skin rewarming devices.[50] The subsequent period of rewarming occurring 2 to 4 hours following extracorporeal cooling is accompanied by marked increases in oxygen consumption, carbon dioxide production, and shivering.[44, 45] Patients who do not exhibit shivering have lower oxygen consumption during this period.[51]

Accidental Hypothermia

Hypothermia is defined as a reduction in core temperature to less than 35° to 36°C. In hospital settings, hypothermia commonly occurs in neonates exposed to cold environmental conditions or in adults anesthetized in cold operating rooms or transfused with unwarmed blood and fluids.[51, 52]

The human body loses heat by radiation, conduction, convection, evaporation, and through the respiratory tract. Decreases in environmental temperature are first sensed by cutaneous cold-sensitive thermoreceptors. Warm-sensitive receptors in the anterior hypothalamus are stimulated by temperatures greater than 44°C, whereas cold-sensitive receptors are inactive until the environmental temperature is less than 24°C.[20]

Anesthetic Effects on Thermoregulation

Effects of General Anesthesia on Thermoregulation. Core temperature usually decreases during the early minutes of anesthesia because of uncovering of the patient, wet and cold preparation solutions, and losses to the anesthetic administration system. Alterations in temperature at various measuring sites are shown in Figure 20-4.

Patients at risk for intraoperative hypothermia include the elderly,[48] and patients with major burns, paraplegia, quadriplegia, cachexia, trauma, hypothyroidism, adrenal insufficiency, diabetes, uremia, epilepsy, and cirrhosis. During anesthesia, temperature decreases about 1.1°C per hour at age 80 versus 0.3°C per hour at age 20 years.[51] Elderly patients are more prone to hypothermia in the perioperative period than younger patients.[53, 54] Aged people are likely to become hypothermic because of immobility, impaired sensation, decreased shivering response, loss of muscle mass, reduced threshold for thermoregulatory vasoconstriction in response to cold (particularly during anesthesia),[55] and inability to maintain their core-to-surface temperature gradient.

Burned patients are unable to limit passage of water vapor through the skin and their peripheral thermoregulatory mechanisms are impaired. Cachectic patients may have lost both muscle mass responsible for heat production and insulating fat. Paraplegia and quadriplegia disrupt the thermosensory pathways as well as the motor pathways responsible for shivering, impairing both autonomic and behavioral thermoregulation. Exposure of large surfaces of the abdominal or thoracic cavities increases intraoperative heat loss.[47, 52, 53] (Table 20-2). Neonates are particularly prone to hypothermia because of their large ratio of body surface area to heat-producing mass, decreased capacity to increase metabolic rate, limited energy stores, lack of insulating fat, and decreased shivering.

About 60% of adult patients have hypothermia on arrival in postanesthetic care units.[56] The duration of recovery is prolonged by approximately 40 minutes in patients whose core temperatures are below 36°C on arrival in postanesthesia recovery.[57] Forced air warming is less effective in warming the body core in the postanesthetic period because of peripheral vasoconstriction limiting heat transfer from periphery to core. However, forced air devices are more effective than blankets in the postoperative period.[58]

Body temperature is reduced to a greater degree during general than during regional anesthesia.[59] During general anesthesia, three phases of heat loss occur. Initially, hypothermia results from redistribution of heat from the central core to the peripheral shell of the body. Core size has also been shown to increase from 66% to 71% of body mass following induction of anesthesia.[60] This initial hypothermia can be minimized by preinduction skin surface warming with an electric blanket for 90 minutes in adult patients[61] (Fig. 20-5). A small amount of heat loss also occurs during surgical

Table 20-2. Causes of Intraoperative Temperature Alterations

Increased Temperature
Malignant hyperthermia, thyrotoxicosis, pheochromocytoma
Infections (endotoxins)
Drugs
Chemical reactions (hardening of plaster casts, methyl methacrylate cement)
Excessive environmental warming (heating lamps, heated humidifiers, blankets, heavy surgical drapes)

Decreased Temperature
Exposure to cold operating room environment
Intravenous, intraperitoneal, intrathoracic administration of cold fluids
Skin preparation with cold solutions
Vasodilation secondary to spinal, epidural, or other regional anesthesia
Hypothyroidism (myxedema)
Trauma or burn with inability to compensate for heat loss
Deliberate hypothermia (surface or extracorporeal cooling)

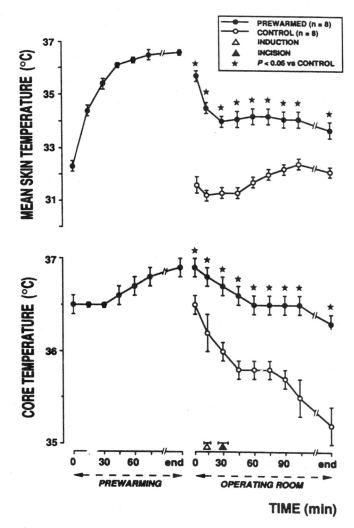

Figure 20-5. Prewarming of the skin of adult patients prior to surgical procedures minimizes the hypothermia which develops after induction of anesthesia. When prewarming is combined with intra-operative surface warming with an electric blanket, near-normothermia is maintained and postoperative shivering is prevented. (From Just B, Trevien V, Delva E, et al: Prevention of intraoperative hypothermia by preoperative skin-surface warming. Anesthesiology 1993; 79:214-218.)

skin preparation, particularly with cold, alcohol-based solutions. Thermal losses during surgical preparation can be minimized by radiant warming, use of water-based solutions, and skin drying after washing.[62]

Heat loss to the environment continues to exceed metabolic heat production during the second phase, reaching a plateau at 34° to 35.5°C in several hours.[63] Normally, thermoregulatory mechanisms respond quickly, causing vasoconstriction to decrease heat loss when decreases in temperature of less than 0.4°C occur.[64] This thermoregulatory threshold is the central temperature at which significant peripheral vasoconstriction occurs.[65] Thermoregulatory vasoconstriction, primarily in the extremities, reduces heat loss and the rate of core cooling in the third phase by 25%.[63, 66] As in unanesthetized humans, the contribution of skin to control of vasoconstriction and shivering remains about 20%.[67]

Anesthetized humans have altered thermoregulatory re-

sponses (determined by skin-to-surface temperature gradients between forearm and fingertip and venous occlusion volume plethysmography[55]) during the third phase of hypothermia during anesthesia with halothane, isoflurane, or fentanyl, and respond only to changes of 2.5° to 4°C.[65, 66, 68] Thus, peripheral thermoregulatory vasoconstriction occurs at a threshold temperature about 2.5°C below normal thermoregulatory levels during general anesthesia in both infants and adults.[69, 70] During isoflurane anesthesia, vasoconstriction induced by thermoregulatory mechanisms also decreases heat loss about 25%.[71] However, shivering intensity decreases and gain of shivering increases during isoflurane anesthesia.[72]

Effects of Regional Anesthesia on Thermoregulation. Peripheral thermal receptors—particularly the warm-sensitive receptors—are blocked by regional anesthesia.[20] Patients receiving regional anesthesia rewarm less readily in the postoperative period because of continued vasodilation and muscle flaccidity.[56] During peridural anesthesia, administration of cold intravenous fluids, alterations in metabolic heat production, and environmental heat loss are insufficient to explain the 1° to 2°C decrease in central temperature. Instead, it is due to redistribution of body heat.[73] Suppression of vasoconstriction by epidural anesthesia increases heat loss to a small extent and compensatory shivering thermogenesis occurs. The gain and maximal intensity of shivering are reduced during epidural anesthesia as the upper extremities cannot compensate for lower extremity blockade.[74] Nevertheless, the body's thermoregulatory mechanisms respond as though metabolic heat production were intact.[74]

Effects of Hypothermia on Organ Systems

Total body metabolism decreases about 7% to 8% per degree Celsius as temperature decreases. Thus, the metabolic rate is about 50% of normal at 28°C. Despite the decrease in metabolic rate, aerobic metabolism continues at low temperatures provided that adequate oxygen is delivered (see Table 20-1).

Heart and Circulatory Effects. In response to sympathetic activation during cooling, heart rate, stroke volume, and peripheral vascular tone increase and shivering occurs. Myocardial substrate use and generation of adenosine triphosphate decrease as temperature decreases.

Changes in the ECG accompany the development of hypothermia. At 34°C, bradycardia, slowed conduction, and Osborne or J waves appear. The duration of the action potential is increased. Below 30°C, atrial fibrillation and ventricular irritability are seen. The threshold for ventricular fibrillation decreases. Below 25°C, ventricular fibrillation occurs, although it may develop at higher temperatures in patients with preexisting myocardial disease.

Ralley and coworkers[51] noted significant reductions in mixed venous oxygen tension even when cardiac output increased in shivering patients after cardiac surgery. This finding indicates an imbalance between whole-body oxygen supply and demand, mandating that shivering patients always receive supplemental oxygen. A greater incidence of myocardial ischemia has been reported in hypothermic patients with peripheral vascular disease on the first postoperative day.[75]

As hypothermia develops, fluid shifts from the vascular space, increasing the hematocrit. Despite the shift of blood to the central compartment, cardiac output decreases, beginning at 32°C. By 30°C, cardiac output is reduced 30% to 40%.[67] Hypovolemia and increased blood viscosity may further reduce cardiac output. Systemic vascular resistance increases with hyperviscosity. Microcirculatory flow is reduced. Because the hemostatic cascade is an enzyme system, coagulation is reduced as hypothermia develops.

Central Nervous System. The effects of hypothermia on the central nervous system include depression of membrane conduction and neurochemical processes. Shivering, the involuntary rhythmic contraction of muscle, is mediated through hypothalamic pathways. Shivering during induction of hypothermia can be characterized by its threshold (temperature triggering shivering), gain (intensity increase associated with increasing hypothermia), and maximum intensity.[72] It ceases at temperatures below 27°C. During shivering, oxygen consumption and calorigenesis are increased, but convective and radiant heat losses are also increased by the increased muscular activity.[76]

As hypothermia progresses, alterations in the electroencephalogram (EEG) occur. The EEG remains normal to temperatures of 35°C. Between 30° and 35°C, the predominant rhythm slows. At temperatures of 32°C responses to stimuli are slowed, ataxia is present, and there is slight clumsiness. The amplitude of the EEG decreases below 32°C. Below 32°C, delirium, followed by stupor and coma, occurs. Pupillary dilatation is seen below 30°C. Slower EEG rhythms predominate between 24° and 29°C. Periods of isoelectricity of ever-lengthening duration develop below temperatures of 22°.[77] Anesthetic requirements decrease so that minimum alveolar concentration decreases about 7% per degree Celsius.[78]

However, aerobic brain metabolism continues at low temperatures, although the cerebral metabolic rate for oxygen ($CMRC_2$) slows concomitantly with temperature reduction. Cerebral blood flow also decreases with hypothermia (about 7% per degree Celsius)[76] due to decreased cardiac output, increased cerebrovascular resistance, and greater viscosity. At electrocerebral silence, there is no further reduction in $CMRO_2$. The preservative effects of hypothermia on the brain are greater than those predicted by decreased $CMRO_2$ alone. The "no reflow" phenomenon after ischemia is prevented by hypothermia.

Respiratory Effects. Respiratory rate initially increases as hypothermia ensues. Between 30° and 34°C, the respiratory response to carbon dioxide decreases (CO_2 response curve shifts to the right). Because carbon dioxide production decreases with hypothermia, respiratory alkalosis is often present. Dead space may increase due to bronchodilatation as temperature decreases if spontaneous respiration continues.

Hypoxic pulmonary vasoconstriction is reduced during hypothermia.[79] The ventilatory response to hypoxia may also be reduced, although it has been incompletely studied.[80] However, respiratory drive does not cease until 24°C.[76] Resistance in the pulmonary circulation increases with hypothermia. There is little change in lung compliance. Hypothermic patients should be fully rewarmed prior to extubation because of these effects on the respiratory system.

The oxyhemoglobin dissociation curve shifts to the left, diminishing release of oxygen at the tissue level. The affinity of oxygen for hemoglobin increases about 6% per degree Celsius. The question of assessment of acid-base disturbances during hypothermia is controversial, addressed in detail in Chapter 19.

Hepatic and Renal Effects. Renal blood flow and oxygen consumption are reduced by hypothermia. Glomerular filtration rate decreases progressively during cooling. Because both renal blood flow and glomerular filtration rate decrease,

filtration fraction is unchanged. Because tubular function requires active enzymatic processes, tubular function is decreased, reducing the concentrating effects of the renal tubules. Antidiuretic hormone release is suppressed because cold-induced vasoconstriction is interpreted by the kidney as volume overload, resulting in diuresis of urine produced by glomerular filtration. Hemoconcentration also results from capillary sequestration of fluid.

Hepatic enzymatic and excretory processes are reduced with hypothermia. Blood flow to the liver is reduced but blood shifts from the periphery to the splanchnic circulation. Drug metabolism is reduced. The liver is also a site for sequestration of platelets during hypothermia. Coagulopathy during hypothermia results from thrombocytopenia, decreased activity of clotting cascade, and slight decrease in platelet function.

Endocrine Effects. Because peripheral utilization of glucose and release of insulin decrease during hypothermia, blood glucose increases.[81] Parenteral insulin has little effect, but the hyperglycemia reverts to normal or near-normal with rewarming. The stress response described previously causes release of adrenocortical and medullary hormones (epinephrine and norepinephrine).[82, 83] In response to cold, the hypothalamus releases thyrotropin-releasing hormone, stimulating secretion of thyroxine and triiodothyronine to increase metabolic rate.

Profound hypothermia is compatible with life for brief periods of time because of the decreased metabolic rate and oxygen demand. However, prolonged hypothermia is not tolerated and usually causes death because of cardiac electrical conduction disturbances. Rewarming in therapeutic applications of hypothermia is usually with extracorporeal circulation at a gradient of no more than 10°C. In accidental hypothermia, surface methods are usually employed, coupled with supportive treatment of associated cardiac, respiratory, and coagulation problems.

Methods to Prevent or Minimize Perioperative Hypothermia

Postoperative hypothermia delays drug clearance, enhances peripheral vasoconstriction, and causes shivering. Shivering may occur because the patient is actually cold or there is a discrepancy between the actual core temperature (normal) and the thermostat set point (elevated) that activates heat generation.[84] For these reasons, both prevention and treatment are mandatory. Modalities to prevent or treat the mild-to-moderate hypothermia seen in the perioperative period include covering the patient with impervious insulation material, increasing the environmental temperature, the use of warmed respiratory gases and intravenous fluids, forced air convection blankets, and pharmacologic agents to reduce shivering (clonidine, ketanserin, meperidine, dexmedetomidine, chlorpromazine, droperidol, and nondepolarizing neuromuscular blockers).[85] The mechanism of improvement with clonidine is by central thermoregulatory impairment, which decreases the thermoregulatory threshold for shivering and peripheral vasoconstriction.[86] Meperidine has been shown to reduce the shivering threshold in humans.[87] Premedication with clonidine has not been shown to reduce the redistribution hypothermia associated with general anesthesia.[88]

Environment Warming. Warmer operating rooms (>21°C) minimize decreases in temperature in adults as compared with unwarmed rooms.[89-91] The "critical ambient temperature" appears to be 21°C (70°F) for stability of patient temperature between 36°C and 37.5°C.[90, 91] Room temperatures of 24° to 26°C are necessary to prevent any heat loss.[20] However, for a naked adult patient to maintain temperature without significant energy use requires ambient temperatures of 27° to 33°C.[20] The room temperatures must also be modified for patients with large surface area to body mass ratios, receiving large volumes of unwarmed intravenous fluids, undergoing body cavity surgery, and in a deeply anesthetized state.[90] However, Roizen and colleagues[92] noted no difference in temperature in the postanesthetic period between patients undergoing surgical preparation and draping in a cold versus a warm operating room. Temperatures at the beginning of surgery were lower in patients in the cold room.[92]

Patient Covering. Since radiation and convection account for as much as 80% of heat loss perioperatively, covering the patient as much as possible is beneficial. Covering the scalp prevents the 50% radiation of heat from the head. Warmed blankets reduce heat loss more than unwarmed blankets, but the effect is transient.[93] Sessler and coworkers[94] noted that reflective paper drapes and unheated paper or plastic quiltlike blankets (blankets of forced air convection devices) prevented heat loss better than did cloth, plastic, or paper drapes.[94] Body heat is conserved when increasing amounts of the patient's body surface area are covered with reflective materials.[94, 95] However, Radford and Thurlow[96] were unable to prevent intraoperative hypothermia with reflective blankets. Prewarming of the skin surface prior to anesthetic induction minimizes early intraoperative hypothermia (see Fig. 20–5).

Forced Air Convection Blankets. The application of forced air warming devices to adults, children, and infants over body surfaces uninvolved in the surgical procedure prevents intraoperative hypothermia more effectively than circulating water mattresses.[97] The efficacy of these devices is maintained when approximately 25% of body surface area is available for warming in adults. In fact, these devices are so effective that continuous monitoring of the patient's core temperature is essential to prevent hyperthermia. Despite initial concerns to the contrary, Zink and Iaizzo[98] failed to demonstrate increased airborne bacterial wound contamination during intraoperative forced air convective warming. Some investigators have suggested that a specific brand of forced air warmer may be more efficient than other similar technology.[99] Because of the effectiveness of these devices, it is important to avoid their use over ischemic tissue such as the extremities during operations involving aortic clamping, as warming might increase tissue oxygen consumption.

Despite availability of effective patient warming devices, the cost-effectiveness of their use remains unclear. Fleisher and coworkers[100] determined that forced air warming reduced time from surgical dressing to tracheal extubation but did not change time to discharge from postanesthesia care. These workers also noted increased costs of $15 per patient if all operating room costs were considered as fixed costs but a $29 per patient savings if all operating room costs could be considered as variable costs.[100]

Radiant Heating. Murphy and coworkers[101] demonstrated that radiant heat lamps stopped postanesthetic shivering (in animals) even without rewarming the core temperature. Sharkey and colleagues[102] showed that radiant heat lamps, but not warm blankets, terminated postanesthetic shivering within 10 minutes of application. Other methods of radiant heat include frequently changed warm blankets or an active warming blanket. Operations in infants can be performed in specially modified radiant warmers to minimize heat loss. However, as shown by Sessler and Moayeri,[103] radiant warming is less effective than forced air convection or circulating-water blankets.

Thermal Mattresses. Thermal mattresses, which circulate thermostatically controlled water, minimize heat loss by increasing the conduction of heat from the environment to the patient. A layer of cotton sheet is placed over the mattress to prevent direct pressure of the fluid cells on poorly perfused skin. The level of the reservoir fluid should be noted before activating the unit. During operation the temperature of the circulating fluid must be noted to prevent excessive temperatures and patient burns.

Although thermal mattresses are efficacious in infants,[104] they fail to maintain body temperature in adults.[89, 90, 105] This finding probably results from the lack of a highly perfused surface area in contact with the blanket.[105] Combination of a thermal mattress (38° to 40°C) and a heated humidifier preserved body heat better than either method alone[105] (Fig. 20–6). The application of the thermal blanket on top of rather than beneath the patient is more effective.

Fluid and Blood Warming. Warming of room temperature intravenous fluids (1000 mL) to body temperature requires about 15 kcal. In the anesthetized patient who is unable to increase caloric production, body temperature decreases.[20, 106] Body temperature decreases about 0.5°C after administration of 1 L of 4°C blood over 15 minutes.[20] The efficacy of various blood warmers to deliver blood at temperatures above 32°C at rates of 150 mL/minute was reviewed by Russell.[53] Active heating of fluid in the delivery tubing (Hotline, Level 1 Technologies, Marshfield, MA) more effectively maintained the temperature of the delivered fluid at flow rates up to 3000 mL/hour than dry-wall warmers.[54] At higher flow rates (3000 to 6000 l/hour), the delivery temperature was similar to that of dry-wall devices.[54] Although fluid warmers reduce postoperative hypothermia, differences in outcome in ambulatory surgery patients have not been demonstrated.[107]

Humidifiers. Heated humidifiers are an excellent way to prevent and treat heat loss in the perioperative pe-

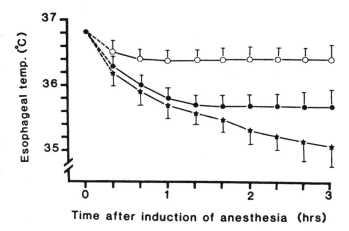

Figure 20–6. Combination of warming mattress and heated humidifier during abdominal aortic surgery (*open circles*) maintains esophageal temperature better than humidifier alone (*closed circles*) or no active warming (*stars*.) (From Tollofsrud SG, Gundersen Y, Anderson R: Peroperative hypothermia. Acta Anaesthesiol Scand 1984; 28:511–515.)

riod.[105, 107-109] They save the patients from warming and humidifying cold dry gases from the anesthetic circuit and, compared with patients receiving unhumidified gases, maintain temperature.[105, 110, 111] Humidified gases minimize damage to the cilia of the respiratory mucosal cells. Preheating of the humidifier prior to use increases its effectiveness. Airway temperature should always be measured and maintained at 38°C or less when humidifiers are used to prevent airway burns or tracheobronchial edema.[109]

A study in outpatients noted that warmed humidified gases during anesthesia resulted in warmer patients arriving in the postanesthetic unit who had shorter postoperative stays.[112] Ralley and coworkers[113] noted the inability of heated humidified gases to prevent decreases in temperature after discontinuation of hypothermic cardiopulmonary bypass. Heated humidifiers are more effective warmers in children than in adults. Even passive, unheated humidifiers (heat and moisture exchangers, artificial "noses") maintain body temperature better than without humidification. However, they fail to provide benefits similar to heated devices.[114] They do limit the intraoperative temperature decrease by about 1°C.[115]

Other Methods. Vasodilator therapy with nitroprusside during extracorporeal rewarming of cardiac surgical patients speeds rewarming, restores core temperatures after cardiopulmonary bypass, and prevents postbypass cooling.[116]

Malignant Hyperthermia

MH is a pharmacokinetic muscle syndrome triggered by stress, succinylcholine, or volatile anesthetic agents; it causes uncontrolled calcium flux in skeletal muscle resulting in increased temperature, muscle rigidity, and respiratory and metabolic acidosis.[117] The disorder occurs in about 1 in 10,000 to 1 in 50,000 anesthetic procedures, but is somewhat more common among populations in West Virginia, Michigan, and Wisconsin. The defect involves an abnormal sensitivity of the calcium channel in the sarcoplasmic reticulum to calcium. Abnormally increased calcium ion in the cellular cytoplasm explains the heat production, muscle rigor, and glycogenolysis associated with the syndrome[118] (see Table 20-2).

Etiology

In susceptible humans, hyperthermia is triggered by various anesthetic agents but can also occur in nonanesthetic settings. Anesthetic agents that trigger MH include succinylcholine, halothane, enflurane, desflurane, sevoflurane, and isoflurane. MH is an autosomal dominantly inherited condition with variable penetrance, and mutations in the ryanodine receptor gene or other proteins controlling calcium release may be responsible, as indicated by genetic linkage and biochemical investigations.[118] An increased incidence has been noted in idiopathic scoliosis, Duchenne's and Becker's muscular dystrophies, strabismus, ptosis, central core disease, sodium channel myotonias, and other musculoskeletal diseases. Susceptibility is suggested by family history, the presence of increased creatine kinase, skeletal muscle contracture to caffeine, and molecular genetic linkage studies.

Symptoms

The earliest symptom of MH may be increased end-tidal carbon dioxide, although masseter muscle rigidity may be seen in children and young adults during attempted tracheal intubation. Other symptoms of MH include general muscular rigidity, tachycardia with dysrhythmias, increased end-tidal carbon dioxide out of proportion to minute ventilation (resulting from increased CO_2 production), tachypnea, peripheral cyanosis, and eventually, hyperthermia. Laboratory studies reveal severe metabolic acidosis with pH less than 7.0, hypercarbia, decreased mixed venous P_{O_2}, and hyperkalemia. Adequate arterial oxygenation is usually present. Hyperphosphatemia, hemoconcentration, hyperglycemia, acute renal failure resulting from acute tubular necrosis caused by excessive myoglobin release from muscle and myoglobinuria, disseminated intravascular coagulation, and central nervous system dysfunction resulting from brain temperatures exceeding the lethal upper limit of 42° to 43°C occur in later stages.[119]

Careful monitoring may be essential to differentiate other causes of hypermetabolism and fever from MH. Patients with sepsis, neuroleptic malignant syndrome, thyrotoxicosis, pheochromocytoma, hypoxic encephalopathy, and faulty temperature monitors can all demonstrate hyperthermia.

Diagnostic Testing

Although the laboratory tests described earlier may be useful in confirming the diagnosis of MH, the only recognized laboratory test for diagnosis is the caffeine-halothane contracture test. [Using a two-component test (≥0.5 g contracture with 3% halothane or ≥0.3 g contracture at 2 mm caffeine, the sensitivity was 97% (95% CI, 84% to 100%) and the specificity was 78% (95% CI, 69% to 85%) when the test was performed according to published standards.[120, 121]]

Therapy

The definitive therapy is dantrolene, given in initial doses of 2.0 mg/kg body weight, with additional increments every 5 to 10 minutes if no reduction in temperature, acidosis, tachycardia, or muscle rigidity occurs, to a total dose of 10 mg/kg. Therapy with dantrolene should commence even while supportive measures are being applied because it must be given while adequate muscle perfusion is present. Dantrolene alters calcium release but does not affect its uptake. It also causes muscle weakness and hepatic dysfunction. General supportive treatment, including hyperventilation with oxygen, intravenous fluids, discontinuation of triggering agents, control of metabolic acidosis with bicarbonate, control of hyperkalemia with dextrose-insulin infusions, and control of dysrhythmias with procainamide or other agents, should accompany dantrolene therapy. Calcium channel blocking drugs should not be used as antiarrhythmic therapy; they may cause hyperkalemia. Attempts to cool the patient with external methods, gastric or peritoneal lavage, or lavage of an open body cavity, or administration of iced intravenous fluids should be made. However, it must be appreciated that bladder irrigation and forced air or circulating-water mattresses have limited cooling potential (0.8°, 1.7°, and 1.6°C per hour, respectively, as compared with immersion in an ice slurry, which lowers temperature by approximately 9.7°C per hour).[122] Monitoring during the episode should include intra-arterial and central venous catheters, urinary bladder catheter, ECG, and if possible, a muscle temperature probe. Otherwise, temperature can be measured in the esophagus or other common sites. Following control of the MH episode, the patient should receive dantrolene 1 mg/kg, every 4 to 6 hours until the signs of MH have been absent for at least 36 hours.

The choices for anesthesia in MH-susceptible patients include local anesthetics given in regional techniques such as epidural or subarachnoid block or thiopental, nitrous oxide, narcotics, benzodiazepines, ketamine, propofol, and nondepolarizing neuromuscular blocking drugs (with the possible exception of curare). An anesthesia machine with clean tubing, new soda lime, and empty vaporizers whose fresh gas flow has been analyzed for absence of volatile anesthetics is satisfactory for administration of anesthesia to an MH-susceptible patient. Pretreatment with intravenous dantrolene to a dose of 1 to 2 mg/kg body weight immediately prior to induction effectively prevents MH.[123]

REFERENCES

1. Chang L: Development and use of the stethoscope in diagnosing cardiac disease. Am J Cardiol 1987; 60:1378–1382.
2. Webster TA: Now that we have pulse oximeters and capnographs, we don't need precordial and esophageal stethoscopes. J Clin Monit Comput 1987; 3:191–192.
3. Petty C: We do need precordial and esophageal stethoscopes. J Clin Monit Comput 1987; 3:192–193.
4. Smith C: An endo-esophageal stethoscope. Anesthesiology 1954; 15:566.
5. Baker AB, McLeod C: Oesophageal multipurpose monitoring probe. Anaesthesia 1983; 38:892–897.
6. Kates RA, Zaidan JR, Kaplan JA: Esophageal lead for intraoperative electrocardiographic monitoring. Anesth Analg 1982; 61:781–785.
7. Parker EO: Electrosurgical burn at the site of an esophageal temperature probe. Anesthesiology 1984; 61:93–95.
8. Maroon JC, Albin MS: Air embolism diagnosed by Doppler ultrasound. Anesth Analg 1974; 53:399–402.
9. Kugler J, Stirt JA, Finholt D, et al: The one that got away: Misplaced esophageal stethoscope. Anesthesiology 1985; 62:643–645.
10. Schwartz AJ, Downes JJ: Hazards of a simple monitoring device, the esophageal stethoscope. Anesthesiology 1977; 47:64–65.
11. Goto H, Hackman LT, Arakawa K: Tracheal insertion of an esophageal stethoscope. Anesth Analg 1977; 56:584–585.
12. Simpson JI, Wolf GL: Flammability of esophageal stethoscopes, nasogastric tubes, feeding tubes, and nasopharyngeal airways in oxygen- and nitrous oxide–enriched atmospheres. Anesth Analg 1988; 67:1093–1095.
13. Himms-Hagen J: Cellular thermogenesis. Annu Rev Physiol 1976; 38:315–351.
14. Benzinger TH: On physical heat regulation and the sense of temperature in man. Proc Natl Acad Sci USA 1959; 45:645–659.
15. Hall GM: Body temperature and anaesthesia. Br J Anaesth 1978; 50:39–44.
16. Imrie MM, Hall GM: Body temperature and anaesthesia. Br J Anaesth 1990; 64:346–354.
17. Adamson K Jr, Gandy G, James L: The influence of thermal factors upon oxygen consumption of the newborn infant. J Pediatr 1965; 66:495–508.
18. Heiser MS, Downes JJ: Temperature regulation in the pediatric patient. Semin Anesth 1984; 3:37–42.
19. Wyon DP, Lidwell OM, Williams REO: Thermal comfort during surgical operations. J Hyg Camb 1968; 66:229–248.
20. Morley-Forster PK: Unintentional hypothermia in the operating room. Can Anaesth Soc J 1986; 33:516–527.
21. Frank SM, Nguyen JM, Garcia CM, et al: Temperature monitoring practices during regional anesthesia. Anesth Analg 1999; 88:373–377.
22. Ramanathan NL: A new weighting system for mean surface temperature of the human body. J Appl Physiol 1964; 19:531–533.
23. Colin J, Timbal J, Houdas Y, et al: Computation of mean body temperature from rectal and mean skin temperatures. J Appl Physiol 1971; 31:484–489.
24. Burton AC: The average temperature of the tissues of the body. J Nutr 1935; 9:264–267.
25. Holdcroft A: Body Temperature Control in Anaesthesia, Surgery, and Intensive Care. London, Balliere Tindall, 1980.
26. Lacoumenta S, Hall GM: Liquid crystal thermometry during anaesthesia. Anaesthesia 1984; 39:54–56.
27. Vaughan MS, Cork RC, Vaughan RW: Inaccuracy of liquid crystal thermometry to identify core temperature trends in postoperative adults. Anesth Analg 1982; 61:284–287.
28. Lees DE, Schuette W, Bull J, et al: An evaluation of liquid-crystal thermometry as a screening device for intraoperative hyperthermia. Anesth Analg 1978; 57:669–674.
29. Shinozaki T, Deane R, Perkins FM: Infrared tympanic thermometer: Evaluation of a new clinical thermometer. Crit Care Med 1988; 16:148–150.
30. Cork RC, Vaughan RW, Humphrey LS: Precision and accuracy of intraoperative temperature monitoring. Anesth Analg 1983; 62:211–214.
31. Benzinger TH: Clinical temperature. JAMA 1969; 209:1200–1206.
32. Benzinger M: Tympanic thermometry in surgery and anesthesia. JAMA 1969; 209:1207–1211.
33. Hickey PR, Andersen NP: Deep hypothermia circulatory arrest: A review of pathophysiology and clinical experience as a basis for anesthetic management. J Cardiothorac Vasc Anesth 1987; 1:137–155.
34. Whitby JD, Dunkin LJ: Cerebral, oesophageal, and nasopharyngeal temperatures. Br J Anaesth 1971; 43:673–676.
35. Kaufman RD: Relationship between esophageal temperature gradient and heart and lung sounds heard by esophageal stethoscope. Anesth Analg 187; 66:1046–1048.
36. Severinghaus JW: Temperature gradients during hypothermia. Ann N Y Acad Sci 1962; 80:515–521.
37. Piironen P: Effects of exposures to extremely hot environments on temperatures of the tympanic membrane, the oesophagus, and the rectum of men. Technical Documentary Report No. AMRL-TDR-63-85, Wright-Patterson Air Force Base, Dayton, OH, 6570th Aerospace Medical Research Laboratory, 1963.
38. Ritter DM, Rettke SR, Hughes RW, et al: Placement of nasogastric tubes and esophageal stethoscopes in patients with documented esophageal varices. Anesth Analg 1988; 67:280–282.
39. Lilly JK, Boland JP, Zekan S: Urinary bladder temperature monitoring: A new index of body core temperature. Crit Care Med 1980; 8:742–744.
40. Bone ME, Feneck RO: Bladder temperature as an estimate of body temperature during cardiopulmonary bypass. Anaesthesia 1988; 43:181–185.
41. Moorthy SS, Winn BA, Jallard MS, et al: Monitoring urinary bladder temperature. Heart Lung 1985; 14:90–93.
42. Stupfel M, Severinghaus JW: Internal body temperature gradients during anesthesia and hypothermia and effect of vagotomy. J Appl Physiol 1956; 9:380–386.
43. Bissonnette B, Sessler DI, LaFlamme P: Intraoperative temperature monitoring sites in infants and children and the effect of inspired gas warming on esophageal temperature. Anesth Analg 1989; 69:192–196.
44. Ramsay JG, Ralley FE, Whalley DG, et al: Site of temperature monitoring and prediction of afterdrop after open heart surgery. Can Anaesth Soc J 1985; 32:607–612.
45. Joly HR, Weil MH: Temperature of the great toe as an indicator of the severity of shock. Circulation 1969; 39:131–138.
46. Matthews HR, Meade JB, Evans CC: Peripheral vasoconstriction after open-heart surgery. Thorax 1974; 29:343–348.
47. Webb GE: Comparison of esophageal and tympanic temperature monitoring during cardiopulmonary bypass. Anesth Analg 1973; 52:729–733.
48. Wallace CT, Marks WE, Adkins WY, Mahafey JE: Perforation of the tympanic membrane, a complication of tympanic thermometry during anesthesia. Anesthesiology 1974; 41:290–291.
49. Rajek A, Lenhardt R, Sessler DI, et al: Tissue heat content and distribution during and after cardiopulmonary bypass at 31°C and 27°C. Anesthesiology 1998; 88:1511–1518.
50. Hohn L, Schweizer A, Kalangos A, et al: Benefits of intraoperative skin surface warming in cardiac surgical patients. Br J Anaesth 1998; 80:318–323.
51. Ralley FE, Wynands JE, Ramsay JG, et al: The effects of shivering on oxygen consumption and carbon dioxide production in patients rewarming from hypothermic cardiopulmonary bypass. Can J Anaesth 1988; 35:332–337.

52. Sladen RN: Temperature and ventilation after hypothermic cardiopulmonary bypass. Anesth Analg 1985; 64:816–820.

53. Russell WJ: A review of blood warmers for massive transfusion. Anesth Intensive Care 1974; 2:109–130.

54. Presson RG, Bezruczko AP, Hillier SC, et al: Evaluation of a new fluid warmer effective at low to moderate flow rates. Anesthesiology 1993; 78:974–980.

55. Kurz A, Plattner O, Sessler DI, et al: The threshold for thermoregulatory vasoconstriction during nitrous oxide/isoflurane anesthesia is lower in elderly than in young patients. Anesthesiology 1993; 79:465–469.

56. Vaughan MS, Vaughan RW, Cork RC: Postoperative hypothermia in adults: Relationship of age, anesthesia, and shivering to rewarming. Anesth Analg 1981; 60:746–751.

57. Lenhardt R, Marker E, Goll V, et al: Mild intraoperative hypothermia prolongs postanesthetic recovery. Anesthesiology 1997; 87:1318–1323.

58. Plattner O, Ikeda T, Sessler DI, et al: Postanesthetic vasoconstriction slows peripheral to core transfer of cutaneous heat, thereby isolating the core thermal compartment. Anesth Analg 1997; 85:899–906.

59. Frank SM, Beattie C, Christopherson S, et al: Epidural versus general anesthesia, ambient operating room temperature, and patient age as predictors. Anesthesiology 1992; 77:252–257.

60. Deakin CD: Changes in core temperature compartment size on induction of general anesthesia. Br J Anaesth 1998; 81:861–864.

61. Just B, Trevien V, Delva E, et al: Prevention of intraoperative hypothermia by preoperative skin-surface warming. Anesthesiology 1993; 79:214–218.

62. Sessler DI, Sessler AM, Hudson S, et al: Heat loss during surgical skin preparation. Anesthesiology 1993; 78:1055–1064.

63. Sessler DI, Moayeri A, Stoen R, et al: Thermoregulatory vasoconstriction decreases cutaneous heat loss. Anesthesiology 1990; 73:656–660.

64. Sessler DI, Olofsson CI, Rubinstein EH: The thermoregulatory threshold in humans during nitrous oxide–fentanyl anesthesia. Anesthesiology 1988; 69:357–364.

65. Rubenstein EH, Sessler DI: Skin-surface temperature gradients correlate with fingertip blood flow in humans. Anesthesiology 1990; 73:541–545.

66. Belani K, Sessler DI, Sessler AM, et al: Leg heat content continues to decrease during the core temperature plateau in humans anesthetized with isoflurane. Anesthesiology 1993; 78:856–863.

67. Lenhardt R, Greif R, Sessler DI, et al: Relative contribution of skin and core temperatures to vasoconstriction and shivering thresholds during isoflurane anesthesia. Anesthesiology 1999; 91:422–429.

68. Stoen R, Sessler DI: The thermoregulatory threshold is inversely proportional to isoflurane concentration. Anesthesiology 1990; 72:822–827.

69. Sessler DI, Olofsson CI, Rubenstein EH, et al: The thermoregulatory threshold in humans during isoflurane anesthesia. Anesthesiology 1988; 68:836–842.

70. Bissonnette B, Sessler DI: The thermoregulatory threshold in infants and children anesthetized with isoflurane and caudal anesthesia. Anesthesiology 1990; 73:1114–1119.

71. Sessler DI, Hynson J, McGuire J, et al: Thermoregulatory vasoconstriction during isoflurane anesthesia minimally decreases heat loss. Anesthesiology 1992; 76:670–675.

72. Ikeda T, Kim J-S, Sessler DI, et al: Isoflurane alters shivering patterns and reduces maximum shivering intensity. Anesthesiology 1998; 88:866–873.

73. Hynson JM, Sessler DI, Glosten B, et al: Thermal balance and tremor patterns during epidural anesthesia. Anesthesiology 1991; 74:680–690.

74. Kim J-S, Ikeda T, Sessler DI, et al: Epidural anesthesia reduces the gain and maximal intensity of shivering. Anesthesiology 1998; 88:851–857.

75. Frank SM, Beattie C, Christopherson R, et al: Unintentional hypothermia is associated with postoperative myocardial ischemia. Anesthesiology 1993; 78:468–476.

76. Roe CF: Temperature regulation in anaesthesia. *In* Hardy JD, (eds): Physiological and Behavioural Temperature Regulation. Springfield, IL, Charles C Thomas, 1970, pp 727–740.

77. Hicks RG, Poole JL: EEG changes with hypothermia and cardiopulmonary bypass in children. J Thorac Cardiovasc Surg 1979; 78:823–830.

78. Vitez T, White PF, Eger EI: Effect of hypothermia on halothane MAC and isoflurane MAC in the rat. Anesthesiology 1974; 41:80–81.

79. Regan MJ, Eger EI: Ventilatory responses to hypercapnia and hypoxia at normothermia and moderate hypothermia during constant-depth halothane anesthesia. Anesthesiology 1966; 27:624–633.

80. Benumof JL, Wahrenbrock EA: Dependency of hypoxic pulmonary vasoconstriction on temperature. J Appl Physiol 1977; 42:56–58.

81. Benzing G, Frances PD, Kaplan S, et al: Glucose and insulin changes in infants and children undergoing hypothermic open heart surgery. Am J Cardiol 1983; 52:133–136.

82. Wood M, Shand DG, Wood AJJ: The sympathetic response to profound hypothermia and circulatory arrest in infants. Can Anaesth Soc J 1980; 27:125–131.

83. Turley K, Roizen M, Vlahakes GJ, et al: Catecholamine response to deep hypothermia and total circulatory arrest in the infant lamb. Circulation 1980; 62(suppl):175–179.

84. Flacke JW, Flacke WE: Inadvertent hypothermia: Frequent, insidious, and often serious. Semin Anesth 1983; 2:183–196.

85. Joris J, Banache M, Bonnet, et al: M: Clonidine and ketanserin both are effective treatment for postanesthetic shivering. Anesthesiology 1993; 79:532–539.

86. Delaunay L, Bonnet F, Liu N, et al: Clonidine comparably decreases the thermoregulatory thresholds for vasoconstriction and shivering in humans. Anesthesiology 1993; 79:470–474.

87. Ikeda T, Sessler DI, Tayefeh F, et al: Meperidine and alfentanil do not reduce the gain or maximal intensity of shivering. Anesthesiology 1998; 88:858–865.

88. Bernard JM, Fulgencio JP, Delaunay L, et al: Clonidine does not impair redistribution hypothermia after the induction of anesthesia. Anesth Analg 1998; 87:168–172.

89. Lewis DG, Mackenzie A: Cooling during major vascular surgery. Br J Anaesth 1972; 44:859–864.

90. Morris RH: Influence of ambient temperature on patient temperature during intra-abdominal surgery. Ann Surg 1971; 173:230–233.

91. Morris RH, Wilkey BR: The effect of ambient temperature on patients monitored during surgery, not involving body cavities. Anesthesiology 1970; 32:102–107.

92. Roizen MF, Sohn YJ, L'Hommedieu CS, et al: Operating room temperature prior to surgical draping: Effect on patient temperature in recovery room. Anesth Analg 1980; 59:852–855.

93. Sessler DI, Shroeder M: Heat loss in humans covered with cotton hospital blankets. Anesth Analg 1993; 77:67–72.

94. Sessler DI, McGuire J, Sessler AM: Perioperative thermal insulation. Anesthesiology 1991; 74:875–879.

95. Bourke D, Wurm H, Rosenberge M, et al: Intraoperative heat conservation using a reflective blanket. Anesthesiology 1984; 60:151–154.

96. Radford P, Thurlow AC: Metallised plastic sheeting in the prevention of hypothermia during neurosurgery. Br J Anaesth 1979; 51:237–239.

97. Kurz A, Kurz M, Pieschl G, et al: Forced-air warming maintained intraoperative normothermia better than circulating-water mattresses. Anesth Analg 1993; 77:89–95.

98. Zink RS, Iaizzo PA: Convective warming therapy does not increase the risk of wound contamination in the operating room. Anesth Analg 1993; 76:50–53.

99. Giesbrecht GG, Ducharme MB, McGuire JP: A comparison of three forced-air patient warming systems. Anesthesiology 1994; 80:671–679.

100. Fleisher LA, Metzger SE, Lam J, Harris A: Perioperative cost-finding analysis of the routine use of intraoperative forced air warming during general anesthesia. Anesthesiology 1998; 88:1357–1364.

101. Murphy MT, Lipton JM, Loughran MB, et al: Postanesthetic shivering in primates: Inhibition by peripheral heating and by taurine. Anesthesiology 1985; 63:161–165.

102. Sharkey A, Lipton JM, Murphy MT, et al: Inhibition of postanesthetic shivering with radiant heat. Anesthesiology 1987; 66:249–252.

103. Sessler DI, Moayeri A: Skin-surface warming: Heat flux and central temperature. Anesthesiology 1990; 73:218–224.

104. Goudsouzian NG, Morris RH, Ryan JF: The effects of warming blanket on maintenance of body temperature in anesthetized infants and children. Anesthesiology 1973; 39:351–353.

105. Tollofsrud SC, Gundersen Y, Anderson R: Perioperative hypothermia. Acta Anaesthesiol Scand 1984; 28:511–515.

106. Boyan CP, Howland WS: Blood temperature: A critical factor in massive transfusion. Anesthesiology 1961; 22:559–563.

107. Stone DR, Downs JB, Paul WL, et al: Adult body temperature and heated humidification of anesthetic gases during general anesthesia. Anesth Analg 1981; 60:736–741.

107a. Smith CE, Gerdes E, Sweda S, et al: Warming intravenous fluids reduces perioperative hypothermia in women undergoing ambulatory gynecological surgery. Anesth Analg 1998; 87:37–41.

108. Pflug AE, Aasheim GM, Foster C, et al: Prevention of postanesthesia shivering. Can Anaesth Soc J 1978; 25:43–49.

109. Tausk HC, Miller R, Roberts RB: Maintenance of body temperature by heated humidification. Anesth Analg 1976; 55:719–723.

110. Shanks CA: Humidification and loss of body heat during anaesthesia. II. Effects in surgical patients. Br J Anaesth 1974; 46:863–865.

111. Bissonnette B, Sessler DI, LaFlamme P: Passive and active inspired gas humidification. Anesthesiology 1989; 71:350–354.

112. Conahan TJ, Williams GD, Apfelbaum JL, et al: Airway heating reduces recovery time (cost) in outpatients. Anesthesiology 1987; 67:128–130.

113. Ralley FE, Ramsay JG, Wynands JE, et al: Effect of heated humidified gases on temperature drop after cardiopulmonary bypass. Anesth Analg 1984; 63:1106–1110.

114. Goldberg ME, Jan R, Gregg CE, et al: The heat and moisture exchanger does not preserve body temperature or reduce recovery time in outpatients undergoing surgery and anesthesia. Anesthesiology 1988; 68:122–123.

115. Haslam KR, Nielsen CH: Do passive heat and moisture exchangers keep the patient warm? Anesthesiology 1986; 64:379–381.

116. Noback CR, Tinker JH: Hypothermia after cardiopulmonary bypass: Amelioration by nitroprusside-induced vasodilation during rewarming. Anesthesiology 1980; 53:277–280.

117. Strazis KP, Fox AW: Malignant hyperthermia: A review of published cases. Anesth Analg 1993; 77:297–304.

118. MacLennan DH, Philips MS: Malignant hyperthermia. Science 1992; 256:789–794.

119. Gronert GA: Malignant hyperthermia. Anesthesiology 1980; 53:395–423.

120. Larach MG, for the North American Malignant Hyperthermia Group: Standardization of the caffeine halothane muscle contracture test. Anesth Analg 1989; 69:511–515.

121. Allen GC, Larach MG, Kunselman AR, and the North American Malignant Hyperthermia Group: Registry of MHAUS. Anesthesiology 1998; 88:579–588.

122. Plattner O, Kurz A, Sessler DI, et al: Efficacy of intraoperative cooling methods. Anesthesiology 1997; 87:1089–1097.

123. Gronert GA, Milde JH, Theye RA: Dantrolene in porcine malignant hyperthermia. Anesthesiology 1976; 44:488–495.

21 Biochemical and Metabolic Indicators

Jonathan T. Ketzler, M.D.
H. Russell Harvey, M.D.
Douglas B. Coursin, M.D.

The integration of patient history, physical examination, and reliable laboratory and radiologic data remains the foundation of the modern scientific practice of medicine. Each year brings greater understanding of the molecular, genetic, and biochemical bases of normal human physiology and of the pathophysiology of disease. For example, the human genome project continues to progress more rapidly to completion than initially projected.[1] Innovations in microchip and computer technologies are dramatically advancing our testing ability, accuracy, and data management resources. With these advances, the clinician continues to be challenged to make rapid, correct, and cost-effective decisions. Therefore, practitioners benefit from understanding some of the techniques in common clinical laboratory practice and the limitations and pitfalls associated with their use.

This chapter provides an overview of current clinically relevant techniques for measurement of commonly acquired laboratory tests. It includes a presentation of available terminology and discusses methods of reporting of data. The recommended container characteristics, methods of sample collection, and handling of specimens are presented. The underlying methodologies of common tests are reviewed, and commentary is made on the advantages and disadvantages of various techniques. Brief comments on newer technologies, such as point-of-care devices (see Chapter 24) and molecular, genomic, and microchip diagnostics, are included. The initial section of this chapter reviews analysis of serum electrolytes. This is followed by a discussion of acid-base chemistry, analysis, and pathology. The final section discusses markers of metabolic activity and methods to evaluate metabolic rate and demands. Intercalated within this review is clinical discussion of the mechanisms of underlying etiologies associated with laboratory abnormalities. Along with this description is a therapeutic approach with rationale based on the underlying pathophysiology.

Basic Concepts

Typically, clinical chemistry data are reported in terms of mass concentration. This is most commonly recorded as mass of solute for a given volume of solvent or volume of solution. In the United States, this has meant that laboratory data were reported in terms of a deciliter as a unit of volume. The international unit system (SI) may be gradually reaching greater acceptance in this country. In this system the unit of volume reference is the liter. In either case, the measure of concentration is essentially the molarity of the solution, defined as the number of moles of solute per liter of solution. The concentration of electrolytes has been traditionally reported as milliequivalents (mEq) per liter. For the monovalent cations and anions, the numeric value for milliequivalents per liter (mEq/L) and moles per liter (mol/L) are the same.

Whatever the units used for reporting, many analytic methods, for example flame photometry or atomic absorption spectrometry, provide a measure of the total ionic concentration.[2-4] Electrochemical methods for analyzing serum electrolytes—direct and indirect potentiometry being the most common—measure the concentration of free unbound ion or perhaps, more accurately, the activity of the ion in solution.[5]

Activity versus Concentration

The activity of an ion is different from, but closely related to, the concentration. The activity takes into account the influence of other ionic species present in the sample and reflects the "effective" concentration. The relationship can be expressed by the equation[5]

$$a = \gamma c.$$

where
a = activity
γ = the activity coefficient
c = the concentration

The value of γ for an ion depends on the total ionic strength of the sample.

Flame Photometry

Flame photometry is a method used to measure ions such as sodium, potassium, and lithium.[3, 4] Flame photometry is performed by introduction of a diluted sample into a high temperature air-propane flame. As the sample undergoes combustion, electrons in the ions are excited. As the electrons return to their ground state, they emit a characteristic light. This light consists of wavelengths that are constant and characteristic for a specific element. This makes flame photometry very specific.

Table 21–1. Advantages and Disadvantages of Selected Tests

Analyte	Most Frequently Used Methods	Advantages	Disadvantages
Sodium	Ion-selective electrode: dilutional	Smaller sample volume	Negative error with decreasing water fraction in sample
	Ion-selective electrode: nondilutional	Can be done on whole blood	Larger sample volume
Potassium	Ion-selective electrode: dilutional	Smaller sample volume	Negative error with decreasing water fraction in sample
	Ion-selective electrode: nondilutional	Can be done on whole blood	Larger sample volume
Chloride	Ion-selective electrode: dilutional	Smaller sample volume	Negative error with decreasing water fraction in sample
	Ion-selective electrode: nondilutional	Can be done on whole blood	Larger sample volume; largest positive interference by Br and I
	Mercuric thiocyanate	Easily automated	Negative interference by lipemia; positive interference by Br and I
	Coulometric	Can measure Cl^- in other body fluids; large range of linearity, minimal interference from Br and I	Not automated, slow
Creatinine	Alkaline picrate, endpoint	Readily automated	Interference by hemoglobin, bilirubin, and ketones
	Alkaline picrate, kinetic	Readily automated	Interference by bilirubin and hemoglobin; positive interference by ketones and cephalosporins
	Enzymatic	Might be most specific method	
Urea	Urease/GLDH	Readily automated to add most instruments	F^- inhibits urease
	Urease/conductivity	Readily automated	F^- inhibits urease
	Urease/dye	Readily automated	F^- inhibits urease
Osmolality	Freezing point depression	Relatively rugged precise instruments	Relatively large sample volume
	Vapor point depression	Smallest sample volume	Relatively imprecise, delicate instruments

GLDH, glutamate dehydrogenase.

The matrix of the specimen does not affect the test. Therefore, it can be performed on aqueous samples such as serum, plasma, urine, or other body fluids. Most clinically available flame photometers are dual-chamber so that potassium and sodium can be measured simultaneously. Flame photometry is the basis for the reference method for sodium and potassium in serum because of its accuracy and precision. A flame photometer, while simple in concept, is a rather complicated device. The flame photometer includes a cylinder of one or more compressed gases, pressure regulators, and atomizers, which all combine to produce the flame or light source, and a monochromomator. The monochromomator isolates the radiant energy given off at a specific wavelength that excludes other, extraneous wavelengths. Monochromators usually consist of a combination of filters, prisms, and various defraction gratings. There are frequently slits or lenses both proximal and distal to the monochromomator to make certain that, when light arrives, it is parallel to the system of gratings and prisms. Several different combinations of gases are used in flame photometry. In clinical laboratories, a propane compressed air flame is used most commonly and provides adequate heat to excite sodium and potassium. In other settings, combinations of acetylene and oxygen or natural gas and acetylene or propane are used with either oxygen or compressed air.

In most clinical laboratories, flame photometers are thought to be the gold standard for the testing of samples for sodium, potassium, lithium, and sometimes magnesium.[3, 6] Flame photometers require calibration on a regular basis.[3] A calibrating solution of sodium and potassium is atomized and aspirated into the flame against which an unknown solution is compared. This is also called a "direct reading method." The use of an internal standard method adds lithium or cesium to all of the calibrator blanks and unknowns in equal concentrations. This is performed because lithium and cesium are normally absent from biologic fluids. The exception is for a patient who receives therapeutic lithium. Lithium is excluded as the internal standard in such patients. Amid a wavelength sufficiently removed from that of sodium, potassium, magnesium, or chloride, this technique permits isolation of the desired spectra. Lithium also acts as a radiation buffer and minimizes the effects of mutual excitation that occurs when samples containing both sodium and potassium are introduced into the photometer. However, the use of flame photometry can be time-consuming and complicated, and is being replaced in most clinical laboratories by other methods such as ion-specific electrode (ISE) potentiometry.[3-6] Table 21–1 shows the advantages and disadvantages of selected tests.

Ion-Specific Electrode Potentiometry

Flame photometry measures substance concentration, while ISEs measure ion activity.[2, 5, 7] ISEs are potentiometers used to measure electrolytes in various body fluids. In most clinical laboratories, the measurement of sodium, potassium, chloride, calcium, and magnesium is almost exclusively performed in various automated ion-selective potentiometers. These devices have largely displaced the use of flame photometry, atomic absorption, spectrophotometry, and coulometry, previously used for the measurement of these electrolytes.[2, 4, 5, 8]

A potentiometer measures the electrical potential difference between two electrodes in an electrochemical or galvanic cell. The electrochemical cell consists of two electrodes of varied composition connected by a solution of electrolytes that acts as an ion conductor. Depending on the type of potentiometer, electrolyte solutions or ionic conductors can be composed of one or more phases and can be physically separated by membranes that are permeable to only specific cations or anions. One of the electrical solutions is commonly an unknown or test solution, and the other is an appropriate reference solution depending on the substance being tested. These devices measure the free unbound ion, or more precisely, the activity of the ion being tested (refer to the previous discussion of activity and concentration). The relative activity of an ion is mathematically related to the molality (the moles per kilogram) times the activity coefficient for that particular ion. Sodium and potassium, for example, are almost completely dissociated in normal plasma; therefore, the difference between free and total ion activity is negligible for these cations. The activities measured by the potentiometer are converted to concentration using appropriate formulas. For sodium and potassium, discrepancies between the concentrations derived from direct potentiometry and the concentrations measured by flame photometry occur only when the mass concentration of water in the sample deviates significantly from normal.[5, 6, 9] This occurs in some patients with various forms of severe hyperlipidemia. In such a patient, the portion of the sample that is water is decreased and the sodium concentration as measured by flame photometry might be low, as it is in the liquid phase of the concentration that is being measured. The potentiometer would show normal sodium activity, and the concentration derived from the measurement of activity would be in the normal range.[5]

Ion-specific or ion-selective potentiometry uses ISEs chosen on the basis of the specific anion or cation tested. The different types of ion-selective sensors include solid phase, fluid membrane, enzyme electrodes coated with immobilized or fixed enzymes, and glass membrane ISEs. The cations, hydrogen (H^+), potassium (K^+), sodium (Na^+), calcium (Ca^{2+}), magnesium (Mg^{2+}), and tritiated hydrogen (H_3^+), and the anions, fluoride (F^-), iodine (I^-), bromide (Br^-), chloride (Cl^-), and bicarbonate (HCO_3^-), are all measured with common ion-selective potentiometers.

The ISE contains a thin membrane of a material chosen for its ability to bind one ion species greater than other ions in the sample. The electrode will develop a small voltage when in contact with a solution containing the specified ion. The membrane is made of glass or an ionophore, a membrane containing large organic molecules with different affinities for various ions. A second electrode is used to complete the circuit that is isolated from the ISE by a "salt bridge."[5] A voltage called the liquid junctional potential (Ej) exists at the interface between the salt bridge and the sample solution. The Ej is the largest cause of error in the ISE method. The composition of the bridge solution can be adjusted to minimize this error.

The imperfect selectivity of an electrode for an ion is another common cause of inaccuracy in this test. This means that the matrix of a sample solution is important in selection of an electrode. For example, measurement of sodium in plasma where sodium's concentration is 30 times greater than potassium would make an electrode that is slightly responsive to potassium acceptable.

Spectrophotometry

A spectrophotometer measures the transmittance of light or, inversely, absorption of light that passes through a solution containing a compound that absorbs light at a specific wavelength. This concept is expressed in Beer's law, which is stated mathematically as $A = abc$, where A is the absorbance, a is the absorbtivity constant, b is the light path in centimeters, and c is the concentration of the absorbing compound. Therefore, absorption increases as the concentration of the solute or the absorbing compound in the solvent increases. Conversely, it is true that the transmittance of light through the solution is inversely related to the concentration of the absorbing substance. For accurate measurement of concentration, it is clear that the solvent must have minimal absorption, the light source must radiate at the correct spectral bandwidth, and the solute concentration tested must be within given limits. This implies that the unknown must be referenced to a sample with a known concentration.

A spectrophotometer consists of a light source through which a beam of light is passed through an entrance slit into a monochromomator (see the explanation of monochromomator under Flame Photometry).[3] In most spectrophotometers, the light is split into two coherent beams so that a sample and a reference solution can be assayed at the same time. The remaining beam minus the wavelength absorbed by the solution is detected, and the intensity is displayed on a meter distal to the detector. The use of spectrophotometry, per se, as a test for quantifying drugs and substances, such as phenytoin, aminoglycosides, and barbiturates, has been largely supplanted by immunochemical-mediated analysis techniques, although spectrophotometry is still important in situations in which immunochemical probes are not available. The mercuric thiocyanate method for determining chloride concentrations is a spectral photometric assay, which remains in use by some laboratories.[3, 4]

Atomic Absorption Spectrophotometry

An atomic absorption spectrophotometer is another device used to measure electrolyte concentrations in body fluids. It is analogous to an absorption spectrophotometer and is essentially the inverse of flame photometry.[3] Test solutions and standards are placed in a lower-energy flame so that the electrons and the atoms are not excited, but dissociated from their chemical bonds and placed in a ground or unexcited state. Then, light of a very specific wavelength is beamed at the flame. Since the neutral atoms are at a very low energy level, they are capable of absorbing radiation with a very specific narrow band that corresponds to their own line spectrum. Say, for example, a sodium or potassium cathode light source was beamed at an unknown in a calibration standard. The light would be emitted by the lamp, enter the flame, and a portion would be absorbed by the ground-state atoms of the flame to a degree proportional to its concentration in the sample. Atomic absorption spectrophotometry is much more sensitive than flame photometry because, even in an excited flame photometric sample, only between 1% and 5% of the sample is actually excited. In addition, because the wavelength from a cathode lamp is very specific, the method is highly specific for each element being tested. Atomic absorption spectrophotometry is subject to interference that can render the test results less accurate.[3] Ionization interference results from atoms being excited rather than simply dissociated in the flame. This causes them to emit light at the same frequency as that being measured. Chemical interference can occur when the flame cannot adequately dissociate the sample into free atoms so that absorption of the individual substances can occur. A third type of interference is referred to as matric interference, which occurs when the solvent has enhanced light absorption.

Coulometry

The coulometric titration method is frequently used to measure chloride in body fluids, especially urine.[4] Coulometry measures the amount of electricity passing between two electrodes in an electrical cell. The amount of electricity is directly proportional to the amount of substance that is either produced or consumed by the reduction process of the electrodes. This is referred to as Faraday's law. In the coulometric assay for chloride (Cl^-), a silver-generating solution produces free silver ions (Ag^{2+}) that complex with Cl^- ions to form insoluble silver chloride ($AgCl_2$). After the chloride is consumed, excess free silver ions are in solution and are sensed by a silver ion–sensing electrode. Because silver ions are produced at a constant rate, the time required to titrate all silver ions is directly proportional to the chloride concentration. This method is subject to interference from other halides, but it remains the gold standard for chloride analysis.[4]

Other Tests

In recent years, another category of testing methods has been developed.[9-11] These are loosely referred to as "biosensors." The exact definition is still in evolution, but for the most part a biosensor consists of a biologic or biochemical component that is often immobile or affixed to a plate. This component interacts with the subject to be studied to produce a signal proportional to the quantity or activity of the analyte in solution. The majority of biosensors are some type of immunochemical-mediated test. Included in this are radioimmunoassay (RIA) tests, enzyme multiplied immunoassay technique or enzyme-linked immunosorbent assay (EMIT or ELISA), and fluorescence polarization immunoassay (FPIA). All of these tests involve the combination of the sample with the specific antibody that is labeled in some way, either with a radioactive substance or an enzyme-labeled antigen, or a flourescein-labeled antigen in the case of FPIA. Examples of these tests are specific, commercially available FPIA measurements of phenytoin, phenobarbital, or gentamicin, while ferritin is measured using an enzyme-linked immunoassay.[12] Point-of-care devices are discussed in Chapter 24.

Terminology of Reporting

Currently, confusion exists regarding the terminology of reporting of laboratory results. Controversy exists over the use of SI units to report laboratory results. In Europe, the laboratory community has readily accepted the use of SI units. However, analogous to the lack of success of the metric system in the United States, the SI system has been adopted incompletely in the United States. The SI unit system is based on seven dimensionally independent units of measurement that were adopted in 1970 by the General Conference of Weights and Measures.[12] In SI units, the amount of known or unknown chemical compound is expressed in moles rather than in grams or milliequivalents. These are then expressed as moles per liter for measurements of mass concentration.

As laboratories change their report and referencing termi-

nology, clinicians need to be aware that some tests may display new numeric values and reference ranges. Some test results will look the same. The concentration of serum sodium, for example, will read 140 mmol/L, whereas before it read 140 mEq/L. The numeric value has not changed. Milliequivalents per liter is the molarity of the solution (the number of moles per liter) times the valence of the substance divided by the milligram molecular weight. Millimoles per liter is simply a statement of the molarity of the solution, milligrams per liter divided by the milligram molecular weight. Because monovalent substances have a valence of 1, the reported value is the same for monovalent substances. Other compounds will be reported differently. This may result in confusion. Glucose results, for example, using the SI system will not be reported as milligrams per deciliter with a reference range of approximately 70 to 110 mg/dL but as millimoles per liter, with a reference range of 3.9 to 6.0 mmol/L. The same is true for reporting cholesterol or creatinine values. When reporting hematology values, the reference range may not change numerically but the field of reference will change. For example, white blood cell counts will be reported as 3.5 to 8.5 $\times$ 10^9 cells per liter as opposed to 3.5 to 8.5 $\times$ 10^3 cells per cubic millimeter. Enzyme levels will be reported as units per liter, which is the same as the standard reference system used in this country prior to the adoption of SI units.[12] So, for example, the reporting of liver transaminases, alanine (ALT) and aspartate (AST) transaminases, will be the same. However, the adoption of SI units is incomplete and rather chaotic in the United States. Therefore it is important to note the terminology of reporting employed by a specific clinic, hospital, or reference laboratory.

Methods of Collection

Types of Tubes

Clinical laboratories use different types of collection tubes for specific tests. The tubes are differentiated by the color of the top. The color of the top indicates the type of additive in the tube, such as an anticoagulant or a serum separator. Tests can be performed only if specimens are collected in the correct tube. The tubes themselves are usually made out of a borosilicate glass or soda lime glass.[12, 13] There are some problems associated with the glass itself. Tubes made from soda lime may release trace elements into solution, particularly calcium and magnesium, so special tubes are available for trace element determination. Stoppers may contain zinc. One of the additives of the rubber stopper, TBEP, may interfere with the measurement of certain drugs.[13] Serum separator tubes contain an inert polymer gel material that may or may not be associated with silica or glass particles. This gel accelerates the clotting of blood so that subsequent centrifugation displaces the gel, like a disk, between the cells and the supernatant serum. The layer of gel situated between the cells and the supernatant prevents release of intracellular components into the supernatant for several hours, or in some cases, a few days. There is some debate about whether free gel particles may persist after centrifugation and affect the function of dialysis membranes or ISEs.

A variety of additives are used in blood collecting tubes. It is important to note the difference. A specimen in the wrong tube with the incorrect anticoagulant may result in invalid test results. A list of tube top colors and the corresponding additive is included in Table 21-2.

Table 21–2. Tube Additives by Color

Color	Additive	Use
Blue	Sodium citrate	Coagulation studies
	Preserves labile procoagulants	Unsuitable for calcium measurements
		Citrate chelates calcium
Gray	Potassium oxalate	Hematologic tests
Green	Sodium heparin	Enzyme and toxicology tests
Lavender	EDTA	Hematologic tests
		Also chelates calcium
Red	No additives	Serum electrolytes

EDTA, ethylenediaminetetraacetic acid.
Data from Merrill B: Clinical Laboratories Handbook 1998–99. Madison, University of Wisconsin Hospital and Clinics, 1998; and Young DS, Bermes EW: Specimen collection and processing; sources of biological variation. *In* Burtis C, Ashwood E (eds): Tietz Textbook of Clinical Chemistry, ed 2. Philadelphia, WB Saunders, 1994, pp 58–101.

Sample Handling

Sample handling is one of the most problematic areas of clinical blood sampling in the hospital. The labeling, preservation, and storing of specimens is specific and important. Clinicians know that there are many times when transport labeling has not been done appropriately, and blood has to be redrawn because test results are invalid.

At the minimum, each specimen container, capillary blood tube, or individually colored topped blood tube should be labeled.[12, 13] The label should have the name of the patient, the identifying number, and the location and date and time of collection. Additionally, some labels might suggest special handling. Some tests require that the specimens receive specific treatment. For example, tests for pyruvate and lactate concentration need to be put on ice immediately and kept at about 4°C; otherwise pyruvate concentration decreases and lactate concentration increases within a few minutes at ambient temperature.[12] Other examples are specimens for blood gas and ammonia determination that change when the sample is at room temperature.

Determination of Electrolytes and Associated Abnormalities

Potassium

Potassium is the most abundant cation in the body, with 98% of the total 4000 mmol contained in the intracellular fluid compartment. The resting membrane potential (RMP) is reflected by the intracellular fluid–extracellular fluid (ICF/ECF) ratio and remains constant.[14] Potassium is kept within the cell primarily by a negative charge created when three sodium ions are exported in exchange for two potassium ions. Most potassium exits the cell via the potassium channel, thus creating most of the RMP. Dyskalemias are rarely related to problems with the potassium channel except in cases such as barium poisoning.

The major hormones promoting the shift of potassium into the cell are insulin and catecholamines. While both result in an exchange for sodium, they work very differently. Insulin exchanges potassium in an electroneutral process with a potassium ion exchanged for a hydrogen ion.[15] Catecholamines probably shift potassium into the cell by activating Na^+, K^+-ATPase using intracellular sodium as the substrate.[16]

Most chronic dyskalemias are related to renal or adrenal abnormalities because the kidney regulates long-term potassium balance. The major site of regulation of the excretion of potassium is the cortical collecting duct (CCD) of the kidney.[17] The rate of excretion of potassium is the product of urine flow rate and urinary potassium concentration. So, to evaluate dyskalemias one should determine why urine flow rate or urinary potassium concentration or both are altered in the CCD.

For potassium to be secreted, potassium channels in the luminal membrane must be present with a negative luminal voltage. To generate a negative luminal voltage, resorption of sodium must be faster than resorption of its accompanying anion, usually chloride.

Sodium is resorbed through renal epithelial sodium channels in the apical membrane of principal cells.[18] Aldosterone causes upregulation of these channels and is the most important determinant in opening these channels. The potassium-sparing diuretics and the antibiotic trimethoprim block these channels, decreasing the negative luminal voltage and thus reducing the net secretion of potassium.

Hyperkalemia

Hyperkalemia is present when the serum potassium is greater than 5.5 mEq/L. Treatment of hyperkalemia is required if there is an abrupt change to greater than 6.5 mEq/L or if associated electrocardiographic (ECG) changes such as peaked T waves, P-R interval lengthening, or a change in QRS morphology are present. However, before hyperkalemia is treated aggressively, laboratory error or pseudohyperkalemia must be ruled out. Pseudohyperkalemia occurs when a specimen is hemolyzed. Because hyperkalemia with even mild ECG changes can rapidly progress to dangerous cardiac arrhythmias, laboratory error or pseudohyperkalemia must be ruled out quickly so that definitive therapy can be provided.[19]

The cardiotoxic effects of hyperkalemia can be ameliorated by administration of intravenous calcium. The effects should be seen in a few minutes and last for 30 to 60 minutes. Methods may then be taken to shift K^+ into the cells acutely and then remove it from the body. Insulin will cause glucose to be shifted into the cell, taking K^+ with it, but glucose must also be administered to prevent hypoglycemia. This will cause $[K^+]$ to fall 1.0 mmol/L within 30 minutes with the effect lasting 1 to 2 hours. Sodium bicarbonate may also be administered intravenously. This will cause H^+ ions to leave cells in exchange for K^+, thus decreasing serum $[K^+]$. Potassium can also be decreased by dilution, expanding the ECF volume with sodium chloride. Giving loop diuretics (furosemide, bumetanide) or ion exchange resins can increase potassium excretion. Because the intracellular stores are not greatly affected above 6 mmol/L, it requires less K^+ loss to lower the serum $[K^+]$ from 7 to 6 mmol/L than is needed to lower serum $[K^+]$ from 6 to 5 mmol/L. In extreme cases emergency hemodialysis may be needed.

Hypokalemia

Hypokalemia is manifested by muscle weakness, hyporeflexia, paresthesias, cardiac abnormalities (arrhythmias and increased sensitivity to digoxin), ileus, mental status changes, and polydipsia. Primary causes of hypokalemia include diuretics, gastrointestinal losses, renal tubular acidosis, inadequate intake, and alkalosis. ECG changes include flat or inverted T waves, depressed ST segments, and prominent U waves.

Slow oral replacement is the optimal means of replacement, but in extreme cases intravenous replacement is required. As potassium must traverse the small extracellular compartment (65 mEq) to replace losses in the large intracellular compartment (4000 mEq), care must be taken to avoid overloading the intravascular compartment, thereby causing transient hyperkalemia.

Sodium

Sodium disturbances are the most common and probably the least understood of electrolyte disorders. The serum sodium concentration $[Na^+]$ is maintained within a very narrow range of 138 to 142 mmol/L despite great variation in water intake. This is achieved with the renal countercurrent mechanism along with osmoreceptors in the hypothalamus that control secretion of antidiuretic hormone (ADH). Hyponatremia results when there is a defect in urinary diluting capacity as well as an excess of water intake. Hypernatremia results from a defect in urinary concentration not accompanied by adequate water intake.

Serum osmolarity is almost completely determined by serum $[Na^+]$ and can be calculated using the following formula:

$$2 \times [Na^+] \text{ mmol/L} + \frac{\text{blood urea nitrogen mmol/L}}{2.8}$$
$$+ \frac{\text{glucose mmol/L}}{18}$$

Although an increased serum $[Na^+]$ always indicates a hypertonic state, a normal or low serum $[Na^+]$ does not necessarily indicate a normal or hypotonic state. Other osmotically active substances can add to serum osmolarity with variable effects on serum $[Na^+]$. Osmotically active substances that freely cross the cell membrane will cause an increase in measured osmolarity without affecting serum $[Na^+]$ or causing cellular dehydration. These substances will cause a difference between measured and calculated serum osmolarity, an osmolar gap. Glucose in the insulinopenic patient will not cross cell membranes and will cause intracellular water to move to the extracellular space, resulting in cellular dehydration. This will cause a hyponatremia that is not reflective of total body water (TBW) increase, but is "translocational." Approximately 15% of inpatient hyponatremia is related to hyperglycemia.[20] For every 100-mg/dL increase in plasma glucose, serum $[Na^+]$ will decrease by 1.6 mmol/L. Mannitol, maltose, and glycine are other osmotically active substances that do not cross the cell membrane.

Hyponatremia

Once it is determined that a state of hyponatremia exists, the next step is to determine whether the plasma osmolarity is increased or decreased (Fig. 21-1).

Hypo-osmolar Hyponatremia. If the hyponatremia is truly hypo-osmolar, it must be determined whether the patient is hypervolemic, euvolemic, or hypovolemic. All hyponatremic states are related to defects in urinary dilution. This is usually due to inappropriate secretion of ADH. Rarely, it is related to a decrease in glomerular filtration rate (GFR). This results in an increased sodium resorption in the proximal tubule or a defect in the NaCl transport in the thick ascending loop of Henle and the distal tubule, which limits urinary dilution.

Hypovolemic Hyponatremia. In this situation, there is a decrease in total body sodium (TBNa) as well as a decrease in TBW. This is caused by dehydration-stimulated secretion of ADH with continued intake of hypotonic fluids. Obtaining urinary electrolytes can facilitate differentiation of renal versus extrarenal causes of dehydration. Gastrointestinal or third space losses are associated with renal sodium retention with a urinary $[Na^+]$ less than 10 mmol/L. Some patients with severe metabolic alkalosis caused by vomiting can secrete bicarbonate in the urine. This causes cations to be excreted as well. This can leave the urinary $[Na^+]$ greater than 20 mmol/L despite severe dehydration. In this case, the urinary chloride will be less than 10 mmol/L.

Use of thiazide diuretics is one of the most common causes of hypovolemic hyponatremia with high urinary $[Na^+]$. Underweight elderly women seem to be the most prone to this complication, which usually happens within 14 days of initiation of therapy.[21] Dehydration with hyponatremia with a urinary $[Na^+]$ greater than 20 mmol/L with elevated serum $[K^+]$, blood urea nitrogen, and creatinine is indicative of mineralocorticoid deficiency.

Hypervolemic Hyponatremia. Heart, liver, kidney failure, and the nephrotic syndrome can cause a state in which TBNa is increased but TBW is more increased, causing hypervolemic hyponatremia. Congestive heart failure (CHF) causes a decrease in mean arterial pressure, leading to a nonosmotic release of ADH.[22] Stimulation of the renin-angiotensin system and release of catecholamines decrease GFR and enhance tubular Na^+ resorption. This decreases distal fluid delivery and contributes to hyponatremia. There is good correlation between the degree of hyponatremia and the degree of left ventricular dysfunction.[23]

Euvolemic Hyponatremia. Most dyskalemic patients in the hospital have a euvolemic hyponatremia. High levels of circulating ADH characterize postoperative hyponatremia. While this is normally attributed to infusion of hypotonic solutions, it can also occur in the presence of isotonic solutions. This develops because of generation of electrolyte-free water by the kidney, much of which is retained because of the high levels of ADH.[24]

Glucocorticoid deficiency can cause impaired water excretion in primary and secondary adrenal insufficiency. High levels of ADH have been noted even in the absence of hypovolemia. Because glucocorticoid deficiency is associated with impaired renal hemodynamics, factors independent of ADH may be involved.[25] In the absence of ADH, glucocorticoid deficiency may increase permeability to water in the collecting tubules.

Hyponatremia can also be associated with severe hypothy-

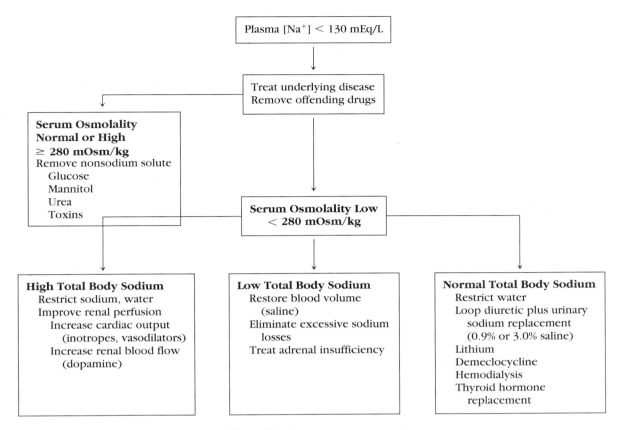

Figure 21-1. Clinical assessment of hyponatremia.

roidism and myxedema. Because cardiac output and GFR can be reduced in severe hypothyroidism, both intrarenal and ADH-mediated mechanisms are involved.

The most common cause of hyponatremia in the hospitalized patient is the syndrome of inappropriate ADH secretion (SIADH). It is, however, a diagnosis of exclusion (Table 21-3). SIADH is most commonly caused by malignancies, pulmonary disease, and central nervous system (CNS) disorders. CNS hemorrhage, tumors, infections, and trauma cause increased ADH from the pituitary itself, while malignancies, usually small cell carcinoma of the lung or duodenum or neuroblastoma of the pancreas or olfactory nerve, cause extrapituitary secretion of ADH.

Diagnosis of Hyponatremia. In many clinical settings there is a specific definable cause of hyponatremia but in

Table 21-3. Diagnostic Criteria for Syndrome of Inappropriate Antidiuretic Hormone (SIADH)

Essential
Osmolality <270 mOsm
Inappropriate urinary concentration (>100 mOsm)
Euvolemia
Elevated urinary [Na$^+$]
Absence of diuretic use or adrenal, thyroid, pituitary, or renal insufficiency
Other Indicators
Plasma ADH inappropriately elevated
Improvement of plasma [Na$^+$] with fluid restriction but not with volume expansion

some cases it may be multifactorial. Patients with hepatic cirrhosis usually have hyponatremia associated with edema or due to excess diuretics, but they may also have essential hyponatremia. Figure 21-1 shows an approach to the diagnosis of hyponatremia.

Treatment of Hyponatremia. Plasma sodium concentration can be raised either by giving NaCl (oral or intravenous) or by restricting fluid intake to below output. The choice is generally determined by the cause and severity of the imbalance. Sodium administration is indicated in hypovolemic and euvolemic states such as true dehydration, diuretic therapy, or adrenal insufficiency, when cortisol replacement is also indicated. Fluid restriction is indicated in hypervolemic states such as CHF, SIADH, primary polydipsia, and end-stage renal failure. In hypovolemic hyponatremia, saline administration will raise the serum sodium by two mechanisms. It will raise the serum sodium by 1 to 2 mEq/L for every liter of saline infused because the saline has a higher sodium concentration than the hyponatremic serum. It will also remove the stimulus for secretion of ADH when volume repletion is reached, allowing excretion of excess water. Once this point is reached, serum sodium may correct quickly.

The optimal rate of correction depends on the clinical state of the patient. In the asymptomatic patient, the plasma sodium should be corrected at 0.5 mEq/L/hour. A more rapid rise increases the risk of osmotic demyelination.

Acute hyponatremia that develops over 2 to 3 days can cause cerebral edema leading to seizures or other severe neurologic disorders.[26] Because the risk of persistent hyponatremia is worse than the risk of rapid correction, the sodium can be raised at an initial rate of 1.5 to 2.0 mEq/L/hour for the first 3 to 4 hours. The amount of sodium needed for a desired increase in serum concentration can be calculated by multiplying the plasma sodium deficit by the TBW. TBW is 0.5 and 0.6 times the lean body weight in women and men respectively. As an example, in an asymptomatic 70-kg man with a serum sodium of 110 mmol/L, if we want to raise it to 120 mmol/L, the sodium deficit = $0.6 \times 70 \times (120 - 110) = 420$ mmol. A loop diuretic can be added if there is concern about fluid overload or if the urine is very concentrated in SIADH.

Severe acute hyponatremia can lead to cerebral edema due to osmotic water movement into the cells. Patients can have asymptomatic severe hyponatremia if the imbalance occurs over several days, allowing the brain to adjust in size. Rapid correction in these patients can lead to central pontine myelinolysis or more diffuse demyelination that does not necessarily involve the pons. The lesions can be seen on CT or MRI, although these tests may not be positive for up to 4 weeks after the initial insult.

Symptoms of osmotic demyelination include mental status changes, dysarthria, dysphagia, paraparesis or quadriplegia, and coma. Patients who have the sodium corrected at a rate greater than 20 mEq/L in the first 24 hours or who are overcorrected to greater than 140 mEq/L are at greatest risk for osmotic demyelination.

Hypernatremia

Hypernatremia can be caused by administration of hypertonic saline or, most commonly, by a decrease in the intake or increase in loss of free water. Figure 21–2 shows an approach to the diagnosis of hypernatremia. Persistent hypernatremia does not exist in normal subjects because a rise in plasma osmolarity stimulates release of ADH and thirst. Therefore, hypernatremia most commonly occurs in patients that cannot express thirst normally: infants, adults with impaired mental status, and the elderly who have diminished osmotic stimulation of thirst. A patient with a serum sodium of 150 mEq/L or greater who is alert but without thirst has

Table 21–4. Causes of Hypernatremia

Unreplaced water loss
  Insensible and sweat loss
  Gastrointestinal losses
  Central or nephrogenic diabetes insipidus
  Hypothalamic lesions affecting thirst or osmoreceptor function
    Primary hypodipsia
    Essential hypernatremia
    Reset osmostat in mineralocorticoid excess
Water loss into cells
  Severe exercise or seizures
Sodium overload
  Intake of hypertonic sodium solution

by definition a hypothalamic lesion affecting the thirst center. The major causes of hypernatremia are listed in Table 21–4.

Symptoms of Hypernatremia. The principal signs of hypernatremia are confusion, altered mental status, increased neuromuscular irritability such as twitching and seizures, obtundation, stupor, and coma. As with hyponatremia, the symptoms depend on the severity and acuity of the imbalance. Severe hyperosmolarity may cause irreversible neurologic deficits apparently due to vascular consequences such as venous sinus thrombosis or hemorrhage from vessels that rupture as a result of the brain's shrinking.

Treatment of Hypernatremia. Hypernatremia is treated with free water, usually by mouth. The free water deficit can be calculated by determining the volume needed to lower the sodium. This is done by multiplying the ratio of actual to desired sodium by the TBW. Thus in a 70-kg man with a sodium of 160 mEq/L and a TBW of $70 \times 0.6 = 42$ L, the

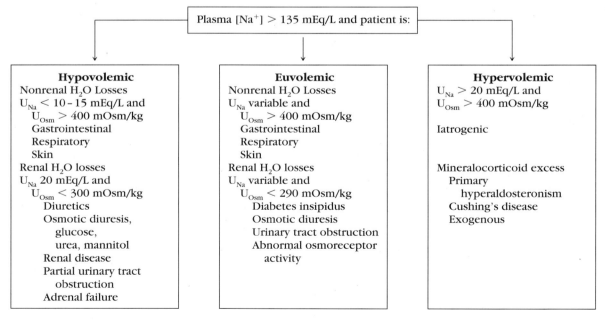

Figure 21–2. Clinical assessment of hypernatremia.

free water deficit is

$$160/140 \times 42 = 48 - 42 = 6 \text{ L.}$$

where
    140 = desired sodium.

As with hyponatremia, rapid correction should be avoided. If the predominant symptom is decreased extracellular volume, 0.9% saline can be used to replenish volume. If the patient has neurologic deficits, 0.45N saline can be used. Patients with hyperosmolar diabetic coma must be volume-resuscitated with 0.9% saline before insulin is given to decrease plasma osmolarity. Once the patient's condition is stable, hypotonic saline can be used to normalize serum sodium.

Calcium

Regulation of extracellular $[Ca^{2+}]$ depends on a complicated relationship between the kidneys, bone, and intestinal tract.[27] The fine regulation is controlled by a calcium receptor and several hormones, the most important of which are parathyroid hormone (PTH) and 1,25-dihydroxyvitamin D_3 $(1,25[OH]_2D_3)$.[28]

Approximately 98% of total body calcium resides in the bone. Roughly 1% of this is exchangeable with serum calcium through physiochemical and cell-mediated mechanisms. Both PTH and $1,25[OH]_2D_3$ stimulate bone-resorbing osteoclasts and result in release of calcium into the ECF. PTH also augments renal hydroxylation of 25-hydroxyvitamin D_3 (25-$[OH]D_3$) into $1,25[OH]_2D_3$ and distal renal tubular calcium resorption.[29]

Serum calcium circulates in three fractions. Half circulates as the biologically active ionized fraction. Ten percent complexes to anions such as bicarbonate, citrate, sulfate, phosphate, and lactate. Forty percent is protein bound and not filtered by the kidney. Most of the protein-bound fraction is bound to albumin but a small fraction is bound to globulins. Hypoalbuminemia is also associated with hypocalcemia but has a lesser effect on ionized calcium. Each gram of albumin per deciliter binds to 0.2 mmol/L of calcium. Approximately 0.2 mmol/dL of $[Ca^{2+}]$ must be added for each 1-g/dL decrease in albumin below the normal of 4.0 g/dL.[30] ECF pH also affects binding of calcium to albumin. For each decrease in pH of 0.1, ionized calcium rises by about 0.05 mmol/L. These corrections for albumin and pH can be avoided by simply measuring ionized calcium.

Hypercalcemia

Hypercalcemia occurs when influx of calcium from the bone or intestine exceeds efflux from intestine, bone, or kidneys. This usually occurs when the renal calcium excretory capacity is exceeded by influx of calcium into the blood from intestine or bone. Excess influx from the intestine may be due to hypervitaminosis D caused by excessive intake or granulomatous disorders such as sarcoidosis. Increased PTH, usually secondary to malignancy, causes increased influx of calcium from bone.[31]

The symptoms of hypercalcemia depend on the magnitude and rapidity of change of serum calcium. Mild hypercalcemia is generally asymptomatic while severe hypercalcemia is associated with neurologic, renal, and intestinal symptoms. Neurologic symptoms range from mild somnolence and weakness to stupor and coma. Renal symptoms include hy-

percalcemia-induced nephrogenic diabetes insipidus, which can result in a reduction in GFR and ECF volume depletion, causing a further increase in $[Ca^{2+}]$. Hypercalcemia may also cause nephrolithiasis and nephrocalcinosis. Intestinal symptoms may include constipation, nausea, vomiting, and anorexia. Peptic ulcer disease may develop.

Primary hyperparathyroidism accounts for 50% of patients who develop hypercalcemia. These patients are usually elderly women with a benign adenoma in a single parathyroid gland. Increased PTH causes enhanced renal calcium absorption and elevated $1,25[OH]_2D_3$, leading to greater intestinal absorption and increased bone turnover. Patients with primary hyperparathyroidism usually have a mild increase in serum calcium, elevated PTH, and normal renal function.

Malignancy-induced hypercalcemia develops from either direct tumor invasion into the bone or release of calcemic factors by malignant cells. Malignancies are the second leading cause of hypercalcemia. Tumors in patients with carcinoma of the breast or squamous cell cancer of the lung release PTH-related peptide (PTH-rP). Although the malignancy has generally been diagnosed when hypercalcemia occurs, there are specific assays for PTH-rP.[32]

Thiazide diuretics increase calcium resorption, causing hypercalcemia. This normally resolves with discontinuation of the medication. Immobilization can lead to an increase in bone resorption and hypercalcemia, especially in the presence of renal insufficiency.

Hypercalcemia can result from granulomatous diseases such as tuberculosis and sarcoidosis. These disorders facilitate tissue conversion of 25-$[OH]D_3$ to $1,25[OH]_2D_3$, leading to hypercalcemia.

Treatment of Mild Hypercalcemia. Management of the asymptomatic hypercalcemic patient is controversial. Indications for surgery include a raised serum calcium, history of life-threatening hypercalcemia, reduced creatinine clearance, kidney stones, raised 24-hour urinary calcium, or substantial reduction of bone mass. In the absence of these findings, medical management is indicated. All patients with symptomatic primary hyperparathyroidism should be referred to a surgeon.

Treatment of Moderate Hypercalcemia. Patients with moderate hypercalcemia are more likely to be symptomatic. Treatment is related to severity of symptoms. In patients with hypercalcemia and altered mental status, other causes must be ruled out. If neurologic or intestinal symptoms are severe, it may be difficult to treat the hypercalcemia with oral fluids and salts. Intravenous saline may be needed to restore intravascular volume. This increases GFR and enhances renal excretion of calcium. Gentle hydration with saline may be sufficient, but in the environment of CHF or if it is necessary to rapidly decrease serum calcium, loop diuretics (furosemide or bumetanide) should be administered to enhance calcium clearance. This combined therapy reduces serum calcium approximately 0.25 to 0.75 mmol/L in 24 to 36 hours.[31]

Treatment of Severe Hypercalcemia. Serum calcium greater than 3.375 mmol/L results in a medical emergency and warrants aggressive intervention even if asymptomatic. Treatment should be aimed at stopping the underlying cause, as well as increasing intravascular volume and renal excretion of calcium, which decreases bone resorption. Initial treatment of severe hypercalcemia entails hydration with saline and loop diuretics. The patient's cardiovascular reserve will dictate how aggressively this can be pursued. Vital signs and electrolytes should be closely monitored, preferably in an intensive care unit. Bisphosphonates or other agents should be administered to reduce bone resorption caused by increased osteoclast activity.[33]

Bisphosphonates are analogs of pyrophosphate and are the primary agents used to decrease osteoclastic bone resorption. They bind firmly to bone mineral and because they resist enzymatic breakdown they have a very long half-life. Precipitation of calcium bisphosphate carries the risk of nephrotoxicity; therefore large volumes of intravenous saline should be administered. Etidronate 7.5 mg/kg/day over 4 hours for 3 to 7 days will start to lower serum calcium by day 2 and reach a nadir at day 7 with the effects lasting for several weeks. To avoid hypocalcemia, therapy should be discontinued if serum calcium drops by more than 0.5 mmol/L within the first 2 days of onset of treatment. Short-term use may cause a transient rise in serum creatinine and chronic use can cause osteomalacia.[33]

A single dose of pamidranate 60 mg over 4 hours for serum calcium less than 3.38 mmol/L (or 90 mg for more severe hypercalcemia) will normally cause serum calcium to fall to normal within 1 week. The effect lasts for over a month.[34] Pamidronate does not appear to worsen renal function, even in patients with severe renal insufficiency. Clodronate 4 to 6 mg/kg/day over 2 to 4 hours is a bisphosphonate commonly used in Europe but is not available in the United States. Alendronate also lowers serum calcium when given intravenously but is currently approved only for oral therapy of osteoporosis.

Plicamycin decreases bone resorption by inhibiting osteoclastic RNA synthesis. It lowers serum calcium more quickly than the bisphosphonates but it has serious side effects, including elevated transaminases, proteinuria, thrombocytopenia, and nausea.[34]

Calcitonin enhances renal calcium excretion and inhibits osteoclastic bone resorption. The effect begins within hours and reaches a nadir within 12 to 24 hours. The effect of calcitonin is transient and minimal so it is not indicated in the treatment of severe hypercalcemia except as an adjunct to other therapy.

Gallium nitrate reduces hydroxyapatite crystal solubility by binding to bone minerals. It takes several days for serum calcium to reach a nadir and the effects last only about a week. Severe side effects, including nephrotoxicity, hypophosphatemia, and anemia, limit the use of this therapy in patients with renal sufficiency.

Hypercalcemia associated with lymphoma, multiple myeloma, and disorders of $1,25[OH]_2D_3$ excess respond to glucocorticoids. Hemodialysis and peritoneal dialysis can be used for hypercalcemic dialysis-dependent patients.

Hypocalcemia

Hypocalcemia results from an efflux of calcium out of the ECF faster than it can be replaced from the bone or reabsorbed from the kidneys. The loss of calcium is usually through the kidney. Pseudohypocalcemia resulting from hypoalbuminemia should be ruled out by measuring the concentration of ionized calcium. As with hypercalcemia, symptoms correlate with the magnitude and rapidity of fall of serum calcium. The most prominent symptoms are related to neuromuscular irritability. Chvostek's sign is a facial twitch elicited by tapping the facial nerve just below the zygoma. Trousseau's sign is elicited when the arterial flow to the arm is occluded with a noninvasive blood pressure cuff for 3 minutes. This results in extension of the fingers with flexing of the thumb and metacarpophalangeal joints in the hypocal-

cemic patient. Symptoms also include dementia and movement disorders. Prolongation of the Q-T interval may develop and may progress to ventricular fibrillation, torsades de pointes, or heart block.[35]

The most common cause of hypocalcemia is idiopathic following parathyroidectomy. Decreased serum PTH levels result in an increase in renal calcium excretion and decreased intestinal absorption. Malignant diseases are often associated with hypoalbuminemia and cause a fall in total calcium, but not ionized calcium (pseudohypocalcemia). Prostate and breast malignancies promote osteoblastic activity and may cause hypocalcemia secondary to increased bone formation.

Renal insufficiency results in decreased excretion of phosphorus. This, combined with intestinal absorption of phosphorus, leads to hyperphosphatemia.[36] This phosphorus binds Ca^{2+} and gives rise to hypocalcemia. Tumor lysis syndrome or rapid crush injuries cause release of cellular phosphorus, which complexes to calcium. Increased serum phosphorus downregulates α-hydroxylase. This enzyme promotes conversion of $25(OH)D_3$ to $1,25[OH]_2D_3$. In renal insufficiency, renal $1,25[OH]_2D_3$ production is decreased. This decrease in $1,25[OH]_2D_3$ causes hypocalcemia secondary to diminished gastrointestinal absorption.

"Hungry bone syndrome" may develop after parathyroid surgical reduction in patients with secondary or tertiary hyperparathyroidism. After reduction of the parathyroid gland, bone is rapidly remineralized, leading to profound hypocalcemia.

The cardiac depression of endotoxic shock may be related to the hypocalcemia that develops with this condition. The mechanism of sepsis-induced hypocalcemia is unknown.

Treatment of Acute Hypocalcemia. Acute symptomatic hypocalcemia generally occurs when total calcium is below 1.875 mmol/L and warrants intravenous replacement until symptoms abate or levels are above 1.875 mmol/L. Intravenous infusion of 15 mg/kg of elemental calcium over 4 to 6 hours will raise the total calcium 0.5 to 0.75 mmol/L.[35] Serum magnesium levels should be measured and corrected when depleted. In the hypocalcemic patient with acidosis from sepsis or renal failure, hypocalcemia must be treated prior to correction of acidosis. Calcium and hydrogen ions compete for binding sites; therefore, increasing the pH will increase the binding sites available for calcium and exacerbate hypocalcemia resulting in cardiac dysfunction, arrhythmias, or arrest. Ten milliliters of 10% calcium gluconate contains 94 mg of elemental calcium. For severe symptomatic acute hypocalcemia, 10 mL can be infused over 4 to 6 minutes followed by infusion of 100 mL of 10% calcium gluconate combined with 900 mL of normal saline. This can be infused as rapidly as 200 to 250 mL/hour. Peripheral infusion of greater than 0.2% calcium gluconate should be avoided because of irritation to veins and tissue damage if extravasation occurs.

Ten milliliters of 10% calcium chloride provide 272 mg elemental calcium and is an excellent source of calcium for rapid replenishment, but can be very irritating to veins so it is not advisable for continuous infusion. Five milliliters of 10% calcium gluceptate contains 90 mg of elemental calcium and is useful for patients who cannot tolerate a large volume load.

Patients with renal failure cannot produce $1,25[OH]_2D_3$, so intestinal calcium absorption remains low. These patients need replacement of vitamin D as well as calcium. $1,25[OH]_2D_3$ is available in oral or parenteral preparations. From 1.0 to 2.0 μg/day may be needed initially followed by a maintenance dose of 0.25 to 1.0 μg/day three times a week. Giving 1,25[OH]$_2$D$_3$ and calcium for several days before parathyroidectomy may prevent postoperative hypocalcemia.

Treatment of Chronic Hypocalcemia. Treatment of chronic hypocalcemia requires both oral calcium as well as vitamin D to enhance absorption. Calcium is generally replaced at 1000 to 2600 mg/day divided into four doses. Calcium citrate is readily available but enhances aluminum absorption so it should be avoided in patients with renal failure who are at risk for aluminum toxicity. Calcitriol is more expensive than the parent vitamin D compounds. Vitamins D$_2$ and D$_3$ are usually adequate to avoid nutritional deficiencies.

Magnesium

Magnesium follows sodium, potassium, and calcium as the fourth most abundant cation in the body. Normal body magnesium content is 22 g. Fifty percent is present in the bone. The normal serum magnesium concentration [Mg^{2+}] is 1.7 to 2.2 mmol/dL. Magnesium is required for cellular energy metabolism and plays an important role in nerve conduction, calcium channel activity, and membrane stabilization. It is important for enzyme activity facilitating the transfer of phosphate groups. These include all reactions that require adenosine triphosphate (ATP). This also includes every step related to the transcription of DNA and the translation of messenger RNA (mRNA). A variety of metabolic abnormalities result from magnesium deficiency.

Magnesium Homeostasis

Serum magnesium depends on flow between bone or muscle and the ECF while total body magnesium (TBMg) depends on absorption from the gastrointestinal tract and excretion from the kidneys. Primarily, the kidney regulates magnesium homeostasis; approximately 100 mg of magnesium is excreted each day. Resorption of magnesium differs from that of other ions in that very little is reabsorbed in the proximal tubule, while 60% to 70% occurs in the thick ascending loop of Henle.[37] Although the distal tubule reabsorbs only about 10% of filtered magnesium, it is the major site of magnesium regulation. Distal tubule and loop of Henle resorption of magnesium is regulated by many factors, including changes in acid-base states, potassium depletion, PTH, calcitonin, glucagon, and vasopressin. The major influence on regulation of magnesium is [Mg^{2+}]. A Ca^{2+}, Mg^{2+} receptor in the capillary side of the loop of Henle senses changes in [Mg^{2+}] where hypermagnasemia inhibits resorption and hypomagnesemia enhances transport.[38] Initially, a negative magnesium balance will result in a rapid fall in serum magnesium. Equilibration with bone stores usually takes several weeks.

Hypomagnesemia

Up to 65% of intensive care unit patients and 12% of medical ward patients are hypomagnesemic.[39] This is usually secondary to gastrointestinal or renal losses (Table 21-5). Magnesium transport in the kidney passively follows sodium so that renal losses can be due to defects in sodium resorption or a primary defect in renal tubular resorption of magnesium. Hypomagnesemia related to gastrointestinal losses can be related to chronic or acute diarrhea or steatorrhea from malabsorption. It can result from extensive bowel resection. It may also be caused by primary intestinal hypomagnesemia, a

Table 21-5. Causes of Hypomagnesemia

Renal Losses
Primary renal tubular magnesium wasting
Hypervolemia
Hypercalcemia with hypercalciuria
Chronic parenteral nutrition
Osmotic diuresis
Renal transplantation
Postobstructive nephropathy
Gastrointestinal Losses
Primary intestinal hypomagnesemia
Malabsorption states
Severe diarrhea
Steatorrhea
Prolonged nasogastric suctioning
Extensive bowel resection
Intestinal fistulas
Acute pancreatitis
Severe malnutrition
Drugs
Diuretics
Alcohol
Aminoglycosides
Cisplatin
Amphotericin B
Cyclosporine
Pentamidine
Other Conditions
Hungry bone syndrome
Hypophosphatemia
Acute correction of chronic acidosis

rare inborn error of metabolism characterized by a selective gastrointestinal defect in magnesium absorption.

Nephrotoxic drugs such as aminoglycosides, cisplatin, cyclosporine, and pentamidine cause hypomagnesemia by damaging the tubule responsible for magnesium resorption. Alcoholism is also implicated as a common cause of hypomagnesemia. As many as 30% of alcoholic patients are hypomagnesemic at the time of hospital admission. Hypomagnesemia resulting from pharmacologically induced acute tubular damage can persist for weeks following reversal of the damage.[40]

Magnesium resorption is inversely related to urine flow so any condition leading to diuresis (diuretic therapy or hyperglycemia) or hypervolemia may cause hypomagnesemia. This hypomagnesemia is usually mild as resorption of magnesium in the proximal tubule is increased. Hypomagnesemia may also be the result of hungry bone syndrome following parathyroidectomy, hypophosphatemia, acute correction of chronic acidosis, postobstructive nephropathy, and renal transplantation.

Signs and Symptoms of Hypomagnesemia. Most symptoms of hypomagnesemia (Table 21-6) are mild or associated with symptoms of abnormalities with other ions such as hypocalcemia, hypokalemia, and alkalosis.[41]

Hypomagnesemic patients are frequently also hypocalcemic. This is especially true when the serum level of Mg^{2+} is less than 0.8 mg/dL. Hypocalcemia is evidenced by Chvostek's and Trousseau's signs or other signs of neuromuscular hyperexcitability. These patients often have decreased PTH levels that normalize quickly upon magnesium replacement. Hypomagnesemia may alter signal transduction from the PTH receptor to catalyze adenylate cyclase, suggesting a primary role for PTH resistance.[42] Forty percent to 60% of patients with hypomagnesemia present with hypokalemia because in

Table 21–6. Signs and Symptoms of Hypomagnesemia

Metabolic
Atherosclerosis
Hyperinsulinemia
Carbohydrate intolerance
Cardiovascular
Widening of QRS complex
Prolongation of P–R interval
Inversion of T wave
U waves
Ventricular arrhythmias
Neuromuscular
Trousseau's and Chvostek's signs
Carpopedal spasm
Seizures
Vertigo and ataxia
Muscular weakness
Depression and psychosis
Bone
Osteoporosis
Osteomalacia

hypomagnesemia, potassium secretion is increased in the loop of Henle and cortical collecting tubules. This hypokalemia does not respond to potassium replacement without magnesium supplementation.

ECG changes associated with hypomagnesemia include widening of the QRS complex and appearance of peaked T waves. With severe depletion, the P–R interval is prolonged and the QRS complex progressively is prolonged with T wave inversion and appearance of U waves. Severe ventricular arrhythmias may develop when hypomagnesemia develops in association with cardiac ischemia.

Profound hypomagnesemia has also been associated with osteoporosis and osteomalacia, especially in patients with diabetes, malabsorption syndromes, or alcoholism.[43]

Treatment. Treatment of hypomagnesemia is determined by the severity of associated signs and symptoms. However, rapid parenteral infusion may decrease magnesium resorption in the loop of Henle with significant renal magnesium loss. Therefore, oral replacement is preferred, especially for asymptomatic patients. Patients with mild asymptomatic hypomagnesemia can be treated with 5 to 15 mmol/day while severe symptomatic cases can be treated with 15 to 20 mmol/day in divided doses.

In severe cases, parenteral replacement is required. In the presence of tetany or ventricular arrhythmias, 25 mmol should be infused over 12 hours. When seizures or acute arrhythmias develop, 4 to 8 mmol should be infused over 5 to 10 minutes followed by 25 mmol over 24 hours. If the patient is also hypocalcemic, treatment should continue for 3 to 5 days.

Magnesium can be used therapeutically in the eumagnesemic patient with preeclampsia, ischemic heart disease, cardiac arrhythmias, and bronchial asthma.[44]

Hypermagnesemia

Hypermagnesemia is rare and usually iatrogenic following replacement or use of large doses of magnesium-containing cathartics or antacids. Elderly patients and those with renal insufficiency are at greatest risk. Hypokalemic metabolic alkalosis with hypomagnesuric hypermagnesemia and severe hypocalciuria has been described recently.[45] Symptoms include hypotension, bradycardia, respiratory depression, and depressed sensorium. Treatment requires discontinuation of replacement therapy and, in severe cases, hemodialysis.

Glucose

The two main energy sources in humans are carbohydrates and fat. Glucose is the primary source of carbohydrates. The minimum requirement for glucose is approximately 200 g/day. This is especially true in the patient with extensive injury. Glucose does offer a "protein-sparing" effect in the unstressed patient, but this effect is less important in the "sick" patient. In the critically ill patient, glucose production and glucose oxidation are enhanced, which serves to limit the glucose supply. The enhanced gluconeogenesis is not suppressed by excess administration of exogenous glucose. Because the maximum rate of glucose oxidation is approximately 7 g/kg/day, excess glucose can become an important factor. Cancer patients, trauma patients, and septic patients were given infusions of glucose of 5 to 6 mg/kg/minute and it was found that oxidation of glucose contributed 60% of carbon dioxide production.[46] Glucagon production, fat synthesis, and storage are also enhanced. About 10% of the energy value of glucose is used to convert it to glucagon for storage. Once glucagon stores are replenished, the glucose is stored as lipids, which uses about 30% of the energy value. When there is overfeeding, energy is expended in storing extra calories. This is exacerbated when feeding is cyclic rather than spread evenly over 24 hours. Insulin administration may improve nitrogen utilization secondary to its effect on skeletal muscle. The effect is not enough to justify using insulin except to regulate serum glucose.

Glucose solutions are available in concentrations from 2.5% to 70%. Solutions greater than 10% should not be infused into peripheral veins.

Acid-Base Abnormalities

There are approximately 350 mmol of bicarbonate (HCO_3^-) available as buffer in the ECF that acts as a buffer. Approximately 1 mmol/kg of acid (H^+) is produced per day. This fixed acid production consists mainly of organic acids along with nonvolatile sulfuric acid from amino acid catabolism and phosphoric and other acids.[47] The kidney resorbs all of the filtered HCO_3^- and generates new HCO_3^- in the collecting duct.

Secretion of H^+ is affected by luminal pH, systemic carbon dioxide tension, mineralocorticoid activity, and the potential electrical difference across the collecting ducts. A major driving force for the secretion of H^+ is the -30- to -60-mV potential across the cortical segment of the renal collecting duct. This is caused by the resorption of sodium.[48] Normally, steady state is maintained because the net secretion of H^+ and the renal production of HCO_3^- equal the rate of H^+ production. Acid-base disturbances result in acidosis or alkalosis.

Acidosis

The consequences of acidosis with pH less than 7.20 include arteriolar dilation, impaired cardiac contractility, sensitization to reentrant arrhythmias, insulin resistance, hyperkalemia, attenuation of response to catecholamines, obtundation, and coma. These can occur whether the acidosis is metabolic, respiratory, or mixed in etiology. The threshold for ventricular fibrillation can be decreased while the defibrillation threshold remains unaltered.[49] Acidemia also triggers a sym-

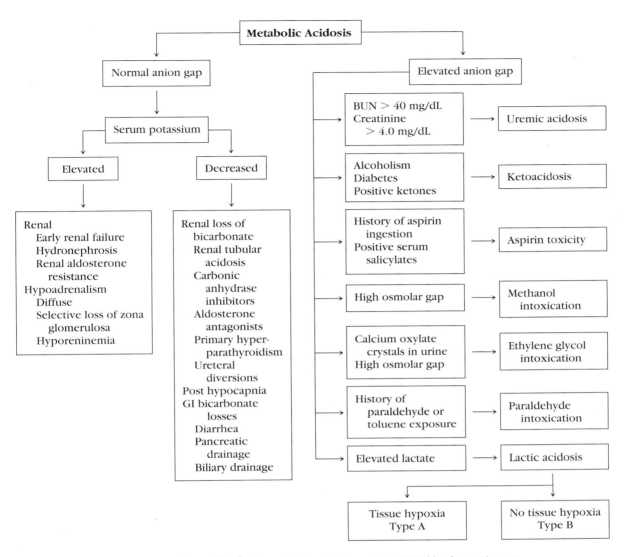

Figure 21-3. Diagnosis of metabolic acidosis. BUN, blood urea nitrogen.

pathetic release but attenuates the effects of catecholamines on the heart and vasculature. Acidemia causes insulin resistance and inhibits anaerobic glycolysis by depressing 6-phosphofructokinase activity.[50] Because anaerobic glycolysis becomes the main source of energy during hypoxia, the consequences of this may be severe. Progressive obtundation and coma may result from severe acidemia because brain metabolism and the regulation of brain volume are impaired.

Lactic Acidosis. Lactic acidosis can be either type A, in which there is impaired tissue oxygenation, or type B, in which no evidence of decreased tissue oxygenation exists. Because evidence of tissue hypoxia is difficult to detect and the pathogenesis of type B lactic acidosis can lead to tissue hypoxia, the distinction between the two is often difficult. Lactic acidosis is most commonly secondary to tissue hypoxia resulting from circulatory failure. Overproduction and underutilization of lactic acid contribute to accumulation. The resulting acidemia contributes to further hemodynamic depression and suppresses lactate metabolism and clearance by the liver and kidneys, thus creating a self-perpetuating cycle.

Treatment is directed at increasing tissue oxygenation and correcting the underlying cause. Increasing tissue oxygenation may require fluid resuscitation, increased fraction of inspired oxygen, and inotropic and vasoactive drugs. Vasoconstrictors should be avoided when possible because vasoconstriction will enhance tissue hypoxia. Correcting the underlying cause may require antibiotics for sepsis, dialysis to remove toxins such as methanol, administration of insulin in diabetic patients, administration of glucose in alcoholic patients or patients with congenital lactic acidosis, and surgery for patients with trauma or vascular compromise.

The prognosis for patients with lactic acidosis is related to the underlying cause.

Diabetic Ketoacidosis. Diabetic ketoacidosis is treated primarily with intravenous insulin. Water, sodium, phosphorus, magnesium, and potassium should be replaced. Because metabolism of keto acids occurs so quickly in response to insulin therapy, bicarbonate is rarely needed. In fact, administration of alkali may augment hepatic ketogenesis. Despite this, patients with impaired myocardial function secondary to severe acidemia (pH <7.00) may benefit from careful titration of bicarbonate. The infusion of insulin should be continued until serum ketones have cleared to prevent reaccumulation of ketones. Once the serum glucose has been corrected to 200 to 250 mg/dL, a glucose infusion should be started to maintain the serum glucose at 250 mg/dL or greater to prevent central pontine myelinolysis.

Alcoholic Ketoacidosis. Alcoholic ketoacidosis induces severe hypobicarbonatemia that will correct quickly with reinstitution of nutritional support. Stimulation of insulin secretion and inhibition of glucagon secretion replenish bicarbonate stores from metabolism of retained keto acids following dextrose infusion. Volume resuscitation will reverse the coexisting lactic acidosis. Multivitamins should be added to treat folate deficiency and thiamine should be given to prevent Wernicke's encephalopathy.

Methanol and Ethylene Glycol Acidosis. Methanol and ethylene glycol intoxication cause a high anion and osmolar gap metabolic acidosis. Treatment often entails large amounts of alkali, gastric lavage, oral charcoal, and rarely hemodialysis.[51] Intravenous or oral ethanol is given to inhibit generation of toxic metabolites from ingested alcohols. Ethanol has a much higher affinity for alcohol dehydrogenase and prevents metabolism of the alcohols that produce toxic metabolites until they can be cleared, unchanged, by the kidneys. Fomepizole (4-methylpyrazole) has recently been approved for use in the United States. It is a potent inhibitor of alcohol dehydrogenase that prevents production of toxic metabolites.

Renal Tubular Acidosis. Renal failure—especially acute renal failure in the patient in a catabolic state—can result in severe metabolic acidosis. This reflects accumulation of endogenous acids, primarily the sulfonates. Type 1 renal tubular acidosis can result in deficits in bicarbonate and potassium. The acidosis may be compounded by inadequate respiration secondary to respiratory muscle paresis caused by potassium depletion.

Aspirin Overdose. Aspirin overdose can lead to a respiratory alkalosis or, more commonly, a mixed respiratory alkalosis and metabolic acidosis. Salicylate works directly on the respiratory center to stimulate respiration causing respiratory alkalosis. The metabolic acidosis is generally due to accumulation of lactic and keto acids. The greatest risk of morbidity and mortality is related to the concentration of salicylate in the CNS. Therefore, therapy is directed at limiting drug absorption by use of activated charcoal. Alkalinizing the blood promotes the exit of toxin from the CNS, so if the patient is not already alkalotic from respiratory alkalosis, alkali should be administered to keep the pH between 7.45 and 7.50. Alkalinizing the urine also inhibits reabsorption of the salicylic acid. Hemodialysis is useful only in severe cases or in patients with renal dysfunction.

Bicarbonate Loss. Excess loss of bicarbonate from the gastrointestinal tract caused by severe diarrhea, or in patients with pancreatic transplants in whom the exocrine system drains into the bladder, can lead to a non-ion gap acidosis. Severe sodium, potassium, and free water deficits usually accompany it. Treatment requires control of the causative factor and replenishment of deficits.

Toluene Exposure. Glue sniffing can cause severe anion gap metabolic acidosis resulting from the metabolism of toluene to benzoic and hippuric acid. In the face of adequate renal function, hippurate, sodium, and potassium are quickly cleared. This can convert an ion gap acidosis to a hyperchloremic acidosis that can be mistaken for a distal renal tubular acidosis.

Dilutional Acidosis. Aggressive fluid resuscitation with a solution that does not contain bicarbonate can lead to dilutional acidosis. Several cases have recently been identified in patients with right ventricular failure secondary to myocardial infarction.[52] Treatment entails replacing bicarbonate during resuscitation.

Respiratory Acidosis. Respiratory acidosis results when production of carbon dioxide exceeds the ability of the lungs to excrete it. The increased carbon dioxide is buffered in the blood and the result is an initial rise in bicarbonate. This response is rapid but very limited. Sustained hypercapnia will cause renal acidification and an increase in serum bicarbonate. Renal correction generally takes 3 to 5 days, resulting in hypochloremic hyperbicarbonatemia.

The morbidity and mortality from respiratory acidosis are generally secondary to acute respiratory failure. Causes of acute respiratory failure are listed in Table 21–7. The alveolar gas equation is

$$PA_{O_2} = FI_{O_2}(Pb - P_{H_2O}) - Pa_{CO_2}/R$$

where

PA_{O_2} = partial pressure of oxygen in the alveolus
FI_{O_2} = fraction of inspired oxygen
Pb = barometric pressure
P_{H_2O} = vapor pressure of water in the alveolus
Pa_{CO_2} = partial pressure of carbon dioxide in arterial blood
R = the respiratory quotient, defined below.

This equation reveals that an acute elevation of Pa_{CO_2} of greater than 80 mmHg for a patient on room air results in a dangerously hypoxic alveolar oxygen content. In this situation it is hypoxia and not hypercapnia that is life-threatening. Because of this, supplemental oxygen is crucial to treatment of respiratory acidosis. Treatment then focuses on correcting the underlying cause of the respiratory failure. If this cannot be done quickly or if the condition is refractory to treatment, the airway should be secured and mechanical ventilation initiated until a normal milieu can be reestablished.

Table 21–8 lists causes of chronic respiratory insufficiency. Infection, narcotic use, or oxygen therapy is usually the cause of acute decompensation in patients with chronic respiratory insufficiency. Treatment depends on severity and rapidity of onset. Antibiotic therapy, bronchodilators, and corticosteroids should be initiated quickly. CNS depressants and high concentrations of supplemental oxygen should be used with great caution. In acute respiratory failure, it is

Table 21–7. Causes of Acute Respiratory Failure

Upper airway obstruction
Lower airway obstruction
Severe alveolar defects
  Pneumonia
  Pulmonary edema
Status asthmaticus
Ventilatory restriction
  Fractured ribs
  Flail chest
Central nervous system depression
Neuromuscular impairment

Table 21–8. Causes of Chronic Respiratory Insufficiency

Chronic obstructive pulmonary disease
Chronic restrictive pulmonary disease
Upper airway obstruction
Central nervous system depression
Neuromuscular impairment
Abnormal chest wall mechanics

important to initiate mechanical ventilation quickly. In patients with chronic respiratory insufficiency, this plan should be undertaken only in selected patients after aggressive non-invasive therapy has failed. Patients with end-stage chronic respiratory insufficiency who require mechanical ventilation have a poor prognosis.

Alkalosis

A blood pH greater than 7.60 can compromise myocardial and cerebral perfusion by causing arteriolar constriction. For unknown reasons, this effect is more pronounced in respiratory alkalosis than it is in metabolic alkalosis. Alkalosis results in a moderate positive inotropic effect on the isolated heart, but it also reduces the anginal threshold that predisposes the heart to supraventricular and ventricular arrhythmias. Neurologic consequences of alkalemia include tetany, lethargy, seizure, headache, delirium, and stupor. These effects are thought to be due to the concurrent reduction in serum ionized calcium. Alkalosis suppresses respiration; this can lead to hypercapnia and hypoxia. Alkalosis may not be a factor in patients with adequate respiratory reserve; however, even mild alkalosis can frustrate efforts to wean patients from mechanical ventilation.

Because of translocation of potassium into the cells and renal losses of potassium, hypokalemia often accompanies alkalosis. Alkalemia stimulates glycolysis and increases the production of lactic and keto acids. Acute alkalemia shifts the oxyhemoglobin curve to the left, increasing the affinity of hemoglobin for oxygen. Chronic alkalemia reverses this effect by increasing the production of 2,3-diphosphoglyceric acid in red blood cells.

Metabolic Alkalosis. If an appropriate respiratory response is elicited to increases in the concentration of bicarbonate, there is no need for treatment until serum bicarbonate levels exceed 45 mmol/L. Treatment is then directed at lowering the bicarbonate to less than 40 mmol/L.

The most severe metabolic alkalosis is hypochloremic, hyperbicarbonatemic. This chloride-responsive alkalosis is generally caused by either gastric losses of hydrochloric acid or excess renal losses of ammonium chloride caused by thiazide and loop diuretics.

A "contraction alkalosis" can occur in patients with massive edema or lung injury after aggressive treatment with diuretics. The diuretic-induced loss of NaCl exacerbates the hyperbicarbonatemia by decreasing the volume of distribution of bicarbonate.

Steps should be taken to stop the ongoing loss of bicarbonate. Nausea and vomiting should be controlled. If gastric drainage is required, acid loss can be lessened by administration of H_2-receptor blockers or gastric H^+, K^+-ATPase inhibitors. These drugs will substitute NaCl loss for hydrochloric acid loss. Loop and thiazide diuretics should be decreased or replaced with potassium-sparing diuretics that limit potassium excretion by decreasing acidification in the distal renal tubules. All exogenous sources of bicarbonate and its precursors, such as lactate, citrate, and acetate, should be stopped.

In severe cases, hydrochloric acid can be administered intravenously in a solution containing 100 to 200 mmol/L. It can be mixed with saline or dextrose without complications. Because hydrochloric acid is sclerosing, it must be infused through a central vein at a rate not greater than 0.2 mmol/kg/hour. Bicarbonate has a volume of distribution of approximately 50% body weight. The equation for calculating the amount of hydrochloric acid needed to decrease bicarbonate to a safe level is

$$\text{Hydrochloric acid (mmol)} = (AB - TB) \times TBW \times 0.5$$

where

AB = actual bicarbonate level
TB = target bicarbonate level
TBW = total body weight in kilograms.

So, to calculate the amount of hydrochloric acid needed to reduce serum bicarbonate from 50 mmol/L to 40 mmol/L in a 70-kg patient,

$$\text{Hydrochloric acid (mmol)} = (50 - 40) \times 70 \times 0.5 = 350$$

Chloride-resistant alkalosis is found in conditions such as severe potassium depletion, mineralocorticoid excess, Bartter's syndrome, and Gitelman's syndrome. Life-threatening alkalemia is very rare in these disorders. The primary treatment of chloride-resistant alkalosis is correction of the underlying condition. The alkalosis usually responds well to aggressive potassium replacement.

Respiratory Alkalosis. Respiratory alkalosis is probably the most common acid-base disorder as it commonly occurs during pregnancy or with anxiety disorders. Respiratory alkalosis is fairly common in critically ill patients and can indicate a poor prognosis, because mortality is directly proportional to severity of hypocapnia.[53] Treatment of respiratory alkalosis is directed toward the underlying cause. Because most cases of respiratory alkalosis are no real risk to health, treatment is not required.

Mixed Alkaloses. Alkalemia in patients with metabolic and respiratory alkalosis can be severe despite the fact that there is not a serious derangement in the plasma bicarbonate or the $Paco_2$. This situation can occur in patients with primary hypocapnia with chronic liver disease who also have metabolic alkalosis from vomiting, nasogastric drainage, and hypokalemia. This can also be seen in patients with primary hypocapnia with renal insufficiency in which the renal response to hypocapnia does not reduce the alkali load. Treatment is aimed at reducing the contributing factors when possible; acid administration is used when needed.

Metabolic Indicators

Clinical questions of metabolism usually center on energy expenditure and supply. Currently no direct measures of cellular metabolic rate are available. The methods used to estimate energy use depend on the correlation between gas exchange or heat production and energy expenditure. For the purpose of this discussion, metabolism is analogous to substrate utilization or energy expenditure.

Parameters to Be Monitored

Estimation of energy expenditure is derived using data about gas exchange or heat production. Alternatively, energy expenditure is estimated by use of standardized formulas (the Harris-Benedict equation is most commonly used). If questions about adequacy (or overabundance) of feeding require measurement and more individual data, the following parameters are required:

Oxygen consumption (Vo_2) is required for predicting energy expenditure. It is obtained from using indirect calorimetry or from the "reverse" Fick method. (For a complete explanation of these methods, see below).

Carbon dioxide production (Vco_2) is calculated for estimating energy expenditure using indirect calorimetry. It is usually *not* calculated when using the Fick method due to the inaccuracy of the result in calculating energy expenditure. In this way, Vco_2 is ignored and the respiratory quotient (R) (see below) is assumed.

Respiratory quotient (R) is the ratio of Vo_2 to Vco_2.

Urea nitrogen excretion is measured over a 24-hour period and used as a correction factor in the Weir equation (the equation which estimates energy expenditure based on Vo_2 and Vco_2 derived from indirect calorimetry). This is often ignored when calculating energy expenditure with indirect calorimetry since the contribution is minor.

Cardiac output (CO) is measured (usually via a thermodilution pulmonary artery catheter) and used in the Fick equation to derive Vo_2.

Content of arterial oxygen (Cao_2) is calculated from measured Pao_2 and used in the Fick equations.

$$Cao_2 \text{ mL/dL} = 1.39 \text{ (Hbg)} \times Sao_2/100 + .0031 \text{ (Pao}_2)$$

Content of mixed venous oxygen ($C\bar{v}o_2$) is calculated from measured Svo_2, used in the Fick equation to derive Vo_2.

$$C\bar{v}o_2 \text{ mL/dL} = 1.39 \text{ (Hbg)} \times Svo_2/100 + .0031 \text{ (Pvo}_2)$$

Two other terms require explanation. The first, basal energy expenditure (BEE), is an assessment of energy expenditure at full repose. It is an estimation of the minimum amount of energy required for homeostasis. BEE can account for 60% to 70% of total energy expenditure in healthy people.[54] Even in hypermetabolic critically ill patients, BEE accounts for 50% of total energy expenditure. This is the reason that estimating nutritional needs is based on calculation of BEE (via the Harris-Benedict equation) plus modifiers for disease states and activity.

The second term is resting energy expenditure (REE). REE is frequently but incorrectly used interchangeably with BEE. REE is BEE plus a factor for the thermogenic effect of feeding.

$^2H_2^{18}O$, a stable isotope of water, is measured in the "doubly labeled water" technique of estimating energy expenditure (see below).

Measurement Methods

Direct Calorimetry. This method is quite cumbersome and used only for research purposes.[54, 55] Direct calorimetry measures heat loss from the subject. It relies on the correlation between heat loss and the known heat of combustion for the specific nutritional milieu of the patient. The various heats of combustion correlate to specific caloric equivalents of the oxygen and gas exchange ratio. An accurate measurement of total heat loss requires thermoneutrality and specialized chambers or suits to measure total body heat loss.

Therefore, this method is highly impractical in a clinical setting.

Doubly Labeled Water Technique. This method estimates energy expenditure by tracking the rate of disappearance of $^2H_2^{18}O$.[54] Measurements are taken over several days and can be done in the "field," in active, nonhospitalized patients. The disappearance of ^2H is proportional to water turnover, but ^{18}O disappearance is due to incorporation into CO_2 as well. Thus, the difference equals Vco_2. In this method, Vo_2 is *not* measured, but estimated based on an assumed R or on FQ (food quotient) which is calculated [FQ = (Vco_2) L sum of Vo_2 for all consumed foods)].

In critically ill, hospitalized patients, this method is impractical due to the time course of the test. Also, no studies elucidating the effect of "ill" metabolism on FQ have been reported.

Fick Method. (This is also known as reverse Fick because it uses the Fick equation to solve for Vo_2 rather than CO.) This method estimates energy expenditure based on Vo_2 derived from the Fick equation.[54-61]

$$Vo_2 = CO \times 10 \ (Cao_2 - C\bar{v}o_2)$$

When Cao_2(mL/dL) = 1.39 (Hb) $\times$ $Sao_2/100$ + .0031 (Pao_2)

$$C\bar{v}o_2(\text{mL/dL}) = 1.39 \text{ (Hb)} \times Svo_2/100 + .0031 \text{ (Pvo}_2)$$

This method is also referred to as circulatory calorimetry. In this method, the Vco_2 (which can be calculated by substituting CO_2 for O_2) is usually not calculated. CO_2 content analysis is more involved, requiring adjustment for temperature and pH. Vo_2 calculation is far more accurate than Vco_2 by the Fick method. A common formula for estimating energy expenditure using Vo_2 derived from the Fick equation is:

$$\text{Energy expenditure (kcal/day)} = Vo_2 \times 7.$$

It would seem that estimating energy expenditure on the basis of data derived from the Fick equation is simple. Why, then, the reliance on cumbersome metabolic carts? First, in this method, Vco_2 is not measured, and the energy expenditure is more of an estimate. Also, correlation between energy expenditure and Vo_2 derived from the Fick method and indirect calorimetry is variable.[56-61] The correlation is less accurate in patients with hemodynamic instability or mechanical ventilation.[56, 57]

Indirect Calorimetry or Metabolic Carts. Indirect calorimetry is the method (other than estimation based on the Harris-Benedict equation) most often used for measuring energy expenditure.[62] Indirect calorimeters measure inspired and expired gas concentrations and volumes that are then used to calculate Vo_2 and Vco_2. There are two types of indirect calorimeters: open and closed circuit calorimeters. The most commonly employed calorimeters are open circuit, in which the inspired gas source is a source other than the calorimeter itself (such as room air or a ventilator).

Because indirect calorimeters measure gas exchange as an analog of metabolism, several assumptions must be made.[54, 55] All O_2 and CO_2 exchange occurs across the lung; oxygen and CO_2 are neither stored nor retained; and all Vo_2 and Vco_2 is associated with ATP synthesis. Of course, not all these assumptions are true. For example, oxygen is involved in free radical production (the oxidative "burst" in neutrophils and in normal cytochromal oxygen metabolism) and CO_2 can be retained out of sync with production. These factors induce error.

There are several types of commercially available indirect calorimeters. All consist of four basic components: an oxygen analyzer, a CO_2 analyzer, a volume measuring device, and a microprocessor. Six quantities are commonly measured: fraction of inspired oxygen (FIO_2), fraction of expired oxygen (FEO_2), fraction of inspired carbon dioxide ($FICO_2$), fraction of expired carbon dioxide ($FECO_2$), volume inspired per minute ($\dot{V}I$), and volume expired per minute ($\dot{V}E$). Volume of oxygen consumed per minute ($\dot{V}O_2$) and volume of carbon dioxide consumed per minute ($\dot{V}CO_2$) are calculated from these parameters.

$$\dot{V}O_2 = (FIO_2 \times \dot{V}I) - (FEO_2 \times \dot{V}E)$$

$$\dot{V}CO_2 = (FICO_2 \times \dot{V}I) - (FECO_2 \times \dot{V}E)$$

Open circuit indirect calorimeters, in fact, do not measure $\dot{V}I$ (as opposed to closed circuit calorimeters where the gas source is part of the calorimeter). Therefore $\dot{V}I$ must be estimated when using an open circuit. This is done via the Haldane transformation formula[54]:

$$\dot{V}I = (1 - FEO_2 - FECO_2/1 - FIO_2) \times \dot{V}E$$

It is because of this "estimation" that an upper limit of FIO_2 is set (usually about 60% to 70% O_2). FIO_2 is the denominator of this formula, and at a higher FIO_2, the denominator approaches zero. This amplifies error.

Energy expenditure is calculated from $\dot{V}O_2$ and $\dot{V}CO_2$ by the Weir equation:

Energy expenditure (kcal/day) =
$$\dot{V}O_2 (3.9) + \dot{V}CO_2 (1.1) - \text{urinary nitrogen} (2.17)$$

(Many indirect calorimeters exclude the urea nitrogen factor, since it has been established that it represents a negligible amount.)

The accuracy of this energy expenditure requires a link between gas exchange and cellular metabolism. This necessitates respiratory and hemodynamic stability prior to and during measurement. This is especially true for the $\dot{V}CO_2$ calculation, as the body pool of CO_2 is very large and changes at the cellular level will take time to be manifest as $\dot{V}CO_2$.[54, 56] Because of this requirement, indirect calorimetry takes time. Some advocate a 30-minute measurement period with frequent testing for variance.[63] Also, many patients whose condition might otherwise beg for accurate energy expenditure and $\dot{V}O_2$ estimations are too unstable or require an excessively high FIO_2 ($>60\%$) that precludes accurate measurement.[54, 55, 64, 65]

Summary

This chapter has reviewed classic techniques used to measure serum electrolytes. Description of common causes of abnormal serum Na^+, K^+, Ca^{2+}, Mg^{2+}, and acid-base homeostasis followed. Diagnostic evaluation and therapeutic intervention were described.

Methods to assess metabolic activity in the critically ill were discussed. These range from empirical formulas to potentially more accurate indirect calorimetric approaches. Unfortunately, direct techniques are cumbersome and not clinically available.

The development of portable and compact point-of-care devices may supplant many of the techniques outlined in this chapter. In addition, increasingly sophisticated application of molecular and genetic testing will enhance laboratory evaluation. Finally, microchip technology will facilitate the acquisition of large quantities of data from relatively miniscule amounts of substrate. This explosion in capability will have major impact on how we care for the critically ill and may enable estimation of risk for the development of various diseases and the therapeutic success of medications.

REFERENCES

1. Collins FS, Patrinos A, Jordan E, et al: New goals for the U.S. Human Genome Project: 1988–2003. Science 1998; 282:682–689.
2. Kruse-Jarres JD: Ion-selective potentiometry in clinical chemistry: A review. Med Prog Technol 1988; 13:107–130.
3. Evenson M: Photometry. In Burtis, C, Ashwood E (eds): Tietz Textbook of Clinical Chemistry, ed 2. Philadelphia, WB Saunders, 1994, pp 104–131.
4. Kaplan L: Renal physiology and water and electrolyte balance. In Tilton RC, Ballows A, Hohnadel DC, et al (eds): Clinical Laboratory Medicine. St Louis, Mosby–Year Book, 1992, pp 84–97.
5. Durst RA, Sigaard-Andersson O: Electrochemistry. In Burtis C, Ashwood E (eds): Tietz Textbook of Clinical Chemistry, ed 2. Philadelphia, WB Saunders, 1994, pp 159–183.
6. Kau N, Gunther M, Fahnenstich H, et al.: Measurements of sodium and potassium in newborns and prematures by ion-selective electrodes and flame photometry: Influence of lipid and protein content of blood. Acta Anaesthesiol Scand Suppl 1995; 39(suppl 107):107–111.
7. Zoppi F, Guagnellini E, Manzoni A: Ion effects in measurement of sodium and ionized calcium in direct potentiometry. Scan J Clin Lab Invest 1993; 53:521–527.
8. Northall H, York GA: Sweat sodium and chloride analysis using Bm/Hitachi 911 ion-selective electrodes. Br J Biomedical Sci 1995; 52:68–70.
9. Hubl W, Wejbora R, Shafti-Keramat L, et al: Enzymatic determination of sodium, potassium, and chloride in abnormal (hemolyzed, icteric, lipemic, paraproteinemic, or uremic) serum samples compared with indirect determination with ion-selective electrodes. Clin Chem 1994; 40:1528–1531.
10. Quiles R, Fernandez-Romero JM, Fernandes E, et al: Automated enzymatic determination of sodium in serum. Clin Chem 1993; 39:500–503.
11. Taylor RP, James TJ: Enzymatic determination of sodium and chloride in sweat. Clin Biochem 1996; 29:33–37.
12. Merrill B: Clinical Laboratories Handbook 1998–99. Madison, University of Wisconsin Hospital and Clinics, 1998.
13. Young DS, Bermes EW: Specimen collection and processing; sources of biological variation. In Burtis C, Ashwood E (eds): Tietz Textbook of Clinical Chemistry, ed 2. Philadelphia, WB Saunders, 1994, pp 58–101.
14. Kamel KS, Quaggin S, Scheich A, et al: Disorders of potassium homeostasis: An approach based on pathophysiology. Am J Kidney Dis 1994; 24:597–613.
15. Zierler K: Insulin hyperpolarizes rat myotube primary cultures without stimulating glucose uptake. Diabetes 1987; 36:1035–1040.
16. Williams ME, Gervino EV, Rosa RM, et al: Catecholamine modulation of rapid potassium shifts during exercise. N Engl J Med 1985; 312:823–827.
17. Wright FS, Giebisch G: Regulation of potassium excretion. In Seldin DW, Giebisch G (eds): The Kidney: Physiology and Pathophysiology. New York, Raven Press, 1992, pp 2209–2247.
18. Rossier BC: Cum grano salis: The epithelial sodium channel and the control of blood pressure. J Am Soc Nephrol 1997; 8:980–992.
19. Gennari JF: Hypokalemia. N Engl J Med 1998; 339:451–458.
20. Zarinetchi F, Berl T: Evaluation and management of severe hyponatremia. Adv Intern Med 1996; 41:251.
21. Sonnerberck M, Friedlander Y, Rosin A: Diuretic induced severe

hyponatremia: Review and analysis of 129 reported patients. Chest 1993; 193:601.

22. Szatalowicz V, Arnold P, Chaimovitz C, et al: Radioimmunoassay of plasma arginine vasopressin in hyponatremic patients with congestive heart failure. N Engl J Med 1981; 305:263.

23. Lee W, Packer M: Prognostic importance of serum sodium concentration and its modification by converting-enzyme inhibitors. Circulation 1986; 73:257.

24. Steele A, Gowrishankar M, Abrahamson S, et al: Postoperative hyponatremia despite near-isotonic saline infusion: A phenomenon of desalination. Ann Intern Med 1997; 126:20.

25. Linas S, Berl T, Robertson G, et al: Role of vasopressin in the impaired water excretion of glucocorticoid deficiency. Kidney Int 1980; 18:58.

26. Berl T: Treating hyponatremia: Damned if we do and damned if we don't. Kidney Int 1990; 37:1006.

27. Bushinsky DA, Krieger NS: Integration of calcium metabolism in the adult. *In* Coe FL, Favus MJ (eds): Disorders of Bone and Mineral Metabolism. New York, Raven Press, 1992, pp 417–432.

28. Monk RD, Bushinsky DA: Treatment of calcium, phosphorous and magnesium disorders. *In* Brady H, Wilcox CS (eds): Therapy in Nephrology and Hypertension. Philadelphia, WB Saunders, 1999.

29. Sutton RAL, Dirks JH: Disturbances of calcium and magnesium metabolism. *In* Brenner BM, Rector FC (eds): The Kidney. Philadelphia, WB Saunders, 1996, pp 1038–1085.

30. Broadus AE: Mineral balance and homeostasis. *In* Favus MJ (ed): Primer on the Metabolic Bone Diseases and Disorders of Mineral Metabolism. Philadelphia, Lippincott-Raven, 1996, pp 57–63.

31. Bilezikaian JP: Management of hypercalcemia. J Clin Endocrinol Metab 1993; 77:1445–1449.

32. Budayr AA, Nissenson RA, Klein RF, et al: Increased serum levels of a parathyroid like protein in malignancy associated hypercalcemia. Ann Intern Med 1989; 111:807–812.

33. Bilezikaian JP: Management of acute hypercalcemia. N Engl J Med 1992; 326:1196–1203.

34. Shane E: Hypercalcemia: pathogenesis, clinical manifestations, differential diagnosis and management. *In* Favus MJ (ed): Primer on the Metabolic Bone Diseases and Disorders of Mineral Metabolism. Philadelphia, Lippincott-Raven, 1996, pp 177–181.

35. Shane E: Hypercalcemia: pathogenesis, clinical manifestations, differential diagnosis and management. *In* Favus MJ (ed): Primer on the Metabolic Bone Diseases and Disorders of Mineral Metabolism. Philadelphia, Lippincott-Raven, 1996, pp 217–219.

36. Bushinsky DA: The contribution of acidosis to renal osteodystrophy. Kidney Int 1995; 47:1816–1832.

37. Quamme GA: Control of magnesium transport in the thick ascending limb. Am J Physiol 1989; 256:F197–F210.

38. Quamme GA: Renal magnesium handling: New insights in understanding old problems. Kidney Int 1997; 52:1180–1195.

39. Wong ET, Rude RK, Singer FR, et al: A high prevalence of hypomagnesemia and hypermagnesemia in hospitalized patients. Am J Clin Pathol 1983; 79:348–352.

40. Mehrotra R, Nolph KD, Kathuria P, et al: Hypokalemic metabolic alkalosis with hypomagnesuric hypermagnesemia and severe hypocalciuria: A new syndrome? Am J Kidney Dis 1997; 29:106–114.

41. Rude RJ: Magnesium metabolism and deficiency. Endocrinol Metab Clin North Am 1993; 22:377–395.

42. Abbott LG, Rude RK: Clinical manifestations of magnesium deficiency. Miner Electrolyte Metab 1993; 19:314–322.

43. Rude RK, Olerich M: Magnesium deficiency: Possible role in osteoporosis associated with gluten sensitive enteropathy. Osteoporos Int 1996; 6:453–461.

44. McLean RM: Magnesium and its therapeutic uses. Am J Med 1994; 96:63–76.

45. Mehrotra R, Nolph KD, Kathuria P, et al: Hypokalemic metabolic alkalosis with hypomagnesuric hypermagnesemia and severe hypocalciuria: A new syndrome? Am J Kidney Dis 1997; 29:106–114.

46. Hammarqvist F, Wernerman J, Ali R, et al: Addition of glutamine to total parenteral nutrition after elective abdominal surgery spared free glutamine in muscle, counteracts the fall in muscle protein synthesis, and improves nitrogen balance. Ann Surg 1989; 209:455.

47. Gluck SL: Acid base. Lancet 1998; 352:474–479.

48. Beyer MD, Jacobson HR: Mechanisms and regulation of renal H^+ and HCO_3^--transport. Am J Nephrol 1987; 7:258–261.

49. Orchard CH, Kentish JC: Effects of changes of pH on the contractile function of cardiac muscle. Am J Physiol 1990; 258:C967–C981.

50. Hood VL, Tannen RL: Maintainance of acid base homeostasis during ketoacidosis and lactic acidosis; implications for therapy. Diabetes Rev 1994; 2:177–194.

51. Garella S: Extracorporeal techniques in the treatment of exogenous intoxications. Kidney Int 1988; 33:735–754.

52. Jaber BL, Madias NE: Marked dilutional acidosis complicating management of right ventricular myocardial infarction. Am J Kidney Dis 1997; 30:561–567.

53. Gennari FJ, Kassirer JP: Respiratory alkalosis. *In* Cohen JJ, Kassirer JP (eds): Acid-Base. Boston, Little, Brown, 1982, pp 349–376.

54. Frankenfield D: Energy dynamics. *In* Matarese JE, Gottslich MM (eds): Contemporary Nutrition Support Practice: A Clinical Guide. Philadelphia, WB Saunders, 1998, pp 79–95.

55. McClave SA. Indirect calorimetry. *In:* Fundamentals II—ASPEN 20th Clinical Congress. Louisville, KY, University of Louisville Press, 1996, pp 1–10.

56. Walsh TS, Hopton P, Alastain L: A comparison between the Fick method and indirect calorimetry for determining oxygen consumption in patients with fulminant hepatic failure. Crit Care Med 1998; 20:1200–1207.

57. Brandi LS, et al: Energy expenditure and gas exchange measurements in postoperative patients: Thermodilution versus indirect calorimetry. Crit Care Med 1992; 20:1273–1283.

58. Bizoman P, Soulard D, Blanveil Y, et al: Oxygen consumption after cardiac surgery: A comparison between calculation by Fick's principle and measurement by indirect calorimetry. Intensive Care Med 1992; 18:206–209.

59. Ogawa AM, Shikora SA, Burke LM: The thermodilution technique for resting energy expenditure does not argue with indirect calorimetry for the critically ill patient. JPEN 1998; 22:347–351.

60. Williams RR, Flemming CR: Circulatory indirect calorimetry in the critically ill. JPEN 1991; 15:509–512.

61. Smithies MN, Roysten B, Makita K, et al: Comparison of oxygen consumption measurements: Indirect calorimetry versus the Reverend Fick method. Crit Care Med 1991; 19:1401–1406.

62. Ferrannini E: The theoretical basis of indirect calorimetry: A review. Metabolism 1988; 37:287–301.

63. Makk LJK, McClave SA, Creech PW, et al: Clinical application of the metabolic cart to the delivery of total parenteral nutrition. Crit Care Med 1990; 18:1320–1327.

64. McClave SA, Snider HL: Understanding the metabolic response to critical illness: Factors that cause patients to deviate from the expected pattern of hypermetabolism. New Horiz 1994; 2:139–145.

65. De Boisblanc BP, McClarity E, Lord K: Oxygen consumption in the intensive care unit: Indirect calorimetry is the way to go, but where? Crit Care Med 1998; 26:1153–1154.

22 Monitoring Coagulation and Hemostasis: Perioperative Assessment of Coagulation and Platelet Function

Gregory A. Nuttall, M.D.
Mark H. Ereth, M.D.
William C. Oliver, Jr., M.D.
Paula J. Santrach, M.D.

Coagulation is a complex, interrelated, and dynamic physiologic process involving enzymatic and cellular mechanisms, many of which interact with other vascular and inflammatory processes. Understanding normal coagulation, its regulation, and the genesis of pathophysiologic processes is necessary in order to make clinical decisions and institute appropriate therapy in the operating room (OR) and intensive care unit (ICU).

Mechanism of Hemostasis

Hemostasis requires the participation and interaction of multiple biologic elements (Fig. 22-1). The elements required for hemostasis are vascular integrity and endothelial function, platelet function, coagulation factors, and fibrinolysis. An overview of thrombosis and fibrinolysis is presented in Figure 22-2.

There are mechanical factors that also affect coagulation. The circulatory system actively maintains the fluid state of blood by constantly moving and mechanically mixing the blood. Polycythemia, sickle cell anemia, or hypoperfusion increases the duration and interaction of cellular and protein elements, greatly enhancing the probability of clot formation. The decreased incidence of deep venous thrombosis with ambulation and the postoperative use of pneumatic compression stockings is most likely related to increased perfusion and reduced physical contact of cellular and protein elements. We are reminded of Virchow's triad for the requirements for clot formation: an alteration in flow, a hypercoagulable state, and a perturbation of a vessel wall or other cellular or tissue element.

Vascular Integrity and the Endothelium

The intimal surface of the entire vascular system is lined by a monolayer of endothelial cells. In concert, these endothelial

---

From the Departments of Anesthesiology and Pathology, Mayo Clinic, Rochester, MN 55905.

cells make up a large body organ weighing only 1.5 kg yet having the surface area of approximately a football field (4260 m²) and covering approximately 600 miles in distance. The endothelium provides for coagulation and anticoagulation activities, vasoconstrictive and vasorelaxing functions, synthesis and degradation of various proteins and mediators, and actively participates in inflammation in addition to providing a blood tissue barrier. The endothelial cells maintain blood fluidity via two primary mechanisms. Physically, endothelial cells act as a barrier to prevent exposure of circulating blood elements to the thrombogenic subendothelial components of the vessel such as von Willebrand's factor (vWF) and collagen. The endothelium is also known to synthesize and secrete a variety of regulatory compounds, many of which have anticoagulant properties[1-3] (Fig. 22-3).

The endothelial cell continuously secretes a coating of proteoglycan containing heparin. The surface of the endothelial cell is covered with hyaluronic acid and branches of linked proteins that electrostatically repel circulating precursors of coagulation factors. These protein complexes are covered with heparin chains, which are constantly being built up and destroyed. The heparin is composed of a heterogeneous group of polysaccharides. A unique pentasaccharide sequence of heparin has been identified that interacts with the serine protease antithrombin III (ATIII).[4] The interaction of heparin with ATIII enhances the anticoagulant activity of ATIII, thereby inhibiting the formation of procoagulants, specifically thrombin (factor IIa), factor IXa, and factor Xa. The endothelial cell can also inhibit the formation of thrombin through protein S, protein C, and thrombomodulin (see Fig. 22-3). The endothelial cell can metabolize fatty acids via cyclooxygenase and other enzymes to produce a number of prostaglandins. The major prostaglandin produced is prostaglandin I_2 (PGI$_2$, prostacyclin) which is the strongest prostaglandin inhibitor of platelet activation. Endothelial cells also synthesize and release nitric oxide (NO). Both prostacyclin and NO are labile molecules that act as autocoids to inhibit platelet activity in the immediate vicinity of their sites of production[5, 6] (Fig. 22-4B).

When platelets are in motion and in proximity to endothelial cells, they become unresponsive to agonists.[7] This platelet unresponsiveness may be due to an ecto-ADPase on the surface of endothelial cells, which metabolizes adenosine

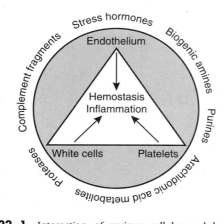

Figure 22–1. Interaction of various cellular and humoral processes. (From Spiess BD (ed): Cardiopulmonary bypass: Coagulation and inflammation issues. J Cardiovasc Pharmacol 1996;27(6).)

diphosphate (ADP) released from activated platelets. This endothelial cell ecto-ADPase, which causes a blockade of the platelet aggregation response, has been described as CD39.[8] Platelets do not adhere to normal vascular endothelial cells but only to those areas of endothelial disruption that provide bonding sites for adhesive proteins, vWF (through the platelet glycoprotein [GP] Ib/Ix complex), fibrinogen, and fibronectin (through the integrin receptors).[9] This ADPase inhibits platelet activity in the immediate vicinity of its site of production (see Fig. 22–4B).

The endothelial cells also are involved in the regulation of vasomotor tone.[2, 3, 10, 11] As already mentioned, the endothelial cells produce and rapidly export NO. NO is an endothelial-relaxing factor, the most potent relaxant of smooth muscle. The response of the vessel to injury and hemorrhage is vasoconstriction and endothelial cell release of vWF. The vWF then binds to the collagen in the vascular basement membrane and acts as an adhesive site for platelets. This process is the first step in the capture of circulating platelets and the initiation of the platelet plug. After initial adherence to subendothelial surfaces, platelets spread out on the surface recruit additional platelets, all delivered by flowing blood, which adhere to the primary layer of platelets in an accelerating manner, rapidly forming a mass of aggregated platelets.

Platelet Function

Platelets are the smallest (2 to 3 μm) of all blood cells. They have RNA but are devoid of DNA and therefore are unable to synthesize new proteins. They are formed in the bone marrow from megakaryocytes, which fragment to produce platelets. The platelets have a plasma half-life of 9 to 10 days. Platelets contain microtubules, alpha granules, and dense granules. Both types of granules contain a number of compounds, factors, and cofactors that enhance coagulation.

The formation of a platelet plug is the initial response to vascular injury. A good hemostatic response is highly dependent on proper platelet adhesion, activation, and aggregation.[12] Blood flow in the capillaries is laminar, resulting in margination of platelets along the vessel wall, producing maximal physical contact and interaction. With injury and denudation of the vessel endothelium, platelets attach to the vWF bound to the exposed collagen of the subendothelium (Fig. 22–5A). GPIb is a platelet membrane component that

attaches to vWF, thus anchoring the platelet to the vessel wall.[13] GPIb is thought to be the receptor most responsible for platelet adhesion to the subendothelial matrix. Platelets also have membrane GPIa and IIa, which may attach directly to exposed collagen.[12]

Upon contact with collagen, platelets release the contents of their alpha and dense granules. The alpha granules contain platelet factor 4 and 4a, β-thromboglobulin, and integrin proteins (fibronectin, fibrinogen, vitronectin, and vWF). Dense granules contain ADP, serotonin, epinephrine, norepinephrine, and calcium. The released ADP acts to recruit additional platelets to the injury site and to stimulate platelet G protein. The G protein activates membrane phospholipase resulting in the formation of arachidonate and eventually thromboxane A$_2$ via platelet cyclooxygenase. Thromboxane and serotonin are both potent vasoconstrictors. Simultaneous with platelet granule release, the platelets undergo a change in shape from disk to sphere (see Fig. 22–5A). The normal equatorial band of microtubules, which maintains the platelet's discoid shape, disappears, the alpha and dense storage granules decentralize, and formation of pseudopodia occurs. This exposes the platelet membrane GPIIb/IIIa receptor, an integrin protein. Aggregation occurs when molecular bridges form between adjacent platelet GPIIb/IIIa receptors via binding to the RGD (arginine-glycine-aspartic acid) sequences of fibrinogen[13] (Fig. 22–5B).[14] Once platelet aggregation has occurred, fibrin cross-linking via the coagulation factor cascade is required to cement the platelets into an aggregate tough enough to withstand pressure and shear forces (Fig. 22–2E). As the network of fibrin is formed, platelets extend cytoplasmic projections out along fibrin strands. The platelets retract these fibrin-adherent pseudopodia, which reduces the clot volume and concentrates the fibrin matrix directly over the site of injury.

Coagulation Factors

The coagulation factor cascade is often presented as a separate process from platelet function, with intrinsic and extrinsic arms joining to form a common final pathway ending with the formation of an insoluble fibrin clot.[14] The coagulation factor pathways actually interact with the platelet membrane. The platelet surface is the site where many of the intrinsic pathway serine protease reactions occur. Fibrin is also known to bind to the platelet GPIIb/IIIa receptors.[15]

The coagulation factors, with a few exceptions, are GPs synthesized in the liver. They circulate as inactive proteins called zymogens. Factor activation proceeds sequentially, with each factor acting as a substrate in an enzymatic reaction catalyzed by the previous factor in the sequence. Enzymatic cleavage of a protein fragment changes the inactive zymogen to an active enzyme. This enzyme is termed a serine protease because the active site for its protease activity is a serine amino acid residue. There are four interrelated groups of coagulation factor cascades: contact activation, and the intrinsic, extrinsic, and common pathways (Fig. 22–2D).

Contact Activation. Disruption of the endothelial cell layer exposes the negatively charged collagen matrix, which initiates coagulation protein contact activation. Factor XII will bind to the negatively charged collagen matrix via high-molecular-weight kininogen, and factor XII autoactivates to factor XIIa. Factor XIIa cleaves both factor XI and prekallikrein to factor XIa and kallikrein, respectively.

Intrinsic Pathway. Contact activation products form factor Xa via the intrinsic pathway. Factor XIa with calcium

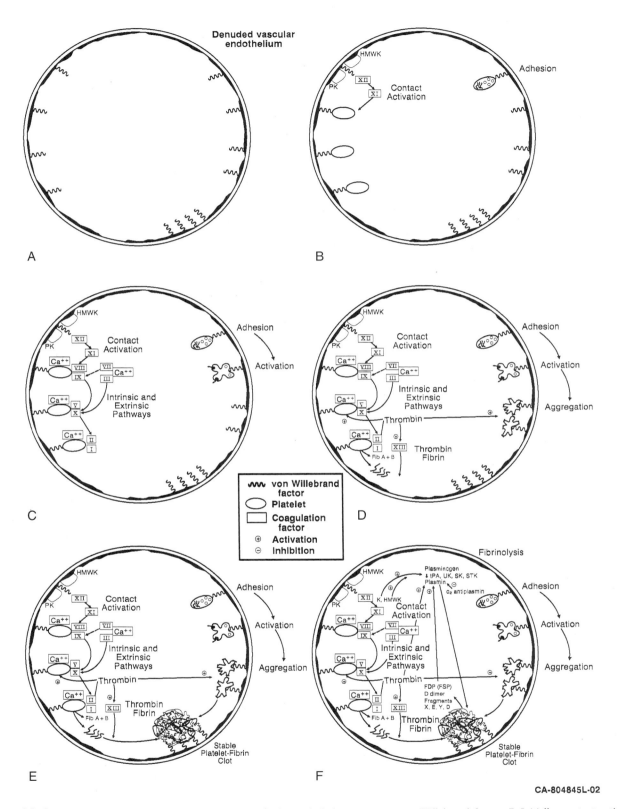

Figure 22-2. Thrombosis and fibrinolysis. *A,* Denuded vascular endothelium exposes von Willebrand factor. *B,* Initially, contact activation occurs, as well as platelet adhesion to von Willebrand factor. *C,* Intrinsic and extrinsic pathways are then activated along with activation of platelets. *D,* Activated platelets recruit and aggregate with other platelets and the final common pathway generates fibrin monomers. *E,* Aggregated platelets and polymerized fibrin form a stable clot. *F,* Initiation of fibrinolysis occurs following conversion of plasminogen to plasmin that initiates clot breakdown (for detailed discussion, see text). HMWK, high-molecular-weight kininogen; PK, protein kinase; tPA, tissue plasminogen activator; UK, urokinase; SK, STK, streptokinase; FDP (FSP), fibrin degradation (split) products.

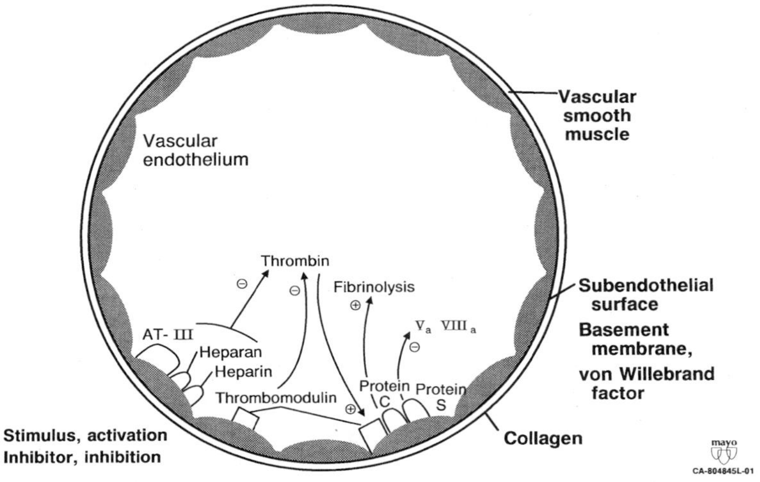

Figure 22-3. Endothelial function contributes to vascular integrity by providing a number of pathways by which thrombin generation is limited (localized antithrombotic and profibrinolytic processes).

cleaves factor IX to IXa. The factor IXa, along with calcium, phospholipid surface, and cofactor VIIIa, splits factor X to factor Xa.

Extrinsic Pathway. Factor X can be activated independently of the contact activation and intrinsic pathway by substances extrinsic to the vasculature. Tissues can release thromboplastin into the vasculature. Thromboplastin acts as a cofactor for factor VII, which activates factor X. Factors VII and X then activate each other with the help of calcium and platelet phospholipid to form factor Xa.

Common Pathway. Factor Xa splits prothrombin (factor II) to thrombin (factor IIa) with the help of cofactor Va, calcium, and platelet phospholipid. Thrombin then cleaves fibrinogen (factor I) to form soluble fibrin monomer and fibrinopeptides A and B. The soluble fibrin monomers then associate to form a soluble fibrin matrix. Factor XIII, which is also activated by thrombin, then cross-links the fibrin strands to form an insoluble (stable platelet-fibrin) clot.

The factors that require calcium for activity (factors II, VII, IX, and X) depend on vitamin K to attach γ-carboxyl groups to glutamic acid residues. The activity of these factors depends on calcium tethering the negatively charged carboxyl groups to the phospholipid surface. The inhibitory proteins, protein C and protein S, are also dependent on vitamin K for their activity.

Mechanisms of Anticoagulation

Coagulation Factor Pathway Modulators

At the site of injury there is active enzymatic control exerted to slow the coagulation reaction and prevent excessive spread. Thrombin is the most important coagulation pathway modulator. It activates cofactors V, VIII, and factors I and XIII and stimulates platelet recruitment (Fig. 22-2D). To prevent excessive clot spread, it induces the release of tissue plasminogen activator (t-PA) and urokinase-type plasminogen activator (u-PA) from endothelial cells, and with thrombomodulin it activates protein C (see Figs. 22-3 and 22-4A).

Serpins and the Protein C System

There are serine protease inhibitors called serpins (*se*rine *p*rotease *in*hibitors) which include ATIII, heparin cofactor II, α_2-antiplasmin, C$\overline{1}$ inhibitor, and others.[16] ATIII is the most important inhibitor of coagulation. It serves as a protease scavenger by forming complexes with many of the coagulation factors that have moved away from the growing clot. It blocks thrombin's (factor IIa) action by covalently binding to its serine-active site. It also blocks the action of other coagulation factors (XIIa, XIa, IXa, and Xa), of kallikrein, and of plasmin. Protein C, along with cofactor protein S, calcium, and phospholipid, degrades factors VIIIa and Va.[17] α_2-Antiplasmin reacts very rapidly with plasmin and is considered a primary regulator of fibrinolysis (see Fig. 22-3).

Fibrinolysis

Fibrinolysis is initiated at the initiation of clot formation (see Fig. 22-4A). Fibrin breakdown is a normal physiologic activity that occurs in the vicinity of a clot. Fibrinolysis remodels formed clot, and removes thrombus when the endothelium heals. Plasminogen is a serine protease synthesized by the liver that circulates as a zymogen. Cleavage of the plasminogen by the proper serine protease forms plasmin. As fibrinogen is being converted to fibrin, plasmin may be incorporated into the fibrin clot. Plasmin splits fibrinogen and fibrin into smaller and smaller fragments. The final breakdown product, the fibrin degradation fragment, the D-dimer, is not able to polymerize. It also acts as a potent serine protease inhibitor. Inhibition of fibrinolysis occurs at the level of the activators (by plasminogen activator inhibitors, PAIs) or the level of plasmin (mainly by α_2-antiplasmin). Plasmin associated with the fibrin surface is protected from rapid inhibition by α_2-antiplasmin and may thus efficiently degrade the fibrin of a thrombus. Plasma normally does not contain any plasmin, because the scavenging protein, α_2-antiplasmin, consumes any plasmin formed from localized fibrinolysis.

Fibrinolysis may also be initiated by intrinsic or extrinsic pathways (see Fig. 22-4A). Both pathways activate plasminogen conversion to plasmin. The intrinsic fibrinolytic pathway occurs when factor XIIa, formed by contact activation, cleaves plasminogen to plasmin. The extrinsic fibrinolytic

Fibrinolysis Ecto ADPase and Nitric Oxide

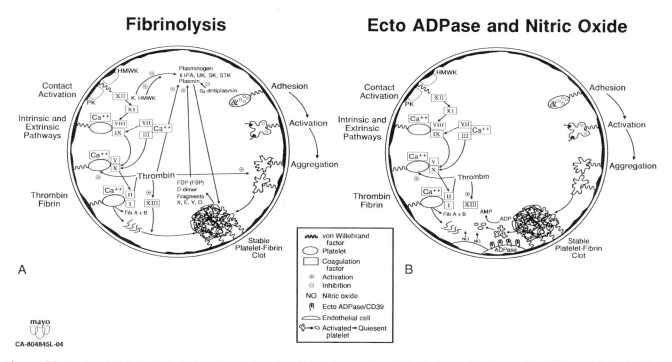

Figure 22–4. *A* and *B*, Both fibrinolysis and ectoadenosine diphosphatase (ecto-ADPase) along with nitric oxide (NO) provide for localized inhibition of clot formation. Ecto-ADPase can convert activated platelets to quiescent platelets. See Figure 22–2 for abbreviations.

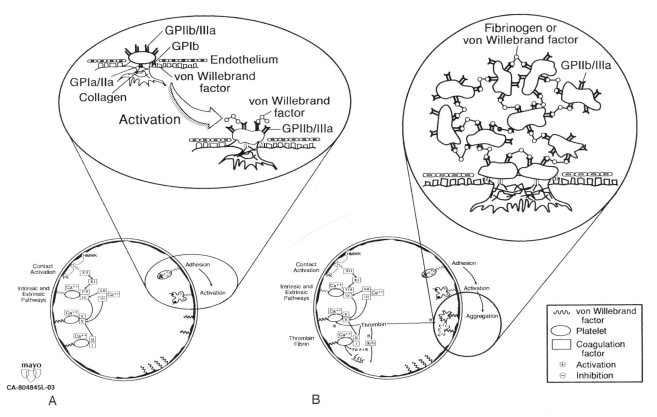

Figure 22–5. *A* and *B*, Platelet glycoprotein receptors (GPIIb/IIIa) are intimately involved in the activation and aggregation processes. During activation the receptors are exposed and provide for cross-linking with receptors on other platelets via fibrinogen or plasmatic von Willebrand factor. HMWK, high-molecular-weight kininogen; PK, protein kinase.

pathway occurs when the endothelial cells release t-PA and u-PA. u-PA and t-PA are serine proteases, which split plasminogen to plasmin. t-PA activity is accelerated by binding with fibrin, concentrating its activity to the thrombus site.

Clinical Relevance

Only 20% to 35% of the basal concentration of most serine protease enzymes is required for normal clot formation (Table 22–1). Greater than 150 mg/dL of fibrinogen should be present for normal clot formation. Normal platelet concentration is 150,000 to 300,000/mm³ of blood. Spontaneous hemorrhage does not occur until the platelet count is below 20,000/mm³. A count of 50,000/mm³ will usually be adequate for surgical hemostasis, if the operant platelet function is normal.[18] There is a wide range of drugs affecting coagulation factor and platelet function that must be considered when clinics assess bleeding and treat coagulopathy. The anticoagulants heparin and warfarin sodium (Coumadin) have obvious effects, as do aspirin and other nonsteroidal anti-inflammatory agents (NSAIDs). The diagnosis and management of coagulopathies are further complicated in the perioperative period in patients who have received thrombolytic drugs, the more potent oral antiplatelet agents ticlopidine and clopidogrel, as well as the GPIIb/IIIa receptor antagonists abciximab, tirofiban, and intrifiban. Many drugs used to treat heart disease, hypertension, and cancer inhibit platelet function (Fig. 22–6).

Pharmacology and Coagulation

Anticoagulants

Heparin

McLean[19] discovered heparin in 1916. In 1939, Brinkhous et al.[20] demonstrated that the anticoagulant activity of heparin is mediated by a cofactor. This cofactor is ATIII, which is a serpin already mentioned[4] (see Figs. 22–3 and 22–6A). The active center serine of thrombin (IIa), and factors Xa, XIIa, XIa, and IXa is inhibited by an arginine-reactive center of the ATIII molecule. Heparin binds to the lysine site on ATIII, which produces a conformational change at the arginine-reactive center. Heparin's catalytic activity depends on a specific pentasaccharide sequence within the molecule. This converts ATIII from a progressive slow inhibitor to a very rapid inhibitor. Following the binding of ATIII to its substrate, heparin dissociates from the complex and can be reused. The ATIII remains covalently bonded to its substrate. Thrombin and factor Xa are the most sensitive to inactivation. Heparin chain length partially determines ATIII substrate specificity. The inhibition of thrombin requires that heparin contain both the pentasaccharide high-affinity binding site and a chain length of at least 13 additional sugars. Only the pentasaccharide high-affinity binding site is required for heparin to catalyze ATIII inhibition of factor Xa.

Standard heparin is a mixture of linear polysaccharides of variable chain lengths (45 to 50 sugars) and molecular weights (5000 to 30,000 Da), with a mean molecular weight of 15,000 Da. The plasma biologic half-life of heparin is between 56 and 152 minutes depending on the size of the loading dose. Multiple randomized clinical trials have established the efficacy of standard heparin anticoagulation for venous thromboembolism prophylaxis. Standard heparin is also used for anticoagulation for cardiopulmonary bypass (CPB) and vascular surgery.

There are high-risk populations for venous thrombosis (patients following total hip and knee replacement) in whom standard heparin therapy is not very effective and may be associated with serious bleeding complications.[21] The ability of low-molecular-weight heparin (LMWH) to safely and effectively prevent postoperative venous thromboembolism has been shown in more than 60 clinical trials including more than 20,000 patients.[22] LMWH has a mean molecular weight of 4000 to 5000 Da and a chain length of 13 to 22 sugars. It is produced by either chemical or enzymatic depolymerization of standard heparin. As already noted, the short chain length of LMWH decreases ATIII affinity to thrombin but maintains its full affinity for factor Xa. The concentration and activity of LMWH is referenced to an international standard and expressed as anti-Xa activity (units per milliliter). Peak anti-Xa levels of 0.1 to 0.2 U/mL provide safe and effective venous thromboembolism prophylaxis after hip and knee replacement surgery.[23] The plasma half-life of LMWH is thought to be 3 to 4 hours.

A serious concern with standard heparin and LMWH therapy is performance of neuraxial blockade. Recommendations have been published for performing neuraxial blockade in patients who have received standard heparin and LMWH.[22]

Warfarin

Dam, in the 1920s, noted the need for a dietary fat-soluble factor to maintain normal blood coagulation.[24] At about the same time as the discovery of vitamin K, a naturally occurring antagonist of vitamin K was discovered in improperly cured sweet clover hay.[25] This compound was dicumarol. A family of dicumarol-related compounds have been developed of which warfarin sodium (Coumadin) is the most common vitamin K antagonist used for anticoagulation therapy in the United States.

As already mentioned, the vitamin K–dependent coagulation factors are prothrombin, factor VII, factor IX, factor X, protein C, and protein S. In the 1970s, it was demonstrated that prothrombin contained a carboxylated form of glutamic acid, γ-carboxylglutamic acid.[26] Vitamin K–dependent carboxylase facilitates the carboxylation of specific glutamic acid residues. These residues allow the Ca^{2+}-dependent interaction of vitamin K coagulation factors with negatively charged phospholipids, a requirement for the activity of these coagulation factors. Warfarin and the other vitamin K antagonists act by inhibiting vitamin K epoxide reductase and possibly vitamin K reductase, which leads to the effective intracellular depletion of vitamin KH_2 and γ-carboxylation of glutamic acid residues of vitamin K–dependent coagulation factors (see Fig. 22–6A). This effect of these vitamin K antagonists on vitamin K–dependent coagulation factor is the basis of therapeutic anticoagulation and explains the prolongation of the prothrombin time (PT) used to monitor therapy.

The clinical effectiveness of oral coumarin therapy for the prevention of venous thromboembolism and with tissue and mechanical heart valves is well established. A regimen that maintains a PT international normalized ratio of 2.5 to 3.5 is recommended for mechanical heart valves.[27] Coumarin therapy has been also shown to be effective in preventing stroke in chronic atrial fibrillation and has been used in the treatment of myocardial infarction. Discontinuation of oral anticoagulants 1 to 3 days prior to major surgery and documentation of the PT being within 20% of normal is recommended.[28] Anticoagulation with heparin is frequently

Table 22-1. Coagulation Cascade Proteins

| Factor | Name | In Vivo Half-Life | Activated/Unactivated | Level Required for Hemostasis | Replacement Choice | Size (mol wt) | Plasma Level | | | Intravascular Recovery (%) | Postransfusion Half-Life (hr) |
							μg/mL	Molality	Minimum* (%)		
I	Fibrinogen	3–4 d		100 mg/dL	Cryoprecipitate (single donor)	340,000	3000	9 μM	25–30	80–100	75
II	Prothrombin	2–5 d		20%–40%	Frozen plasma, concentrates	70,000	100	1.5μM	~40	30–50	60
V		15–36 hr		<25%	Frozen plasma	350,000	0.2	0.5nM	15–20	80–100	12
VII		4–7 hr		10%–20%	Concentrates	50,000	0.5	10nM	10	30–50	6
VIII		9–18 hr		Minimum of 30% for major surgery; less for minor procedures	Concentrates (natural [viral inactivated] or recombinant)	300,000	0.1	0.3nM	30	80–100	10
IX		20–24 hr		25%–30%	Concentrates (cryoprecipitate supernatant)	55,000	5.0	90nM	25–30	30–50	20
X		32–48 hr		10%–20%	Frozen plasma, concentrates	55,000	10	180nM	15–20	30–50	50
XI		40–80 hr		15%–25%	Stored or frozen plasma, concentrates, supernatant from cryoprecipitate	160,000	6.0	40nM	~30	80–100	50–60
XII		48–52 hr		Deficiency not associated with a bleeding tendency	Replacement not necessary						
XIII		12 d		<5%	Stored or frozen plasma, cryoprecipitate	320,000	20	60nM	5	80–100	250
vWF monomer†		A few hours		25%–50%	Cryoprecipitate; factor VIII concentrates of intermediate purity	240,000	10	35nM	40	80–100	~72

vWF, von Willebrand factor.
*Minimum levels for hemostasis reflect lowest or "trough" levels at or below which abnormal surgical bleeding is likely to occur.
†vWF circulates at 800,000 to 12 × 10⁶ mol wt multimers; only the highest molecular weight multimers function in platelet adhesion.
Data from Colman RW, Cook JJ, Niewiarowski S: Mechanisms of platelet aggregation. Colman RW, Hirsh J, Marder VJ, et al (eds): Hemostasis and Thrombosis: Basic Principles and Clinical Practice, ed 3. Philadelphia, JB Lippincott, 1994, pp 508–523.

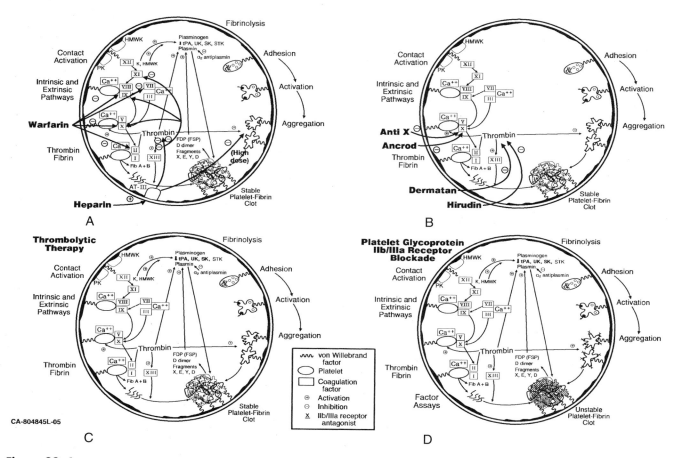

Figure 22–6. Anticoagulant, thrombolytic, and platelet receptor blockade. *A,* Heparin provides anticoagulant properties via antithrombin III and warfarin by inhibition of the production of the hepatic-dependent factors II, VII, IX, and X. *B,* Other agents with anticoagulant properties include hirudin, dermatan, ancrod, and anti–X factor. *C,* Thrombolytic therapy enhances conversion of plasminogen to plasmin, initiating thrombolysis. *D,* Glycoprotein IIb/IIIa receptor antagonists (abciximab, eptifibatide, and tirofiban) inhibit platelet aggregation by competitively displacing fibrinogen or plasmatic von Willebrand factor thus preventing aggregation between platelets. See Figure 22–2 for abbreviations.

used to replace coumarin therapy immediately before surgery. Emergency reversal of coumarin anticoagulation can be achieved with intravenous (IV) vitamin K or fresh frozen plasma (FFP) therapy.

Recombinant desulphatohirudin (r-hirudin) is a small, tight-binding specific thrombin inhibitor that directly inhibits soluble thrombin and thrombin-bound fibrin in clots[29] (Fig. 22–6B). Hirudin is an intense anticoagulant; however, it is not as effective as standard heparin because it does not have the partial attenuation of factor Xa activity seen with heparin therapy. Unfortunately, there is no FDA-approved antidote, analogous to protamine, to hirudin therapy.

Thrombolytic Drugs

Use of plasminogen-activating drugs began in the early 1980s. Thrombolytic therapy has proved to be a major advance in the treatment of acute myocardial infarction, stroke, and venous thromboembolism.[30] As noted above, blood contains an enzyme system, the fibrinolytic system, one of the main functions of which is the dissolution of fibrin clots in the blood vessels. The triggering event in the clinical expression of the acute ischemic phase of myocardial infarction or stroke is not the underlying atherosclerotic lesion but a thrombotic obstruction of the artery in the region of the atheromas from plaque disruption or embolization of the

thrombus. The mainstay of medical treatment for acute arterial thrombosis is the plasminogen-activating agents.

There are multiple plasminogen activating agents in use, all of which must be given intravenously[31] (Fig. 22–6C). Streptokinase, a nonenzyme protein derived from β-hemolytic streptococci, activates the fibrinolytic system indirectly by inducing a conformational change in plasminogen. This change exposes the enzymatic active site of plasminogen and the complex then cleaves a second plasminogen molecule to active plasmin. The half-life of streptokinase is 25 minutes. Anisoylated plasminogen streptokinase complex (APSAC) is a complex of streptokinase already bound to plasminogen. This complex has increased specificity for fibrin and is not inhibited by endogenous inhibitors of plasminogen. APSAC has a 70-minute half-life. Both streptokinase and APSAC are foreign proteins, and repeat doses may induce neutralizing antibody formation. Staphylokinase is a protein produced by *Staphylococcus aureus* that activates plasminogen in the same manner as streptokinase. Staphylokinase is fibrin-specific and its inhibition by α₂-antiplasmin is reduced. Recombinant forms of endogenous agents are in use: t-PA, urokinase, and single-chain urokinase plasminogen activator (scu-PA). These agents have direct enzymatic activity on plasminogen and are not immunogenic.

All plasminogen-activating agents (streptokinase, recombinant t-PA, urokinase, and their derivatives) activate both circulating and fibrin-bound plasminogen, which causes extensive systemic activation of the fibrinolytic system and generation of free plasmin. Unlike endogenous fibrinolysis, which is marked by clot specificity, pharmacologic plasminogen activation is indiscriminate in substrate preference and degrades fibrin, fibrinogen, platelet receptors, and coagulation factors.[32] Bleeding therefore is a substantial problem with all plasminogen activating agents. In the GUSTO (global utilization of streptokinase and tissue plasminogen activator for occluded coronary arteries) trial, severe or life-threatening bleeding occurred in 0.3% to 0.5% of patients.[33] Stroke is one of the most devastating complications of thrombolytic therapy. The GUSTO trial had an overall risk of stroke of 1.4%, with a higher risk in recombinant t-PA–treated patients (1.55%) compared to those treated with streptokinase (1.19%). In those stroke patients, 45% had a fatal stroke, 31% were disabled, and 45% had primary intracranial hemorrhage. Antifibrinolytic drugs can be used to acutely reverse the plasminogen-activating agents.

Aspirin and Nonsteroidal Anti-inflammatory Drugs

Aspirin, after 100 years of use as an anti-inflammatory, antipyretic, and analgesic drug, has become the gold standard for antiplatelet therapy. It is effective in acute myocardial infarction, unstable angina, and in secondary prevention of stroke. Aspirin is a relatively weak antiplatelet agent. Aspirin and other NSAIDs inhibit the isoform 1 of the cyclooxygenase (COX-1) pathway, thus preventing formation of prostaglandin endoperoxides and thromboxane A_2.[34] Since the platelets are unable to synthesize new enzyme, their function is inhibited for the life of the platelet (9 to 10 days). A single 80-mg dose of aspirin administered to patients with coronary artery disease has produced 95% inhibition of platelet thromboxane A_2 generation.[35] Aspirin prevents thromboxane A_2–dependent aggregation, but it does not inhibit thromboxane A_2–independent platelet aggregation. In patients receiving aspirin therapy, other physiologically important mediators of platelet aggregation in circulation such as ADP, thrombin, serotonin, catecholamines, and shear rate provide alternative pathways for platelet aggregation. Alternative pathways for thromboxane A_2 production exist that can limit the effect of aspirin. Thromboxane A_2 can be generated despite full aspirin inhibition of platelet cyclooxygenase and some patients can be aspirin nonresponders. Thromboxane A_2 can be generated by prostaglandin endoperoxides in cells other than platelets or by the isoform 2 of cyclooxygenase (COX-2). COX-2 is inducible in endothelial cells, smooth muscle cells, and monocytes under stimulation by inflammatory mediators.

Ticlopidine and Clopidogrel

The effectiveness of aspirin therapy along with its failure in certain patients has prompted development of other antiplatelet therapies. Ticlopidine and clopidogrel are new antiplatelet agents that may be more effective than aspirin in the prophylaxis of arterial thrombosis.[36] Ticlopidine and clopidogrel when taken orally cause a time- and dose-dependent inhibition of both platelet aggregation and release of platelet granule constituents. They also prolong bleeding time. The mechanisms of action of these drugs are (1) modification of the platelet membrane's affinity for ADP, and possibly for fibrinogen, and (2) interference with platelet membrane function by inhibiting ADP-induced platelet-fibrinogen binding and subsequent platelet-platelet interactions. The effect on platelet function is irreversible for the life of the platelet.

Glycoprotein IIb/IIIa Receptor Antagonists

A variety of strategies have been developed to inhibit platelet aggregation by interfering with fibrinogen binding to the platelet GPIIb/IIIa receptor. The inhibition of platelet function by blockade of the final common pathway of aggregation, fibrinogen binding to platelet GPIIb/IIIa receptor, should produce the greatest antiplatelet effect (Fig. 22–6D). Several types of antagonists have been developed. These include monoclonal antibodies against the GPIIb/IIIa receptor and a variety of peptide and nonpeptide antagonists of the GPIIb/IIIa receptor.

In 1985 Coller[37] produced a mouse monoclonal antibody against the GPIIb/IIIa receptor, called 7E3.[37] The Fab fragment of a mouse-human chimeric version of the murine 7E3 antibody is now called abciximab (ReoPro, Centocor, Inc., Malvern, PA, and Eli Lilly Co. Inc., Indianapolis, IN). Abciximab's antithrombotic effects were demonstrated in animal models,[38] and subsequently in humans.[39] Multiple studies have now demonstrated that abciximab is very effective in preventing abrupt vessel closure by thrombosis and acute myocardial infarction in patients undergoing percutaneous transluminal coronary angioplasty (PTCA).[40, 41] This effect was found to be sustained and durable in patients undergoing PTCA and directional atherectomy. The efficacy and safety of abciximab for other related indications are under study.[42,43] Potential problems with abciximab are the risk of bleeding from IV administration owing to the relatively extended duration of antiplatelet effect (up to 24 hours), immunogenicity, and the rare occurrence of thrombocytopenia.

A number of oral low-molecular-weight GPIIb/IIIa receptor antagonists based on competition for binding with the fibrinogen RGD sequence have been developed. To improve stability and potency of the linear RGD-containing peptides, conformationally constrained cyclic peptides have been synthesized. One inhibitor with a cyclic heptapeptide that contains a KGD (lysine-glycine-aspartic acid) sequence is eptifibatide (Integrilin, COR Therapeutics, Inc., South San Francisco, CA). The KGD sequence makes the agent specific for the GPIIb/IIIa integrin. Eptifibatide has been effective for coronary intervention but has had reduced long-term efficacy compared to abciximab in patients undergoing PTCA and atherectomy.[44] Many nonpeptide mimetics have been developed. These nonpeptide GPIIb/IIIa receptor antagonists have the potential to be orally bioavailable and may be effective for chronic antiplatelet therapy. To inhibit platelet aggregation, these agents mimic the geometric, stereotactic, and charge characteristics of the RGD sequence. A tyrosine derivative, tirofiban (Aggrastat, Merck & Co., Inc., West Point, PA) has reduced the incidence of abrupt vessel closure following PTCA.[44]

The introduction of platelet GPIIb/IIIa receptor antagonists (abciximab, eptifibatide, and tirofiban) has provided for excellent antithrombotic regimens in patients undergoing high-risk coronary angioplasty or atherectomy.[45] These antagonists are platelet-specific, inhibit platelet aggregation induced by all physiologic agonists, and yet may not totally abolish platelet adhesion. Once administered, these agents essentially paralyze platelets for the duration of the agent's activity. Future uses of these agents are likely to include therapy to prevent cerebrovascular and peripheral vascular disease.

Other Antiplatelet Agents

There are multiple drugs such as nitrates, β blockers, calcium channel blockers, chemotherapeutic drugs, and antibiotics that can inhibit platelet function.[46] Dipyridamole, a

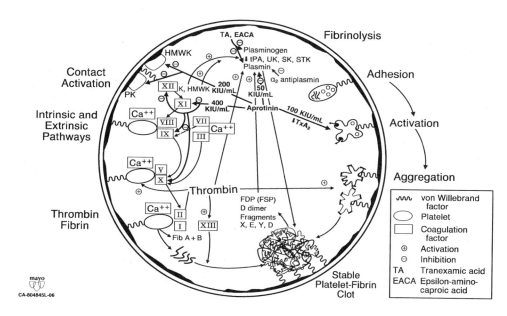

Figure 22-7. Antifibrinolytic agents exert their effects at different locations. Tranexamic acid and ϵ-aminocaproic acid work primarily by limiting the conversion of plasminogen to plasma. Aprotinin works at different concentrations in preventing plasmin generation, as well as decreasing contact and intrinsic pathway activation, and also provides a stabilization of platelet receptor populations. KIU, kallikrein inactivating units; TxA₂, thromboxane A₂; see Figure 22-2 for other abbreviations.

drug which may inhibit platelet function by potentiating the effect of prostacyclin or inhibiting phosphodiesterase activity leading to increased intracellular cyclic AMP (adenosine monophosphate) concentration, is used in combination with warfarin to prevent embolization from prosthetic heart valves. Prostacyclin has vasodilating effects along with producing temporary reversible inhibition of platelets. An analog of prostacyclin, iloprost, has been used to prevent heparin-induced platelet activation in patients with heparin-induced thrombocytopenia.[47] Both prostacyclin and iloprost have been used to protect platelets during CPB with variable effectiveness.[48]

Coagulation-Enhancing Drugs

Aprotinin

Aprotinin is a member of the kinin family of serpins. It is a 58-amino acid peptide derived from bovine lung. It was discovered in 1930 by Kraut et al.[49] The drug has been in clinical use for more than 35 years for a variety of indications such as pancreatitis, hemorrhagic shock, obstetric and gynecologic disorders, urologic surgery, neurosurgery, and fibrinolysis. Recently, aprotinin in high doses has been shown to produce a profound (approximately 50%) reduction in blood loss during cardiac surgery when infused intravenously prior to CPB.[50-52] The drug has also been shown to reduce bleeding in liver transplant patients and patients undergoing reconstructive surgery for aortoiliac occlusive disease and total hip arthroplasty.[53-56] CPB is known to induce fibrinolysis and platelet function inhibition.[57, 58] Liver transplant patients also have fibrinolysis.[53] Aprotinin is known to inhibit multiple proteases such as kallikrein, plasmin, trypsin, and factor XII activation of complement (Fig. 22-7). Aprotinin has been shown to inhibit plasmin formation and decrease fibrinolysis, to preserve platelet GPIb receptor, and to reduce the effects of kallikrein and bradykinin.[59-62]

Aprotinin combined with heparin prolongs the celite-based activated clotting time (ACT) for a given dose of heparin.[63] Graft thrombosis was a problem with early studies of aprotinin therapy. It is now believed this was due to a reduction in heparin dosing based on the false elevation of the celite-based ACT.[64] Prolongation does not occur when kaolin is used as the activator for the ACT. A particularly undesirable effect of aprotinin is immunologic sensitization. The risk of anaphylactic reactions after prior exposure to aprotinin depends on duration of time from prior exposure. If previous exposure occurred less than 6 months before, the risk of anaphylactic reaction was 4.5%. A reexposure to aprotinin after 6 months had an incidence of anaphylactic reaction of 1.5%.[65] A test dose of 1 mL (1.4 mg) of aprotinin is frequently given prior to the loading dose for detection of anaphylactic reactions. Aprotinin undergoes glomerular filtration and is actively reabsorbed by the proximal tubules where it is gradually metabolized by lysosomal enzymes in the kidney. Plasma aprotinin concentrations diminish in a biphasic manner with distribution half-lives of 0.3 to 0.5 hours and elimination half-lives of 5 to 8 hours. Because aprotinin is concentrated in the kidney, there is a concern that use of this agent in patients with renal insufficiency may induce renal failure.[66] Half-doses of aprotinin (140-mg loading dose, 35-mg/hour infusion, and 140-mg priming dose) have been found to be as effective as high doses (280-mg loading dose followed by 70-mg/hour infusion for the duration of the operation and 280 mg added to the priming volume for CPB) in patients having primary coronary artery bypass graft (CABG) surgery.[67]

ϵ-Aminocaproic Acid and Tranexamic Acid

Two commonly used lysine analog antifibrinolytics, ϵ-aminocaproic acid (EACA) and tranexamic acid (see Fig. 22-7), bind to plasminogen and plasmin, and competitively inhibit plasmin's binding to the lysine residue of fibrinogen. Tranexamic acid has a longer half-life, greater efficacy and more potent inhibition of plasmin than does EACA.[68] Each drug is administered either IV or orally with an IV loading dose of 100 to 150 mg/kg for EACA and 10 to 20 mg/kg for tranexamic acid.[69, 70] The loading dose is followed by a constant IV infusion at one-tenth the loading dose per hour for each drug. Up to 10 times the previously mentioned doses have been used.[71] These drugs should not be used in patients with disseminated intravascular coagulation (DIC) because they would prevent clot lysis of the cardiovascular system. They should also be avoided in upper urinary tract bleeding, as they would prevent clot lysis within the ureters.

Patients with hemophilia (factor VIII or IX deficiency) and von Willebrand's disease (vWF deficiency) may have improved clot retraction with the use of antifibrinolytics, especially for oral surgery.[70, 72] Tranexamic acid treatment may reduce the frequency of recurrences in aneurysmal subarachnoid hemorrhage.[73] Use of antifibrinolytics in surgery has had variable results.[74-76] A reduction in blood loss associated with liver transplantation and cardiac surgery has been documented.[68, 69, 77, 78] Pressure to reduce healthcare costs and public concern over the risks of blood transfusion have generated considerable interest in determining the cost-effectiveness of different therapies to reduce bleeding.[79-81]

Desmopressin

Desmopressin, an analog of vasopressin, has greater potency and duration of antidiuretic activity than vasopressin, and little vasoconstrictive activity.[82-84] The drug may actually induce non–histamine-related hypotension when given IV.[82, 85] Desmopressin is known to release multiple coagulation system mediators from the endothelium.[86] Following desmopressin injection, the mean factor VIII levels increase 300%, and the endothelium releases large multimers of vWF. Prostacyclin is also released, but the total effect of desmopressin is procoagulant, probably secondary to the increase in factor VIII and vWF.

Desmopressin can be administered via the IV, subcutaneous, or nasal routes, with the optimal IV dose being 0.3 μg/kg. It has a half-life of 2.3 to 4.0 hours in the plasma, but the increased factor VIII levels persist long after the desmopressin is excreted. Tachyphylaxis occurs because of the depletion of vWF stores within endothelial cells.[87]

The possible indications for desmopressin are coagulopathy secondary to hemophilia, von Willebrand's disease, uremia, cirrhosis, and aspirin therapy. It can be used to treat mild to moderate hemophilia A. Desmopressin has been shown to temporarily correct prolonged bleeding times in uremic patients and patients with von Willebrand's disease.[87-89] The same improvement in prolonged bleeding times has also been demonstrated in cirrhotic patients.[90] Desmopressin may also correct an aspirin-induced prolongation in bleeding time.[91] Some platelet disorders also respond to desmopressin therapy.[92] Desmopressin has had variable effectiveness in treating bleeding associated with different types of surgery.[82, 85, 93-96]

Assessment of Coagulation

The majority of clinically significant bleeding disorders can be detected by clinical examination. A careful history is vital to the detection and diagnosis of coagulation disorders. When properly taken, it also eliminates the need for indiscriminate screening coagulation tests and their associated costs. It is important to determine the frequency of bleeding episodes and to ascertain whether the episodes of bleeding are associated with trauma. Excessive bleeding with surgery is especially pertinent. The documentation of the first episode of bleeding is helpful for differentiation of a hereditary bleeding problem from one that is acquired. A family history is also helpful in establishing the diagnosis of hereditary hemostatic abnormalities. The pattern of inheritance may provide information as to the type of heritable disorder. Since many drugs inhibit coagulation, an accurate drug history is necessary. As an example, aspirin inhibits platelet function. Chlorpromazine and procainamide are known to prolong the activated partial thromboplastin time (APTT) because of to a drug-induced "lupus anticoagulant."[97]

The physical examination also provides useful information. Petechiae are suggestive of abnormal platelet quantity or function, or defects in the integrity of the vascular walls. Fingernail splinter thrombi are evidence of prothrombic processes. Coagulation factor deficiencies may manifest as ecchymoses from subcutaneous bleeding. Deficiency in coagulation factors can also induce hemarthrosis or deep bleeding into the skeletal muscles. The history and physical examination may also highlight coexisting disease processes that induce coagulopathy, such as liver disease, malabsorption, and malnutrition.

Tests and Devices for Evaluation of Coagulation

There is no one single test that provides the perfect evaluation of coagulation. There are a bewildering variety of coagulation tests available to the clinician; therefore, only those tests that provide the best initial assessment of coagulation will be discussed. The vast majority of bleeding problems outside of the OR can be diagnosed with the use of six screening tests. These tests are the peripheral blood smear, the platelet count, the bleeding time (Fig. 22–8C), PT (Fig. 22–8A), APTT (Fig. 22–8B), and thrombin time (TT) (Fig. 22–8D). Coagulation tests for the evaluation of bleeding in the OR usually require that the results be rapidly available. Therefore, point-of-care tests are usually most useful for coagulation testing in the OR.

A detailed discussion of assessment of various specific coagulation factors is beyond the scope of this chapter. However, specific assays of various coagulation factors can be performed in highly specialized hematology laboratories (Fig. 22–8E). These assays are important for the diagnosis of specific hemostatic disorders but have a very limited role in the perioperative setting.

Peripheral Blood Smear and Platelet Count

Evaluation of peripheral blood smear may produce significant information about the patient. The platelet number should be estimated and correlated with the platelet count determined by other means such as an automated instrumentation technique. The platelet estimation should agree with the platelet count. If the platelet count is less than the platelet estimation, then further investigation may be necessary. Some of the common causes of this spurious thrombocytopenia are the presence of giant platelets, cold agglutinins, or platelet satellitosis. The size and morphology of the platelets are also evaluated. Large platelets are younger and more metabolically and physiologically active. An increase in the number of large platelets may be seen with autoimmune thrombocytopenia or with increased peripheral destruction of platelets. Small platelets may be associated with iron deficiency anemia and other disorders.

There are two major methods of determining platelet number: use of a cell-counting instrument, and use of a phase microscope with a hemocytometer. The latter is immensely more time-consuming and is usually reserved for very low platelet count specimens. The platelet count is generally obtained before the bleeding time. Many laboratories do not determine the bleeding time if the platelet count is less than 50,000 cells per microliter (depending on the clinical situation). Patients with thrombocytopenia may be divided into those with decreased bone marrow production of platelets, those with increased peripheral sequestration of platelets, and those with increased peripheral destruction of

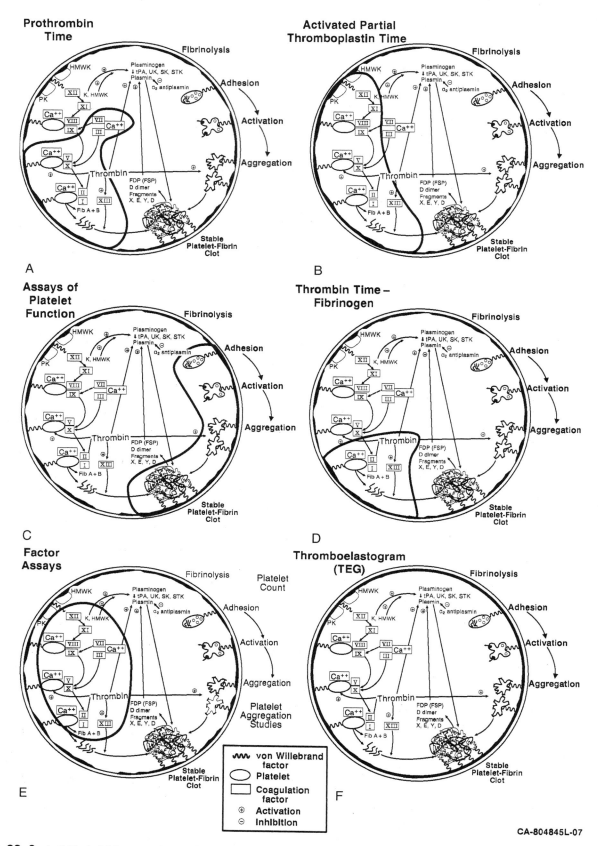

Figure 22–8. *A–F,* Typical laboratory assays of coagulation or platelet function provide only a limited view of parts of the thrombotic and fibrinolytic processes. See Figure 22–2 for abbreviations.

platelets. A bone marrow examination may be indicated for further workup of the disorder.

The Bleeding Time

The bleeding time is the single best test of platelet function that is currently available for patients who are not in the OR or in critical condition. The bleeding time measures the duration of bleeding following a standardized skin incision designed so that only capillary bleeding is affected (only primary platelet-based hemostasis is detected, and a fibrin clot is not required) (see Fig. 22–8C). There are multiple methods of performing a bleeding time.[98] Duke[99] introduced the original bleeding time in 1910 as a global test of hemostasis. Rarely used today, Duke's bleeding time is performed by puncturing the ear lobe and measuring the time required for bleeding to stop. Ivy et at.[100] moved the site of the bleeding time to the forearm in 1935. Ivy also introduced inflating a blood pressure cuff to 40 mmHg throughout the measurement. Multiple triggered blade devices have been introduced to produce uniform bleeding time incisions. To perform the bleeding time testing today, an arm cuff is inflated to 40 mmHg and two standardized parallel skin incisions (9 mm long and 1 mm deep) are made with a template device on the volar surface of the forearm. The resultant laceration is blotted with filter paper every 30 seconds. When the bleeding stops the time is recorded. The results of two cuts are averaged. The normal bleeding time ranges from 4 to 10 minutes and is a function of the type of trigger blade device used and the laboratory. Although the test process has been standardized, it is still very technique-dependent. The test can cause pain and scarring. It also requires that the patient be available for the entire 20 minutes of the test. A normal bleeding time indicates that greater than 100,000 platelets per microliter are present and that they are of normal quality. If the bleeding time is prolonged and the platelet count is normal, then a qualitative abnormality of platelet function is present which requires further evaluation. To further evaluate these patients, additional studies of platelet function are indicated such as platelet aggregation tests and factor VIII complex. Qualitative platelet abnormalities may be hereditary (von Willebrand's disease) or, more commonly, acquired (aspirin use, uremia).

Despite the utility of the bleeding time in diagnosing platelet dysfunction in stable patients (especially those with inherited defects), its use in predicting bleeding and guiding management in patients with various problems has been limited.[101, 102] A large number of drugs affect the bleeding time. Anemia may even affect it. The normal range and the reproducibility of the bleeding time in patients with a variety of diseases have not been determined. Further, the bleeding time in a recent meta-analysis was of no efficacy in predicting bleeding in surgical patients or in patients with a variety of diseases.[103–105]

Special Tests of Platelet Function

Platelet-Rich Plasma Aggregometry. This very popular test of platelet function was first introduced by Born in 1962.[106] Platelet-rich plasma (PRP) is made by centrifugation and is placed in a cuvette. The PRP is stirred in the cuvette and various platelet aggregation agonists (ADP, collagen, epinephrine, ristocetin, thrombin) are added. The test measures the amount of light passing through the sample of PRP. Greater amounts of light pass through the sample as the platelets aggregate. The maximum amount of light transmittance is set on the aggregometer with a platelet-poor plasma sample. The minimum amount of light transmittance is set

with PRP. The rate of aggregation and the maximum amount of aggregation in percent are measured. The test is time-consuming and requires rapid assessment of the blood sample. The test requires training to a high level of technical proficiency and, despite this, there is a large interlaboratory and intertechnician variability in results. There are many sources of variability in the test, such as the platelet count of the PRP, choice of centrifugation speed, time between sampling and analysis, and agonist selection and concentration. Despite its deficiencies, PRP aggregometry is the standard for diagnosis of platelet function defects.

Whole-Blood Aggregometry. Whole-blood aggregometry was developed by Cardinal and Flower in 1980.[107] This test has the advantage of monitoring platelet aggregation and dense granule secretion simultaneously and the platelets are in a more physiologic whole-blood milieu. The time-consuming step of PRP preparation is not needed, which also reduces the amount of specimen handling required. The test measures the electrical impedance (resistance) between electrodes immersed in whole blood. As platelet aggregates build up on the electrodes, impedance increases. Whole blood is placed in the cuvette, as are the electrodes. The agonists of platelet aggregation, as listed above, are added to the blood and the rate of aggregation and the maximum amount of aggregation in ohms are measured. Frequently, the release of adenosine triphosphate (ATP) from the platelet-dense granules is measured concurrently, which is a quantitative measure of platelet activation. Currently, whole-blood aggregometry is used mostly as a research tool.

Fluorescence Flow Cytometry. Flow cytometry detects low concentrations of specific cell surface proteins in large cell populations. The power of this technique has been increased by development of specific monoclonal antibodies. This test has been used to determine the amount of different platelet GP receptors and the state of platelet activation. It is primarily a research tool.

Tests of Plasma Coagulation

The PT and APTT are among the most widely used routine tests of coagulation.[108] The supernatant obtained from centrifugation of anticoagulated blood, plasma, is used as the substrate for these coagulation tests. When the blood sample is collected, citrate anticoagulant sequesters the calcium and coagulation does not occur until calcium is added to the plasma. The coagulation of plasma forms a gel, while blood forms a clot.

Prothrombin Time. The PT is initiated by adding thromboplastin, derived from human or animal brain, placenta, or lung, to citrated plasma. Tissue factor and phospholipid (a platelet surface substitute) are contained in the thromboplastin. The sample is incubated at 37°C. The time elapsed since the addition of calcium to the formation of gel determines the PT test result. In normal plasma with thromboplastin, the addition of calcium enables gel formation in about 10 to 16 seconds (the recalcification time). The plasma sample contains factor VII, which, if in sufficient quantities, will activate the extrinsic and then the common coagulation pathway. The PT is commonly used to study patients with extrinsic pathway coagulation disorders and monitor oral anticoagulant (warfarin) therapy (see Figs. 27–6A and 22–8A).

Partial Thromboplastin Time (PTT). The PTT results when the citrated plasma is incubated for 3 minutes with phospholipid (a platelet substitute) and then initiated with calcium. Treating thromboplastin with alcohol or acetone produces the phospholipid only. The gel forms more slowly under these conditions, because factor XII is autoactivated on the glass surface, and occurs through the intrinsic and common coagulation pathways. The APTT includes a surface activator (celite, kaolin, or others) in the incubation mixture, which speeds the activation of factor XII. The test is frequently performed in duplicate or singly, depending on the device. The mean reference PT or APTT is determined by doing reference value studies and calculating the mean. These reference value studies are frequently performed when reagent manufacturers or lot numbers change. The reference recalcification time ranges vary and are specific for reagent-instrument combinations. The APTT is commonly used to monitor heparin therapy (see Fig. 22-8B).

Because in both tests phospholipid reagent is added, neither test requires, or tests for, adequate platelet number or function. The response of normal plasma to these tests varies with type and lot and quality of the thromboplastin and activator used; therefore, reference ranges and mean reference values must be derived for each instrument-reagent system. Because thromboplastins are produced using different methods and from different sources, the sensitivity of different thromboplastins to reductions in vitamin K–dependent clotting factors also varies. Standardization of the PT has been attempted by comparing the local thromboplastin with a World Health Organization (WHO) standard thromboplastin to produce the International Normalized Ratio (INR).[109] The INR is the PT ratio that would have been produced had the WHO standard thromboplastin, International Reference Preparation (IRP), been used. The reagents used by each laboratory have a specific sensitivity to factor deficiency called the International Sensitivity Index (ISI) relative to the IRP. By definition, the reference WHO preparation has an ISI of 1.0. A more sensitive thromboplastin has an ISI of less than 1.0, and a less sensitive thromboplastin has an ISI greater than 1.0. Each manufacturer provides the ISI for its reagents so that the INR can be reported. The INR result is calculated as follows:

$$INR = (Patient\ PT/mean\ reference\ PT)^{ISI}$$

Small errors in ISI assignment may affect the calculated INR greatly. Although this standardization strategy works well much of the time, there have been several reports of interlaboratory differences in the INR values attributable to incorrect ISI value assignments by manufacturers, differences in citrate anticoagulant concentrations, differences in automated instruments, and unique interactions between specific reagent-instrument combinations.

Thrombin Time. To perform the TT, thrombin is incubated with citrated plasma, and then the recalcification time is determined. A prolongation of the TT indicates a qualitative change in fibrinogen, a fibrinogen deficiency of less than 100 mg/dL, the anticoagulant effect of fibrin degradation products (FDPs), or a heparin effect on thrombin (see Fig. 22-8D). The TT is extremely sensitive to the presence of heparin, and therefore may be useful in monitoring for residual heparin effect.

Tests and Devices for Intraoperative Evaluation of Coagulation

Many hospitals are evaluating point-of-care programs to satisfy the clinical demand for more rapid return of coagulation test results. The development of point-of-care programs requires cooperation between laboratory specialists and clinicians. The laboratory specialist assesses the validity of the methodology and the clinician evaluates the clinical merit of the systems. In many hospitals 45 minutes or more is required to prepare blood products like platelets, FFP, and cryoprecipitate for treatment of the bleeding patient. The time required to receive the results of a coagulation test can prolong the time to treatment. Many point-of-care tests provide results within minutes. Thus, the interest in point-of-care tests, plasma coagulation, viscoelastic tests, point-of-care platelet function tests, and tests of fibrinolysis in the OR environment.

The ideal point-of-care test would be specific, reliable, technically simple, and rapid. The American Society of Anesthesiologists (ASA) task force on blood component therapy has emphasized, and nearly mandated, the need for laboratory testing to guide transfusion therapy.[110]

Use of point-of-care tests and transfusion algorithms may reduce transfusion requirements. A study by Despotis et al.[111] found that using point-of-care coagulation tests (platelet count, whole-blood PT, and APTT) to guide therapy and treatment of microvascular (nonsurgical) bleeding in cardiac surgery patients was effective in reducing allogeneic blood product transfusion. In the aforementioned randomized and controlled study, cardiac surgical patients determined to have microvascular bleeding at the cessation of CPB were assigned to algorithm-driven (n = 30) or standard (n = 36) transfusion therapy. The algorithm to guide transfusion therapy utilized platelet counts of less than 50,000, 50,000 to 100,000, and greater than 100,000 to guide platelet transfusion therapy, and used PT and APTT values greater than 1.5 or 1.8 times control to guide FFP transfusion. The patients treated according to the algorithm received fewer allogeneic hemostatic blood component units ($P = .008$) and had fewer total donor exposures ($P = .007$) during the entire hospitalization period. A retrospective study by Spiess et al.[112] found that after institution of thromboelastograph (TEG)-guided coagulation studies in the perioperative period, there was a significant reduction in the number of blood transfusions and the incidence of mediastinal reexploration for hemorrhage in cardiac surgery patients.[112]

Tests of Plasma Coagulation

There are multiple devices (CoaguChek Plus, Hemochron 801, and Thrombolytic Assessment System Analyzer) that allow bedside or OR determinations of the PT, INR, and APTT on whole blood. The accuracy of different devices for PT and INR depends on how well the ISIs match between the two methods being compared. If the ISIs are not the same, the PT (in seconds) will be significantly different. Comparison of the INRs will reduce this somewhat, but the INRs tend to be more discrepant at levels greater than 3.0. Comparison of APTT results is even more difficult because reagent differences are even greater and there is no standardization currently available. Thus, reference ranges and therapeutic ranges must be established for each reagent and device. Finally, it should be emphasized that a good correlation (r-value) does not always equal good accuracy and difference plots such as those described by Bland and Altman[113] are important to demonstrate how well the two methods compare.

CoaguChek Plus. The CoaguChek Plus (Roche Diagnostics, Indianapolis, IN; previously known as the Biotrack 512 Coagulation Monitor) is the device that was used in the study by Despotis et al.[111] to reduce transfusion requirements in cardiac surgery patients. Before the test is performed, a disposable plastic cartridge is placed in the device and allowed to warm. From the card the device determines the type of test to perform and conversion data for the microprocessor to give the test result. To perform the test, 25 μL (1 drop) of whole blood is placed on the prewarmed disposable plastic cartridge. The blood is drawn by capillary action into the reaction chamber and onto a reaction pathway, where exposure to the reagents occurs. The PT cartridge uses rabbit brain thromboplastin and the APTT cartridge uses soybean phosphatide and bovine brain sulfatide. The device detects clot formation by a laser optical system and this is converted to a ratio of the control value by a microprocessor. The control values are encoded on the cartridge. The PT and INR, or APTT, values are displayed on the face of the device in less than 2 minutes.

The CoaguChek Plus device has been evaluated under several clinical situations. It has been evaluated for monitoring oral anticoagulant therapy using the PT cartridge. The APTT cartridge correlates well with standard laboratory APTT in patients undergoing heparin therapy in the cardiac catheterization laboratory. The accuracy of the CoaguChek Plus PT and APTT has been evaluated in the OR. The CoaguChek Plus PT was accurate relative to the laboratory, but the APTT was inaccurate.[114-117]

Hemochron 801. Another device that performs a PT, APTT, TT, and a heparin-neutralized thrombin time (HNTT) is the Hemochron 801 (International Technidyne Corp., Edison, NJ). The Hemochron system uses glass tubes, which contain a small magnet along with the reagents. A 2-mL whole-blood sample is placed in the tube and mixed with the reagents. The Hemochron PT test tube contains acetone-dried, rabbit brain thromboplastin. The Hemochron APTT test tube contains kaolin activator, sodium citrate, and phospholipase. The Hemochron TT and HNTT test tubes contain lyophilized human thrombin and calcium salts. The HNTT test tube also contains protamine sulfate. The tube is placed in the well of the device, where the tube is warmed and slowly rotated. The firm clot displacing the magnet and triggering a proximity switch determines clot formation. The time to clot formation is converted by a microprocessor to a PT, INR, APTT, TT, or HNTT. Less than 5 minutes is required for the results of each test to become available. Like the previous device, the Hemochron was found to produce an accurate PT relative to the laboratory, but the APTT was inaccurate.[114, 117] The Hemochron TT and HNTT were found to be promising as methods to detect residual heparin following CPB.

Thrombolytic Assessment System Analyzer. The Thrombolytic Assessment System Analyzer (Cardiovascular Diagnostics Inc., Raleigh, NC) is another device that uses a disposable card to determine the PT, INR, APTT, or heparin management test (HMT). There are also cards for performing ecarin clotting time, lysis onset time, and for detection of streptokinase antibodies, but these are not Food and Drug Administration (FDA)–approved yet. Before the test, the disposable card is placed in the device to warm. From the card's magnetic strip the device determines the type of test to perform, conversion data for the microprocessor to give the test result, and a lot number. For the test, 25 μL of either fresh whole blood or citrated whole blood or plasma is placed onto a prewarmed disposable card. The blood is drawn into the reaction chamber where exposure to the reagents and paramagnetic iron oxide particles occurs. The PT card contains thromboplastin from human placenta and calcium chloride, and the APTT card contains chloroform-extracted phospholipid from dried rabbit brain, calcium chloride, and aluminum magnesium silicate. The Thrombolytic

Assessment System Analyzer has two PT cards: one with an ISI of 1.6, the other with an ISI of 1.0. The HMT card was designed to determine heparin effect during high-dose heparin therapy (e.g., during CPB). The HMT card contains celite activator and calcium chloride. While the test is in progress an electromagnet below the card turns on and off every second. The iron oxide particles on the test card stand up and fall down in response to the magnet being on or off, respectively. A light is shown on the reaction chamber and when the iron oxide particles are standing up more intense light is passed onto the photodetector. Conversely, less intense light is passed onto the detector when the particles are down. The device detects clot formation by the cessation of particle movement and detects clot lysis by resumption of particle movement. This information is converted to a ratio of the control value by a microprocessor. The control values are encoded on the card. The PT and INR, or APTT values are displayed on the face of the device in less than 2 minutes.

The accuracy of the Thrombolytic Assessment System Analyzer PT has been studied in patients receiving oral anticoagulant therapy and it has been found to produce accurate PT and INR results.[118, 119] The Thrombolytic Assessment System Analyzer APTT and HMT are useful for monitoring heparin effect in cardiac surgery patients.[120] The correlation of the Thrombolytic Assessment System Analyzer APTT with the laboratory APTT and heparin concentrations was good. Both the Thrombolytic Assessment System Analyzer APTT and HMT results were increased with aprotinin therapy. Our laboratory has found, in an unpublished study, an excellent correlation of the Thrombolytic Assessment System Analyzer PT with the laboratory PT. We also found a good correlation of the Thrombolytic Assessment System Analyzer APTT with the laboratory APTT, but the two tests differed in absolute clotting time results. Therefore, the Thrombolytic Assessment System Analyzer APTT is not directly convertible to the laboratory APTT.

Platelet Function Tests

The ideal point-of-care test of platelet function would be specific, reliable, technically simple, and rapid. None of the current point-of-care tests of platelet function achieves this ideal.[98, 121-125] A clinically effective test of platelet function would be very useful to appropriately guide transfusion therapy. Commonly used and newly introduced tests will be discussed. The only FDA-approved point-of-care platelet function tests are the TEG, the Sonoclot, the PFA 100, and the HemoSTATUS.

Viscoelastic Tests of Platelet Function. Viscoelastic tests measure the change in the physical properties of whole blood with clot formation. There are two commonly used viscoelastic tests, the TEG, and the Sonoclot. Both tests rapidly assess many aspects of hemostasis. These tests have gained popularity because of their use in liver transplantation and cardiac surgery, both intraoperatively and in the ICU.[126-129]

Thromboelastogram. A test first developed in the 1940s, the TEG measures physical properties of clots. To begin the TEG, 0.35 mL of whole blood is placed in a prewarmed cuvette and a piston is lowered into the blood. In the old design, the cup rotated through an angle of 4° 45' and, as the blood clotted, this motion was imparted to the piston, which resulted in the characteristic TEG clot signature. In the new design, the cup is stationary and the piston is rotated through the same angle. When fibrin strands and clot are formed between the cuvette and the piston, rotatory motion is transferred to the piston. This motion is amplified and appears on a computer screen (Fig. 22-9). The TEG assesses clot function from the time of initial clot formation with fibrin formation and platelet aggregation until clot lysis. The entire life of the clot is reflected in grossly, without clear delineation of the individual inputs of each component of the coagulation system (see Fig. 22-8F). The strength of the clot is reflected on the recording as a symmetric deviation from the centerline, and standard parameters may be measured from the recording. The five parameters most frequently discussed in the literature are R, R + K, α angle, MA, and %lysis at 30 minutes (see Fig. 22-9). The R value is the time from sample placement until initial pen deflection, and the R + K is the time from initial sample placement until the pen is deflected 20 mm. The α angle is the angle formed by the tangent of the tracing's amplitude at the initial pen deflection. The MA is the maximal amplitude of the pen deflection, and the %lysis at 30 minutes is the percent decrease in the amplitude of the tracing 30 minutes following the MA. The five TEG parameters are not independent variables. They are interdependent, and a change in one aspect of the coagulation system frequently affects many of the variables.

The three most important variables affecting clot strength, and the subsequent TEG tracing, are fibrinogen concentration, platelet function, and platelet count. The TEG MA is thought to be a function of platelet count and function and fibrinogen concentration.[126, 130] The TEG α angle, MA, and %lysis at 30 minutes correlated well with the fibrinogen concentration and with platelet aggregometry in patients who had undergone cardiac surgery with CPB ($P < .001$).[130] The TEG parameters correlate poorly with other coagulation tests.[127, 131, 132] The TEG %lysis at 30 minutes has been used to detect the presence of fibrinolysis, which results in a teardrop-shaped tracing[133] and may indicate a need for further laboratory analysis.

The TEG has been modified in several ways. In nonactivated whole blood more than 30 minutes are required for TEG MA results. To shorten the time to development of the TEG MA, recombinant human tissue factor or celite is added to the whole blood as an activator. The tissue factor-activated TEG MA is reduced by the GPIIb/IIIa receptor antago-

nist abciximab.[134] The abciximab dose response of the tissue factor-activated TEG clot strength was the same as the thrombin receptor agonist peptide-induced platelet aggregation inhibitory concentration. The inhibition of the TEG MA by abciximab has also been used to separate the effects of fibrinogen concentration on the TEG MA. If high concentrations of abciximab are added to the whole blood, the resultant TEG MA is thought to reflect fibrinogen concentration. The measurement of serum fibrinogen concentration provides useful information in the management of perioperative coagulopathies (see Fig. 22-8D).

Sonoclot. The Sonoclot (Sienco Inc., Morrison, CO) was introduced in 1975 by von Kaulla et al.[135] Like the TEG, the Sonoclot measures the effect of clotting on a piston suspended in a warmed cuvette of whole blood, but with a different mechanism. The disposable plastic piston vibrates up and down at 200 Hz in 0.4 mL of blood and the machine measures the impedance to vibration. As the blood clots, the piston's motion is hindered. This impedance to piston motion is conveyed to a recording pen (Fig. 22-10). Therefore, the Sonoclot follows changes in blood viscosity. The Sonoclot tracing, like the TEG, measures interdependent parameters. The correlation of these parameters with standard coagulation tests is limited, and the parameters have a large coefficient of variation.[136, 137] More recently, Sonoclot time to peak variable has been shown to correlate well with collagen-induced whole-blood aggregation, platelet count, and fibrinogen.[138] The reference range of Sonoclot variables is a function of patient age and sex.[139] Therefore, interpretation of Sonoclot results is difficult.

Newer Tests of Platelet Function

Hemodyne Hemostasis Analyzer. The Hemodyne instrument and technique were initially developed by Carr and Zekert[140] in 1991 to measure the forces produced by platelets during clot formation and retraction. Either whole blood or platelet-rich plasma can be placed between a shallow temperature-controlled cup and an overlying probe. The probe is connected to a transducer that generates a voltage as the probe is moved. A downward force on the probe is generated when the platelets in the clot attempt to shrink

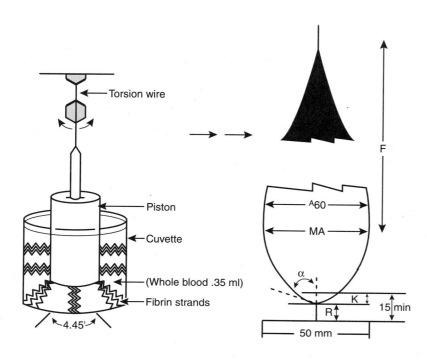

Figure 22-9. In thromboelastography the transfer of rotational force between the piston and the cuvette containing fresh whole blood yields a characteristic tracing which provides specific information about coagulation cascade function, platelet activation, maximal platelet function or clot strength, and fibrinolysis.

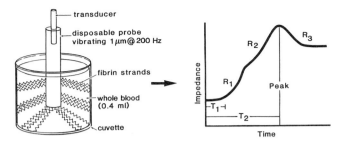

Figure 22–10. A characteristic tracing generated by the Sonoclot coagulation analyzer results when fresh whole blood begins to clot and generates impedance to movement of a vibrating probe. This tracing provides general information on clotting and platelet function as well as fibrinolysis.

the clot. The voltage that is generated is converted to a force (dynes) by a calibration constant. From the force measurements a clot modulus can be calculated.[141] The clot modulus depends on fibrin structure and platelet function, while force development is primarily a platelet function. Reductions in the recovery of peak platelet force development following CPB have been shown to correlate with blood loss following cardiac surgery.[142] At this time, this test is not FDA-approved and is, therefore, available only for research purposes.

HemoSTATUS (Platelet Activating Clotting Test). The HemoSTATUS (Medtronic Inc., Parker, CO) is a newly developed assay of platelet function using a modified Hepcon HMS (Heparin Management System) device. Platelet procoagulant activity is determined by measuring the platelet activating factor (PAF)–induced shortening of the kaolin ACT. PAF is a potent endogenous platelet activator that stimulates in vitro thrombosis indicating platelet responsiveness. There are six channels in the device with increasing doses of PAF in channels 3 to 6. The clot ratio values are thought to reflect platelet function. The clot ratio is calculated by the following formula for each respective PAF concentration:

$$\text{Clot ratio} = 1 - (\text{ACT}/\text{control ACT})$$

The clot ratio in channels 5 and 6 had excellent correlation with blood loss and high sensitivity and specificity for predicting bleeding following cardiac surgery in one study.[143] In other studies, there was poor correlation, sensitivity, and specificity.[144, 145] Differences in heparin concentration are thought to be the reason for the variations in test results. Therefore, the cartridges have been redesigned to remove heparin concentration effects and the test is now called the HemoSTATUS II.

Clot Signature Analyzer (Hemostatometer). The Clot Signature Analyzer, based on the work of Görög and Ahmed in 1984,[146] provides a global assessment of hemostasis using whole non-anticoagulated blood. It is designed to be a point-of-care, in vitro assay of platelet function under conditions similar to those in a blood vessel.[147, 148] This device takes non-anticoagulated whole blood and perfuses it through two polyethylene tubes by paraffin oil displacement at 60 mmHg and 37°C. In one tube holes are punched through the tubing, which results in "bleeding" and a pressure drop distal to the puncture. The pattern of pressure recovery shows the formation of hemostatic plugs in the holes. The initial recovery of the pressure represents platelet plug formation, which results from activation of platelets by shear stress and release

of ADP from shear-damaged platelets and red blood cells (RBCs). The later recovery is due to stabilization of the platelet plug as a result of the formation of thrombin and fibrin, which strengthens the clot and allows it to resist the increasing pressure. The lumen of the tube eventually occludes from propagation of the clot, which results in a pressure drop. The second tube contains a fiber of collagen. The collagen fiber induces thrombus formation, which eventually occludes the lumen and causes a pressure drop to zero distal to the thrombus. This test uses whole blood, preserving interaction between platelets and other formed blood elements. The area of the resultant curve is thought to reflect platelet function but may reflect primary hemostasis.[149, 150] The accuracy of this test is currently being evaluated. The Clot Signature Analyzer was found to be a better preoperative predictor of excessive bleeding in cardiac surgery patients than the routine coagulation tests.[147] In vitro addition of inhibitors of platelet GPIIb/IIIa and GPIb receptor antagonist to normal blood resulted in prolongation of the time for thrombus formation in the collagen channel.[150] The time to recover pressure in the punch channel was prolonged with the GPIIb/IIIa receptor antagonist. At this time, this test is not FDA-approved and is, therefore, available only for research purposes.

PFA-100 (Thrombostat 4000). The PFA-100 (Platelet Function Analyzer-100) is a microprocessor-controlled instrument-cartridge system designed to measure platelet function, especially primary, platelet-related hemostasis in routinely collected citrated whole blood.[151] This automated system is based on an in vitro bleeding test initially called the Thrombostat 4000, developed by Kratzer and Born in 1985.[152] The device uses a disposable test cartridge that contains a biologically active membrane which is coated with collagen and epinephrine or ADP. The instrument aspirates a blood sample under a constant vacuum from the sample reservoir through a capillary and a microscopic aperture cut in the membrane. The biologic stimuli and the high shear rates generated under the standardized flow conditions result in platelet attachment, activation, and aggregation, slowly building a stable platelet plug at the aperture. The time required to fully occlude the aperture is reported as the "closure time." Impairment of vWF, or inhibition of platelet GPIb or IIb/IIIa receptor with monoclonal antibodies, and aspirin therapy resulted in abnormal closure times.[151] The PFA-100 was found to be more sensitive and specific than the Ivy bleeding time for detecting known platelet function defects.[153]

Plateletworks Assay. The Plateletworks Assay (Array Medical, Somerville, NJ), introduced in 1998, is an automated point-of-care test based on a Coulter counter. The test is based on the platelet count ratio.[154] Platelets in whole blood respond to agonist stimulation by forming aggregates, which decrease the number of free platelets. The device is designed to count only free platelets. A baseline platelet count is performed followed by simulation of the platelets with an agonist and a second platelet count. The manufacturer provides tubes with many of the standard aggregometry platelet agonists (i.e., ADP, collagen, epinephrine, ristocetin, and thrombin). The percent of aggregation is calculated as follows:

$$\text{Aggregation (\%)} = 100 \times \frac{(\text{Baseline platelet count} - \text{sample platelet count})}{\text{Baseline platelet count}}$$

Besides possibly measuring platelet function, the device is

also able to provide a measure of complete blood count (CBC). The accuracy of this device is currently being evaluated. At this time, this test is not FDA-approved and is, therefore, available only for research purposes.

Ultegra (Rapid Platelet Function Assay). The Ultegra is a whole-blood automated turbidimetric assay that is designed to assess platelet function based on the ability of activated platelet to bind fibrinogen. The test was developed by Coller et al.[155] in 1997 as an assay of GPIIb/IIIa receptor blockade by receptor antagonists. This point-of-care test consists of a single-use cartridge and instrument with a digital readout, which can produce results in less than 3 minutes with a small sample of citrated whole blood. The cartridge contains fibrinogen-coated microparticles, which will agglutinate in whole blood in proportion to the number of unblocked platelet GPIIb/IIIa receptors. Thrombin receptor–activating peptide is used to activate the platelets without fibrin formation. There is an increase in light transmittance as the activated platelets bind and agglutinate fibrinogen-coated beads. The device measures this change in optical signal from agglutination. There is an excellent correlation of the Ultegra results and the percentage of GPIIb/IIIa receptor blockade.[125] At this time, this test is not FDA-approved and is, therefore, available only for research purposes.

Modified Platelet Adhesion to Glass Bead Columns. Platelet adhesion to glass bead columns is a simple, yet robust assay of platelet adhesiveness and aggregation that was first described in 1963.[156, 157] The assay involves passage of heparinized blood within a few minutes after phlebotomy through a 4-g column of glass beads. Platelet retention is determined as the percentage of platelets not leaving the column, comparing the platelet count pre- and post infusion. Normal volunteers typically have greater than 85% platelet retention onto the glass beads. The assay is dependent on GPIb, GPIIb/IIIa, vWF, shear force, and calcium. Patients with von Willebrand's disease typically have less than 50% platelet adhesion. Addition of either anti-GPIb or anti-GPIIb/IIIa immunoglobulin to whole blood yields less than 5% platelet adhesion. Citrate anticoagulant completely inhibits platelet retention. Platelet glass bead retention obtained while on CPB correlates strongly with post-CPB blood loss.[158] The glass bead retention assay thus provides an expeditious method of identifying dysfunctional platelets. More detailed analysis and modification of the test will probably be used in the perioperative setting.

Conclusions About Platelet Function Assays. There are multiple point-of-care platelet function tests available. However, no studies have been done to determine which of these tests is best for evaluating platelet function in the OR and ICU.

Tests of Fibrinolysis

Fibrinopeptides A and B are produced from the action of thrombin on fibrinogen. They indicate normal coagulation activity (see Fig. 22–4A). Fibrinogenolysis occurs when circulating protease inhibitors are overwhelmed by large mounts of plasmin. Fibrinogenolysis is a pathologic process. The breakdown products of fibrinogen share some antigenic determinants with fibrin breakdown products. The test for fibrin split products (FSPs) measures both fibrinogen and fibrin split products using a latex agglutination technique. A modification of the latex agglutination test, called the D-dimer test, uses a highly specific monoclonal antibody to D-dimers. The D-dimer test and the enzyme-linked immunosorbent assay (ELISA) measure the D-dimer. The D-dimer is

two central D regions of the fibrin molecule joined together, which is a breakdown product of cross-linked fibrin. Positive results are obtained with degradation products of fibrin, but not fibrinogen.

The normal serum level of FSPs is less than 10 μg/mL. With the D-dimer tests, a positive agglutination indicates a concentration of at least 250 ng/mL cross-linked fibrin derivatives containing D-dimer.[159] Semiquantitation can be achieved by determining the dilution of the plasma at which agglutination is seen. Both the FSPs and the D-dimer will be elevated with DIC and with venous and arterial thrombosis within 2 days post surgery, and in late pregnancy. Fibrinolytic therapy may elevate the FSPs.

The euglobulin clot lysis time is a functional test of fibrinolysis. It is rarely used now because it is labor-intensive, slow (normal range, 1.5 to 6.0 hours), and has poor predictive value. The TEG also provides a measure of fibrinolysis.

Monitoring Heparin Therapy

Activated Clotting Time. The ACT[160] is a modification of Lee-White whole-blood clotting time, originally devised in 1975 by Bull et al.[161] Whole blood is added to a glass test tube preloaded with kaolin or celite activator and then placed into a plastic well which rotates with a magnetic indicator stirrer. As the magnet is caught in the clot formation, it is pulled away from a magnetic detector which signals that the clot has formed. The activator (celite or kaolin) concentration is very high, giving a good dose-response relationship to high-dose heparin therapy as needed for CPB. The ACT is a sensitive but not specific assay. Typically, an ACT value greater than 450 seconds is required for CPB. Upon termination of CPB, the ACT can be utilized to confirm the protamine antagonism of heparin therapy. The ACT is not a predictor of abnormal bleeding. The setting of reduced ATIII concentration, reduced factor XII activity, hypothermia, or platelet count less than 50,000/mm^3 or a fibrinogen less than 100 mg/dL can all result in abnormal prolongation of the ACT value.

Modifications of the basic Hemochron 801 system are available in the Hemochron Jr. and Medtronics HemoTec systems. These devices have totally different methods for endpoint detection.

Heparin Concentration. The ACT provides a functional assay of heparin activity in whole blood. However, the exact heparin concentration is not measured. Automated heparin assays based on the ACT technology are available and have been used in many institutions with great success. The Hepcon automated system gives a semiquantitative measurement of heparin by protamine titration and utilizes a series of cartridges with varying amounts of heparin added to various cartridge chambers. Additional cartridges have different aliquots of protamine added to the various chambers. An automated dispenser distributes equal amounts of whole blood to each of the cartridge chambers when activated. Utilizing one or more sets of cartridges, a predictable heparin level can be determined, but this method does not produce the same results as an Anti–Factor Xa method, which is typically used in most reference laboratories. The management of hemostasis with the Hepcon system rather than routinely managed coagulation during CPB improves perioperative bleeding.[162, 163] Other heparin level assays include the use of heparin dose-response (HDR) cartridges, heparinase added to traditional ACT methods, and also the Hemochron RxDx systems.

Thrombolytic Assessment System Coagulation Analyzer. The HMT is one of the components of the thrombolytic assessment system (TAS), described above. The HMT is designed to monitor heparin effect during high-dose heparin therapy. The TAS is a recently introduced device for point-of-care monitoring of coagulation function (Cardiovascular Diagnostics Inc., Raleigh, NC). The TAS system consists of a series of disposable cards that contain all the reagents required for each test (PT, APTT, lysis onset time, detection of streptokinase antibodies, and heparin effect). The movement of paramagnetic iron oxide particles in response to an oscillating magnetic field is the technologic basis for the TAS. The HMT test cards contain calcium chloride and a celite activator. The endpoint is detected by the HMT and APTT tests as the time to clot formation, which is identified by a decrease in the movement of iron oxide particles. The ex vivo addition of heparin to whole blood provided the basis for the comparison between the HMT and heparin concentration.[120] This ex vivo experiment demonstrated a significant correlation ($r^2 = .954$) of the HMT with the natural log of the heparin concentration. In patients undergoing CPB, the coefficient of variation of the HMT was much less than that of the traditional ACT methods. The TAS-HMT system may be a useful monitor of heparin effect in cardiac surgical patients.[120]

Treatment of Coagulopathy

With the use of the history, physical examination, and laboratory analysis, a diagnosis for the cause of coagulopathy can usually be established. The diagnosis will often point to a specific treatment. In acutely bleeding patients, the clinician may have to simultaneously initiate diagnostic tests, treat the presumed cause of bleeding, and replace hemostatic resources depleted by bleeding.

Hemotherapy for Coagulopathy

The goal of hemotherapy should be to replace specific blood components that are deficient, either as the cause of coagulopathy (i.e., thrombocytopenia, hypofibrinogenemia, or anemia), or as a result of the coagulopathy disorder (e.g., DIC). Shotgun therapy, using a number of different coagulation products, should be avoided because unnecessary blood products may be infused, increasing the risk of transfusion-related disease, volume overload, immunosuppression, and production of a possible hypercoagulable state.[164-167]

Whole Blood and Packed Red Blood Cells

RBCs increase oxygen carrying capacity. The primary adverse consequence of whole blood is volume overload. There has been a gradual reduction in the use of whole blood, to the point where it is unavailable in many centers.[168] This resulted from the need to produce factor concentrates, and platelet concentrates to treat oncology and liver transplant patients. The RBC product of whole blood separation is packed red blood cells (PRBCs), which have the same amount of RBCs as whole blood, but with half the volume. Because of this, the problems with volume overload are less frequent, especially when treating anemia in normovolemic patients. In the patient who is bleeding massively and losing plasma as well as RBCs, the use of whole blood would seem logical, since coagulation factors as well as blood volume and RBCs would be replaced.[169] However, because whole blood is no longer available at many institutions, PRBCs plus crystalloid or colloid solutions are typically infused in patients with both anemia and hypovolemia.

The level of hemoglobin at which transfusion becomes necessary is a clinical decision based on the patient's coexisting diseases (e.g., impaired oxygenation or cardiac dysfunction). The lower limit of human tolerance to acute normovolemic anemia has not been determined. A hemoglobin of 7 g/dL or a hematocrit of 21% is frequently used as an absolute minimum in most normovolemic patients.[170] It should be noted that some patients with chronic anemia, such as those with chronic renal failure, have tolerated even lower hemoglobin levels. In patients with coexisting disease, higher levels of hemoglobin or hematocrit should be maintained. Intraoperative and postoperative myocardial ischemia is more likely in elderly patients with hematocrits less than 28% having elective radical prostatectomy, especially with concurrent tachycardia.[171]

In a 70-kg person, a unit of RBCs will increase the hematocrit 3% to 4% (1 g/dL); 1 cc/kg will result in a 1% increase in hematocrit. While it is currently considered good practice to be conservative in transfusion of blood products, the consequences of inadequate or delayed resuscitation must also be considered. Experience with massive trauma has shown that the benefits of timely and adequate restoration of blood volume and tissue oxygenation outweigh the potential deleterious effects of massive transfusion.[169] A study of 125 surgical patients found that operative mortality was greater in patients with a low preoperative hemoglobin.[172] Conversely, a prospective randomized study of 838 critically ill patients who had their hemoglobin concentrations maintained at 7 to 9 g/dL and those with a hemoglobin concentration of 10 to 12 g/dL revealed a lower hospital mortality rate in the restrictive transfusion group.[173]

Transfusion of allogeneic PRBCs has been postulated to have a beneficial hemostatic effect. RBC transfusion decreases the APTT and bleeding time in anemic patients, suggesting a hemostatic effect.[174] The administration of small amounts of platelets (most with little or no functional reserve) and coagulation proteins, which are not fully removed from whole blood during the preparation of PRBC components, may have important benefits. However, the clinical importance of this potential and small hemostatic effect is probably limited compared with the large pathophysiologic insult of surgery or CPB.

An alternative to transfusion therapy for anemia is recombinant human erythropoietin (rEPO).[175] rEPO has been shown to increase hemoglobin levels in patients with renal failure and to reduce transfusion requirements for patients having cardiac surgery.[175, 176] It has also been used to increase preoperative autologous blood transfusions before surgery.[177]

Platelet Concentrates

Platelet concentrates are a collection of platelets separated from whole blood and resuspended in plasma. An individual unit contains 5 to 10 × 10^{10} platelets in 50 to 70 mL of plasma. An apheresis unit contains 3 to 5 × 10^{11} platelets in 200 to 400 mL of plasma.

The platelets are stored at room temperature with use of continuous agitation. They can be stored up to 5 days with the limitation being an increased risk of infection after 5 days. Platelets undergo a number of biochemical changes during storage that reduce their activity. One fourth or more of the platelets will be inactive and a percentage of the remainder will take time to return to normal function after transfusion. Platelet concentrates and other blood products are usually transfused through a 170-μm filter to remove clots or debris.[178]

The indications for platelet concentrate transfusions have been developed by the Consensus Development Conference (CDC) of the National Institutes of Health (NIH),[179] and recommendations for platelet concentrate transfusions by the ASA Task Force on Blood Component Therapy.[110] Indications for platelet concentrate transfusions are significant bleeding with thrombocytopenia (platelet counts < 50,000/mm³) or an abnormality of platelet function (bleeding time more than twice normal), prophylactic treatment of patients with severe thrombocytopenia (platelet counts < 20,000/mm³), replacement of platelets in massive transfusion, and excessive bleeding following CPB.

A dose of 0.1 U/kg is a common starting point for platelet concentrate transfusions in children. The usual adult dose of platelets is 6 to 10 U, depending on the institution. As a rough estimate, a normovolemic 70-kg patient would have an increase in platelet count of between 5000 and 10,000/mm³ after transfusion of 1 U of platelet concentrate.

Fresh Frozen Plasma

The two plasma-based products in common use are FFP and plasma. FFP is plasma that has been separated from the blood of a donor and placed at −18°C or less within 6 hours of collection. Plasma is a comparable product separated from whole blood at any time during storage up to 5 days after expiration of the original unit or prepared from FFP that has become outdated or has had cryoprecipitate removed. Plasma does not contain the labile coagulation factors. "Cryo-poor plasma" is the term used for plasma with cryoprecipitate removed. Cryo-poor plasma has decreased amounts of factor VIII, vWF, fibrinogen, fibronectin, and factor XIII. For patients with multiple coagulation deficiencies, FFP is a valuable source of coagulation factors. FFP is also useful for the emergency treatment of specific coagulation deficiencies when the concentrates are not available or relatively unsafe. Volume overload can be a difficulty in this situation secondary to the volume of FFP (250 mL/U).[180]

The indications for FFP transfusion have been developed by the CDC of the NIH,[181] and recommendations for FFP transfusions by the ASA Task Force on Blood Component Therapy.[110] The indications for FFP therapy are replacement of factors II, V, VII, IX, X, and XI; urgent reversal of warfarin effect or in liver disease patients who are bleeding; replacement of coagulation factors in massive transfusion; ATIII deficiency; treatment of immunodeficiencies (now largely replaced by purified immunoglobulin); and treatment of thrombotic thrombocytopenic purpura. FFP should not be used as a volume expander or as a nutritional source.

Cryoprecipitate

Cryoprecipitate results when FFP is thawed in the cold, and it forms as a white gelatinous precipitate that contains large quantities of factor VIII, vWF, fibrinogen, fibronectin, and factor XIII. Cryoprecipitate is used to treat hemophilia A, von Willebrand's disease, and factor XIII deficiency. It is also used as a source of fibrinogen for the treatment of hypofibrinogenemia, because the usual volume of a unit is 10 to 20 mL with greater than twice the concentration of fibrinogen than plasma.[51, 110] The usual adult dose of cryoprecipitate is 10 to 20 pooled units.

Special Concerns in Coagulation Monitoring

Cardiac Surgery

In 1998 over 500,000 patients in the United States underwent cardiac surgery employing CPB.[182] The majority of these patients (65% to 75%) were transfused with allogeneic

blood.[183] Between 10% and 20% of the approximately 12 million units of RBCs transfused in the United States annually are transfused in cardiac surgical patients.[184] About 50% of the over 7 million units of platelets transfused annually are transfused in patients undergoing cardiac surgery.[185] Approximately 20% of blood transfusions in these patients are inappropriate.[183, 186] Specifically, 47% of platelets, 32% of FFP, and 15% of RBCs are inappropriately transfused.[186] Clinicians are limited in their ability to predict excessive bleeding following CPB and to identify patients who will require blood transfusion. In addition, there is little or no objective evidence that platelet transfusions reduce bleeding.[187]

Excessive Bleeding, Transfusion, and Cardiac Surgery

Excessive bleeding secondary to the deleterious effects of CPB on platelet function and coagulation is well appreciated, occurring in 5% to 25% of patients, and is an important cause of morbidity and mortality.[188, 189] Extracorporeal circulation (ECC) is associated with major hemostatic defects arising from blood exposure to synthetic nonbiologic surfaces.[188, 190] Thrombocytopenia,[191] platelet dysfunction,[58, 192] coagulation factor deficiencies,[193] and fibrinolysis all occur.[194] Insufficient surgical hemostasis accounts for 10% to 20% of excessively bleeding patients; the remaining majority are a result of deficient hemostasis.[57] Platelet activation, sequestration, and dysfunction, contact activation, dilution, and consumption of coagulation factors; fibrinolysis; and a total body inflammatory response (primarily via kallikrein and kininogen) all occur when blood is exposed to the extracorporeal circuit.[195-198] Residual heparin following protamine administration can also cause bleeding.[57] Hypothermia, hemodilution, various medications, and the duration of CPB also are factors that modulate bleeding. During CPB, the platelet count decreases predictably by 30% to 50%.[193, 199-201] Platelet dysfunction, perhaps the critical insult to hemostatic function, correlates directly with postbypass bleeding and increased transfusion requirements.[190, 192, 202]

Following CPB, the PT is prolonged in most patients. In one study, factor X and factor V were reduced by approximately 50% when the PT was 15 seconds.[203] The PT value at which these factors are reduced to 50% is a function of the reagent used to measure the PT. Further evaluation of the effect of the various coagulation factors on the PT in the setting of CPB has not been completed.[115] It is important to know why the PT is elevated because we cannot treat a laboratory value to which many factors contribute. Specifically, the PT is used as an indicator of the extrinsic and common pathways of humoral coagulation. The primary therapy aimed at treating an increased PT is transfusion of FFP, which has normal plasma concentrations of all coagulation factors. Some recombinant factor therapies are now available that avoid the risks of allogeneic FFP transfusion. If we were able to delineate that a specific factor or combination of factors disproportionately accounted for the elevated PT, therapy could be directed more specifically. That is, if factor V was determined to be the primary culprit in post-CPB coagulopathy, then perhaps a single 1-mg dose of recombinant factor V would be all that is needed to treat the excessive bleeding in many patients.

When patients are placed on CPB, hemodilution (plasma dilution) occurs and the importance of hemodilution versus a specific factor deficiency in the outcome of the prolonged PT is unknown. It is unlikely that hemodilution is the sole contributor to this elevated PT. Yet CPB dilutes plasma volume by 25% to 45%. Adequate hemostasis typically occurs in nonsurgical populations with concentrations of a single coagulation factor to levels as low as 15% to 25% of normal.[204] If hemodilution is the most important contributor to inadequate hemostasis, efforts could be made to more aggressively hemoconcentrate (by ultrafiltration) patients during or following CPB, thus concentrating plasma and increasing the serum concentrations of coagulation proteins.

Cardiopulmonary Bypass–Induced Platelet Dysfunction

One major element in post-CPB bleeding is abnormal platelet function, brought about by passage of platelets through the bypass circuit.[58, 205, 206] Immediately after CPB, platelets are less responsive to ADP and collagen and do not adhere well to glass beads.[207]

Platelet factor 4 and β-thromboglobulin, released when platelets are activated, continue to rise during CPB.[208] P-selectin, a marker for release of alpha granules, also confirms ongoing platelet activation during CPB.[209] Significant reductions in platelet GPIIb/IIIa receptor populations (fibrinogen receptor) during and after CPB have been reported in some studies and not in others.[203, 209, 210] In addition, the response of the platelet GPIb receptor (vWF receptor) to CPB is variable.[210] Extended surgical dissections, increased trauma to tissues, and prolonged surgical procedures further enhance platelet activation and may contribute to fibrinolysis and platelet dysfunction.[211, 212] Activated platelets degranulate and attract additional platelets, coagulation proteins, and inflammatory mediators. Atherosclerotic cardiovascular disease has complex interactions with the thrombotic, fibrinolytic, and inflammatory processes.[213] Patients with peripheral atherosclerosis have enhanced platelet reactivity, which is further enhanced by surgical interventions.[214] Progressive platelet activation and subsequent loss of platelet operation or functional platelets is a plausible cause of the coagulopathy associated with CPB. The exact mechanism of this loss of platelet operation is unknown.

The Role of von Willebrand Factor During Cardiac Surgery

vWF participates in hemostasis by mediating the adhesion of platelets to exposed subendothelial and adventitial surfaces and by promoting the formation of platelet thrombi at sites of vascular injury. Both surgery and CPB cause a progressive rise in systemic vWF levels.[215] Smaller multimeric forms of vWF circulate and larger multimers are found in endothelial cells, platelets, and blood vessels.[216] The appearance of larger multimers can be demonstrated in the circulation after acute release induced by stimuli and may result in aggregation of platelets in vivo.[217] The larger multimers of vWF have higher-affinity binding sites and support initial platelet adhesion.[215] The relative contribution of the various vWF multimers to hemostasis after CPB is unknown. The loss of the largest vWF multimers may be of primary importance in the pathogenesis of CPB-induced platelet dysfunction. Recently, a reduced level of vWF was correlated with increased bleeding in patients undergoing CPB.[218] It is thought that CPB induces a vWF disease–like state, with lower levels of vWF a possible mechanism for excessive post-CPB bleeding.[219] Under surgical and CPB conditions some of the platelet and plasma vWF multimers may have a greater role in hemostasis compared to normal. The impact of these various multimers in the setting of CPB is unknown. By documenting the specific nature of the platelet adhesion and aggregation defect associated with CPB, specific clinical interventions and options can be explored.

Transfusion Algorithms May Reduce Transfusion Requirements

Routine coagulation tests (platelet count, PT, APTT) can guide therapy and treatment of microvascular (nonsurgical) bleeding. Incorporated into transfusion algorithms, they have been somewhat effective in reducing blood transfusion.[111, 112]

The transfusion algorithms thus far proposed, however, are complex, not user-friendly, and have limited clinical application.[112, 189] Furthermore, few measurements of platelet function have been included in the algorithms. Platelet count does not correlate with platelet function and is inherently insensitive and nonspecific for predicting bleeding post CPB.[220, 221] In addition, controlled trials of prophylactic platelet transfusion have not demonstrated benefit for patients undergoing CPB.[187]

Vascular Surgery

Most vascular surgery patients are elderly, have generalized atherosclerosis, and have limited physiologic compensatory mechanisms. Most of these patients are taking multiple medications, including aspirin or other antithrombotic agents, and virtually all have diminished platelet function, prolonged bleeding times, and increased risk of perioperative bleeding.[222] The technique and material utilized for vascular surgery procedures are the basis for hemostasis after completion of a vascular anastomosis. Careful balance must be achieved in the immediate postoperative period between thrombosis of a native vessel during clamping and vascular reconstruction and uncontrolled bleeding after restoration of blood flow through the repaired or replaced vascular segment. Acute massive blood loss occurs in rare situations and should be managed as outlined below. Many clinicians advocate the use of a modified transfusion trigger in patients with vascular diseases as compared to other patient populations.[223]

Massive Transfusion

Massive blood transfusion, defined as transfusion of at least 1 blood volume within 24 hours, occurs in many surgical and critical care settings. In addition to the underlying pathophysiology, the transfusion of massive amounts of blood and fluids can cause morbidity. The goal of blood component therapy is to maintain circulation and oxygen transport while avoiding deficiencies of hemostatic factors. Massively transfused patients may require replacement of specific hemostatic factors, including platelets, plasma coagulation factors, or fibrinogen.

Neither whole blood nor PRBCs stored for more than 24 hours contain viable platelets. Furthermore, some dilutional effects are expected during massive transfusion because of these deficiencies. Stored whole blood contains relatively normal levels of most plasma coagulation factors with the exception of the labile coagulation factors V and VIII. However, of interest is the fact that the variability in platelet counts among massively transfused patients cannot be fully explained by simple hemodilution alone.[224] The correlation of the duration of hypotension in massively transfused patients with the development of coagulation abnormalities indirectly suggests that consumption of coagulation factors contributes to the coagulopathy associated with massive transfusion.[225] Significant thrombocytopenia frequently develops after transfusion of 15 to 20 U of whole blood or PRBCs.[226] Significant prolongation of the PT and APTT frequently develops in patients who receive 10 to 12 U or more of RBCs.[226, 227]

Currently, there is no justification for the prophylactic use of platelets or FFP in massively transfused patients.[224] However, transfusion of coagulation components should be guided by frequent monitoring of coagulation laboratory assays (platelet count, PT, APTT, TT, fibrinogen, or TEG) and by signs of clinical coagulopathy.

Liver Transplantation

Patients presenting for orthotopic liver transplantation (OLT) may have abnormalities of the coagulation system, including prolonged PT, APTT, and bleeding time, as well as coagulation factor deficiencies and thrombocytopenia.[228] An ongoing state of fibrinolysis may also be present.[229] During OLT, the most dramatic changes in the coagulation profile are seen at the time of organ reperfusion, including elevation of the PT and APTT, thrombocytopenia, decreased platelet aggregation, and fibrinolysis.[230-235]

Fibrinolysis

Fibrinolysis is a common occurrence in patients with advanced liver disease. Fletcher et al.[229] reported that patients with cirrhosis who were given 100 mg of IV nicotinic acid had an increase in plasma fibrinolytic activity that was two to three times that of normal controls and persisted 2 to 4 hours; the plasma thrombolytic activity in controls returned to normal within 1 hour.

Lewis et al.[236] found significantly shortened euglobulin lysis times (ELTs), which indicates increased fibrinolysis, in 99 patients undergoing OLT, the most dramatic change occurring during reperfusion of the transplanted liver. Fibrinolysis was documented at least once intraoperatively during 80 operations and was most severe in the pre-anhepatic stage in 21 patients, during the anhepatic stage in 19 patients, and in the post-anhepatic stage in 40 patients. Thirty-three patients had the most severe fibrinolysis immediately following reperfusion. Harper et al.[237] reported a rise in D-dimer, reflecting fibrinolysis, in 13 of 14 patients undergoing OLT; from a mean of 220 ng/mL the mean increase was 70 ng/mL immediately following reperfusion, and 6 patients had a mean rise of 220 ng/mL at 1 hour following reperfusion of the graft. Using whole-blood clot lysis time (WBCLT), which is determined by TEG as well as by ELT, Porte et al.[235] divided 20 patients into two groups as having minimal fibrinolysis (n = 7) or severe fibrinolysis (n = 13). Those patients who had severe fibrinolysis had an increase in t-PA that was seen during the anhepatic stage and more than doubled abruptly upon reperfusion of the graft. There was a concomitant decrease in PAI activity, and subsequent increases in fibrinogen and fibrin degradation products (FDPs).

Himmelreich et al.[231] demonstrated decreased platelet aggregation to ADP, collagen, and ristocetin in 10 patients undergoing OLT that began at the anhepatic phase and became marked at reperfusion. The median platelet count of these patients was also significantly reduced at reperfusion. Schalm et al.[238] reported prolonged bleeding time without concomitant thrombocytopenia in nine dogs following liver transplantation. Kalpokas et al.[239] reported a significant reduction in the mean platelet count in 13 patients undergoing OLT.

Platelet activation and platelet adhesive and aggregatory membrane receptors in patients undergoing OLT have not been characterized. Platelet function is affected by fibrinolysis and the action of FDPs,[240, 241] and by plasmin, which can activate platelets[242-244] and alter platelet membrane GPs.[245-247] Other mechanisms could be involved, such as exposure to extracorporeal circuits involved in venovenous bypass.[248-249] Bleeding attributed to platelet dysfunction caused by exposure to extracorporeal circuits is seen in the setting of CPB.

Blood Loss and Transfusion Requirements

Rettke et al.[250] reported mean transfusion requirements of 14.8 U of PRBCs, 13.7 U of platelets, 10.5 U of FFP, and 12.3 U of cryoprecipitate in 83 patients who underwent OLT. In a group of 14 low-risk patients, Harper et al.[237] reported a mean blood loss of 3705 mL (range, 1249 to 8546 mL), and mean transfusion requirements of 6.0 U of PRBCs, 4.2 U of FFP, and all patients save one received 6.0 U of platelets. Lewis et al.[230] reported a mean blood product usage of 25 U of PRBCs, 24 U of FFP, 20 U of platelets, and 9 U of cryoprecipitate in 366 adult liver transplant patients.

Monitoring Blood Loss and Autologous Blood Salvage

Some measures of perioperative coagulation function are quite subjective. Autologous blood salvage can result in retransfusion of a large quantity of RBCs that are deficient in any coagulant factors or platelets and that, in some cases, can introduce profibrinolytic mediators with important effects on surgical patients.

Monitoring Blood Loss

Monitoring blood loss in surgical patients is an inherently subjective activity. In the OR, blood is absorbed into the sterile surgical drapes surrounding the site of incision, collected in sponges that are later discarded, or suctioned into canisters for disposal or processing and reinfusion. Traditionally, some centers have weighed or counted sponges before their disposal in an effort to quantify blood loss. Estimating blood loss that is absorbed into the sterile surgical drapes surrounding the wound is problematic and inaccurate. The most accurate way to assess surgical blood loss is to measure the volume collected in the canisters and then determine RBC mass by completing a hematocrit on the collected blood before its processing or disposal. Because there are sometimes large volumes of irrigation fluid included in this product of suction, the RBC content can be highly variable. Alternatively, if the blood is processed for reinfusion, the autologous procedure results in a 225-mL unit with a hematocrit of 45% to 65%.

In some patients it is more important to monitor the physiologic responses to blood loss than to determine or calculate circulating blood volume and the actual blood loss. Surgical blood loss, like acute hemorrhage, has an immediate impact on blood volume, cardiovascular performance, and tissue oxygen delivery. For many operative procedures blood loss is anticipated and untoward responses are avoided by appropriate volume replacement.

Acute blood loss can be considered to be mild (up to 20% of blood volume), moderate (20% to 40% of blood volume), or severe (over 40% of blood volume).

The initial response to blood loss includes increased heart rate, hyperventilation, vasoconstriction, and increased right ventricular filling. These initial responses result in an increase in cardiac output and the hyperventilation additionally increases arterial hemoglobin saturation. The second response to acute hemorrhage is aimed at restoration of blood pressure by means of secretion of vasoactive hormones and catecholamines. Third, a redistribution of water from the extravascular to intravascular space results in an increase in circulating blood or plasma volume.

Monitoring for acute signs of hypovolemia, including hypotension and tachycardia, are very important in the perioperative period. Monitoring for any additional signs of ischemia (cerebral or myocardial) may be of great benefit (see Chapters 8 and 12). Monitoring urine output and right atrial or pulmonary artery pressures will also help gauge the degree of hemodynamic compromise.

Monitoring Autologous Blood Salvage

Autologous blood transfusion involves the harvesting of blood or blood products for subsequent administration to the same patient. Autologous transfusion was originally used to secure blood replacement when circumstances made conventional transfusion of banked blood impossible. However, safety has become the driving force behind further development and implementation of autologous transfusion procedures.

In 1968, Wilson and Taswell[251] introduced a new apparatus that permitted blood collection, processing, washing, and reinfusion in a continuous process. This development rapidly transformed intraoperative salvage techniques. With this apparatus, blood was collected from the surgical field via a suction aspirator; the blood was then fed into a continuous-flow centrifugation bowl in which the RBCs were selectively separated and extracted from the waste supernatant. These washed RBCs were then resuspended for infusion back to the patient. In 1970, Klebanoff[252] introduced a modified disposable autotransfusion apparatus that was considered to be safe, simple, and efficient. Further refinements in the development of washing with intermittent flow centrifugation devices resulted in a decrease in the coagulopathy associated with intraoperative blood salvage. The removal of thromboplastic material by washing decreased the hemorrhagic complications but also resulted in removing all plasma proteins, including procoagulants.[253, 254] For safety, contemporary autotransfusion practices rely on a combination of reservoirs for collection and washing procedures.

Salvaged blood is known to have low initial hematocrits, elevated free hemoglobin, decreased coagulation factors, increased FDPs, and significant amounts of anticoagulant.[255] Before processing, the hematocrit of shed blood is typically 20% to 30%, with lower levels seen in orthopedic cases[255] and in the later stages of postoperative drainage.[256] Cell salvage instruments can increase the hematocrits to 45% to 65%. Some hemolysis of RBCs occurs secondary to surgical trauma and aspiration from the wound. Resultant free hemoglobin levels are commonly less than 300 mg/dL but may be as high as 2000 mg/dL.[257] Despite these high levels of free hemoglobin, RBC indices and morphology are normal. Washing can remove most free hemoglobin while producing only mild morphologic changes in RBCs. Both processed and unprocessed salvaged RBCs have been shown to have acceptable survival in vivo.[258-260] Variable numbers of platelets and white blood cells (WBCs) are present in salvaged blood. With processing, platelet counts decrease and platelet and WBC function are impaired.

Because thrombosis and fibrinolysis are activated during and after operations, shed blood contains decreased amounts of coagulation factors and increased levels of FDPs.[261] Fibrinogen levels are typically very low in mediastinal and joint drainage; such blood does not usually clot and anticoagulation may not be needed during collection. Concern about the reinfusion of unwashed salvaged blood has focused on the potential of FDPs to initiate coagulopathy. de Haan and colleagues[262] have also suggested that fibrin monomers and t-PA–stimulating activity in shed mediastinal blood potentiate the platelet dysfunction seen after CPB and lead to increased postoperative bleeding. Processing salvaged chest tube blood will further decrease coagulation factors but also effectively remove FDPs and fibrin.

Schaff et al.[263] studied patients receiving shed mediastinal blood and control subjects and found no difference between the groups in PT, APTT, fibrinogen, and FDPs. Others have found increases in fibrinolytic products in the reinfused blood, but the effect on patients was transient.[261] Griffith et al.[264] found extremely high titers of FDPs in mediastinal blood. They compared the level of FDPs in mediastinal blood that was both washed and unwashed. FDP titers were significantly elevated in the unwashed mediastinal blood, but no differences were found in the bleeding or coagulation values of the patients.

Unprocessed blood has also been shown to contain elevated levels of C3a, C5a, and terminal complement complexes[265]; an altered lipid profile; measurable amounts of methyl methacrylate (orthopedic bone cement); and fat particles.[266] The presence of these materials raises concern regarding the safety of infusing unwashed salvaged blood. Faris et al.[267] reported a 22% incidence of febrile reactions accompanying the transfusion of unwashed autologous blood that was collected from joint drainage 6 to 12 hours after operation. However, unprocessed shed blood has been administered to many groups of patients in numerous studies with minimal ill effects. Much of this success may be related to the limited amount of unprocessed blood that is infused (usually <1 L) and to the limited collection periods (usually <6 hours).

Clinical Applications

Blood salvage has been applied most extensively in cardiac operations, such as CABG, valve replacement, repair of congenital heart disease, and other complex cardiac surgical procedures. Blood is typically collected intraoperatively and washed before reinfusion; blood from the CPB circuit may be added to the salvaged blood. As documented by Giordano and colleagues,[268] significant amounts of autologous blood can be harvested in this manner. In their review of 6 years of experience an equivalent of over 3 U of RBCs can be salvaged, with 59% coming from the operative field, 34% from the CPB circuit, and less than 10% from postoperative drainage. Larger amounts of blood are collected in reoperations and in combined CABG and valve replacement operations. Multiple studies have suggested that the use of intraoperative[269-272] and postoperative[272, 273] blood salvage significantly decreased allogeneic transfusion requirements.

Orthopedic surgeons have also been using perioperative blood salvage for spinal operations and hip and knee arthroplasties. In orthopedic procedures, smaller amounts of blood are lost over a longer period of time, and the collected blood contains tissue and bone debris, fat, and methyl methacrylate.

Significant amounts of autologous blood have also been salvaged in vascular, liver transplant, neurosurgical, and trauma operations.[274] Although aortic aneurysm repair commonly uses cell salvage instruments to provide for greater than 50% of the transfusion needs of these patients,[275, 276] reinfusion of unprocessed shed blood has also been reported to be effective.[277] Surgeons performing aortic bifemoral bypass grafting procedures frequently use intraoperative blood salvage, but its efficacy in this setting has recently been questioned.[278] During liver transplantation procedures, blood loss can be both rapid and massive. High-speed cell salvage instruments have been used to provide an average of 4 to 9 U of RBCs per case and 29% to 45% of intraoperative transfusion needs.[279-281] In these instances, blood salvage plays an important role in conserving the allogeneic blood supply. In neurosurgery, shed blood can be salvaged during resection of intracranial arteriovenous malformations. An average of 3.1 U and as much as 16 U have been washed, concentrated, and reinfused in these cases.[282]

Contraindications and Complications

Conditions thought to be contraindications to blood salvage include the use of microfibrillar collagen materials and infection or malignancy at the operative site. Microfibrillar collagen is not removed from the salvaged blood during the washing procedure, and infusion of units containing this material has caused significant morbidity and mortality in animals.[283] Microfibrillar collagen is also not completely removed by passage through the typical 20-μm filter,[284, 285] but recent evidence suggests that WBC depletion filters do eliminate this compound.[285]

Washing of salvaged blood does not reliably remove contaminating microorganisms. Therefore, aspiration of blood from an infected wound or one contaminated by bowel contents has been considered a risk for subsequent sepsis. However, blood salvage, usually with the concurrent administration of broad-spectrum antibiotics, has been used successfully in penetrating abdominal injuries.[286, 287] Even when obtaining cultures from obviously noninfected operative sites, a significant number of routine surveillance cultures of salvaged blood from a wide variety of surgical procedures will be positive. The vast majority of these cases involve very low numbers of organisms (<1 to 2 colony-forming units [CFU]/mL), which are recognized as skin and environmental contaminants (coagulase-negative staphylococci, diphtheroids, and other nonpathogens).[288-291] Clinical infections resulting from the infusion of culture-positive salvaged blood have not been seen.

Malignant cells are also known to survive processing and routine filtering of salvaged blood.[292-295] No consistent correlation exists between the presence of circulating tumor cells and subsequent metastatic disease[296]; furthermore, there have been no reports of cancer dissemination secondary to hematogenous spread by intraoperatively salvaged blood. Studies of the application of blood salvage procedures in urologic cancer operations are ongoing and, thus far, have shown no evidence of increased malignancy recurrence or dissemination.[297, 298] Similar favorable results have been seen in cases of hepatic malignancies[299] and in renal carcinomas with intravascular extension.[279]

Antibiotics not intended for IV use may also end up in salvaged blood if irrigating solutions are aspirated into the collection reservoirs. Topical antibiotics placed in orthopedic wounds can also reach significant levels in postoperative drainage intended for direct reinfusion.[300] Blood salvaged during removal of pheochromocytomas has been shown to cause hypertension in patients after reinfusion,[301] because extensive washing does not eliminate epinephrine and norepinephrine. The direct reinfusion of shed mediastinal blood has been associated with increased serum enzymes (creatine kinase, lactate dehydrogenase, aspartate aminotransferase), and myoglobin and troponin levels in patients undergoing cardiac operations.[302, 303] These elevated laboratory parameters may obscure the diagnosis of postoperative myocardial ischemia. The myocardial band (MB) fraction of creatine kinase is not elevated, however.

The development of clinically significant coagulopathy after infusion of salvaged blood has been a persistent concern. Although it occurred frequently in the past with the administration of large volumes of unwashed blood, coagulopathy is much less common now that modern cell salvage instruments are in use. However, dilutional coagulopathy may still be seen in patients receiving large amounts of washed RBCs. Yawn[304] reported consistent decreases in platelet counts and coagulation factor levels when more than 6 U of washed RBCs were given to patients undergoing complex aortic aneurysm repairs. Moderate to severe abnormalities in PT and PTT were seen in 31% of trauma patients in one large series.[305] In these patients, the coagulopathies developed in patients undergoing massive transfusion (>15 U of salvaged and washed blood, >10 U of salvaged and washed blood in patients with bowel injuries, or > 50 units of salvaged and allogeneic blood). Frank DIC has also been noted, even in patients receiving only 1 to 2 U of salvaged and washed RBCs.[306]

Bull and Bull[307] described the salvaged blood syndrome in which patients develop manifestations of increased capillary permeability (such as adult respiratory distress syndrome or anasarca), intravascular coagulation, or a combination of these complications. Fortunately, salvaged blood syndrome is rare. In some cases of coagulopathy, additional factors such as acidosis, hypotension, hypothermia, and tissue trauma may contribute to the hemostatic abnormalities. Many of these patients require supplemental transfusions of platelets and FFP.

In summary, the ultimate goal of perioperative blood salvage is to minimize the use of allogeneic blood products by providing autologous blood for transfusion. Recent debate has now shifted to the cost-effectiveness of the procedure. For procedures using dedicated cell salvage instruments, that point is 2 to 4 U of salvaged blood.[276, 308] For canister- or reservoir-based systems with subsequent processing it is around 2 U,[308, 309] and for direct reinfusion devices it may be as low as 1 U.[310] One recent retrospective study of patients with spinal operations[311] suggests no benefit with the use of blood salvage when preoperatively donated autologous blood is available in sufficient quantities. Each institution will also have to perform its own cost-benefit analyses when examining the effectiveness of specific autologous programs.

Blood Supply: Cost-Benefit Issues

Each year in the United States, 12 million units of RBCs are transfused in patients at a direct societal cost of $2 billion.[232, 312] Approximately $2 billion is also spent annually on the diagnosis, treatment, and long-term care of transfusion complications.[233]

The U.S. blood supply faces major challenges associated with an aging population and potentially inadequate rates of volunteer donation by healthy citizens.[232, 234, 235, 238] Increasing clinical demands on the banked blood pool may surpass supplies within 10 years. At present rates of RBC utilization, the elderly population alone will require 12 to 13 million units of RBCs per year by the year 2030.[232] If present donation patterns in the United States remain constant, a shortfall of 4 million U of RBCs is projected in the year 2030. While RBC transfusion has leveled out, platelet transfusion continues to grow, placing accelerated demands on the banked blood supply.[249]

Conclusion

The perioperative assessment of coagulation and platelet function, much like hemostasis and thrombosis, is a complex and dynamic process. The use of a single assay or device or even a series of assays provides only partial assessment. In order to provide a specific and appropriate diagnosis, the clinician must observe the surgical field, understand the nature of the pre-existing and ongoing coagulation or hemostatic insult, predict the future insult, and then integrate the results of coagulation or platelet function assays. The integration of both subjective and objective information will then allow the clinician to institute the appropriate pharmacologic or blood product therapy. Perhaps even more important, the summation of all of this information may justify not instituting any therapy in those instances in which the hemostatic insult is limited and it is best to do nothing.

ACKNOWLEDGMENTS

We thank Theresa Hanson for her assistance with manuscript preparation and Ms. Christine Welch for computer graphics.

REFERENCES

1. Mason RG, Sharp D, Chuang HY, et al: The endothelium: Roles in thrombosis and hemostasis. Arch Pathol Lab Med 1977; 101:61–64.
2. Furlong B, Henderson AH, Lewis MJ, et al: Endothelium-derived relaxing factor inhibits in vitro platelet aggregation. Br J Pharmacol 1987; 90:687–692.
3. Griffith TM, Edwards DH, Lewis MJ, et al: The nature of endothelium-derived vascular relaxant factor. Nature 1984; 308:645–647.
4. Hirsh J: Heparin. N Engl J Med 1991; 324:1565–1574.
5. Azuma H, Ishikawa M, Sekizaki S: Endothelium-dependent inhibition of platelet aggregation. Br J Pharmacol 1986; 88:411–415.
6. Mollace V, Salvemini D, Sessa WC, et al: Inhibition of human platelet aggregation by endothelium-derived relaxing factor, sodium nitroprusside or iloprost is potentiated by captopril and reduced thiols. J Pharmacol Exp Ther 1991; 258:820–823.
7. Marcus AJ, Safier LB, Hajjar KA, et al: Inhibition of platelet function by an aspirin-insensitive endothelial cell ADPase. Thromboregulation by endothelial cells. J Clin Invest 1991; 88:1690–1696.
8. Marcus AJ, Broekman MJ, Drosopoulos JH, et al: The endothelial cell ecto-ADPase responsible for inhibition of platelet function is CD39. J Clin Invest 1997; 99:1351–1360.
9. Kunicki TJ, Newman PJ, Amrani DL, et al: Human platelet fibrinogen: Purification and hemostatic properties. Blood 1985; 66:808–815.
10. Furchgott RF, Zawadzki JV: The obligatory role of endothelial cells in the relaxation of arterial smooth muscle by acetylcholine. Nature 1980; 288:373–376.
11. Vanhoutte PM, Lüscher TF, Gräser T: Endothelium-dependent contractions. Blood Vessels 1991; 28:74–83.
12. Colman RW, Cook JJ, Niewiarowski S: Mechanisms of platelet aggregation. In Colman RW, Hirsh J, Marder VJ, et al (eds): Hemostasis and Thrombosis: Basic Principles and Clinical Practice, ed 3. Philadelphia, JB Lippincott, 1994, pp 508–523.
13. Kunicki TJ: Platelet membrane glycoproteins and their function: An overview. Blut 1989; 59:30–34.
14. Furie B, Furie BC: Molecular and cellular biology of blood coagulation. N Engl J Med 1992; 326:800–806.
15. Phillips DR, Charo IF, Scarborough RM: GPIIb-IIIa: The responsive integrin. Cell 1991; 65:359–362.
16. Salvesen G, Pizzo SV: Proteinase inhibitors: α-Macroglobulins, serpins, and kunins. In Colman RW, Hirsh J, Marder VJ, et al (eds): Hemostasis and Thrombosis: Basic Principles and Clinical Practice, ed 3. Philadelphia, JB Lippincott, 1994, pp 241–258.
17. Broze GJ, Miletich JP: Biochemistry and physiology of protein C, protein S, and thrombomodulin. In Colman RW, Hirsh J, Marder VJ, et al (eds): Hemostasis and Thrombosis: Basic Principles and Clinical Practice, ed 3. Philadelphia, JB Lippincott, 1994, pp 259–276.
18. Pisciotto P, Benson K, Hume H, et al: Prophylactic versus therapeutic platelet transfusion practices in hematology and/or oncology patients. Transfusion 1995; 35:498–502.
19. McLean J: The thromboplastic action of cephalin. Am J Physiol 1916; 41:250–257.
20. Brinkhous K, Smith H, Warner E, et al: The inhibition of blood clotting: An unidentified substance which acts in conjunction with heparin to prevent the conversion of prothrombin into thrombin. Am J Physiol 1939; 125:683–687.
21. Clagett GP, Anderson FA Jr, Heit J, et al: Prevention of venous thromboembolism. Chest 1995; 108:312S–334S.
22. Horlocker TT, Heit JA: Low molecular weight heparin: Biochemistry, pharmacology, perioperative prophylaxis regimens, and guidelines for regional anesthetic management. Anesth Analg 1997; 85:874–885.
23. Kessler CM, Esparraguera IM, Jacobs HM, et al: Monitoring the anticoagulant effects of a low molecular weight heparin preparation: Correlation of assays in orthopedic surgery patients receiving ardeparin sodium for prophylaxis of deep venous thrombosis. Am J Clin Pathol 1995; 103:642–648.
24. Dam H: The antihaemorrhagic vitamin of the chick. Occurrence and chemical nature. Nature 1935; 135:652.
25. Link K: The discovery of dicumarol and its sequels. Circulation 1959; 19:97.
26. Stenflo J, Ferlund P, Egan W, et al: Vitamin K dependent modification of glutamic acid residues in prothrombin. Proc Natl Acad Sci U S A 1974; 71:2730–2733.
27. Hirsh J, Dalen JE, Anderson DR, et al: Oral anticoagulants: Mechanism of action, clinical effectiveness, and optimal therapeutic range. Chest 1998; 114:445S–469S.
28. Tinker J, Tarhan S: Discontinuing anticoagulant therapy in surgical patients with cardiac valve prosthesis. Observations in 180 operations. JAMA 1978; 239:738–739.
29. Weitz JI, Hudoba M, Massel D: Clot-bound thrombin is protected from inhibition by heparin-antithrombin III but is susceptible to inactivation by antithrombin III-independent inhibitors. J Clin Invest 1990; 86:385–391.
30. Collins R, Peto R, Baigent C, et al: Aspirin, heparin, and fibrinolytic therapy in suspected acute myocardial infarction. N Engl J Med 1997; 336:847–860.
31. Lijnen HR, Collen D: Development of new fibrinolytic agents. In Colman RW, Hirsh J, Marden VJ, et al (eds): Hemostasis and Thrombosis: Basic Principles and Clinical Practice, ed 3. Philadelphia, JB Lippincott, 1994, pp 625–637.
32. Fitzgerald DJ, Catella F, Roy L, et al: Marked platelet activation in vivo after intravenous streptokinase in patients with acute myocardial infarction. Circulation 1988; 77:142–150.
33. The GUSTO Investigators: An international randomized trial comparing four thrombolytic strategies for acute myocardial infarction. GUSTO-Global utilization of streptokinase and tissue plasminogen activator for occluded coronary arteries. N Engl J Med 1993; 329:673–682.
34. Vane J: Inhibition of prostaglandin biosynthesis as a mechanism of action of aspirin-like drugs. Nature 1971; 231:232–235.
35. Weksler BB, Pett SB, Alonso D, et al: Differential inhibition by aspirin of vascular and platelet prostaglandin synthesis in atherosclerotic patients. N Engl J Med 1983; 308:800–805.
36. CAPRIE Steering Committee: A randomized, blinded trial of clopidogrel versus aspirin in patients at risk of ischemic events. Lancet 1996; 348:1329–1339.
37. Coller BS: A new murine monoclonal antibody reports an activation-dependent change in the conformation and/or microenvironment of the platelet glycoprotein IIb/IIIa complex. J Clin Invest 1985; 76:101–108.
38. Coller BS, Scudder LE: Inhibition of dog platelet function by invivo infusion of F(ab')$_2$ fragments of a monoclonal antibody to the platelet glycoprotein IIb/IIIa receptor. Blood 1985; 66:1456–1469.

39. Ellis SG, Tcheng JT, Navetta FL, et al: Safety and antiplatelet effect of murine monoclonal antibody 7E3 Fab directed against platelet glycoprotein IIb/IIIa in patients undergoing elective coronary angioplasty. Coron Artery Dis 1993; 4:167–175.

40. The EPIC Investigators: Use of a monoclonal antibody directed against the platelet glycoprotein IIb/IIIa receptor in high-risk coronary angioplasty. N Engl J Med 1994; 330:956–961.

41. Topol E, Califf R, Weisman H, et al: Randomized trial of coronary intervention with antibody against platelet IIb/IIIa integrin for reduction of clinical restenosis: Results at six months. Lancet 1994; 343:881–886.

42. Tcheng JE: Platelet glycoprotein IIb/IIIa integrin blockade: Recent clinical trials in interventional cardiology. Thromb Haemost 1997; 78:205–209.

43. Moliterno DJ, Topol EJ: Conjunctive use of platelet glycoprotein IIb/IIIa receptor antagonists and thrombolytic therapy for acute myocardial infarction. Thromb Haemost 1997; 78:214–219.

44. Tcheng JE: Glycoprotein IIb/IIIa receptor inhibitors: Putting the EPIC, IMPACT II, RESTORE, and EPILOG trials into perspective. Am J Cardiol 1996; 78:35–40.

45. Coller BS: Blockade of platelet GPIIb/IIIa receptors as an antithrombotic strategy. Circulation 1995; 92:2373–2380.

46. George JN, Shattil SJ: The clinical importance of acquired abnormalities of platelet function. N Engl J Med 1991; 324:27–39.

47. Addonizio VP, Jr., Fisher CA, Kappa JR, et al: Prevention of heparin-induced thrombocytopenia during heart surgery with iloprost (ZK36374). Surgery 1987; 102:796–807.

48. Janssens M, Hartstein G, David JL: Reduction in requirements for allogeneic blood products: Pharmacologic methods. Ann Thorac Surg 1996; 62:1944–1950.

49. Kraut E, Frey E, Werle E: Über die Inaktivierung des Kallikreins. Z Physiol Chem 1930; 192:1–21.

50. Royston D: The serine antiprotease aprotinin (Trasylol): A novel approach to reducing postoperative bleeding. Blood Coagul Fibrinolysis 1990; 1:55–69.

51. Westaby S: Aprotinin in perspective. Ann Thorac Surg 1993; 55:1033–1041.

52. Royston D: High-dose aprotinin therapy: A review of the first five years' experience. J Cardiothorac Vasc Anesth 1992; 6:76–100.

53. Neuhaus P, Bechstein WO, Lefebre B, et al: Effect of aprotinin on intraoperative bleeding and fibrinolysis in liver transplantation (letter). Lancet 1989; 2:924–925.

54. Mallett SV, Cox D, Burroughs AK, et al: Aprotinin and reduction of blood loss and transfusion requirements in orthotopic liver transplantation (letter). Lancet 1990; 336:886–887.

55. Thompson JF, Roath OS, Francis JL, et al: Aprotinin in peripheral vascular surgery. Lancet 1990; 335:911.

56. Janssens M, Joris J, David JL, et al: High-dose aprotinin reduces blood loss in patients undergoing total hip replacement surgery. Anesthesiology 1994; 80:23–29.

57. Tanaka K, Takao M, Yada I, et al: Alterations in coagulation and fibrinolysis associated with cardiopulmonary bypass during open heart surgery. J Cardiothorac Vasc Anesth 1989; 3:181–188.

58. Harker LA, Malpass TW, Branson HE, et al: Mechanism of abnormal bleeding in patients undergoing cardiopulmonary bypass: Acquired transient platelet dysfunction associated with selective α-granule release. Blood 1980; 56:824–834.

59. Nagaoka H, Innami R, Murayama F, et al: Effects of aprotinin on prostaglandin metabolism and platelet function in open heart surgery. J Cardiothorac Surg 1991; 32:31–37.

60. van Oeveren W, Eijsman L, Roozendaal KJ, et al: Platelet preservation by aprotinin during cardiopulmonary bypass. Lancet 1988; 1:644.

61. Tice DA, Worth MH, Clauss RH, et al: The inhibition by Trasylol of fibrinolytic activity associated with cardiovascular operations. Surg Gynecol Obstet 1964; 119:71–74.

62. van Oeveren W, Harder MP, Roozendaal KJ, et al: Aprotinin protects platelets against the initial effect of cardiopulmonary bypass. J Cardiovasc Surg 1990; 99:788–797.

63. Wendel HP, Heller W, Gallimore MJ, et al: The prolonged activated clotting time (ACT) with aprotinin depends on the type of activator used for measurement. Blood Coagul Fibrinolysis 1993; 4:41–45.

64. Lemmer JH, Stanford W, Bonney SL, et al: Aprotinin for coronary bypass operations: Efficacy, safety, and influence on early saphenous vein graft patency. A multicenter, randomized, double-blind, placebo-controlled study. J Thorac Cardiovasc Surg 1994; 107:543–553.

65. Dietrich W, Spath P, Ebell A, et al: Prevalence of anaphylactic reactions to aprotinin: Analysis of two hundred forty-eight reexposures to aprotinin in heart operations. J Thorac Cardiovasc Surg 1997; 113:194–201.

66. Lemmer JH, Stanford W, Bonney SL, et al: Aprotinin for coronary artery bypass grafting: Effect on postoperative renal function. Ann Thorac Surg 1995; 59:132–136.

67. Levy JH, Pifarre R, Schaff HV, et al: A multicenter, double-blind, placebo-controlled trial of aprotinin for reducing blood loss and the requirement for donor-blood transfusion in patients undergoing repeat coronary artery bypass grafting. Circulation 1995; 92:2236–2244.

68. Horrow JC, Hlavacek J, Strong MD, et al: Prophylactic tranexamic acid decreases bleeding after cardiac operations. J Thorac Cardiovasc Surg 1990; 99:70–74.

69. Horrow JC, Van Riper DF, Strong MD, et al: Hemostatic effects of tranexamic acid and desmopressin during cardiac surgery. Circulation 1991; 84:2063–2070.

70. Verstraete M: Clinical application of inhibitors of fibrinolysis. Drugs 1985; 29:236–261.

71. Bailey K, Karski J, Joiner R, et al: Comparison of the effect of 3 different doses of tranexamic acid on postoperative bleeding in cardiac surgery performed without active systemic cooling (abstract). Anesthesiology 1994; 81:A91.

72. Stern NS, Catone GA: Primary fibrinolysis after oral surgery. J Oral Surg 1975; 33:49–52.

73. Schisano G: The use of antifibrinolytic drugs in aneurysmal subarachnoid hemorrhage. Surg Neurol 1978; 10:217–222.

74. Sindet-Pedersen S, Ramstrom G, Bernvil S, et al: Hemostatic effect of tranexamic acid mouthwash in anticoagulant-treated patients undergoing oral surgery. N Engl J Med 1989; 320:840–843.

75. Auvinen O, Baer GA, Nordback I, et al: Antifibrinolytic therapy for prevention of hemorrhage during surgery of the thyroid gland. Klin Wochenschr 1987; 65:253–255.

76. Smith RB, Riach P, Kaufman JJ: Epsilon aminocaproic acid and the control of post-prostatectomy bleeding: A prospective double-blind study. J Urol 1984; 131:1093–1095.

77. Karski JM, Teasdale SJ, Norman PH, et al: Prevention of postbypass bleeding with tranexamic acid and epsilon-aminocaproic acid. J Cardiothorac Vasc Anesth 1993; 7:431–435.

78. Kang Y, Lewis JH, Navalgund A, et al: Epsilon-aminocaproic acid for treatment of fibrinolysis during liver transplantation. Anesthesiology 1987; 66:766–773.

79. Bennett-Guerrero E, Sorohan JG, Gurevich ML, et al: Cost-benefit and efficacy of aprotinin compared with epsilon-aminocaproic acid in patients having repeated cardiac operations: A randomized, blinded clinical trial. Anesthesiology 1997; 87:1373–1380.

80. Harmon DE: Cost/benefit analysis of pharmacologic hemostasis. Ann Thorac Surg 1996; 61:S21–25.

81. Yost CS: Clinical utility and cost effectiveness of aprotinin to reduce operative bleeding: comparison with other antifibrinolytics. Am J Anesthesiol 1996; 23:233–241.

82. Weinstein RE, Bona RD, Altman AJ, et al: Severe hyponatremia after repeated intravenous administration of desmopressin. Am J Hematol 1989; 32:258–261.

83. Salmenpera M, Kuitunen A, Hynynen M, et al: Hemodynamic responses to desmopressin acetate after CABG: A double-blind trial. J Cardiothorac Vasc Anesth 1991; 5:146–149.

84. Reich DL, Hammerschlag BC, Rand JH, et al: Desmopressin acetate is a mild vasodilator that does not reduce blood loss in uncomplicated cardiac surgical procedures. J Cardiothorac Vasc Anesth 1991; 5:142–145.

85. Jahr JS, Marquez J, Cottington E, et al: Hemodynamic performance and histamine levels after desmopressin acetate administration following cardiopulmonary bypass in adult patients. J Cardiothorac Vasc Anesth 1991; 5:139–141.

86. MacGregor IR, Roberts EM, Prowse CV, et al: Fibrinolytic and haemostatic responses to desamino-D-arginine vasopressin (DDAVP) administered by intravenous and subcutaneous routes in healthy subjects. Thromb Haemost 1988; 59:34–39.

87. Mannucci PM: Desmopressin: A nontransfusional form of treatment for congenital and acquired bleeding disorders. Blood 1988; 72:1449–1455.

88. Williamson R, Eggleston DJ: DDAVP and EACA used for minor oral surgery in von Willebrand disease. Aust Dent J 1988; 33:32–36.

89. Kobrinsky NL, Israels ED, Gerrard JM, et al: Shortening of bleeding time by 1-deamino-8-D-arginine vasopressin in various bleeding disorders. Lancet 1984; 1:1145–1148.

90. Mannucci PM, Vicente V, Vianello L, et al: Controlled trial of desmopressin in liver cirrhosis and other conditions associated with a prolonged bleeding time. Blood 1986; 67:1148–1153.

91. Chard RB, Kam CA, Nunn GR, et al: Use of desmopressin in the management of aspirin-related and intractable haemorrhage after cardiopulmonary bypass. Aust N Z J Surg 1990; 60:125–128.

92. DiMichele DM, Hathaway WE: Use of DDAVP in inherited and acquired platelet dysfunction. Am J Hematol 1990; 33:39–45.

93. Mongan PD, Hosking MP: The role of desmopressin acetate in patients undergoing coronary artery bypass surgery. A controlled clinical trial with thromboelastographic risk stratification. Anesthesiology 1992; 77:38–46.

94. Kentro TB, Lottenberg R, Kitchens CS: Clinical efficacy of desmopressin acetate for hemostatic control in patients with primary platelet disorders undergoing surgery. Am J Hematol 1987; 24:215–219.

95. Czer LS, Bateman TM, Gray RJ, et al: Treatment of severe platelet dysfunction and hemorrhage after cardiopulmonary bypass: Reduction in blood product usage with desmopressin. J Am Coll Cardiol 1987; 9:1139–1147.

96. Kobrinsky NL, Letts RM, Patel LR, et al: 1-Desamino-8-D-arginine vasopressin (desmopressin) decreases operative blood loss in patients having Harrington rod spinal fusion surgery. A randomized, double-blinded, controlled trial. Ann Intern Med 1987; 107:446–450.

97. Triplett DA: Clinical and laboratory approaches to bleeding disorders. In Triplett DA: Hemostasis: A Case Oriented Approach. New York, Igaku-Shoin, 1985, pp 61–71.

98. Carr ME, Jr: In vitro assessment of platelet function. Transfus Med Rev 1997; 11:106–115.

99. Duke W: The relation of blood platelets to hemorrhagic disease: Description of a method for determining the bleeding time and coagulation time and report of three cases of hemorrhagic disease relieved by transfusion. JAMA 1910; 55:1185–1192.

100. Ivy A, Shapiro P, Melnick P: The bleeding tendency in jaundice. Surg Gynecol Obstet 1935; 60:781–784.

101. Barber A, Green D, Galluzzo T, et al: The bleeding time as a preoperative screening test. Am J Med 1985; 78:761–764.

102. Lind SE: The bleeding time does not predict surgical bleeding. Blood 1991; 77:2547–2552.

103. Rodgers RP, Levin J: A critical reappraisal of the bleeding time. Semin Thromb Hemost 1990; 16:1–20.

104. Yardumian DA, Mackie IJ, Machin SJ: Laboratory investigation of platelet function: A review of methodology. J Clin Pathol 1986; 39:701–712.

105. Williams CE, Entwistle MB, Short PE: Platelet function tests: A critical review of methods. Med Lab Sci 1985; 42:262–274.

106. Born G: Aggregation of blood platelets by adenosine diphosphate and its reversals. Nature 1962; 194:927.

107. Cardinal DC, Flower RJ: The electric aggregometer: A novel device for assessing platelet behavior in blood. J Pharmacol Toxicol Methods 1980; 3:135–158.

108. Nichols WL, Bowie EJW: Standardization of the prothrombin time for monitoring orally administered anticoagulant therapy with use of the international normalized ratio system. Mayo Clin Proc 1993; 68:897–898.

109. O'Neill AI, McAllister C, Corke CF, et al: A comparison of five devices for the bedside monitoring of heparin therapy. Anaesth Intensive Care 1991; 19:592–596.

110. Practice guidelines for blood component therapy. A report by the American Society of Anesthesiology Task Force on blood component therapy. Anesthesiology 1996; 84:732–747.

111. Despotis GJ, Grishaber JE, Goodnough LT: The effect of an intraoperative treatment algorithm on physicians' transfusion practice in cardiac surgery. Transfusion 1994; 34:290–296.

112. Spiess BD, Gillies BS, Chandler W, et al: Changes in transfusion therapy and reexploration rate after institution of a blood management program in cardiac surgical patients. J Cardiothorac Vasc Anesth 1995; 9:168–173.

113. Bland J, Altman D: Statistical methods for assessing agreement between two methods of clinical measurement. Lancet 1986; 1:307–310.

114. Reich DL, Yanakakis MJ, Vela-Cantos FP, et al: Comparison of bedside coagulation monitoring tests with standard laboratory tests in patients after cardiac surgery. Anesth Analg 1993; 77:673–679.

115. Nuttall GA, Oliver WC Jr, Beynen FM, et al: Intraoperative measurement of activated partial thromboplastin time and prothrombin time by a portable laser photometer in patients following cardiopulmonary bypass. J Cardiothorac Vasc Anesth 1993; 7:402–409.

116. Samama C, Quezada R, Riou B, et al: Intraoperative measurement of activated partial thromboplastin time and prothrombin time with a new compact monitor. Acta Anaesthesiol Scand 1994; 38:232–237.

117. Despotis GJ, Santoro SA, Spitznagel E, et al: Prospective evaluation and clinical utility of on-site coagulation monitoring in cardiac surgical patients. J Thorac Cardiovasc Surg 1994; 107:271–279.

118. Kitchen S, Preston FE: Monitoring oral anticoagulant treatment with the TAS near-patient test system: Comparison with conventional thromboplastins. J Clin Pathol 1997; 50:951–956.

119. Cachia PG, McGregor E, Adlakha S, et al: Accuracy and precision of the TAS analyser for near-patient INR testing by non-pathology staff in the community. J Clin Pathol 1998; 51:68–72.

120. Gibbs NM, Weightman WM, Thackray NM, et al: Evaluation of the TAS coagulation analyzer for monitoring heparin effect in cardiac surgical patients. J Cardiothorac Vasc Anesth 1998; 12:536–541.

121. Ammar T, Reich DL: Bedside coagulation monitoring (editorial). J Cardiothorac Vasc Anesth 1995; 9:353–354.

122. Fareed J, Bick RL, Hoppensteadt DA, et al: Molecular markers of hemostatic activation. Implications in the diagnosis of thrombosis, vascular, and cardiovascular disorders. Clin Lab Med 1995; 15:39–61.

123. Nicholson NS, Panzer-Knodle BS, Haas NF, et al: Assessment of platelet function assays. Am Heart J 1998; 135:S170–S178.

124. Cox D: Methods for monitoring platelet function. Am Heart J 1998; 135:S160–S169.

125. Frelinger AL III, Hillman RS: Novel methods for assessing platelet function. Am Heart J 1998; 135:S184–S186.

126. Spiess BD, Tuman KJ, McCarthy RJ, et al: Thromboelastography as an indicator of post-cardiopulmonary bypass coagulopathies. J Clin Monit Comput 1987; 3:25–30.

127. Wang JS, Lin CY, Hung WT, et al: Thromboelastogram fails to predict postoperative hemorrhage in cardiac patients. Ann Thorac Surg 1992; 53:435–439.

128. Kang YG, Martin DJ, Marquez J, et al: Intraoperative changes in blood coagulation and thromboelastographic monitoring in liver transplantation. Anesth Analg 1985; 64:888–896.

129. Trentalange MJ, Walts LF: A comparison of thromboelastogram and template bleeding time in the evaluation of platelet function after aspirin ingestion. J Clin Anesth 1991; 3:377–381.

130. Tuman K, McCarthy R, Patel R, et al: Comparison of thromboelastography and platelet aggregometry (abstract). Anesthesiology 1991; 75:A433.

131. Zuckerman L, Cohen E, Vagher JP, et al: Comparison of thromboelastography with common coagulation tests. Thromb Haemost 1981; 46:752–756.

132. Spiess BD, Logas WG, Tuman KJ, et al: Thromboelastography used for detection of perioperative fibrinolysis: A report of four cases. J Cardiothorac Vasc Anesth 1988; 2:666–672.

133. Williams G, Bratton S, Nielsen N, et al: Fibrinolysis in pediatric patients undergoing cardiopulmonary bypass. J Cardiothorac Vasc Anesth 1998; 12:633–638.

134. Khurana S, Mattson JC, Westley S, et al: Monitoring platelet glycoprotein IIb/IIIa-fibrin interaction with tissue factor-activated thromboelastography. J Lab Clin Med 1997; 130:401–411.

135. von Kaulla K, Ostendorf P, von Kaulla E: The impedance machine: A new bedside coagulation recording device. J Med 1975; 6:73–87.

136. Saleem A, Blifield C, Saleh SA, et al: Viscoelastic measurement of clot formation: A new test of platelet function. Ann Clin Lab Sci 1983; 13:115–124.

137. LaForce WR, Brudno DS, Kanto WP, et al: Evaluation of the SonoClot Analyzer for the measurement of platelet function in whole blood. Ann Clin Lab Sci 1992; 22:30–33.

138. Miyashita T, Kuro M: Evaluation of platelet function by Sonoclot analysis compared with other hemostatic variables in cardiac surgery. Anesth Analg 1998; 87:1228–1233.

139. Horlocker TT, Schroeder DR: Effect of age, gender, and platelet count on Sonoclot coagulation analysis in patients undergoing orthopedic operations. Mayo Clin Proc 1997; 72:214–219.

140. Carr ME, Jr., Zekert SL: Measurement of platelet mediated force development during plasma clot formation. Am J Med Sci 1991; 302:13–18.

141. Carr ME, Jr., Carr SL: Fibrin structure and concentration alter clot elastic modulus but do not alter platelet mediated force development. Blood Coagul Fibrinolysis 1995; 6:79–86.

142. Greilich PE Jr, Carr ME, Carr SL, et al: Reductions in platlet force development by cardiopulmonary bypass are associated with hemorrhage. Anesth Analg 1995; 80:459–465.

143. Despotis GJ, Levine V, Filos KS, et al: Evaluation of a new point-of-care test that measures PAF-mediated acceleration of coagulation in cardiac surgical patients. Anesthesiology 1996; 85:1311–1323.

144. Ereth MH, Nuttall GA, Klindworth JT, et al: Does the platelet activated clotting test (HemoSTATUS) predict blood loss and platelet dysfunction associated with cardiopulmonary bypass? Anesth Analg 1997; 85:259–264.

145. Ereth MH, Nuttall GA, Santrach PJ, et al: The relation between the platelet activated clotting test (HemoSTATUS) and blood loss after cardiopulmonary bypass. Anesthesiology 1998; 88:962–969.

146. Görög P, Ahmed A: Haemostatometer: A new in vitro technique for assessing haemostatic activity of blood. Thromb Res 1984; 34:341–357.

147. Ratnatunga CP, Rees GM, Kovacs IB: Preoperative hemostatic activity and excessive bleeding after cardiopulmonary bypass. Ann Thorac Surg 1991; 52:250–257.

148. John LCH, Rees GM, Kovacs IB: Effect of heparin on in vitro platelet reactivity in cardiac surgical patients—a comparative assessment of whole blood platelet aggregometry and haemostatometry. Thromb Res 1992; 66:649–656.

149. John LC, Rees GM, Kovacs IB: Inhibition of platelet function by heparin. An etiologic factor in postbypass hemorrhage. J Thorac Cardiovasc Surg 1993; 105:816–822.

150. Li C, Hoffmann T, Hsieh P, et al: The Xylum Clot Signature Analyzer: A dynamic system that simulates vascular injury. Thromb Res 1998; 92:S67–S77.

151. Kundu SK, Heilmann E, Sio R, et al: Description of an in vitro platelet function analyzer—PFA100. Semin Thromb Hemost 1995; 21:106–112.

152. Kratzer MA, Born GV: Simulation of primary haemostasis in vitro. Haemostasis 1985; 15:357–362.

153. Mammen EF, Alshameeri RS, Comp PC: Preliminary data for a field trial of the PFA-100 system. Semin Thromb Hemost 1995; 21:113–121.

154. Rupwate M, Johnson M: A rapid simple method for the measurement of platelet inhibition by a platelet-specific glycoprotein-IIb/IIIa inhibitor (abstract). Thromb Haemost 1993; 69:706.

155. Coller B, Lang D, Scudder L: Rapid and simple platelet function assay to assess glycoprotein IIb/IIIa receptor blockade. Circulation 1997; 95:860–867.

156. Salzman EW: Measurement of platelet adhesiveness. J Lab Clin Med 1963; 62:724–735.

157. Bowie EJ, Owen CA Jr, Thompson JH, et al: Platelet adhesiveness in von Willebrand's disease. Am J Clin Pathol 1969; 52:69–77.

158. Ereth MH, Nuttall GA, Grubba RN: Platelet retention glass bead assay predicts blood loss after cardiac surgery (abstract). Anesth Analg 1998; 86:SCA25.

159. Tuman KJ, Spiess BD, McCarthy RJ, et al: Comparison of viscoelastic measures of coagulation after cardiopulmonary bypass. Anesth Analg 1989; 69:69–75.

160. Jobes DR, Schwartz AJ, Ellison N, et al: Monitoring heparin anticoagulation and its neutralization. Ann Thorac Surg 1981; 31:161–166.

161. Bull BS, Korpman RA, Huse WM, et al: Heparin therapy during extracorporeal circulation. I. Problems inherent in existing heparin protocols. J Thorac Cardiovasc Surg 1975; 69:674–684.

162. Gravlee GP, Haddon WS, Rothberger HK, et al: Heparin dosing and monitoring for cardiopulmonary bypass: A comparison of technique with measurement of subclinical plasma coagulation. J Thorac Cardiovasc Surg 1990; 99:518–527.

163. Despotis GJ, Joist JH, Joiner-Maier D, et al: Effect of aprotinin on activated clotting time, whole blood and plasma heparin measurements. Ann Thorac Surg 1995; 59:106–111.

164. Stehling LC: Anesthesiology update:19. Adverse reactions to transfusion. Orthop Rev 1986; 15:736–740.

165. Brunson ME, Alexander JW: Mechanisms of transfusion-induced immunosuppression. Transfusion 1990; 30:651–658.

166. Alexander JW: Transfusion-induced immunomodulation and infection (editorial). Transfusion 1991; 31:195–196.

167. Quintiliani L, Buzzonetti A, DiGirolamo M, et al: Effects of blood transfusion on the immune responsiveness and survival of cancer patients: A prospective study. Transfusion 1991; 31:713–718.

168. Gravlee GP: Optimal use of blood components. Int Anesthesiol Clin 1990; 28:216–222.

169. Kruskall MS, Mintz PD, Bergin JJ, et al: Transfusion therapy in emergency medicine. Ann Emerg Med 1988; 17:327–335.

170. Welch HG, Meehan KR, Goodnough LT: Prudent strategies for elective red blood cell transfusion. Ann Intern Med 1992; 116: 393–402.

171. Hogue CWJ, Goodnough LT, Monk TF: Perioperative myocardial ischemic episodes are related to hematocrit level in patients undergoing radical prostatectomy. Transfusion 1998; 38: 924–931.

172. Carson JL, Poses RM, Spence RK, et al: Severity of anaemia and operative mortality and morbidity. Lancet 1988; 1:727–729.

173. Herbert P, Wells G, Blajchman M, et al: A multicenter, randomized, controlled clinical trial of transfusion requirements in critical care. N Engl J Med 1999; 340:409–417.

174. Ho CH: The hemostatic effect of packed red cell transfusion in patients with anemia. Transfusion 1998; 38:1011–1014.

175. Erslev AJ: Erythropoietin. N Engl J Med 1991; 324:1339–1344.

176. Kyo S, Omoto R, Hirashima K, et al: Effect of human recombinant erythropoietin on reduction of homologous blood transfusion in open-heart surgery. A Japanese multicenter study. Circulation 1992; 86:II413–418.

177. Goodnough LT, Price TH, Rudnick S, et al: Preoperative red cell production in patients undergoing aggressive autologous blood phlebotomy with and without erythropoietin therapy. Transfusion 1992; 32:441–445.

178. Simon TL: Platelet transfusion therapy. In Rossi EC, Simon TL, Moss GS (eds): Principles of Transfusion Medicine. Baltimore, Williams & Wilkins, 1991, pp 219–222.

179. National Institutes of Health Consensus Conference: Platelet transfusion therapy. JAMA 1987; 257:1777–1780.

180. Crowley JP: Transfusion of plasma. In Rossi EC, Simon TL, Moss GS (eds): Principles of Transfusion Medicine. Baltimore, Williams & Wilkins, 1991, pp 335–341.

181. National Institutes of Health Consensus Conference: Fresh-frozen plasma. Indications and risks. JAMA 1985; 253:551–553.

182. Edwards FH, Clark RE, Schwartz M: Coronary artery bypass grafting: The Society of Thoracic Surgeons National Database experience. Ann Thorac Surg 1994; 57:12–19.

183. Goodnough LT, Johnston MF, Toy PT: The variability of transfusion practice in coronary artery bypass surgery. JAMA 1991; 265:86–90.

184. Klein HG: Oxygen carriers and transfusion medicine. Artif Cells Blood Substit Immobil Biotechnol 1994; 22:123–135.

185. Wallace EL, Surgenor DM, Hao HS, et al: Collection and transfusion of blood and blood components in the United States, 1989. Transfusion 1993; 33:139–144.

186. Goodnough LT, Soegiarso RW, Birkmeyer JD, et al: Economic impact of inappropriate blood transfusion in coronary artery bypass graft surgery. Am J Med 1993; 94:509–514.

187. Simon TL, Akl BF, Murphy W: Controlled trial of routine administration of platelet concentrates in cardiopulmonary bypass surgery. Ann Thorac Surg 1984; 37:359–364.

188. Bick RL: Hemostatic defects associated with cardiac surgery, prosthetic devices, and other extracorporeal circuits. Semin Thromb Hemost 1985; 11:249–280.

189. Nuttall GA, Oliver WC Jr, Ereth MH, et al: Coagulation tests predict bleeding after cardiopulmonary bypass. J Cardiothorac Vasc Anesth 1997; 11:815–823.

190. Khuri SF, Wolfe JA, Josa M, et al: Hematologic changes during and after cardiopulmonary bypass and their relationship to the bleeding time and nonsurgical blood loss. J Thorac Cardiovasc Surg 1992; 104:94–107.

191. Bick RL, Schmalhorst WR, Arbegast NR: Alterations of hemostasis associated with cardiopulmonary bypass. Thromb Res 1976; 8:285–302.

192. Edmunds LH Jr, Ellison N, Colman RW, et al: Platelet function during cardiac operation: Comparison of membrane and bubble oxygenators. J Thorac Cardiovasc Surg 1982; 83:805–812.

193. Mammen EF, Koets MH, Washington BC, et al: Hemostasis changes during cardiopulmonary bypass surgery. Semin Thromb Hemost 1985; 11:281–292.

194. Gundry SR, Drongowski RA, Klein MD, et al: Postoperative bleeding in cardiovascular surgery. Does heparin rebound really exist? Am Surg 1989; 55:162–165.

195. Holloway DS, Summaria L, Sandesara J, et al: Decreased platelet number and function and increased fibrinolysis contribute to postoperative bleeding in cardiopulmonary bypass patients. Thromb Haemost 1988; 59(1):62–67.

196. Kirklin JK, Westaby S, Blackstone EH, et al: Complement and the damaging effects of cardiopulmonary bypass. J Thorac Cardiovasc Surg 1983; 86:845–857.

197. Wenger RK, Lukasiewicz H, Mikuta BS, et al: Loss of platelet fibrinogen receptors during clinical cardiopulmonary bypass. J Thorac Cardiovasc Surg 1989; 97:235–239.

198. Zilla P, Fasol R, Groscurth P, et al: Blood platelets in cardiopulmonary bypass operations. Recovery occurs after initial stimulation, rather than continual activation. J Thorac Cardiovasc Surg 1989; 97:379–388.

199. Addonizio VP: Platelet function in cardiopulmonary bypass and artificial organs. Hematol Oncol Clin North Am 1990; 4:145–155.

200. Wachtfogel YT, Musial J, Jenkin B, et al: Loss of platelet alpha 2-adrenergic receptors during simulated extracorporeal circulation: Prevention with prostaglandin E_1. J Lab Clin Med 1985; 105:601–607.

201. Martin JF, Daniel TD, Trowbridge EA: Acute and chronic changes in platelet volume and count after cardiopulmonary bypass induced thrombocytopenia in man. Thromb Haemost 1987; 57:55–58.

202. Ray MJ, Hawson GA, Just SJ, et al: Relationship of platelet aggregation to bleeding after cardiopulmonary bypass surgery. Ann Thorac Surg 1994; 57:981–986.

203. Despotis GJ, Santoro SA, Spintznagel E, et al: On-site prothrombin time, activated partial thromboplastin time, and platelet count. A comparison between whole blood and laboratory assays with coagulation factor analysis in patients presenting for cardiac surgery. Anesthesiology 1994; 80:338–351.

204. Edmunds LH, Salzman EW: Hemostatic problems, transfusion therapy, and cardiopulmonary bypass surgical patients. In Colman RW, Hirsh J, Marder VJ, et al (eds): Hemostasis and Thrombosis: Basic Principles and Clinical Practice, ed 3. Philadelphia, JB Lippincott, 1994, pp 956–968.

205. Musial J, Niewiarowski S, Hershock D, et al: Loss of fibrinogen receptors from the platelet surface during simulated extracorporeal circulation. J Lab Clin Med 1985; 105:514–522.

206. George JN, Pickett EB, Saucerman S, et al: Platelet surface glycoproteins. Studies on resting and activated platelets and platelet membrane microparticles in normal subjects, and observations in patients during adult respiratory distress syndrome and cardiac surgery. J Clin Invest 1986; 78:340–348.

207. Muikku O, Kuitunen A, Hynynen M: Effects of organic nitrate vasodilatators on platelet function before and after cardiopulmonary bypass. Acta Anaesth Scand 1995; 39:618–623.

208. Harker LA: Bleeding after cardiopulmonary bypass. N Engl J Med 1986; 314:1446–1448.

209. Rinder CS, Bohnert J, Rinder HM, et al: Platelet activation and aggregation during cardiopulmonary bypass. Anesthesiology 1991; 75:388–393.

210. Vander Kamp KW, Van Oeveren W: Contact, coagulation and platelet interaction with heparin treated equipment during heart surgery. Int J Artif Organs 1993; 16:836–842.

211. Coccheri S, Palareti G: Pro-thrombotic states and their diagnosis. Ann Ital Med Int 1994; 9:16–21.

212. Dahl OE, Pedersen T, Kierulf P, et al: Sequential intrapulmonary and systemic activation of coagulation and fibrinolysis during and after total hip replacement surgery. Thromb Res 1993; 70:451–458.

213. Warkentin TE: Hemostasis and atherosclerosis. Can J Cardiol 1995; 11:29C–34C.

214. Reininger CB, Reininger AJ, Steckmeier B, et al: Platelet response to vascular surgery—a preliminary study on the effect of aspirin and heparin. Thromb Res 1994; 76:79–87.

215. Holdright DR, Hunt BJ, Parratt R, et al: The effects of cardiopulmonary bypass on systemic and coronary levels of von Willebrand factor. Eur J Cardiothorac Surg 1995; 9:18–21.

216. Ruggeri ZM: Structure and function for von Willebrand factor: Relationship to von Willebrand's disease. Mayo Clin Proc 1991; 66:847–861.

217. Moake JL, Rudy CK, Troll JH, et al: Unusually large plasma factor VIII:von Willebrand factor multimers in chronic relapsing thrombotic thrombocytopenic purpura. N Engl J Med 1982; 307:1432–1435.

218. Perrin EJ, Ray MJ, Hawson GA: The role of von Willebrand factor in haemostasis and blood loss during and after cardiopulmonary bypass surgery. Blood Coagul Fibrinolysis 1995; 6:650–658.

219. Williams SB, McKeown LP, Krutzsch H, et al: Purification and characterization of human platelet von Willebrand factor. Br J Haematol 1994; 88:582–591.

220. Mohr R, Goor DA, Lusky A, et al: Aprotinin prevents cardiopulmonary bypass induced platelet dysfunction. A scanning electron microscope study. Circulation 1992; 86:405–409.

221. Shinfeld A, Zippel D, Lavee J, et al: Aprotinin improves hemostasis after cardiopulmonary bypass better than single-donor platelet concentrate. Ann Thorac Surg 1995; 59:872–876.

222. Stein B, Fuster V, Israel DH, et al: Platelet inhibitor agents in cardiovascular disease: An update. J Am Coll Cardiol 1989; 14:813–836.

223. Spence RK, Carson JA: Transfusion decision making in vascular surgery: Blood ordering schedules and the transfusion trigger. Semin Vasc Surg 1994; 7:76–81.

224. Reed RL, Ciavarella D, Heimbach DM, et al: Prophylactic platelet administration during massive transfusion. A prospective, randomized, double blind clinical study. Ann Surg 1986; 203:40–48.

225. Hewson JR, Neame PB, Kumar N, et al: Coagulopathy related to dilution and hypotension during massive transfusion. Crit Care Med 1985; 13:387–391.

226. Leslie SD, Toy PT: Laboratory hemostatic abnormalities in massively transfused patients given red blood cells and crystalloid. Am J Clin Pathol 1991; 96:770–773.

227. Faringer PD, Mullins RJ, Johnson RL, et al: Blood component supplementation during massive transfusion of AS-I red cells in trauma patients. J Trauma 1993; 34:481–485, discussion 485–487.

228. Ritter DM, Owen CA, Jr., Bowie EJ, et al: Evaluation of preoperative hematology-coagulation screening in liver transplantation. Mayo Clin Proc 1989; 64:216–223.

229. Fletcher AP, Biederman O, Moore D, et al: Abnormal plasminogen plasmin system activity (fibrinolysis) in patients with hepatic cirrhosis: Its cause and consequences. J Clin Invest 1964; 43:681.

230. Lewis JH, Bontempo FA, Cornell F, et al: Blood use in liver transplantation. Transfusion 1987; 27:222–225.

231. Himmelreich G, Hundt K, Isenberg C, et al: Thrombocytopenia

and platelet dysfunction in orthotopic liver transplantation. Semin Thromb Hemost 1993; 19:209–212.

232. Kang Y: Clinical use of synthetic antifibrinolytic agents during liver transplantation. Semin Thromb Hemost 1993; 19:258–261.

233. Bohmig HJ: The coagulation disorder of orthotopic hepatic transplantation. Semin Thromb Hemost 1977; 4:57–82.

234. von Kaulla KN, Kaye H, von Kaulla E, et al: Changes in blood coagulation. Arch Surg 1966; 92:71–79.

235. Porte RJ, Bontempo FA, Knot EA, et al: Systemic effects of tissue plasminogen activator–associated fibrinolysis and its relation to thrombin generation in orthotopic liver transplantation. Transplantation 1989; 47:978–984.

236. Lewis JH, Bontempo FA, Awad SA, et al: Liver transplantation: Intraoperative changes in coagulation factors in 100 first transplants. Hepatology 1989; 9:710–714.

237. Harper PL, Luddington RJ, Jennings I, et al: Coagulation changes following hepatic revascularization during liver transplantation. Transplantation 1989; 48:603–607.

238. Schalm SW, Terpstra JL, Achterberg JR, et al: Orthotopic liver transplantation: An experimental study on mechanisms of hemorrhagic diathesis and thrombosis. Surgery 1975; 78:499–507.

239. Kalpokas M, Bookallil M, Sheil AG, et al: Physiological changes during liver transplantation. Anaesth Intensive Care 1989; 17:24–30.

240. Kowalski E, Kopec M, Wegrzynowicz Z: Influence of fibrinogen degradation products (FDP) on platelet aggregation, adhesiveness and viscous metamorphosis. Pol Arch Med Wewn 1965; 35:539–545.

241. Orloff KG, Michaeli D: Inhibition of fibrin-platelet interactions by fibrinogen-degradation fragment D. Am J Physiol 1977; 233:H305–311.

242. Lu H, Soria C, Cramer EM, et al: Temperature dependence of plasmin induced activation or inhibition of human platelets. Blood 1991; 77:996–1005.

243. Puri RN, Zhou F, Colman RF, et al: Plasmin induced platelet aggregation is accompanied by cleavage of agregin and indirectly mediated by calpain. Am J Physiol 1990; 259:C862–868.

244. Puri RN, Hu CJ, Matsueda R, et al: Aggregation of washed platelets by plasminogen and plasminogen activators is mediated by plasmin and is inhibited by a synthetic peptide disulfide. Thromb Res 1992; 65:533–547.

245. Michelson AD, Barnard MR: Plasmin induced redistribution of platelet glycoprotein Ib. Blood 1990; 76:2005–2010.

246. Adelman B, Michelson AD, Loscalzo J, et al: Plasmin effect on platelet glycoprotein IB–von Willebrand factor interactions. Blood 1985; 65:32–40.

247. Stricker RB, Wong D, Shiu DT, et al: Activation of plasminogen by tissue plasminogen activator on normal and thrombasthenic platelets: Effects on surface proteins and platelet aggregation. Blood 1986; 68:275–280.

248. Hennessy VL Jr, Hicks RE, Niewiarowski S, et al: Function of human platelets during extracorporeal circulation. Am J Physiol 1977; 232:H622–628.

249. Fong SW, Burns NE, Williams G, et al: Changes in coagulation and platelet function during prolonged extracorporeal circulation (ECC) in sheep and man. Trans Am Soc Artif Intern Organs 1974; 20A:239–247.

250. Rettke SR, Janossy TA, Chantigian RC, et al: Hemodynamic and metabolic changes in hepatic transplantation. Mayo Clin Proc 1989; 64:232–240.

251. Wilson JD, Taswell HF: Autotransfusion: Historical review and preliminary report on a new method. Mayo Clin Proc 1968; 43:26–35.

252. Klebanoff G: Early clinical experience with a disposable unit for the intraoperative salvage and reinfusion of blood loss (intraoperative autotransfusion). Am J Surg 1970; 120:718–722.

253. Wilson JD, Utz DC, Taswell HF: Autotransfusion during transurethral resection of the prostate: Technique and preliminary clinical evaluation. Mayo Clin Proc 1969; 44:374–386.

254. Kingsley JR, Valeri CR, Peters H, et al: Citrate anticoagulation and on-line cell washing in intraoperative autotransfusion in the baboon. Surg Forum 1973; 24:258–260.

255. Yawn DH: Properties of salvaged blood. *In* Taswell HF, Pineda AA (eds): Autologous Transfusion and Hemotherapy. Boston, Blackwell Scientific, 1991.

256. Eng J, Kay PH, Murday AJ, et al: Postoperative autologous transfusion in cardiac surgery. A prospective, randomized study. Eur J Cardiothorac Surg 1990; 4:595–600.

257. Williamson KR, Taswell HF: Intraoperative blood salvage: A review. Transfusion 1991; 31:662–675.

258. Ray JM, Flynn JC, Bierman AH: Erythrocyte survival following intraoperative autotransfusion in spinal surgery: An in vivo comparative study and 5-year update. Spine 1986; 11:879–882.

259. Kent P, Ashley S, Thorley PJ, et al: 24-hour survival of autotransfused red cells in elective aortic surgery: A comparison of two intraoperative autotransfusion systems. Br J Surg 1991; 78:1473–1475.

260. Davis RJ, Agnew DK, Shealy CR, et al: Erythrocyte viability in postoperative autotransfusion. J Pediatr Orthop 1993; 13:781–783.

261. Fuller JA, Buxton BF, Picken J, et al: Haematologic effects of reinfused mediastinal blood after cardiac surgery. Med J Aust 1991; 154:737–740.

262. de Haan J, Schonberger J, Haan J, et al: Tissue-type plasminogen activator and fibrin monomers synergistically cause platelet dysfunction during retransfusion of shed blood after cardiopulmonary bypass. J Thorac Cardiovasc Surg 1993; 106:1017–1023.

263. Schaff HV, Hauer J, Gardner TJ, et al: Routine use of autotransfusion following cardiac surgery: Experience in 700 patients. Ann Thorac Surg 1979; 27:493–499.

264. Griffith LD, Billman GF, Daily PO, et al: Apparent coagulopathy caused by infusion of shed mediastinal blood and its prevention by washing of the infusate. Ann Thorac Surg 1989; 47:400–406.

265. Bengston JP, Backman L, Stenqvist O, et al: Complement activation and reinfusion of wound drainage blood. Anesthesiology 1990; 73:376–380.

266. Healy WL, Wasilewski SA, Pfeifer BA, et al: Methylmethacrylate monomer and fat content in shed blood after total joint arthroplasty. Clin Orthop 1993; 286:15–17.

267. Faris PM, Ritter MA, Keating EM, et al: Unwashed filtered shed blood collected after knee and hip arthroplasties. A source of autologous red blood cells. J Bone Joint Surg [Am] 1991; 73:1169–1178.

268. Giordano GF, Giordano DM, Wallace BA, et al: An analysis of 9,918 consecutive perioperative autotransfusions. Surg Gynecol Obstet 1993; 176:103–110.

269. Keeling MM, Gray LAJ, Brink MA, et al: Intraoperative autotransfusion. Experience in 725 consecutive cases. Ann Surg 1983; 197:536–541.

270. Breyer RH, Engelman RM, Rousou JA, et al: Blood conservation for myocardial revascularization. Is it cost effective? J Thorac Cardiovasc Surg 1987; 93:512–522.

271. McCarthy PM, Popovsky MA, Schaff HV, et al: Effect of blood conservation efforts in cardiac operations at the Mayo Clinic. Mayo Clin Proc 1988; 63:225–229.

272. Schaff HV, Hauer JM, Bell WR, et al: Autotransfusion of shed mediastinal blood after cardiac surgery: A prospective study. J Thorac Cardiovasc Surg 1978; 75:632–641.

273. Morris JJ, Tan YS: Autotransfusion: Is there a benefit in a current practice of aggressive blood conservation? Ann Thorac Surg 1994; 58:502–507.

274. Yawn DH: Blood salvage for cardiovascular surgery. Perfusion 1990; 5(Suppl):31–37.

275. Hallett JW Jr, Popovsky M, Ilstrup D: Minimizing blood transfusions during abdominal aortic surgery: Recent advances in rapid autotransfusion. J Vasc Surg 1987; 5:601–606.

276. Reddy DJ, Ryan CJ, Shepard AD, et al: Intraoperative autotransfusion in vascular surgery. Arch Surg 1990; 125:1012–1016.

277. Ouriel K, Shortell CK, Green RM, et al: Intraoperative autotransfusion in vascular surgery. J Vasc Surg 1993; 18:16–22.

278. Kelley-Patteson C, Ammar AD, Kelley H: Should the Cell Saver Autotransfusion Device be used routinely in all infrarenal abdominal aortic bypass operations? J Vasc Surg 1993; 18:261–265.

279. Dzik WH, Jenkins R: Use of intraoperative blood salvage during orthotopic liver transplantation. Arch Surg 1985; 120:946–948.

280. Dale RF, Lindop MJ, Farman JV, et al: Autotransfusion, an expe-

rience of seventy six cases. Ann R Coll Surg Engl 1986 68:295-297.

281. Williamson KR, Taswell HF, Rettke SR, et al: Intraoperative autologous transfusion: Its role in orthotopic liver transplantation. Mayo Clin Proc 1989; 64:340-345.

282. Santrach PJ, Williamson KR, Taswell HF, et al: Intraoperative blood salvage in neurosurgery (abstract). Transfusion 1989; 29:23s.

283. Robicsek F, Duncan GD, Born GVR, et al: Inherent dangers of simultaneous application of microfibrillar collagen hemostat and blood-saving devices. J Thorac Cardiovasc Surg 1992; 92:766-770.

284. Niebauer GW, Oz MC, Goldschmidt M, et al: Simultaneous use of microfibrillar collagen hemostat and blood saving devices in a canine kidney perfusion model. Ann Thorac Surg 1989; 48:523-527.

285. Orr MD, Ferdman AG, Maresh JG: Removal of Avitene microfibrillar collagen hemostat by use of suitable transfusion filters. Ann Thorac Surg 1994; 57:1007-1011.

286. Timberlake GA, McSwain NE Jr: Autotransfusion of blood contaminated by enteric contents: A potentially life-saving measure in the massively hemorrhaging trauma patient? J Trauma 1988; 28:855-857.

287. Ozmen V, McSwain NE, Jr., Nichols RL, et al: Autotransfusion of potentially culture-positive blood (CPB) in abdominal trauma: Preliminary data from a prospective study. J Trauma 1992; 32:36-39.

288. Williamson KR, Anhalt JP, Koehler LC, et al: Cultures of intraoperatively salvaged blood in light of FDA guidelines (abstract). Transfusion 1989; 29:23s.

289. Kang Y, Aggarwal S, Virji M, et al: Clinical evaluation of autotransfusion during liver transplantation. Anesth Analg 1991; 72:94-100.

290. Ezzedine H, Baele P, Robert A: Bacteriologic quality of intraoperative autotransfusion. Surgery 1991; 109:259-264.

291. Bland LA, Villarino ME, Arduino MJ, et al: Bacteriologic and endotoxin analysis of salvaged blood used in autologous transfusions during cardiac operations. J Thorac Cardiovasc Surg 1992; 103:582-588.

292. Yaw PB, Sentany M, Link WJ, et al: Tumor cells carried through autotransfusion. Contraindication to intraoperative blood recovery? JAMA 1975; 231:490-491.

293. Homann B, Zenner HP, Schauber J, et al: Tumor cells carried through autotransfusion. Are these cells still malignant? Acta Anaesthesiol Belg 1984; 35:51-59.

294. Miller GV, Ramsden CW, Primrose JN: Autologous transfusion: An alternative to transfusion with banked blood during surgery for cancer. Br J Surg 1991; 78:713-715.

295. Karczewski DM, Lema MJ, Glaves D: The efficacy of an autotransfusion system for tumor cell removal from blood salvaged during cancer surgery. Anesth Analg 1994; 78:1131-1135.

296. Salsbury AJ: The significance of the circulating cancer cell. Cancer Treat Rev 1975; 2:55-72.

297. Klimberg I, Sirois R, Wajsman Z, et al: Intraoperative autotransfusion in urologic oncology. Arch Surg 1986; 121:1326-1329.

298. Hart OJ III, Klimberg IW, Wajsman Z, et al: Intraoperative autotransfusion in radical cystectomy for carcinoma of the bladder. Surg Gynecol Obstet 1989; 168:302-306.

299. Zulim RA, Rocco M, Goodnight JE Jr, et al: Intraoperative autotransfusion in hepatic resection for malignancy. Is it safe? Arch Surg 1993; 128:206-211.

300. Lux PS, Martin JW, Whiteside LA: Reinfusion of whole blood following addition of tobramycin powder to the wound during total knee arthroplasty. J Arthroplasty 1993; 8:269-271.

301. Smith DF, Mihm FG, Mefford I: Hypertension after intraoperative autotransfusion in bilateral adrenalectomy for pheochromocytoma. Anesthesiology 1983; 58:182-184.

302. Wahl GW, Feins RH, Alfieres G, et al: Reinfusion of shed blood after coronary operation causes elevation of cardiac enzyme levels. Ann Thorac Surg 1992; 53:625-627.

303. Hannes W, Keilich M, Koster W, et al: Shed blood after coronary operations. Ann Thorac Surg 1994; 57:1289-1294.

304. Yawn DH: Autologous blood salvage during elective surgery. Transfusion Sci 1989; 10:107-116.

305. Horst HM, Dlugos S, Fath JJ, et al: Coagulopathy and intraoperative blood salvage (IBS). J Trauma 1992; 32:646-652; discussion 652-653.

306. Murray DJ, Gress K, Weinstein SL: Coagulopathy after reinfusion of autologous scavenged red blood cells. Anesth Analg 1992; 75:125-129.

307. Bull BS, Bull MH: The salvaged blood syndrome: A sequel to mechanochemical activation of platelets and leukocytes? Blood Cells 1990; 16:5-20; discussion 20-23.

308. Solomon MD, Rutledge ML, Kane LE, et al: Cost comparison of intraoperative autologous versus homologous transfusion. Transfusion 1988; 28:379-382.

309. Popovsky MA, Devine PA, Taswell HF: Intraoperative autologous transfusion. Mayo Clin Proc 1985; 60:125-134.

310. Kristensen PW, Sorensen LS, Thyregod HC: Autotransfusion of drainage blood in arthroplasty. A prospective, controlled study of 31 operations. Acta Orthop Scand 1992; 63:377-380.

311. Simpson MB, Georgopoulos G, Eilert RE: Intraoperative blood salvage in children and young adults undergoing spinal surgery with predeposited autologous blood: efficacy and cost effectiveness. J Pediatr Orthop 1993; 13:777-780.

312. Starzl TE, Marchioro TL, von Kaulla KN, et al: Homotransplantation of the liver in humans. Surg Gynecol Obstet 1963; 117:659-676.

23 Pulse Oximeter Waveform: Photoelectric Plethysmography

Kirk Shelley, M.D., Ph.D.
Stacey Shelley, B.S.N.

A quiet revolution has occurred in the field of monitoring. Without much fanfare the pulse oximeter waveform has begun to appear routinely on operating room (OR) and intensive care unit (ICU) monitors.[1, 2] Correctly interpreted, the pulse oximeter waveform contains a wealth of information. Once again, as we saw with the introduction of the capnometer,[3] the method of extracting clinically useful information from the pulse oximeter waveform is being left to the clinician to discover. The pulse oximeter has been an ASA (American Society of Anesthesiologists) standard monitor in the OR since January 1, 1990 and is mandated by state law in Massachusetts, New York, and New Jersey before sedation or anesthesia can take place. With this significant investment in monitoring equipment, it seems only sensible that we strive to maximize our understanding of the information presented to us. Previous reviews of this topic can be found in the medical literature.[4-7] This chapter is a summary of those clinical observations with support from published studies. It is hoped that it will be an aid to developing clinically useful algorithms for the analysis of this waveform.

History

The pulse oximeter is based on photoelectric plethysmography. The photoelectric plethysmograph is not a new technology. First described in 1938 by Hertzman,[8] the device has intrigued investigators for quite some time. It was recognized early on that the pulse waveform changes dramatically with cardiovascular shock[9] and sedation.[10] As the mechanisms of control of peripheral circulation came to be understood, there developed a recognition of the fact that the plethysmograph could be used to monitor vascular sympathetic tone.[11, 12] Even before the introduction of the pulse oximeter, plethysmographs found their way to the OR. They were used to monitor the effects of spinal and epidural anesthetics,[13, 14] or to monitor the impact of general anesthetics on vascular tone.[5] With the advent of the pulse oximeter, the photoelectric plethysmograph as an independent monitor has been virtually forgotten in clinical medicine.[4]

Technique

The pulse oximeter, in the process of determining oxygen saturation, must act as a sensitive photoelectric plethysmograph. The photoelectric plethysmograph is a remarkably simple device consisting of a light source (most commonly a light-emitting diode) and light detector (photo diode). The detector can be placed either directly across from the light source for transmission plethysmography or next to the light source for reflective plethysmography. The plethysmographic waveform that is displayed on the pulse oximeter is a highly processed and filtered signal. Of the two wavelengths measured by the pulse oximeter, only the infrared signal (940 nm) is presented. The information from this wavelength is displayed because it is more stable over time. The red signal (660 nm) is more susceptible to changes in oxygen saturation.

In addition, only the pulsatile component or alternating current (AC) portion is displayed. The static component, or direct current (DC) (created mostly by the absorption of light by surrounding tissue), is eliminated by an auto-centering routine used to ensure that the waveform remains on the display screen. With changes in the degree of venous congestion, the waveform can be noted to drift partly off the screen and then return via the auto-centering algorithm. This can be demonstrated by changing the position of the region being studied (e.g., lowering the hand being studied below the level of the right atrium) or by the use of a low-pressure tourniquet. Finally, and most important, all clinical pulse oximeters that display a plethysmographic waveform include an auto-gain function designed to maximize the size of the waveform displayed. Luckily, some manufacturers do include an option to turn off this automatic resizing function. Without this option it would be impossible to analyze the amplitude of the pulse oximeter waveform, an important parameter to measure when analyzing the waveform. The region of the body being measured is important. The finger is a more useful and responsive area than the earlobe when measuring the activity of the sympathetic system.[15]

Beer's law of light (Fig. 23–1) describes the elements that contribute to the pulse oximeter waveform. Conceptually, it is most useful to view the pulse oximeter waveform as measuring the change in blood volume during a cardiac cycle in the region being studied (typically the fingertip or earlobe).[16] There is no calibration procedure possible for the photoelectric plethysmograph. The signal is therefore not given a unit designation. Similar to central venous pressure measurement, the value of the plethysmograph comes from an analysis over time, as opposed to any absolute number. The term *plethysmograph* is derived from the Greek *plethysmos*, increase. There is a close correlation ($r = .9$) between the photoplethysmograph and the more traditional strain gauge plethysmograph.[17] The traditional strain gauge plethysmograph consists of a band wrapped around the limb of interest. A change in electrical resistance or pressure exerted on the band is measured to gauge changes in tissue volume.

Beer's Law of Light

$$A_{total} = E_1C_1L_1 + E_2C_2L_2 + \ldots E_nC_nL_n$$

A_{total} = absorption at a given wavelength

E_n = extinction coefficient (absorbency)

C_n = concentration

L_n = path length

Figure 23-1. Beer's law of light describes the relationship between the extinction coefficient, the concentration of the substance (e.g. hemoglobin), and path length the light has to travel. The path length is the major factor that changes through the cardiac cycle. With each heartbeat the tissue swells with the influx of blood.

A useful technique for deriving the maximum value from the pulse oximeter waveform comes from the study of the waveform amplitude and shifting baseline over time. Changes in waveform amplitude closely correlate to changes in sympathetic tone of the peripheral vessels. The detection of these changes can be facilitated by the use of a slow-moving strip chart recorder to supplement the normal screen trace of the waveform. Important changes in the pulse oximeter waveform often occur slower than the traditional screen scrolling speed. Another useful technique, used by us, is the superimposing of the pulse oximeter waveform over the CO_2 waveform on the monitor screen. This technique allows for easier analysis of the effects of the positive pressure ventilation on the waveform. The traces presented in this chapter were collected with two different computer-based data acquisition systems (BioBench, National Instruments, Austin, TX; and MacLab, AD Instruments, Inc.) and two different pulse oximeters (OxiPleth, Novametrix, Wallingford, CT, and Merlin monitoring system, Hewlett-Packard). Both pulse oximeters have the desirable ability to have their auto-gain function turned off. Table 23-1 gives a list of additional desirable features that pulse oximeter manufacturers might consider adding to their devices.

Amplitude Analysis

One of the most useful and commonly overlooked plethysmographic features is the waveform amplitude (Table 23-2).

Table 23-1. Desirable Characteristics for a Pulse Oximeter Used for Waveform Analysis*

Waveform display
   Ability to change time scales
   Switch between scroll and "erase bar" display modes
   Wavelength selectable (infrared vs. red)
Ability to turn off auto-gain function
Ability to turn off auto-center function
Ability to set the amplitude gain
Numeric display of amplitude and DC signal
Ability to use a wide range of probes (finger, ear, and reflective)
Digital and analog outputs of pulse oximeter waveform for capture
   by data collection equipment

*No pulse oximeter commercially available has this combination of characteristics.

Table 23-2. Features of the Pulse Oximeter Waveform

Rhythm
Amplitude
Wave morphology
   Arterial pulsation
   Venous pulsation
   Dicrotic notch
   Respiratory variability
   Second derivative calculation

Amplitude changes can be concealed by the auto-gain function found on most pulse oximeters. When the auto-gain is turned off, certain observations can be made. For example, over a remarkably wide range of cardiac output, the amplitude of the plethysmograph signal is directly proportional to the vascular distensibility.[5] If the vascular compliance is low, for example during episodes of increased sympathetic tone, the pulse oximeter waveform amplitude is low. With vasodilation, the pulse oximeter waveform amplitude is increased.

Importantly, plethysmography has been shown to be quite sensitive to even small amounts of pulsatile blood flow (as low as 4% of baseline as determined by laser Doppler).[18, 19] One should never confuse a large pulse oximeter waveform amplitude with having a high arterial pressure or vice versa. It is not unusual for the pulse oximeter waveform amplitude to fall during significant increases in blood pressure that are due to increased sympathetic tone. Once a baseline measurement has been established, the pulse oximeter amplitude can be followed as a sensitive gauge of sympathetic tone. Used in this capacity the pulse oximeter can be helpful in a broad range of clinical situations (Table 23-3).

Monitor of Vascular Tone

For example, under general anesthesia, the ungained pulse oximeter signal may be used to determine the extent of attenuation of the sympathetic response to surgical stimulation, as shown in Figure 23-2. Using routine medications for the induction of anesthesia, the patient undergoes a laryngoscopy for intubation. From the arterial line readings it can be seen that the patient's systolic blood pressure increased from 90 to 110 mmHg. During the same period the plethysmograph amplitude decreased by 70%. After the intubation was completed and anesthetic gas started, the amplitude returned to baseline. This pattern of response has been described previously.[15] The responsiveness of the pulse oximeter waveform to surgical stimulation is further demonstrated in Figure 23-3. In this figure a surgical incision has been performed on a patient under general anesthesia. Evidently, even though the patient was "asleep," the sympathetic system was still quite responsive. Once again there was a slight rise in blood pressure, but the response from the plethysmograph was quite dramatic.

Table 23-3. Factors Affecting Pulse Oximeter Waveform Amplitude

Increased amplitude due to vasodilation
   Pharmacologic—nitroprusside
   Physiologic—warming, sedation
   Anesthetic—regional sympathetic blocks (spinal and epidural)
Decreased amplitude due to vasoconstriction
   Pharmacologic—phenylephrine, ephedrine
   Physiologic—cold, surgical stress

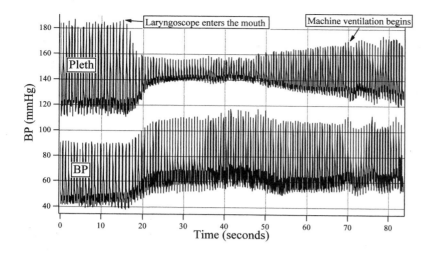

Figure 23-2. Typical pulse oximeter waveform (Pleth) response to intubation. This waveform was obtained from a patient during intubation after routine induction of anesthesia. A rise in the blood pressure (BP) is also demonstrated. This pattern demonstrates the effect of sudden sympathetic stimulation with resulting vasoconstriction on the pulse oximeter waveform.

Figure 23-3. The characteristic response of the pulse oximeter waveform (Pleth) to surgical stimulation. In this case, a patient undergoing general anesthesia experiences the first surgical incision of an operative procedure. The pulse oximeter waveform is noteworthy for the sudden reduction in amplitude. This is believed to be indicative of a sudden increase in sympathetic tone causing peripheral vasoconstriction. A concomitant rise in the blood pressure (BP) supports this explanation.

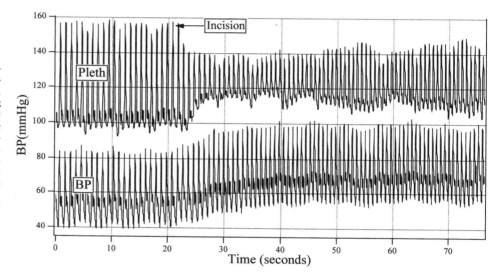

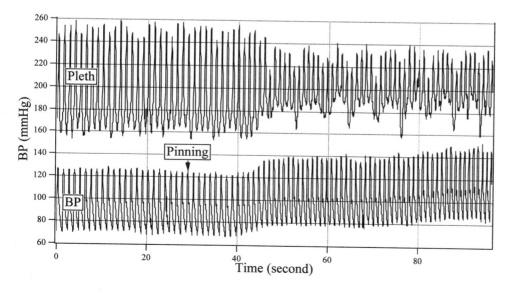

Figure 23-4. A demonstration of the effects of surgical stimulation on the pulse oximeter waveform (Pleth). A patient undergoing a neurosurgical procedure (craniotomy) had a "pinning" performed. Pinning is the process of immobilization of the head in a specially designed headrest. This procedure occurred 30 minutes after the induction of general anesthesia. The reduction in the pulse oximeter waveform amplitude is believed to be an indication of increased sympathetic vascular tone. A rise in blood pressure (BP) at the same time is noted.

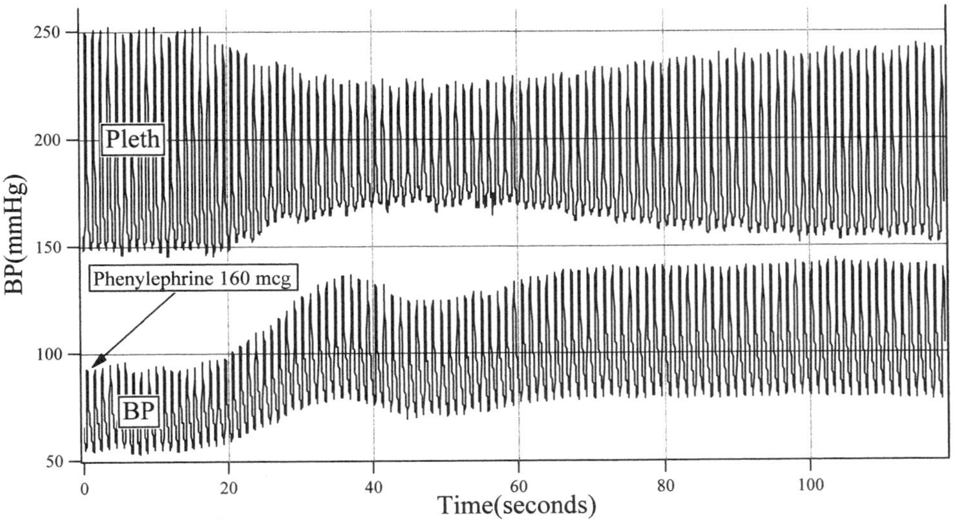

Figure 23-5. An illustration of the effect of phenylephrine on the pulse oximeter waveform (Pleth). An intravenous bolus of phenylephrine is given to a hypotensive patient undergoing a surgical procedure. As expected, the blood pressure (BP) increased. The pulse oximeter waveform first contracted and then expanded back to its original amplitude. (For a detailed analysis of this phenomenon, see Shelley et al.[21])

Finally, in Figure 23-4, the effect of surgical manipulation in preparation for neurosurgery is apparent. In this case, a patient under general anesthesia was "pinned." This process consists of mounting the patient's head into a clamping device to ensure a steady surgical field. Once again, a change in the plethysmograph amplitude can be easily detected. One can speculate that this increase in vascular tone will also be associated with an increase in intracranial pressure.

The responsiveness of the pulse oximeter waveform to changes in sympathetic tone is not limited only to changes caused by catecholamines released by the body. As with the naturally occurring catecholamines, pharmacologic agents cause a predictable reduction in the amplitude of the waveform. Figure 23-5 shows an example of the effect of phenylephrine,[20] a powerful α-adrenergic agonist that directly causes vasoconstriction. Indirect-acting agonists, such as ephedrine, have similar effects (Fig. 23-6). It has been proposed that such changes can be used as the basis for a new vascular tone monitoring device.[21]

As can be predicted, vasodilating pharmacologic agents have the opposite effect. Figure 23-7 demonstrates the effects of nitroprusside, a powerful vasodilator. With the re-

duction in vascular tone the pulse oximeter waveform amplitude increases. This figure also demonstrates that reducing the preload volume to the heart increases the effect of ventilation on the waveform. Increases in amplitude have also been described with both spinal and epidural anesthetics as well as peripheral nerve blocks.[13, 14, 22, 23] This increase in amplitude is thought to be secondary to the block of sympathetic outflow for the central nervous system. As these examples demonstrate, the plethysmograph may be viewed as a sensitive indicator of MAC-BAR.[24] MAC-BAR is the dose of anesthetic required to block adrenergic response in 50% of individuals who have a surgical skin incision. The degree of sympathetic responsiveness a patient retains during an anesthetic may have important clinical implications. This may be particularly true of patients with a compromised coronary circulation, in which dramatic shifts in the hemodynamic status should be avoided. Some investigators have used laser Doppler technology in an attempt to measure the same phenomenon ("skin vasomotor reflex").[25, 26] For example, Shimoda et al.[25] successfully used the detection of vascular reactivity to a fixed stimulation (tetanus nerve simulation) as a predictor of the response to laryngoscopy and intubation.

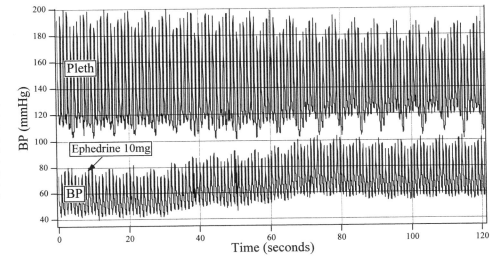

Figure 23-6. The reduction in the pulse oximeter waveform (Pleth) amplitude demonstrates the response to a 10-mg intravenous dose of ephedrine (an indirect-acting adrenergic agonist). Also the effect of positive pressure ventilation on both the arterial pressure (BP) as well as the pulse oximeter waveform is well demonstrated in this figure. This would indicate that hypovolemia was the most likely cause of the patient's hypotension.

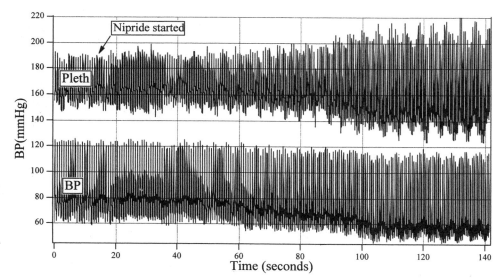

Figure 23-7. The effect of the vasodilator nitroprusside (Nipride) on the pulse oximeter waveform (Pleth). The vasodilation causes the amplitude of the waveform to increase. Interestingly, the vasodilation also causes the effect of positive pressure ventilation to become more pronounced both in the pulse oximeter waveform and the arterial pressure waveform (BP). It is assumed this is due to a reduction in the loading volume of the right ventricle.

The pulse oximeter would appear to be a desirable alternative, representing a much more readily available technology.[27]

Detection of Peripheral Pulsation

A number of creative uses of the pulse oximeter have been developed by clinicians. Most of these uses depend on the ability of the pulse oximeter to detect arterial pulsation. These applications take advantage of the fact that the photoelectric plethysmograph is remarkably sensitive to pulsatile blood flow. The ideal monitoring device would be noninvasive, easy to use and interpret, and it would give an accurate assessment of the adequacy of tissue perfusion. The pulse oximeter has a number of these characteristics.

Blood Pressure Measurement

One clever use of the pulse oximeter has been the determination of systolic blood pressure.[28, 29] This is done by taking advantage of the pulse oximeter's ability to detect a peripheral pulse. Using a manually controlled blood pressure cuff, one inflates the cuff until all signs of peripheral pulsation are

absent from the pulse oximeter waveform. The cuff is slowly deflated until the pulse is once again detected (Fig. 23-8). The pressure at which the pulse is detected corresponds closely to the systolic pressure (r = .880 to .996).[28] This technique is helpful in noisy environments or with neonates in whom the use of stethoscope would be difficult.

Measurement of Regional Tissue Perfusion

A number of studies have been published using the pulse oximeter's plethysmographic capability to detect tissue perfusion. The advantage the pulse oximeter offers is the ability to do noninvasive, continuous monitoring of peripheral blood flow with readily available technology. Using either transmission or reflective plethysmographic techniques, a number of tissues have been studied. The traditional pulse oximeter depends on transmission plethysmography with the light taking a direct path through the tissue being studied (e.g., the fingertip or earlobe). Reflective plethysmography takes advantage of the backscattering of light to the surface (e.g., forehead). Studies using these techniques to determine tissue perfusion have been performed on small bowel,[30, 31] reimplanted fingers,[32] and free flaps.[33] Correctly interpreted, the photoelectric plethysmograph is a viable alternative to

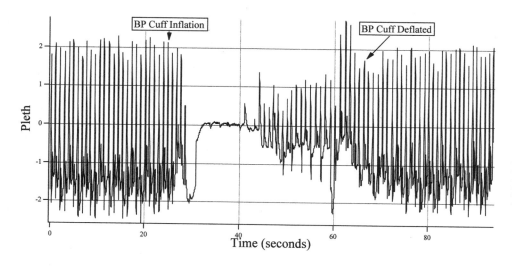

Figure 23-8. The pulse oximeter waveform can be used to determine the systolic blood pressure (BP). In this case the blood pressure cuff is inflated until all pulsation from the pulse oximeter waveform is eliminated. The cuff is then slowly deflated until pulsation is once again detected. The pressure in the blood pressure cuff at the time pulsation first returns corresponds to the systolic pressure.

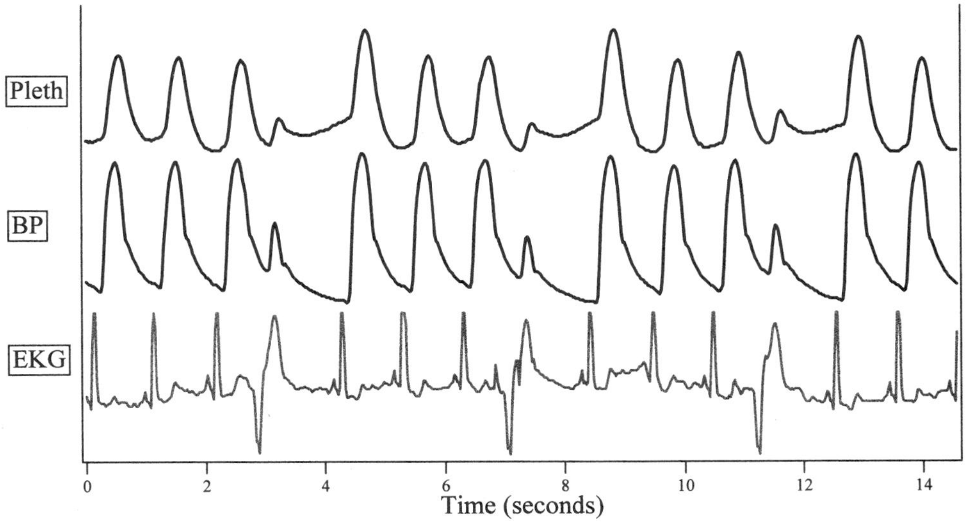

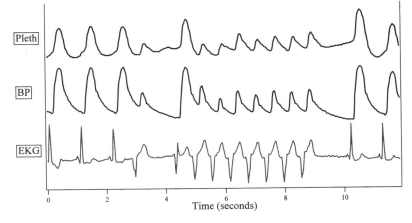

Figure 23-9. The effect of premature ventricular contractions on the pulse oximeter waveform (Pleth), arterial pressure waveform (BP), and electrocardiogram (EKG). The reduction in blood pressure with each premature beat is reflected in the pulse oximeter waveform. This parallel between the arterial pressure and pulse oximeter waveform can be very useful in interpreting cardiac arrhythmias.

the more expensive and less commonly available laser Doppler flowmeter. Key to the interpretation of a pulse oximeter waveform that is being used for the purposes of measuring tissue perfusion is the disabling of any auto-gain function. Changes in the amplitude of the waveform can be very useful in this regard. The loss or reduction of pulsatile blood flow to tissue is reflected by dramatic changes in the pulse oximeter waveform amplitude.

Rhythm Analysis

As can be seen in Figures 23-9, 23-10, and 23-11, the pulse oximeter waveform can be a very useful tool in detecting and diagnosing cardiac arrhythmias.[34] To be used to maximum benefit, the pulse oximeter waveform is used in conjunction with the electrocardiogram (ECG). This can help greatly in correctly interpreting ECG artifacts due to patient movement or electrical cautery. As demonstrated in these figures, the pulse oximeter waveform morphology corresponds remarkably well to the arterial pressure waveform. As expected, after each premature ventricular beat there is a compensatory pause, which gives more time for the ventricle to fill. The next normal heartbeat is therefore associated with an increase in cardiac output. This is reflected in an increase in arterial pressure. Through the same mechanism,

there is an increase in the size of the pulse oximeter amplitude after a compensatory pause. A beat-to-beat shifting of the pulse oximeter amplitude is often the first clue that the patient has developed an irregular heart rhythm. Comparing the pulse oximeter waveform with the ECG is an excellent way to make the correct diagnosis.

Wave Morphology

The study of plethysmographic waveform morphology can be a source of important information regarding cardiovascular function. This form of analysis is still in the process of being refined through continued research. In this section we examine some of the key features that have been studied (Table 23-4).

Respiratory Variability

The effect of positive pressure ventilation on the arterial pressure waveform has been well described.[35] With each positive pressure breath, it is theorized venous return to the heart is impeded, resulting in a temporary reduction in cardiac output.[36] As a patient becomes volume-depleted, with resulting drop in venous pressure, positive pressure ventila-

Figure 23-10. The impact of ventricular tachycardia on the pulse oximeter waveform (Pleth), arterial pressure waveform (BP), and electrocardiogram (EKG). As with isolated premature ventricular contractions the pulse oximeter waveform closely mirrors the arterial pressure. The sudden reduction in the amplitude of the pulse oximeter waveform combined with the typical electrocardiogram pattern should give important warning regarding the presence of a dangerous situation.

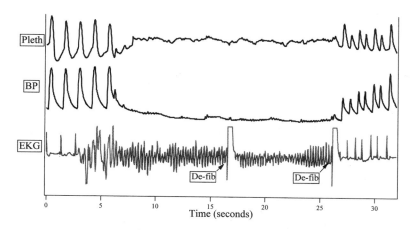

Figure 23-11. Ventricular fibrillation has a dramatic effect on the pulse oximeter waveform (Pleth), arterial pressure waveform (BP), and electrocardiogram (EKG). The sudden loss of the pulse oximeter waveform should always be reason for immediate concern. It should be noted that the pulse oximeter waveform correctly detected the successful cardioversion (De-fib) of the patient back to normal sinus.

tion has an exaggerated impact on the arterial pressure. A similar effect on the plethysmograph has been described.[37, 38] Figure 23-12 demonstrates this phenomenon. Monitoring the respiratory variability seen in the pulse oximeter waveform may be a useful method of detecting occult hemorrhage with its resulting hypovolemia.

Venous Pulse Detection

An often-overlooked feature of the pulse oximeter waveform is the impact of venous pulsation. Even as peripheral as the fingertip is in the circulation, the influence of central venous pulsation can be detected. These pulsations were first described as an artifact causing falsely low oxygen saturation readings on the pulse oximeter.[39] Further investigations have led to the characterization of these venous waveforms.[40] Figures 23-13 and 23-14 show examples of venous pulsation as detected by the pulse oximeter.

The pressures in the venous system are normally low (<20 mmHg), with a detectable pulse pressure of only to 2 to 4 mmHg in the periphery. The fact that such low pressures are detectable in the background of a high-pressure arterial waveform is not remarkable when considering that vascular distensibility is significantly greater (6- to 10-fold) in the venous system than in the arterial system. As already mentioned, the pulse oximeter is very sensitive to vascular tone. The noninvasive detection of the central venous waveform is intriguing. It is important not to overinterpret the presence of the venous waveform in the plethysmograph. A venous waveform is a product of the complex interaction between a number of factors, such as the presence of competent venous valves, vascular tone, right heart function, hand position, and relative blood volume. Once detected, though, changes in the amplitude of the plethysmographic venous pulsation may contain clinically useful information.

It is interesting to speculate about the effect of certain clinical conditions on venous pulsation, as detected by the pulse oximeter. Clinical conditions that increase central venous pressure should increase the amplitude of the venous waveform. Of particular interest would be the ability to non-invasively monitor patients suffering from congestive heart failure or valvular heart disease.

Acceleration Plethysmography

The calculation of the second derivative of the pulse oximeter waveform has been termed "acceleration plethysmography."[41] This type of analysis has been patented (U.S. patent No. 4432374) and has resulted in the development of a new clinical device: the acceleration plethysmograph (Misawa APG 200, Misawa Co., Tokyo). By calculating the rate of change (steepness) in the pulse oximeter waveform through the cardiac cycle, it is hoped an index of vascular elasticity can be measured. So far, the main use of this device has been in the detection of early arteriosclerosis and cardiovascular disease.[42] The determination of the clinical usefulness of this form of analysis awaits controlled studies.

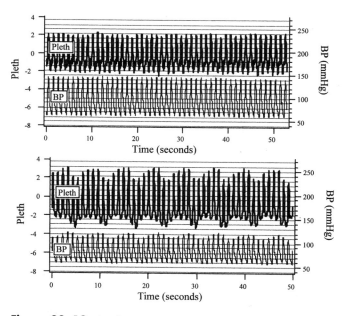

Figure 23-12. An illustration of the effect of blood loss on the pulse oximeter waveform (Pleth) and arterial pressure waveform (BP). The upper diagram shows the baseline waveforms of the patient under general anesthesia with positive pressure ventilation. The lower diagram is after a 1000-mL blood loss. The effect of positive pressure ventilation is apparent.

Table 23-4. Plethysmographic Uses of the Pulse Oximeter

Detection of cardiac arrhythmia
Detection of peripheral pulsation (arterial and venous)
Detection of respiration (controlled and spontaneous)
Monitoring vascular tone
Monitoring cardiovascular function

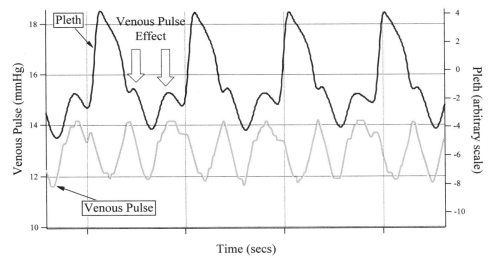

Figure 23–13. This figure demonstrates the typical pattern of peripheral venous pulsation as detected with the pulse oximeter waveform (Pleth). The lower waveform (Venous Pulse) was obtained by measuring the venous pressure in a peripheral vein near the site of the pulse oximeter probe. (For more detail regarding the detection of venous pulsation, see Shelley et al.[21])

Dicrotic Notch Position

It is clear that the dicrotic notch (incisura), as detected in the peripheral circulation, represents more than the timing of the aortic valve closure. It has been noted that when the arterial pressure tracing is measured progressively farther from the heart, the dicrotic notch appears to be increasingly related to reflective pressure from the periphery as opposed to the closure of the aortic valve.[43, 44] From research and clinical observation, it has been speculated that the vertical position of the dicrotic notch, as detected with the pulse oximeter, can be used as an indicator of vasomotor tone.[4] It appears that the dicrotic notch tends to descend toward the baseline during increasing vasodilation and climbs to the apex of the pulse waveform with vasoconstriction. Multiple

"dicrotic notches" can sometimes be detected using the pulse oximeter (Fig. 23–15). Multiple notches are believed to indicate a hyperdynamic circulation with reflective waves from the periphery.[45, 46]

Future Trends

The availability of increasingly powerful computers is allowing for a renaissance in the field of photoelectric plethysmography research. Calculations that once required mainframe computers are now performed almost instantaneously with digital signal processing chips. This fact, combined with the ability to easily capture patient telemetry signals from monitoring equipment, has allowed for detailed reexamination of the plethysmograph. The two leading areas of investigation would appear to be new forms of digital signal processing such as spectral analysis[47] and a combination of the plethysmograph signal with other monitoring signals.[21] It is easy to predict the appearance of "multifunction" pulse oximeters in the near future (Table 23–5).

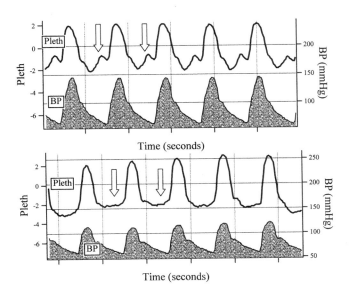

Figure 23–14. The effect of sudden blood loss on the presence of a venous pulse as detected with the pulse oximeter waveform (Pleth). The upper diagram demonstrates the presence of the venous pulse. The *arrows* mark the location of the venous pulse. The lower diagram of the waveforms from the same patient, a short while later, after a sudden and unexpected 500-mL blood loss. As expected, the arterial pressure (BP) dropped and the venous pulse disappeared.

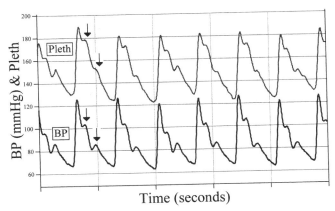

Figure 23–15. This figure demonstrates the existence of multiple dicrotic notches. These multiple notches can be seen in both the pulse oximeter waveform (Pleth) and the arterial pressure waveform (BP). The most common interpretation of the multiple notches is the presence of a hyperdynamic circulation causing reflective waves from the periphery.

Table 23-5. Possible Future Role of Multifunction Pulse Oximeter

Oxygen saturation measurement (arterial and venous)
Respiration monitoring (controlled and spontaneous)
Tissue perfusion monitor
Vascular tone monitor (MAC-BAR)

MAC-BAR, dose of anesthetic required to block adrenergic response in 50% of patients.

REFERENCES

1. Eichhorn JH, Cooper JB, Cullen DJ, et al: Standards for patient monitoring during anesthesia at Harvard Medical School. JAMA 1986; 256:1017-1020.
2. Eichhorn JH, Cooper JB, Cullen DJ, et al: Anesthesia practice standards at Harvard: A review. J Clin Anesthesiol 1988; 1:55-65.
3. Smalhout B, Kalenda Z: An Atlas of Capnography. Netherlands, Kerckebosch - Zeist, 1975, p 222.
4. Murray WB, Foster PA: The peripheral pulse wave—information overlooked. J Clin Monit Comput 1996; 12:365-377.
5. Dorlas JC, Nijboer JA: Photo-electric plethysmography as a monitoring device in anaesthesia. Application and interpretation. Br J Anaesth 1985; 57:524-530.
6. Kelleher J: Pulse oximetry. J Clin Monit Comput 1989; 5:37-62.
7. Partridge BL, Theodore J, Sanford J: Finger plethysmography in anesthesia. Semin Anesth 1989; 8:102-111.
8. Hertzman AB: The blood supply of various skin areas as estimated by the photoelectric plethysmograph. Am J Physiol 1938; 124:328-340.
9. Foster AJ, Neuman C, Rovenstine E: Peripheral circulation during anesthesia, shock and hemorrhage: The digital plethysmograph as a clinical guide. Anesthesiology 1945; 6:246-257.
10. Johnstone M: The effects of sedation on the digital plethysmogram. Anaesthesia 1967; 22:3-15.
11. Dahn I, Jonson B, Nilsen R, A plethysmographic method for determination of flow and volume pulsation in a limb. J Appl Physiol 1970; 28:333-336.
12. Challoner A, Ramsay C: A photoelectric plethysmograph for the measurement of cutaneous blood flow. Phys Med Biol 1974; 19:317-328.
13. Kim JM, Arakawa K, VonLintel T: Use of the pulse-wave monitor as a measurement of diagnostic sympathetic block and of surgical sympathectomy. Anesth Analg 1975; 54:289-296.
14. Kim JM, LaSalle AD, Parmley RT: Sympathetic recovery following lumbar epidural and spinal analgesia. Anesth Analg 1977; 56:352-355.
15. Nijboer JA, Dorlas JC: Comparison of plethysmograms taken from the finger and pinna during anaesthesia. Br J Anaesth 1985; 57:531-534.
16. Kim JM, Arakawa K, Benson K, et al: Pulse oximetry and cirulatory kinetics associated with pulse volume amplitude measured by photoelectric plethysmography. Anesth Analg 1986; 65:1333-1339.
17. Trafford JD, Lafferty K: What does photoplethysmography measure? Med Biol Eng Comput 1984; 22:479-480.
18. Lawson D, et al: Blood flow limits and pulse oximeter signal detection. Anesthesiology 1987; 67:599-603.
19. Palve H, Vuori A: Minimum pulse pressure and peripheral temperature needed for pulse oximetry during cardiac surgery with cardiopulmonary bypass. J Cardiothorac Vasc Anesth 1991; 5:327-330.
20. Hoffman BB, Lefkowitz RJ: Catecholamines and sympathomimetic drugs. In Gilman AG, Hardman JG, Limbird LE, et al (eds): Goodman and Gilman's The Pharmacological Basis of Therapeutics. New York, Pergamon Press, 1996, pp 199-248.
21. Shelley KH, Murray WB, Chang D: Arterial pulse oximetry loops—a new method of monitoring vascular tone. J Clin Monit Comput 1997; 13:223-228.
22. Vegfors M, Tryggvason B, Sjoberg F, et al: Assessment of peripheral blood flow using a pulse oximeter. J Clin Monit Comput 1990; 6:1-4.
23. Okuda Y, Kitajima Y, Asai T: Use of a pulse oximeter during performance of an axillary plexus block. Anaesthesia 1997; 52:717-718.
24. Roizen MF, Horrigan RW, Frazer BM: Anesthetic doses blocking adrenergic (stress) and cardiovascular responses to incision—MAC BAR. Anesthesiology 1981; 54:390-398.
25. Shimoda O, Ikata Y, Sakamoto M, et al: Skin vasomotor reflex predicts circulatory response to laryngoscopy and intubation. Anesthesiology 1998; 88:297-304.
26. Ikuta Y, Shimoda O, Ushijima K, et al: Skin vasomotor reflex as an objective indicator to assess the level of regional anesthesia. Anesth Analg 1998; 86:736-740.
27. Ezri T, Steinmetz A, Geva D, et al: Skin vasomotor reflex as a measure of depth of anesthesia. Anesthesiology 1998; 89:1281-1282.
28. Talke P, Nichols RJ, Traber D: Does measurement of systolic blood pressure with a pulse oximeter correlate with conventional methods? J Clin Monit Comput 1990; 6:5-9.
29. Wallace C, Baker J, Alpent CC: Comparison of blood pressure measurement by Doppler and by pulse oximetry techniques. Anesth Analg 1987; 66:1018-1019.
30. Ferrara J, Dyess D, Lasecki M: Surface oximetry: A new method to evaluate intestinal perfusion. Am Surg 1988; 54:10-14.
31. Stolar C, Randolph J: Evaluation of ischemic bowel viability with a fluorescent technique. J Pediatr Surg 1978; 13:221-225.
32. Graham B, Paulus D, Caffee HH: Pulse oximetry for vascular monitoring in upper extremity replantation surgery. J Hand Surg [Am] 1986; 11:687-692.
33. Stack B, et al: Spectral analysis of photoplethysmograms from radial forearm free flaps. Laryngoscope 1998; 108:1329-1333.
34. Blanc VF, et al: Computerized photoplethysmography of the finger. Can J Anaesth 1993; 40:271-278.
35. Perel A, Pizov R, Cotev S: Systolic blood pressure variation is a sensitive indicator of hypovolemia in ventilated dogs subjected to graded hemorrhage. Anesthesiology 1987; 67:498-502.
36. Cournand A, Motley HL, Werko L, et al: Physiological studies of the effect of intermittent positive pressure breathing on cardiac output in man. Am J Physiol 1948; 152:162-173.
37. Partridge BL: Use of pulse oximetry as a noninvasive indicator of intravascular volume status. J Clin Monit Comput 1987; 3:263-268.
38. Lherm T, Chevalier T, Troche G, et al: Correlation between plethysmography curve variation (dpleth) and pulmonary capillary wedge pressure (pcwp) in mechanically ventilated patients. Br J Anaesth 1995; 74(suppl 1):41.
39. Sami HM, Kleinman BS, Lonchyna VA: Central venous pulsations associated with a falsely low oxygen saturation measured by pulse oximetry. J Clin Monit Comput 1991; 7:309-312.
40. Shelley K, Dickstein M, Shulman S: The detection of peripheral venous pulsation using the pulse oximeter as a plethysmograph. J Clin Monit Comput 1993; 9:283-287.
41. Sano Y, Kataoka Y, Ikuyma T, et al: Evaluation of peripheral circulation with accelerated plethysmography and its practical application. Jpn Sci Lab 1985; 61:129-143.
42. Takada H, Washino K, Harrell JS, et al: Acceleration plethysmography to evaluate aging effect in cardiovascular system. Med Prog Technol 1997; 21:205-210.
43. O'Rourke M, Yaginuma T: Wave reflections and the arterial pulse. Arch Intern Med 1984; 144:366-371.
44. Nichols W, O'Rourke M: Contours of pressure and flow waves in arteries. In McDonald DA (ed): Blood flow in Arteries, Philadelphia, Lea & Febiger, 1990, pp 216-250.
45. Bruner J: Handbook of Blood Pressure Monitoring. Boston, Little, Brown, 1978.
46. Murray W, Gorven A: Invasive vs. non-invasive blood pressure measurement: The influence of the pressure contour. S Afr Med J 1991; 79:134-139.
47. Rusch T, Sankar R, Scharf J: Signal processing methods for pulse oximetry. Comput Biol Med 1996; 26:143-159.

24 Point-of-Care Monitoring and Analysis

Hugh C. Gilbert, M.D.
Jeffery S. Vender, M.D., F.C.C.M.

Point-of-care analysis refers to new technologies that provide clinicians with the capability of obtaining laboratory testing at the bedside. Central to the issue of point-of-care testing is this remarkable advance in technology, allowing complicated analysis to be performed with accuracy, precision, and ease outside the clinical laboratory. This chapter examines the growth and development of point-of-care analysis as it relates to the practice of anesthesiology and critical care medicine.

The clinical laboratory has been and remains an essential component of an acute care hospital. Physicians use laboratory testing to confirm clinical impressions, to make diagnoses, and to guide therapy and management. For the last several decades, availability, accuracy, and optimal turnaround time have been the guiding forces defining the technological and methodological management of hospital laboratories.

In the 1970s, hospitals recognized the importance of laboratory testing in emergency or critical care situations. As critical care units developed, the need for enhanced turnaround time of some laboratory tests became apparent. Tests on arterial blood gases (ABGs), electrolytes, serum glucose, creatinine kinase, and hemoglobin, and coagulation profiles provided essential data for clinical decision making. Today, options such as interruption of regular service, separate "stat" analyzers or near-patient satellite laboratories in critical areas are examples of strategies utilized to ensure that prompt measurement and reporting of the results are available to clinicians caring for unstable or critically ill patients. In 1984, Hall and Shapiro[1] surveyed 227 stat laboratories and found that all of these facilities performed blood gas and pH analysis. Eighteen percent also provided determination of sodium, potassium, calcium, osmotic pressure, and glucose, as well as oxygen saturation, oxyhemoglobin, and hematocrit (Hct) and hemoglobin (Hb) concentration.[1] Currently, stat laboratories and true point-of-care instruments are available offering a wide range of test clusters for analysis. Decentralization using nearby point-of-care hybrid laboratories heralded a transition in laboratory medicine. Today's technology provides the potential for portable, hand-held analyzers to optimize diagnosis and treatment strategies at the bedside or during transport to an acute care facility.[2, 3]

Point-of-care testing (POCT) requires a shift of emphasis from traditional laboratory analysis of plasma to whole-blood analysis. The goal of POCT is to facilitate medical decisions by providing near-instantaneous or rapid measurement of biologic variables. Whole-blood analysis is quicker because centrifugation is unnecessary. Modern whole-blood analysis requires very small volumes compared with traditional plasma testing. Philosophically, POCT should be limited to analytes that mark specific diseases or conditions, or analytes that vary significantly in sickness and in health. Inherent to the POCT paradigm is the ability for rapid diagnoses to result in enhanced decision making, thereby improving medical outcomes. Table 24-1 lists locations where POCT might be utilized to expedite and enhance clinical decisions.

The development of point-of-care options for laboratory medicine required an amalgamation of several divergent technologies. Microdetectors for analytes of interest needed to be invented, bench-tested, and scrutinized. In many instances, laboratory systems could be miniaturized and their performance simplified for bedside use by nontechnicians. New technology was designed that incorporated molecular components of plants and animals bound to electrodes, transistors, or optical fibers. As a group these devices are termed *biosensors*.[4] Practical bedside testing necessitates simple, compact instruments that can be operated by nurses, physicians, and respiratory therapists. Today, tiny "lab on a chip" platforms enable instrument makers to not only design ever-expanding test clusters but also to economize on blood requirements, making point-of-care testing an attractive alternative to traditional stat options.

Biosensors

There is a wide diversity of biologic components that can function as detectors in the design of biosensor systems. For this application biosensors are compact analytic devices that incorporate a biologic or biologically derived sensing element within, or intimately associated with, a physiochemical transducer.[5] Biosensors should have the potential to achieve detection levels with sensitivity and specificity equaling or exceeding standard bench testing. Enzyme electrode systems typically can detect analyte concentrations to micromole per liter levels (10^{-3}). Immunosensors enhance detection levels well below picomole per liter levels (10^{-12}). In the near future, biosensor detection will encompass nanotechnology in which sensitivity to the gene level is possible. Biosensor systems that require the removal of a fluid or tissue function as *analyzers*. If a biosensor is small enough and biologically safe to be placed in an artery, vein, or tissue in vivo, analysis is feasible, permitting the design of instruments which can function as monitors. *Monitors* are devices that are dedicated to a single patient, providing measurements without permanently removing fluid or tissue from the patient.[6]

As a group, biosensors must possess two important properties: *specificity* and *sensitivity*. A *quantitative* biosensor must respond uniquely to the analyte of interest so that the

Table 24–1. Locations Where Point-of-Care Testing Options Are Helpful

Emergency room	Neonatal intensive care unit	Catheterization laboratory
Intensive care unit		Dialysis
Coronary care unit	Burn unit	Mobile intensive care unit
	Trauma unit	
Obstetric suites	Operating room	Helicopter transport

Table 24–2. Agencies and Associations Regulating Point-of-Care Testing

College of American Pathologists (CAP)*
Joint Commission on Accreditation of Healthcare Organizations (JCAHO)
Health Care Financing Administration (HCFA)
State health departments†

*The CAP point-of-care testing (POCT) program does not subclassify tests by complexity and requires on-site inspection. Accreditation of POCT must be inspected as sections of the central laboratory if the POCT is registered under the same Clinical Laboratory Improvement Amendment of 1988 number.
†State and local regulatory agencies may have preferential jurisdiction.
From Gilbert HC, Vender JC: The current status of point-of-care monitoring. Int Anesthesiol Clin 1996; 24,248.

quality of the biosensor response estimates the concentration of analyte present in the sample. This response confers specificity. Specificity is determined by the properties of the biologic component at the analyte-sensor interface. Thus, cofactors, antibodies, receptors, enzymes, membranes, or other cell systems may be incorporated as biologic components of biosensors. Biosensor-analyte interactions produce optical, electrochemical, piezoelectric, calorimetric, mechanical, or even acoustic changes that quantify the concentration of the analyte present at the whole blood–biosensor interface. The sensitivity of a biosensor system depends on both the biologic component and the signal processing components.

Point-of-care instrumentation is designed to provide clinicians with measured and calculated values of analytes that can be linked together in testing clusters. Clustering of biosensors is a strategy used in hybrid laboratory instruments as well as in the design of single-use cartridges. Since the 1990s single-use biosensors such as strip whole-blood glucose testing have in great measure replaced the traditional laboratory for routine glucose testing. On the other hand, single-use cartridge testing is often reserved for special situations. Anesthesiologists often require stat laboratory testing in the emergency room, critical care units, operating room, and delivery room. Other hospital units such as the neonatal intensive care unit (NICU), catheterization laboratory, and renal dialysis may serve patients in whom POCT might be used.

Because remote testing instruments can be engineered to meet virtually any clinical need, it is necessary to consider not only which individual analytes are appropriate for POCT options but also how they might be integrated with one another. Microfabrication of biosensor chips and test strips permits simultaneous direct laboratory analysis using microliters of whole blood. Standard acute care analytic chemistry and ABGs can be measured using various biosensor technology. Sensor systems containing ion-sensitive electrodes are commonly used to measure iCa^{2+}, K^+, Na^+, and Cl^-. Substrate-specific biosensors (SSEs) can be multiplexed to measure glucose, lactate, urea nitrogen, and creatinine. Electrical conductance sensors provide estimates of hematocrit. Optodes or Clark polarographic electrodes are used for quantifying Po_2 and oxygen saturation, and amperometric pH electrodes to quantify Pco_2 and pH. Combinations of these biosensors have been fabricated to interface with hand-held instruments permitting remote laboratory analysis. Hand-held and near-point-of-care instrumentation options often use the same technology as central laboratory bench instruments. The principles of biosensor-based whole-blood measurement have been extensively reviewed by Kost and Hague.[7]

Glucometers were the first point-of-care instruments used widely for clinical decisions. Most bedside blood glucose instruments employ enzymatic biosensors and a chromogenic oxygen acceptor to produce a color change that can be quantified. Instruments using this methodology have been found to be accurate so long as inhibition of the peroxidase reaction is small. An alternative method using an enzyme-electrode sensor has also been designed. Errors in blood glucose measurement have been described using both systems. Kurahashi and colleagues[8] have found that glucose

electrode systems underestimate blood glucose if the Po_2 is high. Because different methods of analysis can be influenced by a variety of factors, it is essential that clinicians be aware of the practical limitations of point-of-care analysis.

Regulation of Point-of-Care Analyzers

Introducing a point-of-care analyzer (POCA) such as a glucose meter or any other point-of-care blood analysis system into a hospital setting requires an understanding of the various agencies and organizations that have a regulatory interest in laboratory testing in the acute care setting. The primary agencies overseeing hospital-based POCT are listed in Table 24–2. Clinical laboratories are certified by the U.S. Department of Health and Human Services (DHHS) and by state health agencies.[9] In the case of hand-held glucose meters, a certificate of waiver has been issued and the prevailing regulations regarding personnel, training, quality assurance, quality control, and calibration are based on each manufacturer's instructions.[10] Table 24–3 lists the salient regulatory guidelines that interact when clinicians introduce POCT into the hospital setting.

The Clinical Laboratory Improvement Amendment of 1988 (CLIA) does not specifically address POCT as a separate form of testing. CLIA regulations are site-neutral and are based on test complexity. Each test or analyzer system is judged on the basis of the skills needed to perform the analysis, the chances of the operator making an error, and the risk of the error causing harm. The DHHS issues waivers for systems in which the method of operation and the analysis is straightforward and inherently dependable. The DHHS requires stat or hybrid laboratories to meet the same requirements as a certified clinical laboratory with respect to quality control and proficiency testing. While there are no specific requirements regarding the education, training, or experi-

Table 24–3. Issues Influencing the Introduction of Point-of-Care Testing

Personnel and training
Quality control
Proficiency testing:
Frequency
Methodology
Calibration verification
Certification and inspection
Records and documentation
Integration with central laboratory

From Gilbert HC, Vender JC: The current status of point-of-care monitoring. Int Anesthesiol Clin 1996; 24,249.

ence of those individuals performing analysis in stat laboratories, significant prerequisites exist regarding documentation, quality assurance, and proficiency testing.[11]

The Joint Commission on Accreditation of Healthcare Organizations (JCAHO) mandates that testing at the bedside must be coordinated by the department of pathology. For POCT to be approved, the College of American Pathologists (CAP) requires that the activities for testing and quality control come under the direction, authority, jurisdiction, and responsibility of the director of laboratories. Therefore, the introduction of hospital-based POCT of moderately or highly complex equipment such as blood gas analyzers, whole-blood electrolytes, and various tests of coagulation require integration with the hospital's clinical laboratory to ensure that issues such as personnel, training, quality control, proficiency testing, and certification are appropriate for the regulatory environment. Often state and local health departments have requirements that may take precedence over federal mandates. Differences in oversight by accrediting bodies and state or federal authorities relate to restrictiveness. Belanger[12] has reviewed the issues regarding alternative-site testing. While one group may be more restrictive, in the final analysis all laboratory regulation involves three basic elements: training of personnel, licensing, and competent mechanisms to assess validity and reliability.[12] For this reason, it is wise to explore regional practices before implementing POCT.

While regulations are enacted to protect the public, current regulations of clinical laboratory testing do not eliminate all risks. Systematic errors may occur and are often inherent to the instrumentation or methodology utilized for analysis. In the case of POCT, biosensor packaging is dated to ensure that reagents and biosensor components are fresh and stable. System checks, single-use biosensor cartridges, cuvettes, test strips, and analyte calibration codes represent design features that can identify with great certainty whether a POCA is functioning within the manufacturer's specifications.

While it is clear that traditional laboratory systems are prone to drift and may require attention and maintenance, point-of-care systems are manufactured for consistent performance. Occasionally, a random analytic error due to a breach of technique or an instability of a biosensor system missed at the time of manufacturing may occur. Well-designed POCAs examine all phases of the testing system before performing a calibration check, thus ensuring that the possibility of a systematic error is small. While POCAs are simple to operate and have built-in quality controls and calibration features, many of these instruments require some judgment and skill with respect to troubleshooting, maintenance, and interpretation. Moderately complex tests lend themselves to point-of-care methods. High-complexity testing, which often requires multiple steps or significant interpretation of endpoints, does not lend itself to POCT unless the technology and design simplify the analysis so that it can be performed outside the laboratory. Table 24–4 lists POCTs currently waived by the Health Care Financing Administration (HCFA).

POCAs are designed to reduce sampling errors. Sampling errors and specimen handling errors are possible whenever samples are collected and transported to a central or nearby POC facility. Sampling errors may still occur as a result of faulty technique.

Regulating bodies require quality-control programs to identify inaccuracy and imprecision. Performance criteria such as accuracy and laboratory precision are statistically validated by enrollment in proficiency testing at regular intervals. *Accuracy* is defined as the nearness of a measurement to the actual value of the analyte. *Bias* defines the consistent difference in the measured value as compared to the meas-

Table 24–4. Summary Listing of Point-of-Care Testing Currently Waived by the Health Care Financing Administration*

Dipsticks for urinalysis and fecal occult blood
Nicotine and metabolites
Ovulation tests by visual color
Urine pregnancy tests†
Erythrocyte sedimentation rate — nonautomated
HemoCue hemoglobin†
Spun micohematocrit†
Blood glucose meters†
Cholesterol, high-density lipoprotein, triglyceride test strips
Rapid microbiologic immunoassays (IgG)
Helicobacter pylori
Group A streptococci
Heterophil antibodies for infectious mononucleosis
Prothrombin time microcoagulation testing systems†
Pending approval
Spuncrit analyzer for hematocrit†
Saliva alcohol test†

*Updated Oct. 30, 1998.
†Indicates test that may be of value to anesthesiologists.

ured value of a known variable. *Precision* defines the closeness of multiple measurements of a stable sample of known value. In the clinical laboratory, accuracy, bias, and precision are closely monitored. For some analytes, such as ABG analyzers, in which accuracy, bias, and precision vary, periodic comparison with other laboratories is performed monthly.[13, 14] Target values are established by calculation of the mean value for the laboratories enrolled.

Most of the regulations that currently apply to point-of-care systems were specifically designed for clinical laboratories. Quality-control regulations serve to detect errors by requiring testing of samples of known composition at frequent intervals. Statistical analysis of quality-control results provides information regarding day-to-day variability. Proficiency testing provides an unbiased assessment of the accuracy of the laboratory's results in relation to its peers.

Unlike a traditional laboratory quality-control program, hand-held POCAs differ in that the only reusable portion of the system is the analyzer. Hand-held instruments do not perform batch runs and their quality-control programs have been designed to test the electrical characteristics of the signals produced by the sensors. Electrical simulators have been designed to produce mock signals consistent with high and low concentrations of analytes, which simplifies quality-control calibration routines. The analytic precision of cartridge-based point-of-care analysis performed by nonlaboratorians compares favorably with laboratory analysis.[15] Point-of-care cartridges have self-contained calibration solutions. Before blood analysis, a pH-buffered solution of the analytes at known concentrations automatically performs a calibration check of the biosensor system.

Point-of-care systems are often used by clinical personnel who are less prone to systematic errors and more likely to make random errors. Quality-control and proficiency-testing programs are not designed to identify random errors. Users of point-of-care systems must be certain that they understand the operation of the instrument, the appropriate handling of biosensor cartridges, and the appropriate method for introducing a sample for analysis. Point-of-care analysis may require documentation of a quality management program and proficiency testing, which may have a significant impact on the cost of offering POCT. The responsibility and authority for quality-control and proficiency-testing programs must be defined within the institution, and the training and continuing education of the end-users must be documented and must demonstrate substantial compliance with the manufacturers' instructions. A policy and procedure plan needs to be established with the advice and consent of the director of the clinical laboratory before a POCT can substitute for or replace an existing certified stat test system.

In the case of portable glucose analyzers, studies have demonstrated substantial variability due to operator technique, disease populations, Hct, state of hydration, and blood sampling technique, as well as instrument performance.[16, 17] The Association of Clinical Biochemists and the Consensus Development Conference on Self-Monitoring of Blood Glucose suggest that point-of-care systems should show agreement within 15% of the central laboratory methodology.[18, 19] Several published reports document their accuracy, precision, and performance when utilized at the bedside.[20-22]

The manufacturers of bedside glucose analyzers recommend that end-users self-monitor the performance of point-of-care glucose testing with accuracy and precision studies. Accuracy is determined by performing duplicate measurements (split sampling) and comparing the means with the reference laboratory method of analysis. Procedural errors are present when differences greater than 30% result. Tables of accuracy are maintained where the percentage differences between the point-of-care meter and the reference method are logged. Precision is analyzed by calculating the standard deviation (SD) of a set of whole-blood glucose values. Calculating the coefficient of variation [CV = (SD/mean) × 100] gives a measure of precision at a specific glucose level for the sample studied. Ideally, precision should be measured for the range of clinically significant values. Whole-blood samples spiked with aliquots of 10% glucose solution can be made to test accuracy and precision over the range of interest. Target values for accuracy and requirements for proficiency testing have been published.[23]

Bedside Point-of-Care Analysis

Point-of-care analysis has developed to permit quick and accurate assessment of an analyte. For anesthesiologists and critical care physicians, the urgency of laboratory analysis is predicated on confirming a diagnosis or establishing that ongoing medical management is appropriate. As an example, many physicians would not consider a point-of-care option of determining Hb or Hct a critical feature for therapeutic options because Hb and Hct values do not usually change rapidly enough to warrant bedside measurements, even in actively bleeding patients. Yet cardiac anesthesiologists welcome the bedside Hb option to determine oxygen-carrying capacity before separation of the patient from bypass because new data suggest that hemodilution may be implicated as contributing to post-bypass cerebral ischemia.[24] Table 24-5 gives our list of point-of-care analyte options and the clinical settings that may warrant POCT.

The following section summarizes pertinent aspects of several point-of-care devices currently available for clinical use. The descriptions have been simplified and are not necessarily inclusive of all point-of-care technologies that can be used for analysis or monitoring. Integration of point-of-care technology with existing operating room (OR) and intensive care unit (ICU) monitoring systems provides the potential for networking of many bedside testing options whereby results can be posted on automated record systems.

Point-of-Care Testing

Hemoglobin, Hematocrit, and Coagulation Testing

Quantitative bedside Hb testing enables clinicians to perform a photometric analysis that estimates the Hb concentration in 1 minute. HemoCue (HemoCue Inc., Mission Viejo, CA) uses 10 μL of whole blood that is introduced into a cuvette containing sodium desoxycholate and sodium nitrite. Once the sample is in the reaction chamber, the erythrocyte walls are disintegrated by the action of the sodium desoxycholate and the free Hb is converted to methemoglobin by the sodium nitrite. An azide dye present in the cuvette reacts with the methemoglobin. The resulting azidemethemoglobin can then be measured by the HemoCue photometer. The HemoCue Hb CV has been determined to be ±1.2% to 1.7% in the ranges of 8 to 18 g/dL. HemoCue also manufactures a different cuvette designed to measure glucose. These capillary collection and detection systems provide multiple analysis using less than 0.2 mL of blood.

Hct is a simple test that has a high probability of blood exposure due to the fragility of capillary tubes and the need to seal them before centrifugation. Spuncrit (Micro Diagnostic Corp., Bethlehem, PA) is a battery-operated, miniature portable optical centrifuge that reduces user contact with

Table 24–5. Point-of-Care Testing (POCT) Options: Locations and Potential Testing Options*

Tests	ER	OR	PACU	ICU/CCU	OB	NICU
Blood sugar	X	X	X	X	X	X
Hb/Hct	X	X	X	X	X	X
Coagulation profile	X	X	X	X	X	
Platelet function testing	X	X	X	X	X	
Creatinine kinase	X	X	X	X	—	—
Troponin T	X	X	X	X		
Arterial blood gases	X	X	X	X	X	X
Electrolytes	X	X	X	X	X	X
iCa^{2+}	X	X	X	X	?	X
Mg^{2+}	—	X	—	X	X	X
Toxicology POCT	X	—	—	—	X	—
Bacteriologic POCT	X	—	—	X	X	X

ER, emergency room; OR, operating room; PACU, postoperative anesthesia care unit; ICU/CCU, all intensive care settings, including trauma units, etc.; OB, obstetric and maternity suites; NICU, neonatal intensive care unit; Hb/Hct, hemoglobin or hematocrit.

*In our opinion, POCT has its greatest potential value in situations in which the immediacy of obtaining the test results influences clinical decision making. This would include situations where delays in needed medical care or surgery could be reduced or eliminated.

From Gilbert HC, Vender JC: The current status of point-of-care monitoring. Int Anesthesiol Clin 1996; 24,251.

blood and measures the Hct employing a diode array and a laser light source to determine the plasma–red blood cell interface. The system estimates Hct in the range of 10% to 60%. Optical centrifugation techniques are currently being developed for platelet counts, Hb, and even potassium. The quality buffy coat (QBC) optical signature technology (Becton-Dickinson, Sandy, UT) is an example of a point-of-care analysis designed for hematologists and primary care physicians. This uses a specially designed capillary tube containing potassium oxalate, monoclonal antibody, and acridine orange coating. During centrifugation, differential staining of whole blood components occurs. Fluorescence scanning permits calculation of Hct, white blood cell count, granulocytes, lymphocytes, monocytes, platelets, and Hb. For the most part, anesthesiologists and critical care physicians are satisfied with the response time of traditional methods of obtaining complete blood counts and platelets. However, point-of-care hematologic options could enhance clinical judgment in high-risk obstetrics, transplantation, trauma, and cardiac surgery. Point-of-care blood gas analyzers calculate total Hb using biosensors that measure Hct electrochemically.

Monitoring the thrombotic response of blood during various medical and surgical procedures often requires quick and accurate tests of anticoagulation. For many years portable systems for evaluating whole blood anticoagulation have been introduced into clinical practice. Recently, microcoagulation instruments (HEMO-CHRON, ITC Corp., Edison, NJ) have been designed to permit evaluation of established tests utilizing a disposable cuvette that precisely delivers 15 μL of blood into a test chamber containing the appropriate regents to determine prothrombin time (PT), activated partial thromboplastin time (APTT), or a silica, kaolin-activated clotting time (ACT⁺). The ACT⁺ reagent system enhances the accuracy of the ACT test when antifibrinolytic therapy (e.g., protease inhibitors such as aprotinin ≤500 KIU/mL blood) has been administered. Microcoagulation tests use a mechanical endpoint to determine clot formation. After whole blood is introduced into a cuvette, a sample is mixed with the appropriate reagents (cuvette-specific) and the mixture is moved back and forth within a test channel. Clot detection is determined by light-emitting diode (LED) optical sensors that track the motion of the sample in the cuvette. Cuvettes are packed in foil pouches and when refrigerated (4° to 8°C) are stable until the marked expiration date. Like any method, microcoagulation testing can be influenced by poor sampling or poor transfer technique. Electronic verification cartridges are available to provide a two-level check of the instrument as well as a check on maintaining the proper temperature for analysis. Whole-blood quality-control kits are available to verify that each box of cuvettes meets performance standards.

POCT of hemostasis is an important area for research and development. Principles for clot detection include particle motion, plunger motion, pattern recognition, fluorescence, hemagglutination, and fluid oscillation. A wide variety of testing protocols have been marketed. Clot detection systems using cartridges, test cuvettes, cards, or strips offer clinicians the ability to perform PT and APTT at the bedside. In addition, thrombotic assessment methods and platelet function can also be quantified at the bedside. Clot detection technologies that provide an absolute number as a result can easily be adapted for point-of-care use. Quantitative detection of platelet dysfunction is also available to monitor the dynamics of platelet plug formation. These tests are often used to augment clinical utility of the PT and APPT. It is possible to detect inherited, acquired, or induced platelet dysfunction in minutes using point-of-care systems.

The PFA-100 (Dade Behring, Miami, FL) is an example of a system that simulates platelet adhesion and aggregation found in a traumatized blood vessel. This system monitors blood flow surrounding a biochemically active membrane, which is mounted under a known shear stress. When platelets adhere and aggregate at the aperture, the elapse time is determined and reported as the closure time. A prolongation of closure time indicates a defect in coagulation. The clinical performance of the PFA-100 system has been evaluated by Kundu and associates.[25] Closure time is principally dependent on the absolute platelet count and the functionality of the platelets. Physiologic testing of platelet function at the bedside often requires evaluation of a timed graphic of physicochemical events. Interpretation of a graphic requires skill. Systems in which abnormalities are quantified by a numeric enhance clinical utility.

Bedside Diagnosis of Myocardial Infarction

As the effectiveness of thrombolysis therapy has been correlated with the timing of treatment, there has been interest in developing point-of-care systems for the early diagnosis of myocardial infarction.[26] Bedside creatine kinase (CK) assay (Reflotron Boehringer Mannheim, Indianapolis), using a microprocessor-controlled reflectance meter and reagent strips to which 32 μL of whole blood is applied, can identify increases in CK activity. Recently, Downie and colleagues[27] found that point-of-care CK had a high specificity and predictive value when studied in patients admitted to the coronary care unit with suspected myocardial infarction. The current technology does not distinguish other potential sources of CK, such as intramuscular injection, polymyositis, or skeletal muscle damage.

To meet the need for a bedside detection system that can identify patients experiencing ongoing cardiac ischemia, a similar system has been designed to measure the cardiac form of troponin T (cTnT) (CARDIAC reader system, Roche Diagnostics). CARDIAC reader quantifies the cardiac markers myoglobin and troponin T. The system uses a test strip and in 8 to 14 minutes displays the result. Early detection using the cTnT assay has been proposed as a sensitive and specific diagnostic indicator of myocardial infarction.[28]

These systems offer clinicians a specific bedside method for the detection of myocardial injury. Because the kinetics of cTnT release are similar for both Q and non-Q wave myocardial infarction, the cTnTc assay may prove helpful in stratifying patients for antithrombotic therapy.[29, 30]

The significance of rapid bedside measurements of cardiac enzymes requires exploration of the time needed to perform a serum cardiac marker on a fully operational random-access chemistry analyzer. In most circumstances, it may take as long as 2 hours, for the managing physicians to obtain a result. Furthermore, not all hospitals are able to support CK-MB analysis on a 24-hour basis. Point-of-care cardiac injury or infarction detection, while considered an appropriate emergency room point-of-care option, may have value in evaluation of patients with chest pain in the post-anesthesia care unit (PACU).

Bedside Blood Chemistry and Arterial Blood Gas Testing

It has been estimated that in the United States alone, 40 million electrolyte and 135 million ABG tests are ordered on a stat basis annually. Blood tests recognized as being essential in emergency or critical care situations include pH, P_{O_2},

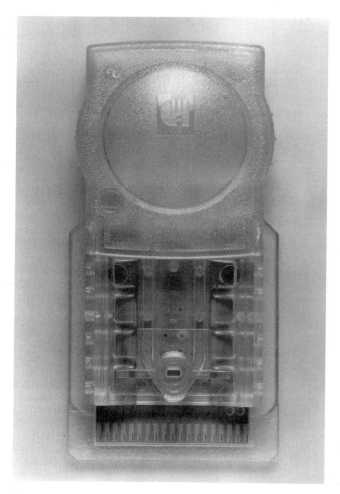

Figure 24–1. Disposable IRMA cartridge for arterial blood gas and electrolyte testing. Biosensor systems used in point-of-care analyzers such as IRMA or i-STAT offer end-users prompt analysis, blood conservation, and safe disposal of all potentially contaminated liquids used in sampling and analysis. (Courtesy of Diametrics Medical Inc., St. Paul, MN.)

PCO_2, Na^+, K^+, and Hct and Hb. Others, such as iCa^{2+}, Mg^{2+}, glucose, lactic acid, and osmolality tests, are commonly ordered on a stat basis. The development and implementation of ion-selective electrodes for analytes such as sodium, potassium, and calcium, coupled with sensor technologies that measure blood gases, permit the design and marketing of a new generation of analyzers that can perform stat analysis at the bedside. Figure 24–1 depicts the simplicity of a single-use sensor array cartridge (IRMA, Diametric Medical Inc., St. Paul, MN).

Bedside testing instrumentation has developed in several directions. Multiuse laboratory analyzers have been miniaturized, made portable, and their operations simplified. They often employ multiuse sensor cartridges packaged with appropriate calibrating and flush solutions. The packaging of the sensor arrays and support solutions simplifies operation so that clinical personnel can perform a stat battery on as many as 50 to 150 sets of measurements because of the modularity of design. Instrumentation often includes autocalibrations, error detection, self-diagnostics, and extensive data management and communication capabilities making it possible to easily integrate these systems with the central labora-

tory's proficiency and quality-control programs.[31, 32] These instruments are suitable for use in stat laboratories. Commonly, this type of equipment is categorized as "transportable" or "near-point-of-care" (NPOC). NPOC analyzers can be distinguished from POCAs in that the sensor design supports *multiple patient testing* using disposable reagents and sensors designed for replacement after a specific number of analyses. Examples include the GEM Premier (Instrumentation Laboratories, Lexington, MA), SenDx 100 (SenDx Medical, Carlsbad, CA), and Nova, (Nova Biomedical, Waltham, MA). These instruments are easily integrated into ongoing quality-control and proficiency-testing programs because of their similarity to laboratory instrumentation. Transportable analyzer systems often permit deselection of a test not ordered or clinically required. This option is particularly desirable because of recent Medicare regulations regarding reimbursement of testing clusters. As a group, NPOC instruments can be operated by nonlaboratory personnel and are easily interfaced with the central laboratory. While they reduce or eliminate the cost of specimen transport, receiving, and accession (e.g., logging-in and assigning a sample to a laboratory workstation), their impact on expenditures depends on the methods utilized to calculate annual laboratory costs and the expiration percentage of test utilization of each disposable cartridge pack.[33]

Bedside POCAs are discrete portable instruments incorporating single-use cartridges that contain sensors and reagents to perform a specific battery of tests on a single sample of whole blood. These systems offer clinicians a true point-of-care option in that the operation of the analyzer is designed to be used by clinical staff who do not have experience or interest in quantitative analysis. Cartridge-based microanalytic methods for measuring ABGs, electrolytes, urea, glucose, and Hct have been approved for clinical use. All of the systems described are subject to the same regulatory requirements that govern the operation of standard analytic instruments. Manufacturers design lockouts and user-identification codes and electronic controls to ensure that quality assurance requirements for tracking machine operations are in place and operational before an end-user can initiate analyte analysis.

POCAs are simple to operate and virtually maintenance-free. Operator training is fast and straightforward. For the most part, discrete sample biosensors incorporate conventional electrochemical or enzyme methodologies, or both, which can be mass-produced and packaged to provide selected test configurations costing from $1.25 to $12.00 per cartridge. For an analysis, the cartridge is inserted into the analyzer and a calibration and equipment check is performed automatically. Cartridges are designed to minimize human exposure to blood. Analyzer systems (e.g., IRMA or i-STAT, i-STAT Corp., Princeton, NJ; OPTI 1, AVL Scientific, Roswell, GA) are battery-operated for portability. All of these systems can provide estimates of ABGs and electrolytes using less than 0.5 mL of blood in approximately 90 seconds. Figures 24–2 and 24–3 depict the i-STAT hand-held and IRMA hand-held analyzers. The analytic performance of these POCAs appears to be reliable based on extensive accuracy and precision testing by the manufacturers.[34–36]

Each of the systems utilizes potentiometric ion-selective membrane electrodes or optical sensors for determining pH and electrolytes in whole blood. Electrochemical instruments measure PCO_2 using micropotentiometric gas sensors in which CO_2 diffuses across a gas-permeable membrane into a thin layer of bicarbonate electrolyte that is in contact with a pH electrode. At equilibrium, the voltage change measured by the pH electrode is directly proportional to the PCO_2 in the sample. PO_2 measurements are performed with Clark polarographic oxygen sensors in which a negative voltage is

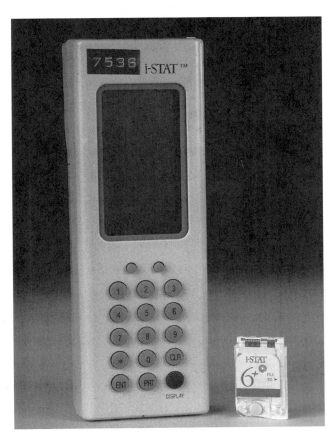

Figure 24–2. Disposable blood chemistry cartridge and hand-held i-STAT analyzer. The number on the cartridge reflects the testing options and biosensors incorporated into the cartridge. (Courtesy of i-STAT Corp., Princeton, N.J.)

applied to a microplatinum electrode; this forces reduction of water to oxygen and hydrogen ions. An outer oxygen-permeable membrane protects the platinum from plasma proteins.

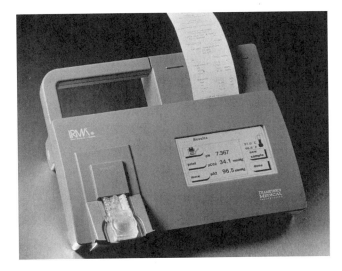

Figure 24–3. IRMA point-of-care analyzer by Diametrics Medical. (Courtesy of Diametrics Medical Inc., St. Paul, MN.)

Optical sensing methods embed fluorescent dyes onto the sensing probe or biosensor. Most fiberoptic systems designed for measuring ABGs use oxygen- and pH-sensitive dyes as indicators. In the case of PO_2 measurements, a fluorescence-based sensor technology has evolved in which the concentration of oxygen in the blood sample "quenches" the intensity of the fluorescence of the dye when it is stimulated by an excitation signal passed through an optical fiber. Similarly, absorbance-based sensors (pH, PCO_2) employ a dye that absorbs incident light in proportion to the concentration of the analyte in question. These types of sensors are generically termed optodes. Optical fluorescence technology has been utilized to design commercially available POCAs and monitors (AVL OPTI, AVL Scientific Corp., Roswell, GA; Paratrend, Diametrix Medical, St. Paul, MN).

Continuous Arterial and Electrolyte Monitoring

If a sensor array is placed within an arterial cannula or is located within an arterial blood sampling sidestream, it is possible for POCAs to function as ABG monitors. Early studies confirm that immediate blood gas results and the trending information from continuous intravenous arterial blood gas measurements (CIABGs) can be clinically relevant and reliable for clinical decision making.[37] In vivo biosensors are designed to be inserted through 20-gauge catheters. Because of their small size, sensor arrays have been limited to pH, PCO_2, PO_2, and temperature. The reliability of in vivo ABG sensors has been extensively studied under many clinical conditions.[38] The precision of PO_2 estimates appears to be dependent on the flow state surrounding the arterial sensor. Mahutte et al.[39] were the first to describe a "down-up-down" pattern of pH and PCO_2 values, which they attributed to clot formation at the sensor tip. Similarly, the author commented on a "down" pattern in PO_2 in which sensor malpositioning against the arterial wall "contaminates" the PO_2 estimate.

For CIABG measurements, outlier samples exhibiting the down-up-down or down patterns often account for those instances in which major differences between CIABG monitoring and standard ABG measurements exceed the usual limits of agreement.[40] In vivo CIABG systems are calibrated before insertion, using tonometry. After insertion, periodic control testing is not feasible.

CIABG has been marketed for real-time respiratory and metabolic information in the most challenging of patients. The Paratrend 7 (Diametrics Medical/Biomedical Sensors, Bucks, U.K.) uses a gamma-irradiated, heparin-coated, single-use sensor that combines an electrode-fiberoptic sensor array that provides on-line, continuous measurements of PO_2, PCO_2, pH, and temperature. Figures 24–4 and 24–5 illustrate the Paratrend sensor and display module. A similar system (Neotrend) is designed for use in neonates; the sensor system is suitable for umbilical insertion. Neotrend uses fluorescent optical technology, providing real-time continuous arterial gas and temperature data without blood sampling. The accuracy and reliability of these patient care systems has been established.[41-46] These systems are "continuously invasive." They reduce variability based on sampling and handling, and in clinical trials appear to provide meaningful data for clinical decisions.

Because CIABG systems have the potential for thrombosis, ex vivo, single-patient sensor arrays have been designed to provide near-continuous bedside analysis of ABGs and selected electrolytes. Ex vivo ABG monitoring incorporating optode sensor technology has also been extensively tested. Placing a sensor array outside of the arterial blood path

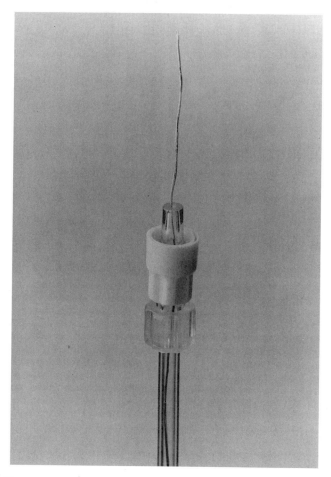

Figure 24–4. Close-up view of the Paratrend 7 in vivo biosensor. This filament is designed to be inserted into a 20-gauge arterial catheter. The filament contains a pH, Pco_2, Po_2, and temperature sensor that can provide continuous monitoring of arterial blood gases. (Courtesy of Diametrics Medical Inc., St. Paul, MN.)

potentially enhances sensor performance, expands the opportunity to include selected biosensors in addition to ABG sensors, permits frequent sampling and trending of ABG values, and permits traditional calibration checks.

A multicentered prospective trial of the ex vivo CDI-2000 system (CDI-3M Healthcare, Tustin CA) has been reported by Shapiro.[47] Clinical studies using CDI-3M technology have demonstrated stability, consistency, and accuracy.[48] In spite of the excellent performance, the manufacturer currently offers systems designed for use during extracorporeal perfusion.

"Paracorporeal" systems can function as on-demand blood gas monitors. Manufacturers of ex vivo systems (e.g., Sensicath, Optical Sensors Incorporated, Minneapolis, MN, Via 1-01 Blood Gas and Chemistry Monitor, Via Medical Corp., San Diego, CA) believe that ex vivo ABG sensors can match the performance of traditional ABG and electrolyte testing while eliminating blood contact and blood loss. These systems have the potential to reduce blood loss in patients requiring frequent blood sampling. Gischler and colleagues[49] have determined that the Sensicath device is cost-effective when at least nine blood gas tests per day are used in pediatric ICU patients. The performance of ex vivo systems mirrors traditional laboratory testing.[50]

The Future of Point-of-Care Testing

POCT has stimulated considerable interest as evidenced by the growth in the number of analyzers approved for clinical use. Advocates of POCT emphasize the potential for enhanced decision making and possible cost savings. While it is clear conceptually that POCT can substantially minimize turnaround time, its impact on quality of care and on hospital costs is still under scrutiny. Because the economics of acute care admissions are changing, it is difficult to ascertain the differences in the annual cost of POCT as compared with central laboratory testing. Nosanchuk and Keefner[51] found that the costs associated with i-STAT POCT analysis exceeded central laboratory stat testing. Furthermore, they contended that augmenting the utilization of POCT glucose and electrolyte testing would increase the annual cost of operation, in contrast to central laboratory testing, in which enhanced utilization lowers the per capita cost.[51] Recent presentations have suggested improved cost-efficiency. The issue of cost-effectiveness has largely not been addressed due to limited experience and institutional variability.

POCT is at a crossroads. Hospital laboratorians must not only be involved in the implementation of point-of-care systems but must endorse the technology and concept. The current regulatory environment may not be synchronous with current controls that manufacturers design into the operation and performance of their systems. Consider the issue of ABG testing at the bedside. Manufacturers perform extensive testing of cartridges prior to distribution. Calibration codes authenticate the efficacy of biosensor-analyzer interfaces, and electronic checks reduce equipment errors. Ana-

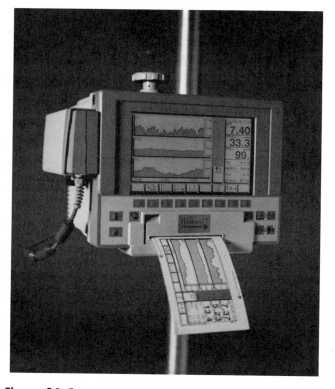

Figure 24–5. The Paratrend 7 arterial blood gas monitor. This system provides clinicians with an updated estimate of arterial blood gases and a real-time plot of pH, Pco_2, and Po_2. Hard-copy print capability is also provided. (Courtesy of Diametrics Medical Inc., St. Paul, MN.)

lyzers perform one-point calibrations before all measurements and monitor biosensor electrolytic characteristics electronically. Single-use biosensor technology has a defined performance.

While the limits of acceptable agreement established for pooled results for ABGs are relatively tight for pH and P_{CO_2}, 3 SD of the pooled P_{O_2} estimates is often acceptable for laboratory instruments.[10, p. 7008] Interinstrument variability of P_{O_2} measurement is very common.[52] Bench testing using split sampling has demonstrated that point-of-care systems (IRMA) for ABG measurements compare favorably with standard ABG analysis.[53]

The crucial issue that needs further study centers on redundancy, cost, and utilization. Most acute care facilities have established procedures to provide reasonable stat testing. In spite of the anxiety clinicians express regarding the time constraints inherent to traditional stat testing, there is very little objective information demonstrating that the expediency inherent to bedside testing fosters an enhancement of therapy unless the clinical care team has been trained to expeditiously alter therapy based on bedside evaluation. On the other hand, there is evidence that laboratory testing in critical care patients often provokes anemia. POCT conserves blood and features biohazard containment.

Laboratorians have implemented programs to deliver essential analysis in a timely manner with appropriate levels of accuracy and control. Point-of-care technology is always faster and has an engineered accuracy that to date appears to meet regulatory scrutiny. Unfortunately, applying the highest level of scrutiny necessary for laboratory certification may disenfranchise potential point-of-care end-users because of the added cost of monitoring split sample analysis and enrolling in proficiency testing. The ultimate success of point-of-care monitoring will be determined by the answers to these questions:

1. Can point-of-care electronic system testing meet regulatory standards for waivers?

2. Are statistically valid differences in cost efficiencies found following the integration of POCT in acute care hospitals?

In spite of the many benefits point-of-care technology may bring, there still remain considerable barriers to its implementation. Clinicians often look on point-of-care technology as streamlining their potential. Laboratorians want to control the process and maintain the central laboratory as the focus for testing. The impact of whole blood analysis using point-of-care technology is still being evaluated. Several hand-held and many portable instruments are currently available. Their test menus, features, analysis time, on-site performance, and information integration have been evaluated.[54] Although there is evidence that progress toward decentralization has been made, most hospitals have heavy investments in laboratory information systems and point-of-care instrument makers have developed strategies to integrate their instruments within these systems. Similarly, POCT can be integrated with OR monitoring systems.

Still, the major issue aside from convenience is the debate over cost. Laboratorians hold fast to conventional analysis, while clinicians claim that traditional laboratory testing is too slow and want the convenience of POCT to streamline their work. In our opinion, the selective use of point-of-care technology can be both clinically useful and cost-efficient. While there are data to suggest that POCT can be less costly than traditional testing, the greatest savings in these analyses appear to be related to the need for fewer laboratory personnel.[55] The cost-effectiveness of POCT is realized through

three potential avenues: a decrease in direct costs, a reduction in personnel costs, and a reduction in turnaround time.[56] Recently, attention has been directed to the potential impact of POCT on anemia seen in critical care patients. POCT has been shown to provide essential laboratory data without substantial losses in circulating blood volume.[57] This is especially important in the NICU.

If POCT furthers clinical decision making, it could ultimately improve healthcare delivery to the critically ill patient. If so, POCT should be embraced as an important component of critical and emergency care medicine.

REFERENCES

1. Hall JR, Shapiro BA: Acute care/blood gas laboratories: Profile of current operations. Crit Care Med 1984; 12:530–533.
2. Herr DM, Newton NC, Santrach PJ, et al: Airborne and rescue point-of-care testing. Am J Clin Pathol 1995; 104:S54–58.
3. Pons PT: Advances in prehospital care: The technology of emergency medical services. Med Instrum 1988; 22:143–145.
4. Rechnitz GA: Biosensors. Chem Eng News 1988; 5:24.
5. Turner APE, Karube I, Wilson GS: Biosensors: Fundamentals and Applications. Oxford, Oxford University Press, 1987.
6. Bone RC, Chernow B, Chiachierini RP, et al (Coalition for critical care excellence: Conclusions Conference on Physiologic Monitoring Devices): Standards of evidence for the safety and effectiveness of critical care monitoring devices and related interventions. Crit Care Med 1995; 23:1756–1763.
7. Kost GJ, Hague C: The current and future status of critical care testing and monitoring. Am J Clin Pathol 1995; 104:S2–17.
8. Kurahashi, K, Maruta H, Usuda Y, et al: Influence of blood sample oxygen concentration measured using an enzyme-electrode method. Crit Care Med 1997; 25:231–235.
9. Baer DM, Belsey RE: The evolving regulatory environment and bedside metabolic monitoring of the acute care patient. Chest 1990; 97:191S–193S.
10. Medicare, Medicaid and CLIA programs: Regulations implementing the Clinical Laboratory Improvement Amendment of 1988 (CLIA '88). Federal Register 1992; 57(Feb 28):7001–7288.
11. Ehrmeyer SS, Laessig RH: Regulatory requirements (CLIA '88, JCHO, CAP) for decentralized testing. Am J Clin Pathol 1995; 104(suppl 1):S40–49.
12. Belanger AC: Alternate site testing—the regulatory perspective. Arch Pathol Lab Med 1995; 119:902–906.
13. Wicker EK, Tenunissen AJ, Van den Camp RA, et al: A comparative study of the electrode systems of three pH and blood gas apparatus. J Clin Chem Biochem 1978; 16:175–185.
14. Interlaboratory Comparison Program Surveys Manual. Section III: Clinical Chemistry. Chicago, College of American Pathologists, 1992, pp 28–29.
15. Jacobs, E., Vadasdi E, Sarkozi L, et al: Analytical evaluation of i-STAT portable clinical analyzer and use by non-laboratory healthcare professionals. Clin Chem 1992; 39:1069–1074.
16. Nichols JH, Howard C, Loman K, et al: Laboratory and bedside evaluation of portable glucose meters. Am J Clin Pathol 1995; 103:244–250.
17. Portable blood glucose monitors: Evaluation. Health Devices 1992; 21:43–78.
18. Price CP, Burrin JM, Nattrass M: Extra-laboratory glucose measurement: A policy statement. Diabetes Med 1988; 5:705–709.
19. Consensus Development Conference. Consensus statement on self-monitoring of blood glucose. Diabetes Care 1987; 10:95–99.
20. Leroux ML, Desjardins PR: Establishment and maintenance of a hospital glucose meter program. Lab Med 1989; 20:97–99.
21. Chu SY, Edney-Parker H: Evaluation of the reliability of bedside glucose testing. Lab Med 1989; 20:93–96.
22. Lee-Lewandrowski E, Laposata M, Eschenbach K, et al: Utilization and cost analysis of bedside capillary glucose testing in a large teaching hospital: Implication for managing point of care testing. Am J Med 1994; 97:222–230.
23. Evaluation of a laboratory's analyte or test performance. Federal Register 1992; 57(Feb 28).

24. Reasoner, DK, Ryu KH, Hindman BJ, et al: Marked hemodilution increases neurologic injury after focal cerebral ischemia in rabbits. Anesth Anal 1996; 82:61–67.

25. Kundu S, Sio R, Mitu A, Ostgaard R: Evaluation of platelet function by PFA-100 (abstract). Clin Chem 1994; 40:1827–1828.

26. ISIS-2 [Second International Study of Infarct Survival] Collaborative Group: Randomized trial of intravenous streptokinase, aspirin, both or neither amount 17,187 cases of suspected acute myocardial infarction. Lancet 1988; 2:349–360.

27. Downie AC, Frost PG, Fielden P, et al: Bedside measurement of creatine kinase to guide thrombolysis on the coronary care unit. Lancet 1993; 341:452, 454.

28. Mair J, Artner-Dworzak E, Lechleitner P, et al: Cardiac troponin T in diagnosis of acute myocardial infarction. Clin Chem 1991; 37:845–852.

29. Katus HA, Remppis A, Neumann FJ, et al: Diagnostic efficiency of troponin T measurements in acute myocardial infarction. Circulation 1991; 83:902–912.

30. Antman EM, Grudzien C, Sacks DB: Evaluation of a rapid bedside assay for detection of cardiac troponinT. JAMA 1995; 273:1279–1282.

31. Misiano DR, Lowenstein E: Evaluation of the Ciba-Corning Diagnostics 278 analyzer (abstract). Clin Chem 1988; 6:1170.

32. Misiano DR, Lowenstein E: Performance characteristic of the Gem-Stat monitor. Proc Int Fed Clin Chem 1988; 10:239–243.

33. Statland BE, Brzys K: Evaluating STAT testing alternative by calculating annual laboratory costs. Chest 1990; 97:198S.

34. Mock T, Morrison D, Yatscoff R: Evaluation of the i-STAT system: A portable chemistry analyzer for the measurement of sodium, potassium, chloride, urea, glucose, and hematocrit. Clin Biochem 1995; 28:187–192.

35. Vender JS, Gilbert HC, Kehoe T: Evaluation of a new point-of-care blood gas monitor (abstract). Crit Care Med 1994; 22:A24.

36. Peruzzi WT, Shapiro BA, Templin R, et al: Comparison of the SenDx point-of-care blood gas and electrolyte analyzer with conventional analysis in both laboratory and clinical settings. Personal communication, 1999.

37. Larson CP, Vender J, Seiver A: Multisite evaluation of a continuous intraarterial blood gas monitoring system. Anesthesiology 1994; 81:543–552.

38. Smith BE, King PH, Schlain L: Clinical evaluation of continuous real time intra-arterial blood gas monitoring during anaesthesia and surgery by fiber optic sensor. Int J Clin Monit Comput 1992; 9:4.

39. Mahutte CK, Sassoon CS, Muro JR, et al: Progress in the development of a fluorescent intravascular blood gas system in man. J Clin Monit Comput 1990; 6:147–157.

40. Bland JM, Altman DG: Statistical methods for assessing agreement between two methods of clinical measurement. Lancet 1986; 1:307–310.

41. Hatherill M, Tibby SM, Durward A, et al: Continuous intra-arterial blood-gas monitoring in infants and children with cyanotic heart disease. Br J Anaesth 1997; 79:665–667.

42. Venkatesh B, Clutton-Brock TH, Hendry SP: Continuous intra-arterial blood gas monitoring during cardiopulmonary resuscitation. Resuscitation 1995; 29:135–138.

43. Venkatesh B, Clutton-Brock TH, Hendry SP: A multi-parameter sensor for continuous intraarterial blood gas monitoring. A prospective evaluation. Crit Care Med 1994; 22:588–594.

44. Weiss IK, Harrison R, Feldman J, et al: Continuous arterial blood gas monitoring in the hypoxemic child; Accuracy of the Paratrend system (abstract). Crit Care Med 1997; 22:A55.

45. Zollinger A, Spahn DR, Singer T, et al: Accuracy and clinical performance of a continuous intra-arterial blood-gas monitoring system during thoracoscopic surgery. Br J Anaesth 1997; 79:47–52.

46. Weiss IK, Fink S, Harrison R, et al: Clinical use of continuous arterial blood gas monitoring in the pediatric intensive care unit. Pediatrics 1999; 103:440–445.

47. Shapiro BA: Evaluation of blood gas monitors: Performance criteria, clinical impact, and cost/benefit. Crit Care Med. 1994; 22:546–548.

48. Mahutte CK, Sasse SA, Chen PA, et al: Performance of a patient-dedicated, on demand blood gas monitor in medical ICU patients. Am J Respir Care Med 1994:150:865–869.

49. Gischler SJ, Albers S, Duvick S, et al: Crit Care Med 1999; 27:A113.

50. Ault ML, Siddal VJA, Templin R, et al: Ex vivo blood gas and chemistry analysis in the intensive care unit versus conventional laboratory analysis (abstract). Anesthesiology 1998; 89:A957.

51. Nonsanchuk JS, Keefner R: Cost analysis of point-of-care laboratory in a community hospital. Am J Clin Pathol 1995; 103:240–243.

52. Scuderi PE, MacGregor DA, Bowton DL, et al: Performance characteristics and interanalyzer variability of PO2 measurements using tonometered human blood. Am Rev Respir Dis 1993; 147:1354–1359.

53. Vender JS, Gilbert HC, Kehoe T: Evaluation of a new point-of-care blood gas monitor (abstract). Crit Care Med 1994; 22:A24.

54. Kost GJ: New whole blood analyzers and their impact on cardiac and critical care. Crit Rev Clin Lab Sci 1993; 30:153–202.

55. Bailey TM, Topham TM, Wantz S, et al: Laboratory process improvement through point-of-care testing. Joint Commission on Quality Improvement 1997; 23:362–380.

56. Guiliano KK, Higgins TL, Pysznik E, et al: Crit Care Med 1999; 27:A115.

57. Salem M, Chernow B, Burke R, et al: Bedside diagnostic testing: Its accuracy, rapidity, and utility in blood conservation. JAMA 1991; 226:382–389.

PART SIX

Monitoring in Special Situations

25 Maternal and Fetal Monitoring in Obstetrics

Andrew M. Woods, M.D.

Once conception has occurred, obstetric monitoring takes on a unique duality in that there are at least two patients (the mother and one or more fetuses) with separate, but interdependent, physiologic systems that require assessment. The ideal of maternal-fetal monitoring is the early detection of physiologic abnormalities that, in the absence of intervention, might progress to serious organ injury in, or death of, the mother or the fetus.

Maternal Monitoring

Maternal Physiology in Normal Pregnancy

Pregnancy is associated with a number of physiologic changes in the mother. All such changes occur to ensure the metabolic needs of the developing fetus or to allow the mother to accommodate the mechanical burden of the fetus during pregnancy and delivery. None of these changes are beneficial to the mother and many are detrimental.

The purpose of antepartum maternal physiologic monitoring in normal pregnancy is to document the normal progression of the various organ system changes and to determine whether the alterations in physiology fall within expected norms. In high-risk pregnancies, the main purpose of physiologic monitoring is to assess the effects of the physiologic changes, whether normal or abnormal, upon maternal organ systems, which may be normal or abnormal. The worst outcomes tend to occur when abnormal maternal physiology interacts with underlying organ system abnormalities, as occurs with preeclampsia in the setting of diabetic renal disease with hypertension. However, even normal physiologic changes may prove disastrous in the presence of preexisting disease; for example, the normal intravascular volume increase associated with pregnancy may precipitate right-sided heart failure and death in patients with pulmonary hypertension.

Cardiovascular Physiology in Normal Pregnancy

Special attention in this chapter is focused upon the maternal cardiovascular system in health and disease. The importance to the fetus of adequate circulatory function in the mother is paramount. The awareness and understanding of the physiology and pathophysiology of the cardiovascular system during pregnancy, coupled with appropriate monitoring, directly affects maternal and fetal morbidity and mortality. Cardiovascular monitoring is also an area in which anesthesiologists providing obstetric care have special expertise; no other specialty spends as much training time in the man-agement of hemodynamic abnormalities as does anesthesiology. Monitoring and management of cardiovascular abnormalities in obstetric patients is an area in which interdisciplinary cooperation is of enormous value. It is also an area in which anesthesiologists can participate in patient care in a manner that more closely resembles the intensivist role in the intensive care unit (ICU) setting than that of the anesthesiologist in the operating room (OR).

Cardiac Output and Vascular Resistance. Tables 25–1 and 25–2 and Figure 25–1 reflect longitudinal hemodynamic data obtained noninvasively during normal pregnancies. Pregnancy is characterized by a 40% to 55% increase in cardiac output that results from a 15% to 30% increase in stroke volume and a 25% increase in heart rate.[1-3] The most rapid rate of increase in cardiac output occurs during the first trimester and most of the increase in cardiac output has occurred by the end of the second trimester. The main variability in findings among studies of cardiac output in pregnancy occurs during the third trimester. Some investigators report a modest decrease in cardiac output, while others find that cardiac output continues to increase. Earlier studies of supine patients invariably found a decrease in cardiac output in the third trimester, but this was caused by impairment of blood return to the heart when the patient lies supine and the uterus compresses the inferior vena cava and possibly the aorta.

There is no correlation between body surface area and cardiac output in normal pregnancies and thus little rationale for reporting cardiac index (cardiac output divided by body surface area) rather than cardiac output.[4] The purpose of normalization of cardiac output for body surface area is to reduce intersubject variability based on differences in body size. However, to do so in pregnant patients results in the inclusion of tissues such as amniotic and edema fluid, as well as the fetal mass and the increased maternal blood volume. Interpatient variations in these tissues account for the lack of correlation between increased body surface area and increased cardiac output in pregnancy.

In comparing pregnancy-related cardiovascular data from two recent studies (see Tables 25–1 and 25–2), the heart rate changes are essentially the same; the baseline rate of approximately 65 bpm increases to 80 bpm by the beginning of the third trimester and remains at this level until delivery. There is a difference in stroke volume between the two studies, with Poppas et al.[1] (see Table 25–1) reporting a larger stroke volume than Mone et al.[5] (see Table 25–2); however, the difference (10 to 15 mL) was fairly consistent at all measuring intervals and is presumably an artifact of measurement of either aortic size or flow. The cardiac output data in Figure 25–1A fall between those in Tables 25–1

Table 25-1. Hemodynamic Changes Over the Course of Pregnancy: Doppler Echocardiography and Subclavian Pulse Tracings

	Trimester of Gestation			Post Partum	
	FIRST	SECOND	THIRD	8 WEEKS	>6 MONTHS
HR (bpm)	70 ±8	77 ±10	80 ±10	66 ±10	65 ±10
CO (L/min)	6.8 ±1.6	7.6 ±1.5	7.9 ±1.6	6.0 ±1.0	6.0 ±1.2
CI (L/min/m²)	3.9 ±0.8	4.3 ±0.8	4.4 ±0.7	3.3 ±0.6	3.4 ±0.5
SV (mL)	95 ±20	99 ±20	99 ±19	87 ±17	90 ±21
TVR (dyne · s · cm⁻⁵)	885 ±193	766 ±157	743 ±131	1040 ±231	992 ±167
MAP (mmHg)	71 ±5	70 ±5	70 ±6	71 ±6	71 ±6
BPS (mmHg)	101 ±6	100 ±8	101 ±8	101 ±8	105 ±8
PS (mmHg)*	87 ±10	87 ±10	90 ±8	88 ±8	96 ±11
PD (mmHg)*	57 ±7	54 ±5	55 ±6	57 ±7	57 ±7
PES (mmHg)*	74 ±6	71 ±8	71 ±6	77 ±8	77 ±6

HR, heart rate; CO, cardiac output; CI, cardiac index; SV, stroke volume; TVR, total vascular resistance; MAP, mean arterial pressure; BPS, systolic blood pressure; PS, peak systolic aortic pressure; PD, minimum diastolic aortic pressure; PES, end-systolic aortic pressure.

*Aortic pressures determined by subclavian pulse tracings.

Modified from Poppas A, Shroff SG, Korcarz CE, et al: Serial assessment of the cardiovascular system in normal pregnancy. Role of arterial compliance and pulsatile arterial load. Circulation 1997; 95:2407–2415. By permission of the American Heart Association, Inc.

and 25-2 and reflect comparable percentage changes over the course of pregnancy.

During pregnancy, approximately 10% of cardiac output goes to the uterus, producing a uterine blood flow (UBF) of approximately 700 mL/minute. Thus, of the 2-L/minute increase in cardiac output during pregnancy, one third goes to the uteroplacental unit and the remaining two thirds go to other maternal tissues to support the increased metabolic needs of pregnancy.

Multiple gestations (twins, triplets) are associated with even greater increases in cardiac output than normal pregnancies.[6] The increase in output appears to be related to increases in contractility and heart rate rather than further increases in chamber size above that in single-gestation pregnancies. Thus, cardiac reserve is reduced in multiple gestations. This may have implications for patients with preexisting cardiac disease.

The large increase in cardiac output during pregnancy results in prominent flow murmurs in almost all pregnant women.[7] Typically, a grade 2/4 systolic murmur is best heard along either the left or right upper sternal border. Such murmurs are almost always related to increased flow, either across the pulmonic or aortic outflow tracts or through the mammary vessels. Murmurs that are diastolic, pansystolic, late systolic, or associated with an abnormal electrocardio-

gram (ECG) cannot be classified as benign and warrant echocardiographic assessment.

Cardiac output and blood pressure are measured directly, either invasively or noninvasively, and vascular resistance is calculated using Poiseille's equation as follows:

$$\text{Resistance} = (\text{pressure/cardiac output}) \times 80 \qquad (1)$$

When invasive techniques are used, the value for pressure is mean arterial pressure (MAP) less central venous pressure (CVP), and resistance is referred to as systemic vascular resistance (SVR). When, as is increasingly frequent in obstetrics, noninvasive techniques are used to measure cardiac output, CVPs are not measured and the value for pressure refers solely to MAP; in this case, resistance is reported as total vascular resistance (TVR). In most circumstances, CVPs are inconsequentially small compared with MAPs and the two measures of resistance are interchangeable.

In normal pregnancy, there are minimal changes in blood pressure (see Tables 25-1 and 25-2). The changes in MAP seen in Figure 25-1B appear striking only because of the scale; the change in pressure from the baseline (postpartum) value of 80 mmHg is only about 5 mmHg in either direction over the course of pregnancy. Thus, the 40% to 50% increase in cardiac output must be accounted for primarily by

Table 25-2. Hemodynamic Changes Over the Course of Pregnancy: Doppler Echocardiography

	Gestation (wk)				Post Partum (wk)	
	9–12	18–20	28–30	36–38	2–4	8–10
HR (bpm)	72 ±10	78 ±11	80 ±10	79 ±13	69 ±11	64 ±9
CO (L/min)	5.9 ±1.0	6.6 ±0.9	6.6 ±1.3	6.2 ±1.3	5.5 ±1.2	4.7 ±1.1
CI (L/min/m²)	3.5 ±0.6	3.8 ±0.7	3.6 ±0.7	3.3 ±0.7	2.9 ±0.6	2.7 ±0.7
SV (mL)	83 ±14	86 ±15	84 ±17	80 ±15	74 ±17	74 ±17
MAP (mmHg)	84 ±9	78 ±10	77 ±8	81 ±11	81 ±9	79 ±12
PSP (mmHg)	107 ±10	103 ±10	102 ±10	105 ±11	102 ±8	101 ±13
DBP (mmHg)	60 ±9	57 ±7	57 ±7	61 ±9	61 ±9	60 ±10
ESP (mmHg)	92 ±12	83 ±12	81 ±11	88 ±13	91 ±10	89 ±14

HR, heart rate; CO, cardiac output; CI, cardiac index; SV, stroke volume; MAP, mean arterial pressure; PSP, peak systolic pressure; DBP, diastolic blood pressure; ESP, end-systolic pressure.

Modified from Mone SM, Sanders SP, Colan SD: Control mechanisms for physiological hypertrophy of pregnancy. Circulation 1996; 94:667–672. By permission of the American Heart Association, Inc.

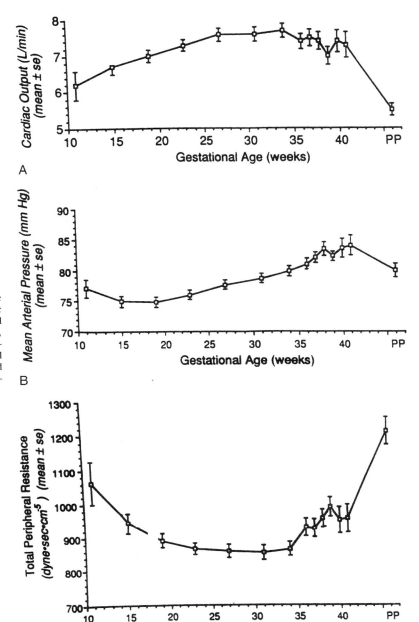

Figure 25-1. Maternal hemodynamics over the course of normal pregnancy (mean ± SEM). *A,* Cardiac output. *B,* Mean arterial pressure. *C,* Total peripheral resistance. (From Easterling TR, Benedetti TJ, Schmucker BC, et al: Maternal hemodynamics in normal and preeclamptic pregnancies: A longitudinal study. Obstet Gynecol 1990; 76:1064-1065. Reprinted with permission from the American College of Obstetricians & Gynecologists.)

a decrease in vascular resistance of similar proportion (Figs. 25-1C and 25-2). The low-resistance uteroplacental circulation accounts for only 20% of the decrease in vascular resistance during pregnancy. The major factor influencing the decrease in vascular resistance is a marked increase in arterial distensibility caused by reduced vascular smooth muscle tone. Estrogen levels are elevated in pregnancy, and estrogen causes vasodilation by potentiating endothelium-dependent (related to acetylcholine) and endothelium-independent (sodium nitroprusside responsive) pathways. In addition, flow-induced shear stress enhances the release of nitric oxide, which enhances vasodilation and blunts the constrictive response to norepinephrine in the myometrial vessels, a maternal vascular bed of utmost importance to the fetus.[8]

Total peripheral resistance is a parameter that describes only one of the components of vascular afterload—the opposition to steady flow. Traditionally, clinicians have modeled the arterial system as a simple hydraulic circuit with a single resistive element (vascular resistance) impeding continuous flow. This model does not account for the pulsatile nature of arterial flow. More complicated models are necessary to explain the arterial mechanical properties that transform the intermittent energy pulses discharged by the heart during systole into an arterial pressure that persists during diastole, even after cessation of arterial inflow.[9]

Use of models that account for both pulsatile and nonpulsatile flow has shown that pregnancy is associated with a significant increase in arterial compliance (AC_A), a measure

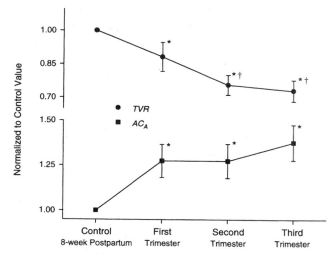

Figure 25–2. Total vascular resistance (TVR) and global arterial compliance (AC$_A$) over the course of normal pregnancy (mean ± SEM; *$P <$ .05, first, second, or third trimester vs. 8-week postpartum control; †$P <$ .05, second or third vs. first trimester). (From Poppas A, Shroff SG, Korcarz CE, et al: Serial assessment of the cardiovascular system in normal pregnancy: Role of arterial compliance and pulsatile arterial load. Circulation 1997; 95(10):2407–2415.)

of the reservoir-like properties of the arterial vascular system (see Fig. 25–2). The increase in AC$_A$ is part of the body's adaptive mechanism to accommodate greater intravascular volume during pregnancy without increasing arterial pressure. Increased compliance offsets the effects of decreased peripheral vascular resistance (PVR) on aortic diastolic pressure, preserving perfusion pressure to the coronary arteries, the uterus, and other vital organs. Now that normative data for AC$_A$ over the course of pregnancy are available, studies to evaluate AC$_A$ in abnormal pregnancies can be expected. Of particular interest will be pregnancies complicated by hypertension.

Cardiac Size and Function. In normal pregnancy, the left ventricle (LV) enlarges and LV mass increases 10% to 12%.[1, 10] Two recent studies have measured the thickness of the LV wall at the end of diastole (EDh) over the course of pregnancy and obtained essentially identical results; EDh increased 0.1 cm, from 0.8 cm to 0.9 cm.[1, 5] The increase in LV mass in pregnancy is similar to the cardiac changes found in long-distance runners, in whom sustained increases in preload due to increased venous return results in a dilated LV with proportionate increases in chamber size and wall thickness.

The issue of ventricular size and thickness of the ventricular wall is important because of the effects on wall tension. The force generated by heart muscle can be approximated by ventricular wall tension (force per unit area). Laplace's law states that wall tension (WT) is directly proportional to both the intracavitary (ventricular) pressure (P) and the ventricular radius (r) and inversely proportional to wall thickness (h).

$$WT \sim Pr/h \qquad (2)$$

Wall tension is elevated in early gestation coincident with the increase in stroke volume before the compensatory increase in cardiac mass. The LV hypertrophy that ensues is temporally related to changes in hemodynamic load; wall tension normalizes by midgestation as LV mass increases. After delivery, wall tension decreases in association with intravascular volume contraction; this induces atrophy of the LV (back to a nonpregnant size) that occurs over a period of several weeks. The cardiac trophic response in pregnancy is a tightly controlled servomechanism that is transduced by wall stress; both ventricular hypertrophy and atrophy have a response time of several weeks.[5]

There is no change in LV end-systolic diameter during pregnancy. Thus, the 15% to 30% increase in stroke volume in pregnant patients is accounted for by a small (5%) increase in ventricular diameter at end-diastole. Volume is proportional to the third power of the radius, so small changes in chamber diameter produce large changes in volume.

Myocardial performance is not significantly changed during normal pregnancy.[1, 11] Most of the previously studied indices of LV performance, such as fractional shortening and velocity of circumferential shortening, are heart rate-, pre-load-, and afterload-dependent. All three of these factors change during pregnancy. The ratio of the rate-corrected velocity of circumferential fiber shortening to LV afterload provides a heart rate- and load-independent assessment of LV contractility; using this measurement, myocardial performance is unchanged by normal pregnancy.[1] The importance of the issue of whether myocardial performance is affected by pregnancy is that, if deterioration in LV function were a normal consequence of pregnancy, then peripartum cardiomyopathy (discussed subsequently) might represent an extreme response of a normal process. This does not appear to be the case.

Studies that measure hemodynamic functions over the course of pregnancy but use early (6 to 8 weeks) or postpartum measurements as equivalent to baseline values tend to underestimate percentage changes. This is because pregnancy-induced changes may persist for several months into the postpartum period.[5, 12] These sustained hemodynamic changes result from structural remodeling that occurs in the LV and the vascular system, that is, larger chamber volume and larger conduit diameters. However, by the end of the second postpartum week, 50% of the changes required to restore cardiac output and stroke volume to prepregnancy values have occurred; thereafter, the change is much more gradual, and probably of no clinical significance in an otherwise healthy patient.[13]

Uterine Vascular Changes. The blood supply to the placenta travels through the uterine musculature (myometrium) and endometrium via an arterial network that includes the uterine, the arcuate, the radial, and the spiral arteries (Fig. 25–3A). There are approximately 150 to 200 spiral arteries in a normal placenta. In pregnancy, the trophoblast (which derives from the fertilized ovum and is thus of fetal origin) invades the wall of the spiral arteries and obliterates the encircling vascular smooth muscle and the internal elastic lamina over an extended length of the vessel, leaving only the external elastic lamina. In essence, the spiral artery structure is changed to that of a vein. Lacking smooth muscle, the modified spiral arteries lose much of their ability to constrict. Smooth muscle is retained in the more proximal myometrial arteries, but their vasoconstrictive responsiveness is blunted in pregnancy. This effect appears to be modulated by flow-induced shear stress along the walls of the myometrial arteries with nitric oxide as the mediator.[8]

The significance of these changes is that, in normal pregnancy, there is a very large increase in the cross-sectional area of the uterine arterial tree; the uterus becomes a low-resistance vascular bed with an impaired ability to constrict

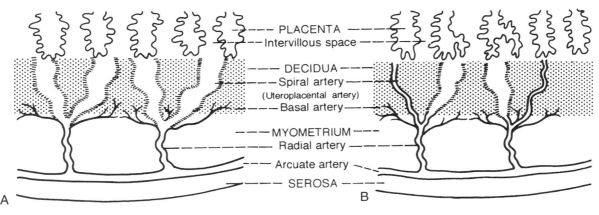

Figure 25–3. Uterine vascular changes during normal and preeclamptic pregnancies. *A,* The spiral arteries uncoil and dilate as they pass through the decidua. *B,* In preeclampsia, there is impaired dilation of the spiral arteries. (From Rurak DW: Anatomy and physiology of the placenta. *In* Bonica JJ, McDonald JS (eds): Principles and Practice of Obstetric Analgesia and Anesthesia, ed 2. Malvern, PA, Williams & Wilkins, 1995, p 161.)

and autoregulate blood flow in response to changes in maternal blood pressure. Because UBF in pregnancy is highly dependent on maternal blood pressure, much attention is paid to preventing even modest hypotension during analgesia and anesthesia for the pregnant patient.

Arterial Pressure. Most studies find a very modest (∼5 mmHg) decrease in MAP during the first half of normal pregnancy; the nadir is reached at midgestation (around 20 weeks).[1–3, 14] By term, the mean blood pressure returns to normal (see Fig. 25–1B). The changes in mean blood pressure are accounted for primarily by changes in the diastolic pressure.

Effects of Patient Position on Arterial Blood Pressure. Blood pressure in the lateral decubitus position is consistently lower (about 15 mmHg) than it is in the supine position, in both the nonpregnant and the pregnant states, when the cuff is placed on the nondependent (up) arm and aortocaval compression by the uterus is avoided. However, this difference is not found when central pressures are measured, indicating that it is due to the elevated position of the brachial artery relative to the heart. The magnitude of the effect is approximately 0.77 mmHg per centimeter of the vertical distance above or below the heart. This positional difference should be considered when evaluating blood pressure in a recumbent patient, as after epidural block; pressures in the dependent arm will be higher than central pressures and pressures in the nondependent arm will be lower. In large patients, this can result in differences of 30 mmHg or greater.[15]

In evaluating the effect of patient position on hemodynamic variables, Clark et al.[16] found no significant changes in blood pressure when comparing the recumbent position to the standing position. However, there were major position-dependent differences in cardiac output and vascular resistance in pregnant patients at term compared to 3 months post partum. Pregnant patients maintained their blood pressure on standing primarily by maintaining cardiac output, whereas the same patients in the postpartum period had a large decrease in cardiac output on standing that was offset by a large increase in vascular resistance (42%). Thus, the hypervolemic and vasodilated state of pregnancy provides some protection against adverse position-related gravitational changes in the distribution of blood volume.

The supine position may have profound effects on cardiovascular function as the enlarged gravid uterus impedes blood return to the heart from the lower body or obstructs blood flow in the distal aorta. Impairment of either aortic or vena caval flow in pregnancy is referred to as the aortocaval compression syndrome and, less descriptively, the supine hypotensive syndrome. It is the impairment in cardiac output that results in adverse consequences for the fetus and possibly the mother; blood pressure changes may be minimal.[17]

The decrease in cardiac output associated with the supine position may be asymptomatic in some patients; others will develop symptoms of shock (dizziness, nausea, vomiting, pallor, sweating, and decreased level of consciousness) if the obstruction is not relieved. Pirhonen and Erkkola[18] reported an increase in maternal blood pressure of 11 mmHg and an increase in heart rate of 23 bpm when pregnant patients with a history of dizziness in the supine position turned to the supine position from the left lateral semirecumbent position (Fig. 25–4A). However, the reported increase in blood pressure is artifactual; it reflects the lower position of the cuffed right arm relative to the heart in the supine position as opposed to the left lateral position. In Figure 25–4B, the data points for blood pressure have been modified (by me) to adjust for the hydrostatic effects upon blood pressure measurement, as previously discussed. The modified data show that the maternal heart rate increased immediately when susceptible patients assumed the supine position from the lateral semirecumbent position. However, mean blood pressure did not change for 5 minutes and then dropped precipitously by 20 mmHg in conjunction with a marked increase in impedance to UBF fetal heart rate (FHR) decelerations that occurred in 2 of 10 subjects. While the blood pressure at which symptoms are present is only about 10 to 20 mmHg below normal, it is clearly associated with a marked decrease in maternal cerebral and uterine blood flows. Modest changes in blood pressure in this situation may give little indication of the marked changes in the underlying components of blood pressure and cardiac output and vascular resistance. Lack of attention to cuff position relative to the heart can thus exaggerate or obscure significant changes in maternal blood pressure. Both maternal symptoms and the uterine hemodynamic disturbances are usually effectively relieved when the pregnant woman shifts from the supine to the lateral recumbent or semirecumbent position.

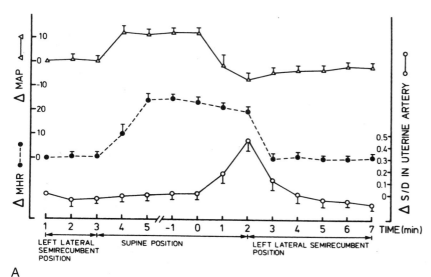

A

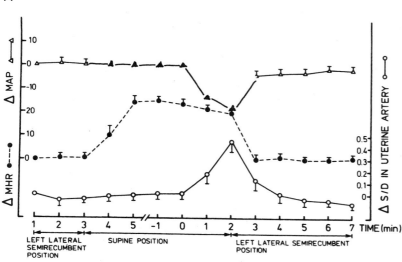

B

Figure 25–4. *A,* Changes in maternal mean arterial pressure, heart rate, and uterine artery systolic-diastolic (S/D) ratios in 10 patients experiencing the supine hypotensive syndrome. Time zero is the point at which blood pressure decreases after a period of stability. The increase in the S/D ratio indicates increased uterine impedance to blood flow. *B,* The mean arterial pressure values are corrected for changes caused by the position of the blood pressure cuff relative to the heart. (Modified from Pirhonen JP, Erkkola RU: Uterine and umbilical flow velocity waveforms in the supine hypotensive syndrome. Obstet Gynecol 1990; 76:177. Reprinted with permission from the American College of Obstetricians & Gynecologists.)

Altered Sensitivity to Vasoactive Compounds. Normal pregnancy is characterized by decreased sensitivity to endogenous and exogenous vasopressors such as phenylephrine, norepinephrine, and angiotensin II.[19, 20] Figure 25–5 plots the dosages of angiotensin II required to increase diastolic blood pressure by 20 mmHg at various intervals over the course of normal pregnancy. At the end of the second trimester, approximately twice the dose of angiotensin II is required as compared with requirements of nonpregnant controls. The decrease in vasopressor sensitivity parallels an increase in plasma renin activity.[21, 22] Increased intravascular volume and increased plasma renin activity are both factors that increase blood pressure in the absence of changes in resistance. Thus, the decrease in pressor sensitivity is important in preventing hypertension in pregnancy.

The attenuated response to vasopressors is in part due to altered baroreflex function in pregnancy.[23] Stretch receptors in the aortic arch and carotid sinus, when stimulated by an increase in blood volume, cause a slowing of heart rate and vasodilation; these changes oppose the increase in blood pressure that would otherwise result. Pregnancy is associated with an increase in baroreflex sensitivity, which allows for more precise short-term regulation of blood pressure. In response to tilt or postural changes that cause a decrease in blood pressure, pregnant patients have a greater increase in heart rate than they demonstrate in the nonpregnant state. In response to increases in blood pressure, patients have a greater decrease in heart rate when pregnant than when nonpregnant. Thus, infusion of vasopressors in normal pregnancy produces less of an increase in blood pressure than in the nonpregnant state because greater compensatory reflex mechanisms are activated to prevent hypertension.

Alterations in vascular responsiveness in pregnancy also occur by other mechanisms. There is downregulation of angiotensin receptor subtypes, particularly in the uterine arteries and placenta, which is mediated by progesterone.[24] Also, basal plasma prostacyclin (a vasodilator) concentrations rise in pregnancy. Interestingly, prostacyclin synthesis can be stimulated by angiotensin II, a potent vasoconstrictor. With its pressor effects blunted, angiotensin II can produce depressor effects during pregnancy by stimulating normal counterbalancing mechanisms.[25]

Altered pressor sensitivity may have implications for obstetric patients in several situations. Patients with uncontrol-

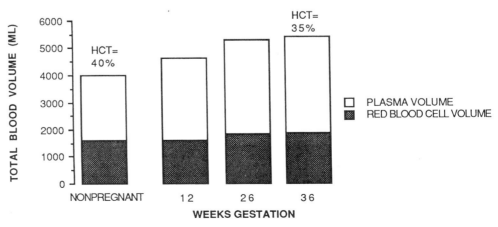

Figure 25–5. Decreased angiotensin II sensitivity over the course of normal pregnancy. The *closed circles* represent the mean dose of angiotensin II (± SEM) required to elicit a pressor response of 20 mmHg in diastolic blood pressure in normotensive pregnant patients. The *broken line* represents the mean for nonpregnant patients. (From Gant NF, Daley GL, Chand S, et al: A study of angiotensin II pressor response throughout primigravid pregnancy. J Clin Invest 1973; 52:2682–2689. By copyright permission of the American Society for Clinical Investigation.)

lable uterine bleeding requiring hysterectomy demonstrate a lack of response to a number of vasoconstrictors,[26] whereas patients with hypertensive pregnancies have increased vasopressor sensitivity.

Venous Pressure. Other than in the lower extremities, venous pressures are unchanged in pregnancy. Venous pressure in the leg increases after the first trimester, reflecting in part the increased hydrostatic load imposed by the expanded blood volume and also the obstruction to venous return caused by the enlarging uterus. These effects are somewhat offset by an increase in venous distensibility in normal pregnancy.[27] This allows an increase in volume without a parallel increase in pressure. To the degree that these conditions promote venous stasis, they place the mother at risk for embolic complications; pulmonary embolism is a leading cause of maternal mortality.[28]

Blood Volume and Oxygen Transport. Maternal blood volume increases by 30% to 40% over the course of normal pregnancy (Fig. 25–6). Red blood cell volume increases 15% and plasma volume increases 40% to 50%, resulting in a dilutional decrease in the hematocrit level from a nonpregnant value of 39% to 41% to 34% to 35% during preg-

nancy.[29-31] Despite the reduced oxygen-carrying capacity associated with a lower hemoglobin concentration, oxygen transport and delivery increase during pregnancy, particularly to vital organs such as the kidneys and the uterus. This increase is the result of increases in both cardiac output and 2,3-diphosphoglycerate (2,3-DPG). The increase in 2,3-DPG causes a rightward shift in the maternal oxyhemoglobin dissociation curve and the oxygen half-saturation pressure of hemoglobin (P-50) increases from 26.7 mmHg to 30.4 mmHg. The availability of oxygen at the tissue level is increased by decreasing the affinity of hemoglobin for oxygen.[32]

Fluid Balance. Total body water increases by 7.5 L during pregnancy, with the increase distributed as described in Table 25–3.[33] Sodium plays a key role in body water balance, and an increase in total body sodium of almost 1000 mmol that is brought about by increased renal reabsorption of sodium drives the expansion in body water. A balanced increase in both salt and water leaves plasma sodium concentration only slightly decreased.

There are changes in osmoregulation, as well as in the secretion and metabolism of the antidiuretic hormone arginine vasopressin (AVP) during pregnancy. Plasma osmolality decreases over the first trimester to a nadir approximately

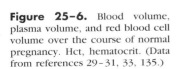

Figure 25–6. Blood volume, plasma volume, and red blood cell volume over the course of normal pregnancy. Hct, hematocrit. (Data from references 29–31, 33, 135.)

Table 25–3. Distribution of Increased Total Body Water in Pregnancy

Tissue	Volume (L)
Interstitial fluid	1.7
Plasma	1.2
Fetus	2.0
Amniotic fluid	1.2
Uterus, placenta, breasts	1.4

Modified from Davison JM: Renal hemodynamics and volume homeostasis in pregnancy. Scand J Clin Lab Invest Suppl 1984; 169:15–27.

10 mOsm/kg below nonpregnant levels, after which a new steady state is maintained until term.[34] Lowered serum osmolality normally causes an increase in AVP, which increases the permeability of the distal and collecting tubules in the kidney to water and concentrates the urine. The osmotic thresholds for thirst and release of AVP decrease in parallel during pregnancy. Lowering the threshold to drink stimulates increased water intake. Lowering the threshold for AVP release allows the ingested water to be retained by the body.

Colloid osmotic pressure (COP) decreases from a range of 25 to 28 mmHg in the nonpregnant patient to 21 to 23 mmHg in the pregnant patient at term.[35] Following delivery, COP decreases still further (13 to 18 mmHg). Pulmonary capillary wedge pressure (PCWP) is unchanged during normal pregnancy. The net result is a modest decrease in the COP–PCWP gradient and a narrowing of the margin of safety against the development of pulmonary edema. Pregnancy is associated with an increased risk and incidence of hydrostatic as well as increased-permeability pulmonary edema in association with maternal heart disease, tocolytic therapy for premature labor, infection, and preeclampsia.[36]

Fluid balance between the capillaries and the interstitium is maintained by opposing forces; capillary and interstitial hydrostatic pressure oppose each other as do capillary and interstitial colloid osmotic pressures. While the capillary hydrostatic pressure cannot be measured directly, it can be calculated when the COP in both plasma and interstitial fluid and the hydrostatic pressure of the interstitial fluid are known. Capillary hydrostatic pressure increases approximately 30% from the first to the third trimester of pregnancy.[37] The increase in capillary hydrostatic pressure coupled with the decrease in plasma COP favors the movement of fluid across the capillary membrane, yet normal pregnancy is not associated with generalized tissue edema. The distribution of fluid between the vascular space and the interstitium is unchanged because interstitial COP decreases markedly over the course of pregnancy, presumably due to increases in local lymphatic flow[38] (Table 25–4). The dependent edema seen in the feet of ambulatory women in the late stages of normal pregnancy is associated with capillary hydrostatic pressures in the ankle region that are 35% higher than capillary pressures in the upper body. The resultant edema reflects an inability of the distribution of plasma and interstitial proteins to counterbalance the increase in hydrostatic pressure in the capillaries, and there is net movement of water across the capillary membrane into the interstitium.

Cardiovascular Changes During Labor, Delivery, and the Puerperium. During active labor, cardiac output increases over prelabor values as a result of catecholamine-mediated increases in heart rate and stroke volume, as long as the patient is not in the supine position. The increase correlates with the degree of cervical dilation[39] (Fig. 25–7). The increase in output reflects an increase in both stroke

volume and heart rate with uterine contractions. The increase in stroke volume is caused by an autotransfusion effect that accompanies each contraction as uterine blood (500 mL) is forced into the central circulation. The peak increase in cardiac output occurs immediately after delivery, as uterine involution relieves the obstruction to venous return and also displaces a large volume of uterine blood into the maternal circulation. Because the uterus is now removed as a parallel circuit in the maternal vascular bed, additional maternal vasodilation is necessary to maintain low PVR and avoid hypertension. Potent vasoconstrictors such as phenylephrine and ergonovine maleate, an oxytocic, can produce severe systemic and pulmonary hypertension if administered in the immediate postpartum period. Endogenous catecholamines, as often accompany tracheal suctioning and extubation, can produce similar results. Such hypertension places the patient at risk for both pulmonary edema and cerebral vascular injury, particularly in the presence of underlying disease.

Summary of Pregnancy-Related Cardiovascular Changes. There is a decrease in vascular tone in very early pregnancy that induces an increase in stroke volume and activation of mechanisms to normalize blood volume in an expanded vascular system.[40] This increase in volume results in an increase in the radius of the LV; this causes an increase in wall tension that induces ventricular hypertrophy. These structural changes result in normal ventricular performance in the face of a dramatic increase in cardiac output that is sustained over the course of pregnancy. Changes in vascular tone and vasopressor sensitivity prevent increases in vascular resistance in response to greatly increased blood volume and blood flow, and also blunt the effects of position-related changes in maternal cardiac output. Changes in oxygen transport and delivery and remodeling of the uterine vasculature contribute further to the ultimate physiologic goal of pregnancy—adequate and sustained oxygen and nutrient delivery to the fetus. These structural changes are gradually reversed in the weeks and months following delivery.

Respiratory Physiology in Normal Pregnancy

Minute ventilation increases 50% during pregnancy to accommodate increased maternal-fetal oxygen consumption and carbon dioxide production. The increase in minute ventilation is due almost entirely to increased tidal volume (Fig.

Table 25–4. Colloid Osmotic Pressures and Hydrostatic Pressures in the Capillaries and Interstitium Over the Course of Pregnancy

	First Trimester (mmHg)	Third Trimester (mmHg)
Colloid Osmotic Pressures		
Capillary	23.2 ± 0.8	21.1 ± 1.2
Interstitial (thorax)	13.1 ± 1.2	8.4 ± 0.8
Interstitial (ankle)	9.6 ± 5.5	5.5 ± 1.4
Hydrostatic Pressures		
Interstitial (thorax)	−1.6 ± 0.7	−1.2 ± 0.9
Interstitial (ankle)	−0.9 ± 0.5	−0.1 ± 0.4
Capillary (thorax)	8.3 ± 1.9	11.5 ± 2.3
Capillary (ankle)	12.7 ± 2.1	15.5 ± 2.3

Modified from Oian P, Maltu JM: Calculated capillary hydrostatic pressure in normal pregnancy and preeclampsia. Am J Obstet Gynecol 1987; 157:104.

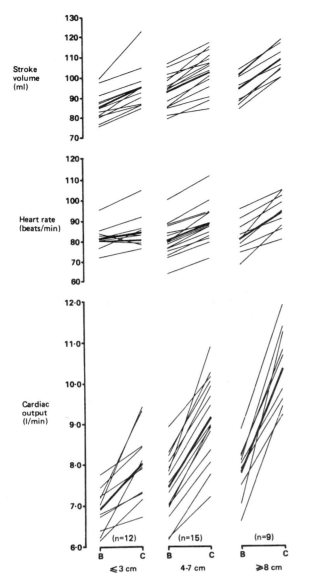

Figure 25-7. Changes in stroke volume, heart rate, and cardiac output during uterine contractions at progressive stages of cervical dilation. Darker lines represent the mean values. (From Robson SC, Dunlop W, Boys RJ, et al: Cardiac output during labor. BMJ 1987; 295:1170.)

25-8); the respiratory rate is unchanged.[41] Carbon dioxide tension in the blood decreases to 30 to 32 mmHg; a decrease in serum bicarbonate to about 22 mEq/L maintains a normal arterial pH. Hyperventilation in pregnancy is caused by increased progesterone. What remains to be elucidated is the site of progesterone action—respiratory centers in the central nervous system (CNS) as opposed to peripheral chemoreceptors—and the influence of factors other than progesterone. Both oxygen consumption and carbon dioxide production increase significantly during the third trimester, a period of accelerated fetal growth, particularly of the brain (Fig. 25-9). The change is proportional, and there is minimal change in the respiratory exchange ratio.

Almost half of all pregnant women with no coexisting cardiopulmonary disease complain of dyspnea by the 20th week of gestation. By 30 weeks, the figure increases to 75%.

Beyond this time period, symptoms of dyspnea tend to plateau or improve in many cases. There is increased sensitivity to CO_2 and hypoxia in pregnant patients who experience dyspnea compared with those who do not.[42] The monitoring challenge is to identify those patients with pathologic dyspnea when most patients have physiologic dyspnea.

Dynamic lung volumes are unaffected by pregnancy; forced vital capacity (FVC) and forced expiratory volume in 1 second (FEV_1) and hence the ratio of FEV_1 to FVC, are unchanged. The static lung volumes that are most affected by pregnancy are functional residual capacity (FRC) and residual volume (RV), both of which may decrease as much as 25% by the 36th week of gestation (see Fig. 25-8). The decrease in FRC results in part from a 4-cm cephalad displacement of the diaphragm by the enlarging uterus, an effect that is somewhat offset by a 2-cm increase in the anteroposterior diameter of the chest cavity.

The decrease in FRC does not result in a significant decrease in total lung capacity (TLC) because of an offsetting increase in the inspiratory capacity (IC), recalling that FRC + IC = TLC. Thus, as compared with the nonpregnant patient, the pregnant patient has decreased lung volumes at the end of exhalation when breathing at normal tidal volumes. However, if the pregnant patient then takes a large breath, she is able to take in almost 3 L of air; this is 500 mL greater than the maximum volume that she can inspire following a normal breath in the nonpregnant state. The physiologic explanation for this is that, even though the diaphragm is displaced upward in pregnancy, its excursion is enhanced by the mechanical changes that have already been described.

The supine position results in an additional 20% decrease in FRC. The change in FRC with the supine position is present by the end of the first trimester and persists throughout pregnancy; by the third trimester, the supine position causes a 50% decrease in FRC.[43] The decrease is independent of the elevation of either the right or the left hip, suggesting that caval compression has no effects on FRC in the supine position.[44] The occurrence of this phenomenon early in pregnancy indicates that factors other than the upward displacement of the diaphragm affect FRC during pregnancy.

Pregnancy does not protect against the deleterious effects of cigarette smoking on lung function, and smokers have a 25% impairment of flow in small airways.[45] Pregnancy has no predictable effects on airway function in patients with preexisting asthma. Peak expiratory flow rate (PEFR) is not affected in normal pregnancy, and thus this measurement tool can be used in asthmatic patients without regard to gestational status.[46]

Closing volume refers to the lung volume at which airway closure begins to occur in dependent zones of the lungs, resulting in areas that are perfused but not ventilated. If the lung volume at end-expiration is less than the closing volume, closure occurs; this causes an increased oxygen alveolar-arterial (P_{AO_2}–Pa_{O_2}) gradient because of intrapulmonary shunting.[47, 48] Half of all pregnant women develop airway closure in the supine position. In the healthy parturient, this produces only a modest decrease in oxygen saturation, as the decrease in Pa_{O_2} occurs along a portion of the oxyhemoglobin dissociation curve that has a relatively flat slope.[49]

The decreased FRC and the tendency toward airway closure in the supine position have particular significance for the pregnant patient during anesthesia. Both conditions effectively decrease the time to hypoxia in the event of an interruption of oxygen delivery to the alveoli, as might result from airway obstruction associated with induction of general anesthesia. Preoxygenation in the 45-degree head-up position prior to assuming the supine position has been shown to improve the FRC of nonpregnant subjects and prolong the

MATERNAL ANATOMIC AND PHYSIOLOGIC ALTERATIONS DURING PREGNANCY AND PARTURITION

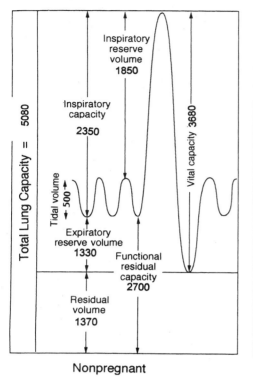
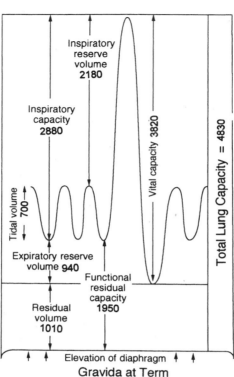

Figure 25-8. Pulmonary volumes and capacities at term compared with the nonpregnant state.

time to desaturation during apnea. However, this position change is of no benefit to the parturient.[50]

Alterations in the maternal vascular bed affect the respiratory system in two ways. There is a modest decrease in total pulmonary resistance during pregnancy that is mediated by progesterone, a known smooth muscle relaxant. There is capillary engorgement of both the nasal and laryngeal mucosa. Nasal engorgement increases the likelihood of bleeding if that route is used for the passage of tubes. Engorgement of laryngeal tissues may complicate laryngoscopy and tracheal intubation. The narrowed upper airway in the pregnant patient may require use of an endotracheal tube that is smaller than one would normally use.

During labor, hyperventilation that accompanies painful contractions may result in pronounced hypocarbia (PaCO$_2$ <20 mmHg) and respiratory alkalemia. The hypoventilation that may occur between contractions when the mother is extremely alkalotic can cause maternal and fetal hypoxemia.[51] These ventilatory abnormalities are not seen if effective epidural analgesia is employed during parturition.

Pregnancy increases the likelihood of hydrostatic pulmonary edema from a variety of causes. Treatment with β-adrenergic drugs for tocolysis of preterm labor is associated with pulmonary edema; treatment of nonpregnant patients for asthma with the same drugs is not. The risk of hydrostatic pulmonary edema is increased in pregnant patients with valvular heart disease causing pulmonary congestion. Increased-permeability pulmonary edema also occurs in pregnancy in association with preeclampsia and maternal infection. DiFederico et al.[52] reported a 20-year-old pregnant woman who developed an unusual case of increased-permeability pulmonary edema following surgery for the in utero repair of a fetal congenital diaphragmatic hernia. The postoperative protocol to prevent premature labor following fetal surgery included intravenous (IV) nitroglycerin (NTG) and

aggressive volume support. Two days after surgery, the patient developed acute respiratory failure and diffuse alveolar edema, and required tracheal intubation and positive pressure ventilation for 5 days. The diagnosis of increased-permeability pulmonary edema was confirmed by the ratio of pulmonary edema fluid to plasma protein (0.99). The authors postulated that NTG, as a nitric oxide donor, may have combined with exogenous oxygen to form peroxynitrite, a known impediment to alveolar epithelial cell function. Sampling of pulmonary fluid can differentiate the type of edema formation and in some cases may help to identify mechanisms of acute lung injury.

Renal Physiology in Normal Pregnancy

Pregnancy induces a state of sustained renal vasodilation caused by decreased vascular tone in both afferent and efferent arterioles.[53, 54] Renal plasma flow and glomerular filtration rate are 50% above normal by the end of the second trimester, resulting in lower values for blood urea nitrogen (8 mg/dL) and creatinine (0.46 mg/dL). A creatinine level in the normal range for the nonpregnant state (0.8 mg/dL) may be indicative of significant renal disease during pregnancy. During the third trimester, renal plasma flow and glomerular filtration rate tend to return toward nonpregnant levels. Both mild glucosuria and moderate proteinuria (<300 mg/day) are very common during pregnancy. Neither condition necessarily indicates underlying disease.

There is dilation of the renal calices, pelvis, and ureters during pregnancy. Subsequent compression of the ureters by the enlarged uterus as well as other enlarged vascular structures may cause obstruction to urine flow and stasis, which increases the risk for infection of the kidney and bladder. Pyelonephritis is a particular concern because it is associated with the premature onset of labor. The changes in renal

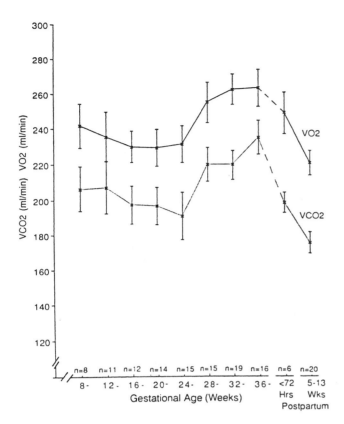

Figure 25-9. Variation in oxygen consumption ($\dot{V}O_2$) and carbon dioxide production ($\dot{V}CO_2$) over the course of normal pregnancy. The number (n) of subjects studied at each stage of gestation is shown. (From Rees GB, Pipkin FB, Symonds EM, et al: A longitudinal study of respiratory changes in normal human pregnancy with cross-sectional data on subjects with pregnancy-induced hypertension. Am J Obstet Gynecol 1990; 162:827.)

water handling, namely altered osmoregulation involving thresholds for thirst and AVP release, have already been discussed.

Gastrointestinal Physiology in Normal Pregnancy

Pregnancy is associated with a loss of competence of the gastroesophageal junction, leading to reports of heartburn and esophagitis in roughly half of all pregnant patients. This effect occurs early in pregnancy, and is caused in part by increased levels of progesterone, a smooth muscle relaxant. Gastric acidity and volume are elevated in late pregnancy as a result of increased gastrin levels. Gastric emptying is minimally affected by pregnancy.[55] However, the onset of labor has a profound retardant effect on gastric emptying. Ultrasound examination of parturients in active labor has shown that two thirds of patients have solid food present in the stomach independent of the time between the last intake of food and the examination.[56] Systemic opiate medications used for labor analgesia further decrease gastric emptying times. While the risk associated with pulmonary aspiration of nonparticulate gastric fluid, irrespective of the pH, is controversial and undefined, there is a high morbidity associated with aspiration of partially digested food. This is an event that continues to contribute to maternal morbidity and mortality in association with general anesthesia in the pregnant patient, particularly in the setting of emergency cesarean

delivery for fetal distress during labor. It is noteworthy that most cases of obstetric pulmonary aspiration in the American Society of Anesthesiologists (ASA) Closed Claims Project Database reflect poor anesthetic management, such as general anesthesia by face mask, excessive sedation, and failure to employ cricoid pressure during induction of anesthesia.

Nervous System Physiology in Normal Pregnancy

Anesthetic requirement, or minimal alveolar concentration (MAC), is decreased approximately 40% during pregnancy. This change is most likely mediated through maternal opioid receptors, because the decrease in MAC is reversible with narcotic antagonists. The decrease in MAC has been demonstrated in humans for isoflurane, halothane, and enflurane; most of the change has occurred by the end of the first trimester.[57]

A smaller amount of local anesthetic drug is required for epidural and subarachnoid blockades in pregnancy. As with MAC, the onset of the decrease in local anesthetic requirement occurs during early pregnancy, before the mechanical effects of uterine enlargement affect the vascularity of the neuraxial column. The nerve membrane is altered to make it more easily penetrated by local anesthetic molecules.[58] This effect, as well as the effects on MAC, appears to be under the influence of progesterone and possibly other pregnancy-related compounds. Progesterone potentiates the effects of both endogenous and exogenous opiates.[59]

Hemostasis in Normal Pregnancy

The blood of pregnant patients becomes slightly hypercoagulable as gestation progresses, a useful adaptation that decreases blood loss at delivery. The enhanced clotting is associated with increased platelet turnover and increased fibrinolysis. Normal pregnancy can be viewed as a state of accelerated but compensated intravascular coagulation; fibrin degradation products are increased.

Factor I (fibrinogen) levels and factor VIII (antihemophilic factor) activity are increased 50% to 100%. Other coagulation factors increase moderately (VII, IX, X, XII), are unchanged (II, V), or decrease (XI, XIII). Plasminogen levels are increased in pregnancy, but plasmin activity is decreased. There is increased platelet reactivity to epinephrine and arachidonic acid during the third trimester which contributes further to the hypercoagulable state and increases the risk of thromboembolic complications.[60] Although the platelet count decreases 20% in pregnancy, no clinically significant change in bleeding occurs.

Maternal Monitoring in Low-Risk Pregnancy

Antepartum Monitoring

Routine maternal antepartum (before the onset of labor) monitoring in low-risk pregnancies consists of periodic examinations with particular attention to blood pressure, weight, uterine size, hematocrit, blood glucose, urinalysis (particularly for protein), and cultures and blood serology for sexually transmitted diseases. Increasingly, ultrasonography is included in routine antepartum monitoring, although the maternal indications are rather limited. The image produced by ultrasound can identify a gestational sac as early as 3 weeks following conception (Fig. 25-10). This can help in the diagnosis of an ectopic pregnancy. Placental problems such as placenta previa, abruption, and abnormally adherent pla-

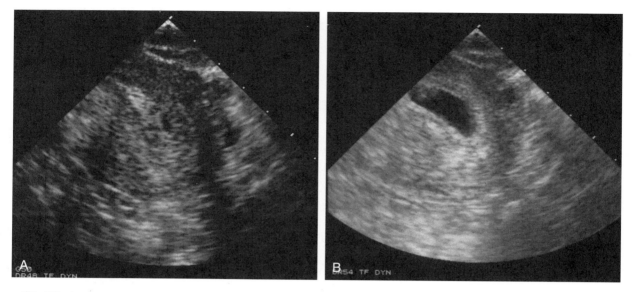

Figure 25–10. *A,* Ultrasound image of intrauterine gestational sac (small black spot in the center of the scan) 3 weeks following conception. The dark shadows on either side of the sac outline the uterus. *B,* Same patient, 12 days later. The gestational sac is much larger, and a tiny fetus is visible. Real-time ultrasonography is able to document the beating of the fetal heart at this early stage.

centas (accreta, increta, and percreta) can be diagnosed using ultrasound. An unsuspected placenta accreta, increta, or percreta may result in massive hemorrhage (44 U of blood intraoperatively in one patient who survived). Placental position (laterally versus centrally located within the uterus) may be a risk factor for the development of preeclampsia and fetal growth retardation.[61]

Blood Pressure. Blood pressure monitoring is important, because maternal hypertension in pregnancy is a major risk factor affecting both maternal and fetal morbidity and mortality. A large study involving almost 15,000 patients found that each 5-mmHg increase in MAP recorded during the fifth and sixth months of gestation was associated with an increase in perinatal mortality, with the largest increase in mortality occurring when the MAP was 90 mmHg or higher.[62] Routine antenatal blood pressure monitoring is the primary surveillance method for the hypertensive disorders of pregnancy,

Unfortunately, this extremely important vital sign is subject to considerable error in measurement.[63] Interobserver variability arises from observer bias (expecting certain pressures), lack of standard technique (fourth versus fifth Korotkoff sound as the diastolic value), observer terminal digit preference (values ending in zero occurring at a frequency many times higher than values ending in a digit other than zero), and improper technique (letting the mercury column fall too fast). Interobserver variability increases with length of gestation and is greater for diastolic pressures than systolic pressures.

In pregnancy, there is a particular lack of reproducibility of the fourth Korotkoff sound when measuring blood pressure using a mercury sphygmomanometer, the most commonly used technique. This is important because many obstetric protocols call for the use of the fourth sound (muffling) to determine diastole and many protocols use a diastolic reading of 90 mmHg as the cutoff for initiating antihypertensive therapy in patients with preeclampsia. In one study, experienced pairs of observers identified the fourth sound in only 52% of measurements in pregnant patients, and there was interobserver agreement on its detection in

only 19% of patients.[64] In this study, the disappearance of sound, Korotkoff phase V, was identified in all patients, and systolic blood pressure was perceived more clearly than either indicator of diastolic pressure. Nevertheless, the debate in this area continues, with valid arguments from both those who advocate the use of the fourth sound and those who would use the fifth.[65, 66]

Some of the problems with observer bias can be corrected by use of a random-zero sphygmomanometer. This device masks the true zero level of the mercury, and the correct pressure is determined by adding or subtracting the baseline value from the measured value. However, this device does not eliminate observer digit preference and has not proved to be superior to standard devices.

Use of automated oscillometric devices such as the Dinamap can eliminate much of the bias of manually measured blood pressure. The MAP is the most reliable of the pressures reported by the Dinamap. Both the systolic and the diastolic pressures are derived from calculations based on the mean pressure using proprietary algorithms, and are less accurate. Unfortunately, studies that utilize automated oscillometric devices often *calculate* the mean pressure from the systolic and diastolic pressures rather than simply use the directly measured value.[3, 67] In most formulas, mean blood pressure approximates the diastolic pressure plus one third of the pulse pressure (the difference between the systolic and diastolic pressure). It is difficult to understand the use of inherently inferior data when the machine reports a directly measured value.

Confusion in blood pressure monitoring also arises when results obtained from manual sphygmomanometry are compared with results from automated devices. There are often very substantial differences in pressures obtained by the different monitoring modalities. Part of the explanation for this is that the events measured by auscultation, that is, the sound of the pulsatile blood progressively "snapping" open the collapsed artery just distal to the cuff until the full volume is restored, are not the same as the events measured by oscillometric devices. Furthermore, most automated devices are manufactured to correlate with invasively measured intra-

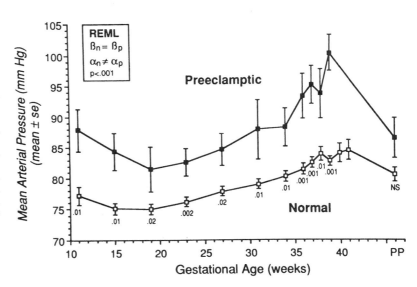

Figure 25–11. Mean arterial pressure (± SEM) over the course of pregnancy in normotensive and preeclamptic nulliparous pregnancies as measured by an automated oscillometric device. Measurements were made with subjects in the left lateral recumbent position with the cuff on the left arm. Differences are significant at all gestational ages but not in the postpartum period (PP). (From Easterling TR, Benedetti TJ, Schmucker BC, et al: Maternal hemodynamics in normal and preeclamptic pregnancies: A longitudinal study. Obstet Gynecol 1990;76:1064. Reprinted with permission from the American College of Obstetricians & Gynecologists.)

arterial blood pressure, and these devices measure different events than does oscillometry or sphygmomanometry.

When automated devices are validated for clinical use, it is by repeat comparison with blood pressure obtained using a manual sphygmomanometer, according to the protocols of the Association for the Advancement of Instrumentation (American) and the British Hypertension Society. Thus, when there is discrepancy between manually obtained pressures and automated pressures, the variation is attributed to the machine, despite the fact that the reproducibility of automated measurements is superior. When automated devices from different manufacturers are compared, there is a very high degree of correspondence in readings of mean blood pressure, but much less in systolic and diastolic pressures, presumably due in part to different algorithms.[68, 69]

Another major problem with blood pressure measurements is lack of uniformity in patient position and cuff height relative to the heart. The data in Figure 25–11 were obtained using an automated oscillometric device with patients in the left lateral recumbent position and with the cuff on the left (down) arm. In Figure 25–12, measurements

were made using the same type of device but with the patient in the sitting position. The data depicted in Figure 25–13 were obtained from the right (up) arm in patients in the left lateral recumbent position using a manual sphygmomanometer. Thus, if one asks the question, 'What is a normal MAP at 20 weeks' gestation?', the answer is 65, 75, or 85 mmHg, depending on patient and cuff position. There may be a measured difference of 20 mmHg in an important physiologic parameter in a situation in which there is no true difference, and in which differences do matter.

The importance of accurate and precise blood pressure measurements is illustrated by studies that, early in gestation, find abnormally increased blood pressures in women who are destined to become preeclamptic[3, 13, 70-72] (see Figs. 25–11, 25–12, and 25–13). A large multicenter study of 2503 women at risk (diabetes mellitus, chronic hypertension, multifetal gestation [twins, triplets], or preeclampsia in a previous pregnancy) found that in the second trimester, MAP less than 75 mmHg was associated with an 8% risk of developing preeclampsia, while a MAP greater than 85 mmHg was associated with a risk of preeclampsia of 27%.[73] Patients with

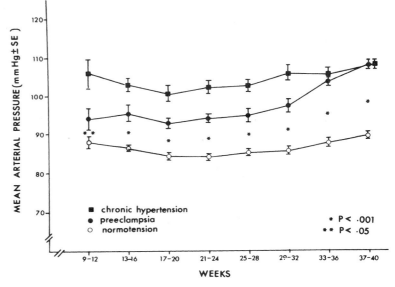

Figure 25–12. Mean blood pressures over the course of pregnancy in normal, nulliparous preeclamptic, and chronically hypertensive patients. Measurements were made with patients in the sitting position using a cuff on the right arm and an automatic oscillometric device. (From Moutquin JM, Rainville C, Giroux L, et al: A prospective study of blood pressure in pregnancy: Prediction of preeclampsia. Am J Obstet Gynecol 1985; 151:192.)

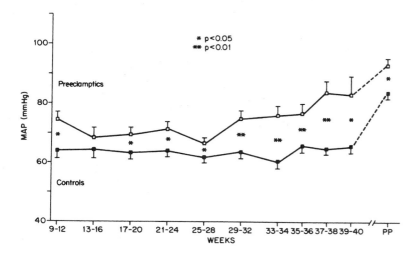

Figure 25–13. Mean blood pressures over the course of normal and preeclamptic pregnancies. Measurements were made with patients in the left lateral recumbent position with the cuff on the right arm using a manual sphygmomanometer. (From Reiss RE, O'Shaughnessy RW, Quilligan TJ, et al: Retrospective comparison of blood pressure course during preeclamptic and matched control pregnancies. Am J Obstet Gynecol 1987; 156: 895.)

MAP in the range of 75 to 85 mmHg had a 16% risk (Table 25–5). Thus, a variation in MAP of only 10 mmHg was associated with a threefold increase in the risk of preeclampsia. In the study, blood pressure measurements were made with patients in the sitting position and the fifth Korotkoff sound was used to determine diastolic blood pressure.

Ambulatory blood pressure monitoring, using an automated device that is worn at home 24 hours a day, has proved superior to clinic blood pressures obtained using conventional methods, even when the clinic measurements are done by a single trained and experienced individual. Patients wearing ambulatory devices are instructed to stand still or sit at times when the machine is making measurements. Results are reported as the mean of the various pressures taken over the 24-hour period. In a study by Churchill et al.,[74] an increase in mean 24-hour diastolic blood pressure of 5 mmHg (1 SD) at 28 weeks' gestation was associated with a 108-g decrease in birth weight. A 5-mmHg increase in pressure at 36 weeks' gestation was associated with a 121-g decrease in birth weight. Clinic measurements of blood pressure using auscultation in the same patients did not show this relationship because of the greater intrapatient variability in the measurements. Even a modest elevation in maternal blood pressure has consequences for the fetus, and conventional sphygmomanometry lacks the precision of a reliable predictive value. The results of Churchill et al. have been validated in another study in which 24-hour ambulatory blood pressure monitoring showed major increases in sensitivity, with only minor decreases in specificity, compared with conventional methods, in predicting the development

of severe preeclampsia.[75] However, even this study did not take full advantage of the power of the automated device to accurately measure MAP, and results were based on systolic and diastolic pressures derived from the manufacturer's algorithms.

Brown et al.[76] compared blood pressure measurements obtained using an automated ambulatory device with clinic blood pressures obtained using standard sphygmomanometry performed in triplicate by different and highly skilled practitioners. Figure 25–14 displays the upper limits of normal (2 SD above the mean) of systolic and diastolic awake blood pressures obtained over the course of pregnancy in women who were both "low risk" and "at risk" for pregnancy complications but nevertheless had a normal pregnancy and delivery. After 31 weeks' gestation, the upper limits for ambulatory awake blood pressure were 135 mmHg systolic and 86 mmHg diastolic; these values were higher than the upper limits from the clinic using the Korotkoff fourth (126/85 mmHg) or fifth sound (126/82 mmHg). Table 25–6 presents similar data obtained from sleeping patients using the ambulatory device. The comparable upper limits are 123 mmHg systolic and 72 mmHg diastolic. The ambulatory device documents the sleep-related variations in blood pressure that occur in both pregnant and nonpregnant women.

On the basis of the combined results from the studies by Brown et al.,[76] Easterling et al.,[3] and Reiss et al.,[71, 72] a mean blood pressure in excess of 85 mmHg prior to the 36th week of gestation, measured in the standing, seated, or left recumbent position with the cuff on the left arm, should raise the suspicion of pregnancy-induced hypertension. Be-

Table 25–5. Impact of Mean Arterial Pressure (MAP) on the Incidence of Preeclampsia in 2503 High-Risk Patients Stratified by Risk Factor

	Incidence of Preeclampsia			
Risk Factor	ENTIRE GROUP (%)	MAP <75 mmHg (%)	MAP 75–85 mmHg (%)	MAP >85 mmHg (%)
Diabetes	20	10	17	27
Hypertension	25	13	15	28
Multifetal gestation	14	7	15	21
Previous preeclampsia	18	8	15	27
All patients	19	8	16	27

Modified from Caritis S, Sibai B, Hauth J, et al: Predictors of pre-eclampsia in women at high risk. National Institute of Child Health and Human Development Network of Maternal-Fetal Medicine Units. Am J Obstet Gynecol 1998; 179:946–951.

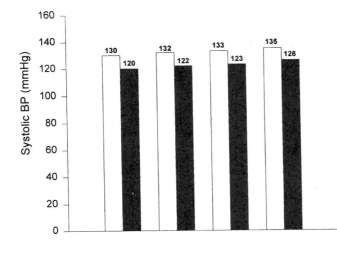

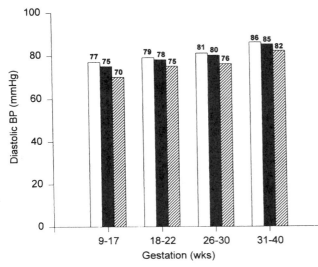

Figure 25-14. Upper limits of normal (2 SD > mean) of awake blood pressures (BP) obtained over the course of pregnancy in women who were both "low risk" and "at risk" for pregnancy complications but nevertheless had a normal pregnancy and delivery. BP determined by ambulatory blood pressure monitoring (*white bars*) and by resting mercury sphygmomanometry (*dark bars*) using phase 4 diastolic BP (*black bars*) or phase 5 diastolic BP (*shaded bars*). (From Brown MA Robinson A, Bowyer L: Ambulatory blood pressure monitoring in pregnancy: What is normal? Am J Obstet Gynecol 1998; 178:840.)

main normotensive and those destined to become preeclamptic can be optimized.

Heart Rate. Maternal heart rate is monitored to detect abnormalities that may be of consequence to the mother or the fetus. For example, extremes of heart rate may be associated with maternal thyroid disease. An increase in maternal heart rate in the supine position is associated with the supine hypotensive syndrome.

Temperature. Once pregnancy is established, the major significance of maternal body temperature variations is as a marker for infection. During the first trimester particularly, maternal infection carries a risk of fetal morbidity, particularly of such disorders as cytomegalovirus infection, toxoplasmosis, rubella, herpes, and syphilis. Later in pregnancy, and particularly once there has been rupture of the membranes, increases in maternal body temperature may be a sign of chorioamnionitis, an intrauterine infection that has consequences for both the mother and the fetus.

Uterine Activity. The usual pain associated with uterine contractions allows the mother to be a very good monitor of uterine activity. When such activity occurs prior to term it is an ominous sign, and premature labor and subsequent delivery of immature infants is still the leading cause of perinatal morbidity and mortality. Once detected, the uterine activity of premature labor may be closely monitored to assess the efficacy of tocolytic therapy, if initiated.

Intrapartum Monitoring

Because low-risk pregnancies can abruptly attain high-risk status without prior identifiable factors, these guidelines apply to all parturients. Blood pressure should be monitored at least every hour in all patients in labor. Hypertension is usually asymptomatic and can be detected only by measurement. Hypotension that is caused by aortocaval obstruction is usually accompanied by clinical signs of lightheadedness

tween 36 weeks and term, but prior to the onset of labor, a mean blood pressure greater than 90 mmHg is roughly 2 SD above normal, and patients with mean pressures in this range should be considered at risk for preeclampsia. While these pressures do not establish a diagnosis, they identify patients who need closer follow-up.

Routine use of automated devices to record mean blood pressures in a standard manner would allow for more reliable data with less variability, and would also facilitate cross-study comparisons. When one study uses the fourth Korotkoff sound to determine diastolic pressure and another uses the fifth sound, and then diastolic pressures are used to calculate MAPs, comparisons are meaningless. To the degree that accuracy in blood pressure determinations can be maximized and variability minimized, zones of overlap can be minimized and distinctions between patients who will re-

Table 25-6. Normal Sleep Ambulatory Blood Pressure in Pregnancy According to Gestational Age

Gestational Age	Mean (±SD)	Range	Upper Normal (Mean + 2 SD)
9-17 wk (n = 9)			
SBP	100 ±5	93-109	110
DBP	56 ±4	50-64	64
MAP	71 ±4	65-78	79
18-22 wk (n = 83)			
SBP	100 ±7	88-120	114
DBP	56 ±5	46-68	66
MAP	72 ±5	61-84	82
23-30 wk (n = 140)			
SBP	103 ±7	87-125	117
DBP	58 ±5	46-76	68
MAP	74 ±5	62-90	84
31-40 wk (n = 44)			
SBP	105 ±9	85-131	123
DBP	60 ±6	47-77	72
MAP	75 ±6	61-91	87

SBP, systolic blood pressure; DBP, diastolic blood pressure; MAP, mean arterial pressure.

Modified from Brown MA, Robinson A, Bower L, et al: Ambulatory blood pressure monitoring in pregnancy: What is normal? Am J Obstet Gynecol 1998; 178:836-842.

or nausea. Heart rate and respiratory rate should be monitored along with blood pressure. Temperature is measured every 4 hours. Once maternal membranes are raptured, the frequency of temperature measurement is increased to every 2 hours for detection of chorioamnionitis. An initial urine examination for protein, glucose, and cellular elements should be performed.

Uterine contractions can be monitored noninvasively by manual palpation of the abdomen or an external tocodynamometer. These noninvasive techniques can document the frequency and duration of contractions, but not the intensity. Internal monitoring of the uterine cavity pressure is necessary to accurately assess the quality of contractions; this requires that the membranes be ruptured in order to place a catheter in the uterus (Fig. 25–15).

Monitoring During Lumbar Epidural Analgesia.

Monitoring during lumbar epidural analgesia (LEA) is focused on detection of the possible complications of the technique: hypotension, intravascular injection, and subarachnoid injection. The risk of all these events is increased in the pregnant patient.

Hypotension. Maternal hypotension is infrequent in patients who are adequately prehydrated (500 to 1000 mL of crystalloid), maintained in the lateral recumbent position, and given limited amounts of local anesthetic (8 to 10 mL of 0.25% bupivacaine, 0.2% ropivacaine, or 1% lidocaine). However, blood pressure should be monitored once every 5 minutes after initiation of LEA for at least 15 minutes, and then once every 15 minutes for the duration of the block. Epidural catheter migration in the subarachnoid space is an ever-present risk; hypotension not associated with catheter dosing may be an early sign of such a problem.

In the absence of regional anesthesia, hypotension may still occur because of vena caval obstruction or maternal hemorrhage. However, these conditions usually present with other symptoms indicative of maternal compromise.

Intravascular Injection. The incidence of blood vessel cannulation is higher in pregnant than in nonpregnant patients due to engorgement of the veins in the epidural plexus. Intravascular injection of large amounts of local anesthetic can result in loss of consciousness, seizures, arrhythmias, and cardiovascular collapse. This risk is avoided by the incremental injection of doses of local anesthetic that, even if given IV, are below the toxic threshold. Incremental doses (3 to 5 mL) of 0.25% bupivacaine or 0.2% ropivacaine will

produce blood levels well below the threshold for toxicity if accidentally injected intravascularly during performance of an epidural block.

An aspiration test should be performed before every injection of local anesthetic, including repeat doses through an indwelling catheter. It is possible for a catheter to migrate into an epidural vein at any time. Gentle pressure or gravity-dependent drainage should be used to check for blood return through the catheter; excessive aspiration pressure can collapse an epidural vein around the catheter and mask an intravascular position. Patient complaints of tinnitus, perioral tingling, or mental confusion should raise concern over an intravascular catheter. Failure of a previously functioning catheter is another possible presentation for intravascular catheter migration.

The use of epinephrine in an epidural test dose to detect an intravascular injection has proponents as well as detractors.[77] Particularly in a laboring patient, any increase in heart rate caused by epinephrine may be difficult to distinguish from increases due to the pain of uterine contraction.[78] The use of low doses of epinephrine (40 to 50 μg) in the epidural space may contribute to systemic hypotension through its β_2-agonist properties (splanchnic dilation). Epinephrine may also decrease UBF. In one study, 2 of 10 healthy laboring patients who received 15 μg of epinephrine, a standard test dose, developed new ominous FHR changes lasting 10 to 12 minutes.[78] This dose of epinephrine causes a decrease in UBF in pregnant sheep lasting 2 minutes.[79]

The introduction of multiorifice epidural catheters has improved the reliability of a simple aspiration test to detect intravascular injection. Norris et al.[80] reported that aspiration alone was effective in detecting 47 of 48 intravascular catheters. Epinephrine as a test dose was given in 535 cases in which there was an initial negative aspiration test. In only one case was there a proven intravascular location detected by use of epinephrine that was undetected by simple aspiration. In 7 cases, a positive epinephrine test (maternal tachycardia) was a false positive; the catheter was reaspirated, incrementally injected, and bilateral epidural blockade obtained. There is no proven benefit to the use of epidural test doses when other standards of modern obstetric anesthesia are observed, and there are potentially deleterious effects in certain cases. However, those who still advocate the test dose do so based on the rationale that, *if* an emergency cesarean section is required, *and* one uses an in situ catheter in which a test dose has not been performed, *and* the correct location of the catheter has not been verified by proven nerve block accomplished through the catheter

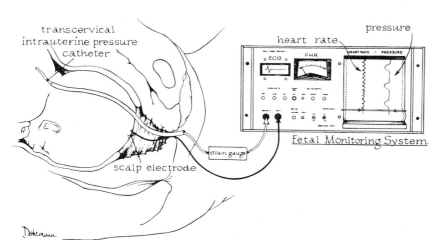

Figure 25–15. Fetal heart rate and intrauterine pressure are recorded from a fetal scalp electrode and a transcervical pressure catheter in the uterus. (From: Parer JT: Biophysical evaluation of fetal status: Fetal heart rate. *In* Creasy R, Resnik R (eds): Maternal-Fetal Medicine. Philadelphia, WB Saunders, 1984, p 292.)

rather than by injection through the epidural needle, then there is a tiny but real possibility that the catheter may be intravascular despite negative aspiration tests.

Those who practice otherwise would point out the following. There is always a risk of catheter migration into a vessel or the subarachnoid space, regardless of a prior test dose possibly hours earlier. Safe practice always requires the use of *fractionated doses* when using large volumes of local anesthetic and *continuous monitoring* of both the patient (through verbal contact) and the ECG (widening of the QRS complex) for evidence of cardiac toxicity. Last, the standard drug (2% lidocaine) used for cesarean section anesthesia has a cardiotoxicity profile that has four times the margin of safety of bupivacaine. Bupivacaine is the drug that initially drew attention to the problem of local anesthetic toxicity in pregnancy and which, in the 0.75% formulation, is now banned by the Food and Drug Administration. The consequences of an intravascular injection of lidocaine are much less severe than those that occur following an equal amount of intravascular bupivacaine.

Isoproterenol has also been evaluated for detection of intravascular injections. Studies in sheep have shown no evidence of neurotoxicity.[79, 81] In humans, IV doses of isoproterenol reliably increase maternal heart rate and increase UBF[82]; the change in maternal heart rate with IV epinephrine is not as reliable and decreases UBF. The use of isoproterenol beyond the test dose has been shown to decrease the duration of analgesia produced by epidural 0.125% bupivacaine.[83] This is of no consequence if one is using continuous infusions as opposed to bolus dosing techniques. It is of note that preeclamptic parturients are five times more sensitive to the chronotropic effects of isoproterenol than are normal parturients.[84]

A very sensitive technique for the safe detection of an intravascular catheter during attempted epidural analgesia or anesthesia is injection of 1 to 2 mL of vigorously shaken saline. The microbubbles created by shaking just prior to injection through the epidural catheter will cause an obvious audible change in heart sounds detected over the sternum using a Doppler ultrasound device.

Because of the unreliability of changes in heart rate as a marker for intravascular injection, many obstetric anesthesiologists who do not use chronotropic agents in their test dose solutions see no need for continuous maternal heart rate monitoring during LEA.

Subarachnoid Injection. Unsuspected subarachnoid injection of a volume of drug sufficient for epidural blockade can produce a total spinal anesthesia and loss of protective airway reflexes in a patient who likely has partially digested food in her stomach. Diaphragmatic function may also be impaired. The possibility of this occurring can be greatly reduced by the incremental administration of small doses of local anesthetic and testing for evidence of subarachnoid block between each injection.

Continuous Epidural Infusions. When epidural analgesia is administered by continuous infusion, the lack of need for frequent redosing does not eliminate the requirement for periodic reassessment by the anesthesiologist. The fact that the patient has no pain complaints is not a sufficient level of assessment. Development of significant lower extremity weakness or sensory loss above the T8 level warrants slowing the rate of infusion. Loss of previous analgesia despite an adequate rate of infusion requires aspirating the catheter for blood before administering a supplemental bolus injection, because the catheter may have migrated to an intravascular

location. Rapid increases in the level of block may be due to subarachnoid catheter penetration. Infusion pumps must be frequently checked to make sure the correct infusion rate is set and that the correct volume of drug is being delivered. As stated in the ASA guidelines for obstetric anesthesia, the safety of continuous infusion techniques is increased by the use of the lowest effective concentration of local anesthetic, often supplemented with small concentrations of epidural narcotics.[85, 86]

Temperature. A 1997 retrospective study suggested a causal relationship between epidural analgesia during labor and maternal fever, leading to a high incidence of neonatal sepsis workups.[87] There was no randomization and patients who received epidural analgesia were not similar to the group that did not. In the epidural group, induced labor was twice as likely, a fact that indicates that the progress of labor was not the same and thus the risk status for the fetus was not the same. As in almost all nonrandomized studies involving epidural analgesia in labor, patients with painful, dysfunctional labor are more likely to receive epidural analgesia than patients without these complicating factors; patients with dysfunctional labor are more likely to have abnormalities of presentation that increase the risk for the fetus. The authors of the study acknowledged that the neonatal infection rate was exceedingly low; only 4 of 1657 infants had documented sepsis; 3 were born to mothers who were receiving epidural analgesia, and one to a mother who was not. The temperature used to define fever was greater than 100.4°F. Astonishingly, 25% of all infants at the reporting institution were evaluated for sepsis. One third of the septic workups were done because of maternal temperature; 9.5% of mothers developed a fever greater than 100.4°F. Unfortunately, this report attracted a great deal of media attention and caused much unnecessary anxiety in expectant mothers, who were given reason to fear that optimal pain relief in labor would increase the risk of infection in their babies.

Prior experience elsewhere has not supported a relationship between epidural anesthesia, maternal fever, and neonatal sepsis. Recently, a prospective trial has confirmed that there is no difference in the rate of fever between parturients receiving epidural analgesia and those receiving patient-controlled IV analgesia, and no evidence for an association of epidural analgesia and maternal or fetal infection.[88] What was found was that epidural analgesia was associated with fever in cases of nulliparity and dysfunctional labor, both of which are independent risk factors for intrapartum fever. There was no association of epidural analgesia and fever in multigravidas. The authors postulated that the occurrence of temperature elevation in nulliparous women having difficult labor may reflect altered thermoregulation and an inability to dissipate an abnormal degree of heat production. Epidural analgesia may in fact contribute to this; however, the mechanisms have nothing to do with maternal infection. Both the ASA and the American College of Obstetricians and Gynecologists (ACOG) continue to endorse epidural analgesia as the most effective method of pain relief in labor.

Monitoring During Routine Cesarean Section. Many cesarean sections are performed on an elective basis, most frequently because of a prior cesarean delivery. This practice is decreasing, and trials of labor to permit vaginal delivery following prior cesarean sections are becoming common. The second most common reason for elective cesarean section is because of fetal concerns (macrosomia in the fetus of a mother with diabetes, fetuses with congenital abnormalities such as meningomyelocoele, gastroschisis, or omphalocoele).

Regional Anesthesia for Cesarean Section. Anesthesia for cesarean delivery requires a much higher level of sensory blockade than analgesia for vaginal delivery. Even though the standard low-transverse (Pfannenstiel's) incision is made in the lowest thoracic dermatomal region (T12), adequate regional anesthesia for cesarean delivery requires a sensory blockade at or above the level of T4. This is because peritoneal retraction involves nerve fibers that originate at much higher thoracic levels, and this is most apparent in situations in which the surgeon exteriorizes the uterus. This degree of blockade (above T4) is associated with a high incidence of maternal hypotension due to vasodilation of all vascular beds below the level of the block, particularly the splanchnic circulation.

Maternal heart rate monitoring is essential during regional anesthesia, regardless of whether a chronotropic test dose is employed. This is because the first sign of an unintended intravascular injection of local anesthetic will be widening of the QRS complex on the ECG. As discussed, epinephrine is not reliable as a marker for intravascular injection during active labor. It is more reliable in nonlaboring patients undergoing cesarean delivery because there is less heart rate variability in these patients. If a drug such as epinephrine is used, the patient should be asked if she has symptoms of adrenergic stimulation (sudden pounding heart and anxiety) in order to detect intravascular injection. This is more reliable than asking about sensations related to local anesthetic effects, because the 50 to 60 mg of lidocaine in a test dose may not be readily detectable to some patients.

Abrupt decreases in maternal heart rate shortly after regional blockade (epidural or spinal) usually immediately precede patient complaints of nausea; the next recorded blood pressure is almost invariably in the hypotensive range. The heart rate decrease is due to the "right atrial reflex."[89] Because the right side of the heart is a passive filling system, the only way it can accommodate a sudden decrease in venous return is slowing the rate of contraction to allow increased time for diastolic filling. If this heart rate slowing fails to allow adequate filling for the maintenance of cardiac output, the various receptor systems in the systemic circulation will, after some delay, initiate the compensatory responses of adrenergically mediated vasoconstriction and tachycardia. Thus, as soon as significant decreases in heart rate occur (usually a drop of 15 bpm or greater), corrective measures should be instituted, including left uterine displacement and elevation of both legs (not Trendelenburg's position). The head-down position is of no benefit to patients with an intravascular volume deficit, presumably because there is already redistribution of blood flow to the brain.[90, 91] Use of elasticized Esmarch's bandages to wrap the legs, coupled with 30 degrees of leg elevation, resulted in a fivefold decrease in the incidence of hypotension following spinal anesthesia (18% vs. 53%).[92] All patients were volume-loaded with crystalloid prior to spinal anesthesia for elective cesarean section. Leg elevation alone did not significantly reduce the incidence of hypotension (39%). An alternative practice is leg elevation to at least 60 degrees and continual left uterine displacement at the first sign of hypotension (bradycardia, nausea). This higher degree of leg elevation increases the hydrostatic pressure column that displaces blood back into the dilated splanchnic circulation and improves the return of blood to the heart. No technique or combination of techniques has been shown to reliably prevent hypotension following spinal block in all cesarean section patients. The necessity for close monitoring and prompt treatment remains.

Because larger volumes and higher concentrations of local anesthetic are required for surgical anesthesia compared with analgesia for labor, the risk of toxicity from intravascular injection is greater. As with epidural analgesia, safe epidural anesthesia requires frequent patient contact, eliciting symptoms of intravascular or subarachnoid injection, as well as frequent monitoring of blood pressure and heart rate. Pulse oximetry should be available in all delivery suites and should be used during regional anesthesia.

ECG monitoring during cesarean section frequently detects changes in the ST segments. This phenomenon has been evaluated in healthy parturients using transthoracic two-dimensional (2-D) echocardiography and myocardial-specific creatine kinase levels.[93] Although the incidence of ST segment changes is greater when using epidural anesthesia than when using spinal anesthesia, the difference may relate to the presence of epinephrine in the epidural solution. No evidence of myocardial ischemia has been found and the phenomenon is presumed to be benign.

General Anesthesia for Cesarean Section. In healthy parturients receiving general anesthesia for cesarean delivery, monitoring considerations must include pregnancy-related risk factors: the uncertainty of gastric contents, especially if labor has begun; shorter times to hypoxia if gas exchange is interrupted; potential difficulties in intubation due to obesity, breast engorgement, or airway mucosal swelling; decreased anesthetic requirement; and the possibility of pulmonary embolism. The unconscious, anesthetized patient is at risk for pulmonary embolism from venous thrombi or amniotic fluid but is unable to communicate the usual symptoms of extreme shortness of breath and chest pain. A *sudden* decrease in expired carbon dioxide, particularly in association with other signs such as severe hypotension, oxygen desaturation, and abnormal breath sounds, suggests a pulmonary embolus. Essential OR monitoring includes ECG, blood pressure measurement, pulse oximetry, and capnography for the detection of unsuspected esophageal intubation as well as for assessment of adequacy of cardiac output. As in all ORs where general anesthesia is administered, the capability for temperature monitoring and assessment of neuromuscular blockade must be available. The decrease in plasma cholinesterase associated with pregnancy is not clinically significant; however, for the occasional patient with a plasma cholinesterase deficiency, a nerve stimulator will be necessary to explain the inability to resume spontaneous respirations following a dose of succinylcholine for a rapid intubation sequence.

Monitoring of Obstetric Patients Receiving Neuraxial Opiates. Epidural and intraspinal narcotics are used extensively in obstetrics, primarily for postoperative analgesia following cesarean section, and usually in combination with local anesthetics, labor analgesia, and anesthesia for cesarean section. The advantages of neuraxial opiates include good pain relief without motor blockade, longer duration of action than other routes of administration, and negligible narcotic blood levels in the fetus when used in appropriate doses. The disadvantages include pruritus, nausea, dizziness, urinary retention, and the potential for respiratory depression. All of these side effects are reversible with drugs that have an antagonist action at the μ receptor, including both pure agonists such as naloxone and mixed agonists-antagonists such as nalbuphine. These antagonists usually do not reverse analgesia when used at recommended dosages; however, their use may shorten the duration of analgesia.[94] The mechanism of analgesic action of neuraxial (epidural and intraspinal) opiates appears to predominantly involve μ receptors in the dorsal horn of the spinal cord, whereas the undesirable side effects predominantly involve receptors in the brain. Presumably, systemic μ antagonists displace opiate compounds from brain receptors more readily than from spinal cord receptors.

One questionable approach to the problems inherent in μ agonists such as morphine and fentanyl is the use of butorphanol, a κ agonist with partial μ antagonism. However, butorphanol has been shown to cause irreversible neurologic injury in sheep when administered intrathecally.[95] Because unsuspected intrathecal injection is always a possibility during epidural drug administration, use of butorphanol in the neuraxis in humans would appear to involve an as yet unspecified risk. This serves to underscore the importance of waiting until good histologic studies are performed in animals and adequate clinical trials are performed in humans before administering a new drug into the epidural or subarachnoid space of patients.[96]

After injection of an epidural opiate, there is some systemic absorption through the epidural vessels that is related to the lipophilicity of the particular opiate and is roughly equivalent to an intramuscular injection of the same dose of drug. There is also the potential for an unsuspected intravascular or intrathecal injection when administering epidural opiates. Thus, patients should be continuously observed following each injection for the possibility of immediate respiratory depression, in the same manner that patients should be monitored after parenteral narcotic administration.

However, it is the potential for delayed respiratory depression that has been the greatest concern in the use of neuraxial narcotics.[97] This effect is thought to be caused by the interaction of the narcotic with respiratory centers in the fourth ventricle of the brain. The narcotic reaches this area of the CNS through the cerebrospinal fluid rather than the systemic circulation, and the flow characteristics of spinal fluid are such that it takes several hours for usual doses of lumbar epidural morphine to reach the brain.[98] Because pruritus and nausea are also centrally mediated, these side effects exhibit the same delay. While the peak time period for delayed respiratory depression is from 4 to 8 hours after epidural morphine administration, Abboud et al. demonstrated a 30% to 50% depression of ventilatory response to CO_2 beginning 90 minutes after 5 mg of epidural morphine and lasting 24 hours.[99]

Other narcotics that are more lipid-soluble than morphine, such as fentanyl, sufentanil, and meperidine, are more extensively bound to lipid tissues near the site of injection; consequently, a smaller proportion of the drug is available for rostral migration to the brain compared to morphine. However, sufficient quantities of highly lipid-soluble agents do reach the brain via the cerebrospinal fluid to cause depression of the CO_2 response in a dose-dependent manner.[100] The onset (15 minutes) of respiratory depression with epidural lipid-soluble opiates is much more rapid than that seen after epidural morphine, and the duration of action is shorter. One case report described apnea and hypoxemia 100 minutes after epidural administration of 100 μg of fentanyl to a healthy 27-year-old woman undergoing cesarean section.[101]

Use of the more lipid-soluble agents does reduce the likelihood of delayed respiratory depression occurring after the patient has left the OR and the postanesthesia recovery area. Unfortunately, it also reduces the duration of analgesia. For example, epidural fentanyl 75 μg has a duration of analgesic action of approximately 6 hours, while epidural morphine 3 to 5 mg has a duration of 18 to 24 hours.

One solution to the problem of delayed respiratory depression is the use of a naloxone infusion. Rawal and

Wattwil[102] demonstrated that a naloxone infusion of 5 μg/kg/hour reversed the ventilatory depression produced by 10 mg of epidural morphine in volunteers. This dose of morphine is at least twice that used clinically and the amount of naloxone used was almost 0.4 mg/hour, the standard volume of an ampule of naloxone. In clinical practice, the addition of one or two ampules (0.4 or 0.8 mg) of naloxone to postoperative IV fluids at a maintenance rate (125 mL/hour) provides 50 to 100 μg/hour of naloxone. If continued for 16 hours, the risk of delayed respiratory depression in patients receiving epidural morphine 3 to 5 mg is extremely unlikely. An additional benefit of the naloxone infusion is that it lessens the severity of nausea and pruritus if initiated shortly after the administration of epidural morphine.[94] Other μ antagonists, particularly nalbuphine, may be superior to naloxone in this regard.[103] Naloxone and nalbuphine infusions are not standard practice at many leading obstetric centers; this in part reflects a cost-benefit ratio that imposes an expense on every patient receiving epidural morphine to prevent the rare (probably < 1 in 1000) case of significant respiratory depression. Postpartum patients receiving epidural morphine are presumably at even less risk for delayed respiratory depression than other patients due to the respiratory stimulant effects of elevated progesterone levels that accompany pregnancy. Also, obstetric patients tend to be young and free of concurrent lung disease, factors that affect the likelihood of delayed respiratory depression.

All cases of clinically significant respiratory depression attributable to epidural narcotic administration have been accompanied by somnolence on the part of the patient. Thus, monitoring of patients receiving epidural opiates should include an assessment of their state of arousal. Excessive sedation should be a cause for concern. Likewise, sedating drugs such as systemic opiates, antihistamines, and benzodiazepines should be used with caution, because their use may mask an early indication of excessive respiratory depression. Sedative drugs may potentiate respiratory depression in a setting in which the patients already have a depressed ventilatory response. It is essential to note that merely documenting the respiratory rate does not ensure against respiratory depression in patients receiving epidural opiates. In contrast to systemic opiates, which decrease minute ventilation primarily by decreasing respiratory rate, epidural opiates decrease tidal volumes. Thus, minute ventilation may be markedly impaired in sleeping patients who appear to be breathing at a normal rate.

Even though all patients receiving neuraxial opiates have a depressed response to CO_2, very few will have any significant changes in respiratory parameters, such as minute ventilation. It is only those patients who are asleep or very sedated that are at risk; in the healthy parturient that risk is still very low. There are as yet no studies that compare either the efficacy or the cost of dealing with this low-risk situation through the use of naloxone infusions as opposed to electronic monitors (capnography, pulse oximetry, impedance respiratory monitors) or frequent nursing assessment.

Maternal Monitoring in High-Risk Pregnancies

Preeclampsia

No other disorder of pregnancy involves such extensive maternal physiologic derangement as that associated with preeclampsia. Most invasive hemodynamic monitoring in obstetric units takes place in patients with severe preeclampsia.

Table 25–7. Classification of Hypertensive Disorders of Pregnancy

Hypertension: systolic blood pressure >140 mmHg or diastolic blood pressure >90 mmHg
Chronic hypertension: hypertension without proteinuria occurring before the 20th week of gestation and persisting more than 6 wk post partum.
Preeclampsia: hypertension and proteinuria occurring after the 20th week of gestation in a previously normotensive woman.
Eclampsia: new onset of seizures or coma in a woman with preeclampsia in the absence of other central nervous system abnormality.
Gestational hypertension: hypertension in the 2nd half of pregnancy or within 24 hr of delivery; no proteinuria or generalized edema; blood pressure returns to normal within 10 days

Modified from American College of Obstetrics and Gynecology Committee on Technical Bulletins: Hypertension in pregnancy. Int J Gynaecol Obstet 1996; 53:175–183.

Worldwide, preeclampsia is still the number one cause of maternal mortality in pregnancy.

Definition and Etiology. *Hypertension* during pregnancy is defined as a sustained blood pressure greater than 140 mmHg systolic or 90 mmHg diastolic (Table 25–7). Hypertension without proteinuria occurring before the 20th week of gestation and persisting more than 6 weeks post partum is classified as *chronic hypertension. Preeclampsia* is defined as hypertension and proteinuria occurring after the 20th week of gestation in a previously normotensive woman. *Eclampsia* refers to the new onset of seizures or coma in a woman with preeclampsia in the absence of other CNS pathologic conditions. *Gestational hypertension* develops in the second half of pregnancy or within 24 hours of delivery; there is no proteinuria or generalized edema and the blood pressure returns to normal within 10 days.[104] The HELLP syndrome (*h*emolysis, *l*iver enzyme abnormalities, and *l*ow *p*latelets) is considered a manifestation of severe preeclampsia. However, the occurrence of this disorder in the absence of hypertension or proteinuria (15% of cases) raises the possibility that it is a distinct entity.[105]

Preeclampsia may be mild or severe. Table 25–8 lists the criteria for the diagnosis of severe preeclampsia. The degree of hypertension in preeclampsia does not necessarily correlate with the severity of the disease, and 20% of patients who become eclamptic (i.e., have generalized seizures) do not have preeclampsia by the above definition. On the other hand, some patients will present as true hypertensive emergencies, with blood pressures as high as 250/150 mmHg.

The classification of hypertensive disorders is a clinical, not a pathophysiologic, classification. It focuses on a universally measurable parameter—blood pressure—and overt signs and symptoms—mainly proteinuria, edema, and seizures—that present in the second half of pregnancy and represent organ injury. Pathophysiologically, preeclampsia begins just after conception with abnormal implantation of the placenta, and patients destined to develop preeclampsia have measurable hemodynamic abnormalities as early as the 10th week of gestation.[3] Of the three interdependent hemodynamic variables—blood pressure, cardiac output, and vascular resistance—cardiac output and vascular resistance display greater deviations from nonpregnant norms than does blood pressure (see Fig. 25–1). However, problems with ease, reliability, and reproducibility of measurements of cardiac output or vascular resistance have precluded the use of these variables in the *clinical* classification of preeclampsia. Over the next decade, this situation will likely change.

If preeclampsia is a single disease, it presents along a spectrum of severity, and subclassifications based on differences in hemodynamic profiles, plasma volumes, and fetal size have more relevance to clinical management and pregnancy outcomes than the present categories based primarily upon the degree of hypertension and proteinuria.

Remarkably little is truly understood regarding the cause of preeclampsia. It may be that there are heterogeneous causes constituting the single syndrome of preeclampsia. Ness and Roberts[106] hypothesize that there are distinct maternal and placental origins for the disease, and that the combination of maternal and placental factors is particularly damaging. In terms of maternal factors, the risk of preeclampsia is related to preexisting hypertension, diabetes, and obesity. Interestingly, each of these factors is predictive of vascular disease later in life. Independently, there are factors associated with abnormal placentation (the interaction between the placenta and the uterus) that result in abnormalities of placental perfusion. The disease is "cured" only by removal of the placenta.

For many years there has been a focus on the imbalance between prostacyclin (from the vascular endothelium) and thromboxane A_2 (from platelets) in preeclampsia. Such an imbalance would favor platelet aggregation, vasoconstriction, and decreased uteroplacental blood flow—key features in the pathophysiology of preeclampsia. Subsequent longitudinal studies have not consistently found abnormalities in the ratio of prostacyclin to thromboxane A_2 in preeclamptic pregnancies.[107, 108] Paarlberg et al.[108] found thromboxane dominance over prostacyclin in patients with *severe* preeclampsia (but not with mild or moderate preeclampsia) and in those with *severe* gestational hypertension. This suggests that the prostacyclin–thromboxane A_2 abnormalities are *secondary and adaptive* to the failure of vasodilation early in pregnancy, and not primary. The lack of prostacyclin–thromboxane A_2 imbalance accounts in part for the failure of aspirin therapy in preeclampsia. It was initially theorized that the vasoconstriction and platelet aggregation seen in preeclampsia might be reversible with low-dose aspirin, a drug that inhibits thromboxane production but spares prostacyclin. While aspirin does produce a favorable effect on the ratio of these compounds in hypertensive pregnancies,[109] large clinical trials have shown aspirin therapy to be of no benefit in altering the course of preeclampsia.[110, 111] However, this is still an area of controversy, and it may be that different treatment protocols in selected patients may yet prove to be of some benefit.[112-114]

The placenta and the uterus are genetically dissimilar; the uterus is genetically maternal, whereas the placenta is genetically fetal and thus contains both paternal and maternal genetic material. This is the basis for the theorized immunologic mechanisms that mediate what some consider a graft-versus-host disease. In normal pregnancy, the mother (the host) tolerates the presence of an allograft (the trophoblast). In preeclampsia, the mechanisms that allow this state are impaired, and the normal uterine vascular remodeling

Table 25–8. Criteria for Severe Preeclampsia

Blood pressure at rest >160 mmHg systolic or >110 mmHg diastolic
Proteinuria (>5 g in 24 hr)
Oliguria (<500 mL urine in 24 hr)
Cerebral or visual disturbances
Epigastric pain
Pulmonary edema
Cyanosis

does not occur because the trophoblast has been "rejected" immunologically.

The convergence point for both the maternal and placental factors that cause preeclampsia is at the lining of the maternal vasculature, the endothelium. The endothelial dysfunction (which may be endothelial activation rather than injury) is mediated by unidentified circulating factors that do not appear to be directly cytotoxic. The clinical manifestations of preeclampsia are the result of different degrees of endothelial dysfunction in different organs (brain, kidney, liver, and so on). The endothelial dysfunction is progressive, and in severe preeclampsia results in vasoconstriction, enhanced capillary permeability, and intravascular coagulation.[115] It appears that vasospasm occurs in tiny end-arteries first and local ischemia causes compensatory vasodilation of the more proximal arteries in an effort to improve perfusion of the ischemic tissue. Overdistention of the conductance arteries occurs, leading to compensatory vasoconstriction to reduce arterial damage. When this occurs, the larger-diameter vessels will demonstrate the elevated resistance that is almost always present in severe preeclampsia.

Cardiovascular Physiology. Noninvasive assessment of cardiac output continues to provide new insight into the cardiovascular abnormalities associated with preeclampsia. Pulsed Doppler ultrasound measurements of cardiac output have been validated in both nonpregnant and pregnant subjects and have consistently demonstrated high degrees of correlation with thermodilution techniques using pulmonary artery catheters.[116]

Cardiac Output and Vascular Resistance. Cardiac output and vascular resistance may be extraordinarily high or extraordinarily low in patients with preeclampsia. Patients with vastly different hemodynamic profiles in terms of cardiac output and vascular resistance may be indistinguishable based solely on blood pressure and clinical appearance. For many years, preeclampsia was considered a disease characterized by decreased cardiac output in the face of increased blood pressure due to high vascular resistance. Hemodynamic data to support this view were primarily obtained from parturients with preeclampsia requiring pulmonary artery catheterization (PAC); hence, most patients had severe preeclampsia. In one important study from the Netherlands by Groenendijk et al.,[117] 10 patients with moderate to severe preeclampsia underwent PAC for hemodynamic measurements before volume or antihypertensive therapy was instituted. MAP ranged between 110 and 135 mmHg (Fig. 25–16). In all patients, cardiac output was abnormally low and SVR was abnormally high. After initial measurements, the patients were given a colloid infusion until the PCWP, which was low in all cases, increased to 8 mmHg. Volume therapy alone insignificantly changed MAP but increased cardiac output and decreased SVR. At this point, vasodilator (dihydralazine) therapy was instituted, and SVR decreased further into the normal range for pregnant patients; MAP decreased as well. A marked improvement in cardiac output with no change in PCWP occurred primarily because of decreased afterload. This study has been one of the cornerstones of current management principles for patients with severe preeclampsia and has reinforced the view of preeclampsia as a disease of an intensely vasoconstricted vascular bed clamped down around a reduced intravascular volume.

However, at the same time, there were other studies involving patients who were not as ill in which the hemodynamic findings displayed much more heterogeneity, with cardiac outputs ranging from 4 to 13 L/minute.[116, 118–123] In Figure 25–17A, the hemodynamic profile of 36 untreated

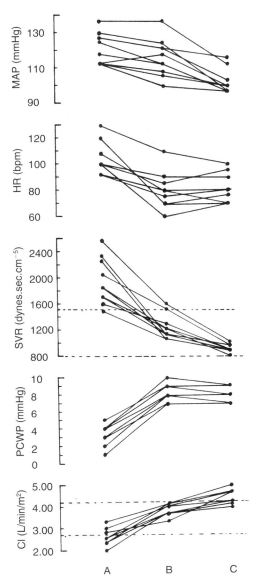

Figure 25–16. Hemodynamic responses in patients with severe preeclampsia. *A,* Before treatment. *B,* Following volume expansion. *C,* After vasodilation. MAP, mean arterial pressure; HR, heart rate; SVR, systemic vascular resistance; PCWP, pulmonary capillary wedge pressure; CI, cardiac index. (From Groenendijk R, Trimbos JBMJ, Wallenburg HCS: Hemodynamic measurements in preeclampsia: Preliminary observations. Am J Obstet Gynecol 1984; 150:234.)

preeclamptic patients monitored noninvasively is compared with data from patients with normal pregnancies. Figure 25–17B provides similar hemodynamic data in preeclamptic patients monitored with pulmonary artery catheters. Most patients in these studies were treated either with volume therapy or vasodilators before hemodynamic measurements were made and thus the hemodynamic picture in the untreated state was not known.

Visser and Wallenburg[124] measured hemodynamic variables using a pulmonary artery catheter in 87 untreated and 47 treated (volume therapy and vasodilators) patients with preeclampsia between 25 and 34 weeks' gestation (Table 25–9). Consistent with almost all other studies, treatment resulted in an improvement in cardiac output (27%) with a

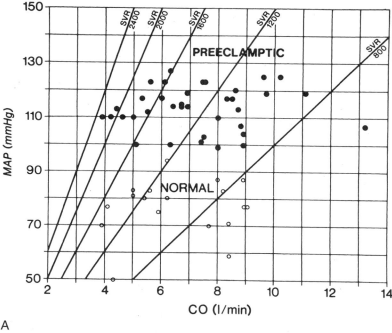

A

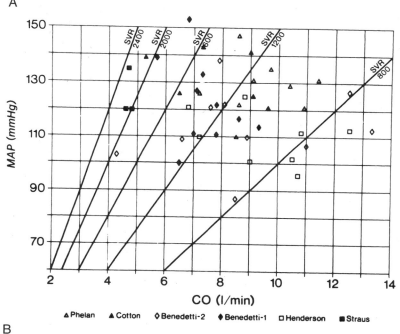

B

▲ Phelan   ▲ Cotton   ◇ Benedetti-2   ◆ Benedetti-1   ☐ Henderson   ■ Straus

Figure 25–17. *A*, Cardiac output (CO), mean arterial pressure (MAP), and systemic vascular resistance (SVR) in normal (*open circles*) and untreated preeclamptic (*black circles*) pregnancies. CO was measured noninvasively using Doppler ultrasound. The variation in MAP among preeclamptic patients is limited (range 95 to 125 mmHg), but there is a wide variation in CO and SVR, with over a threefold increase from the lowest to the highest values. *B*, CO, MAP, and SVR in 46 preeclamptic patients monitored with pulmonary artery catheters. (Data are from six different studies that are differentiated by the various symbols: Phelan JP, Yurth DA: Severe preeclampsia. I. Peripartum hemodynamic observations. Am J Obstet Gynecol 1982; 144:17; Cotton DB, Gonik G, Dorman KF: Cardiovascular alterations in severe pregnancy-induced hypertension: Acute effects of intravenous magnesium sulfate. Am J Obstet Gynecol 1984; 148:162; Benedetti TJ, Cotton DB, Read JC, et al: Hemodynamic observations in severe preeclampsia with a flow-directed pulmonary artery catheter. Am J Obstet Gynecol 1980; 136:465; Benedetti TJ, Kates R, Williams V: Hemodynamic observations in severe preeclampsia complicated by pulmonary edema. Am J Obstet Gynecol 1984; 150:232; Henderson DW, Vilos GA, Milne KJ, et al: The role of Swan-Ganz catheterization in severe pregnancy-induced hypertension. Am J Obstet Gynecol 1984; 148:570; and Strauss RG, Keefer JR, Burke T, et al: Hemodynamic monitoring of cardiogenic pulmonary edema complicating toxemia of pregnancy. Obstet Gynecol 1980; 55:170.) (From Easterling TR, Watts DH, Schmucker BC, et al: Measurement of cardiac output during pregnancy: Validation of Doppler technique and clinical observations in preeclampsia. Obstet Gynecol 1987; 69:848–849. Reprinted with permission from the American College of Obstetricians & Gynecologists.)

small decrease in MAP (4%) and normalization of PCWP. There was a much wider range of hemodynamic values in treated patients as compared with untreated patients. The authors concluded that much of the variability in the published data on the hemodynamics of preeclampsia is an artifact of treatment.

Longitudinal hemodynamic studies over the course of pregnancy have helped reconcile the conflicting data obtained from cross-sectional studies (i.e., done at one point in time). Mild to moderate preeclampsia appears to be a disease of high cardiac output and low or normal peripheral resistance. This is just the opposite of the hemodynamic profile found in patients with severe preeclampsia. Easterling et al.[3] measured a number of hemodynamic variables in women during their first pregnancy, beginning around the 10th week of conception. Patients destined to develop preeclampsia had a significant increase in MAP detectable in the first trimester that continued throughout the pregnancy with the differences becoming even greater at term (Fig. 25–18A). More important, women who eventually developed preeclampsia had higher cardiac outputs compared with normotensive pregnant controls at almost every measuring interval (monthly) over the course of gestation; cardiac output was on the average about 1.5 L/minute greater in preeclamptic patients than in normals (Fig. 25–18B). Peripheral resistance was lower in preeclamptic patients than normals (Fig. 25–18C). The pathophysiologic basis for the higher blood pressure in the preeclampsia group was an increase in car-

Table 25-9. Hemodynamic Profile of Untreated and Treated Preeclamptic Patients and Normotensive Pregnant Women*

	Untreated Preeclamptic Patients (n = 87)	P†	Normotensive Controls (n = 10)	P‡	Treated Preeclamptic Patients (n = 47)
Systemic Circulation					
Heart rate (beats · min⁻¹)	74 (51–110)	<.05	82 (68–93)	NS	85 (62–135)§
Mean intra-arterial pressure (mmHg)	125 (92–156)	<.001	83 (81–89)	<.001	120 (80–154)§
Cardiac index (L · min⁻¹ · m⁻²)	3.3 (2.0–5.3)	<.001	4.2 (3.5–4.6)	NS	4.3 (2.4–7.6)§
Stroke volume index (mL · beat⁻¹ · m⁻²)	46 (25–75)	NS	51 (38–61)	NS	52 (32–82)§
Systemic vascular resistance index (dyne · s · cm⁻⁵ · m⁻²)	3003 (1771–5225)	<.001	1560 (1430–2019)	<.005	2212 (1057–3688)§
Left ventricular stroke work index (J · beat⁻¹ · m⁻²)	0.70 (0.40–1.16)	<.005	0.54 (0.43–0.64)	<.001	0.79 (0.48–1.27)
Pulmonary Circulation					
Mean pulmonary arterial pressure (mmHg)	12 (3–26)	<.05	9 (7–13)	<.01	13 (0.5–30)
Pulmonary capillary wedge pressure (mmHg)	7 (−1–20)	NS	5 (1–8)	<.05	7 (0–25)
Right atrial pressure (mmHg)	2 (−4–10)	NS	1 (0–2)	NS	1 (−3–12)
Pulmonary vascular resistance index (dyne · s · cm⁻⁵ · m²)	131 (47–379)	<.005	91 (63–128)	NS	101 (8–317)§
Right ventricular stroke work index (J · beat⁻¹ · m⁻²)	0.06 (0.01–0.20)	NS	0.05 (0.04–0.08)	<.05	0.08 (0.01–0.22)§

NS, not significant.
*Values given are median (range).
†Differences between untreated preeclamptic patients and normotensive controls.
‡Differences between pharmacologically treated preeclamptic patients and normotensive controls.
§<.05 vs. untreated multiparous patients.
From Visser W, Wallenberg HC: Central hemodynamic observations in untreated preeclamptic patients. Hypertension 1991; 17:1072–1077.

diac output rather than an increase in vascular resistance. In the postpartum period (PP, Fig. 25-18), even though there was no significant difference in blood pressure between preeclamptic patients and controls, there were persistent differences in both cardiac output and peripheral resistance.

All women in the study of Easterling et al. were delivered once they became overtly preeclamptic (developed hypertension and proteinuria). The authors questioned whether or not some patients, had they not been promptly delivered, might have subsequently crossed over from a high output–low resistance condition to one of low output–high resistance. They reported one patient (Fig. 25-19) who was not part of the study but who was followed with a slightly increased MAP of 90 mmHg (77 mmHg was the normal value at 24 weeks' gestation) who initially presented with a high output–low resistance picture (cardiac output 11.3 L/minute). At 27, 28, 29 and 32 weeks, her cardiac output measured between 8 and 10 L/minute with normal resistance for pregnancy. She was lost to care for approximately 1 month, then presented with an elevation in blood pressure to 160/110 mmHg, proteinuria, and hemolysis. Her cardiac output had decreased to 6.9 L/minute and she had a marked increase in PVR. Her creatinine levels were consistent with renal insufficiency. Post partum, her blood pressure and creatinine returned to normal. The authors used this patient as an illustration of the potential for crossover from a high output state to a high resistance state in association with the progression from mild to severe preeclampsia.[3]

In considering a pregnant patient with a diagnosis of preeclampsia, it is essential to recognize that a mean blood pressure of 100 mmHg can be associated with an extremely wide range of cardiac outputs and vascular resistances. Equation 25-1 may be rewritten and substituted as follows:

$$\text{Mean arterial pressure} = \text{vascular resistance} \times \text{cardiac output}/80 \quad (3)$$
$$100 = 4000 \times 2/80$$

for the case in which there is very high vascular resistance

(4000 dynes · sec · cm⁻⁵) and very low cardiac output (2 L/minute), and

$$100 = 500 \times 16/80$$

for the case in which there is very low vascular resistance (500 dynes · sec · cm⁻⁵) and very high cardiac output (16 L/minute). In preeclampsia, these hemodynamic extremes still present with an identical mean blood pressure of 100 mmHg.

It is still unclear whether all patients with preeclampsia go through a hyperdynamic phase (high cardiac output–low resistance), with some eventually progressing to a low output–high resistance state, or whether this latter group represents a different disease process. Evidence that the difference is important, at least to the fetus, comes from a study of preeclamptic patients that compared the hemodynamic parameters of mothers of infants whose birth weights were appropriate for gestational age (AGA) to those whose infants were small for gestational age (SGA).[125] The mean birth weight of the AGA babies was 3576 g, which was more than 1 kg greater than the 2478-g mean birth weight of the SGA infants (Table 25-10). The mothers of the AGA babies had higher mean blood pressures than the mothers of the smaller babies, which would suggest that the mothers of the AGA babies had more severe preeclampsia. However, the hypertension of the AGA mothers was due to increased cardiac output (8.2 L/minute); the SGA mothers had low cardiac outputs (5.8 L/minute) and elevated vascular resistance. Another, more recent study has confirmed that preeclamptic patients with low cardiac output–high peripheral resistance are more likely to have small-for-dates babies than preeclamptic mothers who, despite their hypertension, have a normal or supranormal cardiac output.[126]

Cardiac Size and Function. In preeclampsia, modest increases in LV wall thickness and LV mass parallel those of

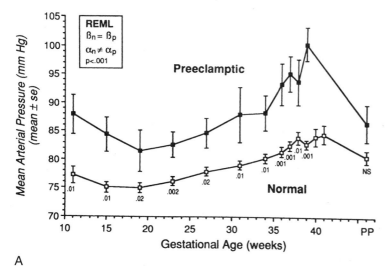

A

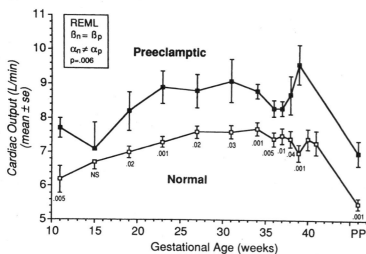

B

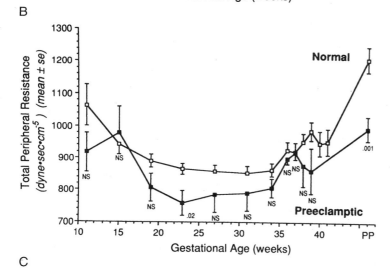

C

Figure 25–18. Hemodynamic changes over the course of normal and preeclamptic pregnancies. *A,* Mean arterial pressure. *B,* Cardiac output. *C,* Total peripheral resistance. Levels of statistical significance are given for each gestational age. To control for the effects of multiple comparisons, the curves for the normotensive (n) and the preeclamptic (p) group were analyzed by the technique of restricted maximal likelihood (REML) where β indicates the slope and α indicates the intercept of the line. The hypothesis that the slopes are equal ($\beta_n = \beta_p$) but the intercepts are different ($\alpha_n \neq \alpha_p$) was significant at the $P = .006$ level. (From Easterling TR, Benedetti TJ, Schmucker BC, et al: Maternal hemodynamics in normal and preeclamptic pregnancies: A longitudinal study. Obstet Gynecol 1990; 76:1065. Reprinted with permission from the American College of Obstetricians & Gynecologists.)

normal pregnancy. Significant LV hypertrophy usually indicates the presence of preexisting hypertension.

LV performance is usually well maintained in patients with pregnancy-induced hypertension; the decrease in cardiac output that does occur represents a mechanically appro-

priate response to increased afterload rather than an abnormality in the ventricular contractile state.[127] In one study of 43 patients with preeclampsia, all but 3 had normal indices of LV performance; of the 3 who had depressed ventricular function, only 1 had clinically apparent heart failure.[128] The

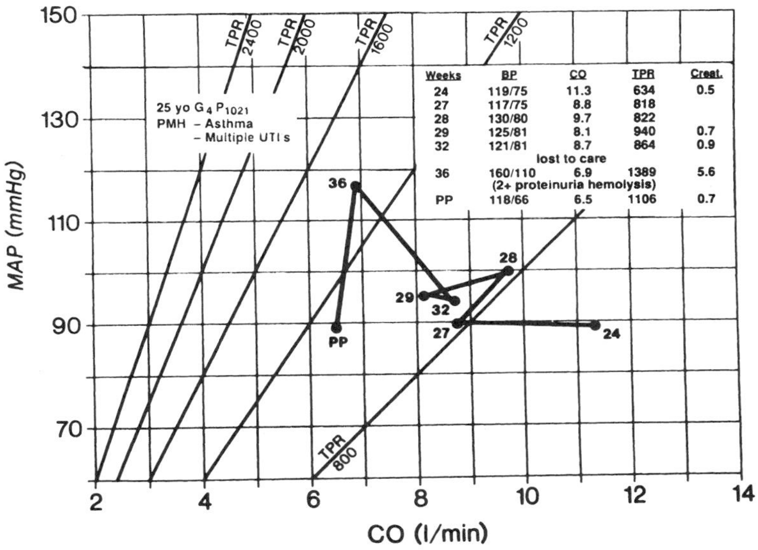

Figure 25-19. Serial hemodynamic data from a single patient who presented initially with a high cardiac output (CO)-low vascular resistance (TPR) profile, and who subsequently developed low cardiac output and high vascular resistance. Numbers adjacent to each point indicate gestational age in weeks; PP, postpartum; MAP, mean arterial pressure, creat., creatinine (mg/dL). (From Easterling TR, Benedetti TJ, Schmucker BC, et al: Maternal hemodynamics in normal and preeclamptic pregnancies: A longitudinal study. Obstet Gynecol 1990; 76:1067. Reprinted with permission from the American College of Obstetricians & Gynecologists.)

previously cited study by Visser and Wallenburg found normal to hyperdynamic LV function in all of 87 untreated preeclamptic patients.[124] In a separate cohort of 34 treated patients, all were normal or hyperdynamic except 3; in these a low LV stroke work index (LVSWI) in association with a high PCWP indicated impending LV failure (Fig. 25-20). Cardiac function is usually normal in patients with preeclampsia but cannot be taken for granted. Because these patients are on bed rest, abnormal LV function may not be apparent until the ventricle is stressed either by increased volume (preload) or increased PVR (afterload).

Uterine Vascular Changes. In normal pregnancy, a large increase in the cross-sectional area of the uterine arterial tree results from obliteration of vascular smooth muscle in the spiral arteries. There is also an interruption of the autonomic innervation of these vessels. In preeclampsia, the normal invasion of the spiral arteries by the trophoblast is impaired and the vessels maintain much of their encircling smooth muscle and autonomic innervation and, hence, the ability to constrict. The myometrial arteries, which are proximal to the spiral arteries, demonstrate loss of endothelium-dependent relaxation in preeclampsia.[129] Nitric oxide is synthesized in the endothelium and is the key mediator of this

process; however, the role of nitric oxide in the pathophysiology of preeclampsia is still unclear.[130]

The failure of appropriate uterine vascular changes in preeclampsia results in increased uterine vascular resistance. It is very common in tertiary treatment centers to avoid treatment of maternal hypertension until the diastolic pressure is greater than 110 mmHg. The underlying, and incorrect, rationale for this practice is the belief that the deleterious effects of increased uterine vascular resistance can be offset by higher maternal blood pressure. Irrespective of maternal blood pressure, preeclamptic patients with high uterine vascular resistance have a greatly increased likelihood of small, premature babies and fetal death compared with preeclamptic patients with lesser increases in uterine vascular resistance.[131] This study serves to underscore the previous discussion of maternal hemodynamics in preeclampsia; the blood pressure measurement per se is much less important than the value of the parameters that underlie the blood pressure—cardiac output and vascular resistance.

Arterial Pressure Measurement. Hypertension is the result of the hemodynamic abnormalities in preeclampsia, not the cause. Even though it is only an indirect indicator of the seriousness of the disease, arterial pressure measurement is still the basis for the diagnosis of preeclampsia. There are often very substantial differences in results obtained by invasive arterial monitoring when compared with manual sphygmomanometry or automated devices; this creates a situation in which the diagnosis depends on the monitoring device chosen rather than the physiologic state of the patient. There is clearly variability in systolic and diastolic pressures obtained by human beings using auscultatory methods, and there is no auscultatory correlate for mean blood pressure. Automated devices measure MAP, most often using oscillatory methods, and then derive systolic and diastolic pressures using an algorithm. Thus, people and machines are not really measuring the same phenomena. Furthermore, most automated devices including the Dinamap, are manufactured to conform as closely as possible to invasively measured intra-arterial blood pressure, the values of which are different from both simultaneous and sequential pressure measurements in the same individual using auscultatory method. To further confound the issue, the Dinamap XL 9301 (Johnson & Johnson Medical, Tampa, FL) and the SpaceLabs Scout

Table 25-10. Maternal Hemodynamic Variables and Neonatal Birth Weights in Pregnancy-Induced Hypertension

Variable	AGA (n = 16)	SGA (n = 5)	P
Mean arterial pressure (mmHg)	115 ±3	102 ±3	.05
Cardiac output (L/min)	8.2 ±0.3	5.8 ±0.2	<.01
Stroke volume (mL)	100 ±5	76 ±7	<.01
Heart rate (bpm)	82 ±2	79 ±5	NS
Systemic vascular resistance (dynes · cm · s⁻⁵)	1450 ±80	1770 ±80	NS
Birth weight (g)	3576 ±76	2478 ±220	<.01

AGA, appropriate for gestational age; SGA, small for gestational age; NS, not significant.

Modified from Nisell H, Lunell N, Linde B: Maternal hemodynamics and impaired fetal growth in pregnancy-induced hypertension. Obstet Gynecol 1988; 71:165–165.

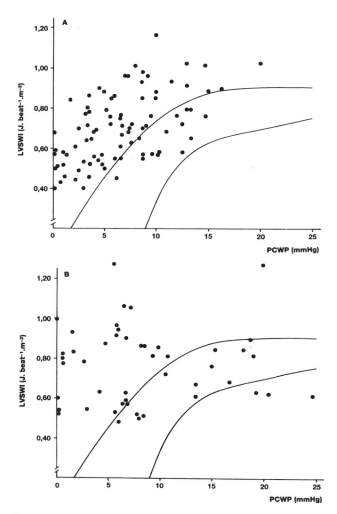

Figure 25-20. Left ventricular function in preeclampsia. *Curved lines* represent borders of normal range of left ventricular stroke work index (LVSWI) in relation to pulmonary capillary wedge pressure (PCWP). *A,* Untreated patients (n = 87). All patients displayed normal to hyperdynamic left ventricular function. *B,* Treated patients (n = 34). In a separate cohort of treated patients, all were normal or hyperdynamic except three; in these a low LVSWI in association with a high PCWP (19 to 24 mmHg) indicated impending left ventricular failure. (From Visser W, Wallenburg HCS: Central hemodynamic observations in untreated preeclamptic patients. Hypertension 1991; 17:1072–1077.)

(SpaceLabs, Redmond, WA), which are designed to reproduce invasively monitored pressures, recorded mean blood pressures that were 14.5 mmHg (Dinamap) and 11.6 mmHg (SpaceLabs) higher than intra-arterial pressures in patients with severe preeclampsia.[132] Using conventional sphygmomanometry to calculate MAP from the systolic and diastolic pressure underestimated MAP by 2 mmHg compared with intra-arterial values. This study involved a small number of patients (nine), but it indicates the need for evaluation of each model of automated device in the specific population of patients for which it will be used. Because of the variability in blood pressure measurements, there is very little scientific basis for treatment protocols in preeclampsia based solely on blood pressure.

Altered Sensitivity to Vasoactive Compounds. Preeclampsia is associated with increased responsivity to vaso-

pressors such as epinephrine, norepinephrine, and angiotensin II, whereas in normal pregnancy vasopressor responsiveness decreases. In Figure 25-21, the response of preeclamptic patients to angiotensin II is compared with the normal response in pregnancy. Despite this differential sensitivity, the angiotensin II infusion test has not proved helpful in the early identification (28 weeks' gestation) of pregnant patients destined to develop preeclampsia.[133] Platelet angiotensin II binding has likewise been found to be of no value as a possible test for the early identification of preeclampsia.[134] The enhanced vascular responsiveness of preeclamptic patients requires careful titration of all vasopressor drugs.

Fluid Balance. In preeclampsia, the expected increase in plasma volume seen in normal pregnancy is impaired, and the degree of impairment is related to the severity of disease.[29, 135] Two studies using different techniques found plasma volume increases of 10% to 15% in patients with preeclampsia compared to increases of 45% to 50% in normal pregnancies.[29, 31] The increase in red blood cell mass that occurs in normal pregnancy is decreased in preeclampsia; it parallels the 10% to 15% increase in plasma volume. Thus, the hematocrit may be unchanged, and preeclamptic patients may have a "normal" hematocrit value.

Preeclamptic patients have the same increase in total body water as is seen in normal pregnancies. However, because less of this volume is distributed to the intravascular space, it must be accounted for by abnormal increases in interstitial or intracellular water. Increases in both interstitial and intracellular water contribute to the edematous, puffy appearance of some patients. The edema is generalized, in contrast to the dependent edema that is typical of normal pregnancy. This has been one reason for suboptimal management of patients with severe preeclampsia; the usual treatment of edema is fluid restriction and diuretics, which is inappropriate treatment in severe preeclampsia. Although these patients are edematous, their intravascular volume is decreased. One of the mechanisms that contribute to this problem is that, in comparison to normal pregnancy, there is no increase in venous distensibility in preeclampsia.[27] Capillary permeability is increased in patients with preeclampsia, regardless of whether or not proteinuria is present.

Capillary hydrostatic pressure increases 30% over the course of normal pregnancy and in mild preeclampsia as well (see Table 25-4). In severe preeclampsia, capillary hydrostatic pressure does not increase despite increased blood pressure (Fig. 25-22). The reason for this is that the arteriolar vasoconstriction of severe preeclampsia results in decreased capillary flow. To some extent, this helps to defend against further fluid losses to the interstitium, because higher capillary pressures coupled with the decreased osmotic pressures associated with preeclampsia would favor fluid movement out of the capillaries. However, very high precapillary resistance, while resulting in lower capillary hydrostatic pressure and potentially less edema, is detrimental to the fetus and maternal organ systems. Brown et al.[38] reported a mean fetal birth weight of 3180 g in 10 infants born to preeclamptic mothers with edema; in a corresponding group of preeclamptic parturients with similar arterial pressures and plasma volumes but without edema, the mean birth weight was 715 g lower.[38]

The significance of the decreased maternal plasma volume in preeclampsia is that it correlates strongly with fetal size, the single most important determinant of outcome. Hays et al.[29] found that normotensive mothers had an increase in plasma volume from 1600 mL/m² to over 2300 mL/m² (Fig. 25-23). Parturients with preeclampsia and AGA babies had an increase to only 1900 mL/m². Preeclamptic patients with

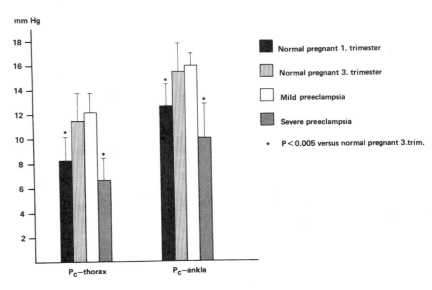

Figure 25-21. Increased angiotensin II sensitivity in patients with preeclampsia. Whereas normal pregnancy (*closed circles*) is associated with a decreased sensitivity to vasopressors such as angiotensin II, patients with preeclampsia have an increased sensitivity, such that small doses produce a marked pressor response. (From Gant NF, Daley GL, Chand S, et al: A study of angiotensin II pressor response throughout primigravid pregnancy. J Clin Invest 1973; 52:2682–2689.) By copyright permission of the American Society for Clinical Investigation.)

SGA babies had a slight contraction in plasma volume. Plasma volume abnormalities are much more central to the pathophysiology and fetal morbidity of preeclampsia than increased blood pressure, which bears no predictable relationship to fetal outcomes.

The decrease in COP seen in normal pregnancy is even more pronounced in preeclampsia.[136] This decrease results in a greater likelihood of pulmonary edema should PCWP increase. The COP continues to decline in the immediate postpartum period when there is an increase in central blood volume due to involution of the uterus. Overly zealous volume administration in this period can elevate the PCWP and result in pulmonary edema.[137, 138]

VOLUME AND VASODILATOR THERAPY IN SEVERE PREECLAMPSIA. The usual hemodynamic response to intravascular volume expansion in patients with *untreated* severe preeclampsia is presented in Table 25-11. Cardiac output improves as a result of increased filling pressures (normalization of PCWP, which is most often very low) and decreased vascular resistance; blood pressure is minimally affected.

Vasodilator therapy after volume expansion produces an additional increase in cardiac output, an additional decrease in SVR, a significant decrease in blood pressure, and minimal effects on PCWP.[117, 139] Volume expansion is essential prior to treatment of severe hypertension, because acute vasodilation in a hemoconcentrated, hypovolemic, hypertensive patient may result in cardiovascular collapse.[138] Volume expansion and vasodilator therapy have been shown to allow expectant management of preeclamptic patients remote from term, an important benefit in terms of fetal maturity.[140]

OLIGURIC PREECLAMPTIC PATIENTS: HEMODYNAMIC SUBSETS. Clark et al.[141] have further characterized the range of hemodynamic abnormalities found in severe preeclampsia and the role of fluid therapy in the oliguric patient. Studies were made in patients who were oliguric (less than 30 mL of urine per hour for 3 consecutive hours) in spite of maintenance fluid therapy of 100 to 125 mL/hour and a fluid bolus of 300 to 500 mL of crystalloid. Three subsets of patients were identified (Table 25-12). Category I (five patients) had low PCWP (4 mmHg), moderately elevated SVR

Figure 25-22. Capillary hydrostatic pressure (P_c) at the thorax and ankle in normal pregnancies, mild preeclampsia, and severe preeclampsia. (From Oian P, Maltau JM: Calculated capillary hydrostatic pressure in normal pregnancy and preeclampsia. Am J Obstet Gynecol 1987; 157:105.)

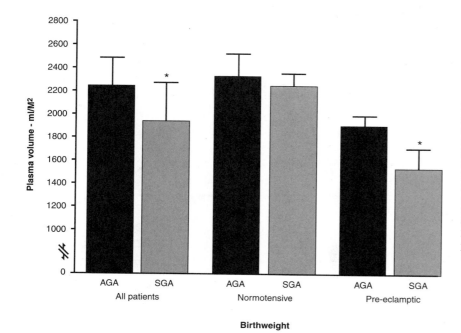

Figure 25–23. Plasma volume in normal and preeclamptic pregnancies. 1600 mL/m² represents a normal nonpregnant plasma volume. Patients with preeclampsia and AGA babies had a lesser expansion in plasma volume than normotensive patients, regardless of the size of the baby. Severe preeclampsia was associated with a contraction in plasma volume and small-for-dates babies. *$P < .05$; AGA, appropriate for gestational age; SGA, small for gestational age. (From Hays PM, Cruikshank DP, Dunna LJ: Plasma volume determination in normal and preeclamptic pregnancies. Am J Obstet Gynecol 1985; 151:962.)

(1330 dynes · s · cm⁻⁵), and a cardiac index of 3.8 L/minute/m². These parameters were consistent with hypovolemia and additional volume therapy resulted in an increase in PCWP (10 mmHg), decreased SVR (1150 dynes · s · cm⁻⁵), an increase in cardiac index (4.5 L/minute/m²), and resolution of the oliguria. These results are similar to the findings of Groenendijk et al. in the Netherlands study of severe preeclamptic patients following fluid therapy but prior to vasodilator therapy.[117]

Category II (three patients) had a normal or elevated PCWP, a normal SVR, and a normal cardiac index. In two of these, the administration of hydralazine and additional fluid was followed by resolution of the oliguria. It was postulated that selective renal artery vasoconstriction maintained the oliguric state in these patients. Abnormalities of the renal vasculature do occur in preeclampsia; other investigators have found dopamine efficacious in preeclamptic oliguria. These results may reflect dopaminergic receptor–mediated decreases in renal vascular resistance as well as improved preload from modest venoconstriction.[142]

The other category II patient had an abnormally high PCWP (18 mmHg) and a cardiac index of 6.1 L/minute/m². The diagnosis of volume overload was made and the patient treated with a nitroglycerin infusion to decrease both preload and afterload. The blood pressure decreased and the

oliguria resolved. NTG is usually an inappropriate vasodilator for patients with preeclampsia because the vasoconstriction of preeclampsia is primarily *arteriolar* and nitroglycerin acts on the *venous* side of the circulatory bed to a greater degree than the arterial side. Venous dilation decreases blood return to the heart and normally decreases cardiac output. Although this may be desirable in a patient with volume overload, it is poorly tolerated by patients with intravascular volume depletion, which is the situation in most patients with severe preeclampsia. Use of NTG in severe preeclampsia impairs maternal cardiac output and may result in fetal distress, presumably because of impaired placental perfusion and fetal hypoxemia.[143]

The third subset in the Clark study included only one patient, but one who helps to illustrate an important aspect of preeclampsia. This oliguric patient had a MAP of 140 mmHg; a very low cardiac index (2.6 L/minute/m²); an elevated PCWP (18 mmHg); and very high SVR (2790 dynes · s · cm⁻⁵). This patient demonstrated LV dysfunction and was managed with fluid restriction and aggressive afterload reduction.

Cardiovascular Physiology During Regional Analgesia and Anesthesia in Patients With Preeclampsia. Epidural or spinal blockade can produce profound hypotension in patients with severe preeclampsia, as in any patient with a severe intravascular volume deficit. Although this concern has resulted in the blanket condemnation by some of epidural blockade,[144] regional analgesia and anesthesia in patients with severe preeclampsia has been proved safe for both the mother and fetus when there is recognition of the underlying maternal hemodynamic status and appropriate management is undertaken.[145–150]

LEA increases UBF while decreasing maternal blood pressure. Most vasodilators affect both the maternal systemic and uterine circulations fairly equally, so that the flow relationships remain relatively constant. LEA (maximum height, T8) selectively blocks the sympathetic innervation of the uterus without blocking sympathetic innervation of other vascular beds, particularly the splanchnic bed. This preferentially reduces uterine vascular resistance relative to maternal periph-

Table 25–11. Hemodynamic Response to Volume and Vasodilator Therapy in Severe Preeclampsia

	Following Volume Therapy Alone	Following Volume and Vasodilator Therapy
Mean arterial pressure	No change	↓
Heart rate		No change
Systemic vascular resistance	↓↓	↓
Pulmonary capillary wedge pressure	↑	No change
Cardiac output	↑	↑

Table 25-12. Hemodynamic Data From Nine Preeclamptic Patients With Persistent Oliguria

Patient No.	Category I (n = 5)					Category II (n = 3)			Category III (n = 1)
	1	2	3	4	5	6	7	8	9
Following Unsuccessful Fluid Challenge									
Mean arterial pressure (mmHg)	120	110	101	118	107	117	129	130	140
PCWP (mmHg)	7	3	4	5	1	9	10	18	18
CVP (mmHg)	6	1	0	2	2	5	9	9	3
Cardiac index (L · min^{-1} · m^{-2})	3.5	4.2	3.5	4.1	4.0	4.8	5.1	6.4	2.6
SVR (dynes · cm · s^{-5})	1378	1245	1393	1497	1135	1093	1043	921	2790
Left ventricular stroke work index	54	90	54	66	59	88	94	89	33
Therapy	Fluid	Fluid	Fluid	Fluid	Fluid	Fluid/ hydralazine	Fluid/ hydralazine	Nitroglycerin	Hydralazine
Following Therapy and Resolution of Oliguria									
Mean arterial pressure (mmHg)	117	123	120	107	107	110	107	105	104
PCWP (mmHg)	11	7	11	9	11	9	15	2	8
CVP (mmHg)	11	5	4	—	—	8	10	—	—
Cardiac index (L · min^{-1} · m^{-2})	4.6	4.5	4.1	5.0	4.4	5.4	5.1	5.6	4.0
SVR (dynes · cm · s^{-5})	961	1237	1367	1138	1049	884	843	910	1867
Left ventricular stroke work index	66	111	65	59	50	65	60	65	51

PCWP, pulmonary capillary wedge pressure; CVP, central venous pressure; SVR, systemic vascular resistance.
Modified from Clark SL, Greenspoon JS, Aldahl D, et al: Severe preeclampsia with persistent oliguria: Management of hemodynamic subsets. Am J Obstet Gynecol 1986; 154:490–499.

eral resistance, thereby increasing the fraction of flow through the low-resistance bed. In one study of severely preeclamptic patients in labor, LEA resulted in a 77% increase in intervillous blood flow over controls when maternal blood pressure was maintained at pre-LEA levels.[147] The modest drop in blood pressure that is usually seen following LEA in adequately hydrated severely preeclamptic patients results from uterine vasodilation and, as maternal pain is relieved, lower levels of endogenous catecholamines.

The same beneficial effect on maternal blood pressure seen with epidural analgesia has been documented for epidural anesthesia in severely preeclamptic patients[149] (Fig. 25-24). In adequately hydrated patients, there is a modest decline in mean blood pressure with no change in PCWP. Cardiac output is well maintained following epidural anesthesia in spite of the decrease in blood pressure[145] (Fig. 25-25). As in all obstetric patients, proper uterine displacement is essential if cardiac output is to be maintained in the supine position.

Spinal anesthesia is increasingly used for anesthesia for

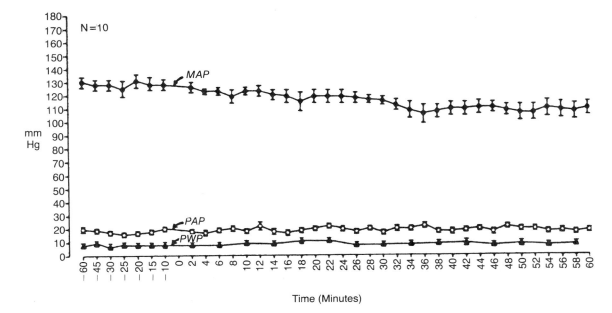

Figure 25-24. Hemodynamic response to lumbar epidural anesthesia for cesarean section in patients with severe preeclampsia. Injection of epidural anesthetic was at time zero. MAP, mean arterial pressure; PAP, pulmonary artery pressure; PWP, pulmonary wedge pressure. (From Hodgkinson R, Husain FJ, Hayashi RH: Systemic and pulmonary blood pressure during caesarean section in parturients with gestational hypertension. Can Anaesth Soc J 1980; 27:392.)

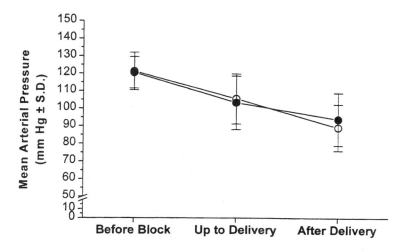

Figure 25-25. Lowest mean blood pressure in patients with severe preeclampsia receiving regional anesthesia for cesarean section. *Open circles,* spinal anesthesia (n = 103); *closed circles,* epidural anesthesia (n = 35). (From Hood DD, Curry R: Spinal versus epidural anesthesia for cesarean section in severely preeclamptic patients. Anesthesiology 1999; 90:1276–1282.)

cesarean delivery of patients with severe preeclampsia. Concerns about precipitous decreases in maternal blood pressure have led many to choose epidural anesthesia under the assumption that the block level could be increased slowly, thus allowing time for hemodynamic adjustments. One prospective study and one large retrospective study found little difference between the two techniques in terms of blood pressure, and both regional techniques were associated with only moderate decreases (15% to 25%) in MAP.[145, 146]

Our knowledge of the wide range of underlying hemodynamic patterns that may be present in preeclamptic patients clearly has implications for management of regional analgesia and anesthesia in such patients. For example, in patients with a high cardiac output–low PVR profile, modest volume supplementation (about 500 mL) is adequate to attenuate the vasodilating effects of epidural analgesia, and 1000 to 1500 mL is adequate for regional anesthesia for cesarean section. These patients have moderately decreased intravascular volumes relative to normal pregnant patients, despite the presence of high cardiac outputs. In patients with low cardiac output–high PVR profiles, much more careful attention

to volume replacement is required, because this pattern may reflect either a severe intravascular volume deficit or cardiac dysfunction. In either case, a more careful program of volume and vasodilator therapy is required for optimal patient management.

Cardiovascular Physiology During General Anesthesia in Patients With Preeclampsia. General anesthesia is associated with potentially dangerous increases in maternal blood pressure and cardiac filling pressures in patients with preeclampsia. The most extreme elevations are related to tracheal intubation and extubation. Hodgkinson et al.[149] documented a 45-mmHg increase in MAP and a 20-mmHg increase in PCWP during both intubation and extubation of the trachea in patients with severe preeclampsia (Fig. 25-26). These changes reflect the increased sensitivity to vasopressors, including endogenous catecholamines, seen in preeclamptic patients. Severe and abrupt pulmonary and systemic hypertension of the magnitude documented by Hodgkinson et al. has been associated with acute heart failure, pulmonary edema, and cerebral hemorrhage in patients with

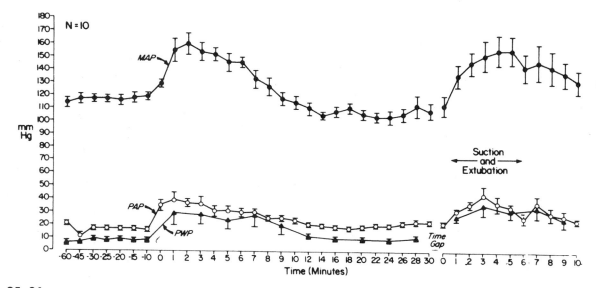

Figure 25-26. Hemodynamic responses in patients with severe preeclampsia receiving general anesthesia for cesarean section. The first zero indicates induction; the second indicates suctioning and extubation. (From Hodgkinson R, Husain FJ, Hayashi RH: Systemic and pulmonary blood pressure during caesarean section in parturients with gestational hypertension. Can Anaesth Soc J 1980; 27:392.)

preeclampsia. A recent report used transcranial Doppler to measure the flow in the middle cerebral artery (MCA) during induction of general anesthesia; in comparison with normals, patients with severe preeclampsia had a significant increase in mean flow velocity in spite of pretreatment with labetalol.[151] The increase in MCA flow paralleled increases in maternal MAP, which increased from 113 mmHg to 134 mmHg. These findings suggest an impairment of normal autoregulation of cerebral blood flow in preeclampsia, and should heighten one's concern for abrupt increases in maternal blood pressure in hypertensive pregnancies.

Optimal patient management requires continuous monitoring of cardiovascular changes and carefully titrated drug therapy to prevent adverse hemodynamic changes. In most patients with severe preeclampsia, this requires invasive intra-arterial monitoring. Bolus doses of sodium nitroprusside (SNP) 100 to 200 μg in adequately hydrated patients are effective in blunting the hypertensive response to tracheal intubation. This is not true for NTG.[152] Longmire et al.[152] used volume expansion to produce a PCWP of 10 to 15 mmHg and a COP greater than 17 mmHg in patients with severe preeclampsia prior to general anesthesia. IV NTG was then administered. Endotracheal intubation still produced a change in the heart rate from 104 to 133 bpm and an increase in MAP from 134 to 164 mmHg. Alternatively or in combination with other antihypertensive agents, short-acting narcotics, particularly alfentanil, decrease the central reflex responses that occur with tracheal intubation and extubation. While labetalol is not sufficient in this setting as the sole antihypertensive agent, its effects on heart rate and blood pressure are useful as adjunctive therapy to narcotics and SNP. It is essential to recognize that the risk of extreme hypertension carries more risk for the patient with severe preeclampsia during induction of anesthesia than the hypotension that may occur with IV narcotics and incremental bolus doses of SNP. At this stage, minutes before delivery, decreases in UBF because of maternal hypotension are of lesser concern.

Treatment of Maternal Hypertension. Treatment of hypertension in pregnancy is directed toward preventing maternal complications. As yet, there is no evidence that long-term control of blood pressure significantly improves fetal outcome and the drugs chosen to treat maternal hypertension may have adverse effects on the fetus. For example, although angiotensin-converting enzyme inhibitors would appear to be ideal agents in a disease in which there is an enhanced and deleterious response to angiotensin, the use of this class of drug has been associated with major adverse effects in the fetus and newborn, including oligohydramnios, renal tubular dysgenesis, neonatal anuria, pulmonary hypoplasia, intrauterine growth retardation, persistent patent ductus arteriosus, and death.[153]

A lack of understanding of the relationship between maternal blood pressure and UBF may lead to suboptimal management of patients with preeclampsia. The standard of practice on many obstetric services is that maternal hypertension is not treated until the diastolic pressure exceeds 105 to 110 mmHg and pharmacologic intervention at pressures above this is primarily to prevent intracranial bleeding. Hypertension is maintained at a level that provides "a margin for maternal safety (95–100 mmHg) without compromising adequate uterine perfusion."[154] The upper limit of cerebral blood flow autoregulation occurs at a mean perfusion pressure of 150 mmHg; above this level, the blood-brain barrier begins to break down and cerebral injury results. Maternal diastolic blood pressures in the range of 105 to 110 mmHg are usually associated with mean pressures of 125 to 130 mmHg. Thus, there is only a *narrow* margin of maternal safety for potential cerebral injury. It is unclear to what the 95 to 100-mmHg safety margin referred to above applies. Furthermore, in preeclampsia, *maternal hypertension does not ensure adequate uterine perfusion.* Despite elevated blood pressure, UBF is reduced 50% to 70% and the highest blood pressures are often associated with the lowest UBF.[155] The use of vasodilators to reduce maternal blood pressure by decreasing PVR usually dilates the uterine vessels as well, and placental flow is not impaired as long as maternal hypotension is avoided.[156] Untreated hypertension increases the workload on the LV. Preeclamptic patients may develop acute left-sided heart failure during the stress of labor or in association with endotracheal intubation and surgery. Thus, there is a very good rationale for reducing maternal blood pressure using therapies that do not compromise UBF. All recent studies on the treatment of severe preeclampsia using appropriate volume and vasodilator therapy demonstrate a normalization of maternal hemodynamic status with no evidence of fetal compromise.[126, 157–159]

SNP is the drug of choice for *acute* control of *extreme* hypertension in preeclampsia. The acceptance of SNP in obstetric practice was delayed in part because of misinterpretation of animal studies in which supraclinical doses were given to pregnant ewes to produce acidosis in the fetuses.[160] However, SNP has been shown to have no detectable adverse effects upon the human fetus when used in the usual clinical doses.[161, 162] Even when SNP is infused at a rate of 25 $\mu g/kg$/minute for 4 hours, which is far in excess of the dosages used clinically, the coinfusion of sodium thiosulfate prevents the development of fetal or maternal cyanide toxicity in sheep (the model that gave rise to the initial concerns over fetal cyanide toxicity).[163] SNP is a potent dilator of both the arterial and venous vascular beds; used in cases of uncorrected severe intravascular volume depletion, as occurs in severe preeclampsia, it is likely to produce extreme hypotension. Preeclamptic patients who receive SNP and develop severe hypotension have an associated and compounding decrease in heart rate. Wasserstrum[164] found that preeclamptic patients fell into two groups, defined by whether the hypotensive effect of SNP was accompanied by a fall or a rise in heart rate. In response to moderate and gradual decreases in MAP (32 mmHg) elicited by an SNP infusion at a rate of 1 $\mu g/kg$/minute, one group of patients showed the expected sinoaortic-baroreceptor reflex elevations in heart rate (17 bpm). However, in the other group of patients, very low doses of SNP (0.35 $\mu g/kg$/minute) caused steep reductions in MAP (75 mmHg). In these patients, hypotension was accompanied by a decrease in heart rate of 21 bpm. This paradoxical response is indicative of severe circulatory compromise with cardiac and vasomotor depression, as is seen in severe hemorrhage and other forms of acute or severe hypovolemic hypotension.

Remote from term, methyldopa is the drug most frequently used to treat maternal hypertension. In hospitalized patients, the main drugs in current use are calcium channel blockers (nifedipine, nimodipine, nicardipine), labetalol, and hydralazine. All of these drugs reduce maternal blood pressure in most patients with preeclampsia. When single-drug therapy fails, a second drug of a different type may be added. In addition to the effects on the mother, the effects of antihypertensive treatment may have an impact on the fetus. All of the calcium channel blockers and magnesium sulfate dilate the vessels in the umbilical cord, an efficacious effect; hydralazine does not have this effect.[165] There are now convincing data that hydralazine is associated with a much higher incidence of precipitating fetal distress than any of the other agents used to treat preeclamptic hypertension.[166-168] Hydralazine is available in both IV and oral preparations, and it is possible that there are different effects depending on route of administration. There are conflicting data over the effects of labetalol on placental and umbilical blood flow.[169, 170] Labetalol should be used cautiously when the infant is stressed, because it may interfere with the normal cardiovascular responses to stress. No differences were seen when labetalol was compared to hydralazine for treatment of hypertension in preeclamptic patients with low-birth-weight fetuses.[171]

In a comparative study of the treatment of maternal hypertension in severe preeclampsia, nifedipine was a more efficacious antihypertensive drug than hydralazine and was associated with a much lower incidence of fetal distress.[158] Infants of nifedipine-treated mothers spent an average of 11 days in intensive care as opposed to 33 days for the hydralazine group. The overall maternal-infant cost in the nifedipine group was 31% lower than in the hydralazine group. Using Doppler technology, nifedipine has been shown to have no adverse effects on fetal or uteroplacental hemodynamics when used in the treatment of preeclampsia.[172] In the postpartum period, nifedipine lowers maternal MAP while enhancing urine output.[173]

As previously stated, NTG has a very limited role in the treatment of hypertension in the setting of preeclampsia. However, it is a useful agent for rapid and transient relief of increased uterine tone; it has been used to treat fetal distress resulting from uterine tetany, to facilitate extraction of a retained placenta, to manage uterine inversion, and to facilitate external version of a twin. In these cases, NTG is used in bolus doses of 50 to 100 μg, and the effect lasts just minutes. However, in the setting of severe preeclampsia with a stressed fetus, it would appear that SNP, which is an equally potent uterine relaxant, would be a safer agent.

An important finding in the studies of antihypertensive therapy in preeclampsia is that drugs have different hemodynamic effects in the mother and the fetus. This information, coupled with new insights into the range of different hemodynamic profiles found in patients with preeclampsia, requires the use of sophisticated noninvasive monitoring techniques, such as Doppler flow velocimetry of the maternal and fetal circulations, to more accurately define the hemodynamic state of preeclamptic patients. With the goal being to stabilize maternal hemodynamics and sustain adequate uteroplacental blood flow, volume management and antihypertensive therapy can then be tailored to the specific hemodynamic pattern. For example, patients with high output and low resistance do not require major volume resuscitation and would be better candidates for treatment with drugs to lower cardiac output, such as β-adrenergic blockers. Patients with low output and high resistance would be better treated with volume expansion and peripheral vasodilation using such drugs as nifedipine. In all cases, it is important to be aware of potential effects upon the fetus.

Invasive Cardiovascular Monitoring in Patients With Preeclampsia. The risk-benefit ratio of invasive cardiovascular monitoring in patients with preeclampsia, as well as with other cardiovascular disorders, must incorporate the skill and experience of the physicians and nursing staff as well as the severity of the patient's disease. Placement of intra-arterial and pulmonary artery catheters in patients with preeclampsia is not warranted, regardless of maternal status, if the obstetric and anesthetic decision makers are either unable or unwilling to incorporate the information obtained into the medical and anesthetic management of the patient. Recognition of the significance of various pulmonary artery waveforms, such as a continuously wedged position, requires

specially trained individuals; pulmonary artery catheters should not be used without the continuous presence of personnel experienced in their use.

In patients with documented coagulation problems, as may occur in preeclampsia, introduction of central venous and pulmonary arterial catheters through an internal jugular vein approach carries a risk of a neck hematoma in the event of carotid artery cannulation. The median basilic vein in the antecubital fossa or an external jugular vein minimizes this risk. The blood of preeclamptic patients may be hypocoagulable or hypercoagulable; in the latter case, the risk of axillary vein thrombosis is increased with prolonged use of brachial venous catheters long enough to reach the central circulation.

Arterial Pressure. In severe preeclampsia, an indwelling arterial catheter is warranted for beat-to-beat assessment of maternal blood pressure. This is especially important during general anesthesia because of the precipitous and extreme systemic and pulmonary hypertension that occurs in association with tracheal intubation and extubation (see Fig. 25–26). Direct intra-arterial monitoring is necessary to guide antihypertensive therapy with rapid-acting agents during general anesthesia. During epidural or spinal anesthesia, direct arterial monitoring allows for earlier correction of possible hypotension. Such prompt therapy is mandated in the setting of a compromised fetus with minimal cardiovascular reserve, as is the usual case in severe preeclampsia. In addition, the waveform of the arterial pressure tracing provides useful information on the volume status of the patient, both in the shape of the waveform and its variation with respiration.

Central Venous Pressure. A central venous catheter may be useful in cases of moderate to severe preeclampsia in which there is reduced urine output. If the initial central venous pressure (CVP) is low (0 to 3 mmHg), and the patient has a normal chest examination and good oxygen saturation on room air, it is appropriate to assume that the oliguric patient has persistent intravascular volume depletion and to continue with fluid and possibly arteriolar vasodilator therapy. However, it must be recognized that in patients with preeclampsia, CVPs may not reliably predict left-sided cardiac filling pressures, either in absolute values or trends.[174] Figure 25–27 indicates that for any level of CVP, the PCWP may be equal to or two to three times greater than the measured CVP. Thus, while a very low CVP will usually indicate a low PCWP, there will be an occasional patient in whom a very low CVP will be associated with a PCWP high enough to pose a risk for pulmonary edema. If the CVP is high (6 to 12 mmHg) in a patient with preeclampsia, one must assume that the PCWP is at least this high, and probably much higher. Such patients have much less tolerance for aggressive volume therapy.

DiFederico et al. reported on a series of pregnant patients who developed pulmonary edema, including several with preeclampsia[36] (Fig. 25–28). The mean CVP for patients developing pulmonary edema was 8 mmHg (the normal value for CVP was 3.6 mmHg in both normal pregnant and nonpregnant subjects). All of the causes of both hydrostatic and increased-permeability pulmonary edema were associated with elevated CVPs.

Disparities between right-sided and left-sided heart filling pressures may occur in the absence of any underlying cardiac abnormality, and are primarily due to differences in afterload. For example, the LV in severe preeclampsia is required to pump against an abnormally high peripheral resistance, whereas the right side of the heart usually sees a normal afterload. Pulmonary vascular resistance is not in-

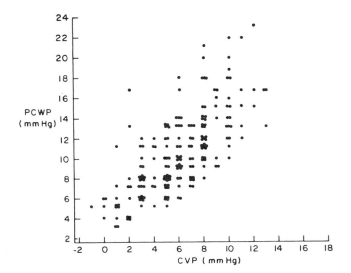

Figure 25-27. Relationship of central venous pressure to pulmonary capillary wedge pressure in patients with severe preeclampsia. (From Cotton DB, Gonik B, Dorman K, et al: Cardiovascular alterations in severe pregnancy-induced hypertension: Relationship of central venous pressure to pulmonary capillary wedge pressure. Am J Obstet Gynecol 1985; 151:763.)

PULMONARY ARTERY PRESSURE. The most frequent indication for monitoring pulmonary artery pressures in patients with preeclampsia is persistent oliguria in the face of presumably adequate fluid therapy. Although most oliguric patients will be found to have a low to normal PCWP, indicative of a persistent intravascular volume deficit, a minority will have markedly increased wedge pressures.[141] Increased wedge pressures in the absence of aggressive fluid therapy usually indicate LV dysfunction. PAC allows for measurement of cardiac output and calculation of SVR, and preeclampsia is associated with widely disparate values for these variables, as seen in Figure 25-17 and Tables 25-9 and 25-12. Knowledge of cardiac output and SVR is essential to optimal hemodynamic management in patients with severe preeclampsia and oliguria.[176]

Another indication for PAC is when a central venous catheter is placed and the initial CVP is greater than 12 mmHg. Such pressures indicate either volume overload or heart failure; additional hemodynamic data are necessary for further assessment and management.

A pulmonary catheter is recommended for management of preeclamptic patients with pulmonary edema to determine the cause of the pulmonary edema and the underlying hemodynamic state. Because COP is decreased in pregnancy and further decreased in preeclampsia, pulmonary edema can occur at "normal" levels of PCWP in these patients. Even when the PCWP is much lower than COP, pulmonary edema may still be present on the basis of increased capillary permeability.[36, 121] Particularly in the immediate postpartum period, pulmonary edema with increased PCWP and cardiac output and normal SVR, coupled with a history of aggressive fluid therapy, is most often due to volume overload. Pulmonary edema with increased PCWP and SVR and decreased cardiac output is most consistent with acute left-sided heart failure.

Volume loading prior to epidural or spinal anesthesia can be guided by CVP if oliguria is not present. However, if there is no increase in the CVP following 1500 mL of crystalloid or 500 mL of colloid, and the catheter position is confirmed, it is likely that there is poor correlation between the CVP and the PCWP. Further fluid management should be based on careful clinical assessment or PAC.

In a preeclamptic patient with decreased oxygen saturation immediately after tracheal intubation or extubation,

creased in preeclampsia, even in the face of precipitous increases in SVR.[175] Thus, pressure differences between the right and the left sides of the heart are to be expected, with the differences being more pronounced the greater the differences in afterload in the pulmonary and systemic circulations.

The limitations of CVP measurements in preeclampsia do not require that every patient have a pulmonary catheter to guide volume therapy. However, one should not rely entirely on a CVP measurement, particularly in the face of persistent oliguria. If fluid and vasodilator therapy is ineffective in establishing adequate urine output, and particularly if the CVP is above 6 to 8 mmHg, a measurement other than CVP is required to assess cardiac filling. The two options available are PAC and echocardiography.

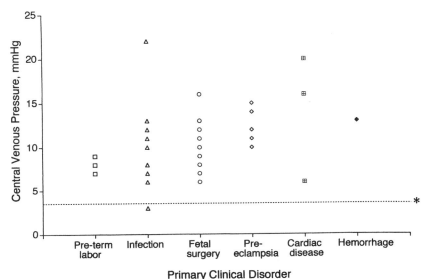

Figure 25-28. Central venous pressure (CVP) in pregnant patients with pulmonary edema from a variety of causes. The mean CVP for patients developing pulmonary edema was 8 mmHg (the normal value for CVP was 3.6 mmHg in both normal pregnant and nonpregnant subjects). All of the causes of both hydrostatic and increased-permeability pulmonary edema were associated with elevated CVPs. (From DiFederico EM, Burlingame JM, Kilpatrick SJ, et al: Pulmonary edema in obstetric patients is rapidly resolved except in the presence of infection or nitroglycerin tocolysis after open fetal surgery. Am J Obstet Gynecol 1998; 179:925-933.)

acute heart failure must be considered in the differential diagnosis. After problems with oxygen delivery have been ruled out, PAC is useful for diagnosis and treatment of the cardiac dysfunction.

NONINVASIVE ASSESSMENT OF CARDIAC FUNCTION. Noninvasive cardiovascular monitoring is increasingly used in patients with preeclampsia, obviating the need in many cases for PAC. Numerous studies have now validated this technique; there is a very high degree of correlation between measures of cardiovascular function determined noninvasively as compared to invasively, even in critically ill obstetric patients.[177, 178] The ability to measure stroke volume, cardiac output, cardiac index, LV filling pressure, pulmonary artery systolic pressure, and right atrial pressure in a noninvasive manner contributes to patient safety, particularly in patients with coagulation defects. Noninvasive 2-D and Doppler echocardiography can readily differentiate patients with high cardiac output and low vascular resistance from those with low cardiac output and high resistance; this information is of great significance in the management of anesthetic and obstetric care.

Renal Alterations. Monitoring of renal function is crucial in preeclampsia, with the most important parameter being urine output. Maintenance of good urine output equates with adequacy of both the cardiovascular system and intravascular volume. Patients in this condition at the time of anesthesia, whether regional or general, usually present minimal challenges in terms of maintenance of cardiovascular hemostasis.

Renal function in preeclampsia is affected adversely by numerous factors. Decreased cardiac output in severe preeclampsia decreases renal blood flow and glomerular filtration rate. There may also be selective renal artery vasoconstriction that further impairs renal perfusion.[141] Uric acid levels are significantly increased in preeclampsia compared with normotensive pregnancy, but the levels are also increased in other forms of pregnancy-related hypertension[179] (Fig. 25-29). An increase in serum uric acid is a marker for renal injury. Unfortunately, the test is neither sensitive enough nor specific enough to diagnose preeclampsia in the setting of new-onset hypertension. However, in women with chronic hypertension, an elevated serum uric acid level identifies those with an increased likelihood of having superimposed preeclampsia. In chronically hypertensive women, a serum uric acid level of 5.5 mg/dL (normal being 4.3) increased the likelihood of superimposed preeclampsia 2.5 times. If the uric acid level is 6.5 mg/dL, the risk is increased eight-fold.

Preeclampsia results in a combination of changes in the glomerulus that produce a characteristic appearance and permit differentiation of preeclamptic nephropathy from other glomerular alterations associated with hypertension in pregnancy.[180] In preeclampsia, the glomerulus is diffusely enlarged and bloodless due to hypertrophy of the intracapillary cells. Endothelial cells undergo marked enlargement and vacuolization due to accumulation of free neutral lipids. These reactive changes have been termed "glomerular capillary endotheliosis" and are specific to preeclampsia. Other lesions that are seen in preeclampsia probably predate the preeclampsia. Fortunately, the renal lesions appear to be fully reversible in the absence of additional injury to the kidney. Clinically, the injury to the glomerulus is reflected by significant proteinuria, which is defined as 0.1 g/L of protein in a random sample or 0.3 g/L in a 24-hour specimen. Severe preeclampsia is diagnosed in the presence of proteinuria of 5 g or more in a 24-hour period. Injury to the glomeruli or

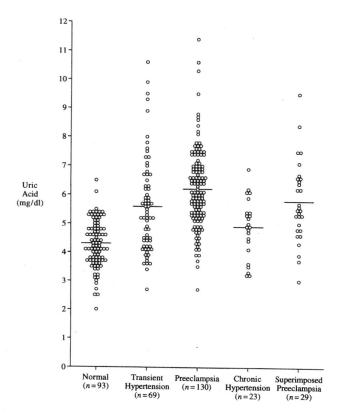

Figure 25-29. Uric acid levels in normal and hypertensive pregnancies. Levels are significantly increased in preeclampsia compared to normotensive pregnancy, but the levels are also increased in other forms of pregnancy-related hypertension and do not permit differentiation. (From Lim KH, Friedman SA, Ecker JL, et al: The clinical utility of serum uric acid measurements in hypertensive diseases of pregnancy. Am J Obstet Gynecol 1998; 178:1067–1071.)

renal tubules in preeclampsia may be so severe as to require dialysis, but this is uncommon. Fetal mortality is directly related to the degree of proteinuria and the uric acid levels, suggestive of a common cause of injury to both the kidney and the placenta.[181] However, the presence and severity of proteinuria do not correlate with the occurrence of seizures (eclampsia), suggesting an alternative mechanism for CNS injury.

Women with impaired renal function and preexisting permanent hypertension have a 50% to 80% risk of developing superimposed preeclampsia during pregnancy, and many patients with preeclampsia have preexisting subclinical renal disease. One study, using phase-contrast microscopy to examine urine for dysmorphic erythrocytes (which has a high specificity for glomerulonephritis), found that two thirds of preeclamptic patients presenting before 37 weeks' gestation had underlying renal disease, with mesangial IgA nephropathy being the most common finding.[182] Another study found a high incidence of preeclampsia (33%) in women with a history of asymptomatic bacteriuria in childhood but with renal scarring demonstrated by an IV pyelogram.[183] Women with a history of childhood bacteriuria but a normal subsequent pyelogram had a preeclampsia incidence of less than 5% (1 in 22 patients), not significantly different from a control group of women without a history of bacteriuria. A study of 345 pregnancies in 137 patients with reflux nephropathy found an incidence of preeclampsia of 24% in those with bilateral renal scarring and only 7% in those with unilateral scarring.[184] Unanswered is the question as to what extent preeclampsia injures the kidney as opposed to kidney disease contributing to the development or severity of preeclampsia.

Decreased urine output is a usual feature of severe preeclampsia and correlates with the severity of the disease. In most patients, volume and vasodilator therapy, guided by sophisticated cardiovascular monitoring when required, will correct the prerenal causes of oliguria. If not, the diagnosis of acute renal failure must be considered. This diagnosis may be difficult to establish, because urinary diagnostic indices, such as the fractional excretion of sodium and urinary sodium concentration, may not correlate with measurements of effective intravascular volume as determined by the PCWP.[185] Management of a preeclamptic patient in renal failure is very challenging and usually demands prompt delivery and possibly renal dialysis for the mother.

Central Nervous System in Preeclampsia. Generalized CNS irritability is a common feature in preeclampsia. Mild degrees of irritability are manifested by the presence of hyperreflexia or clonus on physical examination; extreme irritability results in convulsions, a condition referred to as eclampsia. In England, the death rate for women with eclampsia is 1.8%; fortunately, the incidence of eclampsia is low (4.9 per 10,000 parturients).[186]

Routine management of preeclampsia involves minimizing stimulation of the patient to decrease the risk of convulsions. Seizures may occur in patients with seemingly mild disease in terms of blood pressure, proteinuria, and edema.

Patients with preeclampsia are at risk for cerebral edema, most likely on the basis of endothelial dysfunction and capillary permeability. However, cerebral edema is not the main cause of eclamptic convulsions. One report of seven eclamptic patients with repetitive seizures while receiving IV magnesium sulfate found only one with cerebral edema; computed axial tomography showed that two patients had venous thrombosis, two had a finding of low-density white matter, and two were normal.[187] In another study using cranial magnetic resonance (MR) imaging, 8 of 16 women with severe preeclampsia had abnormal scans with nonspecific foci of increased signal in the deep cerebral white matter on T2-weighted images.[188] All 10 patients with eclampsia had either multifocal areas of increased signal at the gray-white matter junction on T2-weighted images or cortical edema and hemorrhage; basal ganglion lesions were also common. Angiography in preeclampsia patients with severe cerebral symptoms has documented constriction and narrowing of proximal and peripheral vessels suggesting vasculitis with extensive areas of impaired regional cerebral blood flow.[189] There is also evidence of loss of autoregulation in the posterior cerebral circulation; this may result in transient blindness in patients with preeclampsia and eclampsia.[190]

Other types of CNS injury may be misdiagnosed as eclampsia in a pregnant patient, especially in the presence of hypertension. For example, in one series of 24 pregnant women with a variety of cerebrovascular disorders (14 with infarction, 6 with intracranial hemorrhage, 3 with hypertensive encephalopathy, and 1 with an unruptured aneurysm), the presumption of eclampsia delayed the diagnosis in 10 women (41.7%).[191] A subdural hematoma should be considered in any preeclamptic patient demonstrating lateralizing neurologic symptoms.

Magnesium sulfate is the most commonly used drug in the United States for seizure prophylaxis in patients with preeclampsia.[192] It is also the most efficacious in preventing recurrence of seizures in women with eclampsia. In a large international multicenter trial, magnesium sulfate therapy

1 g/hour resulted in 52% fewer recurrent seizures than diazepam and 67% fewer seizures than phenytoin[193] (Fig. 25–30). Magnesium sulfate is a potent dilator of the cerebral vasculature. Because there is direct and indirect evidence of cerebral vasospasm involving small-diameter vessels in preeclampsia,[194] the efficacy of magnesium sulfate in preventing eclamptic seizures may be due its vasodilating effects. Because excessive dosages of magnesium sulfate can produce profound muscle weakness to the point of respiratory arrest, close clinical monitoring is essential. Magnesium affects the neuromuscular junction; reduced dosages of both depolarizing and nondepolarizing neuromuscular blockers are indicated in the presence of magnesium.

A report from South Africa described a large series of hypertensive pregnant patients who were managed during labor with LEA and without anticonvulsant medications.[195] In 1106 patients, there were no convulsions in patients treated with effective LEA. Two patients experienced seizures after catheter placement but before onset of analgesia and four patients had seizures in the postpartum period, hours after termination of the local anesthetic effect. One explanation is that, at the low systemic blood levels that result from epidural analgesia, lidocaine is a mild CNS depressant and thus exerts anticonvulsant effects. It is only at very high doses that the capacity for local anesthetics to cause seizures is manifested. Another explanation is that maternal epinephrine levels are increased during labor and epinephrine enhances platelet aggregation. This may contribute to the CNS ischemia and the likelihood of seizures. Effective epidural analgesia during labor decreases maternal epinephrine levels.[196]

(i) Magnesium sulphate versus diazepam

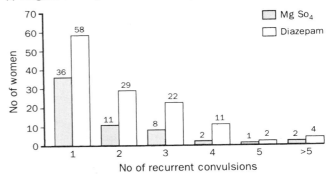

(ii) Magnesium sulphate versus phenytoin

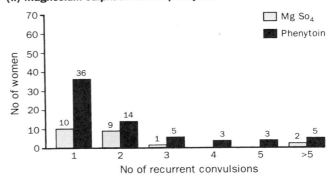

Figure 25–30. Comparison of anticonvulsive agents in the prevention of recurrent seizures in eclamptic patients. (From The Eclampsia Trial Collaborative Group: Which anticonvulsant for women with eclampsia? Evidence from the Collaborative Eclampsia Trial. Lancet 1995; 345:1455–1463.)

This may in turn decrease the adverse effects of platelet aggregation in the brain vessels of patients with preeclampsia. This is not a recommendation for epidural analgesia for seizure prophylaxis, but support for its beneficial concurrent effects.

Should a seizure occur, it can normally be readily terminated with a small dose of barbiturate or benzodiazepine. More common on obstetric units is the administration of IV magnesium sulfate in 2-g increments. Oxygen by mask should be given, and cricoid pressure maintained to protect the airway. This is one instance of an unconscious patient with a potentially full stomach in which prompt tracheal intubation may not be indicated. The extreme hypertensive response associated with tracheal intubation in an unanesthetized patient may pose a greater hazard to the mother than the risk of aspiration, and the seizure can usually be terminated rapidly using IV drugs.

Hemostasis. The gamut of coagulation abnormalities in preeclampsia ranges from the hypercoagulable state of normal pregnancy to the opposite extreme of disseminated intravascular coagulation. Fortunately, clinical bleeding is rarely the basis for patient morbidity or mortality.

A decreased platelet count is the most frequent hematologic abnormality found. Katz et al.[197] reported platelet counts below 150,000/mm³ in approximately one half of 237 patients with preeclampsia, and counts below 100,000/mm³ were seen in one fourth of patients. In 100 patients with severe preeclampsia, Leduc et al.[198] found 36 with platelet counts below 100,000/mm³ and 14 with platelet counts below 50,000/mm³. Standard tests of coagulation (prothrombin time, partial thromboplastin time) usually yield normal results except in severe preeclampsia with thrombocytopenia. Thromboelastography (TEG) is a test of whole-blood coagulation that provides information about the adequacy of platelet function as well as all other clotting factors. Using TEG, Sharma et al.[199] found that patients with preeclampsia were more hypocoagulable than healthy pregnant women, particularly when the platelet count was less than 100,000/mm³, but only patients with severe preeclampsia and platelet counts below 75,000/mm³ had TEG results that were in the abnormal range (Fig. 25–31).

Bone marrow analysis in preeclamptic patients demonstrates a hypercellular marrow with a proliferation of megakaryocytes and increased platelet production, which occurs in response to increased platelet consumption. A decreasing platelet count indicates worsening disease as platelet consumption exceeds replacement. Platelet activation, which results in aggregation and consumption, is favored by the imbalance between thromboxane and prostacyclin and by increased sympathetic nervous tone associated with elevated plasma catecholamines. Endothelial dysfunction, which is a key element in the pathophysiology of preeclampsia, promotes platelet adherence and accelerates platelet consumption.[200] In some cases, platelet destruction may involve immunologic mechanisms.[201] Thrombocytopenia in pregnancy, with or without hypertension, may also be associated with diseases other than preeclampsia, such as hemolytic uremic syndrome, thrombotic thrombocytopenic purpura, immune thrombocytopenic purpura, and systemic lupus erythematosus. The HELLP syndrome is a manifestation of severe preeclampsia or possibly a separate disease entity.[202]

Impaired platelet function increases the risk of an epidural or subarachnoid hematoma, as do other coagulation defects. There are insufficient data to even suggest the risk associated with epidural analgesia and anesthesia in preeclamptic patients with clotting abnormalities. One case report describes epidural bleeding (but no hematoma) in a patient with the HELLP syndrome and a bleeding time in excess of 15 minutes in association with an epidural catheter.[203] No treatment was required. It is important to be aware that epidural hematomas may occur spontaneously in patients with impaired clotting mechanisms, and that the avoidance of an epidural needle neither prevents this complication nor removes the need for vigilance. It is crucial that the symptoms of back pain in association with neurologic deficits in the legs or urogenital region not be ignored, because prompt evacuation of an intraspinal hematoma must be done to avoid permanent injury. Long-term neurologic sequelae are unlikely when high-risk patients are properly observed and evaluated.

There is no consensus on the minimum acceptable platelet count prior to performing regional anesthesia. In the study by Sharma et al., 183 women with preeclampsia and platelet counts below 100,000/mm³ received epidural anesthesia with no bleeding or neurologic sequelae.[199] Although it would seem that a bleeding time might be a more meaningful test than a simple platelet count, because it is an in vivo test of platelet function, there is no correlation between skin bleeding, as measured by the bleeding time test, and organ bleeding during surgery.[204] Ramanathan et al.[205] reported that 2% of normal pregnant patients had abnormal bleeding times in spite of normal numbers of platelets; 20% of patients with preeclampsia had abnormal bleeding times. Because the true incidence of preeclampsia in the United States is less than 5%, there are, if the data of Ramanathan et al. are valid, more normal pregnant patients with prolonged bleeding times (2% of 97%, or 19 in 1000) than there are preeclamptic patients with prolonged bleeding times (20% of 5%, or 10 in 1000). Data from the same study (Fig. 25–32) show that, in preeclampsia, when a platelet count of 100,000/mm³ is used as a cutoff, more patients with platelet counts above this value will have bleeding times in excess of 15 minutes than will patients with platelet counts below 100,000/mm³. Even though some institutions still use bleeding time as an absolute criterion for determining the suitability of preeclamptic patients for regional anesthesia, there are no scientific or clinical data to support the validity of this practice. The fact that regional anesthesia is the preferred anesthetic technique for operative delivery in preeclamptic pregnancies, as well as in normal pregnancies, and the fact that bleeding complications are so rare support the clinical irrelevance of bleeding time tests. The clinical laboratory at our institution no longer performs bleeding time tests because of the proven lack of specificity of the test.

A more rational policy is to base the decision regarding regional anesthesia in the preeclamptic patient on a number of factors, the most significant being not the platelet count but the clinical status of the patient. For example, is there bruising around IV catheter sites? Is there gum bleeding with toothbrushing? Patients with clinical evidence of abnormal bleeding must be considered at increased risk for regional anesthesia bleeding complications, regardless of the absolute platelet count or the results of a bleeding time test. Patients with such symptoms often receive platelet transfusions prior to cesarean section on the basis of surgical considerations; if so, regional anesthesia can be performed after the platelet transfusion with a presumably increased margin of safety, assuming that the clinical bleeding is corrected by the platelet transfusion.

It must be emphasized that the bleeding risks associated with regional anesthesia in severe preeclampsia must be viewed as relative risks. Ramanathan et al.[206] reported a maternal death due to an inability to secure an airway following

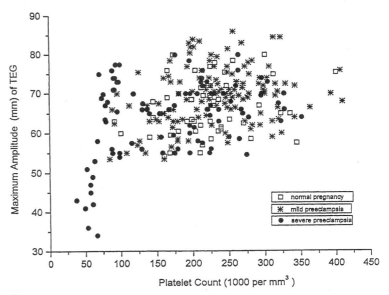

Figure 25-31. Thromboelastography in relation to platelet count. *A,* Normal pregnancy, mild preeclampsia, and severe preeclampsia. Maximum amplitude (MA) <54 mm is the lower limit of normal for pregnant women in the study. *B,* Data points from study patients with severe preeclampsia. A negative exponential curve of best fit indicates that hypocoagulability increases as the platelet count decreases below 100,000/mm³. Only patients with platelet counts below 75,000/mm³ had abnormal MA values. (From Sharma SK, Philip J, Whitten CW, et al: Assessment of changes in coagulation in parturients with preeclampsia using thromboelastography. Anesthesiology 1999; 90:385–390.)

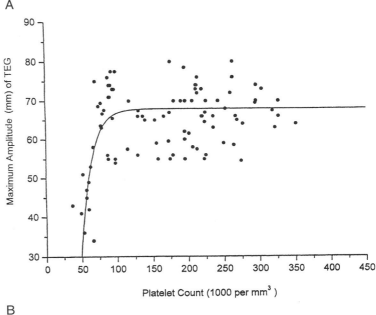

induction of general anesthesia; in this patient, regional anesthesia was thought to be contraindicated because of thrombocytopenia (platelet count, 55,000/mm³) and an abnormal bleeding time (>15 minutes). The authors believed that laryngeal edema contributed to the failure to ventilate or intubate. Thus, the decision to avoid regional anesthesia must be weighed against the potential risks associated with general anesthesia in patients with preeclampsia. These include pulmonary edema, heart failure, cerebral hemorrhage, and the ever-present risk of pulmonary aspiration of gastric contents in patients who may present challenges to tracheal intubation due to edema of the head and neck, including the larynx. Cerebral hemorrhage still ranks as the leading cause of maternal mortality in preeclampsia and is a much more serious bleeding complication than an epidural hematoma. To date, the ASA Closed Claims Project Database does not have a *single case* of a maternal epidural hematoma. Thus,

potential bleeding complications are associated with both regional and general anesthesia, and choices in anesthetic management should reflect these risks.

Maternal Cardiovascular Disease

The normal hemodynamic changes associated with pregnancy may have severe adverse consequences for patients with cardiovascular disease, even those with previously asymptomatic lesions. Increases in blood volume (40% to 50%) and cardiac output (40% to 50% during pregnancy and 80% during labor and delivery) may precipitate pulmonary edema and heart failure in patients with mitral valve disease. Patients with aortic stenosis or right-to-left shunt are most imperiled by systemic hypotension, as might occur during episodes of the supine hypotensive syndrome or following regional anesthesia. Obstetric anesthetic management of pa-

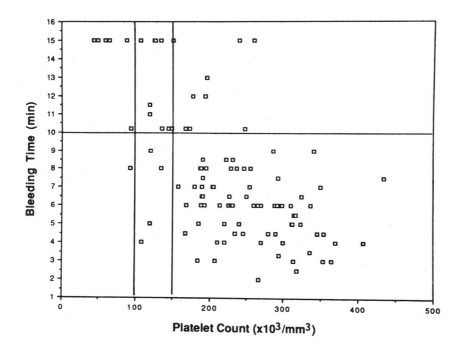

Figure 25-32. Bleeding times plotted against platelet counts in parturients with preeclampsia. (From Ramanathan J, Sibai BM, Vu T, et al: Correlation between bleeding times and platelet counts in women with preeclampsia undergoing cesarean section. Anesthesiology 1989; 71:190.)

tients with cardiac disease is lesion-specific. Thus, it is essential that one know the exact nature of the heart lesion, the expected physiologic impact of the lesion during pregnancy, labor, and delivery, and the hemodynamic consequences of anesthetic interventions.

Indications for Invasive Cardiovascular Monitoring in Parturients With Heart Disease. Because most of the increase in cardiac output occurs before the 24th week of gestation, the parturient presenting with a viable fetus has already undergone a prolonged and quite strenuous cardiac stress test. A careful history and physical examination can usually ascertain the response of the mother to the stress of pregnancy. In many cases, this information alone is sufficient to determine the need for invasive cardiovascular monitoring. Asymptomatic patients who have had an uneventful pregnancy without worsening of their cardiopulmonary status can be expected to tolerate the additional stress of labor and delivery as long as obstetric and anesthetic management is appropriate for the specific cardiac lesion. In such cases, invasive hemodynamic monitoring is usually not required. Some suggested exceptions to this rule include any parturient with a right-to-left shunt, pulmonary hypertension, severe coarctation of the aorta, or severe aortic stenosis. A recent review[207] of pulmonary hypertension found a maternal mortality rate of 30% in case of primary pulmonary hypertension, 36% in Eisenmenger's syndrome (right-to-left shunt secondary to pulmonary hypertension in lesions normally causing left-to-right shunts), and 56% in secondary vascular pulmonary hypertension. Except for three antepartum deaths due to Eisenmenger's syndrome, all fatalities occurred within 35 days *after* delivery. Neonatal survival was similar in the three groups[207] (87% to 89%).[207] Invasive and intensive monitoring are standard in parturients with cardiovascular disease undergoing surgery requiring cardiopulmonary bypass (CPB). The results of a review found an overall maternal mortality of 10% and morbidity of 30%.[208] The corresponding fetal outcomes were 30% mortality and 9% morbidity.

Some form of invasive monitoring is usually required in all parturients with significant cardiovascular disease. Direct intra-arterial pressure monitoring is essential to management during periods of rapid hemodynamic change, that is, labor, delivery, regional or general anesthesia, and the puerperium. Use of data obtained from PAC requires an understanding of the limitations inherent in measurements made in patients with structural or functional cardiac abnormalities. Particularly in patients with heart disease, trends provide more reliable information than any one absolute value, underscoring the importance of frequent observation and early recognition of ominous trends.

Mitral Stenosis

Pathophysiology. Mitral stenosis may be asymptomatic until the sudden development of life-threatening pulmonary edema in pregnancy. Because the incidence of rheumatic fever in the United States has decreased, the patients in this country most likely to present with mitral stenosis in pregnancy are immigrants from the developing world, many of whom may be unaware that they have heart disease. Worldwide, mitral stenosis remains one of the leading causes of death in pregnancy.

In mitral stenosis, there is an impediment to filling of the LV due to narrowing of the mitral valve orifice (Fig. 25-33). The normal gradient of 3 to 5 mmHg across the valve is increased; gradients in excess of 25 mmHg are present in patients with severe mitral stenosis.

The obstruction to left atrial outflow increases pressures in the left atrium, pulmonary veins, and pulmonary capillaries. Pulmonary congestion accounts for the symptoms of dyspnea and orthopnea that occur as the disease progresses in severity. Chronic volume overload usually presents as right ventricular (RV) failure with hepatic congestion, and the presence of RV hypertrophy on the ECG carries a significant risk of cardiac failure. Acute volume overload in pregnant patients with mild to moderate mitral stenosis is more likely to overstress the LV.

Atrial contraction contributes 33% of LV filling in mitral stenosis, compared with 20% in the normal heart. Hence, sinus rhythm is important for maintaining cardiac output in patients with mitral stenosis. The distention of the left

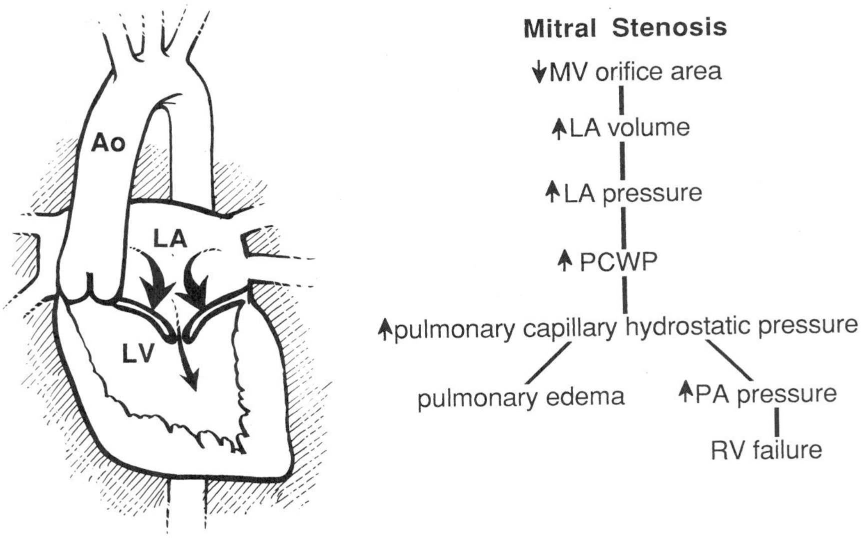

Figure 25-33. Mitral stenosis (diastole). Restricted flow through the narrowed mitral valve orifice results in elevated blood volumes in the cardiopulmonary circuit proximal to the mitral valve. MV, mitral valve; LA, left atrium; PCWP, pulmonary capillary wedge pressure; PA, pulmonary artery; RV, right ventricle; LV, left ventricle; Ao, aorta.

Mitral Stenosis

↓MV orifice area

↑LA volume

↑LA pressure

↑ PCWP

↑pulmonary capillary hydrostatic pressure

pulmonary edema   ↑PA pressure

RV failure

atrium in mitral stenosis predisposes patients to atrial fibrillation, which can rapidly result in pulmonary edema and cardiac insufficiency for two reasons: the loss of atrial contraction and decreased diastolic filling time if the heart rate increases during atrial fibrillation. The sluggish flow of blood through the distended left atrium in patients with mitral stenosis greatly increases the risk of thrombus formation. Atrial fibrillation further increases the likelihood of systemic embolization from a left atrial thrombus.

Patients with mitral stenosis may not tolerate the normal physiologic changes of pregnancy, particularly the increase in pulmonary blood volume. Labor, delivery, and the immediate puerperium are considered the times of maximum risk. Each uterine contraction increases central blood volume by 15% to 25%, worsening any pulmonary congestion. The further distention of the left atrium by this increased blood volume increases the probability of atrial fibrillation. The greatest increase in central blood volume occurs immediately after delivery as a result of uterine involution and relief of vena caval obstruction. Clark et al.[209] documented a 10-mmHg (± 6 mmHg) increase in PCWP after vaginal delivery in a series of patients with severe mitral stenosis (Fig. 25-34). However, the range (0 to 18 mmHg) was wide, and the greatest increases occurred in patients beginning labor with high wedge pressures. Cunningham et al.[210] reported a series of 28 patients with unsuspected and asymptomatic cardiac disease who developed peripartum congestive heart failure; 4 of these patients were found to have mitral stenosis and all 4 became symptomatic after delivery (within 48 hours). Thus, careful monitoring of patients with mitral stenosis must continue for several days post partum.

The risk of cardiac decompensation during delivery is increased by tachycardia, as can be expected with painful uterine contractions. The rapid rate allows less time for ventricular filling through the stenotic mitral orifice; as forward flow decreases, pulmonary congestion increases.

Worldwide, the preferred management of severe mitral stenosis in pregnancy is balloon valvotomy.[211-213] Radiation exposure to the fetus and the mother can be limited by the use of transesophageal echocardiography (TEE) to image the valve.[214, 215] In most published series of balloon valvotomy, the average cross-sectional area of the mitral orifice is less than 1.0 cm² before balloon dilation; afterward, the cross-sectional area increases to approximately 2.0 cm² in most patients. Almost all patients exhibit functional improvement following valvotomy, moving from New York Heart Association class III or IV to class I or II. There was one report of a patient experiencing severe mitral regurgitation following

Figure 25-34. Intrapartum changes in pulmonary capillary wedge pressure (PCWP) in eight patients with mitral stenosis. Delivery is consistently associated with an abrupt increase in PCWP and the risk of pulmonary edema. (From Clark SL, Phelan JP, Greenspoon J, et al: Labor and delivery in the presence of mitral stenosis: Central hemodynamic observations. Am J Obstet Gynecol 1985; 152:984-988.)

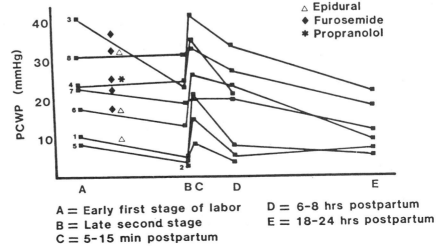

△ Epidural
◆ Furosemide
✳ Propranolol

A = Early first stage of labor
B = Late second stage
C = 5-15 min postpartum

D = 6-8 hrs postpartum
E = 18-24 hrs postpartum

balloon valvotomy requiring emergency valve replacement.[211] Given the efficacy of this procedure during pregnancy, the incidence of pregnant patients with symptomatic mitral stenosis presenting for delivery will be mainly confined to parturients lacking modern prenatal care. Also, this procedure should reduce the frequency of emergent delivery of premature infants necessitated because of worsening maternal condition associated with mitral stenosis.

Monitoring. Parturients with mild mitral stenosis without episodes of pulmonary edema or atrial fibrillation do not require invasive monitoring during labor and delivery. However, the ECG should be monitored continually during this period, specifically to detect atrial fibrillation or flutter. Equipment for external cardioversion must be available. All patients with mitral stenosis should be considered to be at risk for development of pulmonary edema, regardless of the severity of their lesion. This is particularly true immediately post partum, and volume status must be carefully assessed during this time period. Pulse oximetry is useful for early detection of worsening pulmonary congestion.

Symptomatic patients should be monitored with both a peripheral arterial and a pulmonary artery catheter; CVP monitoring is not sufficiently reliable in this situation. In patients with mitral stenosis, there is very poor correlation between CVPs and PCWP, with differences of 10 mmHg or greater in 85% of patients in one study.[209] Clark[216] recommended maintaining the PCWP in the 14-mmHg range. This value is based on the expected increase in PCWP following delivery being somewhat less than 18 mmHg in most patients, and the observation that clinically significant pulmonary edema does not usually occur with wedge pressures below 28 to 30 mmHg. Attaining a PCWP of 14 mmHg may require diuresis in some patients; this must be done with extreme caution, as the PCWP does not accurately reflect LV filling volumes in the presence of mitral stenosis.[217] Treating increased PCWP when in fact the LV end-diastolic volume is decreased may severely impair cardiac output; many patients with mitral stenosis require elevated left atrial pressures for adequate ventricular filling. It is essential that therapeutic alterations in intravascular volume be guided by additional information, such as blood pressure, urine output, weight change, and noninvasive measurement of stroke volume and cardiac output.

Anesthetic Considerations. Because of the severity of the consequences of atrial fibrillation, pregnant patients with mitral stenosis usually receive prophylactic digitalis. Drugs causing tachycardia, such as atropine, ketamine, and pancuronium, should be avoided. If tachycardia does occur, it may be treated with adenosine, verapamil, or β-blocking drugs such as propranolol or esmolol.

Epidural analgesia helps to prevent increases in heart rate associated with painful uterine contractions. Perineal analgesia blocks the urge to push. This is beneficial because the Valsalva maneuver is detrimental; the increased intrathoracic pressure impedes venous return and markedly reduces cardiac output.[218] The venodilation resulting from epidural anesthesia is helpful in reducing central blood volume.[219] Hypotension should be treated with a pure α_1 agonist such as phenylephrine rather than ephedrine, a mixed agent that produces tachycardia by virtue of its β_1 properties. The addition of epinephrine to solutions of local anesthetics for epidural injection also increases the risk of tachycardia.

One report described the use of the Trendelenburg position to adjust PCWP during epidural anesthesia in patients with severe mitral stenosis.[220] The initial PCWP of 37 mmHg decreased to 15 mmHg following epidural blockade; associated with this decrease in preload was a decrease in cardiac index, from 2.4 to 1.8 L/minute/m². By selecting the appropriate angle of the Trendelenburg position, the authors were able to optimize cardiac output; at a PCWP of 25 mmHg, the mean cardiac index was 3.1 L/minute/m². Again, the proven efficacy of percutaneous balloon valvotomy in this group of patients should make an anesthetic for a parturient in decompensated mitral stenosis a rare event.

General anesthesia utilizing a standard rapid intubation sequence and a potent inhalational agent is acceptable only for patients with mild disease. This regimen may precipitate rapid cardiac decompensation as a result of tachycardia. Increased pulmonary artery pressures associated with tracheal intubation worsen any preexisting RV dysfunction. Patients with severe stenosis and cardiac compromise requiring general anesthesia with the complicating factor of a difficult airway are more safely managed with regional blockade of the glossopharyngeal and superior laryngeal nerves and topical anesthesia of the trachea,[221, 222] followed by assessment of the airway using direct laryngoscopy in the awake patient. From this point, narcotic induction and then tracheal intubation are appropriate if the glottic opening appears accessible; if not, flexible fiberoptic bronchoscopy is probably the safest technique, with a large dose of IV narcotic being given just before the endotracheal tube is advanced over the bronchoscope into the trachea. The short duration of alfentanil permits a high-dose narcotic anesthetic, yet with prompt extubation at the end of the surgical procedure; this drug has been used successfully in patients with severe mitral stenosis and pulmonary hypertension.[223] Antagonism of narcosis in the neonate may be required. If so, it should be done with very small, incremental doses of naloxone (1 to 2 μg/kg). As in all patients with significant valvular disease, TEE with color Doppler capability provides information about cardiac function and the effects of valve lesions on blood flow.

Mitral Regurgitation

Pathophysiology. Incompetence of the mitral value permits regurgitant flow from the LV into the left atrium (Fig. 25–35). The compliant atrial walls readily distend to accommodate the increased blood volume and there is no significant pressure increase in the pulmonary vascular bed until late in the course of the disease. Forward flow through the aortic valve depends on the resistance across this valve compared to the resistance across the incompetent mitral valve. Factors that lower PVR tend to favor forward flow and improve cardiac output. For this reason, normal pregnancy is usually well tolerated by individuals with isolated mitral regurgitation. However, parturients with long-standing mitral regurgitation may have increased left atrial pressures and LV dysfunction based on chronic volume overload. The elevated left atrial pressures are transmitted to the pulmonary circulation, predisposing the patient to pulmonary congestion. In such patients, labor can be quite hazardous because enhanced sympathetic nervous system activity increases vascular resistance and worsens regurgitant flow, and further pulmonary blood volume overload occurs with the autotransfusion associated with each uterine contraction. This combination of factors may precipitate acute left-sided heart failure and pulmonary edema.

Atrial fibrillation may occur, but has less of an adverse effect on cardiac output than that seen in patients with mitral stenosis. Mild degrees of tachycardia may be beneficial, as this decreases the regurgitant fraction. Bradycardia, on the other hand, is associated with decreased cardiac output because stroke volume tends to be fairly fixed.

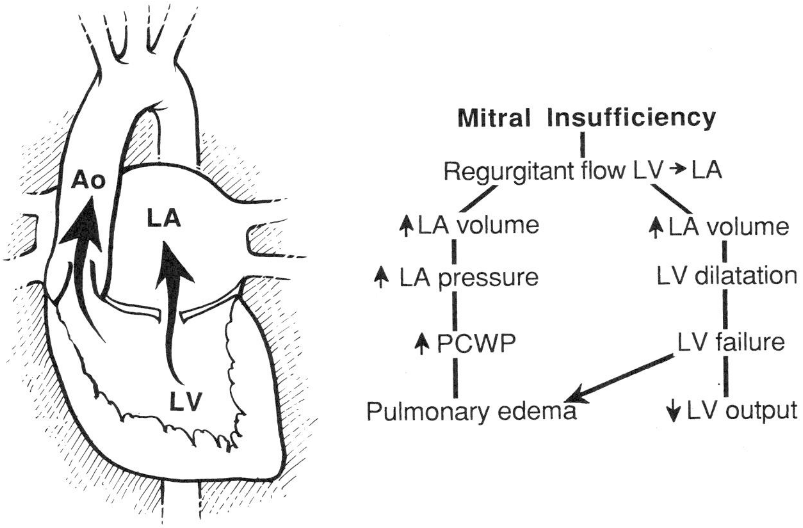

Figure 25-35. Mitral regurgitation (systole). A portion of the left ventricular output is ejected retrogradely into the left atrium, resulting in increased blood volume in the pulmonary venous circuit. During diastole, this extra volume overloads the left ventricle, resulting in chamber enlargement. LV, left ventricle; LA, left atrium; PCWP, pulmonary capillary wedge pressure; Ao, aorta.

Monitoring. Monitoring concerns are similar to those for mitral stenosis. The amount of regurgitant flow parallels the intensity of the insufficiency murmur as well as the size of the v wave on the PCWP tracing. These findings may be a better guide to hemodynamic management than PCWP, because there may be little correlation between left atrial pressure and left atrial volume in a chronically dilated atrium. Such lack of correlation precludes any valid estimate of LV end-diastolic volume.

Anesthetic Considerations. Epidural anesthesia is beneficial in decreasing peripheral resistance, which is very desirable in patients with mitral regurgitation. One potential concern with epidural anesthesia is the bradycardia that usually accompanies the sharp decrease in blood pressure resulting from extensive venodilation and decreased cardiac return. Contrary to what one might expect, the normal response of the right side of the heart and the sinoatrial node to acute hypovolemia is bradycardia.[89] This hemodynamic impairment occurs in normal patients, and frequently results in nausea. When the patient has mitral regurgitation, the combination of hypotension and bradycardia is of particular concern, as it may cause myocardial ischemia and heart failure. Hypotension is minimized by judicious volume administration as the epidural anesthetic is being administered, maintaining the patient in the left lateral decubitus position until the block reaches the upper thoracic dermatomes, and by steeply elevating the patient's legs (while maintaining uterine displacement) at the first sign of hypotension (nausea, slowing of heart rate). Small doses of ephedrine are also useful, providing both inotropic and chronotropic support without an excessive increase in afterload. A direct-acting chronotropic drug such as isoproterenol is also useful, since it increases heart rate without increasing afterload.

The same concerns for hypertension with tracheal intubation apply as discussed for mitral stenosis. The capability for careful titration of a rapid-acting vasodilator such as SNP must be present. Potent agents may cause excessive myocardial depression in already compromised patients.

Mitral Valve Prolapse. Pathologic mitral valve prolapse is a connective tissue abnormality of the leaflets, annulus, and chordae tendineae of the mitral valve, and it must be distinguished from the normal superior displacement of the mitral valve leaflets. The latter condition is very common, occurring in 5% to 15% of healthy patients examined using 2-D echocardiography.[224] Diagnostic criteria for identifying patients with pathologic mitral valve prolapse are given in Table 25-13. One or more major criteria are necessary and sufficient to establish the diagnosis. Patients with one or more minor criteria do not warrant this diagnosis, but they may still have cardiac abnormalities, particularly in the presence of a holosystolic murmur.

Fortunately, mitral valve prolapse remains asymptomatic in most patients, and pregnancy, labor, and delivery are well tolerated.[225, 226] Pregnancy may present complications for the small percentage of patients who present with significant mitral regurgitation.

Pathophysiology. In mitral valve prolapse, the chordae tendineae are elongated, allowing the mitral valve leaflets to prolapse into the left atrium when the ventricular volume decreases during systole. This accounts for the mid- to late systolic click and murmur of mitral regurgitation that are characteristic of mitral valve prolapse. The volume status of the LV affects the degree of regurgitant flow and is a variable that is subject to some therapeutic manipulation. Conditions that augment LV volume tend to decrease regurgitant flow and include hypervolemia, increased afterload, bradycardia, and decreased myocardial contractility. Regurgitant flow increases when LV volume decreases, which can be caused by hypovolemia, sustained increases in intrathoracic pressure, or tachycardia with resultant decreased cardiac filling times. Thus, patients with mitral valve prolapse and severe preeclampsia may be at increased risk for cardiac compromise owing to the hypovolemia and tachycardia that are commonly seen.

Monitoring. Invasive cardiovascular monitoring is rarely necessary in patients with isolated mitral valve prolapse. The most common problem is dysrhythmias, particularly supraventricular tachyarrhythmias; thus, continuous ECG monitoring during labor is recommended to facilitate prompt treatment of significant dysrhythmias.

Anesthetic Considerations. Preload should be maintained in patients with mitral valve prolapse. Epidural anesthesia is appropriate as long as sympathetic blockade (de-

Table 25–13. Criteria Related to the Diagnosis of Mitral Valve Prolapse

Major Criteria

Auscultation

Mid- to late systolic clicks and a late systolic murmur at the cardiac apex

Mobile mid- to late systolic clicks at the cardiac apex

Late systolic murmur at the cardiac apex in the young patient

Auscultation plus echocardiography

Apical holosystolic murmur of mitral regurgitation plus echocardiographic criteria

Two-dimensional/Doppler echocardiography

Marked systolic displacement of mitral leaflets with coaptation point at or on the left atrial side of the annulus

Marked systolic displacement of mitral leaflets, at least moderate mitral regurgitation, chordal rupture, and annular dilation

Two-dimensionally targeted M-mode echocardiography

Marked (<3 mm) late systolic buckling posterior to the C-D line (annular plane)

Minor Criteria*

History

Focal neurologic attacks or amaurosis fugax in the young patient

First-degree relatives with major criteria

Recurrent supraventricular tachycardia (documented)

Auscultation

Soft, inconstant, or equivocal mid- to late systolic sounds at the cardiac apex

Other physical signs

Low body weight, asthenic habitus

Low blood pressure

Thoracic bony abnormalities

Two-dimensional/Doppler/color flow echocardiography

Moderate superior systolic displacement of mitral leaflets with Doppler mitral regurgitation

Two-dimensionally targeted M-mode echocardiography

Moderate (2 mm) late systolic buckling posterior to the C-D line (annular plane)

Holosystolic displacement (3 mm) posterior to the C-D line (annular plane)

---

* Minor criteria arouse suspicion but do not establish the diagnosis of mitral value prolapse.

Modified from Perloff JK, Child JS: Clinical and epidemiologic issues in mitral valve prolapse. Am Heart J 1987; 113:324.

creased SVR) is induced slowly and intravascular volume is carefully evaluated. Ephedrine is not advisable for treating hypotension because its inotropic and chronotropic properties are undesirable in the setting of mitral valve prolapse. Antibiotic prophylaxis against subacute bacterial endocarditis is recommended for all patients with pathologic mitral valve prolapse. Antiarrhythmic medications should be continued, regardless of anesthetic technique. The hyperdynamic cardiac response to tracheal intubation can worsen the degree of prolapse. Control of tachycardia and hypertension is important for optimal management.

Aortic Stenosis

Pathophysiology. Aortic stenosis is rarely symptomatic during the childbearing years. However, in symptomatic patients, pregnancy causes severe hemodynamic derangements. As the aortic valve narrows from a normal cross-sectional area of 2.6 to 3.5 cm² to less than 1 cm², ever-increasing LV pressures are required to maintain cardiac output (Fig. 25–36). This leads to concentric hypertrophy of the LV. The elevation in end-diastolic pressure combined with a thickened LV wall impairs subendocardial blood flow, resulting in myocardial ischemia.

The outlow tract obstruction results in a relatively fixed stroke volume, so that increases in cardiac output are determined primarily by increases in heart rate. However, decreased diastolic compliance may be the major pathophysiologic abnormality in many patients with aortic stenosis, and tachycardia with resultant decreased ventricular filling times worsens cardiac output.[227]

Because of the risk to the fetus of surgical repair of the aortic valve during pregnancy, balloon dilation of compliant aortic valves has been used as a temporizing measure in pregnant patients with severe aortic stenosis.[228]

Monitoring. Invasive hemodynamic monitoring is indicated in patients with severe stenosis (gradient >50 mmHg), symptoms of congestive failure, angina, or a history of syncopal episodes. However, because of decreased LV compliance, LV end-diastolic pressure (LVEDP) may be elevated even though actual chamber volume is low. Higher-than-normal PCWP may be necessary to maintain cardiac output, but such increases in pressure increase the likelihood of pulmonary edema. ECG monitoring is recommended to detect evidence of myocardial ischemia.

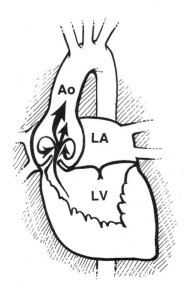

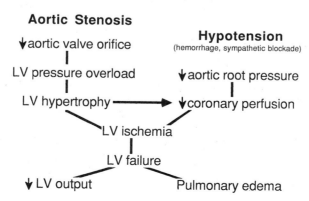

Aortic Stenosis

↓aortic valve orifice

|

LV pressure overload

|

LV hypertrophy ⟶ ↓coronary perfusion

LV ischemia

LV failure

↓LV output   Pulmonary edema

Hypotension
(hemorrhage, sympathetic blockade)

↓aortic root pressure

↓coronary perfusion

Figure 25–36. Aortic stenosis (systole). The narrow aortic valve orifice requires elevated left ventricular pressures to overcome the resistance to ejection. There is turbulent flow just distal to the valve, resulting in dilation of the aortic root. LV, left ventricle; LA, left atrium; Ao, aorta.

Anesthetic Considerations. Pregnant patients with aortic stenosis may not tolerate large decreases in preload (filling volumes), afterload (PVR), or heart rate. Thus, epidural anesthesia, which has the potential for causing all three of these undesirable responses, must be administered carefully, with attention given to adequate fluid pretreatment and prompt correction of hypotension. The recommended treatment for hypotension is administration of a predominantly α-adrenergic agent, such as phenylephrine, to elevate aortic root pressures as a consequence of arteriolar vasoconstriction.

Light general anesthesia such as that typically used for cesarean section is usually tolerated quite well, because both blood pressure and heart rate are well maintained. The hemodynamic response to laryngoscopy and tracheal intubation can precipitate LV dysfunction, and a narcotic-based anesthetic using alfentanil 35 μg/kg has been recommended for blocking this response.[229] The expected side effects of this dose include maternal hypotension and neonatal respiratory depression. Regional and topical anesthesia of the airway prior to induction, as described for patients with mitral stenosis, coupled with reduced dosages of IV induction agents, offer another option for minimizing excessive hemodynamic alterations. In patients with evidence of LV failure, the use of potent inhalational agents should be avoided, owing to their propensity for myocardial depression.

Aortic Regurgitation

Pathophysiology. In aortic regurgitation, the incompetent valve allows blood in the aorta to flow back into the LV (Fig. 25–37). This "runoff" lesion reduces diastolic pressure and widens pulse pressure. Regurgitant blood causes LV volume overload and, if chronic, LV dilation. Thus, LVEDP may remain normal despite an increased LV end-diastolic volume. With progressive distention, the LV eventually fails and LVEDP increases. Bradycardia allows more time for regurgitant flow during diastole and should be avoided. Increased SVR enhances regurgitant flow and may precipitate congestive heart failure.

Pregnancy is well tolerated in patients with mild to moderate aortic regurgitation because the decrease in SVR associated with pregnancy decreases the ratio of regurgitant volume to total stroke volume. However, in patients with severe aortic regurgitation and myocardial dysfunction, the increased blood volume of pregnancy worsens pulmonary congestion, and the increase in SVR associated with labor can cause acute decompensation.

In severe aortic regurgitation, there are abnormalities of coronary flow with phasic flow occurring mainly during systole rather than diastole, reversal of flow during part of diastole, and redistribution of coronary flow from the endocardium to the epicardium. Systemic hypotension will additionally impair coronary flow and precipitate myocardial ischemia and cardiac failure in patients with severe aortic regurgitation.[230]

Monitoring. Isolated aortic regurgitation is usually asymptomatic in patients of childbearing age. Patients with LV dysfunction or echocardiographic evidence of a significantly dilated LV often require invasive hemodynamic monitoring to guide titration of vasodilator and inotropic therapy. The dilated ventricle accommodates a large end-diastolic volume without an increase in pressure, and thus PCWP fails to accurately assess LV volume. However, any increase in PCWP must be investigated and promptly treated, if necessary, because such a change may herald a rapid deterioration in cardiac function.

Anesthetic Considerations. The anesthetic considerations in aortic regurgitation are similar to those for mitral regurgitation: avoid increases in peripheral resistance, bradycardia, and myocardial depression. Carefully administered epidural anesthesia is usually hemodynamically beneficial in patients with aortic regurgitation.

Intracardiac and Extracardiac Shunt

Left-to-Right Shunts

PATHOPHYSIOLOGY. Atrial septal defect, ventricular septal defect, and patent ductus arteriosus differ in the location of the shunt site, yet they have in common an increase in pulmonary blood flow due to a left-to-right shunt. Small defects produce small shunts and minimal symptoms, whereas large defects, in which pulmonary blood flow may be four to five times systemic flow, eventually overload the pulmonary circuit, leading to pulmonary hypertension and RV failure. Increases in SVR normally worsen the shunt.

The increased blood volume associated with pregnancy

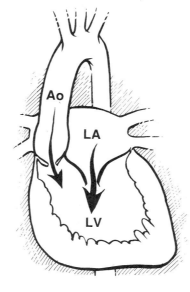

Figure 25–37. Aortic regurgitation (diastole). The incompetent aortic valve allows ejected blood to flow back into the left ventricle during systole at the same time that the ventricle is being filled from the left atrium. This volume overload causes the left ventricle to enlarge and possibly fail. Ao, aorta; LV, left ventricle; LA, left atrium.

adds to the already excessive pulmonary blood flow, but this effect is offset somewhat by the decrease in SVR occurring in normal pregnancy. Maternal and fetal outcomes are usually satisfactory.[231]

MONITORING. Invasive hemodynamic monitoring is not required in patients with small defects and no symptoms. However, patients with pulmonary hypertension and RV dysfunction warrant pulmonary and peripheral arterial monitoring; in the case of patients with either condition in the presence of an atrial septal defect, right atrial pressure monitoring is recommended. Cardiac output determined by thermodilution methods will be unreliable in situations in which pulmonary flow is much greater than systemic flow.[232] Doppler echocardiography is preferable if cardiac output must be measured.

ANESTHETIC CONSIDERATIONS. Patients with shunts are always at risk for systemic embolization of any air introduced into a blood vessel, regardless of the normal direction of the shunt. For example, in patients with an atrial septal defect with a left-to-right shunt, air bubbles introduced into the right atrium may nonetheless traverse the septal defect in a right-to-left direction and gain access to the systemic circulation, notably the cerebral vessels and the coronary arteries. This phenomenon is referred to as "paradoxical" shunting.

Epidural and spinal anesthesia result in peripheral vasodilation and decreased peripheral resistance, conditions that generally benefit patients with left-to-right shunts. Extreme arterial hypotension, however, can cause shunt reversal and hypoxemia. Conversely, general anesthesia and the necessity for tracheal intubation carry the risk of sharp elevations in peripheral resistance and worsening of the left-to-right shunt.

Right-to-Left Shunts

PATHOPHYSIOLOGY. In right-to-left shunts, deoxygenated blood bypasses the pulmonary capillary bed, resulting in systemic arterial desaturation and cyanosis. The shunt can occur at any level in the cardiopulmonary circuit—atrial, ventricular, aortopulmonary, or intrapulmonary. Right-to-left shunts also develop as a consequence of pulmonary hypertension in lesions normally resulting in left-to-right shunting. This reversal of shunt flow is known as Eisenmenger's syndrome. Cyanosis and reversed shunt flow carry a high risk of both maternal and fetal morbidity and mortality.

There are a number of congenital cardiac lesions that produce cyanosis, including transposition of the great vessels, pulmonary atresia, tricuspid atresia, and tetralogy of Fallot. In tetralogy of Fallot, the pulmonic stenosis can be either fixed or dynamic, the latter involving infundibular hypertrophy. In cases of fixed obstruction, increased RV contractility is necessary to maintain adequate pulmonary blood flow. On the other hand, if there is dynamic infundibular obstruction, increases in RV contractility tend to worsen the outflow obstruction, as do hypovolemia and tachycardia.

Pregnancy can be very deleterious to patients with right-to-left shunts, and even more so in the presence of pulmonary hypertension. One study found a deterioration of cardiac status in all pregnant patients with pulmonary artery pressures greater than 50 mmHg.[233] The thickened pulmonary vessels in patients with pulmonary hypertension are minimally responsive to the factors producing vasodilation in pregnancy, and pulmonary vascular resistance does not decrease. The imbalance between pulmonary and systemic vascular resistance in pregnancy worsens the right-to-left shunt. Severe cyanosis can result, with detriment to both the mother and the fetus. In patients with tetralogy of Fallot and RV infundibular hypertrophy, the sympathetic nervous sys-

tem response to labor increases RV contractility and leads to increased pulmonary vascular resistance, conditions that worsen the degree of right-to-left shunt.

MONITORING. Pulse oximetry is the most useful monitor in patients with right-to-left shunts. These patients tend to be on the steep portion of the oxyhemoglobin dissociation curve, and thus they are very sensitive to any of the factors adversely affecting oxygen saturation (SaO_2): (1) decreased inspired fraction of oxygen; (2) increased right-to-left shunting; (3) increased oxygen consumption; (4) decreased cardiac output; and (5) decreased mixed venous oxygen tension.[234] Pulse oximeters calibrated to function over an SaO_2 range of 35% to 95% reliably measure SaO_2 in patients with cyanotic heart disease.[235] Measurement of CVP is helpful in patients with tetralogy of Fallot and infundibular hypertrophy, in whom it is important to maintain an adequate central volume.

ANESTHETIC CONSIDERATIONS. Epidural and spinal anesthesia carry the risk of decreased peripheral resistance with consequent worsening of right-to-left shunting. Peripheral resistance can be controlled with careful volume and appropriate vasopressor therapy. Ephedrine, with its β_1 enhancement of cardiac contractility and inotropy, should not be used to correct venodilation in patients with tetralogy of Fallot and infundibular hypertrophy. Rather, a more selective α_1 agent is preferable.

Light general anesthesia for cesarean section tends to maintain peripheral resistance, a desirable goal in patients with a right-to-left shunt. Halothane is particularly efficacious in reducing RV contractility in patients with tetralogy of Fallot and dynamic outflow tract obstruction, but may be deleterious in patients with tetralogy and a fixed obstruction. Factors that increase pulmonary vascular resistance, such as hypercarbia, hypoxia, and extremes of lung volume, must be assiduously avoided in patients with right-to-left shunts. All of these deleterious conditions arise whenever patients with right-to-left shunts have prolonged coughing while an endotracheal tube is in place.

Peripartum Cardiomyopathy. Peripartum cardiomyopathy is an uncommon form of heart disease of unknown cause. However, an average of 1000 women in the United States develop this condition each year, and many die from it.[236] *Peripartum cardiomyopathy* is defined as the onset of heart failure in the last month of pregnancy or in the first 6 months post partum in the absence of a determinable cause of cardiac failure and absence of demonstrable heart disease before the last month of pregnancy. The main evidence for the existence of peripartum cardiomyopathy as a distinct clinical entity is the clustering of cases in the peripartum period. However, the presence of a temporal relationship does not prove causality, and it may be that the disorder reflects an unmasking of previously undiagnosed heart disease by the hemodynamic stress of pregnancy. Data on 28 patients with a diagnosis of peripartum cardiomyopathy are presented in Table 25–14. Of note is the high association with other disorders, particularly chronic hypertension and preeclampsia, and the dismal outcome of the disease.[237, 238]

Pathophysiology. In peripartum cardiomyopathy, the heart is dilated and contractility is impaired. Pregnancy-induced decreases in vascular resistance may compensate for the ventricular dysfunction by reducing afterload and thereby delaying clinical manifestations of congestive heart failure. In patients with concurrent diseases associated with compromised intravascular volume or increased SVR, as is the case

Table 25-14. Echocardiographic Data (Mean ± SD) in Patients With Cardiomyopathy of Pregnancy

Parameter	All (N = 28)	Survivors Without Disease (n = 2)	Survivors With Disease (n = 18)	Survivors With Transplant (n = 3)	Nonsurvivors (n = 5)
FS (%)	17.5 ± 6.75	20 ± 4.24	16 ± 5.03	13.3 ± 2.52	15.5 ± 4.99
LVIDd (mm)	64.9 ± 6.76	55 ± 4.24	64.5 ± 4.53*	73.3 ± 10.26	69.75 ± 7.14*
LVIDs (mm)	54.4 ± 7.88	44 ± 5.66	53.9 ± 6.33*	67.5 ± 2.12*	62.67 ± 6.43*
LAD (mm)	42 ± 6	35.5 ± 7.78	43.3 ± 5.4	40.7 ± 5.03	44.7 ± 7.37
PWTd (mm)	10.6 ± 1.81	9 ± 1.41	11.2 ± 1.77	8.5 ± 0.71	10.5 ± 0.71
IVSTd (mm)	9.71 ± 1.62	9.5 ± 0.71	10.27 ± 2.15	7.5 ± 2.12	9 ± 1.41

FS, fractional shortening; LVIDd, left ventricular end-diastolic dimension; LVIDs, left ventricular end-systolic dimension; LAD, left atrial dimension; PWTd, posterior wall thickness in diastole; IVSTd, intraventricular septal thickness in diastole.
* Values are significant ($P < .05$) compared with survivors without disease.
From Witlin AG, Mabie WC, Sibai BM: Peripartum cardiomyopathy: An ominous diagnosis. Am J Obstet Gynecol 1997; 176:182–188.

in both severe preeclampsia and chronic hypertension, the workload on the LV is increased earlier in pregnancy and LV dysfunction will present earlier and with greater severity.

The signs and symptoms of peripartum cardiomyopathy are the same as for any other dilated cardiomyopathy—fatigue, shortness of breath, orthopnea, peripheral edema, chronic cough, left upper quadrant pain, rales, wheezes, and extra heart sounds (S_3, S_4) may be present to varying degrees (Table 25-15). One patient who was 6 weeks post partum presented to our OR for cholycystectomy; her abdominal pain was thought to be related to gallbladder disease. She was obese. On physical examination, the patient had rales over both lung fields. On further questioning, she stated that she had been very active during pregnancy but had been in bed almost continuously since delivery because of extreme fatigue. An echocardiographic study confirmed the diagnosis of dilated biventricular cardiomyopathy, and she was placed on a heart transplant list. Her abdominal pain was due to hepatic congestion secondary to heart failure, not gallbladder disease. As discussed previously, the normal dyspnea and edema of pregnancy may be difficult to distinguish from the same symptoms in patients with heart failure. Echocardiography is the diagnostic tool of choice when there is uncertainty of diagnosis; once the diagnosis of failure is confirmed, echocardiography is recommended to exclude valvular heart disease as the cause of failure. Echocardiographic findings always involve LV dilation and dysfunction; there may be two-chamber (left atrium and LV) or four-chamber enlargement.

Rapidly changing hemodynamic conditions during labor and delivery increase the workload of the LV and are detrimental to patients with dilated cardiomyopathies. Preload may go up and down as much as 10% with each uterine contraction; 500 mL of blood is ejected into the maternal circulation as the uterus contracts and then the blood rapidly returns to the low-resistance uterine vascular bed as the contraction subsides. Afterload is increased as the result of

catecholamine-induced (pain) vasoconstriction and the lithotomy position of vaginal delivery. Valsalva's maneuvers during the second stage of labor also cause major changes in both preload and afterload. Increased vascular resistance and increased cardiac filling pressures resulting from uterine constriction immediately after delivery will worsen LV dysfunction. Why women develop peripartum cardiomyopathy well past the time of pregnancy-related hemodynamic changes is unknown; this indicates how little is actually understood about the cause of this disease.

Monitoring. The monitoring requirements in peripartum cardiomyopathy are determined by the patient's clinical status combined with echocardiographic assessment of cardiac function. Intravascular pressure monitoring of both the peripheral and pulmonary circulations is often necessary. Management of dilated cardiomyopathies consists of afterload reduction, preload reduction (fluid restriction, diuresis), and inotropic support for the heart. The management goal is to optimize cardiac output. Although there may be very little correlation between PCWP and LV volume in cases of dilated cardiomyopathies, cardiac output measurements (both invasively and noninvasively obtained) are reasonably reliable.

Anesthetic Considerations. Regional analgesia is beneficial in most patients with dilated cardiomyopathies. The decrease in afterload helps improve LV function as long as preload is not severely impaired. Thus, patient positioning and volume status are extremely important. Compared with normals, patients with dilated cardiomyopathies are less likely to have an intravascular volume deficit because of the congestive nature of the disease. More often than not, therapy is directed at decreasing intravascular volume and venous pressure by the use of venodilators (e.g., NTG) and diuretics. Thus, vigorous volume loading without evidence of an intravascular volume deficit is unwise.

The effects of general anesthesia and tracheal intubation tend to be the reverse of those of regional anesthesia and may be disastrous. The increase in LV work associated with the reflexive responses to tracheal stimulation (hypertension and tachycardia) will worsen cardiac dysfunction in patients with dilated cardiomyopathies; this may produce ischemia, decreased ventricular compliance, and an irreversible series of deleterious changes leading to cardiac arrest. Techniques to blunt the adverse cardiovascular reflexes associated with laryngoscopy and tracheal intubation include topical and regional anesthesia of the airway, high-dose narcotic techniques with short-acting agents, and potent arteriolar dilators such as SNP. Any beneficial effects of potent anesthetic agents on vascular resistance may be offset by the deleteri-

Table 25-15. Cardiomyopathy of Pregnancy: Symptoms and Signs

Symptoms	Signs
Fatigue	Rales
Shortness of breath	Wheezes
Dyspnea on exertion	Jugular venous distention
Orthopnea	Edema
Abdominal pain	Extra heart sounds (S_3, S_4)
Chronic cough	Apical holosystolic murmur
Palpitations	

ous myocardial depressant effects of these agents in patients with severe LV dysfunction.

Diabetes in Pregnancy

Many of the hormones of pregnancy have anti-insulin effects, and even though insulin levels rise progressively during pregnancy, a state of insulin resistance develops. In susceptible pregnant women, this may cause impaired glucose tolerance (gestational diabetes) or, in diabetic women, a worsening of metabolic control.

Insulin-dependent diabetes mellitus (IDDM), also identified as type 1 diabetes, is a chronic autoimmune disease resulting from destruction of the pancreatic beta cells. Predisposition is genetically determined; the relevant genes are located on chromosome 6 in association with the major histocompatibility complex. These patients are prone to the development of ketoacidosis. Their weight is usually normal, although some patients are obese. *Non-insulin dependent diabetes* (type 2) usually occurs in obese patients. Although not insulin-dependent, these patients may require insulin during pregnancy to prevent hyperglycemia. These patients are not ketosis-prone. *Gestational diabetes* (type 3) occurs only in pregnancy and is diagnosed on the basis of abnormal glucose tolerance tests. Type 4 diabetes occurs secondary to another condition such as cystic fibrosis or endocrine disorders (acromegaly, Cushing's syndrome).

Fetal Effects of Maternal Diabetes. The major impact on the fetus of maternal diabetes is a marked increase in the rate of major congenital anomalies and late-term in utero fetal death. The risk of neural tube defects is increased 10-fold in pregnancies complicated by IDDM.[239] A rarer complication is the caudal regression syndrome, which can include a range of abnormalities, from agenesis of the lumbosacral spine to sirenomelia (fusion of the lower extremities). Cardiac abnormalities occur in 4% of IDDM pregnancies (five-fold increase) and include ventricular septal defects, transposition of the great vessels, and coarctation of the aorta. The fetus in IDDM pregnancies may develop a severe hypertrophic cardiomyopathy characterized by a thick intraventricular septum; this can lead to LV outflow obstruction and cardiac failure. Gastrointestinal anomalies such as duodenal or anal atresia are more likely, as are renal anomalies. The anomalies in the various organ systems result from a disruption of organogenesis in early pregnancy, which is presumably caused by the metabolic effects of diabetes. Tight control of maternal blood glucose concentrations in the early weeks of pregnancy is associated with a highly significant reduction in the risk of serious congenital anomalies.[240] As hemoglobin A_{1C} concentrations at the time of conception exceed 8%, the risk of congenital anomalies increases commensurately.[241]

Infants of mothers with both IDDM and gestational diabetes are at high risk for macrosomia (birth weight of ≥4500 g) if the pregnancy goes to term. Macrosomia greatly increases the risk of birth injury (shoulder dystocia causing neurologic injury, fractures, and perinatal asphyxia). Although poor maternal glucose control increases the risk for macrosomia, tight control does not reliably prevent macrosomia. An overly large fetus also increases the maternal risk for uterine atony and hemorrhage following delivery. Until recently, delayed lung maturity was another problem ascribed to infants of diabetic mothers. However, this is not the case, as lung development reflects the gestational age of the fetus in both IDDM and normal pregnancies. Fetal adaptive responses to chronic hypoxia are impaired by hyperglycemia

and lactic acidosis, which are the consequences of inadequate maternal glucose control.

Preeclampsia is a frequent complicating factor in diabetic pregnancies and increases the risks for the mother and the fetus; the degree of uteroplacental insufficiency caused by preeclampsia correlates with growth retardation in the fetus (IUGR). Uteroplacental insufficiency also occurs in pregnant woman with diabetic vasculopathy and causes similar fetal growth impairment. IUGR is present in 20% of IDDM pregnancies and can be assumed to reflect maternal vascular compromise, either from diabetes or another condition.

In the newborn period, hyperinsulinemia (of fetal origin) caused by in utero hyperglycemia (of maternal origin) may result in severe hypoglycemia unless the infant is given glucose or a glucose source. This is true of both IDDM and gestational diabetes. Hypocalcemia is an additional problem in infants of diabetic mothers.

Maternal Complications Associated With IDDM Pregnancy. There are four prognostically bad signs of diabetic pregnancy that are related to maternal complications: diabetic ketoacidosis, preeclampsia, pyelonephritis, and maternal neglect. Apart from preeclampsia, their incidence can be reduced by tight metabolic control.

Ketoacidosis. Ketoacidosis in pregnancy is one of the factors that correlate with poor fetal outcome, particularly when it occurs in the first trimester. Risk factors for ketoacidosis are infection, β-adrenoceptor agonists such as terbutaline (used for tocolysis of preterm labor), hyperemesis gravidarum, and corticosteroid use for fetal lung maturation. Patient noncompliance with insulin therapy and insulin pump failure may also result in ketoacidosis. Prompt correction of the metabolic, acid-base, and intravascular volume alterations is crucial to the fetus as well as the mother.[242, 243]

Preeclampsia. Preeclampsia complicates almost 14% of type 1 diabetic pregnancies, compared with 5% of nondiabetic pregnancies.[244] The incidence increases in parallel with the severity and duration of the underlying diabetes. As with ketoacidosis, the presence of preeclampsia is a marker for poor fetal outcome, with a 20-times greater risk for perinatal mortality. In diabetic parturients with nephropathy and hypertension, the diagnosis of preeclampsia may be problematic, as many of these patients will have marked proteinuria and hypertension. The combination of IDDM with renal disease and hypertension, which is usually present in IDDM nephropathy, is associated with a 60% to 80% risk for the diagnosis of superimposed preeclampsia.

Maternal Infections. Maternal infections occur more frequently in IDDM than in normal pregnancies; 80% of IDDM pregnancies are complicated by at least one episode of infection, compared with 26% in nondiabetic women.[245] Urogenital, respiratory, wound, and endometrial infections predominate. The rate of postpartum infection is five times higher in IDDM patients. Pyelonephritis is a particular concern, because it occurs four times more frequently in IDDM pregnancies and is associated with an increased incidence of premature rupture of the membranes, preterm labor, and perinatal mortality.

Diabetic Nephropathy. Diabetic nephropathy is present in 5% of IDDM pregnancies. Patients with diabetic nephropathy may have large increases in proteinuria, with 24-hour totals in the 5- to 20-g range. Renal failure is one of the most dreaded complications of IDDM, ultimately afflicting 30% to

40% of all patients and accounting for as many as one half of all deaths in women of childbearing age. Understandably, the question of whether pregnancy increases the risk of diabetic renal disease or accelerates the progression of preexisting nephropathy is of major concern for women of reproductive age with IDDM. Most patients with IDDM nephropathy regain prepregnancy renal capacity, despite having greatly increased proteinuria during pregnancy.[246] The risk of accelerated and nonreversible renal injury is primarily related to the degree of underlying renal disease.[247] Although there is no absolute value of serum creatinine that identifies pregnant patients who will have accelerated progression to end-stage renal disease and dialysis, a serum creatinine level above 2 mg/dL, which is about three times the normal value for pregnancy, puts patients in a high-risk range. During pregnancy, a serum creatinine level of 2.8 mg/dL, or a creatinine clearance of less than 25 mL/minute/1.73 m², in the presence of severe hypertension or heavy proteinuria and systemic disease with glomerulonephritis, as occurs in IDDM, will result in irreversible renal failure in most patients.[54]

Diabetic Retinopathy. The issue of diabetic retinopathy is particularly problematic during pregnancy because there is evidence that pregnancy worsens proliferative retinopathy and that retinopathy *may* be worsened by improved glycemic control in early pregnancy, a practice that has positive benefit for the mother and fetus in so many other areas.[239] Proliferative retinopathy is characterized by capillary growth over the surface of the retina, a process referred to as neovascularization. As in prematurely born infants with proliferative retinopathy, laser photocoagulation therapy is useful in the prevention as well as treatment of this deleterious process. Background retinopathy presenting with microaneurysms and punctate hemorrhages may worsen in pregnancy. It would seem that Valsalva maneuvers during labor would pose an additional risk for such patients; however, cesarean section has not been shown to be an advantage in decreasing the incidence of vitreous hemorrhage.

Diabetic Neuropathy. Peripheral neuropathies are uncommon in diabetic patients of childbearing age. Autonomic neuropathy in IDDM pregnancy, which is more common, contributes to postural hypotension and diminished catecholamine response to hypoglycemia. Diabetic gastropathy during pregnancy causes nausea and vomiting leading to nutritional problems that can complicate glucose control.

Monitoring and Anesthetic Considerations. The most important monitoring concern in diabetic patients is the blood glucose level. The perioperative management of blood sugar in patients scheduled for elective cesarean section is the same as in nonpregnant diabetic patients. The major difference between these two groups is that in diabetic patients removal of the placenta removes most of the factors responsible for the insulin resistance that occurs. Thus, diabetic patients are at increased risk for hypoglycemia following delivery, and insulin levels must be adjusted downward accordingly.

Peripartum glucose management may likely be complicated by maternal drug therapy directed at other conditions (most often β-adrenoceptor agonists and corticosteroids). Calcium channel blockers are increasingly used as the primarily tocolytic agents in IDDM patients because of their lack of effect on glucose metabolism.

Regional analgesia and anesthesia are beneficial in parturients. Earlier studies found that babies born to IDDM mothers under regional (spinal or epidural) anesthesia were more acidotic than those born to mothers receiving general anesthesia.[248, 249] However, Datta et al.[250] subsequently showed that this was the effect of using glucose-containing solutions for volume expansion prior to regional anesthesia. When IDDM parturients with well-controlled glucose levels are volume-loaded with Ringer's lactated solution without glucose, the acid-base status of the newborns is the same with either regional or general anesthesia. These reports serve to underscore the importance to the fetus of strict glucose control in the mother. Also, it is important to be aware of the increased likelihood of preeclampsia and the derangements in volume status and vascular responsiveness that this disease may superimpose on the diabetic woman.

Fetal Monitoring

Fetal monitoring consists of assessments of fetal well-being and developmental progress. This process begins in early pregnancy and continues until delivery.

Fetal Cardiovascular Physiology

An understanding of fetal cardiovascular physiology is important in the interpretation of FHR patterns and noninvasive studies of blood flow dynamics in different areas of the fetal circulation (umbilical cord, vena cava, aorta, and cerebral arteries). The physiologic responses of the cardiovascular and central nervous systems of the fetus are gestation-dependent. A 26-week gestation fetus responds differently to the stress of hypoxemia than does a 38-week gestation fetus.

The Fetal Circulation

Oxygenated blood from the placenta has a normal oxygen tension of about 30 mmHg. However, owing to the presence of fetal hemoglobin, this represents a saturation of 80%. The saturated blood is carried by the umbilical vein (Fig. 25–38). A portion goes to the liver, but the majority bypasses the liver by traversing the ductus venosus and empties into the inferior vena cava. Streaming occurs, so that much of the oxygenated blood from the placenta is directed across the foramen ovale into the left atrium and, subsequently, the LV. This oxygenated blood is then preferentially supplied to the brain and myocardium. Desaturated blood from the head and upper body returns via the superior vena cava and is directed into the RV, where it mixes with saturated blood from the placenta. Because of the high pulmonary vascular resistance, most of the RV output crosses the ductus arteriosus and enters the descending aorta. A portion of this blood then goes to the placenta via the umbilical arteries to be reoxygenated. The normal oxygen tension of this desaturated umbilical artery blood is 20 mmHg, with a saturation of approximately 55%. The fetal circulation is gestation-dependent. For example, from 20 weeks to 30 weeks of gestation, the ratio of foramen ovale blood flow to the combined cardiac output of both the RV and LV decreases almost 50%, while the proportion of combined cardiac output to the lung through the pulmonary arteries increases almost 50%[251] (Fig. 25–39).

Fetal Asphyxia

Asphyxia may be defined as insufficient exchange of respiratory gases, and in the fetus it is almost always caused by inadequate umbilical (fetal) or uterine (maternal) blood flow.

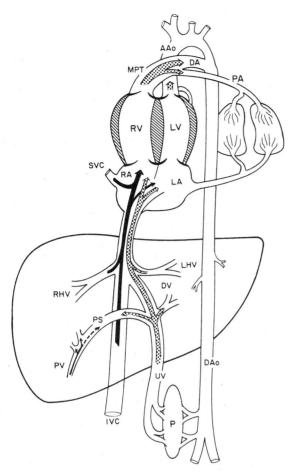

Figure 25–38. The fetal circulation. *Dark arrows* indicate oxygenated blood; *stippled arrows,* deoxygenated blood. P, placenta; UV, umbilical vein; IVC, inferior vena cava; DV, ductus venosus; RHV, right hepatic vein; LHV, left hepatic vein; PV, portal vein; PS, portal sinus; RA, right atrium; LA, left atrium; SVC, superior vena cava; RV, right ventricle; LV, left ventricle; MPT, main pulmonary trunk; DA, ductus arteriosus; AAo, ascending aorta; PA, pulmonary artery; DAo, descending aorta. (From Heymann MA: Biophysical evaluation of fetal status. *In* Creasy R, Resnik R (eds): Maternal-Fetal Medicine. Philadelphia, WB Saunders 1984, p 260.)

This causes a reduction in oxygen content (hypoxemia) and elevation of CO_2 (hypercarbia) in fetal blood. The fetal response to hypoxemia and hypercarbia consists of a redistribution of blood flow to essential organs, decreased oxygen consumption, and anaerobic glycolysis. The favored organs are the brain, heart, placenta, and adrenal glands. Blood flow to the adrenal gland increases markedly during periods of asphyxia and there is a 10-fold increase in plasma norepinephrine. The redistribution of blood flow is accomplished by vasoconstriction of certain vascular beds and alterations in downstream impedance. Increased impedance in the descending aorta favors blood flow to the cerebral and coronary circulation.

With hypoxia, the heart rate decreases because of increased vagal stimulation, and overall oxygen consumption decreases. Fetal pH decreases as a result of metabolic acidosis caused by lactic acid production in vascular beds receiving inadequate oxygen for aerobic metabolism. Impaired CO_2 exchange at the level of the placenta contributes a respira-

tory component to the acidosis. As the oxygen supply continues to decrease, the physiologic compensatory mechanisms themselves fail; myocardial performance deteriorates and cardiac output decreases. This decreases umbilical blood flow even further, and the asphyxia worsens. Eventually, the fetus has regional hypoxia and organ (brain, heart, kidney) damage at the cellular level.[252]

The assessment of fetal well-being, both antepartum (before labor begins) and intrapartum (during labor and delivery), consists primarily of methods to *infer* the absence of asphyxia by documenting the absence of features of the fetal hypoxic response—heart rate slowing, acidosis, and alterations in patterns of fetal blood flow.

Antenatal Monitoring

Antenatal monitoring consists of efforts to assess fetal well-being, as well as to assess developmental progress. Fetal well-being and fetal maturity are not the same thing. A fetus can be mature and not well or be immature and quite well as long as it continues an intrauterine existence. Ultrasound technology is the key modality for the assessment of fetal growth, structural development, and, in high-risk pregnancies, well-being. During the third trimester, the most important aspect of fetal development becomes maturation of the lungs. In preterm fetuses, pulmonary maturity is inferred by evidence of lung surfactant production.

Certain high-risk fetuses warrant frequent (twice-weekly) assessment of well-being before the onset of labor. The most frequent pregnancies so monitored are those complicated by diabetes mellitus, hypertension, cardiac disease, renal disease, hyperthyroidism, collagen-vascular disease, sickle cell disease, a growth-retarded fetus, a prior in utero fetal death, or a postdates fetus (>40 weeks' gestation). The benefits of frequent antepartum testing in such patients are so significant that the likelihood of fetal death in high-risk tested populations is lower than that in low-risk untested populations.[253]

Noninvasive Antenatal Monitoring

Nonstress Test (NST). The NST monitors FHR variability and accelerations with fetal movement over a 20-minute period. The NST is considered *reactive* if there is both normal variability and accelerations with movement. If there is no fetal movement or no acceleration of FHR with movement over the 20-minute test period, the test is classified as *nonreactive*. The test is classified as *uncertain reactivity* in cases in which there are less than two fetal movements in the test period, accelerations with movement are less than 15 bpm, or long-term variability amplitude is less than 10 bpm. In some cases, a vibroacoustic stimulator is used over the maternal abdomen to elicit FHR accelerations. A nonreactive NST does not necessarily indicate a depressed fetus but does require further evaluation.

Oxytocin Challenge Test (OCT). The OCT evaluates the FHR pattern in response to uterine contractions induced by oxytocin. Ultrasonography is used to record the heart rate. The appearance of abnormal heart rate slowing (late decelerations) with contractions indicates a *positive* test. Doppler velocimetry (see below) has shown that a positive OCT is associated with increases in resistance in the fetal umbilical arteries (an undesirable finding), whereas there is no change in cases of a negative OCT. Thus this test, by inducing uterine contractions, will stress a compromised fe-

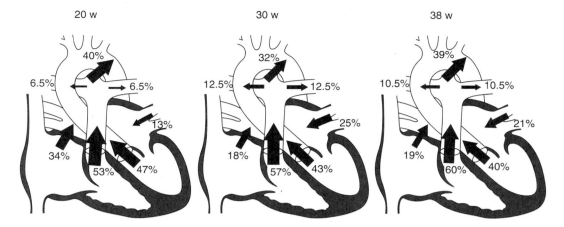

Figure 25–39. Changes in patterns of blood flow through the heart and great vessels at different stages of gestation. Values are given as percentages of combined cardiac output of both the right and left ventricles. Most of the significant changes occur between 20 and 30 weeks' gestation. Over this period, the ratio of foramen ovale blood flow to the combined cardiac output decreases from 34% to 18%; the proportion of flow to the lungs through the pulmonary arteries increases almost 50%. (From Rasanen J, Wood DC, Weiner S, et al: Role of the pulmonary circulation in the distribution of human fetal cardiac output during the second half of pregnancy. Circulation 1996; 94(5):1068–1073.)

tus, and many testing protocols no longer use this test. A *nonreactive* NST (absent variability and accelerations) coupled with a *positive* contraction stress test (late decelerations) is indicative of a distressed fetus and demands immedi-

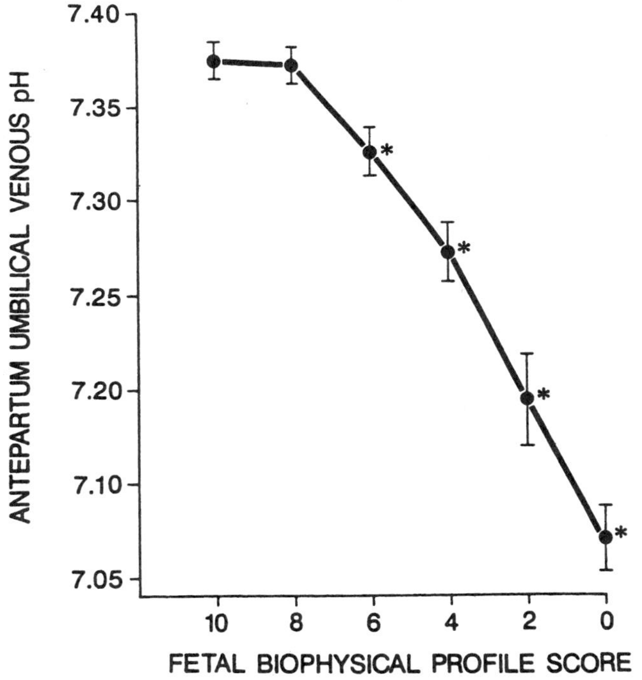

Figure 25–40. Antepartum umbilical vein pH (mean ± 2 SD) per last fetal biophysical profile score. Blood samples for pH were obtained by ultrasound-guided percutaneous umbilical vessel puncture (cordocentesis). Every biophysical profile score below 8 was associated with a significantly lower mean pH compared to the immediately higher biophysical score. * $P < 0.01$. (From Manning FA, Snijders R, Harman CR, et al: Fetal biophysical profile score. VI. Correlation with antepartum umbilical venous fetal pH. Am J Obstet Gynecol 1993; 169:755–763.)

ate intervention to either reverse the condition causing the distress or to deliver the fetus.

Fetal Biophysical Profile (BPP). Fetal BPP scoring is a method of antepartum fetal risk assessment that, in addition to the NST, uses real-time ultrasonography for fetal assessment. The BPP score is based on a composite survey of four biophysical variables (fetal breathing, gross body movements, tone, and heart rate reactivity) that reflect immediate well-being and one variable (amniotic fluid volume) that reflects fetal condition for the previous 7 to 10 days. The latter is a marker for the longer-term adequacy of placental function.[254] For amniotic fluid volume, the deepest vertical cord-free pocket of amniotic fluid is measured in each quadrant of the uterus, and the amniotic fluid index is the sum of the four measurements. An amniotic fluid index less than or equal to 5 cm is considered abnormal, and all women with such a finding require hospitalization for extended evaluation or delivery. A range of values is possible for each component of the BPP, and a total score is reported. The last BPP score correlates highly with fetal acidemia (Fig. 25–40), Apgar scores, the need for neonatal resuscitation, extended intensive care, the incidence of cerebral palsy, and perinatal death.[255, 256] The incidence of perinatal death is significantly reduced in high-risk pregnancies in which fetal BPP scoring is used in management.

In a study of malformed fetuses, those with a musculoskeletal anomaly were more likely to lose points for fetal movement; fetuses with a genitourinary system anomaly lost points for amniotic fluid, tone, and breathing; fetuses with a CNS anomaly lost points for tone and breathing; and fetuses with a thoracic anomaly lost points for breathing.[257]

A modified BPP, which includes only an NST and amniotic fluid index, is used in many testing protocols, and the complete BPP evaluating fetal breathing, tone, and movement is reserved for cases in which the NST is nonreactive. In a very large series that used a modified fetal BPP test, the rate of cerebral palsy in 26,290 high-risk tested patients was 1.33 per 1000 (35 cases) compared with a rate of 4.74 per 1000 live births in 8657 untested mixed low-risk–high-risk patients (278 cases); the difference was highly significant[254] (Fig. 25–41). In the tested population the relationship be-

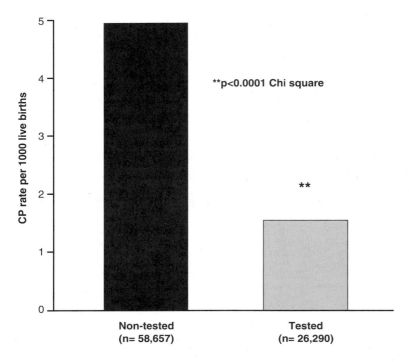

Figure 25–41. Incidence of cerebral palsy (CP) in tested (modified biophysical profile) high-risk patients and untested mixed low-risk–high-risk patients. There were 35 cases of cerebral palsy in 26,290 tested patients and 278 cases in 58,657 untested patients. (From Manning FA, Bondaji N, Harman CR, et al: Fetal assessment based on fetal biophysical profile scoring. VIII. The incidence of cerebral palsy in tested and untested perinates. Am J Obstet Gynecol 1998; 178:696–706.)

tween the incidence of cerebral palsy and the last test fetal BPP score was inverse and exponential (Fig. 25–42). Antenatal asphyxia is one important and potentially avoidable cause of cerebral palsy.

Doppler Flow Velocimetry. Combination real-time and Doppler ultrasonography allows noninvasive hemodynamic evaluation of the fetus and its supporting circulation. Doppler flow velocimetry is now used to evaluate blood velocity waveforms in the pulsatile fetal and uteroplacental vessels and is a powerful new tool for the identification of fetal distress in pregnancy.[258, 259]

One specific application of Doppler velocimetry involves computation of the ratio of systolic-to-diastolic (S/D) flows in specific vessels. As downstream resistance to flow increases, diastolic flow is disproportionately impeded, and the S/D ratio increases. This allows an indirect, but reproducible, estimate of vascular resistance. These techniques are limited in reliability prior to 26 weeks' gestation.[260]

Use of *ratios* rather than *values* for flow permits assessments that are independent of the angle of incidence of the ultrasound beam. The S/D ratio is also identified as the A/B ratio and compares the peak systolic flow to the end-diastolic flow (Fig. 25–43). The resistance index (RI) is computed as the peak systolic minus end-diastolic frequencies divided by the peak systolic frequency. The pulsatility index (PI) is computed by subtracting the nadir of the diastolic frequencies from the peak systolic frequencies and dividing this value by the mean maximum frequency over one cardiac cycle (Fig. 25–44).

Uterine Artery Doppler Velocimetry. After the 26th week of gestation, a uterine artery S/D ratio greater than 2.6 is highly suggestive of increased resistance to uterine artery blood flow and correlates with increased maternal and fetal morbidity (Figs. 25–45 and 25–46). Fleischer et al.[131] have documented the power of uterine S/D ratios to identify the at-risk fetus in hypertensive pregnancies; infants born to hy-

pertensive mothers with S/D ratios greater than 2.6 were delivered 5 weeks earlier and weighed 1125 g less than infants born to hypertensive mothers with S/D ratios less than 2.6. The 17 stillbirths in the study all occurred in mothers with abnormal uterine S/D ratios. In spite of the dramatic differences in fetal outcomes, the difference in mean blood pressure between the two groups (mothers with high vs. mothers with normal S/D ratios) was 5 mmHg and not statistically or clinically significant. Because Doppler flow velocimetry estimates vascular resistance, it is a more powerful tool for predicting the outcome of pregnancy than blood pressure.[261, 262]

Not only is the S/D ratio significant, but, as it reflects the mean of both uterine arteries, divergent ratios between the two sides are also significant. A difference of greater than 1 between the left and right uterine artery S/D ratios is associated with an increased risk of growth retardation, preeclampsia, and premature delivery. This divergence most likely reflects placental laterality, a factor shown to have an adverse outcome upon pregnancy,[61] particularly in diabetic patients.[263]

Umbilical Doppler Velocimetry. In the umbilical circulation, both the arterial and the venous flow can be studied. The umbilical arteries carry desaturated blood from the fetal descending aorta to the placenta. Umbilical artery S/D ratios are calculated as for the uterine circulation; however, the cutoff value for term infants is a ratio of 3.0, while for preterm infants 3.5 is a more appropriate value (Fig. 25–47). In a study of diabetic patients, umbilical artery S/D ratios were better predictors of an adverse fetal outcome than either an NST or fetal BPP.[264]

Systolic-Diastolic Ratio Patterns. Because the umbilical (fetal) and uterine (maternal) vascular structures are independent, there are four different patterns of umbilical and uterine S/D ratios that may arise: (1) uterine greater than 2.6 and umbilical greater than 3.0 (both abnormal); (2) uterine

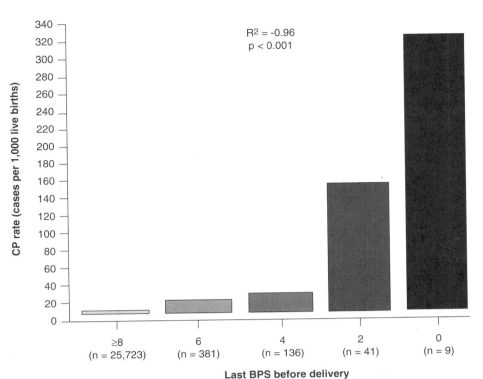

$R^2 = -0.96$
$p < 0.001$

Figure 25-42. The incidence of cerebral palsy in relation to the last biophysical profile score. The relationship is inverse and exponential. (From Manning FA, Bondaji N, Harman CR, et al: Fetal assessment based on fetal biophysical profile scoring. VIII. The incidence of cerebral palsy in tested and untested perinates. Am J Obstet Gynecol 1998; 178: 696–706.)

greater than 2.6 and umbilical normal; (3) uterine normal and umbilical greater than 3.0; (4) uterine and umbilical both normal.

1. *Normal uterine and umbilical circulation.* Hypertensive pregnancies with normal S/D ratios in both circulations (50% of patients) have pregnancy outcomes that are similar to normotensive patients. Thus, once this pattern is documented at the beginning of the third trimester, additional monitoring need only be maternal blood pressure and routine assessment of fetal well-being, as in normal pregnancy, with velocimetry repeated once at 32 to 34 weeks.

2. *Normal uterine and abnormal umbilical circulation.* When the fetal umbilical circulation is abnormal and the maternal uterine circulation is normal, the usual consequence is fetal growth retardation. Even if the mother is normotensive, 70% of infants will be SGA if the umbilical S/D ratio is abnormally high. Conversely, despite the presence of maternal hypertension, if the umbilical flow velocity waveforms are normal, only 3% of cases will be SGA infants. The circumstance of an abnormal umbilical circulation coupled with a normal uterine circulation is usually caused by a decrease in the number of small muscular arteries in the placenta, and probably represents a failure of angiogenesis.

The value of Doppler velocimetry in evaluation of the SGA fetus is illustrated in a study by Hitschold et al.[265] The placentas from SGA fetuses with umbilical S/D ratios less than 3 had no evidence of placental insufficiency; perfusion and diffusion capacities and placental-fetal weight ratios were not different from those in AGA babies. However, SGA babies with S/D ratios greater than 3 were markedly smaller than SGA fetuses with normal flow velocimetry. In the placentas of the high S/D ratio infants, vascularization in the terminal villi was reduced and diffusion conditions were impaired. Thus, Doppler flow velocimetry is able to distinguish fetuses that are genetically small from those that are small due to placental insufficiency. This distinction is important, because, in the study of Hitschold et al., all SGA fetuses with abnormal S/D ratios required cesarean delivery due to additional evidence of fetal distress, whereas the SGA fetuses with S/D ratios less than 3 were all delivered vaginally following spontaneous labor.

3. *Abnormal uterine and normal umbilical circulation.* The pattern of abnormal uterine S/D ratios and a normal umbilical flow pattern occurs in only 10% of hypertensive patients, and is not associated with severe fetal growth retar-

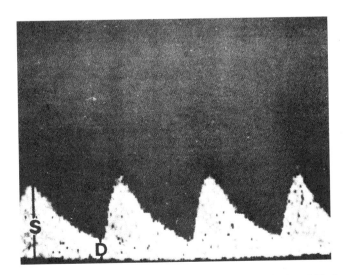

Figure 25-43. Flow velocity waveform from the fetal umbilical artery. The A/B ratio compares the peak systolic (S) flow velocity to the end-diastolic (D) velocity. (From Fleischer A, Anyaegbunam AA, Schulman H, et al: Uterine and umbilical artery velocimetry during normal labor. Am J Obstet Gynecol 1987; 157:41.)

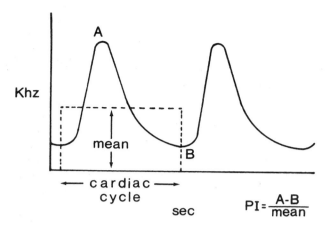

Figure 25–44. Schematic flow velocity waveform indicating the method for calculation of the pulsatility index (PI). Khz, kilohertz; A, peak systolic frequency; B, lowest diastolic frequency. (From McCowan LM, Mullen MB, Ritchie K: Umbilical artery flow velocity waveforms and the placental vascular bed. Am J Obstet Gynecol 1987; 157:901.)

dation or an increased risk of fetal distress during labor. However, the mothers may be symptomatic, with headaches, hypertension, and decreased urine output, and this often prompts premature delivery of the baby.

4. *Abnormal uterine and umbilical circulation.* The 20% of hypertensive pregnancies with both abnormal uterine and umbilical circulations are associated with the highest degrees of maternal and fetal morbidity, and warrant the most intensive surveillance. Fetal growth retardation is most severe for this group (50% of normal), because the increased resistance to maternal UBF is compounded by increased resistance to fetal blood flow through the placenta. This represents true uteroplacental insufficiency, and fetuses under such conditions will most likely display signs of distress—late heart rate decelerations, absent or reverse end-diastolic flow, venous pulsations (see below).[266] Appearance of distress patterns before the onset of labor is particularly ominous.

Absent or Reversed Umbilical Artery Diastolic Flow (AREDF).

AREDF in the fetal aorta (Fig. 25–48) or umbilical artery carries a very high risk for the fetus. In a study of 65 patients with preeclampsia, the presence of AREDF was associated with a mortality rate of 30%, whereas in fetuses without AREDF there was no mortality.[267] Another study of patients with pregnancy-induced hypertension reported that AREDF in the fetal umbilical artery before 30 weeks' gestation had a perinatal death rate of 62%, whereas the same pattern presenting after 30 weeks had a mortality of only 14%.[261] The difference reflects the increased severity of preeclampsia presenting early in gestation. Yet another study of 37 pregnancies with AREDF in the umbilical arteries reported a fetal death rate of 38%.[268] The explanation for the loss of the diastolic waveform is either very high placental resistance or impaired fetal myocardial function, and possibly both. AREDF usually precedes the onset of abnormal FHR patterns in cases of asphyxia; the interval from the occurrence of AREDF to the occurrence of abnormal FHRs ranges from 1 day to several weeks. Once detected, this ominous finding requires intensive monitoring.

Umbilical Vein Pulsations.

The normal Doppler flow pattern obtained from the umbilical vein is seen in Figure 25–49, along with umbilical arterial and venous waveforms.

Pulsations in the umbilical vein are often associated with AREDF in the umbilical arteries. In one study of 21 fetuses with AREDF, 11 had venous pulsations and 10 did not; 6 of the 11 with pulsations died, whereas all but 1 of the 10 without pulsations survived.[269] In another study of fetuses with AREDF in the umbilical arteries, 10 of 16 (62.5%) with pulsations in the umbilical vein died, compared to four deaths in a group of 21 (19%) fetuses without venous pulsations.[268] It thus appears that pregnancies complicated by AREDF can be further subdivided on the basis of the presence or absence of venous pulsations in the umbilical vein, with the presence of pulsations carrying an ominous prognosis.

The venous pulsations are due to large increases in the amount of reverse blood flow from the right atrium into the inferior vena cava, with the waveform being reflected back into the umbilical vein. Venous pulsations are invariably present when there are extremes of fetal heart rate. Rates greater than 180 bpm increase end-diastolic pressure in the ventricles because of either insufficient ejection time or inadequate time during diastole for coronary perfusion with resultant ischemia and decreased compliance. When the right atrium contracts and the ventricular pressure is increased, a portion of the blood will be pumped into the vena cava as it follows the path of least resistance. Venous pulsations also occur with heart rates less than 120 bpm, and the end-diastolic timing is the same as during tachycardia except in cases of complete heart block (Fig. 25–50). The explanation

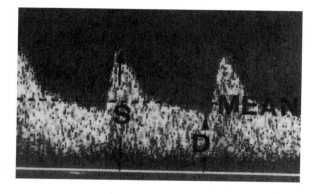

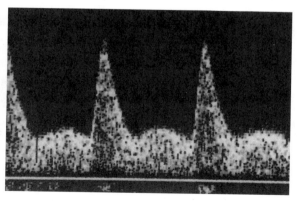

Figure 25–45. *Top,* Normal uteroplacental flow velocity waveform, with peak systolic (S) and end-diastolic (D) frequencies marked. *Bottom,* Abnormal uteroplacental flow velocity waveform characterized by decreased end-diastolic velocity as well as diastolic notching at the beginning of diastolic flow. (From Grab D, Hutter W, Sterzik K, et al: Reference values for resistance index and pulsatility index of uteroplacental Doppler flow velocity waveforms based on 612 uneventful pregnancies. Gynecol Obstet Invest 1992; 34:83.)

Figure 25-46. *Left,* Normal uterine artery flow velocity waveform with systolic-diastolic (S/D) ratio less than 2.6. *Right,* Abnormal uterine artery flow velocity waveform with S/D ratio = 4.0. There is markedly decreased velocity (notching) at the beginning of diastole as well as at end-diastole. (From Ducey J, Schulman H, Farmakides G, et al: A classification of hypertension in pregnancy based on Doppler velocimetry. Am J Obstet Gynecol 1987; 157:682.)

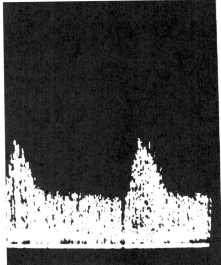
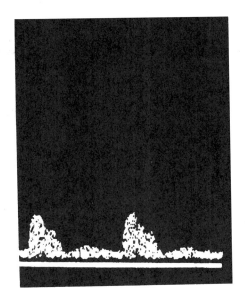

NORMAL
S/D=2.3

ABNORMAL
S/D=4.0

for venous pulsations with slow heart rates is that maximal ventricular filling occurs during the lengthened diastole, and the atrial contraction ejects a portion of blood in a retrograde direction rather than forward into the already full ventricle. During complete heart block, atrial contractions occur independently of ventricular volume changes, and those occurring during ventricular systole will tend to eject blood in a retrograde direction or across the foramen ovale. In the study by Indik et al.,[269] all infants with venous pulsations due to extremes of heart rate survived.

Figure 25-47. *Left,* Normal umbilical artery flow velocity waveform with systolic-diastolic (S/D) ratio less than 3.0. *Right,* Abnormal umbilical artery flow velocity waveform with S/D ratio = 4.0. (From Ducey J, Schulman H, Farmakides G, et al: A classification of hypertension in pregnancy based on Doppler velocimetry. Am J Obstet Gynecol 1987; 157:682.)

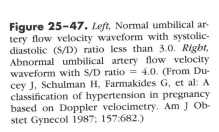
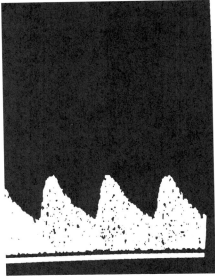
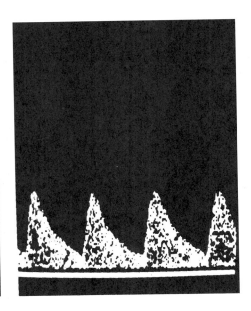

NORMAL
S/D=2.1

ABNORMAL
S/D=4.0

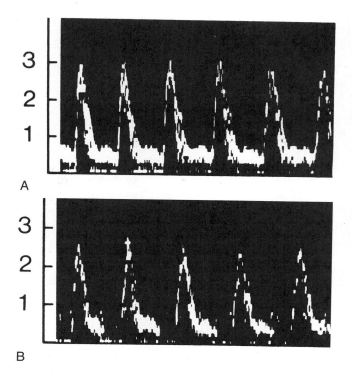

A

B

Figure 25–48. *A,* Normal flow velocity waveform from the descending aorta of a fetus at 39 weeks' gestation. Scale is in kilohertz. *B,* Flow velocity waveform from the descending aorta of a fetus in distress with absent end-diastolic frequencies (150 Hz). (From Jouppila P, Kirkinen P: Blood velocity waveforms of the fetal aorta in normal and hypertensive pregnancies. Obstet Gynecol 1986; 67:857–858. Reprinted with permission from the American College of Obstetricians & Gynecologists.)

In the presence of a normal heart rate and in the absence of fetal breathing movements, which affect intrathoracic pressures, reversal of flow is primarily due to decreased ventricular compliance secondary to ischemia. The vena cava becomes a lower-resistance circuit than the path of forward flow through the ventricle. Retrograde flow decreases the volume of potentially oxygenated blood reaching the coronary arteries, further compromising myocardial blood flow and exacerbating the ischemia and decreased compliance. The pattern of AREDF in the umbilical arteries coupled with venous pulsations in the umbilical vein that are not due to irregularities of heart rate or fetal breathing movements carries an extremely high mortality. Once detected, such a pattern demands intense efforts to improve fetal oxygenation or deliver the fetus if it is at a viable gestational age.

Inferior Vena Cava Waveforms. Pulsed Doppler studies of inferior vena cava flow in the fetus may provide even more sensitive information regarding myocardial function than umbilical artery studies. The ratio of systolic and diastolic peak flow velocities for vena caval flow can be measured just as for other vascular beds, and reverse flow can also be estimated (Fig. 25–51). Rizzo et al.[270] found evidence of decreased cardiac function (increased S/D ratios, increased AREDF) on the basis of vena cava waveforms in fetuses in which there were no significant abnormalities seen in umbilical artery waveforms, and the subsequent clinical course was consistent with uteroplacental insufficiency. Likewise, Indik et al. found a high association between venous pulsations in the fetal umbilical vein and abnormal flow velocities in the inferior vena cava, a result that is not surprising because the two vascular beds are closely linked in series.[269]

Internal Carotid and Cerebral Arterial Waveforms. The fetal response to hypoxia, which involves preferential streaming of blood to the brain at the expense of most other organs and tissues, has a measurable impact on cerebral hemodynamics that can be assessed using color Doppler ultrasonography. Fetal cerebral blood flow increases linearly with decreases in the arterial oxygen tension of umbilical venous blood. Fetal hypoxia is associated with decreased pulsatility indices in the internal carotid (Fig. 25–52) and cerebral arteries (due to cerebral vasodilation or loss of cerebral autoregulation) with simultaneous increases in the pulsatility indices in the umbilical arteries and the descending aorta caused by increases in vascular resistance in these circulations.[271] When the ratio of the pulsatility index in the umbilical artery relative to the middle cerebral artery (MCA) in the fetus is abnormally high, it is indicative of a "brain

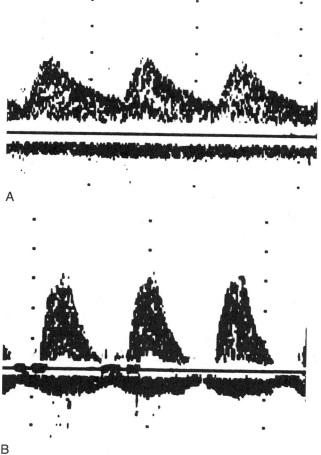

A

B

Figure 25–49. *A,* Umbilical arterial (*upper tracing*) and venous (*lower tracing*) Doppler flow velocity waveform in a normal fetus. The venous velocities have no variation with the cardiac cycle. *B,* Abnormal flow velocity waveform from the umbilical artery and vein of a fetus with absent diastolic umbilical arterial blood flow and pulsations in the umbilical venous flow tracing. (From Reed KL, Anderson CF, Shenker L: Changes in intracardiac Doppler blood flow velocities in fetuses with absent umbilical artery diastolic flow. Am J Obstet Gynecol 1987; 157:775.)

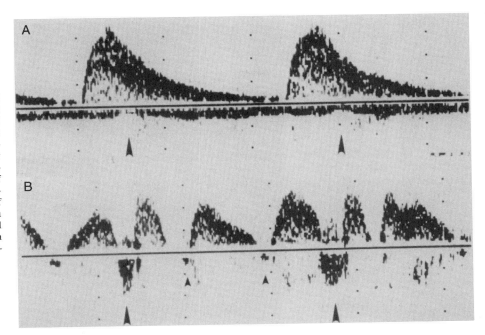

Figure 25-50. *A,* Umbilical arterial and venous flow velocity waveform from a fetus with complete heart block. Atrial contractions *(arrows)* result in venous pulsations when they occur in midsystole. *B,* Inferior vena cava flow velocity waveform in the same fetus. Venous pulsations are associated with reversal of flow in the inferior vena cava. (From Indik JH, Chen V, Reed KL: Association of umbilical venous with inferior vena cava blood flow velocities. Obstet Gynecol 1991; 77:554. Reprinted with permission from the American College of Obstetricians & Gynecologists.)

sparing" state in which the vascular resistance in the umbilical vessels is increased while the vascular resistance in the brain is decreased.[272] This is the reverse of the findings in other vascular beds during periods of hypoxemia and represents a compensated but threatened status for the fetus.

In the face of continuing and severe hypoxemia, the cerebral PI may subsequently increase due to the presence of cerebral edema.[273] In fetuses with absent end-diastolic velocities in the umbilical artery, abnormal FHR patterns occur when the MCA begins to lose its compensatory maximal dilation.[274] The MCA PI increases and there is a significant reduction in LV output (which goes preferentially to the

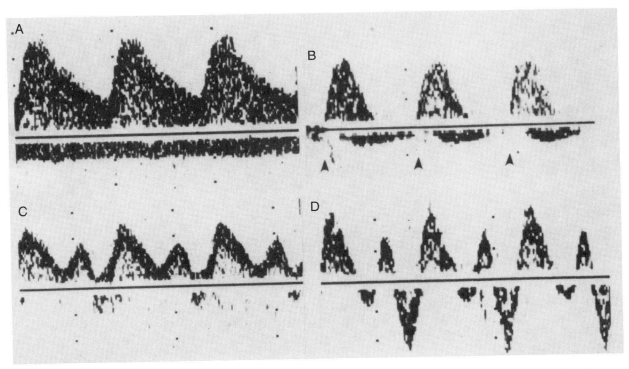

Figure 25-51. *A,* Umbilical arterial and venous flow velocity waveform in a normal 38-week fetus. *B,* Umbilical arterial and venous flow velocity waveform in a 34-week fetus with absent diastolic velocities and venous pulsations. *C,* Inferior vena cava flow velocity waveform from the normal fetus in *A. D,* Inferior vena cava flow velocity waveform from the fetus in *B.* There is reversal of flow during atrial contraction *(arrows).* (From Indik JH, Chen V, Reed KL: Association of umbilical venous with inferior vena cava blood flow velocities. Obstet Gynecol 1991; 77:552. Reprinted with permission from the American College of Obstetricians & Gynecologists.)

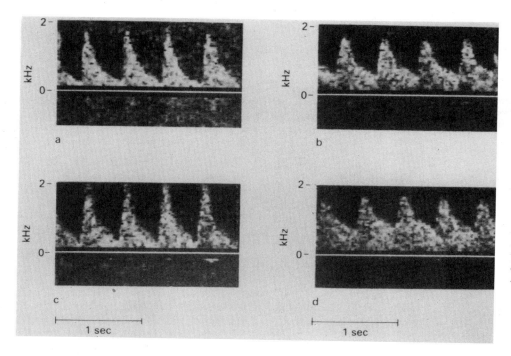

Figure 25–52. Internal carotid artery blood flow velocity waveforms. Waveforms in panel *A* and panel *C* are from a normal fetus at 27 and 37 weeks' gestation. The waveform in panel *B* is from a growth-retarded fetus at both 27 and 37 weeks' gestation. The increase in diastolic flow is abnormal, and is due to decreased cerebral vascular resistance and possible loss of autoregulation. (From Wladimiroff JW, Tonge HM, Stewart PA: Doppler ultrasound assessment of cerebral blood flow in the human fetus. Br J Obstet Gynaecol 1986; 93:471–475.)

brain) without significant changes in RV function. Thus it appears that a loss of autonomic reactivity occurs in the brain first and is followed within a few days by a similar response in the heart, manifested by decreased FHR variation. The finding of reverse end-diastolic flow in the MCA has been reported as an agonal pattern[275] (Fig. 25–53).

The incorporation of the velocity flow S/D ratios of the middle cerebral and umbilical arteries into the modified BPP was shown to reduce the incidence of cesarean section for fetal distress in patients with suspected uteroplacental insufficiency.[276] Evaluation of cerebral vascular resistance provides important additional information in the quest for the answer to the key question in fetal assessment: Is this fetus at risk for asphyxia?

Comparison of Antepartum Tests. The primary measure of the effectiveness of antepartum testing is the false-negative rate, usually defined as the incidence of fetal death within 1 week of a normal test result. The false-positive rate reflects those cases in which the test indicates a distressed fetus and the outcome was a birth with no evidence of short- or long-term fetal compromise. Each currently available method of antepartum testing has unique advantages and disadvantages and different false-positive and false-negative rates. The NST is easy to perform; however, it has a fairly high false-negative rate (3.2 per 1000) and a false-positive rate of approximately 50%. The contraction stress test (CST) is limited to once- rather than twice-weekly testing and may precipitate fetal distress. It has a false-negative rate of 0.4 per 1000. The CST is highly effective; a fetus that survives the stress test is unlikely to die within the next week. However, the CST is more difficult to perform than the NSTs and, as might be expected, has a high false-positive rate.

A report of 15,482 modified BPPs performed in 54,617 high-risk pregnancies had a false-negative rate (fetal death within a week of a reassuring test) of 0.8 per 1000 women tested.[253] In 60% of deliveries following an abnormal antepartum test, there was no evidence of short-term or long-term fetal compromise. These *false-positive* tests resulted in pre-

term delivery in 1.5% of those tested before term and a small increase in the rate of cesarean section (16.7 vs. 13.2%). The rate of neonatal complications in this iatrogenic group (early delivery) was 20%. Two thirds of all patients did not undergo testing until term (post dates, diet-controlled diabetes) and thus had no risk for premature delivery based on a false-positive test. The most impressive statistic, however, was a fetal death rate in tested high-risk patients that was 6.75 times lower than the death rate in the untested population, which consisted primarily of low-risk patients. From the same report, in cases in which the complete BPP was performed, the false-negative rate was 0.6 per 1000 and the false-positive rate was only 40%. However, the complete BPP is usually more time-consuming than the NST or the modified BPP and requires additional experience.

Invasive Antenatal Monitoring

Amniocentesis. Amniocentesis performed early in the second trimester allows the antenatal determination of the cytogenetic constitution of the fetus, the diagnosis of inborn errors of metabolism, and the detection of possible neural tube and abdominal wall defects (identified by elevated alpha-fetoprotein levels in the amniotic fluid). In late pregnancy, amniocentesis is used to estimate fetal lung maturity, assess the severity of Rh isoimmunization, and decompress polyhydramnios.

If amniocentesis is necessary, ultrasound is required to locate fluid for aspiration and to avoid the placenta, the umbilical cord, and the fetus. Fetal death from exsanguination has occurred following undetected injury to the umbilical vessels during amniocentesis.

Assessment of Fetal Maturity. Prematurity is still the most significant cause of perinatal morbidity and mortality. Fetal maturity in present perinatal practice is synonymous with pulmonary maturity, the rate-limiting step in the process that allows the fetus to become independent of the placenta. Because of variability in the timing of lung maturation relative to gestational age, specific markers for lung

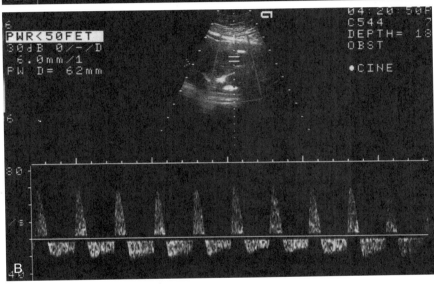

Figure 25–53. Pulsed-wave Doppler ultrasonography preceding fetal death in a severely growth-restricted fetus at 30 weeks' gestation. *Upper panel,* Reverse end-diastolic flow in the umbilical artery. *Lower panel,* Reverse end-diastolic flow in the middle cerebral artery. (From Sepulveda W, Shennan AH, Peek MJ: Reverse end-diastolic flow in the middle cerebral artery: An agonal pattern in the human fetus. Am J Obstet Gynecol 1996; 174:1645–1647.)

maturity have been sought. The most reliable tests at present are those that assess surfactant production in the fetal lung.

A major limitation of all tests of fetal lung maturity is that, although they are quite sensitive in identifying the fetus with mature lungs, they are much less specific in identifying fetuses who will develop respiratory distress syndrome (RDS) of prematurity. Thus, in a high-risk pregnancy in which it is deemed necessary to deliver the fetus as soon as lung maturity is in evidence, tests of lower specificity will result in delay in some cases in which delay is not necessary. For example, in one test described below (the TDx test), the expectation is that only 25% of the tests indicating immaturity will be associated with subsequent RDS. Part of the reason for lower specificity for RDS with a test that indicates lung immaturity is that there may be 3 days between an immature test result and delivery. As seen in Figure 25–54, there is a rapid maturation phase, based on the lecithin-to-sphingomyelin (L/S) ratio, that occurs around 35 weeks of gestation,[277] and this change correlates clinically with a low incidence of RDS after the 34th week[278] (Table 25–16). Testing in high-risk patients does not usually begin until the 34th week of gestation. Thus, in some cases in which the test

indicates immaturity and yet the infant does not develop RDS, it is because the tested parameter changes (matures) over the time between the test and delivery.

In all quantitative tests of fetal lung maturity, picking any one value for a cutoff changes the number of false positives and false negatives for the test. The consequences of a false-positive test (mature study and yet the infant develops RDS because of an elective premature delivery) must be weighed against the risk of a false-negative test. In this case, immature studies may lead to delayed delivery in cases in which there is lung maturity. Because almost all such testing is done in high-risk patients with an increased risk of in utero death, the consequences of delay will be fatal in some cases in which prompt delivery would have allowed survival. Fortunately, exogenously administered surfactant has greatly reduced the incidence and severity of hyaline membrane disease in premature newborns and allows for earlier delivery of high-risk fetuses with much less pulmonary morbidity.

Conditions that result in abnormal increases in amniotic fluid volume (polyhydramnios) result in lowered lung maturity indices (presumably on a dilutional basis).[279] The converse does not hold, and oligohydramnios does not alter test

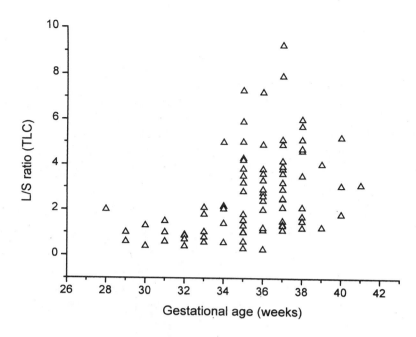

Figure 25–54. Correlation between the lecithin-sphingomyelin (L/S) ratio (determined by thin-layer chromatography) and gestational age. Before gestation week 35, very few tested fetuses have a mature L/S ratio (>2). (From Liu KZ, Dembinski TC, Mantsch HH: Prediction of RDS from amniotic fluid analysis: A comparison of the prognostic value of TLC and infra-red spectroscopy. Prenat Diagn 1998; 18:1267–1275.)

results. Fetal lung maturity, as reflected in amniotic fluid tests, is delayed in hypertensive pregnant patients, and glucocorticoid therapy (usually betamethasone) increases all lung maturity indices except phosphatidylglycerol (see below).[280]

Lecithin-Sphingomyelin Ratio. The standard method of assessing lung maturity is the L/S ratio. This test compares the concentrations of two phospholipids, lecithin and sphingomyelin, in amniotic fluid obtained by amniocentesis. Thin-layer chromatography (TLC) is used to assay the two substances, and the ratio is assessed either by planimetry using calipers or stoichiometrically by measurement of organic phosphorus from the chromatograph spots. Planimetric L/S and stoichiometric L/S can thus give different values. Before 34 weeks, both lecithin and sphingomyelin are present in approximately equal amounts. After 34 weeks, the amount of lecithin increases and the amount of sphingomyelin de-

creases (Fig. 25–55). An L/S ratio of 2:1 is taken as indicative of lung maturity. Figure 25–54 shows the high correlation between L/S ratio and gestational age, the primary determinant of fetal lung maturity. Unfortunately, the utility of the L/S ratio in predicting specific clinical outcomes is less than ideal. A 1992 study found that 20% of infants who developed RDS of prematurity had an L/S ratio greater than 2.[281] Blood or meconium in amniotic fluid invalidates the test. Despite this and other limitations, the L/S ratio remains the gold standard for assessing fetal lung maturity at most institutions.

Phosphatidylglycerol. One reason that a significant number of fetuses with L/S ratios above 2 still, if delivered at that point, develop RDS is thought to be a lack of phosphatidylglycerol. This compound appears to stabilize lecithin in surfactant. Phosphatidylglycerol measurements of 3% or greater in the amniotic fluid indicate functional lung maturity. Phosphatidylglycerol is not present in blood, vaginal secretions, or meconium, so these contaminants do not confuse the interpretation as they do in all surfactant tests.

Shake Test. The shake test is a functional test of surfactant. It is performed by mixing amniotic fluid with 95% ethanol at dilutions of 1:1, 1:1.3, 1:2, and 1:4. The mixtures are shaken for 15 seconds and then left to stand for 15 minutes. The shake test is considered mature if a stable complete foam ring at the meniscus occurs in the 1:2 dilution.

Foam Stability Index. This semiquantitative test, a commercial modification of the shake test, is based on the ability of pulmonary surfactant to generate stable foam in the presence of ethanol, an inhibitor of foaming. Serial tube dilutions of amniotic fluid and ethanol are shaken for 15 seconds and then, after 15 minutes, observed for the presence of stable foam. A complete ring of bubbles in the meniscus constitutes a positive test. Results are reported in terms of the volume fraction of ethanol, and the foam stability index value is the highest ethanol volume fraction (volume of ethanol/volume of ethanol + volume of amniotic fluid) that will

Table 25–16. Neonatal Outcome in Relation to Gestational Age

	Weeks' Gestation		
	34	35	36
N	121	156	139
Birth weight (g)	2358 ±321	2466 ±255	2502 ±398
NICU admissions	24	3*	2*
5-min Apgar score <7	4	0†	0†
Hospital stay >7 d	24	18†	8*
Birth weight <2000 g	9	1†	0*
RDS	18 (14.9%)	1* (0.6%)	0* (0%)
Preterm rupture of membranes	5 (12.2%)	0† (0%)	0† (0%)
Preterm labor	13 (16.3%)	1* (0.9%)	0* (0%)

NICU, neonatal intensive care unit; RDS, respiratory distress syndrome.
* $P < .05$ (compared against 34-week group).
† $P < .001$ (compared against 34-week group).
Modified from Lewis DF, Futayyeh S, Towers CV, et al: Preterm delivery from 34 to 37 weeks of gestation: Is respiratory distress syndrome a problem? Am J Obstet Gynecol 1996; 174:525–528.

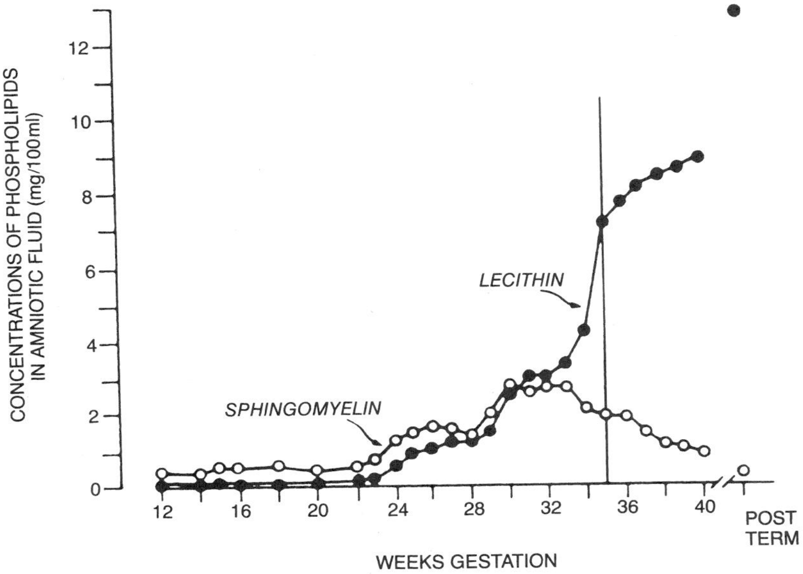

Figure 25–55. Changes in concentrations of lecithin and sphingomyelin in amniotic fluid over the course of a normal pregnancy. (From Gluck L, Kulovich MV: Lechithin/sphingomyelin ratios in normal and abnormal pregnancy. Am J Obstet Gynecol 1973; 115:541.)

allow foam to persist. Thus, a foam stability index of 47 indicates that when 0.443 mL of ethanol was added to 0.5 mL of centrifuged amniotic fluid and shaken, there was a continuous ring of bubbles around the meniscus, but when 0.48 mL of ethanol was added, the meniscal ring was discontinuous.

Fluorescent Polarization Techniques. Two current tests utilize fluorescent dyes that are synthetic derivatives of lecithin and have binding and solubility characteristics similar to those of surfactant-associated phospholipids. One such dye is NBD-phosphatidylcholine (NBD-PC) and the other is PC16; the latter is used in an automated kit marketed as the TDx fetal lung maturity assay (Abbott Laboratories, Abbott Park, IL). The fluorescent dye partitions between albumin and phospholipid in amniotic fluid samples, and the degree of partitioning can be measured using a standard polarimeter, which is available in virtually all laboratories. The polarization measured by the analyzer reflects the ratio of surfactant to albumin in the amniotic fluid sample, and this value correlates with lung maturity. Fetal conditions that result in decreased levels of albumin in the amniotic fluid, such as urinary tract obstruction, can give a normal ratio when, in fact, surfactant production is below normal.

There is no universally agreed-upon maturity value for the surfactant-albumin ratio when using fluorescence polarization. The manufacturer of the TDx test kit has recently lowered the cutoff value for maturity to 55 mg/g. The previous value of 70 mg/g was thought to be associated with too many false-negative tests (showing immaturity when the infant was in fact mature). However, this is still an area of controversy.[282–284]

Lamellar Body Count. Pulmonary surfactant is packaged into structures known as lamellar bodies within type II pneumocytes in the lung, and these lamellar bodies are released by exocytosis into the alveolus. A count of lamellar bodies (LBC) in amniotic fluid can be rapidly performed using standard automated counters. With an LBC cutoff value of 50,000/μL, the diagnostic sensitivity and specificity for estimating fetal lung maturity were 100% and 80% in a recent study of 170 neonates.[285] All cases of RDS had an LBC of 50,000/μL or less.

Refractive Index-Matched Anomalous Defraction (RIMAD). The RIMAD is another tool for assessment of fetal lung maturity. By subtracting the absorbance at 650 nm (A650) of amniotic fluid diluted in glycerol from that of amniotic fluid diluted in water, the total light scattered by the surfactant-containing lamellar bodies is determined; this allows an estimation of the concentration of lamellar bodies and correlation with lung maturity. The test is not significantly affected by such contaminating chromogens as hemoglobin and bilirubin at the usual clinical levels. However, microamounts of erythrocytes result in significant interference. Use of a RIMAD referent value of greater than 0.040 to indicate fetal lung maturity yielded results that were comparable to the TDx assay—the predictive value for RDS was 72% and the predictive value for lung maturity was 100%.[286] However, the study numbers were small, and further testing will be necessary before the test can be recommended.

Infrared (IR) Spectroscopy. IR spectroscopy is a new method for the determination of fetal lung maturity using a commercial spectrometer to analyze amniotic fluid[277] (Fig. 25–56). The IR spectra have been calibrated using TLC-based L/S ratios. In clinical application, IR spectroscopy was highly accurate in predicting the absence of RDS (97%). The prediction accuracy for the presence of RDS was 83%, which compares favorably with all other tests. The test requires only microscopic amounts of amniotic fluid, leaving material for other tests such as alpha-fetoprotein and chromosomal analysis. Also, IR spectroscopy has recently been used to quantitate lactate and glucose in the amniotic fluid.[287] Lactate in amniotic fluid comes from fetal metabolism and is highly indicative of anaerobic glycolysis and fetal hypoxemia. Decreased amniotic fluid glucose is a marker for infection. Thus, if IR spectroscopy proves to be equivalent to other tests of fetal maturity, the additional information that can be obtained from the same microsample will likely result in increased use of this technology.

Evaluation of the Fetal Lung Maturity Tests. Both

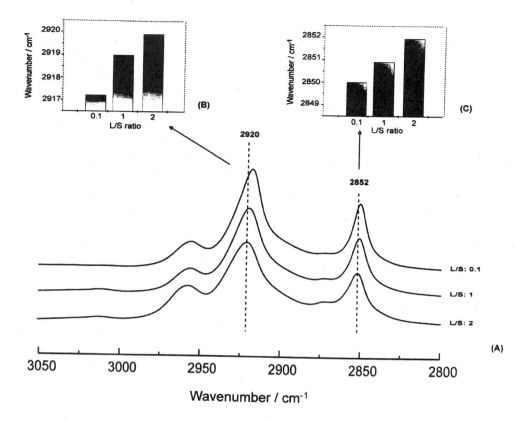

Figure 25–56. Infrared spectra from solutions with lecithin-sphingomyelin ratios of 0.1, 1, and 2. *Insets* show details of band frequency distribution. (From Liu KZ, Dembinski TC, Mantsch HH: Prediction of RDS from amniotic fluid analysis: A comparison of the prognostic value of TLC and infrared spectroscopy. Prenat Diagn 1998; 18:1267–1275.)

L/S and phosphatidylglycerol assays require 2-D TLC, a process that takes 3 to 4 hours. TLC technology is very dependent on the technical skill of the person performing the test. The assignment of quantitative values to a smear on a gel plate is inherently imprecise, and TLC tests suffer from poor precision and poor interlaboratory agreement.[288] The shake test and the foam stability index are faster than TLC (15 to 25 minutes turnaround time) but still require technician expertise and depend on the subjective interpretations of the test. Fluorescence polarization, LBC, and IR spectroscopy are all simple tests that can be done in less than 30 to 45 minutes, with minimal technical skills.[277, 285, 289] Consequently, the tests are very precise and have excellent interlaboratory agreement. Costs are lower with all of the discussed tests compared with TLC tests (L/S and phosphatidylglycerol). Because a positive test, indicating lung maturity, has a very high predictive rate (>96%) regardless of the test used, performing a second test following a positive result contributes very little to improving predictive ability. However, because of the weakness of all tests in correctly predicting RDS when the test indicates immaturity, cascade (sequential) testing does offer the benefit of improving predictive ability in the case of an initial immature test result. Cascade testing requires two or more different tests that indicate immaturity before that determination is made. For all cascade testing, starting with a rapid, high-precision, low-cost test offers the most cost-efficient approach. As medical costs are subjected to greater scrutiny, it is likely that simple and inexpensive tests will be revived and supplement more costly and technologically intense tests that provide no greater predictive value.

Magnetic Resonance Spectroscopy. All present tests for fetal lung maturity require amniocentesis, which is time-consuming, expensive, and not without risk. Lecithin, a marker for lung maturity, can be detected by MR spectroscopy using a whole-body scanner.[290] MR spectroscopy is a noninvasive method for the in vivo localization and identification of molecules with known resonance peaks at specified chemical shifts. It has been recently reported that amniotic fluid at term demonstrates a resonance peak at 3.2 ppm; this is the same as the chemical shift of lecithin in saline. The lecithin peak was not observed in preterm amniotic fluid. If the technology proves to have clinical efficacy, the main advantage will be the noninvasive nature of the test. The disadvantage will be cost and the requirement that the mother be in a whole-body scanner.

Intrapartum Fetal Monitoring

Intrapartum Fetal Heart Rate Monitoring

Evaluation of FHR patterns remains the cornerstone of monitoring for the purpose of assessing fetal well-being during labor. Auscultation of the FHR using a stethoscope provides very limited information other than identifying extremes of heart rate and arrhythmias. Owing to the intermittent nature of this technique, significant abnormalities may be present but not detected. Maximum information from FHR monitoring is obtained with continuous beat-to-beat monitoring for an extended period of time using electronic monitoring equipment. Despite this seemingly obvious statement regarding the information differences between intermittent stethoscopic auscultation and continuous electronic monitoring of FHR, there is a tremendous amount of controversy and confusion in this area.

The original rationale for the introduction of FHR monitoring was that it could allow the recognition of asphyxia at a sufficiently early stage so that timely obstetric intervention would avoid asphyxia-induced brain damage or death. The initial definitions of FHR patterns evolved from large numbers of investigators worldwide in the 1960s. However, four decades later, a National Institute of Child Health and Human Development (NICHHD) Research Planning Workshop[291] produced the following conclusions:

> A major impediment to progress in the evaluation and investigation of FHR monitoring is lack of agreement in definitions and nomenclature of FHR patterns despite the plethora of publications on the subject. Although there are at least 12 controlled trials of the efficacy of FHR monitoring, it is rarely possible to determine from most of the publications exactly what the authors used for definitions and quantification of the various patterns. In addition, the FHR patterns signifying jeopardy for the fetus and the need for immediate delivery are often inexactly stated, and quantitation is rarely included . . . it would be premature to recommend another randomized control trial at this stage because there is not yet a commonly agreed on protocol for intervention. (p 1385)

This lack of precision in the use of FHR monitoring information has led to inconclusive studies and consequently much controversy over the value of the technology. The ACOG guidelines for intrapartum monitoring state that "within specified intervals, intermittent auscultation is equivalent to continuous electronic fetal monitoring in detecting fetal compromise."[292] This applies to both high-risk and low-risk pregnancies. Unfortunately, the basis for this guideline has been the very studies found to be so deficient by the NICHHD. Thus, FHR monitoring is a field in which there is inadequate agreement on the definitions, quantification, and significance of the changes in the FHR so that when separate evaluators review the same FHR tracing, one finds "fetal distress" and the other does not. To compound this, for the ones that find "fetal distress," some would intervene immediately (emergent cesarean section for fetal distress) while others would temporize.

Another problem is that the currently used definitions, however imprecise, fail to take into consideration the fact that the response of the fetus to various conditions is different depending on gestational age. Cibils,[293] in an excellent review of the controversy in this area stated:

> The inappropriate use of FHR monitoring is clear from the conclusions of controlled studies that show intermittent auscultation to be equal to or better than continuous FHR monitoring . . . Under no circumstance can an intermittent recording of a phenomenon give information that is better than its continuous recording; if the conclusions drawn from the latter are not correct it behooves the interpreter to refine his or her understanding of it. To use electronic fetal monitoring properly it is necessary to start a new learning of the physiology of the fetus, its changing evolution as pregnancy advances, its different responses under stress or distress, and the various ways these are represented in electronic fetal monitoring tracings.

The reason that stethoscopic surveillance is acceptable, even though it cannot identify early fetal distress, is that the true incidence of fetal distress is so low — about 2%. Thus, 98% of low-risk mothers monitored in this manner, or in any other manner, can be expected to deliver vigorous infants. Because of the small numbers of affected fetuses (fetal distress), it takes very large numbers to generate meaningful studies. Such numbers (>100,000 births) have been obtained from nonrandomized surveys and the following information was generated. The interpartum stillbirth rate decreased

from 2.4 to 0.5/1000 with monitoring ($P < .0001$), and the neonatal death rate decreased from 8.1 to 3.6/1000 with monitoring ($P < .0001$). The data are suggestive, but not conclusive, that routine fetal monitoring can improve neonatal outcomes. On the basis of these data, Parer[294] in 1984 predicted that future studies should expect to show a benefit of 5 saved lives per 1000 high-risk births through the proper use of electronic monitoring, and 1 saved life per 1000 low-risk births.

A recent randomized study by Vintzileos et al.,[295] while suffering the limitation of numbers in that only 1428 patients were studied, reported that patients monitored electronically had a greater incidence of nonreassuring FHR patterns compared with those monitored by intermittent auscultation (23.4% vs. 10.7%) and a higher rate of cesarean delivery for suspected fetal distress (5.3% vs. 2.3%). There were no differences in 1- and 5-minute Apgar scores, fetal acidosis at birth, need for neonatal resuscitation, neonatal ICU admission, use of assisted ventilation, neonatal hospital stay, or any other neonatal complications between the two groups. This would tend to support the position of those who claim that electronic monitoring leads to increased rates of operative delivery without altering outcomes. However, there was one major difference between the two groups in this study. The perinatal death rate related to fetal asphyxia was significantly less in the electronically monitored group (0 of 746 vs. 6 of 682). This randomized, prospective study confirmed that in the vast majority of cases, the nature of intrapartum fetal surveillance is of little consequence. However, it also provided evidence that in a small number of cases, possibly less than 1%, electronic monitoring detects early fetal hypoxia. Recognition of fetal hypoxia allows accelerated delivery, likely by cesarean section, and thus decreases neonatal mortality when compared to intermittent auscultation, which does not permit detection of early fetal distress. The results of this study confirm the predictions of Parer.[294] Vintzilios et al. stated that intensive training in FHR monitoring was given to the medical staff who participated in Parer's study as one cannot expect to show a benefit with an improperly applied technology.[295]

In addition to decreasing fetal mortality, the early hope for electronic heart rate monitoring was that it would decrease the incidence of cerebral palsy. However, most cerebral palsy (about 80%) is not related to intrapartum events[296-298]; thus, intrapartum monitoring cannot be expected to have an impact on these cases. Also, "the recording of one fetal pathophysiologic response to labor cannot predict what will happen to that fetus later in life when even a most meticulous neonatal examination by neurologists within the first month of life cannot do it. It follows that one cannot ask from a test more than what it can give . . ."[293]

Thus it is unrealistic to expect that the monitoring of intrapartum heart rate can identify with any degree of sensitivity and specificity those fetuses destined to have cerebral palsy at a stage at which intervention could alter the outcome. A recent study estimated that among 100,000 singleton children born at term, 9.3%, or 9300, would be expected to have multiple late decelerations or decreased beat-to-beat variability on fetal monitoring.[299] These findings were shown to greatly increase the risk of cerebral palsy. Of those with these FHR abnormalities, about 18 children (0.19% of 9300) would be expected to have cerebral palsy. If in 20% of these children cerebral palsy might be related to asphyxia during delivery and if there were an intervention that could prevent asphyxia-related cerebral palsy once monitoring abnormalities were recognized, then approximately 4 of 100,000 full-term infants might benefit. However, the authors pointed out that the intervention would be administered in 9296 (9300 minus 4) additional deliveries (2324 nonbeneficial interventions for each child in whom cerebral palsy was prevented).

It is unclear whether electronic monitoring has led to an increase in the rate of cesarean sections. The number has increased, but it reflects factors other than monitoring, such as changed management for genital herpes and breech presentation, as well as the decline of midforceps interventions. However, it is likely that part of this increase has resulted from inadequate interpretation of FHR patterns. The performance of heart rate monitoring as a tool for predicting fetal distress has been shown to be significantly enhanced by the use of computer analysis of heart rate tracings.[274] This supports the position that the tool is valid, and it is the variation in the human observation component that is the main area of weakness.

In a certain portion of cases in which vigorous infants were delivered by emergent cesarean section for suspected fetal distress based on fetal heart tracings, the fetal condition would have deteriorated over time if labor had been allowed to continue. Thus, higher rates of cesarean section for fetal distress do not necessarily equate with unnecessary surgery. In the study by Vintzileos et al. cited above, even though the cesarean rate for *fetal distress* was twice as high in patients monitored electronically, there was a significantly lower incidence of fetal deaths due to intrapartum hypoxia compared with patients monitored by auscultation.[295]

The protocols under which the ACOG find intermittent auscultation acceptable for intrapartum monitoring are stringent.[292] The FHR must be auscultated within 15 minutes of arrival in the delivery suite. The FHR must be auscultated every 15 minutes for a full minute during the first stage of labor and every 5 minutes during the second stage of labor, again for a full minute. The data must also be recorded at the time they are measured. This requires a 1:1 nurse-patient ratio, and consumes a considerable amount of nursing time. When this protocol was applied in a busy university setting, over half the patients had to be initially excluded because 1:1 nursing care was not available. In 19 of 442 patients in whom intermittent auscultation was attempted, auscultation was impossible because of maternal obesity. In the remaining 423 patients, auscultation as the mode of monitoring was discontinued in 392 patients because of inability to maintain the stringent frequency of auscultation and recording.[300] Acceptance of intermittent monitoring without provision of staffing requirements raises standard-of-care concerns, and failure to meet the stringent requirements involves an unacceptable liability exposure.

Fetal Heart Rate Changes. FHR changes consist of baseline changes and periodic changes. Baseline changes include beat-to-beat variability, tachycardia, and bradycardia. Periodic changes refer to deceleration patterns: early, late, and variable accelerations in heart rate. All periodic changes are calculated from the most recently determined portion of the baseline.

Baseline Changes

BEAT-TO-BEAT VARIABILITY. The baseline FHR is normally 110 to 160 bpm. In the healthy fetus, there is a slight difference in the interval between successive heartbeats. This is known as beat-to-beat variability, or short-term variability. Beat-to-beat variability produces the irregular baseline seen in normal FHR tracings (Fig. 25–57). The physiologic origins and significance of this variability are not known with certainty, but clinical evidence suggests that its presence confirms an intact pathway from the cerebral cortex to the midbrain, to the vagus nerve, to the cardiac conduction system.[301] Sporadic input from various areas in the cerebral cortex is transmitted to the cardiac centers in the medulla oblongata. This results in continuously varying levels of vagal stimulation, and the heart rate reflects this uneven input. Cerebral asphyxia causes decreased heart rate variability (Fig. 25–58), possibly because of decreased cerebral input to the midbrain. Absent beat-to-beat variability is seen in anencephalic infants, in whom there is an absence of cerebral cortex. It may also be caused by drugs that depress higher brain centers, such as narcotics and sedatives. Anticholinergic drugs in high doses decrease variability. Defects in the fetal cardiac conduction system also cause loss of variability.

During labor, one should rarely if ever make the diagnosis of fetal asphyxia based solely on a lack of heart rate variability. However, in the presence of other indicators of fetal distress, the presence or absence of heart rate variability is highly significant.

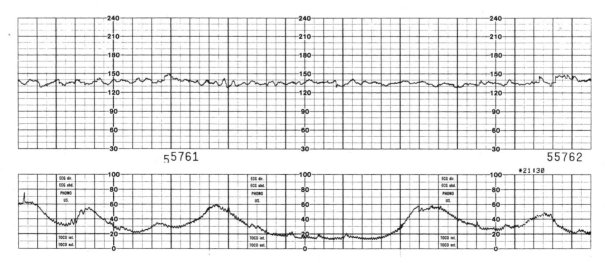

Figure 25–57. Normal fetal heart rate tracing (*upper trace*) showing good beat-to-beat variability, a baseline rate of 135 bpm, and no heart rate changes with uterine contractions (*lower trace*).

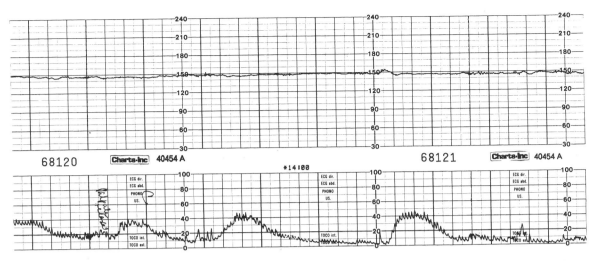

Figure 25–58. Decreased beat-to-beat variability. The fetal heart rate trace is almost a straight line.

FETAL TACHYCARDIA. *Fetal tachycardia* is defined as a heart rate greater than 160 bpm. If normal variability is present, tachycardia does not indicate asphyxia (Fig. 25–59). However, tachycardia may be seen in the recovery phase following a period of asphyxia and the resultant release of catecholamines. Other causes of tachycardia are maternal or fetal infection, especially chorioamnionitis, drugs such as β_2 agonists or parasympathetic blockers, tachydysrhythmias, and thyrotoxicosis.

FETAL BRADYCARDIA. Bradycardia in the fetus is a sustained (>2 minutes) heart rate less than 110 bpm. Bradycardia is the initial response of a normal fetus to acute hypoxia. If normal variability is present, it indicates that the fetus is able to tolerate mild hypoxic states by the compensatory mechanisms already discussed, namely, redistribution of blood flow, decreased oxygen consumption, and anaerobic glycolysis. In some patients moderate bradycardia is idiopathic and benign and does not represent hypoxia.

Other causes of bradycardia are less common. Complete heart block (CHB), a condition associated with a significant incidence of structural heart disease, may be present. Congenital heart block may also be seen in the offspring of mothers with systemic lupus erythematosus. Bradycardia can be caused by maternal medications, such as β blockers or local anesthetics. Of particular note is the high incidence of fetal bradycardia following paracervical block.

Bradycardia due to CHB, in the absence of structural heart disease, is better tolerated than sinus bradycardia (SB) at the same rate (e.g., 50 bpm) because the atrial rate tends to be twice as fast in CHB (see Fig. 25–50). The slow atrial rate of SB is associated with greater abnormalities of blood flow streaming, so that there is greater mixing of oxygenated and deoxygenated blood in the right atrium and, therefore, lower oxygen saturation in blood leaving the LV for the brain and myocardium. Also, there is a greater amount of reverse flow in the vena cava (an undesirable finding) during SB than during comparable episodes of bradycardia due to CHB.[302]

Severe bradycardia, with heart rates below 60 bpm, even-

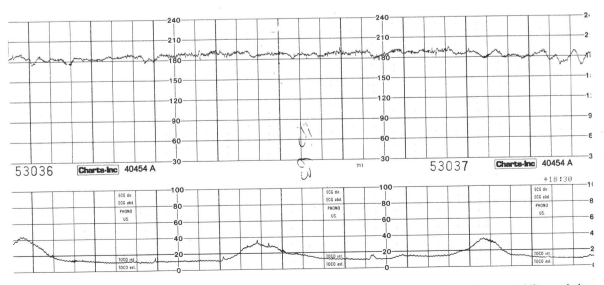

Figure 25–59. Fetal tachycardia. The baseline fetal heart rate is 190 bpm, but there is good beat-to-beat variability and there are no deceleration patterns.

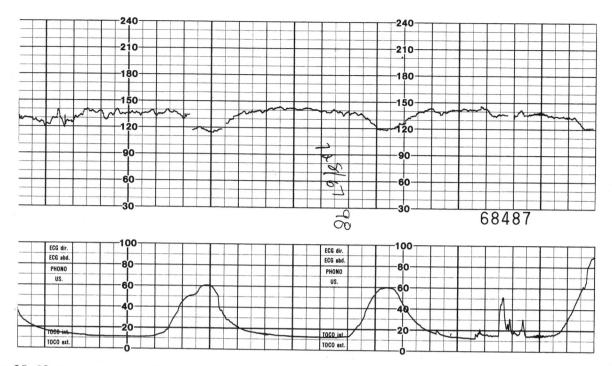

Figure 25-60. Early decelerations. The onset of the fetal heart rate slowing corresponds to the onset of the uterine contraction. Although early decelerations may resemble late decelerations, this pattern is not associated with fetal distress but is attributed to vagal discharge, possibly in response to fetal head compression. This infant was subsequently delivered by cesarean section for prolonged bradycardia. At delivery, the infant had a tight nuchal cord, but Apgar scores of 9 and 9 at 1 and 5 minutes.

tually results in cardiac decompensation and must be managed urgently. In the fetus, because cardiac output is primarily determined by heart rate, a decrease in heart rate signifies a decrease in cardiac output. The decreased cardiac output causes less blood to circulate through the placenta, causing progressively lower oxygen tension in circulating blood and the accumulation of tissue acids. Unless this process is reversed, severe bradycardia will eventually result in insufficient oxygen delivery to support myocardial demand and the fetus will die.

Heart Rate Accelerations. FHR accelerations with fetal movements or maternal contractions correlate highly with fetal well-being. *Acceleration* is defined as a visually apparent abrupt (peak in < 30 seconds) increase in FHR above the baseline. The acme is at least 15 bpm above the baseline, and the acceleration lasts at least 15 seconds but less than 2 minutes from the onset to return to baseline. Before 32 weeks of gestation, accelerations are defined as having an acme of at least 10 bpm above the baseline and a duration of at least 10 seconds. Prolonged accelerations last longer than 2 minutes. If the acceleration lasts 10 minutes or longer, it represents a baseline change.

Periodic Fetal Heart Rate Changes. There are three specific periodic deceleration patterns: early decelerations, late decelerations, and variable decelerations. Heart rate slowing with contractions is not normal. A normal FHR pattern has a baseline rate between 110 and 160 bpm with good beat-to-beat variability and no periodic changes (heart rate decelerations with contractions; see Fig. 25-57). Prolonged deceleration of the FHR is a visually apparent decrease in FHR below the baseline of at least 15 bpm lasting at least 2 minutes but less than 10 minutes. A prolonged deceleration of 10 minutes or greater is a baseline change.

EARLY DECELERATIONS. Early deceleration of the FHR occurs concomitantly with the uterine contraction and is a visually apparent gradual (time to nadir at least 30 seconds) decrease and return to baseline. Early decelerations are coincident in timing, with the nadir of the deceleration occurring at the same time as the peak of the contraction; they are a mirror image of the uterine contraction (Fig. 25-60). Early decelerations are mild (<20 bpm below baseline). The cause is unknown, although the usual explanation is fetal head compression.

LATE DECELERATIONS. Late deceleration of the FHR is a visually apparent gradual (onset of deceleration to nadir at least 30 seconds) decrease and return to baseline associated with a uterine contraction (Fig. 25-61). The deceleration is delayed in timing, with the nadir of the deceleration occurring after the peak of the contraction. In most cases the onset, nadir, and recovery of the deceleration occur after the beginning, peak, and ending of the contraction, respectively.

This pattern is indicative of uteroplacental insufficiency. UBF decreases during the contraction, and fetal blood returning from the placenta is not adequately oxygenated. Chemoreceptors sense the low oxygen tension and trigger a vagal discharge. As long as cerebral oxygenation is maintained, FHR variability should also remain normal, in spite of the late decelerations. However, if the deoxygenation is severe enough, it may affect the CNS. Cerebral hypoxia will cause decreased or absent beat-to-beat variability, as seen in Figure 25-61. The pattern of late decelerations coupled with decreased beat-to-beat variability is the only specific FHR pattern that is associated with increased fetal mortality and long-term neurologic sequelae. Late decelerations often occur in the setting of an already impaired placental reserve, such as preeclampsia or intrauterine growth retardation. The combination of late decelerations with absent variability is an

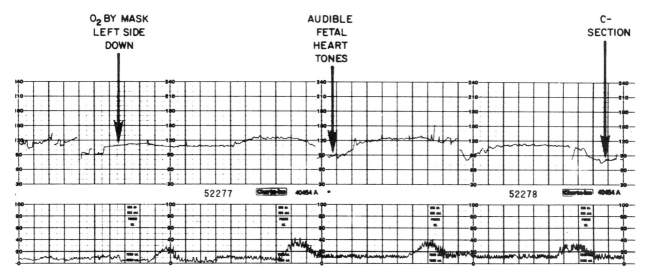

O₂ BY MASK LEFT SIDE DOWN

AUDIBLE FETAL HEART TONES

C-SECTION

Figure 25–61. Late decelerations. The slowing of the fetal heart rate coincides with the peak of the uterine contraction. The absence of beat-to-beat variability is indicative of a decompensated fetus. The persistence of late decelerations and a low baseline heart rate compared to an earlier rate of 145 bpm prompted an emergency cesarean section. The infant was severely depressed; Apgar scores were 1 (1 minute), 2 (5 minutes), and 6 (10 minutes).

ominous pattern, because it indicates that each contraction stresses the fetus beyond its compensatory capacity.[297]

The treatment of the maternal-fetal unit when late decelerations occur consists of efforts to optimize placental blood flow and oxygenation. Maternal position should be changed—particularly if the mother is lying supine—in order to eliminate the mechanical effects of the uterus on the aorta or vena cava. In Figure 25–61, the documented response to the FHR of 110 bpm with absent variability was to administer oxygen, place the patient on her left side, and notify the obstetrician. Maternal hypotension must be corrected by proper positioning and blood pressure support with ephedrine. One hundred percent oxygen should be delivered to the mother by sealed face mask rather than nasal cannula. It takes almost 10 minutes for maternally administered oxygen to reach *maximal* value as measured by fetal pulse oximetry.[303] However, there is a lag between changes in central oxygen values and those in the skin, and maximal value is not necessary for improvement in fetal

oxygen status. Uterine activity can be reduced by stopping oxytocin if it is being infused, or by the use of tocolytic agents, most often terbutaline. Uterine hypertonus can be most rapidly treated by the IV administration of small boluses (50 to 100 μg) of NTG.[304]

Measures to increase uterine perfusion and oxygenation will often correct late decelerations in which good beat-to-beat variability is still present, as the presence of variability indicates a margin of fetal reserve. In a decompensated fetus, these measures, although still important, are less likely to improve the status of the fetus, and immediate delivery is required.

VARIABLE DECELERATIONS. *Variable deceleration* of the FHR is defined as a visually apparent abrupt decrease (onset of deceleration to beginning of nadir < 30 seconds) in FHR below the baseline. The decrease in FHR must be at least 15 bpm, last at least 15 seconds, and return to baseline within 2 minutes. When variable decelerations are associated

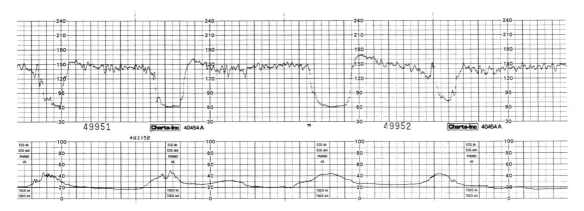

Figure 25–62. Severe variable decelerations. The deceleration tends to mirror the uterine contraction. Fetal heart rate often overshoots the baseline at the termination of the deceleration. Note the variable appearance of each deceleration tracing relative to the preceding tracing. Despite the dramatic appearance of this "severe" pattern, there is still good beat-to-beat variability present, and this infant was delivered vaginally with Apgar scores of 7 (1 minute) and 9 (5 minutes).

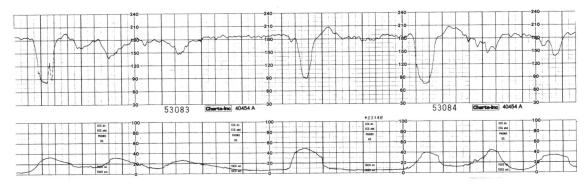

Figure 25–63. Variable decelerations. Compared with Figure 25–62, there is less beat-to-beat variability. This heart rate tracing is from the same infant as in Figure 25–59, but 5 hours later. The baseline tachycardia is still present, but now there is decreased beat-to-beat variability, and persistent variable decelerations, identified by the lack of uniformity of the deceleration tracings. The mother was an insulin-dependent diabetic. She was allowed to deliver vaginally. The infant weighed 3680 g, and had a 1-minute Apgar score of 3 and a 5-minute score of 8.

with uterine contractions, their onset, depth, and duration commonly vary with successive uterine contractions. There is no definite relationship to uterine contractions (Figs. 25–62 and 25–63). When there is a delayed rather than abrupt return to baseline, transient hypoxemia is most likely occurring.

Variable decelerations are believed to represent vagal firing in response to cord compression or sustained head compression, as when the mother is pushing during the second stage of labor. Temporary mechanical occlusion of the umbilical vein causes increased resistance to fetal umbilical arterial flow. If the pressure in the umbilical vein, and hence the placenta vessels, is higher than the diastolic pressure in the umbilical artery, there will be a reversal of flow during part of the cardiac cycle. This results in a to-and-fro movement of blood that is readily recorded using Doppler flow velocimetry. This decrease in arterial perfusion causes a prompt and often dramatic heart rate deceleration.[305] However, in other cases the decrease in perfusion appears to be the result and not the cause of the deceleration of the FHR. This may be the result of a parasympathetic reaction in the CNS caused by either systemic or local hypoxemia; the latter might occur when the head is compressed. Fetal head compression pressures in the range of 38 to 390 mmHg (mean, 158 mmHg) have been measured during the second stage of labor.[306]

The presence or absence of baseline variability in the presence of variable decelerations correlates with oxygenation of central tissues and is indicative of the severity of the stress producing the decelerations. Measures to improve uterine perfusion and oxygenation are the same as those used to treat late decelerations.

Predictive Value of Fetal Heart Rate Patterns. A normal FHR pattern (rate 120 to 160 bpm with good beat-to-beat variability and no late or variable decelerations) during the last 30 minutes of labor is predictive of a vigorous infant at birth greater than 98% of the time, even in high-risk pregnancies, assuming that the delivery is atraumatic and the infant has no congenital malformation inconsistent with extrauterine life, such as tracheal atresia or aplastic lungs.[297] However, the converse is not true. Heart rate patterns of variable or late decelerations do not guarantee a depressed newborn. Earlier studies of late and variable decelerations showed very little correlation between these patterns and depressed newborns; in part this was because of failure to subdivide patient populations on the basis of heart rate variability.[307] Patients with decelerations and adequate variability often have a low 1-minute Apgar score but usually have a 5-minute Apgar score of 8 or above. The presence of decelerations and decreased variability increases the risk for significant neonatal depression. Severe deceleration patterns with absence of variability are almost always associated with an asphyxiated fetus that will likely require active resuscitation. It is the fetus that presents an indeterminate heart rate pattern that causes the most uncertainty; it is in this situation that other testing, such as scalp blood samples for assessment of metabolic acidosis, and fetal Doppler flow velocimetry, can help identify the fetus that needs immediate delivery.

The vast majority of fetuses with major congenital anomalies will have normal FHR patterns. Exceptions are anencephaly and congenital heart disease with CBC.

Techniques of Fetal Heart Rate Monitoring. Meaningful FHR monitoring requires both the FHR pattern plus the pattern of uterine contractions to assess the relationship between the two. There are four methods of obtaining the FHR. Intermittent stethoscopic auscultation remains a main form of surveillance during labor in low-risk pregnancies and continues to be used in high-risk pregnancies despite the fact that there is no auscultatory pattern of early fetal distress. Auscultation is able to identify only the extreme condition. The patterns of variable and late decelerations were only described in 1967 with the advent of electronic monitoring techniques.[308] They were never recognized through the stethoscope by generations of skilled clinicians.

Phonocardiography and Doppler ultrasound are both non-invasive and detect sounds produced by the fetal heart valves. Neither technique is adequate for assessing beat-to-beat variability but each can be used to detect deceleration patterns. ECG can be either indirect from the maternal abdomen or direct from stainless steel spiral electrodes placed in the infant's scalp (see Fig. 25–15). The latter technique is invasive and cannot be performed if the maternal membranes are intact. It carries the risk of fetal scalp infection, facial injury (particularly the eye), and bleeding. However, this technique provides the most precise data on beat-to-beat variability for clinical decision making.

Intrapartum Doppler Velocimetry

Intrapartum Doppler velocimetry may be used to assist in identification of true distress when there are FHR changes of concern. For example, in one study of 102 parturients with a presumptive diagnosis of fetal distress based on FHR patterns, 82 patients had normal S/D ratios and 20 had abnor-

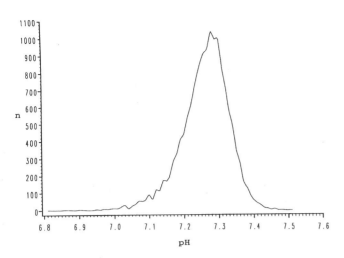

Figure 25–64. Distribution of values for umbilical artery pH in healthy newborns. The mean pH is 7.26. (From Helwig JT, Parer JT, Kilpatrick SJ, et al: Umbilical cord blood acid-base state: What is normal? Am J Obstet Gynecol 1996; 174:1807–1812.)

mal ratios. Eighteen neonates (90%) in the abnormal S/D ratio group had at least one adverse outcome, compared with only 13 (15.8%) of those with a normal S/D ratio.[309] In an interesting observational study, it was found that knowledge of a concurrent Doppler flow study affected the physicians' interpretation of FHR patterns; they were more likely to interpret heart rate changes as benign if they were aware that the fetus had a Doppler study that did not indicate stress.[310]

Fetal Acid-Base Status

When a FHR pattern is suggestive of fetal compromise, blood may be obtained from the fetal scalp for pH and base deficit measurement. The absence of acidosis is strong evidence for the lack of intrapartum fetal asphyxia. The mean umbilical artery pH of blood obtained immediately after delivery of *healthy* infants is 7.26 (Fig. 25–64 and Table 25–17). The umbilical artery carries deoxygenated fetal venous blood, while the umbilical vein carries oxygenated blood from the placenta. In cases of umbilical cord compression or obstruction, umbilical venous blood may not represent the true oxygen–acid-base status of the fetus.[311] The

normal mild acidosis of the healthy intrapartum fetus has both a respiratory component ($PaCO_2$ = 53 mmHg) and a metabolic component (base deficit, 4 mEq/L). An umbilical artery pH of 7.10 is 2 SD below the mean (2.5th percentile). The 2.5th percentiles for $PaCO_2$ and base deficit are 74 mmHg and 11 mEq/L (see Table 25–17). Figure 25–65 shows the relationship between fetal scalp O_2 saturations and fetal scalp pH; in the study, no fetus with a pH above 7.20 had low O_2 saturations (<30%).[312] Almost all fetuses with pH values below 7.20 had low O_2 saturations. Thus, 7.20 is a reasonable cutoff point for defining clinically relevant fetal acidosis. A pH value of 7.10 or less constitutes *severe* acidosis and a pH value of 7.00 constitutes *pathologic* acidosis. As pH levels decrease below 7.10, the risk of newborn mortality and long-term morbidity increases. However, the majority of fetuses with pH values below 7.0 will not require intensive care and have no apparent neurologic sequelae.[313]

When pH values fall in the range from 7.00 to 7.20, clinical interpretation is required. What is the maternal pH? Before a fetus is diagnosed as acidotic on the basis of a scalp sample, the maternal pH should be measured and the maternal-fetal pH difference evaluated. Use of this approach resulted in a 33% reduction in the rate of false-positive scalp samples (vigorous infant with "acidotic" scalp pH before delivery); acidotic babies born to acidotic mothers were all vigorous.[314] Also, what is the type of acidosis? A metabolic acidosis (base deficit >10 mEq/L) is indicative of asphyxia, most often due to uteroplacental failure.[315, 316] Respiratory acidosis (increased $PaCO_2$) is more likely to reflect umbilical cord compression, and has less severe consequences for the fetus.[252, 317] Table 25–18 presents data of the type of acidemia in the fetus at time of delivery by pH group.[313] In acidotic fetuses (pH <7.20) most of the acidosis was respiratory; it was only when the pH decreased to less than 7.00 that a significant metabolic component developed. Sixty-two percent of fetuses with a pH less than 7.00 had a mixed acidosis; of 3419 acidotic fetuses with pH between 7.00 and 7.19, only 2 had a mixed acidosis, and less than 3% had a metabolic acidosis. Was there any preceding maternal event, such as a seizure or anesthetic-induced maternal hypotension, to account for the fetal acidosis? In these cases, treatment of the maternal problem can be expected to correct the fetal acidosis. Also important is the timing of the fetal scalp sampling in relation to maternal contractions. The best information regarding the well-being of the fetus is obtained by sampling just before a contraction.

Increased lactic acid as the result of anaerobic glycolysis

Table 25–17. Umbilical Artery and Umbilical Vein Blood Gas Values Obtained Immediately After Delivery of 15,073 Healthy Infants

	Mean	SD	2.5th Percentile	5th Percentile
Umbilical Artery				
pH	7.26	0.07	7.10	7.13
PCO_2 (mmHg)	53	10	35	37
PO_2 (mmHg)	17	6	6	8
Base excess (mEq · L^{-1})	−4	3	−11	−10
Umbilical Vein				
pH	7.34	0.06	7.20	7.23
PCO_2 (mmHg)	41	7	28	30
PO_2 (mmHg)	29	7	16	18
Base excess (mEq · L^{-1})	−3	3	−8	−8

Modified from Helwig JT, Parer JT, Kilpatrick SJ, et al: Umbilical cord blood acid-base state: What is normal? Am J Obstet Gynecol 1996; 174:1807–1812.

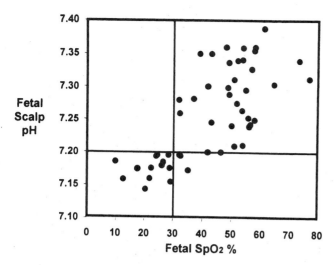

Figure 25–65. Relationship between fetal scalp O_2 saturations and fetal scalp pH. (From Kuhnert M, Seelbach-Goebel B, Butterwegge M: Predictive agreement between the fetal arterial oxygen saturation and fetal scalp pH: Results of the German multicenter study. Am J Obstet Gynecol 1998; 178:330–335.)

is the basis for the metabolic acidosis that accompanies fetal asphyxia. Short periods of hypoxemia (<10 minutes) do not appear to result in lactic acid accumulation.[318] Lactic acidosis is invariably present in severely hypoxemic fetuses. Lactate concentrations in fetal scalp blood correlate well with those in cord arterial and venous blood, and with pH and base deficit in cord blood.[319, 320] There is a new disposable test strip that requires only 5 μL of blood for lactate determination.[321] The small volume requirements make it easier to get an adequate sample compared to scalp pH testing and lactate may well be a better marker for fetal distress than pH.

Sampling volume requirements are significant; the use of scalp pH has been in steady decline for a number of years, in part because of technical problems with obtaining an adequate sample. A report from the hospitals of the University of Southern California, in which over 16,000 deliveries occur annually, found a steady decline in the use of scalp pH sampling over a 4-year period; the rate in 1992 was 0.03% (only five cases).[322] During the period of declining scalp pH usage, there was no increase in the cesarean rate for fetal distress, low Apgar score requiring neonatal ICU admission, or the clinical diagnosis of perinatal asphyxia or meconium aspiration syndrome. It may be that the increased ease and success of obtaining a scalp sample for a lactate strip test will produce a mild resurgence in the use of scalp blood sampling.

However, other factors have also influenced the use of scalp sampling. Better understanding of FHR patterns has in many instances decreased the fear that a fetus is in distress. Mild to moderate decelerations in the presence of good variability do not correlate with fetal acidosis and do not require aggressive interventions. Severe decelerations with decreased baseline variability are highly predictive of an acidotic fetus, and there is little benefit to be gained in scalp sampling when the heart rate pattern is ominous and persistent or when ominous patterns (i.e., umbilical venous pulsations) are present on Doppler flow velocity waveforms. Use of Doppler flow velocimetry has in many cases identified distressed fetuses even before the presence of abnormal changes in the FHR patterns suggests the need for scalp sampling. Use of BPP testing has also resulted in the early delivery of many fetuses that, had pregnancy continued, would likely have exhibited distress patterns during labor and, in cases of indeterminate FHR patterns, has encouraged the assessment of fetal acid-base status by scalp sampling.

Some situations where sampling may be helpful are the presence of *moderate to severe* decelerations with *somewhat decreased* heart rate variability that does not respond to standard treatment (i.e., an indeterminate FHR pattern); the need to monitor a fetus during labor when maternal drug therapy affecting FHR variability is required; and the absence of variability when the monitor is first applied if there is no obvious cause for this. Fetal blood scalp sampling is invasive, and should not be done when there is any known or suspected bleeding disorder such as hemophilia or von Willebrand's disease. Sampling in such cases has resulted in fetal death.

Intrapartum Pulse Oximetry

Conventional pulse oximetry has not been routinely applicable to the fetus during the late stage of labor because of the necessity that the sensor light pass *through* a tissue bed. Because only one surface usually presents itself, conventional absorbance oximetry is not feasible. *Reflectance,* as opposed to *transmission,* pulse oximetry has been assessed in in utero measurement of oxygen saturation (SpO₂).[323, 324] Because the amniochorionic membranes do not absorb light at the wavelengths used by oximeters, reflectance oximetry can be used in the presence of intact membranes, a distinct advantage compared to fetal scalp blood sampling (Fig. 25–66). Best results are obtained when the sensor is placed against the fetal cheek. Reflectance oximetry, like scalp samples, can provide erroneously low oxygen saturation data in the presence of scalp congestion or caput succedaneum.[325] Decreased signal-to-noise ratios, motion artifacts (e.g., contractions, fetal or maternal movement), and impediments to light transmission (e.g., vernix, hair, meconium) all interfere with accurate assessment of SpO₂ in the fetus using reflec-

Table 25–18. Type of Acidemia According to pH Values

	pH Values				
	<7.00 (n = 87)	7.00–7.04 (n = 95)	7.05–7.09 (n = 290)	7.10–7.14 (n = 798)	7.15–7.19 (n = 2236)
Mixed	54 (62.1%)	1 (1.1%)	0	1 (0.1%)	0
Metabolic	4 (4.6%)	12 (12.6%)	23 (7.9%)	16 (2%)	47 (2.1%)
Respiratory	29 (33.3%)	79 (83.2%)	230 (79.3%)	513 (64.3%)	834 (37.3%)
Unclassified*	0	3 (3.2%)	37 (12.8%)	268 (33.6%)	1355 (60.6%)

*Acidemic newborns in whom both PCO₂ and HCO₃⁻ fell within 2 SD of the mean.
From Goldaber KG, Gilstrap LC, Leveno KJ, et al: Pathologic fetal acidemia. Obstet Gynecol 1991; 78:1103–1106.

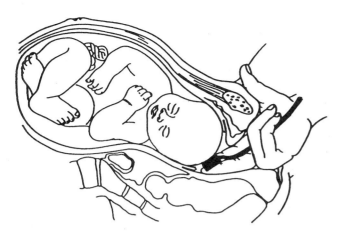

Figure 25-66. Placement of transvaginal probe for fetal reflectance pulse oximetry. (From Haeusler MC, Arikan G, Haas J, et al: Fetal pulse oximetry and visual on-line signal identification in the second stage of labor. Am J Obstet Gynecol 1996; 175:1071–1074.)

tance oximetry. For example, meconium interferes with light transmission at the crucial wavelengths used by the oximeter, and can result in artificially low saturation readings. Modifications in reflectance pulse oximetry sensors for specific fetal use have improved the device considerably; a change in the wavelength of the LED in the red spectrum from 660 nm to 735 nm has been shown to improve sensor precision. Further refinements in equipment design should improve the accuracy of SpO_2 determination and the ability to obtain an adequate signal.

The standard algorithms used in transmission pulse oximeters were clinically derived for use over a range from 70% to 100% oxygen saturation, and pulse oximetry values for oxygen saturations below this level were extrapolated. Assessment of oxygen saturation in the fetus, in which SpO_2 may range from 20% to 80%, required totally new calibration which has been done by several manufacturers of oximeters. The mean and range of SpO_2 values at progressive stages of

labor in *normal,* good-outcome pregnancies are presented in Figure 25–67.[323] Figure 25–68 shows the distribution of mean SpO_2 values of all readings taken continuously over a 30-minute period during the first stage of labor in a study population with *abnormal* FHR patterns; intrapartum abnormalities of heart rate are associated with significantly lower SpO_2 values compared to normals.[326] Mean SpO_2 is around 60% during the first stage of labor in normal cases; when there are FHR abnormalities, mean SpO_2 falls in the range of 35% to 50%.

Multicenter studies from Germany and France have shown that in a high-risk population fetal pulse oximetry is comparable to fetal scalp sampling in terms of identifying distressed fetuses with precision and reliability.[312, 326, 327] These studies are also in agreement that a fetal oxygen saturation of 30% by oximetry is a good cutoff for normal. Unfortunately, neither scalp pH nor oximetry reliably identifies all infants who will be born severely acidotic. In a recent study, the relationship between SpO_2 values in utero and acidosis at birth was present but the correlation was not strong.[328] Infants with metabolic acidosis at birth did not necessarily have low SpO_2 measurements just before delivery. For example, one infant had reassuring SpO_2 values before delivery (>40%), yet had variable decelerations, loss of beat-to-beat variability, thick meconium-stained amniotic fluid, and required low-forceps delivery. The infant was severely depressed at birth, with a pH of 6.84 and a base excess of −23 mmol/L. There are a number of possible explanations for the lack of correlation between SpO_2 and fetal acidosis. It is unlikely that it represents deterioration in fetal oxygenation occurring during delivery since there was no terminal catastrophic event in any of the patients studied. It may be that periodic decreases in fetal oxygenation during uterine contractions with umbilical cord compression can give rise to a *cumulative* acidosis over time that is not predicted by SpO_2 values, either between or during contractions. In support of this notion, the authors noted that a number of patients in the study had variable FHR decelerations, indicative of cord compression, during which time SpO_2 signal quality was unsatisfactory.[328] This is not unexpected, because pulsatile flow of blood (in this case to fetal skin and underly-

Figure 25-67. Fetal scalp oxygen saturations (mean and range) as determined by oximetry at progressive stages of labor in normal pregnancies with normal newborns. (From Dildy GA, Clark SL, Loucks CA: Intrapartum fetal pulse oximetry: Past, present, and future. Am J Obstet Gynecol 1996; 175:1–9.)

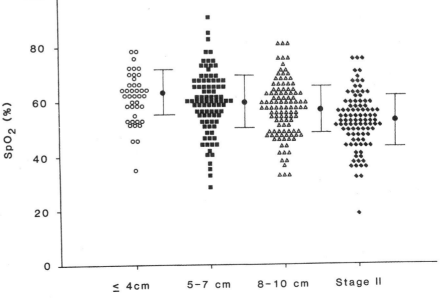

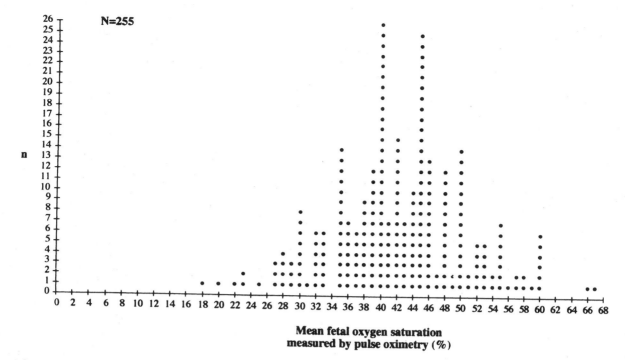

Figure 25–68. Fetal scalp mean oxygen saturations as determined by oximetry during the first stage of labor in a study population with abnormal fetal heart rates. (From Goffinet F, Langer B, Carbonne B, et al: Multicenter study on the clinical value of fetal pulse oximetry. I. Methodologic evaluation. The French Study Group on Fetal Pulse Oximetry. Am J Obstet Gynecol 1997; 177:1238–1246.)

ing muscle) decreases markedly during acutely induced hypoxemia. Another possibility is that, in the hypoxemic fetus with worsening metabolic acidosis, oxygen consumption decreases dramatically and, as oxygen extraction decreases, there is a perceived improvement in the level of oxygenation. This phenomenon has been seen in fetal sheep following several hours of hypoxemia and severe acidemia (arterial pH <7); measured oxygen saturation *increases* when oxygen consumption falls below a critical level of 60% of normal.[329] Finally, newborn acidosis may be caused by factors other than a limitation in oxygenation, such as increased maternal lactate during labor and delivery. Conversely, *low* SpO_2 readings may be encountered in cases in which there is *no fetal acidosis*. The best explanation for this is that low SpO_2 may be well tolerated with no increase in anaerobic metabolism, depending on the duration of labor and the ability of the fetus to initiate compensatory mechanisms.

It is likely that the reliability of fetal pulse oximetry in predicting fetal acidosis will improve as advances in monitoring technology continue. However, to the extent that incongruous data reflect true biologic adaptations or responses, fetal oximetry will not fulfill its promise of providing highly reliable data on the intrapartum status of the fetus.

Table 25–19. Proposed Indications for Amnioinfusion

Prevention or treatment of fetal heart rate decelerations due to oligohydramnios

Dilution of thick meconium-stained amniotic fluid

Prolongation of pregnancy following premature rupture of membranes

Prevention of fetal pulmonary hypoplasia (a consequence of inadequate amniotic fluid volume)

Amniotic Fluid Volume

Real-time ultrasonography is used to estimate amniotic fluid volume (AFV), and an abnormally low AFV increases the risk of fetal distress during labor. This is the reason that AFV is a component of biophysical and modified BPP testing in high-risk patients. Once the fetal membranes are ruptured, oligohydramnios (decreased AFV) increases the likelihood of umbilical cord compression. Amnioinfusion is a new form of therapy designed to reduce the risk of intrapartum complications in selected patients. Some of the proposed indications for amnioinfusion are presented in Table 25–19. In several randomized trials, amnioinfusion has been shown to be beneficial in one or more of the following: reduction in the incidence and sequelae of meconium aspiration syndrome; reduction in FHR decelerations; decreased rate of cesarean sections; fewer low Apgar scores; fewer low umbilical artery pH values; and less postpartum endometritis.[330, 331]

Neonatal Assessment in the Delivery Room

With severance of the umbilical cord at delivery, the infant must rapidly make the transition from intrauterine dependency to extrauterine independency. Careful monitoring of the fetus during this period is essential if one is to intervene promptly in the event of failure of transition, the consequences of which can be devastating and lifelong.

Apgar Score

The standard method of assessing the immediate well-being of a newborn is the Apgar score. While some assume that Apgar is a mnemonic for *a*ppearance, *p*ulse, *g*rimace, *a*ctiv-

Table 25-20. Apgar Neonatal Scoring System*

	Score		
	0	1	2
Heart rate	Absent	>100 bpm	>100 bpm
Respiratory effort	Absent	Slow, irregular	Good, crying
Color	Blue, pale	Acrocyanosis (pink body, blue extremities)	Completely pink
Muscle tone	Limp	Some flexion of extremities	Active motion
Reflex irritability (response to nasal catheter)	Absent	Grimace	Cough, sneeze

* Each sign is evaluated and scored from 0 to 2 at 1 and 5 minutes after birth. The sum of each individual score is the Apgar score for that period.
Modified from Apgar V: A proposal for a new method of evaluation of the newborn infant. Anesth Analg 1953; 32:260–267.

ity, and *r*espiration, others know that it was Dr. Virginia Apgar, an anesthesiologist, who first proposed the scoring system.[332] The Apgar scoring system assigns a score of 0, 1, or 2 in the categories listed above (Table 25-20). For example, an absent heart rate results in a score of 0, any heart rate below 100 bpm gets a score of 1, and a heart rate over 100 bpm gets a score of 2. The Apgar score is measured at 1 and 5 minutes and occasionally at 10 minutes. A 1-minute score of 0 to 2 is indicative of a severely depressed neonate in need of active resuscitation. A score of 3 to 6 is indicative of a moderately depressed infant who will probably respond to oxygen administration by mask, possibly with positive pressure ventilation. Infants with scores of 7 or greater rarely need respiratory assistance. The Apgar score is not a good predictor of long-term neurologic outcome. For any individual infant a very low score at 5 minutes is of little value in predicting either the likelihood of survival or the neurologic outcome. However, a 1-minute Apgar score of 7 or above is good evidence that there was no *recent* severe intrapartum asphyxia.

Clinical Assessment

Newborn assessment in the delivery room requires the same clinical observations used in other critical care settings. Paramount are the ABCs of basic life support: *a*irway, *b*reathing, and *c*irculation. Is the airway patent? Are bilateral breath sounds present? What is the quality of respiratory effort? Are there sternal retractions or nasal flaring? Is the abdomen distended? Is capillary refill adequate? Is the infant cyanotic? Cyanosis in the immediate newborn period is most often brief and a manifestation of residual right-to-left shunting during the transition from fetal to neonatal circulation. In a small percentage of cases cyanosis may be caused by congenital heart disease, such as transposition of the great vessels. Also, for cyanosis to be present, *circulation* is required. Circulatory failure results in extreme pallor; this color signals a medical emergency. Circulatory failure (shock) can result from intrapartum asphyxia and extreme acidosis, intrapartum hemorrhage (usually placental abruption), or overwhelming fetal sepsis. Lack of tone after establishment of adequate circulation and gas exchange may be a manifestation of residual asphyxia, and possibly a harbinger of permanent neurologic injury. In other cases, it may be a maternal drug effect, such as a magnesium overdose. Flaccidity can also be caused by congenital neuromuscular disease, such as Werdnig-Hoffmann disease (infantile spinal muscular atrophy). Regardless of the cause, poor tone is usually indicative of the need for respiratory support.

Pulse Oximetry

Pulse oximetry is increasingly being used in the delivery room to monitor newborn SpO_2.[333-335] This allows an imme-

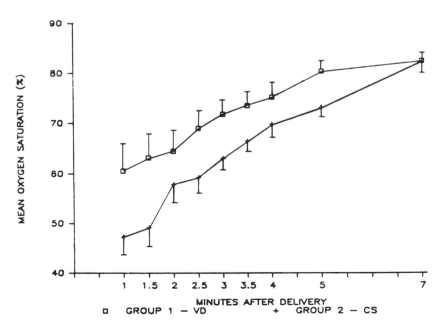

Figure 25-69. Oxygen saturation in the lower extremity in the immediate newborn period as measured by pulse oximetry. *Open squares* represent newborns delivered vaginally (VD); *crosses* indicate cesarean delivery (CS). (From Harris AP, Sendak MJ, Donham RT: Changes in arterial oxygen saturation immediately after birth in the human neonate. J Pediatr 1986; 109:117–119.)

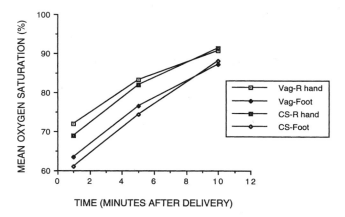

Figure 25-70. Oxygen saturation in the right hand (preductal) and lower extremity (postductal) in the immediate newborn period as measured by pulse oximetry. At 1, 5, and 10 minutes after delivery, measured oxygen saturations in the lower extremity are lower compared with those taken from the right hand, regardless of the mode of delivery. Vag, vaginal delivery; CS, cesarean delivery; R hand, right hand. (From Dimich I, Singh PP, Adell A, et al: Evaluation of oxygen saturation monitoring by pulse oximetry in neonates in the delivery system. Can J Anaesth 1991; 38:985-988.)

diate assessment of the infant's initial oxygen saturation, as well as documentation of the normal transition from the low saturation state found in utero to the much higher saturations associated with pulmonary gas exchange (Fig. 25-69). Oxygen saturation is slightly lower in infants delivered by cesarean section compared with those delivered vaginally. Compression on the fetal chest during delivery compresses some of the fluid from the lungs of the fetus; cesarean babies do not get this "squeeze" benefit and clinically are more likely to have transient tachypnea and other signs of mild respiratory distress (grunting, nasal flaring). Owing to the presence of right-to-left shunting through the ductus arteriosus in the transition period immediately after birth, SpO_2 will be higher in the right hand than in the left hand or lower extremities (Fig. 25-70). These differences steadily narrow in normal newborns and are not significantly different by 24 hours. At 5 minutes after delivery, a SpO_2 of 80% in the hand or 75% in the foot is normal, and does not warrant aggressive respiratory intervention in the absence of clinical signs of respiratory distress. By 10 minutes, infants born vaginally should have an SpO_2 of 90 mmHg and those born by cesarean delivery should have an SpO_2 of 85 mmHg, indicative of a normal newborn PaO_2 of 55 to 60 mmHg. SpO_2 immediately after birth correlates with umbilical vein oxygen tension.[336] This can serve to document the absence of birth asphyxia, information of both clinical and medicolegal value.

Pulse oximetry has been shown to be unreliable at low saturations (<60%) in sick neonates, and should not replace direct arterial blood gas sampling in such infants until better algorithms are incorporated into the monitors.[337] However, it is a valuable trend monitor, and as such can be used in any situation in which a reading can be obtained and in which there is accurate heart rate correlation.

Capnography

While capnography is the standard in care in the OR, particularly to confirm tracheal rather than esophageal intubation, it has not been embraced in other settings where tracheal

intubation is performed. In the neonatal units and delivery room, capnography has been limited in part by technical issues involving sampling. An ideal system would have minimal dead space or would require very small amounts of expired gas for sampling. Improvements in technology in this area can be expected. However, even in its current configuration, end-tidal CO_2 monitoring is useful in assessing neonatal status in cases of severe asphyxia requiring tracheal intubation and cardiopulmonary resuscitation (pharmacologic or chest compressions). The *presence* of a CO_2 waveform provides information concerning both endotracheal tube placement and adequacy of cardiac output; for these purposes, in-line sampling can be used for just a few breaths and then removed. The *absence* of a CO_2 waveform does not necessarily indicate esophageal intubation when used in the setting of cardiac arrest in an asphyxiated neonate. Extremely high pulmonary artery pressures favor shunting of blood through the ductus arteriosus and away from the lung. Thus, there may be minimal CO_2 flux in the trachea for the capnograph to detect even when chest compressions are moving blood through the heart. This is almost always caused by a combination of *extreme systemic hypotension* and *high pulmonary vascular resistance.* The high pulmonary vascular resistance is caused by a combination of hypercarbia, hypoxia, and compressed pulmonary vessels in the unexpanded, fluid-filled lungs of the asphyxiated newborn who has not commenced respiration. The treatment for this situation is *volume resuscitation,* usually with blood or colloid solution, *epinephrine* to increase systemic blood pressure and decrease the right-to-left shunting through the still-patent ductus arteriosus, and ventilatory support with positive pressure ventilation to expand the lungs and express fluid from the alveoli to permit gas exchange.

REFERENCES

1. Poppas A, Shroff SG, Korcarz CE, et al: Serial assessment of the cardiovascular system in normal pregnancy. Role of arterial compliance and pulsatile arterial load. Circulation 1997; 95:2407-2415.
2. Mabie WC, DiSessa TG, Crocker LG, et al: A longitudinal study of cardiac output in normal human pregnancy. Am J Obstet Gynecol 1994; 170:849-856.
3. Easterling TR, Benedetti TJ, Schmucker BC, et al: Maternal hemodynamics in normal and preeclamptic pregnancies: A longitudinal study. Obstet Gynecol 1990; 76:1061-1069.
4. van Oppen AC, van der Tweel I, Duvekot JJ, et al: Use of cardiac index in pregnancy: Is it justified? Am J Obstet Gynecol 1995; 173:923-928.
5. Mone SM, Sanders SP, Colan SD: Control mechanisms for physiological hypertrophy of pregnancy. Circulation 1996; 94:667-672.
6. Veille JC, Morton MJ, Burry KJ: Maternal cardiovascular adaptations to twin pregnancy. Am J Obstet Gynecol 1985; 153:261-263.
7. Mishra M, Chambers JB, Jackson G: Murmurs in pregnancy: An audit of echocardiography. BMJ 1992; 304:1413-1414.
8. Kublickiene KR, Cockell AP, Nisell H, et al: Role of nitric oxide in the regulation of vascular tone in pressurized and perfused resistance myometrial arteries from term pregnant women. Am J Obstet Gynecol 1997; 177:1263-1269.
9. Marcus RH, Korcarz C, McCray G, et al: Noninvasive method for determination of arterial compliance using Doppler echocardiography and subclavian pulse tracings. Validation and clinical application of a physiological model of the circulation. Circulation 1994; 89:2688-2699.
10. Veille JC, Hosenpud JD, Morton MJ: Cardiac size and function in pregnancy-induced hypertension. Am J Obstet Gynecol 1984; 150:443-449.

11. Geva T, Mauer MB, Striker L, et al: Effects of physiologic load of pregnancy on left ventricular contractility and remodeling. Am Heart J 1997; 133:53–59.

12. Capeless EL, Clapp JF: When do cardiovascular parameters return to their preconception values? Am J Obstet Gynecol 1991; 165:883–886.

13. Robson SC, Hunter S, Moore M, et al: Haemodynamic changes during the puerperium: A Doppler and M-mode echocardiographic study. Br J Obstet Gynaecol 1987; 94:1028–1039.

14. Moutquin JM, Rainville C, Giroux L, et al: A prospective study of blood pressure in pregnancy: Prediction of preeclampsia. Am J Obstet Gynecol 1985; 151:191–196.

15. Goldkrand JW, Jackson MJ: Blood pressure measurement in pregnant women in the left lateral recumbent position. Am J Obstet Gynecol 1997; 176:642–643.

16. Clark SL, Cotton DB, Pivarnik JM, et al: Position change and central hemodynamic profile during normal third-trimester pregnancy and post partum [erratum in Am J Obstet Gynecol 1991; 165:241]. Am J Obstet Gynecol 1991; 164:883–887.

17. Kinsella SM, Lohmann G: Supine hypotensive syndrome. Obstet Gynecol 1994; 83:774–788.

18. Pirhonen JP, Erkkola RU: Uterine and umbilical flow velocity waveforms in the supine hypotensive syndrome. Obstet Gynecol 1990; 76:176–179.

19. Gant NF, Jimenez JM, Whalley PJ, et al: A prospective study of angiotensin II pressor responsiveness in pregnancies complicated by chronic essential hypertension. Am J Obstet Gynecol 1977; 127:369–375.

20. Gant NF, Daley GL, Chand S, et al: A study of angiotensin II pressor response throughout primigravid pregnancy. J Clin Invest 1973; 52:2682–2689.

21. Langer B, Grima M, Coquard C, et al: Plasma active renin, angiotensin I, and angiotensin II during pregnancy and in preeclampsia. Obstet Gynecol 1998; 91:196–202.

22. August P, Mueller FB, Sealey JE, et al: Role of renin-angiotensin system in blood pressure regulation in pregnancy. Lancet 1995; 345:896–897.

23. Leduc L, Wasserstrum N, Spillman T, et al: Baroreflex function in normal pregnancy. Am J Obstet Gynecol 1991; 165:886–890.

24. Kalenga MK, De Gasparo M, Thomas K, et al: Down-regulation of angiotensin AT1 receptor by progesterone in human placenta. J Clin Endocrinol Metab 1996; 81:998–1002.

25. Broughton Pipkin F, Baker PN: Angiotensin II has depressor effects in pregnant and nonpregnant women. Hypertension 1997; 30:1247–1252.

26. Nelson SH, Suresh MS: Lack of reactivity of uterine arteries from patients with obstetric hemorrhage. Am J Obstet Gynecol 1992; 166:1436–1443.

27. Sakai K, Imaizumi T, Maeda H, et al: Venous distensibility during pregnancy. Comparisons between normal pregnancy and preeclampsia. Hypertension 1994; 24:461–466.

28. Grimes DA: The morbidity and mortality of pregnancy: Still risky business. Am J Obstet Gynecol 1994; 170:1489–1494.

29. Hays PM, Cruikshank DP, Dunn LJ: Plasma volume determination in normal and preeclamptic pregnancies. Am J Obstet Gynecol 1985; 151:958–966.

30. Gallery ED: Pregnancy-associated hypertension: Interrelationships of volume and blood pressure changes. Clin Exp Hypertens 1982; 1:39–47.

31. Blekta M, Hlavaty V, Trnkova M, et al: Volume of whole blood and absolute amount of serum proteins in the early stage of late toxemia of pregnancy. Am J Obstet Gynecol 1970; 106:10–13.

32. Kambam JR, Handte RE, Brown WU, et al: Effect of normal and preeclamptic pregnancies on the oxyhemoglobin dissociation curve. Anesthesiology 1986; 65:426–427.

33. Davison JM: Renal haemodynamics and volume homeostasis in pregnancy. Scand J Clin Lab Invest Suppl 1984; 169:15–27.

34. Lindheimer MD, Davison JM: Osmoregulation, the secretion of arginine vasopressin and its metabolism during pregnancy. Eur J Endocrinol 1995; 132:133–143.

35. Cotton DB, Gonik B, Spillman T, et al: Intrapartum to postpartum changes in colloid osmotic pressure. Am J Obstet Gynecol 1984; 149:174–177.

36. DiFederico EM, Burlingame JM, Kilpatrick SJ, et al: Pulmonary edema in obstetric patients is rapidly resolved except in the presence of infection or nitroglycerin tocolysis after open fetal surgery. Am J Obstet Gynecol 1998; 179:925–933.

37. Oian P, Maltau JM: Calculated capillary hydrostatic pressure in normal pregnancy and preeclampsia. Am J Obstet Gynecol 1987; 157:102–106.

38. Brown MA, Zammit VC, Lowe SA: Capillary permeability and extracellular fluid volumes in pregnancy-induced hypertension. Clin Sci 1989; 77:599–604.

39. Robson SC, Dunlop W, Boys RJ, et al: Cardiac output during labour. BMJ 1987; 295:1169–1172.

40. Duvekot JJ, Cheriex EC, Pieters FA, et al: Early pregnancy changes in hemodynamics and volume homeostasis are consecutive adjustments triggered by a primary fall in systemic vascular tone. Am J Obstet Gynecol 1993; 169:1382–1392.

41. Rees GB, Pipkin FB, Symonds EM, et al: A longitudinal study of respiratory changes in normal human pregnancy with cross-sectional data on subjects with pregnancy-induced hypertension. Am J Obstet Gynecol 1990; 162:826–830.

42. Garcia-Rio F, Pino JM, Gomez L, et al: Regulation of breathing and perception of dyspnea in healthy pregnant women. Chest 1996; 110:446–453.

43. Norregaard O, Schultz P, Ostergaard A, et al: Lung function and postural changes during pregnancy. Respir Med 1989; 83:467–470.

44. Russell IF, Chambers WA: Closing volume in normal pregnancy. Br J Anaesth 1981; 53:1043–1047.

45. Das TK, Moutquin JM, Parent JG: Effect of cigarette smoking on maternal airway function during pregnancy. Am J Obstet Gynecol 1991; 165:675–679.

46. Brancazio LR, Laifer SA, Schwartz T: Peak expiratory flow rate in normal pregnancy. Obstet Gynecol 1997; 89:383–386.

47. Ang CK, Tan TH, Walters WA, et al: Postural influence on maternal capillary oxygen and carbon dioxide tension. BMJ 1969; 4:201–203.

48. Awe RJ, Nicotra MB, Newsom TD, et al: Arterial oxygenation and alveolar-arterial gradients in term pregnancy. Obstet Gynecol 1979; 53:182–186.

49. Kambam JR, Entman S, Mouton S, et al: Effect of preeclampsia on carboxyhemoglobin levels: A mechanism for a decrease in P50. Anesthesiology 1988; 68:433–434.

50. Baraka AS, Hanna MT, Jabbour SI, et al: Preoxygenation of pregnant and nonpregnant women in the head-up versus supine position. Anesth Analg 1992; 75:757–759.

51. Huch A, Huch R, Schneider H, et al: Continuous transcutaneous monitoring of fetal oxygen tension during labour. Br J Obstet Gynaecol 1977; 84:1–39.

52. DiFederico EM, Harrison M, Matthay MA: Pulmonary edema in a woman following fetal surgery. Chest 1996; 109:1114–1117.

53. Sturgiss SN, Dunlop W, Davison JM: Renal hemodynamics and tubular function in human pregnancy. Baillieres Clin Obstet Gynaecol 1994; 8:209–234.

54. Jungers P, Chauveau D: Pregnancy in renal disease. Kidney Int 1997; 52:871–885.

55. Sandhar BK, Elliott RH, Windram I, et al: Peripartum changes in gastric emptying. Anaesthetist 1992; 47:196–198.

56. Carp H, Jayaram A, Stoll M: Ultrasound examination of the stomach contents of parturients. Anesth Analg 1992; 74:683–687.

57. Chan MT, Gin T: Postpartum changes in the minimum alveolar concentration of isoflurane. Anesthesiology 1995; 82:1360–1363.

58. Datta S, Lambert DH, Gregus J, et al: Differential sensitivities of mammalian nerve fibers during pregnancy. Anesth Analg 1983; 62:1070–1072.

59. Jayaram A, Carp H: Progesterone-mediated potentiation of spinal sufentanil in rats. Anesth Analg 1993; 76:745–750.

60. Louden KA, Broughton Pipkin F, et al: Platelet reactivity and serum thromboxane B_2 production in whole blood in gestational hypertension and pre-eclampsia. Br J Obstet Gynaecol 1991; 98:1239–1244.

61. Kofinas AD, Penry M, Swain M, et al: Effect of placental laterality on uterine artery resistance and development of preeclampsia and intrauterine growth retardation. Am J Obstet Gynecol 1989; 161:1536–1539.

62. Page EW, Christianson R: The impact of mean arterial pressure in the middle trimester upon the outcome of pregnancy. Am J Obstet Gynecol 1976; 125:740-746.

63. Villar J, Repke J, Markush L, et al: The measuring of blood pressure during pregnancy. Am J Obstet Gynecol 1989; 161:1019-1024.

64. Shennan A, Gupta M, Halligan A, et al: Lack of reproducibility in pregnancy of Korotkoff phase IV as measured by mercury sphygmomanometry. Lancet 1996; 347:139-142.

65. Brown MA, Buddle ML, Farrell T, et al: Randomised trial of management of hypertensive pregnancies by Korotkoff phase IV or phase V. Lancet 1998; 352:777-781.

66. Lopez MC, Belizan JM, Villar J, et al: The measurement of diastolic blood pressure during pregnancy: Which Korotkoff phase should be used? Am J Obstet Gynecol 1994; 170:574-578.

67. Danilenko-Dixon DR, Tefft L, Cohen RA, et al: Positional effects on maternal cardiac output during labor with epidural analgesia. Am J Obstet Gynecol 1996;175:867-872.

68. Kaufmann MA, Pargger H, Drop LJ: Oscillometric blood pressure measurements by different devices are not interchangeable. Anesth Analg 1996; 82:377-381.

69. Brown MA, Buddle ML, Bennett M, et al: Ambulatory blood pressure in pregnancy: Comparison of the Spacelabs 90207 and Accutracker II monitors with intraarterial recordings. Am J Obstet Gynecol 1995; 173:218-223.

70. Gallery ED, Hunyor SN, Ross M, et al: Predicting the development of pregnancy-associated hypertension. The place of standardized blood-pressure measurement. Lancet 1977; 1:1273-1275.

71. Reiss RE, O'Shaughnessy RW, Quilligan TJ, et al: Retrospective comparison of blood pressure course during preeclamptic and matched control pregnancies. Am J Obstet Gynecol 1987; 156:894-898.

72. Reiss RE, Tizzano TP, O'Shaughnessy RW: The blood pressure course in primiparous pregnancy. A prospective study of 383 women. J Reprod Med 1987; 32:523-526.

73. Caritis S, Sibai B, Hauth J, et al: Predictors of pre-eclampsia in women at high risk. National Institute of Child Health and Human Development Network of Maternal-Fetal Medicine Units. Am J Obstet Gynecol 1998; 179:946-951.

74. Churchill D, Perry IJ, Beevers DG: Ambulatory blood pressure in pregnancy and fetal growth. Lancet 1997; 349:7-10.

75. Penny JA, Halligan AW, Shennan AH, et al: Automated, ambulatory, or conventional blood pressure measurement in pregnancy: Which is the better predictor of severe hypertension? Am J Obstet Gynecol 1998; 178:521-526.

76. Brown MA, Robinson A, Bowyer L, et al: Ambulatory blood pressure monitoring in pregnancy: What is normal? Am J Obstet Gynecol 1998; 178:836-842.

77. Birnbach DJ, Chestnut DH: The epidural test dose in obstetric patients: Has it outlived its usefulness? Anesthesiology 1999; 88:971-972.

78. Leighton BL, Norris MC, Sosis M, et al: Limitations of epinephrine as a marker of intravascular injection in laboring women. Anesthesiology 1987; 66:688-691.

79. Norris MC, Arkoosh VA, Knobler R: Maternal and fetal effects of isoproterenol in the gravid ewe. Anesth Analg 1997; 85:389-394.

80. Norris MC, Ferrenbach D, Dalman H: Does epinephrine improve the diagnostic accuracy of aspiration during labor epidural analgesia? Anesth Analg 1999; 88:1073-1076.

81. Marcus MA, Bruyninckx FL, Vertommen JD, et al: Spinal somatosensory evoked potentials after epidural isoproterenol in awake sheep. Can J Anaesth 1997; 44:85-89.

82. Marcus MA, Vertommen JD, Van Aken H, et al: Hemodynamic effects of intravenous isoproterenol versus saline in the parturient. Anesth Analg 1997; 84:1113-1116.

83. Marcus MA, Vertommen JD, Van Aken H, et al: The effects of adding isoproterenol to 0.125% bupivacaine on the quality and duration of epidural analgesia in laboring parturients. Anesth Analg 1998; 86:749-752.

84. Leighton BL, Norris MC, DeSimone CA, et al: Pre-eclamptic and healthy term pregnant patients have different chronotropic responses to isoproterenol. Anesthesiology 1990; 72:392-393.

85. Practice guidelines for obstetric anesthesia. A report by the American Society of Anesthesiologists Task Force on Obstetrical Anesthesia. Anesthesiology 1999; 90:600-611.

86. Leighton BL, Gross JB: Air: An effective indicator of intravenously located epidural catheters. Anesthesiology 1989; 71:848-851.

87. Lieberman E, Lang JM, Frigoletto F Jr, et al: Epidural analgesia, intrapartum fever, and neonatal sepsis evaluation. Pediatrics 1997; 99:415-419.

88. Phillip J, Alexander JM, Sharma SK: Epidural analgesia during labor and maternal fever. Anesthesiology 1999; 99:1271-1275.

89. Baron JF, Decaux-Jacolot A, Edouard A, et al: Influence of venous return on baroreflex control of heart rate during lumbar epidural anesthesia in humans. Anesthesiology 1986; 64:188-193.

90. Taylor J, Weil MH: Failure of the Trendelenburg position to improve circulation during clinical shock. Surg Gynecol Obstet 1967; 124:1005-1010.

91. Sibbald WJ, Paterson NA, Holliday RL, et al: The Trendelenburg position: hemodynamic effects in hypotensive and normotensive patients. Crit Care Med 1979; 7:218-224.

92. Rout CC, Rocke DA, Gouws E: Leg elevation and wrapping in the prevention of hypotension following spinal anaesthesia for elective caesarean section. Anaesthetist 1993; 48:304-308.

93. Zakowski MI, Ramanathan S, Baratta JB, et al: Electrocardiographic changes during cesarean section: A cause for concern? Anesth Analg 1993; 76:162-167.

94. Kendrick WD, Woods AM, Daly MY, et al: Naloxone versus nalbuphine infusion for prophylaxis of epidural morphine-induced pruritus. Anesth Analg 1996; 82:641-647.

95. Rawal N, Nuutinen L, Raj PP, et al: Behavioral and histopathologic effects following intrathecal administration of butorphanol, sufentanil, and nalbuphine in sheep. Anesthesiology 1991; 75:1025-1034.

96. Hodgson P, Neal J, Pollack J, Liu S: The neurotoxity of drugs given intrathecally (spinal). Anesth Analg 1999; 88:797-809.

97. Gustafsson LL, Schildt B, Jacobsen K: Adverse effects of extradural and intrathecal opiates: Report of a nationwide survey in Sweden. Br J Anaesth 1982; 54:479-486.

98. Bromage PR, Camporesi EM, Durant PA, et al: Rostral spread of epidural morphine. Anesthesiology 1982; 56:431-436.

99. Abboud TK, Moore M, Zhu J, et al: Epidural butorphanol or morphine for the relief of post cesarean section pain: Ventilatory responses to carbon dioxide. Anesth Analg 1987; 66:889-893.

100. Cohen SE, Labaille T, Benhamou D, et al: Respiratory effects of epidural sufentanil after cesarean section. Anesth Analg 1992; 74:677-682.

101. Brockway MS, Noble DW, Sharwood-Smith GH, et al: Profound respiratory depression after extradural fentanyl. Br J Anaesth 1990; 64:243-245.

102. Rawal N, Wattwil M: Respiratory depression after epidural morphine—an experimental and clinical study. Anesth Analg 1984; 63:8-14.

103. Wang JJ, Ho ST, Tzeng JI: Comparison of intravenous nalbuphine infusion versus naloxone in the prevention of epidural morphine-related side effects. Reg Anesth Pain Med 1998; 23:479-484.

104. American College of Obstetricians and Gynecologists Committee on Technical Bulletins: Hypertension in pregnancy. Int J Gynaecol Obstet 1996; 53:175-183.

105. Stone JH: HELLP syndrome: Hemolysis, elevated liver enzymes, and low platelets. JAMA 1998; 280:559-562.

106. Ness RB, Roberts JM: Heterogeneous causes constituting the single syndrome of preeclampsia: A hypothesis and its implications. Am J Obstet Gynecol 1996; 175:1365-1370.

107. Smith AJ, Walters WA, Buckley NA, et al: Hypertensive and normal pregnancy: A longitudinal study of blood pressure, distensibility of dorsal hand veins and the ratio of the stable metabolites of thromboxane A_2 and prostacyclin in plasma. Br J Obstet Gynaecol 1995; 102:900-906.

108. Paarlberg KM, de Jong CL, van Geijn HP, et al: Vasoactive mediators in pregnancy-induced hypertensive disorders: A longitudinal study. Am J Obstet Gynecol 1998; 179:1559-1564.

109. Vainio M, Maenpaa J, Riutta A, et al: In the dose range of 0.5-2.0 mg/kg, acetylsalicylic acid does not affect prostacyclin production in hypertensive pregnancies. Acta Obstet Gynecol Scand 1999; 78:82-88.

110. Caritis S, Sibai B, Hauth J, et al: Low-dose aspirin to prevent preeclampsia in women at high risk. National Institute of Child Health and Human Development Network of Maternal-Fetal Medicine Units. N Engl J Med 1998; 338:701-705.

111. Darling M: Low-dose aspirin not for pre-eclampsia. Lancet 1998; 352:342.

112. Duley L: Aspirin for preventing and treating pre-eclampsia (editorial). BMJ 1999; 318:751-752.

113. Dumont A, Flahault A, Beaufils M, et al: Effect of aspirin in pregnant women is dependent on increase in bleeding time. Am J Obstet Gynecol 1999; 180:135-140.

114. Riyazi N, Leeda M, de Vries JI, et al: Low-molecular-weight heparin combined with aspirin in pregnant women with thrombophilia and a history of preeclampsia or fetal growth restriction: A preliminary study. Eur J Obstet Gynecol Reprod Biol 1998; 80:49-54.

115. Brown MA: The physiology of pre-eclampsia. Clin Exp Pharmacol Physiol 1995; 22:781-791.

116. Easterling T, Watts D, Schmucker B, et al: Measurement of cardiac output during pregnancy: Validation of Doppler technique and clinical observations in preeclampsia. Obstet Gynecol 1987; 69:845-850.

117. Groenendijk R, Trimbos JB, Wallenburg HC: Hemodynamic measurements in preeclampsia: Preliminary observations. Am J Obstet Gynecol 1984; 150:232-236.

118. Phelan JP, Yurth DA: Severe preeclampsia. I. Peripartum hemodynamic observations. Am J Obstet Gynecol 1982; 144:17-22.

119. Cotton DB, Gonik B, Dorman KF: Cardiovascular alterations in severe pregnancy-induced hypertension: Acute effects of intravenous magnesium sulfate. Am J Obstet Gynecol 1984; 148:162-165.

120. Benedetti TJ, Cotton DB, Read JC, et al: Hemodynamic observations in severe preeclampsia with a flow-directed pulmonary artery catheter. Am J Obstet Gynecol 1980; 136:465-470.

121. Benedetti TJ, Kates R, Williams V: Hemodynamic observations in severe preeclampsia complicated by pulmonary edema. Am J Obstet Gynecol 1985; 152:330-334.

122. Henderson DW, Vilos GA, Milne KJ, et al: The role of Swan-Ganz catheterization in severe pregnancy-induced hypertension. Am J Obstet Gynecol 1984; 148:570-574.

123. Strauss RG, Keefer JR, Burke T, et al: Hemodynamic monitoring of cardiogenic pulmonary edema complicating toxemia of pregnancy. Obstet Gynecol 1980; 55:170-174.

124. Visser W, Wallenburg HC: Central hemodynamic observations in untreated preeclamptic patients. Hypertension 1991; 17:1072-1077.

125. Nisell H, Lunell NO, Linde B: Maternal hemodynamics and impaired fetal growth in pregnancy-induced hypertension. Obstet Gynecol 1988; 71:163-166.

126. Yang JM, Yang YC, Wang KG: Central and peripheral hemodynamics in severe preeclampsia. Acta Obstet Gynecol Scand 1996; 75:120-126.

127. Lang RM, Pridjian G, Feldman T, et al: Left ventricular mechanics in preeclampsia. Am Heart J 1991; 121:1768-1775.

128. Kuzniar J, Piela A, Skret A: Left ventricular function in preeclamptic patients: An echocardiographic study. Am J Obstet Gynecol 1983; 146:400-405.

129. Ashworth JR, Warren AY, Baker PN, et al: Loss of endothelium-dependent relaxation in myometrial resistance arteries in preeclampsia. Br J Obstet Gynaecol 1997; 104:1152-1158.

130. Sladek SM, Magness RR, Conrad KP: Nitric oxide and pregnancy. Am J Physiol 1997; 272:R441-463.

131. Fleischer A, Schulman H, Farmakides G, et al: Uterine artery Doppler velocimetry in pregnant women with hypertension. Am J Obstet Gynecol 1986; 154:806-813.

132. Penny JA, Shennan AH, Halligan AW, et al: Blood pressure measurement in severe pre-eclampsia. Lancet 1997; 349:1518.

133. Kyle PM, Buckley D, Kissane J, et al: The angiotensin sensitivity test and low-dose aspirin are ineffective methods to predict and prevent hypertensive disorders in nulliparous pregnancy. Am J Obstet Gynecol 1995; 173:865-872.

134. Pouliot L, Forest JC, Moutquin JM, et al. Platelet angiotensin II binding sites and early detection of preeclampsia. Obstet Gynecol 1998; 91:591-595.

135. Goodlin RC, Quaife MA, Dirksen JW: The significance, diagnosis, and treatment of maternal hypovolemia as associated with fetal/maternal illness. Semin Perinatol 1981; 5:163-174.

136. Benedetti TJ, Carlson RW: Studies of colloid osmotic pressure in pregnancy-induced hypertension. Am J Obstet Gynecol 1979; 135:308-311.

137. Sibai BM, Mabie BC, Harvey CJ, et al: Pulmonary edema in severe preeclampsia-eclampsia: Analysis of thirty-seven consecutive cases. Am J Obstet Gynecol 1987; 156:1174-1179.

138. Wasserstrum N, Cotton DB: Hemodynamic monitoring in severe pregnancy-induced hypertension. Clin Perinatol 1986; 13:781-799.

139. Belfort M, Uys P, Dommisse J, et al: Hemodynamic changes in gestational proteinuric hypertension: The effects of rapid volume expansion and vasodilator therapy. Br J Obstet Gynaecol 1989; 96:634-641.

140. Visser W, Wallenburg HC: Maternal and perinatal outcome of temporizing management in 254 consecutive patients with severe pre-eclampsia remote from term. Eur J Obstet Gynecol Reprod Biol 1995; 63:147-154.

141. Clark SL, Greenspoon JS, Aldahl D, et al: Severe preeclampsia with persistent oliguria: Management of hemodynamic subsets. Am J Obstet Gynecol 1986; 154:490-494.

142. Kirshon B, Lee W, Mauer MB, et al: Effects of low-dose dopamine therapy in the oliguric patient with preeclampsia. Am J Obstet Gynecol 1988; 159:604-607.

143. Cotton DB, Longmire S, Jones MM, et al: Cardiovascular alterations in severe pregnancy-induced hypertension: Effects of intravenous nitroglycerin coupled with blood volume expansion. Am J Obstet Gynecol 1986; 154:1053-1059.

144. Lindheimer MD, Katz AI: Hypertension in pregnancy. N Engl J Med 1985; 313:675-680.

145. Hood D, Curry R: Spinal versus epidural anesthesia for cesarean section in severely preeclamptic patients. Anesthesiology 1999; 90:1276-1282.

146. Wallace DH, Leveno KJ, Cunningham FG, et al: Randomized comparison of general and regional anesthesia for cesarean delivery in pregnancies complicated by severe preeclampsia. Obstet Gynecol 1995; 86:193-199.

147. Jouppila P, Jouppila R, Hollmen A, et al: Lumbar epidural analgesia to improve intervillous blood flow during labor in severe preeclampsia. Obstet Gynecol 1982; 59:158-161.

148. Newsome LR, Bramwell RS, Curling PE: Severe preeclampsia: Hemodynamic effects of lumbar epidural anesthesia. Anesth Analg 1986; 65:31-36.

149. Hodgkinson R, Husain FJ, Hayashi RH: Systemic and pulmonary blood pressure during caesarean section in parturients with gestational hypertension. Can Anaesth Soc J 1980; 27:389-394.

150. Ramanathan J, Bottorff M, Jeter JN, et al: The pharmacokinetics and maternal and neonatal effects of epidural lidocaine in preeclampsia. Anesth Analg 1986; 65:120-126.

151. Ramanathan J, Angel JJ, Bush AJ, et al: Changes in maternal middle cerebral artery blood flow velocity associated with general anesthesia in severe preeclampsia. Anesth Analg 1999; 88:357-361.

152. Longmire S, Leduc L, Jones MM, et al: The hemodynamic effects of intubation during nitroglycerin infusion in severe preeclampsia. Am J Obstet Gynecol 1991; 164:551-556.

153. Buttar H: An overview of the influence of ACE inhibitors on fetal-placental circulation and perinatal development. Mol Cell Biochem 1997; 176:61-71.

154. Roberts JM: Pregnancy-related hypertension. *In* Creasy R, Resnik R (eds): Maternal-Fetal Medicine, ed 4. Philadelphia, WB Saunders, 1999, p 859.

155. Lunell NO, Lewander R, Mamoun I, et al: Uteroplacental blood flow in pregnancy induced hypertension. Scand J Clin Lab Invest Suppl 1984; 169:28-35.

156. Jouppila P, Kirkinen P, Koivula A, et al: Effects of dihydralazine infusion on the fetoplacental blood flow and maternal prostanoids. Obstet Gynecol 1985; 65:115-118.

157. Belfort M, Akovic K, Anthony J, et al: The effect of acute volume expansion and vasodilation with verapamil on uterine and umbilical artery Doppler indices in severe preeclampsia. J Clin Ultrasound 1994; 22:317-325.

158. Fenakel K, Fenakel G, Appelman Z, et al: Nifedipine in the treatment of severe preeclampsia. Obstet Gynecol 1991; 77: 331–337.

159. Carbonne B, Jannet D, Touboul C, et al: Nicardipine treatment of hypertension during pregnancy. Obstet Gynecol 1993; 81: 908–914.

160. Naulty J, Cefalo RC, Lewis PE: Fetal toxicity of nitroprusside in the pregnant ewe. Am J Obstet Gynecol 1981; 139:708–711.

161. Shoemaker CT, Meyers M: Sodium nitroprusside for control of severe hypertensive disease of pregnancy: A case report and discussion of potential toxicity. Am J Obstet Gynecol 1984; 149:171–173.

162. Stempel JE, O'Grady JP, Morton MJ, et al: Use of sodium nitroprusside in complications of gestational hypertension. Obstet Gynecol 1982; 60:533–538.

163. Curry SC, Carlton MW, Raschke RA: Prevention of fetal and maternal cyanide toxicity from nitroprusside with coinfusion of sodium thiosulfate in gravid ewes. Anesth Analg 1997; 84: 1121–1126.

164. Wasserstrum N: Nitroprusside in preeclampsia. Circulatory distress and paradoxical bradycardia. Hypertension 1991; 18:79–84.

165. Belfort MA, Saade GR, Suresh M, et al: Human umbilical vessels: Responses to agents frequently used in obstetric patients. Am J Obstet Gynecol 1995; 172:1395–1403.

166. Derham RJ, Robinson J: Severe preeclampsia: Is vasodilation therapy with hydralazine dangerous for the preterm fetus? Am J Perinatol 1990; 7:239–244.

167. Visser W, Wallenburg HC: A comparison between the hemodynamic effects of oral nifedipine and intravenous dihydralazine in patients with severe pre-eclampsia. J Hypertens 1995; 13: 791–795.

168. Kirshon B, Wasserstrum N, Cotton DB: Should continuous hydralazine infusions be utilized in severe pregnancy-induced hypertension? Am J Perinatol 1991; 8:206–208.

169. Jouppila P, Kirkinen P, Koivula A, et al: Labetalol does not alter the placental and fetal blood flow or maternal prostanoids in pre-eclampsia. Br J Obstet Gynecol 1986; 93:543–547.

170. Harper A, Murnaghan GA: Maternal and fetal haemodynamics in hypertensive pregnancies during maternal treatment with intravenous hydralazine or labetalol. Br J Obstet Gynaecol 1991; 98: 453–459.

171. Hjertberg R, Faxelius G, Belfrage P: Comparison of outcome of labetalol or hydralazine therapy during hypertension in pregnancy in very low birth weight infants. Acta Obstet Gynecol Scand 1993; 72:611–615.

172. Moretti MM, Fairlie FM, Akl S, et al: The effect of nifedipine therapy on fetal and placental Doppler waveforms in pre-eclampsia remote from term. Am J Obstet Gynecol 1990; 163: 1844–1848.

173. Barton JR, Hiett AK, Conover WB: The use of nifedipine during the postpartum period in patients with severe preeclampsia. Am J Obstet Gynecol 1990; 162:788–792.

174. Cotton DB, Gonik B, Dorman K, et al: Cardiovascular alterations in severe pregnancy-induced hypertension: Relationship of central venous pressure to pulmonary capillary wedge pressure. Am J Obstet Gynecol 1985; 151:762–764.

175. Cotton DB, Lee W, Huhta JC, et al: Hemodynamic profile of severe pregnancy-induced hypertension. Am J Obstet Gynecol 1988; 158:523–529.

176. Fox DB, Troiano NH, Graves CR: Use of the pulmonary artery catheter in severe preeclampsia: A review. Obstet Gynecol Surv 1996; 51:684–695.

177. Rokey R, Belfort MA, Saade GR: Quantitative echocardiographic assessment of left ventricular function in critically ill obstetric patients: A comparative study. Am J Obstet Gynecol 1995; 173: 1148–1152.

178. Belfort MA, Rokey R, Saade GR, et al: Rapid echocardiographic assessment of left and right heart hemodynamics in critically ill obstetric patients. Am J Obstet Gynecol 1994; 171:884–892.

179. Lim KH, Friedman SA, Ecker JL, et al: The clinical utility of serum uric acid measurements in hypertensive diseases of pregnancy. Am J Obstet Gynecol 1998; 178:1067–1071.

180. Gaber LW, Spargo BH, Lindheimer MD: Renal pathology in pre-eclampsia. Baillieres Clin Obstet Gynaecol 1994; 8:443–468.

181. Many A, Hubel CA, Roberts JM: Hyperuricemia and xanthine oxidase in preeclampsia, revisited. Am J Obstet Gynecol 1996; 174:288–291.

182. Ihle BU, Long P, Oats J: Early onset pre-eclampsia: Recognition of underlying renal disease. BMJ 1987; 294:79–81.

183. Sacks SH, Verrier Jones K, Roberts R, et al: Effect of symptomless bacteriuria in childhood on subsequent pregnancy. Lancet 1987; 2:991–994.

184. el-Khatib M, Packham DK, Becker GJ, et al: Pregnancy-related complications in women with reflux nephropathy. Clin Nephrol 1994; 41:50–55.

185. Lee W, Gonik B, Cotton DB: Urinary diagnostic indices in preeclampsia-associated oliguria: Correlation with invasive hemodynamic monitoring. Am J Obstet Gynecol 1987; 156:100–103.

186. Douglas KA, Redman CW: Eclampsia in the United Kingdom. BMJ 1994; 309:1395–1400.

187. Dunn R, Lee W, Cotton DB: Evaluation by computerized axial tomography of eclamptic women with seizures refractory to magnesium sulfate therapy. Am J Obstet Gynecol 1986; 155: 267–268.

188. Digre KB, Varner MW, Osborn AG, et al: Cranial magnetic resonance imaging in severe preeclampsia vs eclampsia. Arch Neurol 1993; 50:399–406.

189. Lewis LK, Hinshaw DB Jr, Will AD, et al: CT and angiographic correlation of severe neurological disease in toxemia of pregnancy. Neuroradiology 1988; 30:59–64.

190. Cunningham FG, Fernandez CO, Hernandez C: Blindness associated with preeclampsia and eclampsia. Am J Obstet Gynecol 1995; 172:1291–1298.

191. Witlin AG, Friedman SA, Egerman RS, et al: Cerebrovascular disorders complicating pregnancy—beyond eclampsia. Am J Obstet Gynecol 1997; 176:1139–1145; discussion 1145–1148.

192. Witlin AG, Sibai BM: Magnesium sulfate therapy in preeclampsia and eclampsia. Obstet Gynecol 1998; 92:883–889.

193. The Eclampsia Trial Collaborative Group: Which anticonvulsant for women with eclampsia? Evidence from the Collaborative Eclampsia Trial. Lancet 1995; 345:1455–1463.

194. Hansen WF, Burnham SJ, Svendsen TO, et al: Transcranial Doppler findings of cerebral vasospasm in preeclampsia. J Matern Fetal Med 1996; 5:194–200.

195. Merrell DA, Koch MA: Epidural anaesthesia as an anticonvulsant in the management of hypertensive and eclamptic patients in labour. S Afr Med J 1980; 58:875–877.

196. Abboud T, Artal R, Sarkis F, et al: Sympathoadrenal activity, maternal, fetal, and neonatal responses after epidural anesthesia in the preeclamptic patient. Am J Obstet Gynecol 1982; 144: 915–918.

197. Katz VL, Thorp JM Jr, Rozas L, et al: The natural history of thrombocytopenia associated with preeclampsia. Am J Obstet Gynecol 1990; 163:1142–1143.

198. Leduc L, Wheeler JM, Kirshon B, et al: Coagulation profile in severe preeclampsia. Obstet Gynecol 1992; 79:14–18.

199. Sharma SK, Philip J, Whitten CW, et al: Assessment of changes in coagulation in parturients with preeclampsia using thromboelastography. Anesthesiology 1999; 90:385–390.

200. Roberts JM, Taylor RN, Musci TJ, et al: Preeclampsia: An endothelial cell disorder. Am J Obstet Gynecol 1989; 161:1200–1204.

201. Burrows RF, Hunter DJ, Andrew M, et al: A prospective study investigating the mechanism of thrombocytopenia in preeclampsia. Obstet Gynecol 1987; 70:334–338.

202. Saphier CJ, Repke JT: Hemolysis, elevated liver enzymes, and low platelets (HELLP) syndrome: A review of diagnosis and management. Semin Perinatol 1998; 22:118–133.

203. Sibai BM, Taslimi MM, el-Nazer A, et al: Maternal-perinatal outcome associated with the syndrome of hemolysis, elevated liver enzymes, and low platelets in severe preeclampsia-eclampsia. Am J Obstet Gynecol 1986; 155:501–509.

204. Channing-Roberts RP, Leven J: A critical reappraisal of the bleeding time. Semin Thromb Hemost 1990; 16:1–30.

205. Ramanathan J, Sibai BM, Vu T, et al: Correlation between bleeding times and platelet counts in women with preeclampsia undergoing cesarean section. Anesthesiology 1989; 71:188–191.

206. Ramanathan J, Khalil M, Sibai BM, et al: Anesthetic management of the syndrome of hemolysis, elevated liver enzymes, and low platelet count (HELLP) in severe preeclampsia: A retrospective study. Reg Anesth 1988; 13:20-24.

207. Weiss BM, Zemp L, Seifert B, et al: Outcome of pulmonary vascular disease in pregnancy: A systematic overview from 1978 through 1996. J Am Coll Cardiol 1998; 31:1650-1657.

208. Weiss BM, von Segesser LK, Alon E, et al: Outcome of cardiovascular surgery and pregnancy: A systematic review of the period 1984-1996. Am J Obstet Gynecol 1998; 179:1643-1653.

209. Clark SL, Phelan JP, Greenspoon J, et al: Labor and delivery in the presence of mitral stenosis: Central hemodynamic observations. Am J Obstet Gynecol 1985;152:984-988.

210. Cunningham FG, Pritchard JA, Hankins GD, et al: Peripartum heart failure: Idiopathic cardiomyopathy or compounding cardiovascular events? Obstet Gynecol 1986; 67:157-168.

211. Martinez-Reding J, Cordero A, Kuri J, et al: Treatment of severe mitral stenosis with percutaneous balloon valvotomy in pregnant patients. Clin Cardiol 1998; 21:659-663.

212. Gupta A, Lokhandwala YY, Satoskar PR, et al: Balloon mitral valvotomy in pregnancy: Maternal and fetal outcomes. J Am Coll Surg 1998; 187:409-415.

213. Ben Farhat M, Gamra H, Betbout F, et al: Percutaneous balloon mitral commissurotomy during pregnancy. Heart 1997; 77:564-567.

214. Poirier P, Champagne J, Alain P, et al: Mitral balloon valvuloplasty in pregnancy: Limiting radiation and procedure time by using transesophageal echocardiography. Can J Cardiol 1997; 13:843-845.

215. Saleh MA, El Fiky AA, Fahmy M, et al: Use of biplane transesophageal echocardiography as the only imaging technique for percutaneous balloon mitral commissurotomy. Am J Cardiol 1996; 78:103-106.

216. Clark SL: Labor and delivery in the patient with structural cardiac disease. Clin Perinatol 1986; 13:695-703.

217. Nadeau SNWH: Misinterpretation of pressure measurements from the pulmonary artery catheter. Can Anaesth Soc J 1986; 33:352-363.

218. Woods AM, Queen JS, Lawson D: Valsalva maneuver in obstetrics: The influence of peripheral circulatory changes on function of the pulse oximeter. Anesth Analg 1991; 73:765-771.

219. Hemmings GT, Whalley DG, O'Connor PJ, et al: Invasive monitoring and anaesthetic management of a parturient with mitral stenosis. Can J Anaesth 1987; 34:182-185.

220. Ziskind Z, Etchin A, Frenkel Y, et al: Epidural anesthesia with the Trendelenburg position for cesarean section with or without a cardiac surgical procedure in patients with severe mitral stenosis: A hemodynamic study. J Cardiothorac Vasc Anesth 1990; 4:354-359.

221. Woods AM, Longnecker DE: Endoscopy. In Marshall BE, Longnecker DE, Fairley HB (eds): Anesthesia for Thoracic Procedure. Boston, Blackwell Scientific, 1988, pp 338-341.

222. Stone DJ, Gal TJ: Airway management. In Miller RD, (ed): Anesthesia, ed 3. New York, Churchill Livingstone, 1996, p 1424.

223. Batson MA, Longmire S, Csontos E: Alfentanil for urgent caesarean section in a patient with severe mitral stenosis and pulmonary hypertension. Can J Anaesth 1990; 37:685-688.

224. Perloff JK, Child JS, Edwards JE: New guidelines for the clinical diagnosis of mitral valve prolapse. Am J Cardiol 1986; 57:1124-1129.

225. Alcantara LG, Marx GF: Cesarean section under epidural analgesia in a parturient with mitral valve prolapse. Anesth Analg 1987; 66:902-903.

226. Shapiro EP, Trimble EL, Robinson JC, et al: Safety of labor and delivery in women with mitral valve prolapse. Am J Cardiol 1985; 56:806-807.

227. Dineen E, Brent BN: Aortic valve stenosis: Comparison of patients with to those without chronic congestive heart failure. Am J Cardiol 1986; 57:19-22.

228. Pesonen E, Banning AP, Pearson JF, et al: Role of balloon dilatation of the aortic valve in pregnant patients with severe aortic stenosis. Br Heart J 1993; 70:544-545.

229. Redfern N, Bower S, Bullock RE, et al: Alfentanil for caesarean section complicated by severe aortic stenosis. Br J Anaesth 1987; 59:1309-1312.

230. Alderson JD: Cardiovascular collapse following epidural anaesthesia for caesarean section in a patient with aortic incompetence. Anaesthetist 1987; 42:643-645.

231. Shime J, Mocarski EJ, Hastings D, et al: Congenital heart disease in pregnancy: Short- and long-term implications [erratum in Am J Obstet Gynecol 1987; 156:1361]. Am J Obstet Gynecol 1987; 156:313-322.

232. Pearl RG, Siegel LC: Thermodilution cardiac output measurement with a large left-to-right shunt. J Clin Monit Comput 1991; 7:146-153.

233. Sugishita Y, Ito I, Kubo T: Pregnancy in cardiac patients: Possible influence of volume overload by pregnancy on pulmonary circulation. Jpn Circ J 1986; 50:376-383.

234. Laishley RS, Burrows FA, Lerman J, Roy WL: Effect of anesthetic induction regimens on oxygen saturation in cyanotic congenital heart disease. Anesthesiology 1986; 65:673-677.

235. Boxer RA, Gottesfeld I, Sharanjeet S, et al: Noninvasive pulse oximetry in children with cyanotic congenital heart disease. Crit Care Med 1987; 15:1062-1064.

236. Brown CS, Bertolet BD: Peripartum cardiomyopathy: A comprehensive review. Am J Obstet Gynecol 1998; 178:409-414.

237. Witlin AG, Mabie WC, Sibai BM: Peripartum cardiomyopathy: An ominous diagnosis. Am J Obstet Gynecol 1997; 176:182-188.

238. Witlin AG, Mabie WC, Sibai BM: Peripartum cardiomyopathy: A longitudinal echocardiographic study. Am J Obstet Gynecol 1997; 177:1129-1132.

239. Garner P: Type I diabetes mellitus and pregnancy. Lancet 1995; 346:1157-1161.

240. Steel JM, Johnstone FD, Hepburn DA, et al: Can prepregnancy care of diabetic women reduce the risk of abnormal babies? BMJ 1990; 301:1070-1074.

241. Hanson U, Persson B, Thunell S: Relationship between haemoglobin A_{1C} in early type 1 (insulin-dependent) diabetic pregnancy and the occurrence of spontaneous abortion and fetal malformation in Sweden. Diabetologia 1990; 33:100-104.

242. Chauhan SP, Perry KG Jr, McLaughlin BN, et al: Diabetic ketoacidosis complicating pregnancy. J Perinatol 1996; 16:173-175.

243. Cullen MT, Reece EA, Homko CJ, et al: The changing presentations of diabetic ketoacidosis during pregnancy. Am J Perinatol 1996; 13:449-451.

244. Garner PR, D'Alton ME, Dudley DK, et al: Preeclampsia in diabetic pregnancies. Am J Obstet Gynecol 1990; 163:505-508.

245. Stamler EF, Cruz ML, Mimouni F, et al: High infectious morbidity in pregnant women with insulin-dependent diabetes: An understated complication. Am J Obstet Gynecol 1990; 163:1217-1221.

246. Miodovnik M, Rosenn BM, Khoury JC, et al: Does pregnancy increase the risk for development and progression of diabetic nephropathy? Am J Obstet Gynecol 1996; 174:1180-1189; discussion 1189-1191.

247. Purdy LP, Hantsch CE, Molitch ME, et al: Effect of pregnancy on renal function in patients with moderate-to-severe diabetic renal insufficiency. Diabetes Care 1996; 19:1067-1074.

248. Datta S, Brown WU Jr: Acid-base status in diabetic mothers and their infants following general or spinal anesthesia for cesarean section. Anesthesiology 1977; 47:272-276.

249. Datta S, Brown WU Jr, Ostheimer GW, et al. Epidural anesthesia for cesarean section in diabetic parturients: Maternal and neonatal acid-base status and bupivacaine concentration. Anesth Analg 1981; 60:574-578.

250. Datta S, Kitzmiller JL, Naulty JS, et al: Acid-base status of diabetic mothers and their infants following spinal anesthesia for cesarean section. Anesth Analg 1982; 61:662-665.

251. Rasanen J, Wood DC, Weiner S, et al: Role of the pulmonary circulation in the distribution of human fetal cardiac output during the second half of pregnancy. Circulation 1996; 94:1068-1073.

252. Richardson BS, Bocking AD: Metabolic and circulatory adaptations to chronic hypoxia in the fetus. Comp Biochem Physiol A Physiol 1998; 119:717-723.

253. Miller DA, Rabello YA, Paul RH: The modified biophysical profile: Antepartum testing in the 1990s. Am J Obstet Gynecol 1996; 174:812–817.

254. Manning FA, Bondaji N, Harman CR, et al: Fetal assessment based on fetal biophysical profile scoring. VIII. The incidence of cerebral palsy in tested and untested perinates. Am J Obstet Gynecol 1998; 178:696–706.

255. Yoon BH, Romero R, Roh CR, et al: Relationship between the fetal biophysical profile score, umbilical artery Doppler velocimetry, and fetal blood acid-base status determined by cordocentesis. Am J Obstet Gynecol 1993; 169:1586–1594.

256. Manning FA, Snijders R, Harman CR, et al: Fetal biophysical profile score. VI. Correlation with antepartum umbilical venous fetal pH. Am J Obstet Gynecol 1993; 169:755–763.

257. Lin CC, Adamczyk CJ, Sheikh Z, et al: Fetal congenital malformations. Biophysical profile evaluation. J Reprod Med 1998; 43: 521–527.

258. Schmidt KG, Di Tommaso M, Silverman NH, et al: Doppler echocardiographic assessment of fetal descending aortic and umbilical blood flows. Validation studies in fetal lambs. Circulation 1991; 83:1731–1737.

259. Kaaja R, Wallgren EI, Hallman M: Value of absent or retrograde end-diastolic flow in fetal aorta and umbilical artery as a predictor of perinatal outcome in pregnancy-induced hypertension. Acta Paediatr 1993; 82:19–24.

260. Farmakides G, Schulman H, Schneider E: Surveillance of the pregnant hypertensive patient with Doppler flow velocimetry. Clin Obstet Gynecol 1992; 35:387–396.

261. Fairlie FM, Moretti M, Walker JJ, et al: Determinants of perinatal outcome in pregnancy-induced hypertension with absence of umbilical artery end-diastolic frequencies. Am J Obstet Gynecol 1991; 164:1084–1089.

262. Bekedam DJ, Visser GH, van der Zee AG, et al: Abnormal velocity waveforms of the umbilical artery in growth retarded fetuses: Relationship to antepartum late heart rate decelerations and outcome. Early Hum Dev 1990; 24:79–89.

263. Bracero LA, Evanco J, Byrne DW: Doppler velocimetry discordancy of the uterine arteries in pregnancies complicated by diabetes. J Ultrasound Med 1997; 16:387–393.

264. Bracero LA, Figueroa R, Byrne DW, et al: Comparison of umbilical Doppler velocimetry, nonstress testing, and biophysical profile in pregnancies complicated by diabetes. J Ultrasound Med 1996; 15:301–308.

265. Hitschold T, Weiss E, Beck T, et al: Low target birth weight or growth retardation: Umbilical Doppler flow velocity waveforms and histometric analysis of fetoplacental vascular tree. Am J Obstet Gynecol 1993; 168:1260–1264.

266. Ducey J, Schulman H, Farmakides G, et al: A classification of hypertension in pregnancy based on Doppler velocimetry. Am J Obstet Gynecol 1987; 157:680–685.

267. Eronen M, Kari A, Pesonen E, et al: Value of absent or retrograde end-diastolic flow in fetal aorta and umbilical artery as a predictor of perinatal outcome in pregnancy-induced hypertension. Acta Paediatr 1993; 82:919–924.

268. Arduini D, Rizzo G, Romanini C: The development of abnormal heart rate patterns after absent end-diastolic velocity in umbilical artery: Analysis of risk factors [erratum in Am J Obstet Gynecol 1993; 169:1073]. Am J Obstet Gynecol 1993; 168:43–50.

269. Indik JH, Chen V, Reed KL: Association of umbilical venous with inferior vena cava blood flow velocities. Obstet Gynecol 1991; 77:551–557.

270. Rizzo G, Arduini D, Romanini C: Inferior vena cava flow velocity waveforms in appropriate- and small-for-gestational-age fetuses. Am J Obstet Gynecol 1992; 166:1271–1280.

271. Veille JC, Hanson R, Tatum K: Longitudinal quantitation of middle cerebral artery blood flow in normal human fetuses. Am J Obstet Gynecol 1993; 169:1393–1398.

272. Mari G, Deter RL: Middle cerebral artery flow velocity waveforms in normal and small-for-gestational-age fetuses. Am J Obstet Gynecol 1992; 166:1262–1270.

273. Vyas S, Nicolaides KH, Bower S, et al: Middle cerebral artery flow velocity waveforms in fetal hypoxemia. Br J Obstet Gynaecol 1990; 97:797–803.

274. Weiner Z, Farmakides G, Schulman H, et al: Central and peripheral hemodynamic changes in fetuses with absent end-diastolic velocity in umbilical artery: Correlation with computerized fetal heart rate pattern. Am J Obstet Gynecol 1994; 170: 509–515.

275. Sepulveda W, Shennan AH, Peek MJ: Reverse end-diastolic flow in the middle cerebral artery: An agonal pattern in the human fetus. Am J Obstet Gynecol 1996; 174:1645–1647.

276. Ott WJ, Mora G, Arias F, et al: Comparison of the modified biophysical profile to a "new" biophysical profile incorporating the middle cerebral artery to umbilical artery velocity flow systolic/diastolic ratio. Am J Obstet Gynecol 1998; 178:1346–1353.

277. Liu KZ, Dembinski TC, Mantsch HH: Prediction of RDS from amniotic fluid analysis: A comparison of the prognostic value of TLC and infra-red spectroscopy. Prenat Diagn 1998; 18:1267–1275.

278. Lewis DF, Futayyeh S, Towers CV, et al: Preterm delivery from 34 to 37 weeks of gestation: Is respiratory distress syndrome a problem? Am J Obstet Gynecol 1996; 174:525–528.

279. Piazze JJ, Maranghi L, Cosmi EV, et al: The effect of polyhydramnios and oligohydramnios on fetal lung maturity indexes. Am J Perinatol 1998; 15:249–252.

280. Piazze JJ, Maranghi L, Nigro G, et al: The effect of glucocorticoid therapy on fetal lung maturity indices in hypertensive pregnancies. Obstet Gynecol 1998; 92:220–225.

281. Chen C, Roby PV, Weiss NS, et al: Clinical evaluation of the NBD-PC fluorescence polarization assay for prediction of fetal lung maturity. Obstet Gynecol 1992; 80:688–692.

282. Bonebrake RG, Towers CV, Rumney PJ, et al: Is fluorescence polarization reliable and cost efficient in a fetal lung maturity cascade? Am J Obstet Gynecol 1997; 177:835–841.

283. Russell JC, Cooper CM, Ketchum CH, et al: Multicenter evaluation of TDx test for assessing fetal lung maturity. Clin Chem 1989; 35:1005–1010.

284. Tait JF, Foeerder CA, Ashwood ER, et al: Prospective clinical evaluation of an improved fluorescence polarization for predicting fetal lung maturity. Clin Chem 1987; 33:554–558.

285. Lee IS, Cho YK, Kim A, et al: Lamellar body count in amniotic fluid as a rapid screening test for fetal lung maturity. J Perinatol 1996; 16:176–180.

286. Rohlfs EM, Chaing SH, Chapman JF: Analytical and clinical evaluation of refractive index-matched anomalous diffraction (RI-MAD) for assessment of fetal lung maturation. Clin Chem 1996; 42:1861–1868.

287. Liu KZ, Mantsch HH: Simultaneous quantitation from infrared spectra of glucose concentrations, lactate concentrations, and lecithin/sphingomyelin ratios in amniotic fluid. Am J Obstet Gynecol 1999; 180:696–702.

288. Statland BE, Sher G: Reliability of amniotic fluid surfactant measurements. Am J Clin Pathol 1985; 83:1629–1641.

289. Ashwood ER, Palmer SE, Lenke RR: Rapid fetal lung maturity testing: Commercial versus NBD-phosphatidylcholine assay. Obstet Gynecol 1992; 80:1048–1053.

290. Fenton BW, Lin CS, Seydel F, et al: Lecithin can be detected by volume-selected proton MR spectroscopy using a 1.5 T whole body scanner: A potentially non-invasive method for the prenatal assessment of fetal lung maturity. Prenat Diagn 1998; 18: 1263–1266.

291. National Institute of Child Health and Human Development Research Planning Workshop: Electronic fetal heart rate monitoring: Research guidelines for interpretation. Am J Obstet Gynecol 1997; 177:1385–1390.

292. American College of Obstetricians and Gynecologists: Fetal heart rate patterns: Monitoring, interpretation and management. ACOG Tech Bull No. 209. Int J Gynaecol Obstet 1995; 51:65–74.

293. Cibils LA: On intrapartum fetal monitoring. Am J Obstet Gynecol 1996; 174:1382–1389.

294. Parer JT: Fetal heart rate. In Creasy R, Resnik R (eds): Maternal-Fetal Medicine, ed 2. Philadelphia, WB Saunders, 1984, p 314.

295. Vintzileos AM, Antsaklis A, Varvarigos I, et al: A randomized trial of intrapartum electronic fetal heart rate monitoring versus intermittent auscultation. Obstet Gynecol 1993; 81:899–907.

296. Perlman JM: Intrapartum hypoxic-ischemic cerebral injury and subsequent cerebral palsy: Medicolegal issues. Pediatrics 1997; 99:851–859.

297. Low JA, Victory R, Derrick EJ: Predictive value of electronic fetal monitoring for intrapartum fetal asphyxia with metabolic acidosis. Obstet Gynecol 1999; 93:285–291.

298. Rosen MG, Dickinson JC: The paradox of electronic fetal monitoring: More data may not enable us to predict or prevent infant neurologic morbidity. Am J Obstet Gynecol 1993; 168: 745–751.

299. Nelson KB, Dambrosia JM, Ting TY, et al: Uncertain value of electronic fetal monitoring in predicting cerebral palsy. N Engl J Med 1996; 334:613–618.

300. Morrison JC, Chez BF, Davis ID, et al: Intrapartum fetal heart rate assessment: Monitoring by auscultation or electronic means. Am J Obstet Gynecol 1993; 168:63–66.

301. Parer JT, Livingston EG: What is fetal distress? Am J Obstet Gynecol 1990; 162:1421–1427.

302. Reed KL, Appleton CP, Anderson CF, et al: Doppler studies of vena cava flows in human fetuses. Insights into normal and abnormal cardiac physiology. Circulation 1990; 81:498–505.

303. McNamara H, Johnson N, Lilford R: The effect on fetal arteriolar oxygen saturation resulting from giving oxygen to the mother measured by pulse oximetry. Br J Obstet Gynaecol 1993; 100:446–449.

304. Axemo P, Fu X, Lindberg B, et al: Intravenous nitroglycerin for rapid uterine relaxation. Acta Obstet Gynecol Scand 1998; 77: 50–53.

305. Weiss E, Hitschold T, Berle P: Umbilical artery blood flow velocity waveforms during variable deceleration of the fetal heart rate. Am J Obstet Gynecol 1991; 164:534–540.

306. Svenningsen L, Lindemann R, Eidal K: Measurements of fetal head compression pressure during bearing down and their relationship to the condition of the newborn. Acta Obstet Gynecol Scand 1988; 67:129–133.

307. Paul RH, Suidan AK, Yeh SY, et al: Clinical fetal monitoring. VII. The evaluation and significance of intrapartum baseline FHR variability. Am J Obstet Gynecol 1975; 123:206–210.

308. Hon EH: Instrumentation of fetal heart rate and fetal electrocardiography. Obstet Gynecol 1967; 30:281–286.

309. Ogunyemi D, Stanley R, Lynch C, et al: Umbilical artery velocimetry in predicting perinatal outcome with intrapartum fetal distress. Obstet Gynecol 1992; 80:377–380.

310. Almstrom H, Axelsson O, Ekman G, et al: Umbilical artery velocimetry may influence clinical interpretation of intrapartum cardiotocograms. Acta Obstet Gynecol Scand 1995; 74:526–529.

311. Helwig JT, Parer JT, Kilpatrick SJ, et al: Umbilical cord blood acid-base state: What is normal? Am J Obstet Gynecol 1996; 174:1807–1812.

312. Kuhnert M, Seelbach-Goebel B, Butterwegge M: Predictive agreement between the fetal arterial oxygen saturation and fetal scalp pH: Results of the German multicenter study. Am J Obstet Gynecol 1998; 178:330–335.

313. Goldaber KG, Gilstrap LC, Leveno KJ, et al: Pathologic fetal acidemia. Obstet Gynecol 1991; 78:1103–1107.

314. Bowen LW, Kochenour NK, Rehm NE, et al: Maternal-fetal pH difference and fetal scalp pH as predictors of neonatal outcome. Obstet Gynecol 1986; 67:487–495.

315. Low JA, Lindsay BG, Derrick EJ: Threshold of metabolic acidosis associated with newborn complications. Am J Obstet Gynecol 1997; 177:1391–1394.

316. Low JA: Intrapartum fetal asphyxia: definition, diagnosis, and classification. Am J Obstet Gynecol 1997; 176:957–959.

317. Wible JL, Petrie RH, Koons A, et al: The clinical use of umbilical cord acid-base determinations in perinatal surveillance and management. Clin Perinatol 1982; 9:387–397.

318. Seelbach-Gobel B, Heupel M, Kuhnert M, et al: The prediction of fetal acidosis by means of intrapartum fetal pulse oximetry. Am J Obstet Gynecol 1999; 180:73–81.

319. Kruger K, Kublickas M, Westgren M: Lactate in scalp and cord blood from fetuses with ominous fetal heart rate patterns. Obstet Gynecol 1998; 92:918–922.

320. Westgren M, Kruger K, Ek S, et al: Lactate compared with pH analysis at fetal scalp blood sampling: A prospective randomised study. Br J Obstet Gynaecol 1998; 105:29–33.

321. Nordstrom L, Ingemarsson I, Kublickas M, et al: Scalp blood lactate: A new test strip method for monitoring fetal wellbeing in labour. Br J Obstet Gynaecol 1995; 102:894–899.

322. Goodwin TM, Milner-Masterson L, Paul RH: Elimination of fetal scalp blood sampling on a large clinical service. Obstet Gynecol 1994; 83:971–974.

323. Dildy GA, Clark SL, Loucks CA: Intrapartum fetal pulse oximetry: Past, present, and future. Am J Obstet Gynecol 1996; 175: 1–9.

324. Dildy GA, Clark SL, Garite TJ, et al: Current status of the multicenter randomized clinical trial on fetal oxygen saturation monitoring in the United States. Eur J Obstet Gynecol Reprod Biol 1997; 72:S43–50.

325. Johnson N, Johnson VA, Bannister J, et al: The effect of caput succedaneum on oxygen saturation measurement. Br J Obstet Gynaecol 1990; 97:493–498.

326. Goffinet F, Langer B, Carbonne B, et al: Multicenter study on the clinical value of fetal pulse oximetry. I. Methodologic evaluation. The French Study Group on Fetal Pulse Oximetry. Am J Obstet Gynecol 1997; 177:1238–1246.

327. Carbonne B, Langer B, Goffinet F, et al: Multicenter study on the clinical value of fetal pulse oximetry. II. Compared predictive values of pulse oximetry and fetal blood analysis. The French Study Group on Fetal Pulse Oximetry. Am J Obstet Gynecol 1997; 177:593–598.

328. Alshimmiri M, Bocking AD, Gagnon R, et al: Prediction of umbilical artery base excess by intrapartum fetal oxygen saturation monitoring. Am J Obstet Gynecol 1997; 177:775–779.

329. Rurak DW, Richardson BS, Patrick JE, et al: Oxygen consumption in the fetal lamb during sustained hypoxemia with progressive acidemia. Am J Physiol 1990; 258:R1108–1115.

330. Mahomed K, Mulambo T, Woelk G, et al: The Collaborative Randomised Amnioinfusion for Meconium Project (CRAMP): 2. Zimbabwe. Br J Obstet Gynaecol 1998; 105:309–313.

331. Persson-Kjerstadius N, Forsgren H, Westgren M: Intrapartum amnioinfusion in women with oligohydramniosis. A prospective randomized trial. Acta Obstet Gynecol Scand 1999; 78: 116–119.

332. Apgar V: A proposal for a new method of evaluation of the newborn infant. Anesth Analg 1953; 32:260–267.

333. Maxwell LG, Harris AP, Sendak MJ, et al: Monitoring the resuscitation of preterm infants in the delivery room using pulse oximetry. Clin Pediatr (Phila) 1987; 26:18–20.

334. Harris AP, Sendak MJ, Donham RT: Changes in arterial oxygen saturation immediately after birth in the human neonate. J Pediatr 1986; 109:117–119.

335. Dimich I, Singh PP, Adell A, et al: Evaluation of oxygen saturation monitoring by pulse oximetry in neonates in the delivery system. Can J Anaesth 1991; 38:985–988.

336. McNamara H, Chung DC, Lilford R, et al: Do fetal pulse oximetry readings at delivery correlate with cord blood oxygenation and acidaemia? Br J Obstet Gynaecol 1992; 99:735–738.

337. Fanconi S: Reliability of pulse oximetry in hypoxic infants. J Pediatr 1988; 112:424–427.

26 Monitoring in Office-Based Anesthesia

Rebecca S. Twersky, M.D.
Melinda Mingus, M.D.

Overview

The office anesthesia environment poses challenges to the anesthesiologist whose practice experience has been established primarily in hospital-based operating rooms.[1-3] It must be emphasized that the standard of care in an office surgical suite should be no less than that of a hospital or an ambulatory surgical unit. The American Anesthesiologists Association (ASA) *Standards for Basic Anesthetic Monitoring*[4] and the *Guidelines for Office-Based Anesthesia*[5] set the foundation for any equipment and monitoring that is used in office-based surgery and anesthesia practice.

The anesthesiologist who administers or medically directs the administration of an anesthesia service should ensure that a means to monitor and evaluate the patient's status will be immediately available for all patients.

There are special problems that must be recognized when administering anesthesia in the office setting. Compared with acute care hospitals and licensed ambulatory surgical facilities, office-based facilities currently have little or no regulation, oversight, or control by federal, state, or local laws. With the exception of California, accreditation by the three major accrediting bodies—the Joint Commission on Accreditation of Healthcare Organizations (JCAHO), the American Association for Ambulatory Health Care (AAAHC), and the American Association for Accreditation of Ambulatory Surgery Facilities (AAAASF)—is not required at this time. Requirements for accreditation are general and nonspecific with regard to anesthesia equipment and monitoring.[6-8] Therefore, anesthesiologists must personally conduct investigation of areas that would be taken for granted in the hospital or ambulatory surgical facility, such as responsibility for facility construction and equipment. Anesthesiologists providing care in the facility should also ensure that established policies and procedures regarding fire, safety, drug usage, emergencies, staffing, training, and unanticipated patient transfers are in place.

The anesthesiologist, as a "guest" in the operating room, may be working with staff unfamiliar with the equipment and its maintenance, and without backup equipment or experienced personnel to assist during emergency or equipment failure. It is imperative that the anesthesiologist be satisfied that the quality and safety of the anesthesia monitoring and equipment used in the office is sufficient to reduce the risk and liability of all members of the office team.

Adherence to the *Standards for Basic Anesthetic Monitoring*,[4] *Standards for Pre- and Post-Anesthesia Care*,[9] *Guidelines for Ambulatory Anesthesia and Surgery*,[10] *Guidelines for Nonoperating Room Anesthetizing Locations*,[11] and *Guidelines for Office-Based Anesthesia*[5] should be the benchmarks for anesthetic delivery in the office. Under extenuating circumstances and according to his or her professional judgment, the anesthesiologist may waive specific requirements noted by the ASA, and the reasons should be documented in writing.

What Should Be Monitored During Office Anesthesia, and With What Equipment?

Intraoperative Care

Following *Standards for Basic Anesthetic Monitoring*[4] during intraoperative care, the anesthesiologist should monitor ventilation, oxygenation, cardiovascular status, body temperature, and neuromuscular function, if appropriate. The patient's positioning and physical safety should also be assessed.

Patient monitoring in the office should incorporate clinical observation, verbal communication, and the use of monitoring devices. As such, it is essential that the anesthesiologist be afforded direct observation of and expeditious access to the patient and anesthesia equipment, regardless of the spatial configuration within the operating area.

At a minimum, all facilities should have a reliable source of oxygen and a means to deliver positive-pressure ventilation and suctioning; resuscitation equipment and emergency drugs should be available.[10, 11] Depending on the type of anesthesia, different equipment may be used to monitor those functions[4] (Table 26-1). The equipment should be portable, reliable, and serviceable. All equipment should be maintained, tested, and inspected according to the manufacturer's specifications, and documentation of such should be readily available.

Ventilation and Oxygenation

For monitoring of ventilation, the anesthesiologist may use a precordial stethoscope, direct observation of the patient, or an in-line capnograph through a nasal cannula during monitored anesthesia care. For patients receiving general anesthesia, adequacy of ventilation should be continually evaluated. Continual monitoring for the presence of expired carbon dioxide (CO_2) shall be used unless invalidated by the nature of the patient's condition, the procedure, or the equipment. Quantitative monitoring of volume of expired gas is strongly encouraged. When an endotracheal tube or laryngeal mask

Table 26–1. Equipment for Office-Based Anesthesia by Anesthesia Type

Equipment	Monitored Anesthesia Care	Regional Anesthesia	General Anesthesia
Oxygen delivery	Nasal cannula; face masks ±	Nasal cannula; face masks ±	Breathing circuit capable of delivering >90% oxygen; anesthesia machine when inhalation agents are used
Pulse oximeter	+	+	+
Electrocardiograph	+	+	+
Blood pressure monitor	+	+	+
Anesthesia machine	—	—	+ (If inhalation agents are used)
Capnograph	Emergency intubation ±	Emergency intubation ±	+
Temperature monitor	±	±	±
Emergency equipment	+	+	+

airway (LMA) is inserted, its correct position must be verified and identified as evidenced by the presence of CO_2 in the expired gas. This can be done by capnography, capnometry, or mass spectroscopy. Many types of in-line devices are available (for example, EasyCap, Nellcor Puritan Bennett, Inc., Pleasanton, CA), and can be found on many kinds of portable equipment.

In addition to direct observation, oxygenation can be measured using pulse oximetry. Several different compact models are available for office surgery.

Cardiovascular Status

Cardiovascular status is commonly measured using a noninvasive blood pressure device, set for every 5 minutes or for intervals determined appropriate by the anesthesiologist. Continuous electrocardiographic (ECG) monitoring with the capability of strip recording is considered standard when anesthesia care is administered by anesthesiologists.

Both pulse oximetry and direct palpation can aid in assessing the patient's cardiovascular status.

Neuromuscular Function

A nerve stimulator should be available as a means of measuring neuromuscular function when paralytic agents are used.

Body Temperature

A way of measuring body temperature must be readily available for any type of anesthesia, when clinically significant changes in body temperature are intended, anticipated, or suspected.

Postoperative Care

Monitoring of the patient for ventilation, oxygenation, and cardiovascular status should be continued during the recovery period, as dictated by the ASA Standards for Postanesthesia Care.[9] Given that many patients complete the first phase of postanesthesia recovery while still in the operating room suite, the second phase of recovery may not require continuous monitoring of ventilation, oxygenation, and cardiovascular status.[12] However, the patient needs to be observed and monitored until criteria for discharge have been met. This includes an assessment of vital signs before discharge. Regardless of the level of patient recovery that is deemed necessary on the day of the procedure, all monitoring and equipment considered essential for phase 1 and phase 2 recovery should already be in place.

Preanesthesia Equipment Check

The primary responsibility for selecting, purchasing, and maintaining the anesthesia equipment, as well as emergency equipment, in an office belongs to the providers. Before any office-based procedure is started, it should be verified that the following are available (see Tables 26–2 and 26–3):

1. A reliable source of oxygen adequate for the length of the procedure; there should also be a backup supply. The anesthesiologist should consider the capabilities, limitations, and accessibility of both the primary and backup oxygen sources.

2. An adequate and reliable source of suction, comparable to standard operating room facilities.

3. A self-inflating hand resuscitator bag capable of administering at least 90% oxygen (Ambu bag) as a means to deliver positive pressure ventilation.

4. Adequate drugs, supplies, and equipment for the intended anesthesia care.

5. Emergency backup power to ensure patient protection for unforeseen circumstances.

6. An emergency cart with a defibrillator, emergency drugs, laryngoscopes, emergency airway devices, airways, masks, and other equipment needed to provide cardiopulmonary resuscitation.

7. Equipment for establishing an emergency airway.

Table 26–2. Basic Equipment and Monitoring for Office-Based Anesthesia

Oxygen source and delivery
Suction
Anesthesia medication and supplies
Blood pressure
Electrocardiograph with paper recorder
Pulse oximeter
Temperature monitoring when clinically indicated
Stethoscope

Table 26-3. Emergency Equipment

Positive pressure ventilation capable of delivering 90% oxygen, and self-inflating Ambu bag
Defibrillator
Resuscitative drugs (age-appropriate)
Appropriate-sized airways, masks, and endotracheal tubes; laryngeal mask airway
Laryngoscope blades
Emergency airway equipment
Telephone or other means of communication
Intravenous catheters and fluids
Dantrolene, if triggering agents are used
In-line capnograph or equivalent for emergency intubation

8. A reliable means of communication to request assistance.

9. Sufficient electrical outlets and backup power to satisfy anesthesia machine and monitoring equipment requirements.

10. Adequate means to illuminate the patient, anesthesia machines (when present), and monitoring equipment.

11. Adequate space to accommodate necessary equipment and personnel and to allow unhindered access to the patient and the anesthesia equipment.

12. Age- and size-appropriate equipment to care for pediatric, adult, and obese patients.

13. In any location in which inhalation anesthetics are administered, there should be anesthesia machines and equipment with monitoring consistent with current operating room standards (e.g., oxygen analyzer, disconnection alarm, oxygen fail-safe system, gas evacuation system, an accepted method of identifying and preventing inadvertent mixture of different gases, and a reliable and adequate system for scavenging waste anesthetic gases).

Anesthesia Machines

Whereas anesthesia machines are ubiquitous in hospital and surgicenter settings, office practice requires an anesthesia machine only when inhalation anesthesia is administered. Some specially designed anesthesia machines are available from several manufacturers. They contain built-in monitors that are compatible with the constraints of small office space. Regardless of whether the anesthesia machine is new or refurbished, the monitoring and equipment used during the conduct of a general anesthetic should be consistent with ASA *Standards for Basic Anesthetic Monitoring,*[4] and regular preventive maintenance as recommended by the manufacturer should be implemented and documented.

Optional Equipment

Use of the bispectral index (BIS) monitor in offices is currently being evaluated to aid in providing rapid emergent fast-track recovery, essential to the success of office anesthesia practice. This monitor measures the depth of anesthesia in relation to the anesthetic administered. The BIS monitor may allow the anesthesiologist to more precisely titrate the anesthetic under varying levels of surgical stimulation, and thereby time the emergence from anesthesia with more accuracy.[13] The latest model, the A-2000 (Aspect Medical Systems, Inc., Natick, MA), is more compact so that it may be comfortably placed in the small operating room of an office.[14]

Summary

Faced with this important and fast-growing subspecialty, anesthesiologists involved in office-based anesthesia are challenged to uphold and deliver the highest-quality patient care. It is important to recognize that delivery of care in the small and often isolated environment of the surgical office imposes special constraints on anesthesia monitoring and use of equipment. However, by adhering to ASA guidelines and standards, practitioners are equipped with the necessary tools to successfully meet that challenge.

REFERENCES

1. Twersky RS: Anesthetic and management dilemmas in office based surgery. Ambulatory Surg 1998 (6):79-83.
2. Twersky RS, Koch ME: Considerations in setting up an office-based practice, ASA Newsletter 1997; 61(9):30-32.
3. Twersky RS, Showan AM: Office-based anesthesia update: Guidelines, education and support are invaluable, ASA Newsletter 1999; 63(4):22-24.
4. Standards for Basic Anesthetic Monitoring (last amended October 21, 1998). Park Ridge, IL, American Society of Anesthesiologists, 1999.
5. Guidelines for Office-Based Anesthesia. (Approved by House of Delegates October 13, 1999.) Park Ridge, IL, American Society of Anesthesiologists, 1999.
6. Accreditation Handbook for Ambulatory Health Care. Accreditation Association for Ambulatory Health, Skokie, IL, 1998.
7. Manual for Accreditation of Ambulatory Surgery Facilities. American Association for Accreditation of Ambulatory Surgery Facilities, Mundelein, IL, 1997.
8. A Crosswalk between the American College of Surgeons' Guidelines for Optimal-Based Surgery and the Joint Commission's Ambulatory Care Standards. Oakbrook Terrace, IL, Joint Commission on Accreditation of Healthcare Organizations, 1998.
9. Standards for Pre- and Post-Anesthesia Care (last amended October 19, 1994). Park Ridge, IL, American Society of Anesthesiologists, 1999.
10. Guidelines for Ambulatory Anesthesia and Surgery (last amended October 21, 1998). Park Ridge, IL, American Society of Anesthesiologists, 1999.
11. Guidelines for Nonoperating Room Anesthetizing Locations (approved by House of Delegates October 19, 1994). Park Ridge, IL, American Society of Anesthesiologists, 1999.
12. Twersky RS: Fast tracking in ambulatory surgery: Choice of anesthetic technique. Anesth Analg 1998(suppl):1-9.
13. Rosow C, Manberg PJ: Bispectral index monitoring. Anesth Clin North Am 1998; 2:89-107.
14. Gan TJ, Glass PS, Windsor A, et al: Bispectral index monitoring allows faster emergence and improved recovery from propofol, alfentanil, and nitrous oxide anesthesia. Anesthesiology 1997; 87: 808-818.

27 Monitoring in Unusual Environments

Kirk Shelley, M.D., Ph.D.
Stacey Shelley, B.S.N.
Charlotte Bell, M.D.

Monitoring patients has always been an integral part of the operating room (OR) and critical care setting. However, in recent decades it has become necessary to monitor patients in other areas as well. The most common reason to monitor a patient in an unusual environment (non-OR or non–critical care unit) is because a procedure is being performed. The reason that the procedure is not done in the traditional OR environment normally involves one of the following three factors:

1. *Equipment.* The growth of noninvasive diagnostic and therapeutic techniques has been achieved through the introduction of sophisticated technology. This technology often comes in the form of large, bulky, and yet delicate devices. The prototype of such devices is the magnetic resonance (MR) imaging system. Currently, this device is too large to be moved but is very effective in diagnosing disorders and guiding therapy. For this type of equipment, the site is often designed around the device, to facilitate its use, and not for the convenience of the patient care provider. This equipment is often placed in crowded, poorly lighted, and out-of-the-way locations in the hospital; therefore, providing adequate monitoring for patients in these locations can be a significant challenge.

2. *Convenience.* Modern medicine has seen remarkable changes in where care is provided. Early in the 20th century, home-based care was the standard. With increasing technical sophistication came centralization and hospital-based care. Now, with increasing marketplace competition has come a degree of decentralization. Medicine is moving toward an office- or clinic-based medical practice. Increasingly, complex procedures are being offered on a convenient, local outpatient basis. Cosmetic surgery is a leading example of this trend. While those locations are convenient for the surgeon and the patient, practice in them can be inconvenient for the responsible anesthesiologist.

3. *Cost.* There is a perception that care rendered outside the traditional OR environment is less expensive. It is a credit to modern anesthesia techniques and equipment that sophisticated procedures can be performed in these nontraditional environments. How much these shifts in location will affect the true overall cost of the procedures is still unclear. However, it is true that it is not financially feasible at this time to equip all ORs with large, expensive diagnostic equipment (i.e., MR or sophisticated radiology scanners, and the like) or to physically bring such equipment to the operating suite as needed. Therefore, it is necessary that the patient be outside the controlled environment of the OR or intensive care unit (ICU) for the equipment to be used.

Familiarity with basic monitoring principles is vital to the safe observation of a patient in any environment, but it is especially important in a nontraditional one. It should be determined well in advance what equipment is essential in certain extreme environments. Thought must also be given to backup systems and the minimum essential equipment that will suffice should all else fail. An appreciation of the technical problems related to monitoring is only half the battle. Monitoring in certain extreme environments (e.g., MR imaging and extracorporeal shock wave lithotripsy [ESWL]) requires an understanding of the underlying principles of these techniques in order to select appropriate equipment and thereby safely monitor the patient.

As already mentioned, the number of procedures performed outside the OR has continued to rise sharply over the past couple of decades, due mainly to increasing technical advances in diagnostic imaging, the aggressive pursuit of minimally invasive therapeutic techniques, and cost-effectiveness. Although many of the patients who undergo these procedures are healthy, one must keep in mind that children, the mentally retarded, psychiatric patients, and the critically ill also undergo these procedures. These patients can make a "routine" procedure quite challenging. Even healthy patients can find the requirements of physical immobility during radiologic procedures very demanding. In addition to equipment, an anesthesiologist or critical care specialist may be necessary for a number of reasons, including airway management, sedation, analgesia, the patient's inability to cooperate, and the need for close hemodynamic monitoring.

In order to aid the clinician in managing patients, the American Society of Anesthesiologists (ASA) first established recognized standards for monitoring in 1986, and they have been updated periodically.[1] The ASA and other societies have further delineated specific standards for monitoring and caring for patients away from the OR suite.[2] These standards were expanded in 1996 to cover nonanesthesiologist care providers.[3] The American Academy of Pediatrics (AAP) has published guidelines for monitoring children during procedures.[4] In addition, the American College of Emergency Physicians (ACEP)[5] and the American Academy of Pediatric Dentists (AAPD) have published guidelines as well. The Joint Commission on Accreditation of Healthcare Organizations (JCAHO) has also mandated regulations pertaining to uniformity of monitoring, and documentation of monitoring at locations throughout the hospital. It is now necessary to recognize standards imposed not only by the hospital but

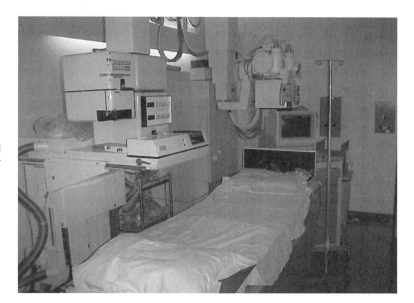

Figure 27-1. Radiology suites are often dark and cramped. They do not make the ideal monitoring environment.

also by states, the JCAHO, multiple societies, and individual departments. The result of these overlapping standards is that most institutions and clinicians attempt to provide for full monitoring in nontraditional environments. Many of the seemingly overwhelming problems first encountered when providing such monitoring in extreme environments have been greatly reduced, if not eliminated altogether, with subsequent technical advances. Equipment is now available for use in the proximity of MR imaging scanners, and newer ESWL machines no longer require that the patient be immersed in water. The following discussion concerns some of the general problems encountered with equipment and monitoring in non-OR sites and more specific recommendations for extreme environments such as MR imaging and ESWL.

This chapter examines the special considerations that must be taken when monitoring and caring for patients in three unique environments: the radiology suite (including

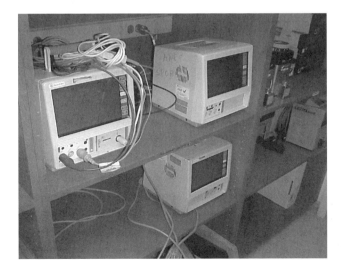

Figure 27-2. Lightweight, portable monitors can serve dual functions. Often purchased as transport monitors, they can function well as stand-alone systems. Always remember to plug them in. Most have less than 1-hour battery power available.

stereotactic radiosurgery—the so-called gamma knife), the MR imaging suite, and lithotripsy.

Basic Monitoring and Patient Care Issues in Radiology Suites

In caring for patients in nontraditional environments, one must make sure that the requirements for basic patient care are met. It is easy to overlook obvious essentials when coming from the equipment-rich environment of the OR or critical care unit. Remote locations using radiation (e.g., computed tomography [CT] scanner, angiography, and cardiac catheterization laboratory) do not normally impose physical limitations on the type of monitoring equipment that can be used. The department may limit where clinical personnel can work safely, and the physical space available for extra monitoring equipment may be at a premium. While modern radiology suites often have some type of basic patient monitors, this equipment must compete with a multitude of x-ray cameras, display devices, and mobile tables. Figure 27-1 shows a typical radiology suite with monitoring equipment competing for space. All commonly used monitors and machines can be safely used in any radiology suite, although adaptations necessary for size, electrical requirements, and scavenging systems (for anesthesia machines) may be problematic.

Electrical Considerations

While all portable monitoring systems have battery backup, a source of power must be found if one must monitor a patient for more than a few minutes. A common error when a patient is brought to an area for a procedure is to forget to plug in the portable monitor (Fig. 27-2). Almost none of the portable systems give any warning about pending battery failure. It is also important to note the type of electrical outlet that is available (Fig. 27-3). While the OR and ICU will undoubtedly have grounding precautions (i.e., isolated systems or ground fault interruption), this feature may not be present in the nontraditional settings.[6, 7] In addition, electrical outlets may not accommodate the plugs of standard

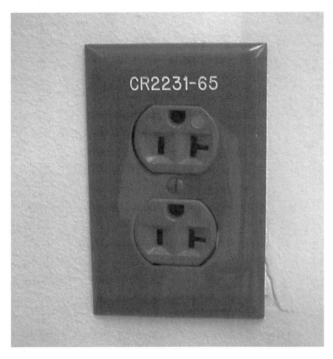

Figure 27–3. Standard three-pronged wall outlet. This was color-coded to indicate that it has emergency backup generator power available.

OR equipment, or be in sufficient supply. Historically, the use of flammable agents made it necessary to supply anesthesia machines and monitoring equipment with "explosion-proof" plugs (Fig. 27–4). These plugs are large, round, slotted disks that fit only into explosion-proof outlets. When the disk is rotated clockwise in the outlet, the contacts in the receptacles are engaged, preventing the plug from being pulled out of the outlet (Fig. 27–5). This technique also seals the system from any flammable vapors in order to prevent the escape of sparks (even static sparks) that might cause an explosion. OR equipment fitted with these explosion-proof plugs will not fit into traditional three-pronged outlets. The solution to this problem is to take an adapter and extension cords to the remote location when necessary (Fig. 27–6). At the other extreme, one may be faced with attempting to give care in an area with the old-style two-pronged wall outlet. Given the fact that the monitoring equipment is attached to the patient and that procedures are often done in "wet environments," the use of a three-pronged adapter or "cheater plug" is unacceptable.[8] Without precautions the risk of electrical shock and burns is significant.[9, 10]

Electrocardiographic Monitoring

Electrocardiography (ECG) has been the de facto standard for patient monitoring for many years. Its value has been well established and a part of published monitoring standards.[1] Although heart rate can be measured by a pulse oximeter, the ECG remains a first-line monitor for detection of arrhythmias or ischemia. Many radiologic procedures rely on the use of contrast dyes or intravascular wires to manipulate catheters. The incidence of life-threatening reactions associated with angiography or other studies utilizing contrast is approximately 1 in 1000.[11, 12] Arrhythmias are frequently

the harbinger of an untoward reaction,[13, 14] making ECG of paramount importance in remote locations. When placing the ECG electrodes, care must be taken to avoid interfering with radiologic imaging. The skin should be well prepared and the leads placed on the arms and legs, especially during angiography or CT scans of the thorax and abdomen. A brief consultation in advance with the radiologist will confirm the areas to be imaged.

Noninvasive Blood Pressure Monitoring

Automated oscillometry is advisable because it allows personnel to move away from the patient during periods of either extremely high radiation exposure (CT, radiation therapy) or of prolonged radiation exposure (cinematography during an angiogram or cardiac catheterization). An automated system will provide continuous blood pressure monitoring, and its display may be viewed through a leaded window or on a remote video monitor. It also allows the clinician greater freedom to attend to the patient.

Pulse Oximetry

Although the AAP accepts pulse oximetry as the sole monitor during conscious sedation procedures in children, caution is advised in accepting this minimum for daily practice. Although oximetry is a real-time monitor, it does not provide beat-to-beat response; it does provide averages over time. Depending on probe placement, delays in desaturation and resaturation may approach 60 seconds.[15, 16] Furthermore, accuracy is affected by common interferences, including light, motion, some intravenous dyes, and probe placement.[17] Finally, oximetry does not monitor ventilation, and oxygen saturations may be unaffected by intermittent airway obstruction or rising carbon dioxide levels. It has been said that attempting to monitor ventilation with the pulse oximeter is similar to attempting to monitor the altitude of an airplane by using its wheels. By the time you hear the bump, you are

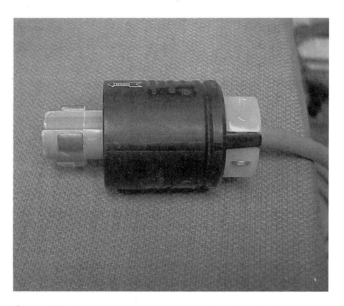

Figure 27–4. An operating room–type plug originally designed for an environment with flammable gases. These are still common in older hospitals.

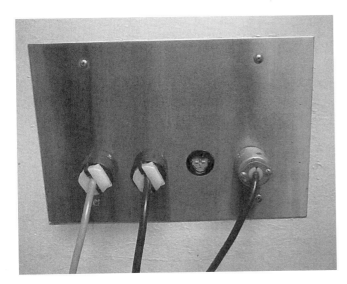

Figure 27–5. A bank of operating room outlets found commonly in older hospitals.

too low. However, most oximeters do offer the additional monitors of heart rate and plethysmography, particularly useful in some environments where ECG usage is problematic. With advances in pulse oximeter probe design, pulse oximeters are presently remarkably stable in an environment with intensive radio frequencies (RFs) (e.g., electrocautery).

Temperature

The value of temperature monitoring, well recognized in anesthesiology, is of particular significance in remote locations. Radiology suites, like ORs, are maintained at colder temperatures to accommodate the computer systems, which reconstruct images in CT, angiography, and MR imaging. These systems are sensitive to atmospheric temperature and can easily overheat. However, warming techniques commonly used in the OR cannot be utilized. For instance, radiant heat lamps or warming blankets usually interfere with imaging. Finally, cold fluids that come into contact with the patient's skin further contribute to evaporative heat loss. Use of a standard thermistor is strongly advised to enable prompt recognition and treatment of hypothermia or hyperthermia, because recent studies indicate that hypothermia may also adversely affect recovery.[18] Liquid crystal thermometers are not as accurate and may be difficult to observe in these settings.[19]

Auscultation

Auscultation of heart and breath sounds has long been the mainstay of monitoring. However, the distance between the patient and the clinician often complicates auscultation in remote locations. The remote FM wireless transmitter may be suited for remote monitoring of heart and breath sounds.[20] However, this system will not operate in the MR imaging suite, due to interference from the RF waves. The FM signal will not transmit well through shielded walls but will transmit through glass.

An infrared remote auscultation unit may be used if the clinician remains in the procedure room.[21] These units are ideal if the clinician needs freedom of movement or wishes to avoid use of an excessive amount of extension tubing. Infrared systems will not transmit through walls (they rely on a beam of light) and therefore cannot be used when the clinician must remain outside the patient room. The infrared system is well suited to angiography, fluoroscopy, or cardiac catheterization. However, in the MR imaging suite, interference may be caused by magnetic saturation of the transmitting system. The special difficulties encountered in the MR imaging suite are dealt with later.

End-Tidal Carbon Dioxide

Monitoring of end-tidal CO_2 is a simple and efficacious method of ensuring that ventilation is adequate.[22] End-tidal CO_2 monitoring is also possible in the sedated, spontaneously ventilating patient who is not tracheally intubated. Respiratory gas analysis sampling and aspirating systems can be attached to a shortened intravenous catheter and placed inside nasal oxygen prongs. An oxygen nasal cannula is available with an integral port for a sidestream anesthesia gas analyzer (Salter Labs, Arvin, CA). These cannulas are commercially available in small sizes for use with pediatric patients. Increased tubing length, particularly in small patients, may affect accuracy.

The Easy Cap (Nellcor, Hayward, CA) colorimetric disposable end-tidal CO_2 detector changes color in the presence of CO_2. It is available in adult and pediatric sizes and will give some quantification of the amount of CO_2 present.[23] Although not as accurate as gas analysis,[24] It is easily portable and can be used even in difficult environments (MR imaging).

Compact Monitoring Systems

Many of the currently available compact monitoring systems are ideal for monitoring in remote locations because they decrease the amount of equipment that must be transported. If routine OR monitors are used, they are commonly stacked for transport, which entails the risks of serious damage to

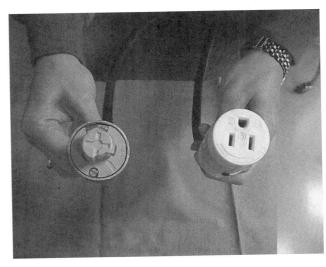

Figure 27–6. An extension cord designed to adapt older operating room (OR) electrical outlets for use with newer conventional equipment in the OR.

expensive equipment and injury to the personnel responsible for transport (Fig. 27–7). Many compact transport monitors weigh less than 10 lbs and may contain in one small box equipment for the following: ECG, two invasive pressure channels, noninvasive blood pressure, oximetry, respiratory rate, end-tidal CO_2, gas analysis, oxygen concentration, and temperature.

Monitoring and Patient Care Issues in the Magnetic Resonance Imaging Suite

First described by Rabi in 1939, (MR imaging) is one of the most significant developments in medical diagnosis. It was utilized for biologic purposes in 1946 separately by Bloch and Purcell and their colleagues,[25, 26] but several decades passed before it was refined sufficiently for clinical use. The simultaneous advances in computer and superconductor technology served to make MR imaging a practical reality. It was not until 1977 that Damadian was able to produce the first human images with this technology.[27]

The use of MR imaging for precision diagnosis is continuing to increase in popularity. When the process is used for imaging only, sedation requirements are usually minor because the imaging is painless and, because of faster technology, usually brief. On the other hand, the requirement of being still for an extended period in a claustrophobic, noisy environment can be trying for many normal adults or impossible for small children or adults with diminished mental capacity. In addition, open magnets have been designed so that intricate neurosurgical procedures can be performed within the MR imaging suite with the patient inside the magnet bore. The very nature of these procedures increases the need for precise, and at times invasive, monitoring. The monitors also need to be in close proximity to the magnet bore where the greatest magnetic field is present. General Electric maintains a website with detailed information on vendors that market equipment specifically designed for use in the delivery of anesthesia, and performance of surgical procedures, within the MR imaging scanner (http://www.ge.com/medical/mr/iomri/vendors2.htm).

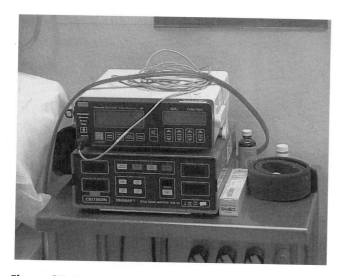

Figure 27–7. The pulse oximeter combined with the automatic blood pressure cuff is considered by many as the bare minimum monitoring system. Consideration must be given to the proposed procedure and risk of morbidity to the patient when deciding on the level of monitoring required.

The difficulties associated with using standard monitors in the presence of a powerful magnetic field have required considerable ingenuity and flexibility. The principles of MR imaging must be understood, as well as its physiologic and electronic effects on both patient and equipment, in order to adapt old equipment or design new equipment while still maintaining the same monitoring standards currently used in other locations.

Magnetic Resonance Imaging Process

The creation of an image involves six sequential steps[27–29]:

1. *Magnetic field.* First, a powerful uniform magnetic field is created, which aligns all randomly oriented nuclei. The field strengths used for medical imaging are usually 1.5 tesla (1 T = 10,000 gauss), with magnets used for human research having field strengths up to 4.0 T.[28] The earth's magnetic field is just under 1 G.

2. *Radiofrequency pulses.* Next, RF pulses are directed at the patient. In the presence of an external magnetic field, cell nuclei absorb more energy. The so-called magnetic resonance is created when these cells are superenergized by RF waves in a magnetic field.

3. *Recovery of alignment.* After nuclei have been superenergized with RF, they will recover their original alignment within the magnetic field. Each tissue will emit an RF signal proportional to the difference between the energized magnetic resonance state and the original alignment. Tissue contrast develops as a result of the different rates of realignment.

4. *Time-varied magnetic fields.* Time-varied magnetic fields (TVMFs), the contribution of Lauterbur in 1973,[30] finally made MR imaging a practical imaging modality. Magnetic field gradients are briefly applied to spatially encode the RF signals emitted from the patient. Prior to this development, two (2-D)- or three-dimensional (3-D) images had not been possible.

5. *Signal readout.* Signal readout times must be determined for each patient prior to examination, for the recording of the RF signal after initial excitation. This process is done before the actual MR imaging, after the patient is anesthetized or sedated.

6. *Fourier transform.* The signal from the patient is collected by the RF coil that surrounds the patient and is then transformed by computer into a 2- or 3-D image.

The difficulties encountered when monitoring in the MR imaging environment are related to three of these processes. They are the powerful magnetic field, RF pulses, and the TVMFs. The implications of each are discussed separately.

Magnetic Interference

The most obvious hazard of the high-static magnetic field created by MR imaging (usually 1.5 T) is the attraction of ferromagnetic objects into the magnet. An early survey revealed that up to 24% of all MR imaging centers experienced a projectile-related accident.[31] Even a ballpoint pen or metal jewelry can present a hazard. Before selecting an installation site for an MR imaging center, all potential sites must be thoroughly surveyed since all environmental iron is magnetized. It may be necessary to reroute pipes and electrical wiring and remove all stationary environmental iron (i.e., structural steel, floor decking, and concrete reinforcing rods). In spite of such precautions, it is still not possible to isolate the field completely. There is always some magnetization of the environment immediately surrounding the magnet.

Three criteria exist when evaluating equipment for use in the MR scanner. These are whether

1. The effect of the magnetic fields on the equipment presents a danger to the patient (i.e., heat creation)[32]
2. The equipment functions properly within the magnetic fields
3. The equipment has no intrinsic effects on the quality of imaging produced[33]

The influence of the scanner on equipment depends on the strength of the magnet, the proximity to the magnet bore, the amount of ferromagnetic material present, and the design of equipment circuitry. Newer MR imaging machines are shielded, so that the effects of the magnetic field decrease significantly only a few feet from the magnet bore, albeit in a deceptively nonlinear manner. It is recommended that the 50-G line be marked on the floor by a biomedical engineer, representing the point in the MR imaging suite at which the magnetic field falls to 30 to 50 G.[34, 35] At this point, some standard ferromagnetic equipment is not substantially affected by the magnet and can be used safely. Although for most newer MR imaging models the 50-G line is only 7 to 8 ft from the magnet bore, it remains critically important that no equipment be brought into the MR imaging vicinity without being checked by the biomedical engineer responsible for the area.[36] This system will not only ensure patient and personnel safety but also prevent damage to expensive equipment and prevent utilization of equipment that interferes with successful imaging.

Considerable creativity and flexibility have been necessary to adapt anesthesia equipment for use in the MR imaging environment. In general, replacing the machine's ferrous material with stainless steel, brass, or aluminum will enable its placement within the imaging room. However, even with the reduced ferrous load, much of the equipment's smaller, more delicate instrumentation is still ferromagnetic and subject to torque, the alignment of ferromagnetic material within a magnetic field. Constant torque can cause serious damage to sophisticated precision electronic equipment. Therefore, all equipment should be removed from the site when not being used. In addition, all equipment should undergo routine calibration procedures.

Another hazard of working in the magnetic field is the erasure of all magnetic media such as credit cards, passkeys, floppy disks, and videotapes. Most centers provide lockers outside the most damaging magnetic field for storage of such items and all potential projectiles. Quartz-driven analog watches will stop running in a magnetic field but will resume function once outside the field. Digital clocks are not affected and most MR imaging units include one in the control panel. This can be useful for patient record-keeping.

Magnetic interference may affect the functioning and accuracy of equipment within the immediate vicinity. Computer or oscillometric images are distorted by the bending of electronic beams into circular arcs. MR imaging–compatible equipment is designed to compensate for these distortions.

MR imaging interference also causes transformers to be saturated. Any piece of equipment powered by alternating current (AC) can be damaged in a high magnetic field.[37] Saturation of the transformer prevents the production of inductive voltage and excessive currents can burn out the power transformer.

Radiofrequency Interference

The two large RF coils that surround the patient present some of the more significant challenges to monitoring in the MR imaging suite. The outer coil transmits the RF while the inner one receives the RF emitted from the patient. The scanning room must be shielded from outside RF interference, such as television transmitters, beeper paging systems, two-way radios, and commercial radio stations, which may affect RF transmission and reception. In addition, any cables or leads can behave as antennae for the RF. The MR imaging suite can be RF-shielded by lining the walls and windows with thin continuous sheets of copper, and by using waveguides in the walls.

RF pulses are also capable of inducing electrical eddy currents and short-circuiting electrical equipment, necessitating that monitors and cables are shielded. For passive shielding, cables can be wrapped in a thin layer of aluminum foil, and small copper boxes can be used to house electrical equipment. At present, two RF-shielded nonferromagnetic monitoring systems developed by Magnetic Resonance Equipment Corporation (Bay Shore, NY) and In-Vivo Research (Winter Park, FL) are approved for use in MR imaging suites.

Time-Varied Magnetic Field

With the introduction of TVMF gradients, MR imaging became clinically useful. TVMF enables the computer to spatially encode the RF emitted from the patient to construct 2-D or 3-D images. TVMF can induce electrical eddy currents in both biologic tissue and electrical wiring. Although the biologic effects are usually minimal, very large TVMFs ($>$10,000 T/second) have the potential to interfere with nerve conduction, induce seizures, or cause ventricular fibrillation. For this reason, coils in any cables or leads should be avoided. However, since the TVMF for currently available units is well within the range of biologic current densities (1 to 10 mA/m²),[38] this particular risk is minimal.

An innocuous, albeit annoying, effect of TVMF to personnel is the presence of flickering illuminations known as magnetophosphenes. These are caused by the torque from the magnetic field gradients on the retinal cones. This effect has been completely reversible thus far, and no long-term effects have been reported.[39]

Monitoring in the Magnetic Resonance Imaging Suite

Basic Setup

Systems for central wall gases (oxygen, nitrous oxide, and air) are now commercially available for MR imaging centers.[40] It is advisable to have these installed during construction of the MR imaging suite after consultations with biomedical engineers and architects.

Electrical power sources for monitoring systems are usually available in the magnet room itself. These consist of isolated duplex power circuits with filtered 120 V (AC) to prevent electrical noise artifacts from interfering with the images.[33] Any monitors that are plugged into these outlets should be located as far from the core of the magnet as possible, beyond the gauss line. In addition, they should have little or no ferromagnetic material, and be RF-shielded. If possible, monitors should be kept outside the magnet room, and an external power source used. When thus located, only the cables should be passed through wave-guides in the wall to limit the effects of magnetization, RF, and TVMFs on the equipment.

Wave-guides. Wave-guides are necessary for pipes, cables, ducts, and electrical wires entering an RF-shielded room. Wave-guides prevent both leakage of RF pulses from the magnet room and interference from outside RF (beepers, radio, or TV signals). Additionally, electrical wiring and cables of monitoring equipment can act as antennae for RF, causing interference.

Several different types of wave-guides are available depending on the intended use. A low-pass filter is necessary for passing electrical signals through an RF-shielded wall, including electrical lighting and outlets. These filters were originally placed low in the wall, at the position farthest from the magnetic field and RF coils. The filter consists of an RF-shielded copper box covering the external passage into the room. Cables or wires pass through this box and then zigzag into the wave-guide.[37] When possible, wave-guides for monitoring systems should be included during construction of the MR imaging suite. Newer magnets are now installed with wave-guides available in the control panels in the wall so that monitoring systems can be added conveniently after construction.

An easy and economical solution to a lack of commercially installed wave-guides is to simply have a large copper pipe placed in the wall. It must be large enough to accommodate all the cables, circuits, hoses, and electrical extensions that must pass through the wall for monitors and anesthetic equipment.

Specific Monitoring Concerns

Electrocardiography. ECG is always problematic within a static magnetic field. Maximum voltage charges are induced in any column of conducting fluid (e.g., blood within the transverse aorta) when the fluid flow is 90 degrees to the field (supine patient in MR scanner).[35] The superimposed potentials are greatest in ST segments and T waves of leads I, II, V_1, and V_2 and increase with field strength. Also, spike artifacts that mimic R waves are often produced due to the changing magnetic fields of the imaging gradients. These changes in the ECG waveform are present to some degree, even in filtered systems designed for MR imaging use and essentially make it impossible to reliably monitor for ischemia or to interpret arrhythmias. Plethysmography can be used as a heart tachometer but is not useful for ischemia or arrhythmia detection.[41, 42] Telemetry units have been used with low magnetic fields (0.6 T), but generally their use interferes with the RF needed for imaging.[43, 44] In patients highly susceptible to ischemia, a 12-lead ECG pre- and post-MR imaging is recommended.

Several MR-compatible ECG systems are currently available. They use ECG electrodes made of carbon graphite to lower resistance, eliminate ferromagnetism, and minimize RF interference. In order to optimize the ECG signal, the skin must be adequately prepared (dried or abraded). ECG cables are coaxialized to avoid any coils and subsequent burning of the skin. As an extra precaution, a small towel is folded and placed on the patient's chest, to avoid lead wire contact with the skin.[45]

Blood Pressure. Automated oscillometric blood pressure monitoring eliminates the problems of electromagnetic interference, because it is based on pneumatic principles. Several manufacturers have marketed units that have been used successfully in MR imaging suites.[46] These units should be placed well away from the magnet's core, and the tubing extended to accommodate this distance using plastic connectors when required. A conventional noninvasive blood pressure unit is not shielded from either RF or the magnetic field and uses a 120-V electrical outlet. Consequently, there is usually some interference with RF during scanning, and if the patient's condition is stable, blood pressures may be recorded using the manual mode between RF pulses. Manual mercury sphygmomanometers have been adapted in a similar manner for use in MR imaging by replacing all ferromagnetic hardware with brass or aluminum pieces.[33] This enables more frequent measurement of systolic blood pressure by the "bounce" method, as well as permitting closer proximity of the blood pressure unit to the magnet.

Invasive blood pressure monitoring in the MR imaging center has certain practical limitations. Conventional disposable transducers may function adequately outside of the 50-G line, although their accuracy should be determined by a biomedical engineer. Because disposable transducers have a predictably high natural frequency, a modest addition of tubing to move the transducers away from the patient is unlikely to cause damping. Self-contained multiple-monitor systems designed for MR imaging suites are now built with modes for invasive monitoring (Magnetic Resonance Equipment, Bay Shore, NY).

Ventilation. Because the magnet depth is nearly 2 m, it is virtually impossible to visualize the patient's face and chest for adequacy of ventilation during scanning. Multiple techniques can be used simultaneously to replace direct observation.[47] Respiratory capnography is available in both conventional systems placed beyond the gauss line and MR-compatible systems. Flow-through systems are not recommended as the sensor is within the magnet bore and will likely interfere with imaging even if it is not ferromagnetic.

In anesthetized or deeply sedated spontaneously breathing patients, the Jackson Rees circuit can be attached to either the endotracheal tube or a tight-fitting mask (using a mask strap). When the circuit is placed on the chest, visualization of bag movement outside of the magnet reinforces adequacy of ventilation. In patients who are not tracheally intubated, adding continuous positive airway pressure (CPAP) has been shown to maintain airway patency during MR imaging in adults receiving propofol.[48] Direct visualization of the airway by observing the scan image is also useful to confirm airway patency.[47, 48]

Acoustic noise produced by the rapidly changing electric current pulsing through a static magnetic field makes auscultation during scanning almost impossible. Noise levels of 95 dB are frequently appreciated in 1.5-T scanners, equivalent to light roadwork.[34] Alternative monitoring techniques for confirmation of heart rate and ventilation should be used. A system for remote auscultatory monitoring using microphones to pick up heart and breath sounds has been described.[49] The sounds are transmitted to a remote receiver and headphone set as infrared light which does not interfere with imaging.

Oxygenation. Although many commercially available pulse oximeters function well in the magnet, complications have been reported with their use. Severe burns to extremities have been caused by the induction of current within a loop of wire in the presence of magnetic flux with resultant heating of the wires.[32, 50] MR-specific pulse oximeters use heavy fiberoptic cables which do not overheat and cannot be looped. Although complications are avoided, these cables are expensive and easily damaged. If conventional oximeters are used, burns can usually be avoided by placing the sensor on the extremity distal to the magnet, keeping the sensor wires free of coils, and protecting the digits with clear plastic wrap.[47]

Quench monitors are usually present within each MR imaging suite. The magnet superconductors are kept cool in liquid nitrogen. Should this coolant evaporate due to leaky housing ("quench"), the ambient oxygen supply of the room can drop precipitously, causing hypoxia and the potential for thermal injury.

Anesthesia Equipment. Until recently, existing anesthesia machines required modification before they could be used in a magnetic field.[33] By replacing the machine's ferromagnetic components with brass, aluminum, and plastic, the ferromagnetic content can be reduced to less than 2% of the total weight. The back bars and vertical supports are among the largest components that should be replaced. An MR-compatible machine, the Excel-210 MRI (Ohmeda, Madison, WI) is 99.8% stainless steel, brass, aluminum, and plastic. A similar model has recently been marketed by Dräger (Doylestown, PA). The position of the machine in the scanner suite should be determined by a biomedical engineer. Medical gas cylinders constructed from aluminum should be used exclusively in the MR imaging suite. Vaporizers, however, are affected little by the powerful magnetic field, and function accurately in this environment.

For tracheal intubation, plastic battery-operated laryngoscopes may be used. One such laryngoscope is manufactured by North American Medical Products (Londonville, NY). Batteries will last longer if shielded with a paper casing or if plastic-coated. If MR-compatible laryngoscopes are not available, the airway can be secured outside the magnet room using conventional ferromagnetic laryngoscopes before the patient is moved into the scanner.

Both circle and rebreathing anesthesia systems can be used for ventilation in the MR imaging suite but may require additional lengths of tubing. Nonferromagnetic ventilators powered by compressed oxygen are commercially available for use with MR imaging (Omnivent, Topeka, KS). Standard ventilators on anesthesia machines can be modified by reducing the ferromagnetic content. A standard Air Shields Ventimeter Controller II (Hatboro, PA) has been used successfully at a distance of 12 ft from the core of the magnet at the 70-G line.[33]

The difficulties of administering general anesthesia with an anesthesia machine can be avoided by using total intravenous anesthesia with a continuous infusion of propofol. However, all commercially available infusion pumps contain ferromagnetic circuitry that can be damaged and malfunction in the presence of a high magnetic field. Several pumps have been tested and found to be accurate in the MR imaging environment outside the gauss line, including the IVAC 530 33, the IVAC 710/711 35, the IMED 960/960A 35, and the Medfusion 2010.[51] As previously stated, each of these models should be checked on site by the biomedical engineer.

Temperature. Temperature monitoring is necessary during MR imaging because RF raises body temperature. While no biologic damage has been documented to date, tissues which dissipate heat poorly are at risk (e.g., the eye lens and the scrotum). Thermistors are not practical because of the ferromagnetic content of the cables. Consequently, liquid crystal thermometers are employed routinely, although their accuracy is limited.[52] Intermittent temperature monitoring has been recommended to reduce the possibility of skin burns from the thermistor.[53]

Monitoring and Patient Care Issues With Lithotripsy

Since the early 1980s, the use of lithotripsy to fragment renal stones has become common. This noninvasive technique is now the treatment of choice, because it removes most renal stones safely and effectively without the morbidity and prolonged recovery usually associated with open operative procedures.

Despite the continued development of lithotriptors which now offer greater convenience and less pain than the prototypes, the role of monitoring with lithotripsy is essential. In order to avoid the hazards associated with anesthetic management in remote locations, the responsible clinician must be familiar with the type and model of lithotriptor being used to anticipate patient needs and design appropriate monitoring. This section includes a discussion on the different types of lithotriptors currently available, specific monitoring needs and modifications, and environmental hazards.

The Lithotriptor

The original lithotriptor was marketed for patient use by Dornier Medical Systems (Marietta, GA), an aerospace company, which discovered that jets traveling at speeds greater than Mach 1 sustained fuselage damage from the shock waves of raindrops.[54] The subsequent application of shock waves for the bursting of calculi was based on the following principles: (1) the mechanical stress from the shock waves is greater than the strength of the renal calculus; (2) shock waves can be transmitted through water (and therefore body tissue) without losing energy until they encounter a nontissue substance (air or stone); (3) shock waves can be focused using reflectors to direct the point of impact; and (4) shock waves can be reproduced reliably.[55]

The Dornier HM-3, the prototype lithotriptor, was designed on the basis of these principles of shock waves and is still being used today in many facilities. In this spark-gap–type lithotriptor, an electric spark is generated under water and the resultant shock wave is focused with the help of an ellipsoid dish.[54, 56, 57] The shock wave is transmitted approximately three times more effectively in water than in air. Water also provides the same acoustic impedance (density) as body tissue. Consequently, no energy is lost by the shock wave until it reaches a non-tissue (non-water) interface (water-stone or water-air). Upon impact with the particular focal point, a burst of short-term high energy is released, which is greater than the tensile strength of the calculus. Repeated shock waves will pulverize or disintegrate the stone into smaller particles that subsequently can be eliminated through the ureter.

The force of the shock wave varies from 18 to 24 kV and is determined by the voltage across the electrode.[54, 58] Depending on this voltage, as much as 15,000 psig of pressure may be generated by the shock wave.[59] The Food and Drug Administration (FDA) has placed a limit on the maximum number of shocks (2000) within the 18- to 24-kV range permissible for each treatment episode on the HM-3.[54]

The original Dornier HM-3 requires that the patient be immersed to the level of the clavicles to keep both the entrance and exit of the shock waves below water. Either general or regional anesthesia is necessary with this method because pain is caused when the waves enter and exit the skin.

Several improvements have been made in the newer generations of spark-gap–type lithotriptors. With the Dornier HM-4 and Med Stone 1000, the water bath has been replaced by a water cushion, although fluoroscopy is still necessary for focusing the shock wave.[54, 55] The intentionally lower pressure generated by the shock waves of these machines reduces the pain of the procedure and therefore reduces the anesthetic requirement.

In 1986, Siemens (Siemens-Lithostar, Erlangen, Germany) introduced its second-generation Lithostar, which utilized an electromagnetic shock wave source allowing the shock wave head to be coupled to the patient without the use of a water bath. In this machine a high-voltage pulse from a capacitor is passed through an electromagnetic coil discharging 15 to 20 kV. The energy pulse passes through a thin isolating layer to a metal membrane that actually generates the shock wave. The shock waves move at the speed of sound through water to an acoustic lens system; this system focuses the waves. Coupling of the shock wave to the patient is accomplished by the use of a soft silicone coupling head which abuts the patient's flank. The stone is localized using biplanar fluoroscopy units.[60, 61] The relatively low shock wave pressure and large coupling area between the shock head and the skin produces less pain, allowing the procedure to be completed usually with only intravenous sedation on an outpatient basis.[62]

There is less need for general or regional anesthesia with this new-generation lithotriptor. In fact, an increasing need for sedation or analgesia may alert the clinician to the occurrence of complications. Patient-controlled analgesia has been advocated, as have continuous infusions.[63-65] However, neither of these methods dispenses with the need for continuous patient monitoring by a clinician.

The piezoelectric lithotriptor does not require a special water tub or any patient positioning devices. It can be placed easily in a mobile unit with no special room adaptations necessary, using standard power and water sources.[66] However, the lower pressure of the shock wave may also necessitate the use of more shock waves, or even repeat procedures, to achieve stone dissolution.

Patient Monitoring

Monitors of Cardiovascular Function

The first-generation lithotriptors (Dornier HM-3) required that the patient be immersed in warm water up to the level of the clavicles while seated semiupright in a hydraulic chair (gantry). Before appropriate monitors of cardiovascular function for use during lithotripsy are selected, it is vital to have a basic understanding of the physiologic changes during immersion and shock wave therapy. Physiologic changes with immersion are compounded by the use of anesthesia, and by having the patient seated in an upright position. Peripheral venous pooling and hypotension caused by vasodilation is even more pronounced with regional than with general anesthesia because of the resultant sympathetic blockade.[67, 68]

During immersion, increased hydrostatic pressure on the legs and abdomen compresses the peripheral capacitance vessels, causing the intravascular volume to shift to the intrathoracic compartment.[54, 59, 67] The increased intrathoracic pressure manifests itself as an increase in central venous pressure, right atrial pressure, mean pulmonary capillary wedge pressure, and peak airway pressure during positive pressure ventilation.[59, 67, 68] Acute changes in right atrial and right ventricular wall tension caused by a rapid increase or decrease in preload may result in arrhythmias.[69] The warm water temperature of the bath may heighten peripheral vaso-

dilation and increase the difficulty of maintaining hemodynamic stability. Metabolic changes produced by immersion include kaliuresis, natriuresis, diuresis secondary to decreased antidiuretic hormone (ADH), and renin production.[59]

Anesthesia, by blocking normal physiologic reflexes, may inhibit the patient's usual ability to compensate for these changes. Although such changes are generally well tolerated by young healthy patients, they may not be tolerated by patients with coronary artery disease, congestive heart failure, or significant valvular disease. Some of the cardiovascular changes caused by immersion can be lessened by immersing the patient slowly and for a brief period.[70]

Unfortunately, it is not always possible to predict the magnitude to which the cardiovascular system will be altered by immersion. In addition, it may be necessary to increase intravascular fluid, as well as administer diuretics to eliminate all stone fragments. Therefore, a pulmonary artery catheter may be required for patients with cardiac disease to detect and treat acute changes in ventricular wall tension caused by rapid changes in intravascular fluid.[54] Because patients are immersed to the level of the clavicle, it is important that the catheter insertion site be covered and protected adequately with a sterile plastic adhesive dressing to reduce the risk of infection. The presence of any catheter within the heart also increases the risk of microshock; consequently all equipment that may come in contact with either the patient or the intracardiac catheter should be carefully checked for leakage current.

The shock wave generated by lithotripsy may affect cardiac conduction. When lithotriptors were first being used, arrhythmias were frequently seen if the shock waves were delivered during the cardiac repolarization phase. Consequently, a cardiac gating capability (synchronization) was added to the original machine which enabled recognition of the QRS complex so that the shock could be delivered approximately 20 ms later, during the refractory period of the cardiac cycle. The number of shocks per minute was determined by the heart rate. Cardiac gating is used to reduce the incidence of serious arrhythmias, particularly ventricular tachycardia. Several authors have found that nonsynchronized or nongated ESWL can be safely performed in most patients.[71] These studies used the second-generation lithotriptors. With the advent of the upgraded systems (Siemens shock wave system C) that have more precise focal zones, and greater energy density in the focal zone, with overall lower average energy settings and pressure, nonsynchronized ESWL continues to be used without a concurrent rise in arrhythmias.[71]

It is still recommended that the ECG lead system be free from interference, which might trigger the shock wave and inhibit recognition of the actual QRS complex, although this risk has diminished with newer systems. Amplitude and slope criteria are utilized to assess the QRS complex and thereby prevent inadvertent recognition of noise.[72] Materials and objects capable of emitting a significant electrical charge should be kept away from the ECG to prevent random shock waves. Interference has been reported from pacemakers, shivering, peripheral nerve stimulators, electrode movement, defective wires, and signals from other equipment. Static electrical charges caused by a technician accidentally hitting the Styrofoam supports reportedly produced high-amplitude energy spikes which interfered with cardiac gating.[72]

The following steps will help to ensure that the ECG is free from interference. ECG leads should be attached to dry skin for good contact and to maintain an accurate signal. The electrode leads must be appropriately covered with a dry adhesive dressing to maintain good contact throughout the procedure. Maintaining a five-lead system for ischemia detection may be technically difficult. The Prince Henry ECG montage has been used in Australia and reportedly has a reasonable sensitivity and specificity using a three-lead system during immersion procedures.[73] In this system, the right arm electrode is placed at the manubrium, the left arm at the xiphoid, and the left leg electrode at the V_5 position. This system will give a larger P and R wave than usually seen in the lead II position and decreased muscle and respiratory artifact. When the ECG is turned to lead I, the P wave appears almost as big as when an esophageal electrode is utilized.

The safety of ESWL for patients who are pacemaker dependent remains controversial. The pacemaker spike may be erroneously perceived as a QRS complex by the lithotriptor.[74] If this occurs, the shock might not be generated during the quiescent period of the heart, causing ventricular arrhythmias. Conversely, pacemaker malfunction may occur if the shock wave is recognized as a QRS complex. Some authors believe that contemporary pacemakers sufficiently filter extraneous electrical energy and therefore shock waves would have little effect on pacemaker function.[54] Nevertheless, it has been suggested that before treatment is begun, the lithotripsy team should ensure that the pacer is at least 10 cm from the "blast path" to avoid possible damage to timing crystals. Patients with rate-responsive pacemakers undergoing ESWL should have the pacer programmed in the VVI (ventricular demand inhibited) code, in which interference is less likely to occur.[75] For patients who are not in failure, the pacer can be reprogrammed to VOO (ventricular asynchronous) at a higher rate to facilitate stone removal. This should be done just prior to lithotripsy and then reprogrammed to original settings prior to discharge. As in all situations involving pacer-dependent patients and possible interference, the anesthesiologist should have access to backup assistance, including an appropriate magnet, programmer, cardiologist, noninvasive transthoracic pacemaker, or have an emergency transvenous pacemaker kit immediately available. Medications for hemodynamic support such as isoproterenol, ephedrine, phenylephrine, and epinephrine should also be readily available.[76]

Blood pressure monitoring must be accurate and reliable during ESWL because of the anticipated hemodynamic changes brought on by immersion. Furthermore, significant postoperative hypertension has been documented in approximately 4% of patients as a result of perirenal hematoma or renal vascular damage.[77] This hypertension is usually seen during the postanesthesia recovery phase but may occur much later, and might not be recognized in outpatients who have been discharged.

An automatic (oscillometric) blood pressure device is recommended because of the patient's remoteness from the anesthesiologist.[68] Elevation of the arms may change oscillometric blood pressure readings by as much as 15 mmHg. This inaccuracy may be a problem with older gantry devices in which the arms were suspended above the patient's head out of the water bath. More recently, most institutions have elected to float the patient's arms loosely in the water to avoid peripheral neuropathy. Although the ulnar nerves may be spared with this procedure, the problem is now that of a wet blood pressure cuff. Transducers or microphones in some automatic blood pressure cuffs will not function when wet.[68] Blood pressure cuffs with Velcro may lose their adhesive ability when immersed for extended periods. A blood pressure cuff with a metal band and clip is more likely to remain correctly positioned on the patient's arm.[54]

An intra-arterial catheter with continuous waveform monitoring is recommended for patients in whom blood pressure lability is anticipated, for those whose hemodynamic status

requires continuous monitoring, or for those who may require frequent blood sampling. The catheter insertion site can be covered with a sterile plastic adhesive dressing to prevent possible contamination or infection.

Respiratory Monitoring

Immersing the patient to the level of the clavicles results in a decrease in both functional residual capacity and vital capacity because of increased hydrostatic pressure.[54, 59, 78] Perfusion shifts to the upper lobe of the lung, causing a mismatch in the ventilation-perfusion ratio. Intrapulmonary shunt is also increased because closing capacity exceeds tidal ventilation, which in turn increases the work of breathing.[59, 78] Finally, many consider the danger of airway obstruction to be greater with the lithotripsy patient simply by virtue of being remote from the anesthesiologist during general anesthesia or sedation.[59] As a result of this respiratory compromise, Vegfors and colleagues[78] noted a 2% decrease in oxygen saturation (measured by oximetry) in ASA status I and II patients undergoing immersion lithotripsy. A decrease of up to 4% was noted in patients classified as ASA III. The authors also found that premature ventricular contractions occurred more frequently in patients whose oxygen saturations decreased to 92% and that ectopy was resolved by administering higher concentrations of oxygen. There is apparently little difference in lung function regardless of whether regional or general anesthesia is used for immersion procedures.[79]

The compromised respiratory physiology and technical difficulties of patient management make it particularly important that adequate systems be available for ventilation as well as for respiratory monitoring. The precordial stethoscope is useless during lithotripsy because the loud shock wave occurs at the same time as the QRS complex, which obscures the heart tones. Furthermore, with immersion-type lithotriptors, it is difficult to secure the precordial stethoscope to the chest wall. Although the esophageal stethoscope can be placed with general anesthesia, the heart sounds cannot necessarily be auscultated over the shock waves.[54] Radiotelemetry overcomes the problem of remoteness by eliminating the need to extend the stethoscope with additional tubing but does not provide improved acoustics when shock waves are firing. None of these auscultatory methods is very useful because of the noise levels typical during lithotripsy; therefore, another means of monitoring respiration is essential.

Pulse oximetry and capnography are particularly important in remote and hostile environments where resuscitation is difficult and early information about respiratory malfunction is crucial. Ohmeda produces a fully immersible oximeter probe (Softprobe, Ohmeda, Boulder, CO) which offers a bright light-emitting diode (LED), can be molded to fit almost any size of patient, and is electrically safe in the water bath. Furthermore, the probe can be adapted to fit on the ear, nasal septum, or tongue, and thus be accessible outside the water bath. Placing the oximeter sensor on the ear offers the additional advantage of decreased lag time during desaturation or resaturation.[16, 80]

Infrared capnography systems are available in efficient portable units and can be adapted easily to a remote environment or even a mobile van. A nasal oxygen cannula can be used for CO_2 monitoring in the spontaneously breathing patient. In patients who are undergoing lithotripsy without immersion, apnea monitoring by impedance will enable the remote monitoring of respiratory rate. Impedance apnea monitoring does not indicate, however, that ventilation is adequate, or that it is actually occurring, because it detects chest movement only and does not monitor exhalation of CO_2.

The goal of mechanical ventilation during lithotripsy is to minimize stone movement while maximizing respiratory function. Deep "sigh" breaths may decrease intrapulmonary shunting, but they also increase movement of the diaphragm and therefore the kidney. This may expose parts of the lung field to shock waves resulting in pulmonary parenchymal injury and hemoptysis. More commonly, increased movement of the kidney causes shock waves to be fired with decreased precision of focus, impeding the accuracy of the shock waves. This results in longer procedures and possible incomplete stone destruction because less energy is delivered to the stone. Also, more energy reaches non-stone tissue or surrounding perirenal parenchyma.[81] The stone must be within 1 cc of the shock wave to be completely disintegrated.

Because of these problems with conventional mechanical ventilation, high-frequency jet ventilation has been advocated to decrease stone movement. It has been shown that stones may move as much as 15 to 68 mm with conventional positive pressure ventilation or spontaneous ventilation.[82] Several studies have shown that mean stone movement can be decreased by as much as 90% with high-frequency jet ventilation.[82, 83] Either high-frequency jet ventilation or high-frequency positive pressure ventilation using a conventional ventilator will minimize the stone movement.[83] This provides for better disintegration with fewer shock waves, shorter fluoroscopy time, less trauma to surrounding tissue, shorter immersion time, and the need to use fewer spark plugs.[59, 83] However, some investigators reportedly found no statistically significant difference in the number of shock treatments with either conventional mechanical ventilation or high-frequency jet ventilation.[84]

The use of high-frequency jet ventilation is attended by its own set of problems. Special equipment is required, which may or may not be available at a given institution, along with personnel specially trained and comfortable with the use of that equipment. System alarms become more important when unconventional equipment is being used in areas remote from the anesthesiologist and other backup support personnel.[68] The system must be specially modified for use with anesthetic agents, to scavenge gases, or to successfully monitor end-tidal CO_2.[83] However, during jet ventilation, end-tidal CO_2 can be measured intermittently by periodically shutting off the jet and giving manual deep-sigh breaths.[83, 85] Shock waves should be suspended during this short procedure to ensure they stay focused on the stone. Finally, the jet ventilator may fail to ventilate adequately in patients with bronchospasm, because increased airway resistance will necessitate higher inflation pressures, which eventually stalls the jet, halting gas flow. This may compromise ventilation markedly and may necessitate changing to conventional ventilatory techniques.[85] Regardless of the benefit-risk ratio of using high-frequency ventilation, the use of general anesthesia cannot be justified simply to minimize stone movement if the regional technique would be more appropriate for a given patient and procedure.[83]

Another technique that has been used to decrease stone movement is ECG-synchronized ventilation.[81] With this technique, the mechanical breath and therefore stone displacement occur at a fixed interval after the shock wave. Because the shock wave hits the stone during end-expiration only, the stone is totally motionless and does not leave the area of primary focus.[86] Furthermore, this type of ventilation will eliminate shock waves during aortic pulsation, which may cause movement of stones located on the left side.[81] QRS complex–activated ventilation requires the ECG to be connected to a heart rate meter and a trigger delay unit.[86] Be-

sides ventilation, shock waves are still triggered by the QRS complex to prevent arrhythmias. Therefore, a low tidal volume mechanical breath (3 Ml/kg) starts 50 to 100 ms after the shock wave is fired and ends 20 to 50 ms before beginning the next QRS complex.[87]

It has been argued that there is less stone movement with ECG-synchronized ventilation simply because the tidal volume is lower.[88] In either case, the higher ventilatory frequency increases dead space, raising the gradient between end-tidal and arterial CO_2. Consequently, monitoring arterial blood gases may be more effective than monitoring end-tidal CO_2. Alternatively, the high-frequency ventilation could be interrupted with a period of conventional ventilation, after which intermittent end-tidal CO_2 readings could be obtained. Shock waves again would be suspended during this time. Patients with pulmonary disease may be especially susceptible to greater arterial-to-end-tidal gradients. With these patients, one should consider using higher concentrations of inspired oxygen and larger ventilatory volumes.

Temperature Monitoring

Even though it is assumed that the temperature of the water bath is reliably constant, aberrations of core temperature are not uncommon. Therefore, precise temperature monitoring of both the patient and the water bath is imperative. Significant hyperthermia may be manifested as increased sweating, increased minute ventilation, decreased urine output, and increased heart rate and cardiac output.[89] If this condition is left untreated, multiple organ system failure can occur. Conversely, immersion may cause hypothermia even when the water bath is maintained at 36°C.[68] In addition to the common complications of hypothermia, including decreased peripheral perfusion and cardiac ectopy, shivering may also be a problem, affecting stone movement and shock wave accuracy. Shivering from hypothermia appears to be worse with epidural anesthesia but usually stops when the patient is placed in the heated water bath.[58]

Liquid crystal temperature strips can be placed on the forehead of the immersed patient. However, this technique is more accurate for trending than for precise monitoring and also requires that the anesthesiologist be close enough to the patient to be able to read the temperature strip. Esophageal, nasopharyngeal, or tympanic membrane probes can be used with general anesthesia. Care must be taken to avoid submerging the connection of the temperature probe to the main cable, which often causes malfunction. A skin disk can be used above the level of the clavicle with regional anesthesia. A rectal probe can also be used as long as connections are either covered with waterproof wrap or kept out of the water bath.

Mobile Lithotripsy Units

In an effort to contain costs and make expensive lithotripsy units more accessible, mobile trailers or vans with self-contained units are being used in many areas. Usually, these vans become modular extensions of the hospital interior for convenient transport of patients and personnel. Mobile units are subject to the same standards as any OR with regard to oxygen, suction, and scavenging of anesthetic gases. Some even have separate hookups connecting the van to the hospital central supply for nitrous oxide and air. To avoid having multiple gas hoses along the floor, which might constitute a potential environmental hazard, hoses are supported by rings or hooks along the ceiling.

Full electrical capabilities, as in a regular OR or radiology suite, should be present along with access to the hospital backup generator. An isolated electrical power supply with a line isolation monitor should be considered, particularly for water bath–type units. The specific details of electrical, architectural, pneumatic, and electronic interfacing with the main hospital from the mobile unit are beyond the scope of most clinicians and demand the expertise of biomedical engineers. However, an anesthesiologist should be part of the planning and design committee to ensure that all safety and risk management principles are observed.

Having a separate monitoring system located in the mobile van along with a fully stocked anesthesia cart is not only convenient but also decreases the wear and tear that occurs when equipment is transported to the van on a daily basis. Many companies now manufacture small, efficient multifunctional monitoring units that can be mounted easily on an anesthesia machine, which is especially convenient in areas with limited space. These units should be selected on the basis of a number of factors, including financial constraints and the company's previous service record with the hospital or department. The new systems offer software for all the capabilities of basic monitoring, including ECG, invasive pressure transduction, noninvasive blood pressure monitoring, oximetry, and temperature monitoring, as well as end-tidal CO_2 and apnea monitoring.

The patient is usually distant from the anesthesiologist because of either the size and shape of the lithotripsy unit or the need to protect the anesthesiologist from radiation exposure. For this reason, the monitoring unit will likely be near the anesthesiologist and distant from the patient, which will require some modification of connections or extension tubing. On the other hand, the monitoring equipment can be placed near the patient and away from the anesthesiologist. In this scenario, the monitor screen should be easy to read from a distance of 6 ft, and may have a keyed function pad which can be used separately. A monitor with extended battery pack is useful for transporting patients from the van to recovery areas or if further procedures are necessary (e.g., stent placement).[54]

Environmental Hazards in the Lithotripsy Unit

Unfortunately, much of what is required for successful stone pulverization is also the source of potential hazard for both patients and personnel. The room itself may have less direct lighting than the usual OR suite, making it difficult to see the patient, monitors, and chart. The light is often dimmed during fluoroscopy to enhance imaging, further reducing visibility.[58]

Noise pollution is of the "high-impact" type, which, though irritating, is not likely to cause permanent damage to hearing.[54] Because the HM-3 lithotriptor is louder than newer models, ear plugs can be useful for the anesthesiologist. Providing the patient with earphones can reduce noise pollution as well as improve the effectiveness of sedation or analgesia. Earphones that provide a musical background may be a worthwhile addition but may pose an electrical hazard if the patient is seated in a water bath. Commercially available earphones that use batteries would be less hazardous than those that require electrical wiring, but both types should be checked and approved by the biomedical engineers before using them with immersion-type lithotriptors. Noise pollution also interferes with monitoring by making it more difficult to perceive breath sounds, heart tones, monitoring pitches on oximetry and ECG units, and alarms.

Electrical safety for both patients and medical personnel is of paramount concern when using the immersion-type lithotripsy unit. The tank and all monitors must be carefully grounded and the entire suite electrically isolated whether in a mobile unit or not.[72] Hepp[90] used a model to show that electrical hazards are minimal as long as the patient does not touch the ellipsoid rim of the water bath while simultaneously grounded.

When defibrillation is necessary, it can be a potential hazard if the person delivering the countershock has wet hands and is also standing on the wet floor. In this situation, one must rely for protection on the internal safety devices of the defibrillator. When the skin is wet, the delivered countershock follows the path of least resistance along the skin and the amount of energy that actually reaches the heart may be inadequate.

It is difficult to position the patient in the water bath in a way that will avoid nerve injuries.[69] During the procedure, the patient must be suspended in a hydraulic chair (gantry), which presents the two-fold problem of possibly unrecognized pressure points and the difficulty of removing the patient quickly should resuscitation be required.[58] Malhotra[57] has described an adaptation of the Surgilift Stretcher Lifter (Trans-D Corporation, Carson, CA) to assist in the placement of anesthetized patients in the gantry as well as in their prompt removal. This system prevents the patient's monitors or catheters from being dislodged, reduces the risk of back injuries to personnel, and minimizes exposure of personnel to water with its attendant electrical hazards.[57] Pressure injuries can also be minimized by floating the patient's arms in the water bath rather than securing them either laterally or above the head. With the increased use of monitored anesthesia care for patients undergoing piezoelectric or electromagnetic lithotripsy, awake patients can position themselves prior to receiving sedation to alleviate pressure points and reduce pressure injuries. Of course, vigilant observation of these patients once they have received analgesia and sedation is necessary because they may not have sufficient pain or awareness to reposition themselves during the procedure.

The use of biplanar fluoroscopy to localize stones adds radiation exposure to the list of potential hazards.[56] In addition, spot films that require more radiation exposure are necessary to monitor the location and disintegration of the stone. The actual amount of radiation to which the patient is exposed depends on a number of factors, including the imaging technique used (fluoroscopy versus spot pictures), the x-ray tube output (voltage and amperage), total exposure time, patient weight and body surface area, and stone size and position. Tube collimators are used to reduce the field size and therefore the amount of exposure.[56] Although not studied, the increasing number of lithotripsy procedures performed with conscious sedation may cause an increase in the number of inadvertent or reflex movements by the patients necessitating increased imaging and therefore increased radiation exposure.

It is almost impossible to successfully shield patients from radiation within the water bath. However, shielding of the genitalia, thyroid, and eyes may be accomplished with other types of lithotriptors. Exposure of medical personnel to radiation appears to be negligible at a distance of approximately 3 ft from the lithotriptor.[54] Regardless, all personnel should be appropriately protected with lead shielding or stand behind leaded glass, and those exposed on a routine basis should wear dosimeters.[56]

Summary

The key to successfully monitoring a patient in an unusual environment is flexibility. The clinician must be prepared to adapt to whatever resources may be available (Fig. 27–8). It

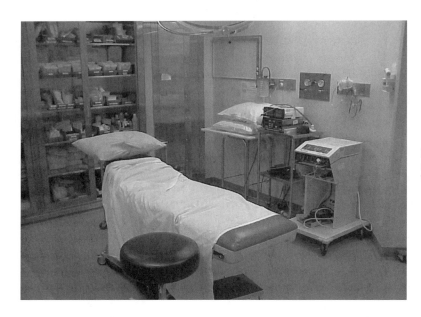

Figure 27–8. A nicely arranged procedure room with supplies and monitoring equipment nearby. Note that wall oxygen and suction are readily available.

is particularly important to recruit whatever local expertise may be available. While it may be impossible to duplicate the level of monitoring available in the OR or critical care unit, adequate monitoring for short procedures should be attainable anywhere.

REFERENCES

1. Standards for Basic Anesthesia Monitoring, Directory of Members, ed 63. Park Ridge, IL, American Society of Anesthesiologists, 1998, pp 438–439.
2. Guidelines for Nonoperating Room Anesthetizing Locations, Directory of Members, ed 63. Park Ridge, IL, American Society of Anesthesiologists, 1998, pp 438–439.
3. Practice guidelines for sedation and analgesia by non-anesthesiologists. A report by the American Society of Anesthesiologists Task Force on Sedation and Analgesia by Non-Anesthesiologists. Anesthesiology 1996; 84:459–471.
4. American Academy of Pediatrics Committee on Drugs: Guidelines for monitoring and management of pediatric patients during and after sedation for diagnostic and therapeutic procedures. Pediatrics 1992; 89:1110–1115.
5. Sacchetti A, Schafermeyer R, Geradi M, et al: Pediatric analgesia and sedation. Ann Emerg Med 1994; 23:237–250.
6. Hull CJ: Electrical hazards in monitoring. Int Anesthesiol Clin 1981; 19:177–195.
7. Albisser A, Parson I, Pask B: A survey of the grounding systems in several large hospitals. Med Instrum 1973; 7:297–302.
8. Ehrenwerth J: Lasers and electrical safety in the operating room. *In* Ehrenwerth J, Eisenkraft JB (eds): Anesthesia Equipment: Principles and Applications. St Louis, Mosby–Year Book, 1993, pp 445–468.
9. Uyttendaele K, Grobstein S, Svetz P: Monitoring instrumentation. Isolated inputs, electrosurgery filtering, burns protection: What does it mean? Acta Anaesthesiol Belg 1978; 29:317–330.
10. Harpell TR: Electrical shock hazards in the hospital environment. Their causes and cures. Can Hosp 1970; 47:48–53.
11. Ansell G, Tweedie MC, West CR, et al: The current status of reactions to intravenous contrast media. Investigative Radiology 1980; 15:S32–39.
12. Shehadi WH, Toniolo G: Adverse reactions to contrast media: A report from the Committee on Safety of Contrast Media of the International Society of Radiology. Radiology 1980; 137:299–302.
13. Goldberg M: Systemic reactions to intravascular contrast media. A guide for the anesthesiologist. Anesthesiology 1984; 60:46–56.
14. Harding MB, Davidson CJ, Pieper KS, et al: Comparison of cardiovascular and renal toxicity after cardiac catheterization using a nonionic versus ionic radiographic contrast agent. Am J Cardiol 1991; 68:1117–1119.
15. Broome IJ, Harris RW, Reilly CS: The response times during anaesthesia of pulse oximeters measuring oxygen saturations during hypoxaemic events. Anaesthesia 1992; 47:17–19.
16. Reynolds LM, Nicolson SC, Steven JM, et al: Influence of sensor site location on pulse oximetry kinetics in children. Anesth Analg 1993; 76:751–754.
17. Trivedi NS, Ghouri AF, Shah NK, et al: Effects of motion, ambient light, and hypoperfusion on pulse oximeter function. J Clin Anesth 1997; 9:179–183.
18. Lenhardt R, Marker E, Goll V, et al: Mild intraoperative hypothermia prolongs postanesthetic recovery. Anesthesiology 1997; 87:1318–1323.
19. Lees DE, Schuette W, Bull JM, et al: An evaluation of liquid-crystal thermometry as a screening device for intraoperative hyperthermia. Anesth Analg 1978; 57:669–674.
20. Mizutani AR, Ozaki G, Benumof JL: A low-cost, high-fidelity FM wireless precordial radiostethoscope for continuous monitoring of heart and breath sounds. J Clin Monit Comput 1990; 6:61–64.
21. Moretti EA, Monti RA, Zeig NJ: A cordless infrared headphone system for monitoring heart and breath sounds. Anesth Analg 1990; 71:309.
22. Murray IP, Modell JH: Early detection of endotracheal tube accidents by monitoring carbon dioxide concentration in respiratory gas. Anesthesiology 1983; 59:344–346.
23. Kelly JS, Wilhoit RD, Brown RE, et al: Efficacy of the FEF colorimetric end-tidal carbon dioxide detector in children. Anesth Analg 1992; 75:45–50.
24. Ping ST, Mehta MP, Symreng T: Accuracy of the FEF CO_2 detector in the assessment of endotracheal tube placement. Anesth Analg 1992; 74:415–419.
25. Purcell E, Torry H, Pound C: Resonance absorption by nuclear magnetic moments in a solid. Phys Rev 1946; 69:37.
26. Bloch F, Hansen W, Packard M: Nuclear induction. Phys Rev 1946; 69:127.
27. Edelman R, Kleefield J, Wentz K, et al: Basic principles of magnetic resonance imaging. *In* Edelman R, Hesselink J (eds): Clinical Magnetic Resonance Imaging. Philadelphia, WB Saunders, 1990.
28. Edelman RR, Warach S: Magnetic resonance imaging. N Engl J Med 1993; 328:708–716.
29. Menon DK, Peden CJ, Hall AS, et al: Magnetic resonance for the anaesthetist. Part I: Physical principles, applications, safety aspects. Anaesthesia 1992; 47:240–255.

30. Lauterbur P: Image formation by induced local interactions: Examples employing nuclear magnetic resonance. Nature 1973; 242:190–191.

31. Pavlicek W: Safeguarding against MRI hazards. Diagn Imaging 1985; 2:166.

32. Brown TR, Goldstein B, Little J: Severe burns resulting from magnetic resonance imaging with cardiopulmonary monitoring. Risks and relevant safety precautions. Am J Phys Med Rehabil 1993; 72:166–167.

33. Karlik SJ, Heatherley T, Pavan F, et al: Patient anesthesia and monitoring at a 1.5-T MRI installation. Magn Reson Med 1988; 7: 210–221.

34. Gangarosa RE, Minnis JE, Nobbe J, et al: Operational safety issues in MRI. Magn Reson Imaging 1987; 5:287–292.

35. Peden CJ, Menon DK, Hall AS, et al: Magnetic resonance for the anaesthetist. Part II: Anaesthesia and monitoring in MR units. Anaesthesia 1992; 47:508–517.

36. Jorgensen NH, Messick JM Jr, Gray J, et al: ASA monitoring standards and magnetic resonance imaging. Anesth Analg 1994; 79:1141–1147.

37. Koskinen M: Site planning. *In* Edelman R, Hesselink J (eds): Clinical Magnetic Resonance Imaging. Philadelphia, WB Saunders, 1990.

38. Pavlicek W: Safety considerations. *In* Stark D, Bradley W (eds): Magnetic Resonance Imaging. St Louis, Mosby–Year Book, 1988.

39. Budinger T: Thresholds for physiologic effects due to RF and magnetic fields used in NMR imaging. Trans Nucl Sci 1979; 26: 2821–2825.

40. Holshouser BA, Hinshaw DB Jr, Shellock FG: Sedation, anesthesia, and physiologic monitoring during MR imaging: Evaluation of procedures and equipment. J Magn Reson Imaging 1993; 3: 553–558.

41. Selldén H, de Chateau P, Ekman G, et al: Circulatory monitoring of children during anaesthesia in low-field magnetic resonance imaging. Acta Anaesthesiol Scand 1990; 34:41–43.

42. Volgyesi GA, Doyle DJ, Kucharczyk W, et al: Design and evaluation of a pneumatic pulse monitor for use during magnetic resonance imaging. J Clin Monit Comput 1991; 7:186–188.

43. Barnett GH, Ropper AH, Johnson KA: Physiological support and monitoring of critically ill patients during magnetic resonance imaging. J Neurosurg 1988; 68:246–250.

44. McArdle CB, Nicholas DA, Richardson CJ, et al: Monitoring of the neonate undergoing MR imaging: Technical considerations. Work in progress. Radiology 1986; 159:223–226.

45. Dimick RN, Hedlund LW, Herfkens RJ, et al: Optimizing electrocardiograph electrode placement for cardiac-gated magnetic resonance imaging. Invest Radiol 1987; 22:17–22.

46. Patteson SK, Chesney JT: Anesthetic management for magnetic resonance imaging: Problems and solutions. Anesth Analg 1992; 74:121–128.

47. Bell C, Conte AH: Monitoring oxygenation and ventilation during magnetic resonance imaging: A pictorial essay. J Clin Monit Comput 1996; 12:71–74.

48. Mathru M, Esch O, Lang J, et al: Magnetic resonance imaging of the upper airway. Effects of propofol anesthesia and nasal continuous positive airway pressure in humans. Anesthesiology 1996; 84:273–279.

49. Henneberg S, Hok B, Wiklund L, et al: Remote auscultatory patient monitoring during magnetic resonance imaging. J Clin Monit Comput 1992; 8:37–43.

50. Shellock FG, Slimp GL: Severe burn of the finger caused by using a pulse oximeter during MR imaging (letter). AJR 1989; 153:1105.

51. Pope KS: An infusion pump that works in MRI (letter). Anesth Analg 1993; 77:645.

52. Marsh ML, Sessler DI: Failure of intraoperative liquid crystal temperature monitoring. Anesth Analg 1996; 82:1102–1104.

53. Hall SC, Stevenson GW, Suresh S: Burn associated with temperature monitoring during magnetic resonance imaging (letter). Anesthesiology 1992; 76:152.

54. Moyer MK, O'Gara JP, Burrus LE: General anesthesia for extracorporeal shock wave lithotripsy. AANA J 1988; 56:121–126.

55. Jocham D, Brandl H, Chaussy C, et al: Treatment of nephrolithiasis with ESWL. *In* Gravenstein J, Peter K (eds): Extracorporeal

Shock-Wave Lithotripsy for Renal Stone Disease. Boston, Butterworths, 1986.

56. Carter HB, Näslund EB, Riehle RAJ: Variables influencing radiation exposure during extracorporeal shock wave lithotripsy. Review of 298 treatments. Urology 1987; 30:546–550.

57. Malhotra V: A modified stretcher-lifter device for transfer of patients during extracorporeal shock wave lithotripsy (ESWL) (letter). Anesth Analg 1989; 68:699–700.

58. Silbert BS, Kluger R, Dixon GC, et al: Anaesthesia for extracorporeal shockwave lithotripsy at the Victorian Lithotripsy Service—the first 300 patients. Anaesth Intensive Care 1988; 16: 310–317.

59. London RA, Kudlak T, Riehle RA: Immersion anesthesia for extracorporeal shock wave lithotripsy. Review of two hundred twenty treatments. Urology 1986; 28:86–94.

60. Grace PA, Gillen P, Smith JM, et al: Extracorporeal shock wave lithotripsy with the Lithostar lithotriptor. Br J Urol 1989; 64: 117–121.

61. Staritz M, Rambow A, Mildenberger P, et al: Electromagnetically generated extracorporeal shock waves for gallstone lithotripsy: In vitro experiments and clinical relevance. Eur J Clin Invest 1989; 19:142–145.

62. Anderson KR, Keetch DW, Albala DM, et al: Optimal therapy for the distal ureteral stone: Extracorporeal shock wave lithotripsy versus ureteroscopy. J Urol 1994; 152:62–65.

63. Schow DA, Jackson TL, Morrisseau PM, et al: Use of alfentanil sedation anesthesia with the Dornier HM3 lithotripter. J Endourol 1993; 7:445–448.

64. Uyar M, Ugur G, Bilge S, et al: Patient-controlled sedation and analgesia during SWL. J Endourol 1996; 10:407–410.

65. Arroyo CS, Michaels EK, Laurito CE, et al: Use of continuous-infusion alfentanil for analgesia during spark-gap lithotripsy. J Endourol 1995; 9:41–43.

66. Marberger M, Türk C, Steinkogler I: Painless piezoelectric extracorporeal lithotripsy. J Urol 1988; 139:695–699.

67. Frank M, McAteer EJ, Cohen DG, et al: One hundred cases of anaesthesia for extracorporeal shock wave lithotripsy. Ann R Coll Surg Engl 1985; 67:341–343.

68. Abbott MA, Samuel JR, Webb DR: Anaesthesia for extracorporeal shock wave lithotripsy. Anaesthesia 1985; 40:1065–1072.

69. Roth RA, Beckmann CF: Complications of extracorporeal shock-wave lithotripsy and percutaneous nephrolithotomy. Urol Clin North Am 1988; 15:155–166.

70. Behnia R, Shanks CA, Ovassapian A, et al: Hemodynamic responses associated with lithotripsy. Anesth Analg 1987; 66:354–356.

71. Greenstein A, Kaver I, Lechtman V, et al: Cardiac arrhythmias during nonsynchronized extracorporeal shock wave lithotripsy. J Urol 1995; 154:1321–1322.

72. Schiller EC, Heerdt P, Roberts J: Life-threatening ECG artifact during extracorporeal shock wave lithotripsy (letter). Anesthesiology 1988; 68:477–478.

73. Wicks M, Hunt J, Walker R, et al: An electrode montage for electrocardiographic monitoring. Anaesth Intensive Care 1989; 17:74–77.

74. Walts LF, Atlee JL: Supraventricular tachycardia associated with extracorporeal shock wave lithotripsy. Anesthesiology 1986; 65: 521–523.

75. Madsen GM, Andersen C: Rate-responsive pacemakers and extracorporeal shock wave lithotripsy: A dangerous combination? (letter; comment). Anesth Analg 1993; 76:917.

76. Eide TR: Anesthetic considerations for extracorporeal shock wave lithotripsy. Int Anesthesiol Clin 1993; 31:47–56.

77. Peterson J, Finlayson B: Effects of ESWL on the blood pressure. *In* Gravenstein J, Peters K (eds): Extracorporeal Shock-Wave Lithotripsy for Renal Stone Disease. Boston, Butterworths, 1986.

78. Vegfors M, Gustafson M, Sjöberg F, et al: Pulse oximetry during extradural analgesia for extracorporeal shock wave lithotripsy. Br J Anaesth 1988; 61:771–772.

79. Kelly RE, Binion M, Malhotra V, et al: Pulmonary function after extracorporeal shock wave lithotripsy—a comparison of general and regional anaesthesia. Can J Anaesth 1989; 36:137–140.

80. Young D, Jewkes C, Spittal M, et al: Response time of pulse oximeters assessed using acute decompression. Anesth Analg 1992; 74:189–195.

81. Jansson L, Bengtsson M, Carlsson C: Heart-synchronized ventilation during general anesthesia for extracorporeal shock wave lithotripsy. Anesth Analg 1988; 67:706–709.
82. Warner MA, Warner ME, Buck CF, et al: Clinical efficacy of high frequency jet ventilation during extracorporeal shock wave lithotripsy of renal and ureteral calculi: A comparison with conventional mechanical ventilation. J Urol 1988; 139:486–487.
83. Perel A, Hoffman B, Podeh D, et al: High frequency positive pressure ventilation during general anesthesia for extracorporeal shock wave lithotripsy. Anesth Analg 1986; 65:1231–1234.
84. Finlayson B, Newman R, Hunter P, et al: Efficacy of ESWL for stone fracture. In Gravenstein J, Peter K (eds): Extracorporeal Shock-Wave Lithotripsy for Renal Stone Disease. Boston, Butterworths, 1986.
85. Berger JJ, Boysen PG, Gravenstein JS, et al: Failure of high frequency jet ventilation to ventilate patients adequately during extracorporeal shock-wave lithotripsy. Anesth Analg 1987; 66:262–263.
86. Perel A, Segal E, Pizov R, et al: QRS-activated ventilation during general anesthesia for extracorporeal shock wave lithotripsy. J Clin Anesth 1989; 1:268–271.
87. Segal E, Perel A: Heart synchronized ventilation during extracorporeal shock wave lithotripsy (letter). Anesth Analg 1989; 69:139.
88. Pond WW, Lindsey RL, Weaver GA: Value of heart-synchronized ventilation during extracorporeal shock wave lithotripsy remains unproven (letter). Anesth Analg 1989; 68:823.
89. Higgins TL, Miller EV, Roberts J: Accidental hyperthermia as a complication of extracorporeal shock-wave lithotripsy under general anesthesia. Anesthesiology 1987; 66:389–391.
90. Hepp W: Electrical safety of the Dornier lithotriptor. In Gravenstein J, Peter K (eds): Extracorporeal Shock-Wave Lithotripsy for Renal Stone Disease. Boston, Butterworths, 1986.

28 Monitoring Pain Management Procedures

James D. Helman, M.D.

Concerns and Issues for Utilization of Interventional Pain Procedures

Interventional procedures to alter or impede the transmission or perception of painful stimuli by patients are appealing. The application of diagnostic and, potentially, therapeutic neural blockade for the care of patients with acute or chronic malignant or nonmalignant pain, when appropriately implemented, may reduce the patient's discomfort. However, numerous factors limit the successful application of interventional procedures. Pain is a subjective entity that poorly correlates with the severity of the patient's medical condition. The dynamic state of disease processes (e.g., growth or invasion of tumor) and anatomic variability may mitigate the technical success of interventional procedures. In addition, forces of psychological, sociologic, financial, and legal sources may confound the uncertain pathophysiology of pain mechanisms. Hence, Carron's astute observation, that "minimal pathology with maximum dysfunction remains the enigma of chronic pain," succinctly summarizes the predicament.[1] However, information obtained from neural blockade may provide insight into the pathophysiology and location of nociception. The prior information is incorporated into a multidisciplinary approach to care of the patient with pain syndromes, which may include oral or parenteral medications, therapeutic blocks, or surgical procedures, complemented by psychological therapies.[2]

Application and interpretation of diagnostic and therapeutic interventional neural blockade are difficult. Limitations include the accurate selection of the diagnostic technique for the pain syndrome, the exact implementation of the technique, and the appropriate interpretation of the efficacy of the technique by both the patient and the practitioner.[3] Monitoring is imperative to assess physiologic homeostasis, safety, and efficacy during the implementation and interpretation of interventional procedures. This chapter discusses the utilization of monitoring for patients with pain syndromes who are being treated with interventional pain procedures.

Monitoring and Equipment Utilized in an Interventional Pain Management Procedure Clinic

An interventional pain management facility should have procedure rooms that have adequate space and equipment for both diagnostic and resuscitative care. The following equipment should be included:

1. Monitors: electrocardiography (ECG), blood pressure, pulse oximetry

2. Procedure bed(s) that can be adjusted to various positions in order to facilitate the procedure and, if necessary, resuscitation

3. Oxygen source (tank and wall, if available) with self-inflating bag-valve-mask to provide positive pressure ventilation

4. Suction machine and catheter with tubing

5. Emergency resuscitation cart with medication and airway intubation equipment

6. Cardiac defibrillator

7. Nerve stimulator

8. Intravenous fluids and catheters

9. Apparatus to hang intravenous fluids for administration

10. Radiography viewing device (light source, computer [digital images], and the like)

11. Fluoroscopy equipment and lead-impregnated garments for practitioners and patients

Adjuvant Agents and Modalities for Diagnostic or Therapeutic Intervention

Local Anesthetics

Surgical anesthesia, acute pain relief, and diagnostic and therapeutic treatment of chronic pain syndromes have been achieved with local anesthetic agents. Von Gaza,[4] Braun,[5] and Mandl[6] introduced these agents as alternative treatments for chronic pain as early as 1914. In order to determine which monitoring modalities are appropriate when using these agents, it is necessary to describe the actions and side effects resulting from the administration of local anesthetics.

Local anesthetics block sodium channels of nerve fibers by binding protein receptors in the sodium channel and impeding neuronal conduction. The duration of action is primarily related to the extent of protein binding. The onset of local anesthetic effect is correlated with the pK_a of the specific anesthetic and the frequency of nerve stimulation. Lipid solubility is also a primary determinant of intrinsic anesthetic potency and onset of action, perhaps because the site of action is the nerve membrane, which is composed primarily of lipids. Absorption of local anesthetics from various body locations relates to the proximity and distribution of the adjacent vascular blood supply. The rate of systemic absorption ranges from slowest to fastest uptake in the following locations: subarachnoid, brachial plexus, lumbar epidural, caudal epidural, subcutaneous, intercostal, and interpleural. Vasoconstrictive agents (epinephrine, norepinephrine) added to local anesthetic agents may deter systemic absorption and protract the clinical duration of anesthesia and analgesia.

The systemic and toxic effects of local anesthetics affect the central nervous system (CNS), the peripheral nervous system, and the cardiovascular system. The systemic effects are based on dose, site, and agent-specific metabolism. The CNS is extremely susceptible to the action of local anesthetics. The low molecular weight and high lipophilicity facilitate the agents' passage across the blood-brain barrier. Whereas at low concentrations local anesthetics elevate seizure thresholds, at increased concentrations they promote convulsant activity. They initially impede inhibitory neural pathways that manifest as excitation, muscle fasciculations, and tonic-clonic seizures. With increasing CNS anesthetic concentrations, respiratory arrest and coma are precipitated due to depression of inhibitory and facilitory neural pathways. Local anesthetics inhibit the peripheral nervous system through both direct peripheral and central mechanisms. Loss of sympathetic autonomic tone is evidenced by hypotension, increased gastrointestinal motility, and reduced uterine contractile tone.

Anesthetic-induced alterations in the cardiovascular system include effects on vascular smooth muscle tone, myocardial contractility, and cardiac electrophysiology. The threshold for cardiovascular toxicity exceeds CNS threshold values by 3.5- to 6.5-fold, depending on the anesthetic agent. Vasomotor tone varies from vasodilation to vasoconstriction in an agent- and dose-specific manner. An increase in sympathetic tone with CNS stimulation will result in vasoconstriction and, subsequently, vasodilation with higher anesthetic levels. The magnitude of myocardial contractile force reduction is inversely related to local anesthetic concentration. Mechanistically, myocardial dysfunction develops due to local anesthetic obstruction of cation channels (sodium, calcium, potassium) and inhibition of cyclic adenosine monophosphate (cAMP) production. Finally, automaticity in pacemaker cells (phase 4 depolarization) is depressed with local anesthetics and the effect is amplified by hypoxia and acidosis. Conduction alterations manifest due to cation flow impedance. The alterations manifest as prolongation of ECG indices (e.g., P-R, atrioventricular, and QRS time intervals). The conduction abnormalities may progress to conduction blockade (sinoatrial), reentry dysrhythmias, and, potentially, ventricular fibrillation.

Direct local anesthetic toxicity affects both neural and muscular structures. Cytotoxic inflammatory changes (edema, myelin, and Schwann cell injury) follow in vivo exposure of nerves to clinical concentrations of anesthetics.[7] Myonecrosis from local anesthetics occurs secondary to nonspecific release of intracellular calcium into the myoplasm. The immediate destruction of the adult myocytes is amplified by the addition of epinephrine and steroids.[8]

The safe and efficacious utilization of local anesthetics requires sensible selection of monitoring. Considerations should include the following:

1. Patient's medical and physical condition
2. Patient's pain syndrome (differential diagnosis)
3. Interventional procedure selected
4. Site of anesthetic administration
5. Local anesthetic compound selected (concentration, dose, metabolism)
6. Addition of adjunctive medications (adrenergic agents, opioids, and the like)[9]

Monitoring includes frequent assessment of signs of neurologic toxicity (circumoral numbness, diplopia, vertigo, fasciculations, and obtundation) and electronic monitoring (ECG, blood pressure measurement, pulse oximetry). The differential diagnosis for a local anesthetic reaction includes local anesthetic toxicity, reaction to an adjunctive vasoconstrictor, vasovagal reaction, allergic reaction (immediate or delayed anaphylaxis), extended neural blockade (e.g., subarachnoid or epidural block), or exacerbation of a concurrent medical condition (e.g., myocardial ischemia, cerebrovascular disease, pulmonary disease).[9-11]

α_2-Adrenergic Receptor Agonists

α_2-Adrenergic receptor agonists, alone or in combination with other pharmacologic agents, are gaining increased utility in the management of perioperative and chronic pain. They affect neuronal excitability and transmitter release by the action of numerous G proteins at both pre- and postsynaptic neural membrane sites. Their mechanisms of action include activation of potassium channels to hyperpolarize cells, inhibition of adenyl cyclase, inhibition of voltage-sensitive calcium channels, stimulation of phosphatidylinositol phosphate, and acceleration of sodium-hydrogen exchange. α_2-Adrenergic agonists can impede the noradrenergic cells of the locus caeruleus in the brainstem at presynaptic receptor sites by activating a G_i protein to inhibit adenyl cyclase. The locus caeruleus is associated with regulation of the sympathetic nervous system. The stimulation of central α_2 receptors may lead to bradycardia, hypotension, sedation, decreased salivation, decreased adrenocorticotropic hormone (ACTH) release, altered temperature regulation, and elevation of seizure thresholds.[12]

α_2-Adrenergic agonists have been utilized in interventional pain management by administration at neuroaxial locations (epidural or intrathecal techniques). The α_2 agonists inhibit A delta– and C nerve fiber–induced firing of wide-dynamic-range neurons in the spinal cord dorsal horn. The most favorable results for the use of α_2 agonists are in patients with deafferentation and sympathetically mediated pain in both malignant and nonmalignant states. Agents include clonidine, guanabenz, medetomidine, and dexmedetomidine. Monitoring for the principal side effects of hypotension, bradycardia, and sedation include assessment of mental status, heart rate, blood pressure, and pulse oximetry (dose >300 μg). Chronic administration of α_2 agonists (case report as short as 6 days) may result in the development of hypertension upon withdrawal of therapy. Gradual tapering of the α_2 agonists may mitigate this untoward development.[13]

α_2-Adrenergic Receptor Antagonists

Phentolamine is a nonselective α_2-adrenergic receptor antagonist that is administered by intravenous infusion to diagnose and treat sympathetically mediated pain conditions. The agent has no effect on central α_2 receptors owing to its inability to cross into the brain. There are no selective α_2 antagonists available for clinical use. The advantage of phentolamine administration over local anesthetic conduction blockade in the diagnosis of sympathetically maintained pain is phentolamine's lack of impedance of somatic and visceral neural conduction. Clinical effects of systemic phentolamine include hypotension and tachycardia and warrant monitoring with ECG and blood pressure measurement.[14] Many trials have been limited by their inadequate administration of phentolamine to a specified dose as compared with appropriate administration to physiologic effects (nasal congestion, hypotension, subjective or objective warmth of skin). In addition, no studies that have determined the response to intravenous phentolamine predict the efficacy of systemic or local anesthetic sympathetic blockade.

GABA Receptor Agonists

The amino acid γ-aminobutyric acid (GABA) is the dominant inhibitory transmitter of the spinal cord and brain. It is synthesized by GABA decarboxylase and its action is terminated by degradation (GABA transaminase) or active uptake. Three GABA receptor types exist and each has unique properties (GABA$_A$, -$_B$, and -$_C$). GABA$_A$ is a chloride-regulated ion channel receptor with 13 subunits that causes neural suppression or inhibition. The GABA$_A$ receptors are found in the spinal cord primarily at laminae I and II and with moderate density in laminae III and IV. The ion channel complex has discrete sites for binding numerous classes of sedative and hypnotic compounds to include GABA, picrotoxin, barbiturate, benzodiazepine, and neurosteroid sites.[15] The GABA$_B$ receptor is a seven-segment complex that is coupled to a G protein and uses a second messenger to cause an increase in potassium conductance or decrease in calcium conductance. The greatest density of GABA$_B$ receptors is on monosynaptic Ia afferents and descending fibers. They mediate slow inhibition of polysynaptic potentials and act presynaptically to decrease the release of substance P and other primary sensory afferent transmitters. GABA$_B$ receptors have minimal baseline activity until pathologic conditions arise.[16] GABA$_B$ agonists, such as baclofen, are effective analgesics in acute pain conditions but are inadequate for persistent pain syndromes. This inconsistency may be explained by the excess release and saturation of GABA$_B$ receptors in chronic pain syndromes. GABA$_C$ receptors have been recently detected in the spinal cord, and further study is pending.

GABA$_B$ agonists, such as baclofen, have been used for interventional pain procedures to suppress spasticity associated with spinal cord injury and multiple sclerosis.[17, 18] Baclofen inhibits excitatory amino acid release from spinal interneurons and primary afferents that subsequently depress mono- and polysynaptic spinal motor reflexes and result in muscle relaxation. It can be administered through an indwelling intrathecal catheter and implanted pump and reservoir. Adverse effects include weakness, nausea, emesis, drowsiness, dizziness, ataxia, and mental confusion. Abrupt withdrawal of baclofen may precipitate seizures. Monitoring during initial intrathecal baclofen trial includes serial neurologic evaluations of spasticity, and hemodynamic (blood pressure measurement) and respiratory (ventilatory rate and effort, pulse oximetry) function.

Opioids

Neuraxial opioids have been implemented in the treatment of acute perioperative pain and malignant and nonmalignant chronic pain conditions for two decades. Opioids may be administered to reduce or eliminate pain, which may have a positive impact on perioperative morbidity and mortality in at-risk surgical patient populations.[19] Adverse effects from the neuraxial administration of opioids include acute and delayed symptoms. Acute effects of opioids include nausea and emesis, urinary retention, pruritus, and respiratory depression. Delayed phenomena include constipation, reduced libido, amenorrhea, myoclonus, edema, facial flushing, arthralgias, diaphoresis, and nail bed discoloration. The duration of monitoring for the respiratory depressant effects of the neuraxially administered opioids depends on the chosen agent's lipophilicity (e.g., morphine, 6 to 12 hours; fentanyl, minutes to 4 hours).[20] However, studies do not suggest a significantly greater risk of respiratory depression with hydrophilic opioids (e.g., morphine, 0.1% to 0.5% incidence) as compared with lipophilic opioids (e.g., fentanyl, 0.6% incidence).[21-23] Monitoring should include hourly assessments of respiratory rate and level of sedation. Assessment of patients' respiratory performance by clinicians has demonstrated greater application than the use of apnea, carbon dioxide, or oxygen saturation monitors.[24]

Neurolysis

Neuroablative techniques have been utilized as an adjunct in the management of intractable pain secondary to malignancy and, infrequently, in nonmalignant pain syndromes. The application of lytic techniques should be restricted to pain that is discrete and expected to persist. Somatic and visceral origins of pain syndromes are more amenable to neurolysis than is neuropathic pain. The implementation of these techniques should be reserved for patients for whom trials of aggressive pharmacologic therapy and other conservative modalities have been unsuccessful. Neurolytic modalities include chemical, thermal, and surgical approaches. Appropriate monitoring of patients undergoing neurolytic procedures is determined by the lytic agent chosen, the site of administration, adjacent tissue structures at risk for injury, and the level of sedation utilized for the procedure. Surgical interventions and the coincidental monitoring implications during surgery are not discussed in this chapter.

Chemical Neurolysis

Neurolytic chemical agents used to treat pain syndromes include alcohol, phenol, and, infrequently, ammonium sulfate, chlorocresol, or glycerol. Absolute alcohol acts by extracting cholesterol, phospholipids, and cerebrosides from the nervous tissue and causes precipitation of lipoproteins and mucoproteins (wallerian degeneration).[25] Alcohol diffuses rapidly from the injection site after injection. The volume of the agent administered is usually small and hence the effects of ingested alcohol are not observed. However, complications, including local tissue injuries that range from irritation to cellulitis and necrosis, may occur. This injury may be avoided by flushing the injection needle with normal saline before removal of the needle. Alcohol neurolysis is occasionally associated with pain at the site of injection, neuralgia of variable duration (weeks to months), or hypoesthesia in the distribution of the chemically lysed nerve(s). Appropriate patient counseling may mitigate the patient's distress if these conditions occur. Lumbar and sacral intrathecal alcohol administration may result in bowel and bladder incontinence. Appropriate patient positioning and the hypobaricity of alcohol may be considered to avoid this complication. Somatic neuralgia and paraplegia secondary to vascular spasm may occur during lumbar sympathetic neurolysis with alcohol.[26] Preferential sites for administration of alcohol neurolysis include intrathecal, celiac plexus, lumbar sympathetic chain, cranial neural, paravertebral, and epidural locations.

Phenol, or carbolic acid, is a monohydroxy benzene compound that is poorly soluble and diffuses slowly from tissues. Phenol acts by nonselectively denaturing the proteins in axons and perineural blood vessels. Neural degeneration takes approximately 14 days and recovery occurs in 14 weeks. Phenol, in comparison with absolute alcohol, yields a less pronounced neurolytic block of reduced duration. Combined with glycerin or contrast solutions, phenol produces a hyperbaric mixture. Phenol acts as a local anesthetic at lower concentration and as a neurolytic agent at higher concentration. Hence it causes less pain with injection than does alcohol. Phenol's high affinity for vascular tissue must be considered when it is applied near major blood vessels (e.g., celiac plexus). The injury to blood vessels may be a factor in the pathogenesis of the neurotoxicity (i.e., paraplegia) inherent in the use of phenol. In addition, like alcohol, subcutaneous administration of phenol may cause ulceration.[26] Preferential sites for administration of phenol neurolysis include epidural, paravertebral, peripheral, intrathecal, and cranial nerves.

Monitoring during the administration of chemical neurolytic agents includes appropriate patient positioning with regard to agent baricity, precise attention to selection of injection site with serial aspiration through the needle to avoid intravascular or intrathecal injection (unless it is the proposed procedure), utilization of contrast agents and radiologic modalities to verify needle position, and serial neurologic evaluations during and following the interventional procedure.

Cryolysis and Cryoanalgesia

Neurolysis of variable duration can be achieved by hypothermia-induced nerve injury. The administration of cold results in the removal of pure water from solution. The subsequent formation of ice crystals causes changes in tissue osmolarity, cell wall permeabilty, and disruption of neural myelin.[27] The axons are damaged at the site of injury with this process. However, the epineurium, perineurium, and endoneurium are preserved. The technique is quite safe, but unfortunately the duration of analgesia may be variable.

Cryoprobes operate using two refrigeration methodologies, which include gas expansion of compressed gas (e.g., nitrous oxide, carbon dioxide, helium) or change-of-phase liquified gas (e.g., nitrogen). Cryoprobes incorporate a nerve stimulator to localize the nerve to be lysed and a thermocouple to measure the probe temperature. The area of tissue injury is approximately two to three times the diameter of a gas expansion probe ($-60°C$) and three to five times the diameter of a liquid nitrogen probe ($-180°C$). The efficacy of nerve cryolysis is predicated on the generation of a lesion greater than 4 mm in length and attainment of a tissue temperature of less than 20°C.[27]

Cryolysis may be applied to any nerve that can be precisely isolated. It may be utilized in the treatment of pain disorders involving peripheral nerves, pelvic pain, spinal facet pain, intercostal neuralgia, and facial pain. The nerves are initially blocked by the application of local anesthesia and then allowed to return to baseline function before lysis. This facilitates careful identification of sensory innervation in order to avoid motor nerve lysis. In addition, precise location of the distal tip of the cryoprobe may be facilitated by the use of fluoroscopy. Cryolysis equipment may leak along the shaft of the cryoprobe during the treatment and must be examined prior to use on the patient. Cryoprobe design includes insulation but may be augmented by the placement of the probe through a large-gauge intravenous catheter. Finally, the application of cryolysis may be extremely painful during the initial freeze cycle. Hence patients must be appropriately counseled and, perhaps, may need analgesia and sedation. Hence monitoring for cryolysis includes careful isolation of the sensory nerve roots with nerve stimulation, fluoroscopy assistance to precisely position the cryoprobe, diagnostic application of local anesthetics, and utilization of

appropriate hemodynamic and ventilatory monitoring if sedation is administered.[28]

Radiofrequency Neurolysis

Electrical current has been used to ablate neural structures and pain pathways. A radiofrequency-derived thermal injury occurs when the temperature of neural tissue exceeds 45°C. The increase in temperature is a product of frictional heat derived from molecular movement in a field of alternating current (AC). The current is derived from radio wave frequencies that form an electromagnetic field around an active electrode. The active probe is placed in the preferential location for neural lesioning, and a dispersive or indifferent electrode is placed to minimize current delivery across the heart. Heat is not generated by the active electrode itself but from current movement through adjacent tissues. Gradually increasing the wattage results in the development of heat in the tissues and the thermocouple attached to the active electrode. The temperature is monitored and wattage adjusted to a desired temperature to produce the desired lesion size. The radiofrequency equipment specifications must include the ability to (1) measure impedance, amperage, and voltage; (2) stimulate a wide range of frequencies; and (3) accurately measure the duration of a specified probe tip temperature. Hence the needle-thermocouple apparatus used for radiofrequency ablation allows injecting, lesioning, and monitoring with one apparatus. Other advantages include a low incidence of neuroma formation, a decreased incidence of adjacent tissue trauma due to temperature control of the lesion size and probe placement verification by prelesion electrical stimulation, the ability to perform the procedure under local or sedative anesthesia, and the ability to repeat the procedure if regeneration occurs.[29-31]

Indications for radiofrequency ablation have included pain syndromes involving ganglia at all levels (stellate, sphenopalatine, trigeminal, cervical, thoracic, lumbar, and sacral) and facet joints from the cervical to sacral vertebral regions. Percutaneous cordotomy is a commonly used procedure for the treatment of cancer pain, especially for pain in the contralateral torso. Complications of radiofrequency lysis have included neuralgia, incomplete sympatholysis, pneumothorax, Horner's syndrome, and motor paralysis. Monitoring to mitigate these complications includes (1) inspection of equipment for potential fractures in the needle insulation that may cause tissue injury anywhere along the course of the needle, (2) fluoroscopic or computed tomography (CT) guidance to facilitate placement of the needle, and (3) stimulation with a wide range of frequencies to accurately position the tip of the probe and avoid motor nerve injury. Patients with sensing pacemakers represent a specific situation that warrants ECG monitoring. Patients with implanted stimulators may be at increased risk of injury with radiofrequency lesioning.[29-31]

Adjuvant Techniques to Increase Efficacy and Safety of Interventional Procedures

Sedation and Analgesia

Sedation and analgesia may be administered to permit patients to undergo unpleasant interventional pain procedures. Additionally, the relief of anxiety, discomfort, or pain with analgesia or sedation may facilitate the safe, rapid, and precise conduct of the procedures. However, it is imperative to maintain adequate neurologic and cardiorespiratory function during the administration of the sedation and performance of the procedure. Guidelines for the safe conduct of sedation and analgesia have been suggested by various organizations.

Recommendations from these groups[32, 33] include the following:

1. A focused history and physical examination to assess any underlying medical conditions that would affect the administration of sedation (e.g., cardiorespiratory disease, airway abnormalities)

2. Appropriate patient counseling on the indications and risks of the interventional procedure, sedation, and preprocedure fasting

3. Appropriate monitoring before, during, and following the procedure (level of consciousness, pulmonary ventilation, oxygenation, and hemodynamics)

4. Appropriate documentation of the medications administered to the patient and the patient's contemporaneous level of consciousness, pulmonary ventilation, oxygenation, and hemodynamics

5. Administration of supplemental oxygen

6. Intravenous access to facilitate titration of sedatives and analgesics to achieve the desired effect, and the administration of pharmacologic antagonists or resuscitative adjuncts, if indicated

7. Availability of emergency equipment to establish a patent airway, provide positive pressure ventilation with supplemental oxygen, and administer pharmacologic antagonists to the analgesics and sedatives administered

8. Monitoring the patient following the procedure until the risk of cardiorespiratory depression is negligible and the patient can be discharged

Patients receiving sedation should be monitored by a medical caregiver competent in titration of sedation and able to implement airway support and resuscitation as needed. The caregiver should not be performing the interventional procedure; he or she should provide focused attention to the patient and the response to the medications administered. Patient monitoring includes periodic assessment of the level of consciousness, pulmonary ventilation (respiratory rate and depth), oxygenation (skin color, pulse oximetry), and hemodynamics (heart rate and blood pressure).[32, 33]

Radiography

Fluoroscopy and, occasionally, CT are crucial adjuncts to the performance of interventional pain procedures in the cranial, cervical, thoracic, abdominal, and pelvic regions. Radiographic technology is most pertinent to the safe and successful completion of neuroablative procedures. In addition, the instillation of opaque contrast material augments the precision of needle (probe) placement provided by radiography. Contrast dyes used in radiography are either ionic or nonionic compounds formed from a triiodinated benzene ring. Nonionic formulations (iopamidol [Isovue], iohexol [Omnipaque]) have a lower risk of CNS toxicity when administered near the neuraxis than ionic agents (diatrizoate meglumine [Renografin, Hypaque], iothalamate meglumine [Conray]). Ionic agents may be safely used when they are injected in regions other than the neuraxis. However, contrast agents may precipitate local and systemic toxicity. Signs of toxicity may range from urticaria or skin ulceration (infrequent) to

bronchospasm and possible anaphylaxis. Monitoring and treatments include therapies for hypoxemia, hypotension, and bronchospasm.[34-36]

Monitoring During Peripheral Nerve Blocks

Peripheral nerve blockade is used as a diagnostic procedure to obtain a correct differential diagnosis by blocking a particular nerve or pathway.[37] Therapeutic blocks with local anesthetics result in pain relief in accordance with the duration of the specific agents selected. Consequently, repetition of the procedure may be necessary. The beneficial effects of repeated infiltration of nerve may facilitate the implementation of physical therapy by relieving pain-induced immobilization.

The application of peripheral nerve blockade for either diagnosis or therapy must be interpreted cautiously because chronic pain may not be solely caused by a nociceptive mechanism.[38] Chronic pain resulting from peripheral nerve damage may no longer be dependent on peripheral input. Spontaneous neural activity or altered spinal and supraspinal processing (central sensitization) of stimuli may produce the patient's pain syndrome. Subsequently, a partially successful diagnostic procedure may provide more uncertainty than information. In addition, peripheral nerve blockade has limited diagnostic utility to predict successful outcome for nerve transection or neuroablative procedures. Therefore, diagnostic peripheral nerve blockade must be performed in the context of multidisciplinary assessment and management of chronic pain.

Trigger Point Injections

Palpable, discrete muscle tenderness is characteristic of myofascial pain. The pain is associated with other painful disorders, which include radiculopathy and joint arthropathy. Diagnosis includes clinical examination and electromyography (inconsistent). Conclusive, controlled therapeutic trials of the outcome of intramuscular injections are unavailable. Monitoring is applicable to the particular agents selected (local anesthetics, steroids, neurolytic techniques) and adjacent tissue structures at risk for injury (neural, muscular, vascular).

Intravenous Regional Anesthesia

Intravenous regional anesthesia (IVRA) has been used for both diagnostic and therapeutic treatment of sympathetically mediated pain syndromes. Adjuncts utilized in IVRA include local anesthetics combined with either guanethidine or bretylium. The purported mechanisms of action of local anesthetics via the IVRA technique are temporary and include (1) conduction impedance of small nerves and nerve endings, (2) conduction impedance of nerve trunks at a proximal location, (3) ischemia to neural structures, and (4) direct compression of nerve fibers. IVRA application of guanethidine and bretylium demonstrates prolonged effects in patients with sympathetically mediated pain by inhibiting the release of norepinephrine from nerve terminals and by guanethidine's effect of depleting tissues of norepinephrine.[39]

Monitoring during IVRA includes verification of the proper function of the tourniquet system, continuous evaluation for signs of neurologic toxicity, continuous hemodynamic monitoring (ECG, blood pressure measurement) because of the risk of hypotension during and following the procedure, and intravenous access to treat untoward neurologic and cardiorespiratory events.[3, 39]

Somatic Nerve Block

Somatic nerve blocks are performed for perioperative pain control and diagnostic and therapeutic relief of chronic pain disorders. In addition, the procedure may determine the efficacy of neurolysis, cryoanalgesia, or surgical nerve division. Unfortunately, the nociceptive source of the pain may be proximal to the site of the diagnostic intervention and yield the incorrect diagnosis for the origin of the pain. In addition, neuroablative procedures demonstrate poor long-term relief despite resolution of pain with local anesthetic injection. Accurate needle placement may be confirmed by knowledge of the anatomy and adjacent structures, use of radiographic adjuncts, use of a nerve stimulator, or detection of paresthesias with needle placement. Considerations for the selection of monitoring modalities utilized during the performance of interventional procedures are determined by the following:

1. Patient's medical and physical condition (e.g., impaired hemostasis)[40]
2. Patient's pain syndrome (differential diagnosis)
3. Interventional procedure selected
4. Site of the somatic nerve procedure selected
5. Adjacent tissue structures at risk for injury or adverse effects
6. Chemical agent (e.g., local anesthetic, opioid [concentration, dose, metabolism]), or neurolytic technique (chemical, cryoanalgesia, radiofrequency ablation) selected
7. Addition of adjunctive medications (adrenergic agents, opioids, and so on)

Refer to Table 28–1 for specific pain syndromes, possible neural contributions to the pain condition, and monitoring suggested for interventional procedures.[41-45]

Monitoring During Major Neuraxial Interventional Procedures

Neuraxial diagnostic and therapeutic interventional pain procedures, their associated risks, and suggested monitors are listed in Table 28–2. Interventional procedures include the following: autonomic (sympathetic and visceral) blockade of the sphenopalatine ganglion,[31] the cervicothoracic (stellate) ganglion,[46] the thoracic sympathetic ganglion,[47] the celiac (splanchnic) plexus,[48] the lumbar sympathetic ganglion,[47] the superior hypogastric plexus,[49] and the ganglion impar (ganglion of Walther),[49, 50] subarachnoid techniques,[22, 41, 52-55] epidural techniques,[41, 52, 55, 56] epidural steroid injection techniques (e.g., cervical, lumbar),[57-59] spinal cord stimulation techniques,[60-62] lysis techniques for epidural adhesions,[63] and interventional discography.[64]

Neuromodulation of the Spinal Cord

Spinal cord stimulation was initially implemented for the treatment of chronic pain in 1967.[65] The original proposed mechanism of action was stimulation of large myelinated fibers (A beta) in the dorsal column of the spinal cord.

Subsequently, additional proposed mechanisms have included activation of descending inhibitory systems, dorsal root modulation, antidromic stimulation, central inhibition of sympathetic efferent neurons, and activation of neurotransmitters (neuromodulators).[66] The success of this modality has improved with advances in the implantable electrodes (arrays of multiple electrodes),[60] computer-controlled pulse generators, and radiofrequency-coupled devices with appropriate patient selection.[61] North et al.[62] reviewed their clinical experience over 2 decades and noted that 52% of patients continued to report at least 50% pain relief with implanted spinal cord stimulators (7-year mean follow-up). Patient factors that were associated with successful treatment outcomes in their review included (1) female sex, (2) deafferentation or neural injury (versus nociceptive pain), and (3) those patients with fewer prior operations.[62] Other patient screening criteria prior to consideration of a percutaneous stimulation trial include objective pathologic findings, failure of all conservative therapies, and no evidence of major psychiatric illness or drug habituation. Presently, diagnostic indications for trial stimulation include (1) perineural fibrosis (postlaminectomy syndrome), (2) sympathetically maintained pain, (3) adhesive arachnoiditis, (4) peripheral nerve injury (neuralgia), (5) peripheral vascular disease with ischemic pain, (6) phantom limb pain, (7) spinal cord lesions with defined segmental pain, and (8) angina.

The complications of spinal cord electrode and pulse generator or receiver implantation include wound infection, electromechanical failure (electrode, receiver, pulse generator), electrode migration, and, infrequently, catheter fibrosis.[61] The neuromodulation modality may also fail if the patients are inappropriately screened during the percutaneous trial (adequate duration of trial to assess efficacy) or the patients have inappropriate expectations or comprehension with regard to the capabilities and effects of the technology.[62] Monitoring implications for spinal cord stimulator placement are noted in Table 28–2.

Monitoring to Determine Therapeutic Efficacy

Psychological and Subjective Assessment of Efficacy

In an attempt to encourage standardization of methodology that can facilitate treatment outcome monitoring, it is imperative to perform a thorough evaluation of the patient who presents with a painful condition.[67, 68] Acquired information may be used for baseline assessment and subsequent interval responses to therapeutic interventions with waxing or waning of the pain disorder. The evaluation should include the acquisition of information through a medical pain history: (1) chief complaint and associated symptom characteristics of the pain condition (characteristics of pain; date of onset; conditions at onset; quality, severity, and persistence of the pain; associated symptoms; and provocative and mitigating factors); (2) past medical history; (3) medication history; (4) systems review; (5) family history; and (6) occupation and social history. The physical examination should include a thorough evaluation and specifically a focused evaluation of three particular areas: pain behavior during the examination, and neurologic and musculoskeletal structures. The inclusion of pertinent diagnostic modalities to include radiographic tests of structure, electrodiagnostic tests of somatic function, and tests of hematologic and metabolic status augment the formulation of a differential diagnosis.

Table 28–1. Location of Pain With the Appropriate Interventional Procedure and Associated Risks

Location of Pain	Intervention	Risks	Monitors
Head			
Face	Trigeminal NB	CSF, vascular injection Hypo-, hypertension Bradycardia, asystole	IV access Fractionated dosing BP, ECG Respiratory function Pulse oximetry Fluoroscopy/CT
Orbit, ethmoid cells, sphenoid sinus, eyelid, forehead, root of nose	Ophthalmic NB	CSF, vascular injection Injury to globe	Fractionated dosing Pulse oximetry
Forehead	Supraorbital/supratrochlear NB	Vascular injection	Fractionated dosing
Upper jaw, antrum of maxilla	Maxillary NB	Vascular injection	Fractionated dosing
Lower eyelid, cheek, upper lip, temple, lateral aspect of nose	Infraorbital NB		
Lower jaw, lower lip, anterior two thirds of tongue, floor of mouth, mental nerve distribution	Mandibular NB	Vascular injection	Fractionated dosing
Lower jaw and lower lip	Mental NB		
Palate, nose	Sphenopalatine NB	Vascular injection	Fractionated dosing
Posterior one third of tongue, parotid gland, soft palate to larynx	Glossopharyngeal NB	Vascular injection	Fractionated dosing
Scalp, back of neck	Greater occipital NB	CSF, vascular injection	Fractionated dosing
Neck			
Shoulder and upper neck	Cervical plexus block	CSF, vascular injection Phrenic n. paresis	Fractionated dosing Respiratory function
	Cervical paravertebral (C1–4) block	CSF, vascular injection Phrenic n. paresis	Fractionated dosing Respiratory function Fluoroscopy
Larynx, trachea	Laryngeal NB	Glottic dysfunction	Respiratory function
	Deep cervical plexus block	CSF, vascular injection Phrenic n. paresis	Fractionated dosing Respiratory function
Structures superficial to deep fascia	Superficial cervical plexus block		
Back of neck	Greater occipital NB	CSF, vascular injection	Fractionated dosing
	Spinal accessory NB		
	Cervical facet block	CSF, vascular injection Epidural injection Nerve root paresis	Fractionated dosing Fluoroscopy
Upper extremity			
Upper extremity, including shoulder	Brachial plexus block Interscalene	CSF, vascular injection Pneumothorax Phrenic n. paresis	Fractionated dosing CXR Respiratory function
	Supraclavicular	CSF, vascular injection Pneumothorax	Fractionated dosing CXR
	Subclavian perivascular	Vascular injection Pneumothorax	CXR
	Suprascapular	Pneumothorax	CXR
Shoulder and scapular region	Brachial plexus block Suprascapular	Pneumothorax Pneumothorax	CXR CXR
Mid-upper arm to hand	All techniques	CSF, vascular injection Pneumothorax	Fractionated dosing CXR
Elbow, forearm	All techniques	CSF, vascular injection Pneumothorax	Fractionated dosing CXR
	IV regional anesthesia	Tourniquet failure (CNS, cardiac effects)	BP, Oximetry
Lower forearm, wrist, hand	Brachial plexus block, all techniques	CSF, vascular injection Pneumothorax	Fractionated dosing CXR
Lower forearm, wrist, hand	IV regional anesthesia	Tourniquet failure (CNS, cardiac effects)	
	Elbow block		
Hand	Brachial plexus block, all techniques	CSF, vascular injection Pneumothorax	Fractionated dosing CXR BP, ECG
	Elbow block, wrist block		
Digits	Wrist block, digit block		
Thorax			
Chest, parietal and visceral pleura	Intercostal NB (ribs 1–6)	Pneumothorax Vascular injection	CXR Fractionated dosing BP, ECG
	Thoracic epidural block	Hypotension CSF, vascular injection	Fractionated dosing BP, ECG
	Thoracic paravertebral block	Hypotension CSF, vascular injection Pneumothorax	Fractionated dosing CXR BP, ECG
Chest, parietal and visceral pleura, upper abdominal viscera	Interpleural block	Hypotension Vascular absorption Pneumothorax	Monitor dosing CXR

Table continued on following page

Table 28–1. Location of Pain With the Appropriate Interventional Procedure and Associated Risks *Continued*

Location of Pain	Intervention	Risks	Monitors
Back			
Back, thoracic vertebrae	Thoracic facet block	CSF, vascular injection Epidural injection Nerve root paresis Pneumothorax	Fractionated dosing Fluoroscopy CXR
Back, lumbar vertebrae	Lumbar facet block	CSF, vascular injection Epidural injection Nerve root paresis	Fractionated dosing BP, ECG Fluoroscopy
Sacroiliac joint	Sacroiliac joint block	Vascular injection Sacral nerve root paresis	Fractionated dosing
Abdomen			
Abdominal wall and abdominal and pelvic viscera	Thoracic/lumbar epidural block	Hypotension CSF, vascular injection	BP, ECG Fractionated dosing
	Subarachnoid block	Hypotension	BP, ECG
	Lumbar paravertebral block	Hypotension CSF, vascular injection Pneumothorax	BP, ECG Fractionated dosing CXR
	Intercostal NB (ribs 6–12)	Vascular injection Hypotension	Fractionated dosing BP, ECG
	Field block for upper and lower abdomen with celiac plexus and splanchnic NB	Vascular injection	Fractionated dosing Fluoroscopy
Inguinal region	Field block for inguinal region Ilioinguinal/iliohypogastric NB		
Greater pelvis, including hips, pelvic viscera, perineal floor	Subarachnoid block Lumbar epidural block	Hypotension Hypotension CSF, vascular injection	BP, ECG BP, ECG Fractionated dosing
Lesser pelvis (pelvic viscera, renal tract, genital structures, overlying dermatomes)	Subarachnoid block Lumbar epidural block Caudal epidural block	Hypotension Hypotension CSF, vascular injection Hypotension CSF, vascular injection	BP, ECG BP, ECG Fractionated dosing BP, ECG Fractionated dosing
Perineum and urinary tract	Transacral NB, caudal epidural block	Hypotension CSF, vascular injection	BP, ECG Fractionated dosing
Cervical os	Pudendal NB Paracervical NB	Vascular injection	Fractionated dosing
Penis	Penile block		
Pelvic viscera, perineal floor, rectum, bladder, genital tract	Caudal epidural block	Hypotension CSF, vascular injection	BP, ECG Fractionated dosing
Lower extremity			
Entire extremity, including hip	Subarachnoid block Lumbar epidural block Lumbosacral plexus and femoral NB Caudal epidural block	Hypotension CSF, vascular injection Hypotension CSF, vascular injection Vascular injection Hypotension CSF, vascular injection	BP, ECG Fractionated dosing BP, ECG Fractionated dosing Fractionated dosing BP, ECG Fractionated dosing
Hip joint	Sciatic, femoral NB Lumbar paravertebral block (T12–L3)	Hypotension CSF, vascular injection Vascular injection	BP, ECG Fractionated dosing Fractionated dosing
Hip and anterolateral thigh	Femoral NB Obturator NB Lateral femoral cutaneous NB		
Knee and leg	Sciatic, femoral, obturator NB		
Knee	Sciatic, femoral, obturator NB		
Leg	Common peroneal and tibial NB at knee		
Medial aspect of leg	Saphenous NB at knee		
Ankle, foot	Common peroneal and tibial NB at knee Saphenous NB at knee Ankle block IV regional anesthesia	Vascular injection	Fractionated dosing
Distal one third of foot and toes	Metatarsal block IV regional anesthesia	Vascular injection	Fractionated dosing

NB, nerve block; CSF, cerebrospinal fluid; IV, intravenous; BP, blood pressure; ECG, electrocardiogram; CT, computed tomography; CXR, chest radiograph; CNS, central nervous system.

Note: (1) Potential risk of vascular injection (CNS and cardiac morbidity) and nerve and adjacent tissue injury with all procedures warrants hemodynamic and respiratory monitoring and resuscitation equipment immediately present. (2) Monitoring infers constant clinical examination by the physician performing the interventional procedure. (3) IV access is desirable for procedures involving administration of agents in or near the neuraxis or large masses of local anesthetics at any location. (4) Monitoring for conscious sedation is discussed elsewhere in this chapter.

Adapted from references 29, 41–45, and Raj PP: Techniques. *In* Raj PP (ed): Pain Medicine: A Comprehensive Review. St Louis, Mosby–Year Book, 1996, pp 177–178.

Table 28–2. Neuraxial Procedures, Risks, and Monitors

Intervention	Risks	Monitors
Autonomic (sympathetic and visceral) blockade		
Sphenopalatine[31]	Vascular injection	IV access Fractionated dosing BP, ECG Respiratory function Pulse oximetry Fluoroscopy/CT
Cervicothoracic (stellate) sympathetic[46]	Subarachnoid injection Vascular injection Phrenic n. paresis Pneumothorax	IV access Fractionated dosing BP, ECG Respiratory function Pulse oximetry CXR ± Fluoroscopy/CT
Thoracic sympathetic[47]	Pneumothorax Subarachnoid injection	IV access Fractionated dosing BP, ECG Respiratory function Pulse oximetry Fluoroscopy/CT CXR
Celiac plexus[48]	Vascular injection Hypotension Diarrhea Paraplegia Pneumothorax Renal puncture Lumbar somatic nerve paresis	IV access Fractionated dosing BP, ECG Pulse oximetry Respiratory function Fluoroscopy/CT CXR
Lumbar sympathetic[47]	Vascular injection Hypotension Renal puncture Lumbar somatic nerve paresis	IV access Fractionated dosing BP, ECG Respiratory function Pulse oximetry Fluoroscopy/CT
Superior hypogastric plexus[49]	Vascular injection Hypotension Ureter injury Lumbar and sacral somatic nerve paresis	IV access Fractionated dosing BP, ECG Respiratory function Pulse oximetry Fluoroscopy/CT
Ganglion impar (ganglion of Walther)[50, 51]	Vascular injection Caudal epidural injection Rectum perforation	Fractionated dosing Fluoroscopy
Central neuraxial procedures		
Subarachnoid technique		

Temporary duration[11, 41, 52]
  Acute pain
  Differential block
  Diagnostic trial (morphine, baclofen)
	Hypotension
	Respiratory compromise
	Nerve injury
		IV access
		BP, ECG
		Respiratory function
		Pulse oximetry

Chemical neurolysis (e.g., alcohol, phenol)[26]	Same as above + Somatic nerve injury	Same as above + Fractionated dosing Baricity considerations in patient positioning ± Fluoroscopy

Continuous intrathecal infusions[11, 53–55]	Same as above +
	Equipment malfunction:
	  Catheter: dislodgment, leak, obstruction
	  Subdural hematoma
	  Infection
	
	Pump failure
		Includes above monitors
		
		Catheter contrast study
		
		CT
		
		Examination, complete blood count (CBC)
		Interrogate pump

Epidural technique		

Temporary duration[41, 52, 56]
  Acute pain
  Differential block
  Diagnostic trial—chronic pain (e.g., bupivacaine)
	Hypotension
	Respiratory compromise
	Nerve injury
	Dural puncture/injection
	Vascular injection
	Infection
		IV access
		Fractionated dosing
		BP, ECG
		Respiratory function
		Pulse oximetry
		Examination, CBC

Table continued on following page

Table 28–2. Neuraxial Procedures, Risks, and Monitors *Continued*

Intervention	Risks	Monitors

Continuous epidural infusions
  Acute or chronic pain [55, 56]
	Same as above +
	Permanent catheter placement:
	  Catheter: dislodgment, leak, obstruction
	Epidural hematoma
	Infection
	Pump failure
	Dural puncture/injection
	Nerve injury
	Vascular injection
		Includes above monitors
		± Fluoroscopy
		Catheter contrast study
		CT
		Examination, CBC
		Interrogate pump
		± IV access
		± Fluoroscopy

Epidural steroid injections (e.g., cervical, lumbar)[57-59]		
Spinal cord stimulation[60-62]	Epidural hematoma Infection Dural puncture Nerve injury Stimulation lead: dislodgment, fracture Epidural hematoma Infection	CT Examination, CBC IV access Fluoroscopy Interrogate system, radiography CT Examination, CBC
Lysis of epidural adhesions[63]	Pump failure Dural puncture Nerve injury Vascular injection Spinal cord compression from saline Paralysis Bowel/bladder dysfunction Infection Epidural hematoma Catheter shearing	Interrogate system IV access Fluoroscopy and water-soluble contrast BP, ECG Respiratory function Pulse oximetry
Discography (e.g., cervical, thoracic, lumbar)[64]	Dural puncture/injection Nerve injury Vascular injection Epidural hematoma Infection (discitis)	IV access Fluoroscopy and water-soluble contrast BP, ECG Respiratory function Pulse oximetry

For abbreviations, see footnote to Table 28–1.

Note: (1) Potential risk of vascular injection (CNS and cardiac morbidity) and nerve and adjacent tissue injury with all procedures warrants hemodynamic and respiratory monitoring and resuscitation equipment immediately present. (2) Monitoring infers constant clinical examination by the physician performing the interventional procedure. (3) Monitoring for conscious sedation is discussed elsewhere in this chapter.

The measurement of pain is a difficult task given its subjective variability among patients with similar disorders. Nonetheless, various tools and modalities are used in the assessment of pain and the subsequent impact of therapy. Single descriptor pain measurement scales are simple to administer and include (1) numeric pain scales, (2) visual analog scales, and (3) facial drawings. These tools are easily understood by patients, easily used by pain clinic personnel, demonstrate reliability, and permit the assessment of analgesic efficacy. However, they are restricted by the limited response choices and occasionally by reduced comprehension by the elderly, mentally handicapped, and patients with poor communication skills.

Self-reporting of pain using multidimensional pain scales is commonly used in practice today (e.g., McGill Pain Questionnaire).[69] These devices provide a mechanism to evaluate pain in more than one dimension and detect the motivational-affective components that may be missed on a single-descriptor pain assessment scale. In addition, the information may facilitate the identification of patients with functional pain. However, they are more time-consuming to administer than single-descriptor assessments. Interval assessment of the impact of therapy for pain syndromes requires that patients be unaware of previous descriptor ratings.[70] A complicating factor to the interpretation of interventional procedures includes a significant incidence of a placebo response. Patients obtain pain relief from placebo interventions in approximately one third of acute pain conditions and in upward of two thirds of chronic pain syndromes. Hence initial and subsequent pain assessment modalities are useful, but their interpretation must be cautiously individualized for each patient.[67, 68]

Stimulus Application to Assess Efficacy

Quantitative assessment of either reduction or elimination of pain in the clinical setting is desirable to validate the efficacy of interventional procedures. Their utility includes the collection of objective outcome data to guide the continuation, revision, or deletion of present clinical therapies for painful conditions. However, the significant association of placebo response in both acute and persistent pain conditions warrants guarded interpretation of the efficacy of all interventional procedures. In addition, the contribution of subjective psychological factors is difficult to measure. Modalities for the assessment of the alteration in pain thresholds by interventional procedures should include the following features: (1) a defined, adjustable stimulus; (2) an easily implemented stimulus that mimics the production of the pain; (3) a stimulus that does not produce tissue trauma; and (4) a stimulus that is reproducible under similar clinical conditions. Techniques available for assessment of interventional efficacy include controlled mechanical stimulation (e.g., algometer, algesimeter, dolorimeter, Frey's fibers, palpatometer) and quantitative sensory testing devices.

Mechanical stimulation tests are inexpensive and easy to implement in the evaluation of the efficacy of interventional pain procedures. The pressure algometer (algesimeter, dolorimeter) consists of a pressure gauge combined with a 1-cm-diameter firm rubber tip. The device is applied manually, using steadily increasing pressure at the site of inquiry. Patients are instructed to comment when pain is perceived and the pressure value is noted. Nociceptors stimulated with algometry include A delta mechanoceptors and C-polymodal nociceptors. Unfortunately, the rate of force application with the algometer is not standardized.[71] Calibrated Frey's fibers of increasing rigidity are easy to implement in the serial assessment of pain and the response to therapy.[72] The latter techniques are limited by their lack of reproducibility and variability in the rise and maintenance of a constant stimulus intensity. The palpatometer is a force-sensing resistor that can quantify the magnitude of force application to tissues by either an algometer or the examiner's fingers. This device provides a measurable and reproducible assessment of the efficacy of therapy.[73]

Quantitative sensory testing (QST) devices employ controlled electrical or thermal stimulation of the skin to reproducibly quantify sensory nerve function of nociceptive pathways. The tests depend on the subjective report of the patient when he or she perceives the testing stimulus. Abnormal patterns have been associated with pathophysiologic changes in the central or peripheral sensory nervous system. QST measurements are useful in documenting and quantifying hypoesthesia, hyperesthesia, hypalgesia, and hyperalgesia. QST testing devices include the thermal stimulation test (TST) and current perception threshold (CPT) test. The TST is performed by applying a regulated ramp of descending or ascending thermal energy through a Peltier electrode (surface area 3 to 13 cm²).[74] The patient is instructed to note the first sensation of cold, warmth, cold pain, and heat pain by depressing an inactivation switch. The stimulator subsequently returns to baseline and data points are graphically recorded. The test uses standardized thermode size, stimulation sites, rate of change in stimulus temperature, between-stimulus intervals, and pretest skin temperatures. The TST evaluates the entire peripheral and central contributions of the sensory nervous system that participate in the transmission of painful hot or cold stimuli (C-fiber and A delta nociceptors).[75, 76] Wahren et al.[77, 78] have utilized this modality to follow patients' clinical course and response to therapy. The CPT is measured by an electrical neurostimulator and two gel-coated electrodes applied within the distribution of a cutaneous nerve or dermatome. The device delivers a sinusoidal, constant AC at three different frequencies (5, 250, and 2000 Hz) and intensities ranging from 0.01 to 9.99 mA.[79] The electrical current is insufficient to directly stimulate receptors in the skin. The CPT technique appears to be neuroselective in its ability to evaluate three different types of nociceptive nerve fibers. The three different stimulation frequencies activate different groups of sensory nerve fibers (5 Hz, C; 250 Hz, A delta; 2000 Hz, A beta).[80, 81] Although QST provides a reproducible measurement of nociceptive nerve dysfunction, it cannot precisely localize the site of injury. It can be used for initial assessment and evaluation of therapeutic interventions for pain syndromes (medications, interventional procedures). In addition, experience with the testing devices has provided clues to nonphysiologic and psychogenic abnormal testing patterns.

Assessment of Efficacy of Treatment for Spasticity

Spasticity may develop subsequent to an insult to the CNS. The prolonged restriction of patient movement or the ability to change body position contributes to the development of pain and discomfort. Interventional therapies for this condition include neurodestructive techniques (subarachnoid alcohol and phenol, dorsal rhizotomies, and dorsal root entry zone lesions), central nervous stimulation, and continuous infusions of neuraxial opioids (e.g., morphine) and antispasmodics (e.g., baclofen). Methodologies to assess the efficacy of these interventions include subjective clinical assessment by clinicians or self-reporting by the patients.[82] These are easy to implement but are limited by observer bias and lack of a standardized reference system. External technical monitors include the use of time-lapse photography to record both gait and ambulatory movement. This modality is limited to patients with spasticity who are ambulatory.[83] Electromyography directly measures muscular activity. It is limited by its assessment of monosynaptic reflex activity that may not correlate with the complex pathophysiology comprising spasticity. An externally applied device (dynamic flexometer) has been developed that measures the force necessary to move an extremity through its maximum range of motion. It extends the spastic limb distal to the joint at a constant velocity (30 degrees/second) and digitally records the angle position and forces necessary to move the limb. Digitization of angle and force data from serial evaluations objectively document the efficacy of treatment.[84] Thus various approaches to monitor therapies for spasticity are available but are limited by either subjective bias or cost.

Assessment of Efficacy to Alter Sympathetic Activity

Sympathetically maintained pain may arise from ganglia in the head (e.g., carotid, sphenopalatine, submandibular), from paravertebral ganglia along the spine, and from prevertebral plexuses anterior to the spine (e.g., celiac, mesenteric, superior hypogastric). Assessment of interventional procedures to treat painful conditions from either known (e.g., tumor, trauma) or idiopathic (CRPS [chronic regional pain syndrome] I) causes is limited. Assessment alternatives include the patient's perception of complete or partial resolution of pain or technologic detection of reduction in sympathetic activity with sympathetic blockade. Methodologies suggesting a reduction in sympathetic activity to an affected limb or head have included changes in temperature, sympathogalvanic response, the quantitative sudomotor axon reflex test (QSART), or thermography. However, the resolution of the pain may be due to a placebo response or pharmacologic inhibition of somatic innervation to the region of the pain disorder. Hence an erroneous application, performance, or interpretation of the test may yield the incorrect diagnosis and subsequent therapy.[47]

An increase in skin temperature is the most commonly used clinical sign of sympathetic blockade. A temperature probe is applied to the affected region and the contralateral site as a control measure both prior to and during the sympathetic nerve block. However, different magnitudes of temperature change have been described to indicate an effective sympathetic blockade (increases of 1.5° to 7.5°C).[46, 85, 86] Benzon[87] noted that the greatest magnitude of temperature increase after sympathetic blockade was observed in patients with lower preprocedure skin temperatures. Additionally, Horner's syndrome is acceptable to indicate a sympathetic block in the cephalic region only and not the upper extremity.[88] However, neither relief of pain nor temperature change verifies complete sympathetic interruption or that the patient's pain is solely due to sympathetically maintained causes.

Alternatively, assessment of the skin conductance response or sympathogalvanic reflex (SGR) provides a method to determine complete sympatholysis. ECG leads (right [white] and left [black] arms) are placed on the plantar and dorsal surfaces of the affected extremity. All other leads are placed on the contralateral extremity. The ECG lead selector is placed on lead I and a stimulus (loud noise, pinprick, or deep breath) is provided. The response generated is a monophasic or biphasic ECG signal in a partial sympathetic blockade and abolished in settings of complete sympathetic interruption. Unfortunately, the SGR is limited by rapid habituation and variable ECG responses in patients of different age and by skin temperature and mental stress.[85]

The QSART evaluates the function of the postganglionic sudomotor axon and sweat gland.[89] Iontophoresis of acetylcholine with a 2-mA constant current activates the nerve terminal. The stimulus impulse travels antidromically and, subsequently, orthodromically to other nerve terminals to stimulate sweat formation. The sweat volume is determined using nitrogen gas and a multicompartmental sweat capsule firmly attached to the skin. The QSART coupled with assessment of resting sweat output is useful in providing an objective indication of pathophysiology.[90] However, it may not necessarily be a causative factor for the neurogenic pain. In addition, its efficacy as a serial monitor of therapy is poorly documented.

Although thermography is useful in the evaluation of neuropathic pain syndromes, it should not be considered as an absolute diagnostic test or a sole criterion for invasive therapies. Thermography reflects the degree of thermal asymmetry between extremities in patients as a result of cutaneous vasoconstriction or vasodilation. The thermal emission profile may be due to physiologic or pathophysiologic neural and non-neural processes. Hence, not all abnormal thermographic evaluations suggest altered sympathetic activity. Thermographic information must be interpreted with consideration of the patient's history, physical examination, and other diagnostic studies.[91] Thermography includes either contact thermography with plates of heat-labile cholesterol esters or infrared thermography with conversion of radiated thermal energy to electronic signals. Sherman et al.[92] noted that infrared thermography is less expensive and equally accurate as videothermography, whereas contact thermography is markedly inaccurate and difficult to implement reliably. There are no controlled studies available that utilize thermography monitoring to determine the efficacy of interventional pain therapy.

Functional Assessment of the Efficacy of Interventional Procedures

Resolution of painful conditions and subsequent improvement or return to premorbid activity may be determined following interventional pain procedures. However, the evaluation of neuromuscular function is complex. Clinical evaluation of neuromuscular performance in patients with painful conditions includes manual muscle testing, functional index measures, one-leg or tandem stance for balance, and ability to ambulate. Other objective performance technologies include force dynamometry and clinical gait analysis. Objective estimation of muscle strength or force can be evaluated through computerized force dynamometers. Assessment of upper or lower extremity muscle performance is performed under isometric, isotonic, and isokinetic loading conditions. Unfortunately, the results are potentially biased by patient compliance and motivation, and the reliability is partly determined by the mechanical efficiency and position adjustments

of the dynamometer. The variability may be markedly attributed to the range of machine motion used and to age and sex differences. Examples of dynamometers in use include the Cybex II (Lumex Inc., Bay Shore, NY), Kinetic Communicator (Chattex, Inc., Chattanooga, TN), and the Lido system (Loredan Biomedicals, Sacramento, CA). Gait analysis derived from clinical observations has been found to be unreliable and subjective. Objective gait analysis warrants the measurement of gait velocity, stride length, cadence, and stance and swing time. This may be accomplished with a video gait analysis system that includes a gait path with pressure-sensitive switches, video camera or recorder, time code generator, and piezoelectric accelerometers. Alternatively, an in-sole pressure system measures force distribution on an elastic synthetic mat consisting of an intersecting row and column matrix. The sensor-condenser plates convert the load exerted into a digitized video signal. The abnormal pressure distribution recorded over time provides insight into a patient's gait abnormalities. The reliable implementation of objective technologies is presently limited by patient compliance and lack of acceptable standardization. Future assessment techniques need to be sensorial, dependable for acute and persistent pain conditions, cost-effective, and not limited by the patient's age, sex, and physical size.[93]

Summary

The management of pain, whether acute or chronic, warrants careful technical implementation and cautious interpretation and application of interventional procedures. Pain, as defined by the International Association for the Study of Pain (IASP), is "an unpleasant sensory and emotional experience associated with actual or potential tissue damage or described in terms of such damage." Besides pathophysiologic mechanisms for the generation of pain, perception of pain is modified by subjective and affective processes. The interpretation of interventional procedures may be confounded by the improper use of pain measurement scales, placebo effects, incorrect clinician observations, and skewed patient expectations. Nonetheless, monitoring for both patient safety and efficacy of interventional pain procedures remains justified. Finally, the future of interventional pain management requires the development of sensitive and specific monitors of efficacy and carefully conducted clinical trials.[3, 94]

REFERENCES

1. Carron H: The changing role of the anesthesiologist in pain management. Reg Anesth 1989; 14:4–9.
2. Rowlingson JC: Interventional cancer pain management. Anesth Analg 1998; 86(S):106–113.
3. Hogan Q: Neural blockade for diagnosis and prognosis: A review. Anesthesiology 1997; 86:216–241.
4. Von Gaza W: Die Resektion der paravertebralen Nerven und die isolierte Durchschneidung des Ramus communicans. Arch Klin Chir 1924; 133:479.
5. Braun H. (ed): Local Anesthesia: Its Scientific Basis and Practical Use. Philadelphia, Lea & Febiger, 1914.
6. Mandl F: Die Wirkung der paravertebralen Injektion bei "Angina pectoris." Arch Klin Chir 1925; 136:495.
7. Myers RR, Kalichman MW, Reisner LS, et al: Neurotoxicity of local anesthetics: Altered perineural permeability, edema, and nerve fiber injury. Anesthesiology 1986; 64:29–35.
8. Hogan Q, Dotson R, Erickson S, et al: Local anesthetic myotoxicity: A case and review. Anesthesiology 1994; 80:942–947.
9. Lema MJ: Monitoring epidural local anesthetic actions during the postoperative period. Reg Anesth 1996; 21(6S):94–99.

10. Hogan Q: Local anesthetic toxicity: An update. Reg Anesth 1996; 21(6S):43–50.

11. Hodgson PS, Neil JM, Pollock JE, et al: The neurotoxicity of drugs given intrathecally (spinal). Anesth Analg 1999; 88:797–809.

12. Kamibayashi T, Harasawa K, Maze M: Alpha-2 adrenergic agonists. Can J Anaesth 1997; 44:R1–R18.

13. Eisenach JC, De Kock M, Klimscha W: Alpha-2 adrenergic agonists for regional anesthesia: A clinical review of clonidine (1984–1995). Anesthesiology 1996; 85:655–674.

14. Raja SN, Treed R-D, Davis KD, et al: Systemic alpha-adrenergic blockade with phentolamine: A diagnostic test for sympathetically maintained pain. Anesthesiology 1991; 74:691–698.

15. Canavero S, Bonicalzi V: The neurochemistry of central pain: Evidence from clinical studies, hypothesis and therapeutic implications. Pain 1998; 74:109–114.

16. Bowery NG: GABA-B receptor pharmacology. Annu Rev Pharmacol Toxicol 1993; 33:109–147.

17. Kerr DIB, Ong J: GABA$_B$ receptors. Pharmacol Ther 1995; 67:187–246.

18. Penn RD, Savoy SM, Corcos D, et al: Intrathecal baclofen for severe spinal spasticity. N Engl J Med 1989; 320: 1517.

19. Yeager MP, Glass DD, Neff RK, et al: Epidural anesthesia and analgesia in high-risk surgical patients. Anesthesiology 1987; 66: 729–736.

20. Bromage PR, Camporesi EM, Durant PAC, et al: Rostral spread of epidural morphine. Anesthesiology 1982; 56:431–436.

21. De Leon-Cassola OA, Parker B, Lema MJ, et al: Postoperative epidural bupivacaine-morphine therapy: Experience with 4,227 surgical cancer patients. Anesthesiology 1994; 81:368–375.

22. Gourlay GK, Murphy TM, Plummer JL, et al: Pharmacokinetics of fentanyl in lumbar and cervical CSF following lumbar epidural and intravenous administration. Pain 1989; 38:253–259.

23. Scott DA, Beilby DSN, McClymont C: Postoperative analgesia using epidural infusions of fentanyl with bupivacaine—A prospective analysis of 1,014 patients. Anesthesiology 1995; 83:727–737.

24. Ready LB, Loper KA, Nessly M, et al: Postoperative epidural morphine is safe on surgical wards. Anesthesiology 1991; 75: 452–456.

25. Waller A: Experiments on the section of the glossopharyngeal and hypoglossal nerves of the frog and observations of the alterations produced thereby in the structure of their primitive fibres. Philos Trans R Soc Lond 1850; 140.

26. Jain S, Gupta R: Neurolytic agents in clinical practice. *In* Waldman SD, Winnie AP (eds): Interventional Pain Management. Philadelphia, WB Saunders, 1996, pp 167–171.

27. Evans PJD, Lloyd JW, Green CJ: Cryoanalgesia: The response to alteration in freeze cycle and temperature. Br J Anaesth 1981; 53:1121–1127.

28. Saberski LR: Cryoneurolysis in clinical practice. *In* Waldman SD, Winnie AP (eds): Interventional Pain Management. Philadelphia, WB Saunders, 1996, pp 172–184.

29. Taha JM, Tew JM: Treatment of trigeminal neuralgia by percutaneous radiofrequency rhizotomy. Neurosurg Clin North Am 1997; 8:31–39.

30. Lord SM, Barnsley L, Wallis BJ, et al: Percutaneous radiofrequency neurotomy for chronic cervical zygapophyseal joint pain. N Engl J Med 1996; 335:1721–1726.

31. Kline M (ed): Stereotactic Radiofrequency Lesions as Part of the Management of Pain. Orlando, FL, Paul M Deutsch Press, 1992.

32. Practice guidelines for sedation and analgesia by non-anesthesiologists: A report by the American Society of Anesthesiologists Task Force on sedation and analgesia by non-anesthesiologists. Anesthesiology 1996; 84:459–471.

33. Holzman RS, Cullen DJ, Eichhorn JH, et al: Guidelines for sedation by non-anesthesiologists during diagnostic and therapeutic procedures. J Clin Anesth 1994; 6:265–275.

34. Gangi A, Dietmann J-L, Mortazavi R, et al: CT-guided interventional procedures for pain management in the lumbosacral spine. Radiographics 1998; 18:621–633.

35. Thomsen HS, Bush WH Jr: Adverse effects of contrast media: Incidence, prevention and management. Drug Saf 1998; 19:313–324.

36. Cohan RH, Bullard MA, Ellis JH, et al: Local reactions after injection of iodinated contrast material: Detection, management, and outcome. Acad Radiol 1997; 4:711–718.

37. Amer S, Lindblom U, Myerson BA, et al: Prolonged relief of neuralgia after regional anesthetic blocks: A call for further experimental and systematic clinical studies. Pain 1990; 43:287–297.

38. Wall PD, Devo M: Sensory afferent impulses originate from dorsal root ganglia as well as from the periphery in normal and nerve injured rats. Pain 1983; 17:321–329.

39. Rosenberg PH: Intravenous regional anesthesia: Nerve block by multiple mechanisms. Reg Anesth 1993; 18:1–5.

40. Stafford-Smith M: Impaired haemostasis and regional anesthesia. Can J Anaesth 1996; 43:R129–R135.

41. Cousins MJ, Bridenbaugh PO (eds): Neural Blockade in Clinical Anesthesia and Management of Pain, ed 3. Philadelphia, Lippincott-Raven, 1998.

42. Gouda JJ, Brown JA: Atypical facial pain and other pain syndromes. Neurosurg Clin North Am 1997; 8:87–100.

43. Jho H-D, Lunsford LD: Percutaneous retrogasserian glycerol rhizotomy. Current technique and results. Neurosurg Clin North Am 1997; 8:63–74.

44. Maldjian C, Mesgarzadeh M, Tehranzadeh J: Diagnostic and therapeutic features of facet and sacroiliac joint injection. Anatomy, pathophysiology, and technique. Radiol Clin North Am 1998; 36: 497–508.

45. Link SC, El-Khoury GY, Guilford WB: Percutaneous epidural and nerve root block and percutaneous lumbar sympatholysis. Radiol Clin North Am 1998; 36:509–521.

46. Carron H, Litwiller R: Stellate ganglion blockade. Anesth Analg 1975; 54:567–570.

47. Boas RA: Sympathetic nerve blocks: In search of a role. Reg Anesth Pain Med 1998; 23:292–305.

48. Mercadante S, Nicosia F: Celiac plexus block. Reg Anesth Pain Med 1998; 23:37–48.

49. Plancarte R, de Leon-Casasola OA, El-Helaly M, et al: Neurolytic superior hypogastric plexus block for chronic pelvic pain associated with cancer. Reg Anesth 1997; 22:562–568.

50. Plancarte R, Amescua C, Patt RB: Presacral blockade of the ganglion of Walther (ganglion impar) (abstract). Anesthesiology 1990; 73:A751.

51. Plancarte R, Amescua C, Patt RB: Sympathetic neural blockade. *In* Patt RB (ed): Cancer Pain. Philadelphia, JB Lippincott, 1993, pp 377–425.

52. Renck H: Neurological complications of central nerve blocks. Acta Anaesthesiol Scand 1995; 39:859–868.

53. Abram SE: Continuous spinal anesthesia for cancer and chronic pain. Reg Anesth 1993; 18:406–413.

54. Nitescu P, Sjoberg M, Appelgren L, et al: Complications of intrathecal opioids and bupivacaine in the treatment of "refractory" cancer pain. Clin J Pain 1995; 11:45–62.

55. Dahm P, Nitescu P, Appelgren L, et al: Efficacy and technical complications of long-term continuous intraspinal infusions of opioid and/or bupivacaine in refractory nonmalignant pain: A comparison between the epidural and the intrathecal approach with externalized or implanted catheters and infusion pumps (review). Clin J Pain 1998; 14:4–16.

56. Mulroy MF, Norris MC, Liu SS: Safety steps for epidural injection of local anesthetics: Review of the literature and recommendations. Anesth Analg 1997; 85:1346–1356.

57. Rowlingson JC: Epidural steroids: Do they have a place in pain management? American Pain Society (APS) J 1994; 3:20–27.

58. Ryedevik BJ, Cohen DB, Kostuik JP: Spine epidural steroids for patients with lumbar spinal stenosis. Spine 1997; 22:2313–2317.

59. Abram SE, O'Connor TC: Complications associated with epidural steroid injections. Reg Anesth 1996; 21:149–162.

60. North RB, Ewend MG, Lawton MT, et al: Spinal cord stimulation for chronic, intractable pain: Superiority of "multi-channel" devices. Pain 1991; 44:119–130.

61. Holsheimer J: Effectiveness of spinal cord stimulation in the management of chronic pain: Analysis of technical drawbacks and solutions. Neurosurgery 1997; 40:990–999.

62. North RB, Kidd DH, Zahurak M, et al: Spinal cord stimulation for chronic, intractable, pain: Experience over two decades. Neurosurgery 1993; 32:384–395.

63. Racz GB, Holubec JT: Lysis of adhesions in the epidural space. *In* Racz GB (ed): Techniques of Neurolysis. Boston, Kluwer Academic, 1989, pp 57–72.

64. Tehranzadeh J: Discography 2000. Radiol Clin North Am 1998; 36:463–496.

65. Shealy CN, Mortimer JT, Reswick J: Electrical inhibition of pain by stimulation of the dorsal column: Preliminary clinical reports. Anesth Analg 1967; 46:489–491.

66. Shetter A: Spinal cord stimulation in the treatment of chronic pain. Curr Rev Pain 1997; 1:213–222.

67. Turk DC, Marcus DA: Assessment of chronic pain patients. Semin Neurol 1994; 14:206–212.

68. Rucker KS, Metzler HM, Kregel J: Standardization of chronic pain assessment: A multiperspective approach. Clin J Pain 1996; 12:94–110.

69. Melzack R: The McGill pain questionnaire: Major properties and scoring methods. Pain 1971; 1:277–299.

70. Chapman CR, Syrjala KL: Measurement of pain. *In* Bonica JJ. (ed): The Management of Pain, ed 2. Philadelphia, Lea & Febiger, 1990, pp 580–594.

71. Hogeweg JA, Langereis MJ, Bernards ATM, et al: Algometry: Measuring pain threshold, method and characteristics in healthy subjects. Scand J Rehabil Med 1992; 24:99–103.

72. Von Frey M: Untersuchungen über die Sinnesfunctionen der menschlichen Haut. Erste Abhandlung: Druckempfindung und Schmerz. Abhandlungen Sachs Gesamte Wiss Math Phys Cl 1896; 23:175–266.

73. Bendtsen L, Jensen R, Jensen NK, et al: Muscle palpation with controlled finger pressure: New equipment for the study of tender myofascial tissues. Pain 1994; 59:235–239.

74. Fruhstorfer H, Lindblom U, Schmidt WG: Method for quantitative estimation of thermal thresholds in patients. J Neurol Neurosurg Psychiatry 1976; 39:1071–1075.

75. Dotson RM: Clinical neurophysiology laboratory test to assess the nociceptive system in humans. J Clin Neurophysiol 1997; 14:32–45.

76. Verdugo RJ, Ochoa JL: Use and misuse of conventional electrodiagnosis, quantitative sensory testing, thermography, and nerve blocks in the evaluation of painful neuropathic syndromes. Muscle Nerve 1993; 16:1056–1062.

77. Wahren LK, Torebjork E: Quantitative sensory tests in patients with neuralgia 11 to 25 years after injury. Pain 1992; 48:237–244.

78. Wahren LK, Torebjork E, Nystrom B: Quantitative sensory testing before and after regional guanethedine block in patients with neuralgia in the hand. Pain 1991; 46:23–30.

79. Smith PJ, Mott G: Sensory threshold and conductance testing in nerve injuries. J Hand Surg [Br] 1986; 11:157–162.

80. Katims JJ, Rouvelas P, Sadler BT, et al: Reproducibility and comparison with nerve conduction in evaluation of carpal tunnel syndrome. Trans Am Soc Artif Intern Organs 1989; 35:280–284.

81. Liu SS, Kopacz DJ, Carpenter RL: Quantitative assessment of differential sensory nerve block after lidocaine spinal anesthesia. Anesthesiology 1995; 82:60–63.

82. Ashworth B: Preliminary trial of carisoprodol in multiple sclerosis. Practitioner 1964; 192:540–542.

83. Neuhluser G: Methods of assessing and recording motor skills and movement patterns. Dev Med Child Neurol 1975; 17:369–386.

84. Chabal C, Schwid HA, Jacobson L: The dynamic flexometer: An instrument for the objective evaluation of spasticity. Anesthesiology 1991; 74:609–612.

85. Breivik H, Lofstrom JB Cousins MJ: Sympathetic neural blockade of upper and lower extremity. *In* Cousins MJ, Bridenbaugh PO (eds): Neural Blockade in Clinical Anesthesia and Management of Pain, ed 3. Philadelphia, Lippincott-Raven, 1998, pp 411–445.

86. Benzon HT, Avram MJ: Temperature increases after complete sympathetic blockade. Reg Anesth 1986; 11:27–30.

87. Benzon HT: Importance of documenting complete sympathetic denervation after sympathectomy. Anesth Analg 1992; 74:599–601.

88. Hogan QH, Taylor ML, Goldstein M, et al: Success rates in producing sympathetic blockade by paratracheal injection. Clin J Pain 1994; 10:139–145.

89. Low PA, Caskey PE, Tuck RR, et al: Quantitative sudomotor axon reflex test in normal and neuropathic subjects. Ann Neurol 1983; 14:573–580.

90. Low PA: Laboratory evaluation of autonomic failure. *In* Low PA (ed): Clinical Autonomic Disorder: Evaluation and Management. Boston, Little, Brown, 1993, pp 169–195.

91. Sherman RA, Karstetter KW, Damiano M, et al: Stability of temperature asymmetries in reflex sympathetic dystrophy over time and changes in pain. Clin J Pain 1994; 10:71–77.

92. Sherman RA, Woerman AL, Karstetter KW: Comparative effectiveness of videothermography, contact thermography, and infrared beam thermography for scanning relative skin temperature. J Rehabil Res Dev 1996; 33:377–386.

93. Jaweed MM, Monga TN: Neuromuscular function assessment. *In* Walsh NE (ed): Rehabilitation of Chronic Pain. Physical Medicine and Rehabilitation-State of the Art Reviews, vol 11. Philadelphia, Hanley & Belfus, 1997, pp 205–237.

94. Raja SN: Nerve block in the evaluation of chronic pain: A plea for caution in their use and interpretation. Anesthesiology 1997; 86:4–6.

Index

Note: Page numbers in *italics* refer to illustrations; page numbers followed by (t) refer to tables. *Color Figures* appear as an insert in Chapter 15.

ISBN 0-7216-8698-2